Lecture Notes in Artificial Intelligence 5315

Edited by R. Goebel, J. Siekmann, and W. Wahlster

Subseries of Lecture Notes in Computer Science

Caihua Xiong Honghai Liu Yongan Huang
Youlun Xiong (Eds.)

Intelligent Robotics and Applications

First International Conference, ICIRA 2008
Wuhan, China, October 15-17, 2008
Proceedings, Part II

Springer

Series Editors

Randy Goebel, University of Alberta, Edmonton, Canada
Jörg Siekmann, University of Saarland, Saarbrücken, Germany
Wolfgang Wahlster, DFKI and University of Saarland, Saarbrücken, Germany

Volume Editors

Caihua Xiong
Yongan Huang
Youlun Xiong
Huazhong University of Science and Technology
School of Mechanical Science and Engineering
Wuhan 430074, China
E-mail: {chxiong, yahuang, ylxiong}@mail.hust.edu.cn

Honghai Liu
University of Portsmouth
Institute of Industrial Research
Burnaby Building, Portsmouth PO1 3QL, UK
E-mail: honghai.liu@port.ac.uk

Library of Congress Control Number: 2008936489

CR Subject Classification (1998): I.2.9, J.3, I.4, I.2.10, I.5.4

LNCS Sublibrary: SL 7 – Artificial Intelligence

ISSN 0302-9743
ISBN-10 3-540-88516-1 Springer Berlin Heidelberg New York
ISBN-13 978-3-540-88516-0 Springer Berlin Heidelberg New York

Springer is a part of Springer Science+Business Media

springer.com

Printed in Germany

Typesetting: Camera-ready by author, data conversion by Scientific Publishing Services, Chennai, India
Printed on acid-free paper SPIN: 12538850 06/3180 5 4 3 2 1 0

Preface

The 2008 International Conference on Intelligent Robotics and Applications (ICIRA 2008) was the first event in this conference series. It was advocated by the International Workshop on Robotic Grasping and Fixturing in June 2007, Wuhan, China. Robotics research, however, involves a wide spectrum of research and applications from the first industrial manipulator to Mars rovers, and from surgery robotics to cognitive robotics. Industrial and real-world applications are the force driving the research frontier further forward. The aim of the ICIRA 2008 conference is to promote interactions and collaborations between disciplines, which are beneficial in bringing fruitful solutions to the forefront, and to be an international forum that brings together those actively involved in intelligent robotics and applications.

These volumes of Springer's *Lecture Notes in Artificial Intelligence* and *Lecture Notes in Computer Science* contain papers accepted for presentation at ICIRA 2008, held in Wuhan, China, October 15–17, 2008. The conference received 552 submissions from all over the world, which were subsequently peer refereed by the Program Committee, with the assistance of external referees. Among them, 265 high-quality papers were accepted for presentation at the conference, covering the most active topics in intelligent robotics such as robot cognition, robot learning, robot vision, motion planning, multifingered manipulation and intelligent control. Advances in robotized equipments applied in rehabilitation and medical robotics, health care and artificial limbs, digital manufacturing, electronic manufacturing, and manufacturing automation are also reported. The authors come from the following countries and regions: Australia, Austria, China, France, Germany, Hong Kong, Iran, Italy, Japan, Korea, Malaysia, Poland, Romania, Singapore, Slovakia, Spain, Sweden, Switzerland, Taiwan, UK, and USA. In addition, ICIRA 2008 held a series of plenary talks, where we were fortunate to have such keynote speakers as *Peter Luh, Tianmiao Wang, Jiping He, and Jun Wang,* who shared their expertise with us in diverse topic areas spanning the range of intelligent robotics and application activities.

We would like to thank all who made this conference possible: the authors for submitting papers, the external referees for their scrupulous work, the invited speakers for their excellent talks, the International Advisory Committee for their guidance and advice. We are also especially grateful to the Program Committee members for their rigorous and efficient work, and to the Organizing Committee members for their enormous efforts. In addition, we greatly appreciate Huazhong University of Science and Technology (HUST), National Natural Science Foundation of China (Grant No. 50810305023), State Key Laboratory of Digital Manufacturing Equipment and Technology, State Key Laboratory of Robotic Technology and Systems, State Key Laboratory of Robotics and State Key Laboratory of Mechanical Systems and Vibration for their financial support and assistance. Sincere thanks also go to the editors of the Lecture Notes and Springer for their support in publishing this volume in a timely manner.

It has been our pleasure to organize ICIRA 2008. We believe that ICIRA 2008 provided an interesting opportunity to present and discuss the latest theoretical advances and real-world applications in this multidisciplinary research field. We hope it is your pleasure to read these selected papers by high-quality researchers and practitioners in the field of intelligent robotics. We also hope that they also provide inspiration for your own research and help advance the state of the art in the multidisciplinary field of robotics and its applications.

October 2008

Youlun Xiong
Caihua Xiong
Honghai Liu
Xinyu Shao
Han Ding

Organization

Honorary Chair

Peigen Li	HUST, China

Advisory Committee Chairs

Hegao Cai	Harbin Institute of Technology, China
Peihua Gu	University of Calgary, Canada
Toshio Fukuda	Nagoya University, Japan
Jun Ni	University of Michigan, USA
Huosheng Hu	University of Essex, UK
Peter Luh	University of Connecticut, USA
Shuguo Wang	Harbin Institute of Technology, China
Christian Freksa	University of Bremen, Germany
Shigeki Sugano	Waseda University, Japan
Lotfi Zadeh	University of California, USA

General Chairs

Youlun Xiong	HUST, China
Michael Wang	Chinese University of Hong Kong, China

Program Chairs

Caihua Xiong	HUST, China
Honghai Liu	University of Portsmouth, UK

Program Co-chairs

Tianmiao Wang	Beihang University, China
Lining Sun	Harbin Institute of Technology, China
Guang Meng	Shanghai Jiao Tong University, China
Miroslav Karny	Academy of Sciences, Czech Republic
Naoyuki Kubota	TMU, Japan
Mikael Ericsson	University West, Sweden
Xiaorong Xiong	Intel Co., USA
Ming Tan	Chinese Academy of Sciences, China
Rosemary Gault	University of Sheffield, UK
Sebastian Thrun	University of Stanford, USA
Weiliang Xu	Massey University, New Zealand
Zengqi Sun	Tsinghua University, China

Organizing Committee Chairs

Xinyu Shao	HUST, China
Guobiao Wang	NSFC, China
Han Ding	HUST, China
Yuechao Wang	Chinese Academy Sciences, China

Organizing Committee Co-chairs

Gary Feng	City University of Hong Kong, China
Chenghong Wang	NSFC, China
Tao Mei	Chinese Academy of Sciences, China
J.S. Dai	King's College, London University, UK
Y.F. Li	City University of Hong Kong, China
Qiang Huang	Beijing Institute of Technology, China
Jie Zhao	Harbin Institute of Technology, China
Ming Xie	Nanyang Technological University, Singapore
Kevin Y. Rong	WPI, USA
X.H. Huang	HUST, China

Local Chairs

Zhongqin Lin	Shanghai Jiao Tong University, China
Jianbin Luo	Tsinghua University, China
Jrgen Leopold	IWU, Germany
Stefano Nolfi	CNR, Italy
Hong Qiao	Chinese Academy of Sciences, China
Tian Huang	Tianjin University, China
Gurvinder S. Virk	Massey University, New Zealand
Zhouping Yin	HUST, China
Dongbing Gu	University of Essex, UK
Puren Ouyang	Ryerson University, Canada

Program Area Chairs

Xiangyang Zhu	Shanghai Jiao Tong University, China
L. Kroll	Chemnitz University of Technology, Germany
Pingyu Jiang	Xi'an Jiao Tong University, China
S. Nahavandi	Deakin University, Australia
Wenyu Yang	HUST, China
M.C. Zhou	New Jersey Institute of Technology, USA
H. Zhang	University of Alberta, Canada
Jianda Han	Chinese Academy of Sciences, China
Loulin Huang	Massey University, New Zealand
Yunhui Liu	Chinese University of Hong Kong, China

The 2008 International Conference on Intelligent Robotics and Applications was sponsored by Huazhong University of Science and Technology (HUST) and National Natural Science Foundation of China (NSFC), organized by the School of Mechanical Science and Engineering of HUST and State Key Laboratory of Digital Manufacturing Equipment and Technology; coorganized by State Key Laboratory of Robotic Technology and System, State Key Laboratory of Robotics and State Key Laboratory of Mechanical System and Vibration; and supported by 973 National Basic Research Program of China under grants 2003CB716200, 2004CB719400, 2005CB724100, 2006CB705400, 2007CB714000.

Table of Contents – Part II

Keynote Speeches

Human-Machine Interaction and Coordination

Micro/Nano Mechanical Systems

Manufacturing Automation

Multi-axis Surface Machining

Realworld Applications

Table of Contents – Part I

Robot Control

Cognitive Robotics

Health Care and Artificial Limb

Robot Learning

Robot Vision

Mobile Robotics

Human-Machine Interaction and Coordination

Modeling and Optimization of Crowd Guidance for Building Emergency Evacuation

Peng Wang[1], Peter B. Luh[1], Shi-Chuang Chang[2], and Jin Sun[3]

[1] Department of Electrical and Computer Engineering, University of Connecticut, Storrs, CT 06269-2157, USA
[2] Electrical Engineering Department, National Taiwan University, Taipei, Taiwan
[3] Center for Intelligent and Networked Systems, Department of Automation, Tsinghua University, Beijing, China
Peng.Wang@uconn.edu, Peter.Luh@uconn.edu, scchang@cc.ee.ntu.edu.tw, sunjin00@mails.tsinghua.edu.cn

1 Introduction

Effective building evacuation in case of emergencies such as fires, chemical spills, or spreads of biological agents has long been recognized as an important issue, and effective crowd guidance can improve egress efficiency, occupant survivability, and mitigate or prevent undesirable consequences such as blocking or stampeding. To effectively guide crowds, however, is a challenging issue because emergency events may propagate in uncertain ways and affect the availability of egress paths; egress path capacities may constrain the speed of crowd movement; and crowd could be stressed making their behaviors different from their normal modes. Although good results have recently been obtained on microscopic behaviors of individuals such as the social force model of Helbing [1-3], there is a major gap between these microscopic models of individuals evacuating from rooms and the macroscopic models of crowd flows needed to evacuate them from a building. Most existing egress guidance methods assume that crowd behaviors are independent of emergency situations and are fully controllable under guidance. These assumptions make it difficult to capture important features such as stampeding or blocking.

2 The Probabilistic Graphical Model

To bridge the gap between microscopic and macroscopic crowd models, a probabilistic graphical model is established in this paper to characterize the nonlinear interactions among the states of the emergency events, crowd stresses, egress capacities, and crowd flow rates. As shown in Fig. 1, there are several major components in the model:

- There is a "desired flow rate" for an individual, similar to the "desired velocity" of Helbing et al. [1]. If an emergency becomes urgent, people become more impatient, and the desired flow rate increases in a probabilistic manner.
- If the aggregate desired flow rate of a crowd is smaller than the egress capacity of a passage, then the crowd flow rate is equal to the desired flow rate

C. Xiong et al. (Eds.): ICIRA 2008, Part II, LNAI 5315, pp. 1–6, 2008.

without blocking. However, if the aggregated desired flow rate is larger than the passage capacity, then the crowd flow rate decreases drastically in a probabilistic and nonlinear fashion, resulting in the "faster-is-slower" scenario of Helbing et al. [1], and eventually leading to blocking and stampeding.

- Whether an individual would follow guidance is probabilistic and depends on his/her trust on the guidance provided, and his familiarity with the evacuation paths and whether other people follow the guidance.

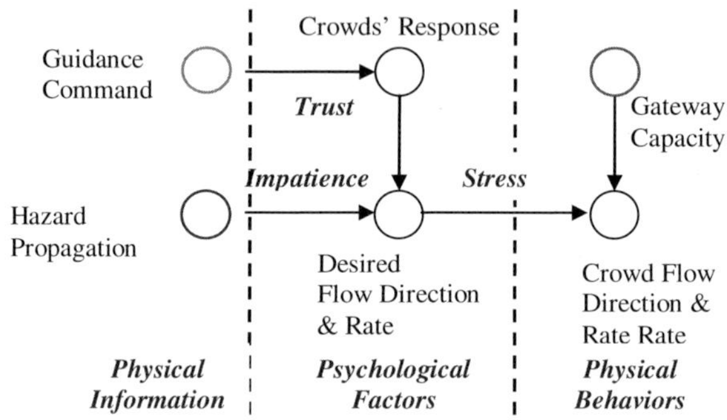

Fig. 1. The Probabilistic Graphical Model

This probabilistic graphical model incorporates two insightful psychological factors: impatience and trust, where impatience is the cause of blocking events, and trust reflects how crowds respond to guidance. An individual's trust in guidance evolves with how effective the guidance has been and affects one's egress direction. The high pressure derived from the state of the emergency event causes people to become impatient, and want to move through a passage fast, however, the actual flow rate is constrained by the passage capacity. If the desired flow rate is below the passage capacity, it can be achieved. The more it exceeds the capacity, the higher is the blocking probability, causing drastic decrease of the crowd flow rate. At a higher level, this model can be characterized by the energy balance concept, where the state of the emergency drives the desired flow rate and therefore the "Stress Energy." This stress energy is "balanced" between the "Static Energy" captured by the crowd density (affected by the passage capacity) and the "Dynamic Energy" represented by the flow rate. Such a macroscopic model thus provides a theoretical foundation for linking crowd stress behaviors to the situation, enables us to predict potential blockings in emergency evacuation, and provides a foundation to optimize crowd guidance.

3 The Overall Optimization Formulation

The above guided crowd behavior model can be combined with the egress network and the emergency event dynamics to form an optimization problem with the goal to evacuate as many people and as fast as possible while reducing the relevant risks through appropriate guidance of the crowds. The egress network can be modeled as a room-and-path structure by using a directed graph with egress path capacity constraints. Fig. 2 illustrates a sample room-and-path structure and how it is converted to a direct graph.

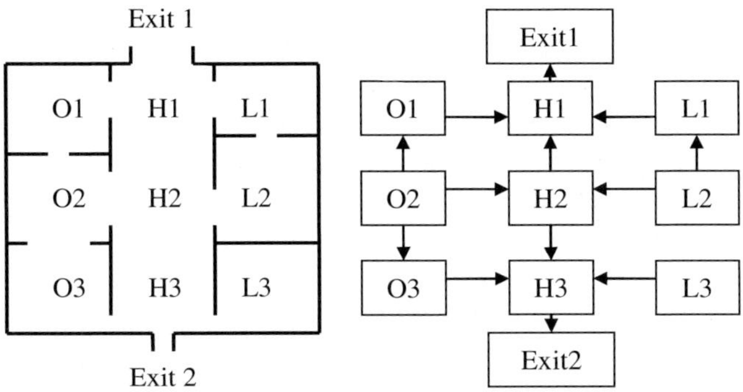

Fig. 2. An Egress Network

For the propagation of emergence events such as fire and smoke in buildings, many models have been established, including field models [4, 5]; NIST's Fire Dynamics Simulator [6]; and McGrattan et al. [7], zone models [8], and cellular automaton models [9, 10]. These models can simulate fire propagation in a building. In this paper, the fire propagation dynamics is simplified as a state transition model, where the transition is governed by conditional probabilities that fire propagates from one room to its "adjacent" rooms. The probabilistic graphical models, the egress network, emergency event dynamics, and crowd guidance then generate the crowd flow rates.

The goal of crowd guidance is to evacuate as many people and as fast as possible while reducing the relevant risks. This translates to maximizing a weighted sum of the expected number of total people evacuated, expected cumulative number of people evacuated, and the negative values of the corresponding semi-variances considered as a risk measure.

4 Solution Methodology

The problem thus formulated is a Markov decision problem, and to obtain an optimal solution, computation complexity is a major challenge. To reduce the computational requirements, Lagrangian relaxation is used. This is based on the insight that groups of crowds are mostly independent except when they compete for small passages, and such interactions are described by a set of nonlinear egress capacity constraints as described in Section 2. The problem is thus solved by using the "divide and conquer" approach. After the coupling nonlinear egress capacity constraints are "approximately relaxed" based on the sum of individual flow rates, individual group subproblems are solved by using stochastic dynamic programming with the rollout scheme [11]. Individual groups are then coordinated by the iterative updating of Lagrangian multipliers by using the surrogate subgradient method [12].

5 Numerical Testing Results

The above method has been implemented in Matlab and run on an Intel Core™2 Duo CPU with 2G memory for scenarios with fire as the emergency event. An example is tested where 50 people are evacuated in a structure of 6 rooms, a lobby area, 9 paths and 2 exits as depicted in Fig. 2. Two groups of evacuees are considered where Group 1 consists of 30 people locating in Office 3 initially; and Group 2 consists of 20 people locating in Lab 2 initially. A fire starts at Lab 3 and its propagation is based on a state transition model. For each discrete decision point we look ahead five time steps.

Fig. 3 shows the optimal paths at the initial time. These paths are obtained because the probabilistic graphical model foresees a potential blocking for the path from Office 3 to Exit 2. Thus Exit 2 is not used and people are guided to use Exit 1. At time 5, the guidance is updated due to fire propagating to the lounge area affecting the availability of the previous paths as shown in Fig. 4.

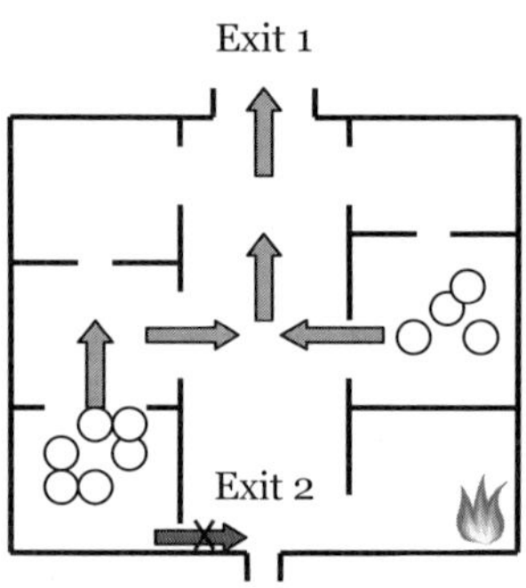

Fig. 3. Initial guidance at t = 1

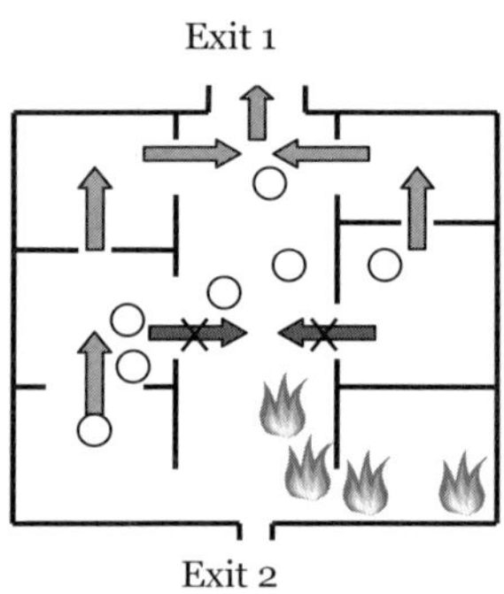

Fig. 4. Guidance updated at t = 5

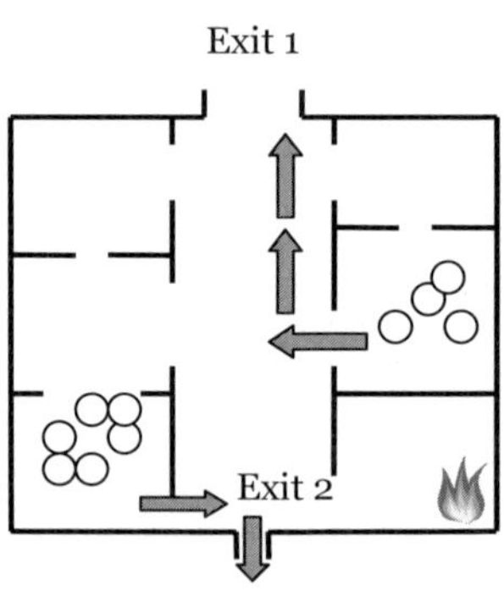

Fig. 5. Initial guidance ignoring nonlinear behaviors

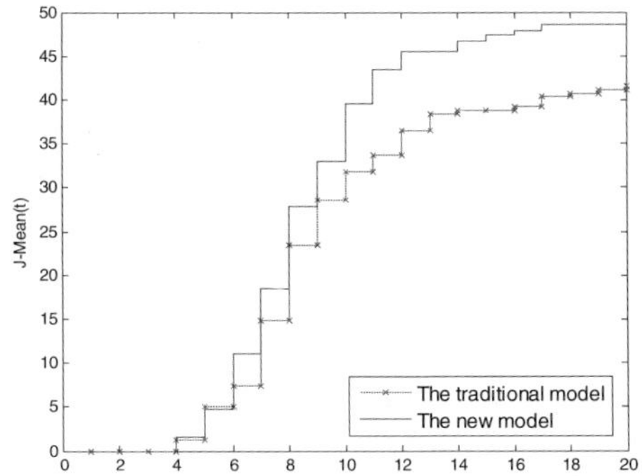

Fig. 6. Comparison of the new vs. the traditional methods

If the nonlinear crowd behaviors are not considered while other conditions remain the same, the guidance at the initial time is shown in Fig. 5 where Group 1 is guided to use Exit 2. However, this would lead to blocking as the crowd try to rush through the narrow passage of Exit 2, resulting in a much slower egress. The average objective functions of 25 Monte Carlo simulation runs are summarized in Fig. 6, showing the superiority of the new model and the method.

6 Conclusion

This paper investigates the crowd guidance problem for building emergency evacuation. A probabilistic graphical model is established to bridge the gap between microscopic models and macroscopic models while capturing the characteristics of crowd behaviors in emergencies. Then the guidance is obtained by using stochastic dynamic programming with rollout within the Lagrangian relaxation framework. Compared with results obtained by the traditional model, the guidance obtained by the new model can help prevent or mitigate potential blockings, improve evacuation efficiency, and manage risks. A different way to look at our approach is to provide crowds with expected times to safety as egress advices while considering crowd behaviors and the corresponding effects.

Acknowledgments. This work was supported in part by the National Science Foundation under grants DMI-0423607 and by the SNET Endowment Fund.

References

1. Helbing, D., Farkas, I., Vicsek, T.: Simulating Dynamical Features of Escape Panic. Nature 407, 487–490 (2000)
2. Helbing, D.: Traffic and Related Self-Driven Many-Particle Systems. Reviews of Modern Physics 73(4), 1067–1141 (2001)
3. Helbing, D., Johansson, A.: Dynamics of Crowd Disasters: An Empirical Study. Physical Review E75, 046109 (2007)

4. Novozhilov, V., Harvie, D.J.E., Green, A.R., Kent, J.H.: A Computational Fluid Dynamic Model of Fire Burning Rate and Extinction by Water Sprinkler. Combustion Science and Technology 123(1-6), 227–245 (1997)
5. SMARTFIRE V2.0 User Guide and Technical Manual, Doc Rev 1.0 (July 1998)
6. NIST: Final Report on the Collapse of the World Trade Center Towers (September 2005), http://wtc.nist.gov/reports_october05.htm
7. McGrattan, K.B., Klein, B., Hostikka, S., Floyd, J.: Fire Dynamics Simulator (Version 5) User's Guide. NIST Special Publication 1019-5 (February 2008), http://fdssmv.googlecode.com/svn/trunk/FDS/trunk/Manuals/All_PDF_Files/FDS_5_User_Guide.pdf
8. Janssens, M.L.: An Introduction to Mathematical Fire Modeling, 2nd edn. Technomic Publishing Company, Inc. (2000)
9. Duarte, J.: Bushfire Automata and Their Phase Transitions. International Journal of Modern Physics C 8, 171–189 (1997)
10. Ohgai, A., Gohnai, Y., Watanabe, K.: Cellular Automata Modeling of Fire Spread in Built-Up Areas - A Tool to Aid Community-Based Planning for Disaster Mitigation. Computers, Environment and Urban Systems 31, 441–460 (2007)
11. Bertsekas, D.P.: Dynamic Programming and Optimal Control, 3rd edn., vol. 1, 2. Athena Scientific (2005)
12. Zhao, X., Luh, P.B., Wang, J.: The Surrogate Gradient Algorithm for Lagrangian Relaxation Method. Journal of Optimization Theory and Applications 100(3), 699–712 (1999)

Peter B. Luh received his B.S. degree in Electrical Engineering from National Taiwan University, Taipei, Taiwan, in 1973; M.S. degree in Aeronautics and Astronautics Engineering from M.I.T., Cambridge, MA in 1977; and Ph.D. degree in Applied Mathematics from Harvard University in 1980. Since then he has been with the University of Connecticut, and currently is the SNET Professor of Communications & Information Technologies and the Head of the Department of Electrical and Computer Engineering. He is also a member of the Chair Professors Group at the Center for Intelligent and Networked Systems, the Department of Automation, Tsinghua University, Beijing, China. He is interested in planning, scheduling, and coordination of design, manufacturing, and supply chain activities; configuration and operation of elevators and HVAC systems for normal and emergency conditions; schedule, auction, portfolio optimization, and load/price forecasting for power systems; and decision-making under uncertain or distributed environments. He is a Fellow of IEEE, Vice President of Publication Activities for the IEEE Robotics and Automation Society, an Associate Editor of *IIE Transactions on Design and Manufacturing*, an Associate Editor of *Discrete Event Dynamic Systems*, and was the founding Editor-in-Chief of the *IEEE Transactions on Automation Science and Engineering* (2003-2007), and the Editor-in-Chief of *IEEE Transactions on Robotics and Automation* (1999-2003).

Designing Interactive and Intelligent Control for Rehabilitation Robots

Jiping He[1,2], S. Balasubramanian[1], and Ruihua Wei[1,3]

[1] Harrington Department of Bioengineering and Center for Neural Interface Design, Arizona State University, Tempe, AZ, USA
[2] Huazhong University of Science and Technology, Wuhan, China
[3] Tongji University, Shanghai, China
jiping.he@asu.edu

Abstract. The control system design for rehabilitation robotics requires certain special considerations: interactive nature with highly adaptive neural muscular system of a human user, ability to accommodate spastic and slow responses from patients with neurological disorders, and less stringent accuracy and precision specifications. In developing a control scheme for the Robotic Assisted Upper Extremity Repetitive Therapy (RUPERT™), we reviewed and implemented an interactive and adaptive control structure that satisfies the special consideration and also takes advantage of the less stringent performance specifications. The RUPERT™ is developed to provide a low cost, safe, easy-to-use robotic-device to assist the patient and therapist to achieve more systematic therapy at home or in the clinic. Because the device is wearable and lightweight, it can be worn standing or sitting or even walking around, providing therapy tasks that better mimic activities of daily living.

Keywords: interactive control, pneumatic muscle, rehabilitation robot, stroke, neuromotor function, intelligent control.

1 Introduction

Continued improvement of longevity and survival rate of neural trauma demands improved service for neural rehabilitation to improve quality of life in aging population and survivors of neural trauma. Functional maps from brain imaging show that motor cortical representation shrinks with inactivity following lesions and may expand with subsequent intensive activity [1-6]. Recent research has shown that induced neural plasticity in the brain may help stroke survivors to recover certain control ability for motor functions. Combination of these observations suggests that intensive and repetitive physical exercises relevant to tasks of daily living may be a viable therapy to induce desirable neural plasticity to overcome brain damage caused by stroke. However, to make the therapy effective repetition is the key and the rehabilitation process may need to last for many months. This will be costly and labor intensive if the therapy requires full attention and non-interruptive physical therapist assistance.

During rehabilitation the pattern of physical activity does not need to be precise or accurate in trajectory and position. As a matter of fact the research has shown that

C. Xiong et al. (Eds.): ICIRA 2008, Part II, LNAI 5315, pp. 7–16, 2008.

variation is desirable and may be more effective in inducing neural plasticity [29]. This nature of repetition for a set of fixed physical exercises with relatively low precision and accuracy requirement is very attractive for robotic assisted therapy. A very good review of robotic devices to assist in these therapies is presented in [7].

There is clearly a need for affordable, practical and multi-dimensional devices to assist therapists in rehabilitation. Before rushing to modify robots or developing new robots for rehabilitation application, we need to understand the special need and consideration in rehabilitation. Aside from cost and safety consideration, technical specifications for a rehabilitation robot present both ease and challenge for design, especially control system for such systems.

It is important to note that most tasks of activities of daily living (ADL) are practiced in a natural setting. This will require mobility and one attractive solution is wearable exoskeleton type of robot for upper extremity or lower extremity. The wearable type of rehabilitation robot will have to be light weight and solve several challenges in control. The users of these robots are people who have neurological disorders and impaired motor and/or sensory/perception functions. They respond and react slow and move slow. The control system design has to accommodate these existing conditions, be adaptive to improved or continued deteriorating conditions. Furthermore, the system needs to have features to motivate voluntary participation in the rehabilitation process so that the robot is to assist not replace voluntary control for a movement.

Many important ADLs, such as grooming, dressing and eating, depend on two-handed function [8]. It is important to design the robots and the control systems to assist the patient to practice coordinated bi-manual activities at clinic or at home to take full advantage of the repetitive therapy.

2 Special Consideration on Control Design of Rehabilitation Robot

The experience from the development of a wearable and interactive rehabilitation robot: Robot assisted UPper Extremity Repetitive Therapy (RUPERT™) is valuable for the general guidelines of rehabilitation robot design. RUPERT is an exoskeleton robot for arm function. The device is compact and lightweight for portability, relatively easy to use for self donning and doffing, capable of interacting with a biofeedback system to capture the interest of the user, and can provide adequate torque at the shoulder, elbow, and wrist during training of functional reaching and feeding tasks. The device can also provide measurement of functional performance for evaluation purposes, guiding the progress of each therapy session. One specific requirement in this research is to develop an inexpensive device that can assist the therapist at the clinic and can be used for supplemental in-home therapy. It is based on the design principle of Hand Mentor™ an air-muscle driven wrist/hand device [9] and a gait trainer, both using pneumatic muscles as actuators and only uni-direction drive on each joint [10].

The "McKibben" type pneumatic actuators used in RUPERT provide compliant actuation and thus reduce the complexity of the control system compared to usually stiffer motor drives. They can naturally extend or yield to prevent injury if a spastic response from the user occurs during the rehabilitation task. These pneumatic muscles (PMs) have a venerable history of use in rehabilitation devices [14-17]. However, the compliance also presents challenges in design and control, in a different way: slower response time in force generation and the dependence of the position and movement speed on external load or resistance, the nonlinearity similar to natural muscles. Further, the dynamic range of PMs for required range of motion also depends on the anchor position and the length. We used modeling and simulation to guide the design and selection of parameters for the pneumatic muscles. To prepare for a safe and effective closed-loop feedback controller we are investigating dynamic relationships among applied pressures, muscle sizes and material properties, and external loads [30].

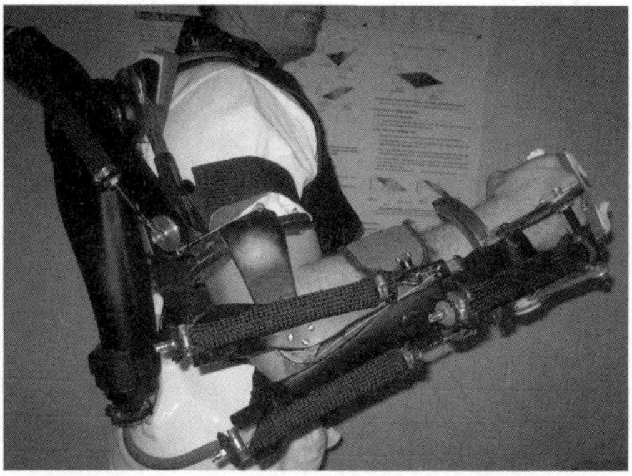

Fig. 1. RUPERT is powered by five pneumatic muscles on five actuated degrees of freedom (2 at the shoulder, 2 at the elbow and 1 at the wrist). Shown here is the version for the right arm. Lengths of both upper and lower arm segments can be adjusted to fit a wide range of patient body sizes. It is easy to put on and take off.

RUPERT incorporates coordinated elbow and shoulder motions and provides active assistance at five degrees of freedom (DOF): shoulder elevation (flexion), elbow extension, humeral external rotation, forearm supination, and wrist/hand extension. Since the activation provided by RUPERT is uni-directional at each DOF voluntary control by the user has to be asserted for the device to work effectively. Such enforcement of patients voluntary involvement during the therapy and rehabilitation process of the affected upper extremity is oriented toward restoring the normal sensorimotor relationships between the joints for actually performing activities of daily living [11].

To limit the stimulation of spastic synergy motions, RUPERT is designed to restrict certain motions and promote "reflex-inhibiting" motions that are incorporated in many everyday tasks. This strategy is recommended by many stroke therapy programs [23].

Many stroke survivors initiate early motion of the scapula in shoulder elevation either because of synergistic interactions or for compensatory reasons. To assist in training desired motions, the scapula is restricted by the support pad that is part of the attachment structure. The RUPERT IV shoulder design restricts the elevation of the humerus to a plane rotated 30° clockwise from the sagittal plane. This plane is also the most common plane of humeral elevation for activities of daily living [25, 26, 27].

3 Adaptive and Intelligent Control

System Overview

The hardware of control system for the robot consists two major components, (i) a control box housing a PC104 single board computer, and five pressure regulators that actuate each of the DOF in RUPERT IV, (ii) a main PC (mPC) which acts the terminal for the physician/therapist/operator to interact with the robot.

Overall Controller Structure

The general structure of the closed-loop controller for RUPERT IV is shown in Fig. 2. The control law consists of two loops, namely (i) Inner Loop (IL) and (ii) Outer Loop (OL). The IL consists of five independent joint controllers, one for each DOF, and the OL controller is basically a trajectory planning module that generates the trajectory command for the IL.

Closed-Loop Controller Design

The current closed-loop controller for RUPERT IV is developed for assisted therapy mode.

1) Outer Loop Controller: The OL controller is currently a simple trajectory planning module that generates a command trajectory in the joint space for the controllers in the IL. It will be gradually evolved into a rule based command center for specifying therapy tasks and control parameters on individual patients and individual therapy sessions.

Given an initial and target position in joint space, the OL generates a smooth reference trajectory for each joint using the following equations,

$$\theta^c(t) = \theta_i + (\theta_t - \theta_i) \times \left(15\left(\frac{t}{T}\right)^4 - 6\left(\frac{t}{T}\right)^5 - 10\left(\frac{t}{T}\right)^3 \right) \tag{1}$$

Where, θ^C is the command angle, θ_i is the initial angle, θ_t is the target angle, T is the task duration, and t is time. The above equation is the minimum jerk equation in the Cartesian space [31], but we use it in the joint space in our reaching tasks to train coordinated movement

2) Inner Loop Controller: Each of the five joint controllers consists of a modified PID feedback controller with nonlinear filter. Additionally, three of the joint controllers (Shoulder flexion/extension, Elbow flexion/extension, and Humeral rotation) have a feedforward controller built upon Iterative Learning algorithm (ILC) in parallel (Fig. 3). Because of the highly nonlinear nature of the plant (robot + Stroke subject's arm) with high variability in spastic resistance there is a need for an adaptive control scheme that can accommodate for these nonlinearities to ensure a consistent performance. An ILC is a very attractive option for this application because of the following reasons,

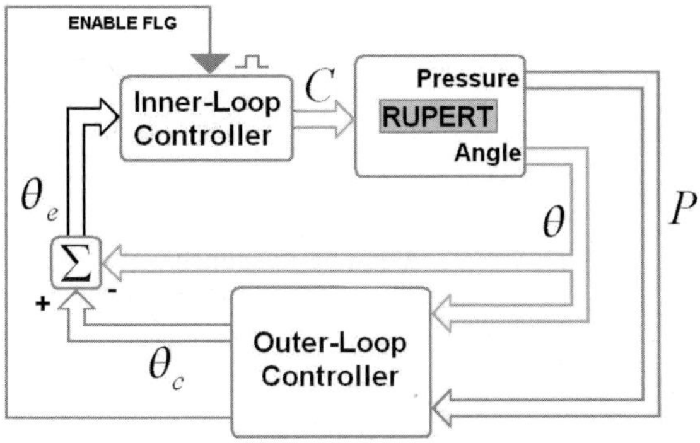

Fig. 2. Overall Closed-Loop Control Structure

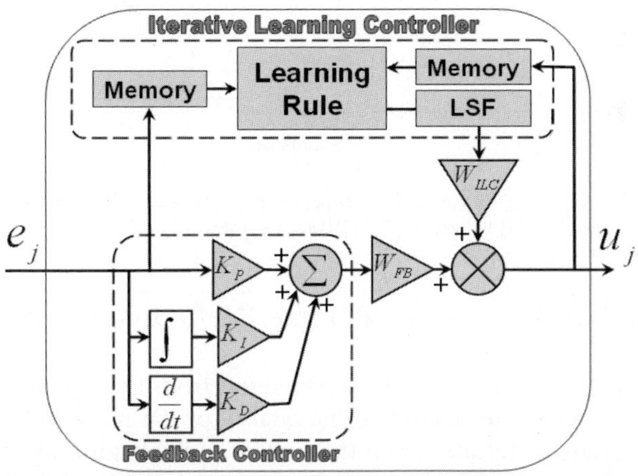

Fig. 3. Individual Joint Controller with PID and ILC Controller (Shoulder Flexion/Extension, Elbow Flexion/Extension and Humoral Rotation have PID+ILC controller; Elbow Supination/Pronation and Wrist Flexion/Extension have only PID controllers)

1. Highly repetitive nature of the therapeutic training tasks.
2. ILC is a model-free scheme that requires no prior knowledge of the system being controlled.
3. A simple and economical method to implement.

ILC improves the performance of the system by learning from the previous executions [32].

The PID gains for PID+ILC controllers are set to low values to ensure an overdamped response from the controller for slow and smooth action and for safety considerations. The ILC helps the IL adapt to different subjects by learning from the previous performance of the controller.

Figure 4 shows the effect of ILC in shaping the feedforward control commands and overall performance of the RUPERT in assisting a reaching movement.

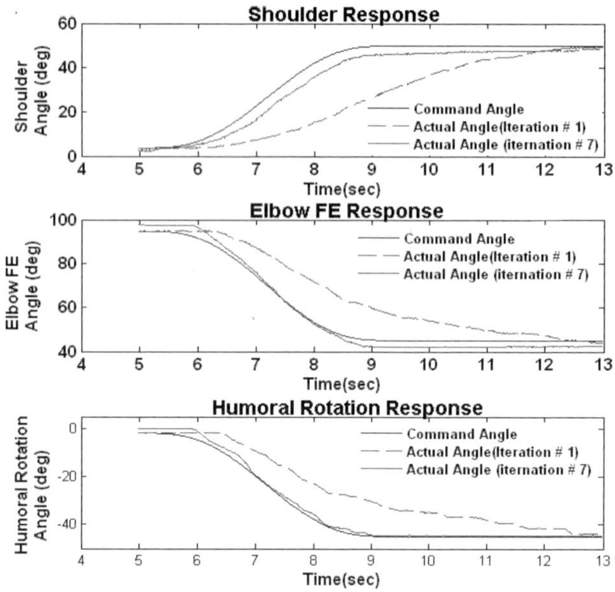

Fig. 4. Closed-Loop Responses for a Reaching Task (Subject1). The plots show the response of the controller for the 1st (PID) and the 7th (PID+ILC) iteration.

4 Biofeedback to Provide Real-Time Performance Evaluation

Together with the pressure sensors the information from the position sensors is used in the biofeedback system to determine the quality of the movement and for estimation of voluntary muscle torques from the patient in evaluation of recovery and improvement of motor function. The performance assessment is then displayed and provide the real-time quantative assessment to assist the therapist and patient during the therapy. The integrated biofeedback system in Figure 5 directly interacts with the Controller shown in Figure 2. He inverse dynamic model of combined arm and RUPERT assists the assessment of how well coordinated in muscle control by the patient for each movement. Once the dynamic torque is estimated for each joint by SimMechanics, the amount of torque supplied by the PMAs is determined. The nonlinear properties of each PMA are empirically measured and derived for a more accurate dynamic model for PMA torque estimation. The biofeedback system estimates the voluntary muscle activity on each joint of the subject by subtracting the estimated dynamic torque from the torque supplied by the PMA. In real-time, the clinician can get an estimate of the amount of voluntary muscle activity of the patient. The goal is to provide only the required pressure in the PM and motivate the voluntary control and initiation of the movement by the patient to promote desired neuroplasticity.

The information provided in the biofeedback currently includes: actual trajectory, movement smoothness, joint synergy, amount of voluntary force, and time to complete the task.

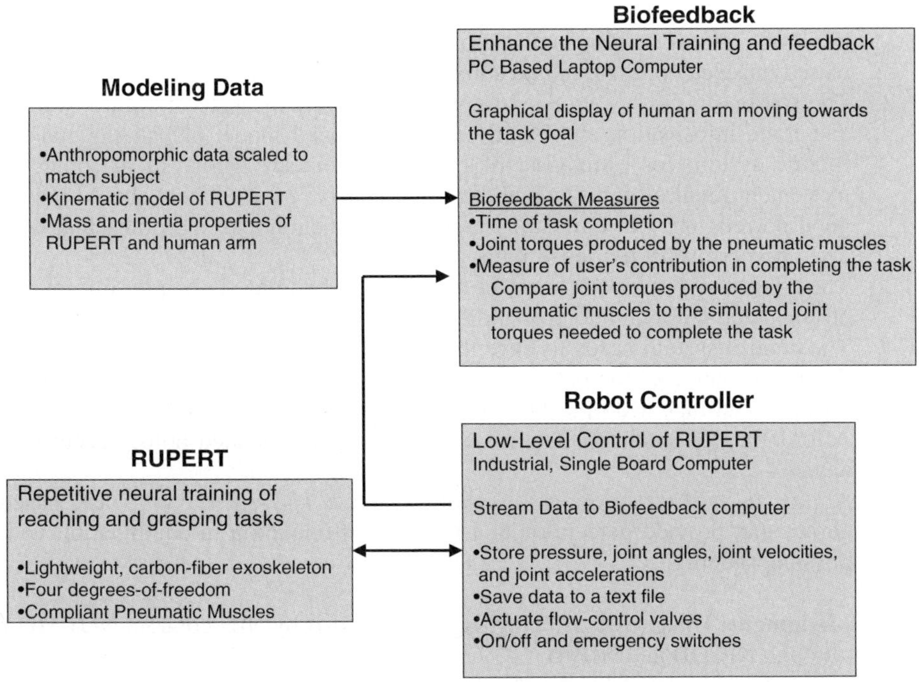

Fig. 5. The integrated biofeedback system directly interacts with the Robot Controller shown in Figure 2. The pressure, joint angles, joint velocities, and joint accelerations are streamed to the biofeedback system for analysis. Anthropomorphic data and RUPERT data are used to determine the inertia and mass of each arm segment. The biofeedback system then estimates the voluntary muscle activity of each joint segment of the subject. The time of task completion is also measured. Lastly, the data is stored in a database for follow-up analysis by the clinician.

5 Discussion

Stroke is the leading cause of adult disability in the United States and efficient and cost-effective rehabilitation therapy is needed to alleviate the social and economical burden. Robotic devices that provide assistance to professional therapists for safe, convenient and standardized treatment in the home and clinic offer a way. Using a robot assistance device, extra therapy can be achieved, reducing the strenuous physical requirements demanded of the therapists.

The existing robotic devices and experience accumulated in many years of developing industrial and other robots provide the technical foundation for more effective rehabilitation robots. However, it is important for the community to realize many special features and unique requirements of a safe, compliant, easy to use, and easily adjustable system setup and control algorithm for rehabilitation robots.

Using the development and testing of RUPERT as an example this presentation summarizes several key features and requirements for practical rehabilitation robots. It also presents some unique challenges for the control system design for such systems.

1. The mechanical structure of the system needs to accommodate varying conditions of patients in terms of anatomical and impaired range of motion, impaired muscle coordination and sometimes spastic movement pattern;
2. The sensors in the system need to provide accurate measure of both positional and force information and based on the combined model of patients and the robotic system for estimation of patient's voluntary ability to generate the movement required for a task under training. This measurement should have a good correlation with clinical assessment of function and neuromuscular condition to perform activities of daily living;
3. The control system needs to adapt to patient's changing, hopefully improving, physical and voluntary control ability to generate the movement;
4. The control system needs to have the capability to promote and encourage active participation of the patients during therapy and interact with the patient in a way to facilitate neuroplasticity by providing only necessary assistance;
5. Affordable, low maintenance and easy to use for expanded home based therapy.
6. Ability to interact or integrate with attractive and entertaining task based games that provide perception and cognitive stimulation in combination with physical training.

Acknowledgment. This project is being supported in part by NIH contract NO1-HD-3-3353 through NICHD and NIBIB.

References

1. Jenkins, W.M., Merzenich, M.M.: Reorganization of neocortical representations after brain injury: a neurophysiological model of the bases of recovery from stroke. Prog. Brain Res. 71, 249–266 (1987)
2. Nudo, R.J., Milliken, G.W.: Reorganization of movement representations in primary motor cortex following focal ischemic infarcts in adult squirrel monkeys. J. Neurophysiol 75, 2144–2149 (1996)
3. Nudo, R.J., Milliken, G.W., Jenkins, W.M., Merzenich, M.M.: Use-dependent alterations of movement representations in primary motor cortex of adult squirrel monkeys. J. Neurosci. 16, 785–807 (1996)
4. Nudo, R.J., Plautz, E.J., Frost, S.B.: Role of adaptive plasticity in recovery of function after damage to motor cortex. Muscle Nerve 24, 1000–1019 (2001)
5. Nudo, R.J., Wise, B.M., SiFuentes, F., Milliken, G.W.: Neural substrates for the effects of rehabilitative training on motor recovery after ischemic infarct. Science 272, 1791–1794 (1996)
6. Pons, T.P., Garraghty, P.E., Ommaya, A.K., Kaas, J.H., Taub, E., Mishkin, M.: Massive cortical reorganization after sensory deafferentation in adult macaques. Science 252, 1857–1860 (1991)
7. Reinkensmeyer, D., Lum, P., Winters, J.: Emerging Technologies for Improving Access to Movement Therapy following Neurologic Injury Emerging and Accessible Telecommunications. In: Winters, J., Robinson, C., Simpson, R., Vanderheiden, G. (eds.) Information and Healthcare Technologies - Emerging Challenges in Enabling Universal Access. IEEE Press, Los Alamitos (2002)

8. van der Lee, J.H., Wagenaar, R.C., Lankhorst, G.J., Vogelaar, T.W., Deville, W.L., Bouter, L.M.: Forced use of the upper extremity in chronic stroke patients: results from a single-blind randomized clinical trial. Stroke 30, 2369–2375 (1999)
9. Koeneman, E.J., Schultz, R.S., Wolf, S.L., Herring, D.E., Koeneman, J.B.: A pneumatic muscle hand therapy device. In: The 26th Annual International Conference of the IEEE EMBS, San Francisco, CA (presented 2004)
10. Bharadwaj, K., Sugar, T.G., Koeneman, J.B., Koeneman, E.J.: Design of a robotic gait trainer using spring over muscle actuators for ankle stroke rehabilitation. J. Biomech. Eng. 127, 1009–1013 (2005)
11. Levin, M.F.: Interjoint coordination during pointing movements is disrupted in spastic hemiparesis. Brain 119(Pt 1), 281–293 (1996)
12. Hogan, N., Bizzi, E., Mussa-Ivaldi, F.A., Flash, T.: Controlling multijoint motor behavior. Exerc. Sport. Sci. Rev. 15, 153–190 (1987)
13. Lemay, M.A., Hogan, N., van Dorsten, J.W.: Issues in impedance selection and input devices for multijoint powered orthotics. IEEE Trans. Rehabil. Eng. 6, 102–105 (1998)
14. Caldwell, D.G., Tsagarakis, N.: Biomimetic actuators in prosthetic and rehabilitation applications. Technol. Health Care 10, 107–120 (2002)
15. Klute, G.K., Czerniecki, J.M., Hannaford, B.: McKibben artificial muscles: pneumatic actuators with biomechanical intelligence. In: IEEE/ASME 1999 International Conference on Advanced Intelligent Mechatronics (AIM 1999), Atlanta, GA (1999)
16. Nickel, V.L., Perry, J., Garrett, A.L.: Development of Useful Function in the Severely Paralyzed Hand. Journal of Bone and Joint Surgery 45(A), 933–952 (1963)
17. Tondu, B., Boitier, V., Lopez, P.: Naturally compliant robot-arms actuated by McKibben artificial muscles. In: 1994 IEEE International Conference on Systems, Man and Cybernetics, San Antonio, TX (1994)
18. He, H., Ingalls, T., Olson, L., Ganley, K., Rikakis, T., He, J.: Interactive Multimodal Biofeedback for Task-Oriented Neural Rehabilitation. In: The 27th Annual International Conference of the IEEE EMBS (2005)
19. He, J., Koeneman, E.J., Schultz, R.S., Huang, H., Wanberg, J., Herring, D.E., Sugar, T., Herman, R., Koeneman, J.B.: Design of a robotic upper extremity repetitive therapy device. In: 9th International Conference on Rehabilitation Robotics (2005)
20. Huang, H., He, J.: Utilization of Biomechanical Modeling in Design of Robotic Arm for Rehabilitation of Stroke Patients. In: 26th Annual International Conference of the IEEE EMBS, San Francisco, CA (2004)
21. Byl, N., Roderick, J., Mohamed, O., Hanny, M., Kotler, J., Smith, A., Tang, M., Abrams, G.: Effectiveness of sensory and motor rehabilitation of the upper limb following the principles of neuroplasticity: patients stable poststroke. Neurorehabil. Neural Repair 17, 176–191 (2003)
22. Baer, H.R., Wolf, S.L.: Modified Emory Functional Ambulation Profile: An Outcome Measure for the Rehabilitation of Poststroke Gait Dysfunction. Stroke 32, 973–979 (2001)
23. Carr, E.K., Kenney, F.D.: Positioning of the Stroke Patient: a Review of the Literature. Int. J. Nurs Stud. 29(4), 355–369 (1992)
24. Fugl-Meyer, A.R., et al.: The post-stroke hemiplegic patient: a method of physical performance. Scandinavian Journal of Rehabilitation and Medicine 7, 13–31 (1975)
25. Jones, A., Carr, E.K., Newham, D.J., Wilson-Barnett, J.: Positioning of Stroke Patients: Evaluation of a Teaching Intervention with Nurses. Stroke 29, 1612–1617 (1998)
26. Pearl, M.L., Harris, S.L., Lippitt, S.B., et al.: A System for Describing Positions of the Humerus Relative to the Thorax and its use in the Presentation of Several Functionally Important Arm Positions. J. Shoulder Elbow. Surg. 1(2), 113–118 (1992)
27. Simon, S.R., Alaranta, H.A., An, K.-A., et al.: Kinesiology. In: Simon, S.R., Wilson, J. (eds.) Orthopaedic Basic Science, pp. 519–622. American Academy of Orthopaedic Surgeons, Chicago (1994)

28. Wolf, S.L., Catlin, P.A., et al.: Assessing the Wolf Motor Function Test as an Outcome Measure for Research with Patients Post-stroke. Stroke 32, 1635–1639 (2001)
29. Patton, J.L., Stoykov, M.E., Kovic, M., Mussa-Ivaldi, F.A.: Evaluation of robotic training forces that either enhance or reduce error in chronic hemiparetic stroke survivors. Exp. Brain Res. 168(3), 368–383 (2006)
30. Balasubramanian, S., Ward, J., Sugar, T., He, J.: Characterization of the Dynamic Properties of Pneumatic Muscle Actuators. In: Proc. ICORR (2007)
31. Flash, T., Hogan, N.: The coordination of arm movements: an experimentally confirmed mathematical model. J. Neurosci. 5, 1688–1703 (1985)
32. Bristow, D.A., Tharayil, M., Alleyne, A.G.: A survey of iterative learning control. Control Systems Magazine. IEEE 26, 96–114 (2006)

Jiping He was born in Shanghai, China. He received the B.S. degree in control engineering from Huazhong University of Science and Technology, Wuhan China, in 1982, the M.S. and Ph.D. degrees in electrical engineering from the University of Maryland, College Park, in 1984 and 1988, respectively. He then spent one and a half years as a postdoctoral fellow in the Center for Biological Information Processing and Artificial Intelligence Laboratory, Massachusetts Institute of Technology, Cambridge.

In 1990, he joined Functional Neurosurgery Division of Thomas Jefferson University (TJU), Philadelphia, PA, as a Research Assistant Professor and Adjunct Professor of Physical Therapy. He was a Visiting Scientist at Human Information Processing Program of Princeton University, Princeton, NJ during 1991 and 1992. He has been a faculty at Arizona State University, Tempe, since 1994 and is now Professor of Bioengineering, Director of Center for Neural Interfaces Design. His primary research and teaching interests include the application of advanced control theory to the analysis and control of neuromuscular systems for posture and movement, implantable neural interface technology, cortical and spinal cord recording and stimulation for sensorimotor adaptation and control, application of robotics and virtual reality research to neural rehabilitation and prosthetic devices. He is also actively involved in the curriculum development of bio-control and neural engineering, and reform in interdisciplinary graduate education and research training.

Dr. He is a Senior Editor for the *IEEE Transaction on Neural Systems and Rehabilitation Engineering*. He is active in professional services by organizing and chairing international conferences.

Architecture of Multi-Agent-Based Multi-Operator Multi-Mobile-Manipulator Teleoperation System

Zhenzhong Yu, Jihong Yan, Jie Zhao, Yongsheng Gao, and Hegao Cai

State Key Laboratory of Robotics and System, Harbin Institute of Technology, 150080 Harbin, China
yzzrobot@126.com, 2002paradise@163.com, jzhao@hit.edu.cn, gao_ys@hit.edu.cn, hgcai@hope.hit.edu.cn

Abstract. Being characteristics of motion, coordination, distribution, non-determinism etc, multi-operator multi-mobile-manipulator teleoperation system has difficulties in controlling and implementation. Multi-Agent-Based architecture of the system can distinctly describe the information interactive relationship between components of the system, and optimize intelligence distribution between human and robot, so it helps to reduce difficulties in controlling and implementation of the system. After the physical structure of the system was analyzed, the system was divided into several sub-systems with given function, and then a Multi-Agent-Based layered architecture with shared control mode of the system was proposed and the function of each Agent was planned. Multi-Agent's mixed communication structure was designed by both of blackboard model and Peer-to-Peer model. According to characteristics of the system, a kind of general mixed architecture for Agent was proposed, and an example of implementation method of Agent was given, then the validity of the mixed architecture was verified by designing experiment.

Keywords: Architecture, multi-agent, multi-mobile-manipulator, teleoperation.

1 Introduction

Multi-operator multi-mobile-manipulator (MOM^3) teleoperation system has the characteristics of mobility, cooperation, distribution, fault tolerance, redundancy etc, it can enlarge working scope of robots and enhance the ability of the system to fit into more complex task. And MOM^3 teleoperation technology becomes the forefront of teleoperation technological development. However, due to the layers of the structure of the system and the interactive information between components of the system are very complex, the system is more difficult to be controlled and established.

Suzuki proposed a three-layers operational functions of the human-machine interaction of multiple robots to achieve the organization and coordination [1] and [2]. However, these are simple command consultations, dynamic coordination can not be made for operation orders. Danel discussed an interactive method between agents and blackboard model, and a common control model was presented in terms of it [3]. L.X ZHANG built a kind of control model of a single remote control robot welding

C. Xiong et al. (Eds.): ICIRA 2008, Part II, LNAI 5315, pp. 17–26, 2008.

system in the base of Mulit-Agent technology [4]. At present, few scholars research on the architecture of MOM^3 teleoperation system at domestic and international.

Multi-Agent has the characteristics of autonomy, distribution, coordination, and self-organizing, learning and reasoning abilities [5]. The use of Multi-Agent technology to build the architecture of MOM^3 teleoperation system, can divide the entire system into a number of functions scattered components that described by Agent, which have certain intelligence that is capable of finishing some work independently and improving interactive and synergic ability of system. Fully make use of the Multi-Agent technology can greatly reduce the system's difficulties in controlling and implementation and can improve the stability and the ability to coordinate operation of the system.

On the basis of analyzing the characteristics of the physical structure of MOM^3 teleoperation system, a Multi-Agent-based layered architecture with shared control mode [6] for the system was built. According to the characteristics of MOM^3 teleoperation system, a kind of mixed architecture for Agent which adapt to MOM^3 system was designed. An example of describing Agent's specific implementation method was given, and an experiment to validate the efficiency of the designed mixed architecture of Agent was made.

2 Physical Structure of MOM^3 System

The physical structure of MOM^3 teleoperation system is shown in Fig. 1. Several mobile-manipulator located in the same physical space. A number of operators in different geographical location cooperate with each other by virtual environment to finish teleoperation tasks on the assistant of real-time video transmitted from the remote side. In accordance with the function, system can be divided into six subsystems, User Interaction Sub-system, Real-time Video Sub-system, Communication Sub-system, Security Sub-system, Coordination and Control Sub-system and Robotics Sub-system.

(1) User Interaction Sub-system: It Includes Distributed Virtual Environment, user interactive equipments (master hand, mouse, keyboard, etc.), and it gives supports for the operators to interact with MOM^3 teleoperation system.

(2) Real-time Video Sub-system: The vidicons capture remote robots' whole or part scene information, and the information is disposed in Video Collection and Disposal PC, and then being transmitted to operators by network. It provides operators with real-time video assistance.

(3) Communication Sub-system: It can implement the information communication between components of the system. There are several communication modes in the Communication Sub-system. It provides master and slave side with TCP/IP protocol and implements communication between them by client / server communication mode. The robots and network server exchange information with each other by WLAN.

(4) Security Sub-system: It is used to keep the system working safely and no collision. On the one hand, inhibit operator's misoperation by software tools in distributed virtual environment. On the other hand, Coordination and Control Sub-system fusing the control information of the system to detect abnormity and making quick response, and Robotics Sub-system with its own sensors to achieve real-time obstacle avoidance.

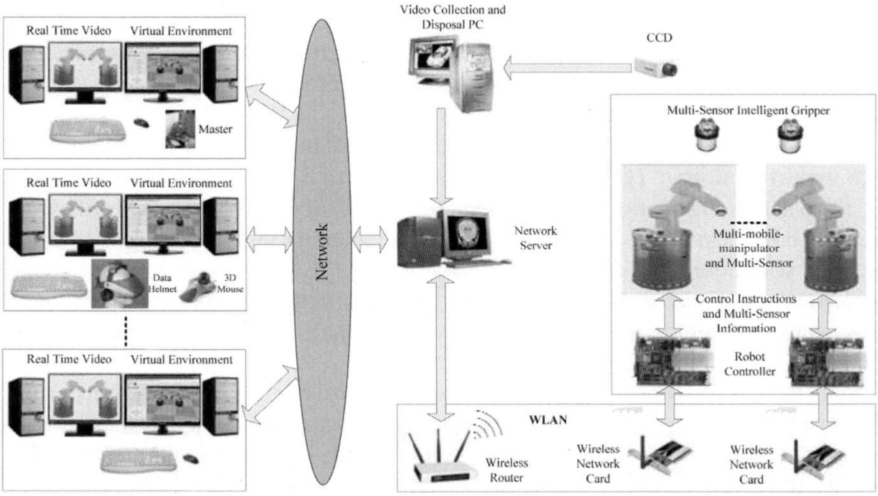

Fig. 1. Physical structure of MOM^3 system

(5) Coordination and Control Sub-system: It fuses the operators' control orders, robot's movement prior knowledge, multi-sensor information etc, to plan and make decision, and then control several robots to work efficiently and no collision.

(6) Robotics Sub-system: It is the implementation part of the MOM^3 teleoperation system. Robots are smart in a certain extent, able to respond quickly to dangerous conditions, and can use its intelligence to give operators with operation support on sophisticated teleoperation tasks. Robots can communicate with each other through wireless network, and then achieve some certain autonomy collaboration to some extent.

3 Multi-Agent Based Architecture of MOM^3 System

In accordance with the characteristics of MOM^3 teleoperation system, combining with the advantages of Multi-Agent, a Multi-Agent based, layered and shared control architecture for the system is proposed, shown in Fig. 2. Functions of each Agent are described as follows:

Sub-system Administration Agent administers the transmitted information between the sub-system and external components of the MOM^3 system and launched Agents in the sub-system. The full name and feature list of the launched Agents are stored in the Agent's Database in the sub-system.

System Administration Agent operates in the network server that is located in the robot side. The Agent has two main functions : *1)* Communicating with each Sub-system Administration Agent to get all the activated Agent's name, sub-system belongingness and functional description, which may be used by other Agent to invite public bidding use Contract Net Protocol [7]. *2)* Administrating operators' logging, withdraw and roles (team leader, team members, candidate etc) distribution. When an operator logged successfully, the System Administration Agent will stored the name and functional info of all the Agents in sub-system in which the operator locates into the Database. And the information of the Agents stored in the Database will be written off along with the operator's withdrawing.

Operation Administration Agent belongs to User Interaction Sub-system, and has three main functions : *1)* Providing software tools to operators such as virtual guides [8], to make the operation task conveniently. *2)* Carrying out the path planning of virtual robot, to give the operators support on incident-class operation. *3)* Providing operators with coordination between them.

Consistency Control Agent cooperates with Consistency Control Agent of other sub-systems in keeping the DVE's virtual model state consistency and the consistency between virtual model and physical model.

Abnormality Detection Agent in all sub-systems has similar functions, such as monitoring emergency events and network communication status and making a rapid response to solve the problems. According to the specific requirements of sub-systems, the achievement of the Agent is slightly different.

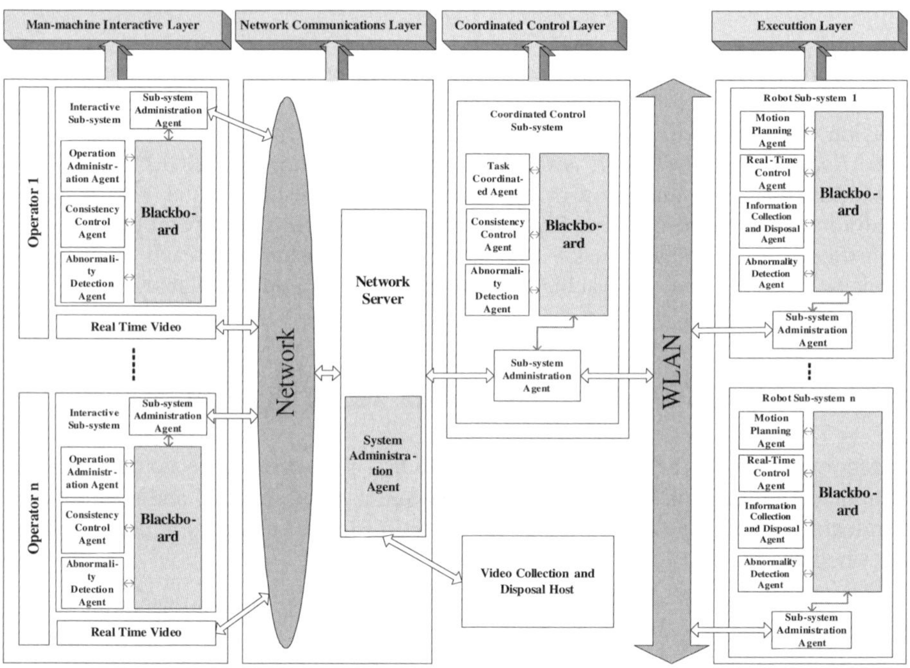

Fig. 2. Multi-Agent based and layered architecture of MOM^3 system

Task Coordinated Agent operates in Coordination and Control Sub-system, has four main functions : *1)* Syncretizing the intelligence of operators and robots. *2)* Achieving task allocation. *3)* Fusing the operation orders of operators and multi-sensor information of the robots, and replanning the task if it is necessary. *4)* Coordinating with Abnormality Detection Agent to make sure that the system works safely.

Motion Planning Agent operates in Robotics Sub-system. It receives the control tasks from coordinated control layer and in accordance with the knowledge (Planning Algorithm) of itself to make a real-time motion planning, and coordinating with Real-Time Control Agent to achieve operational tasks.

Real-Time Control Agent operates in Robotics Sub-system. It receives the motion information planned by Motion Planning Agent, and generates control orders to control the robot in real time. The Results of the implementation were sent back to Task Coordinated Agent cyclically.

Information Collection and Disposal Agent collects and disposes the information of sensors of robot in real time, and then provides it to other Agent.

Communication between Agents adopts the mode of the combination of blackboard structure and peer-to-peer structure. Agents in the same sub-system work under the same software running environment, is easily to implement information-sharing, should adopt the blackboard structure to achieve communications. Agents between different sub-systems have the characteristic of distribution, and there were the network delay, should adopt peer-to-peer communications structure. In addition, System Administration Agent and Sub-system Administration Agents communicate with each other using peer-to-peer structure also.

4 Realization of Agent

4.1 Design Architecture of Agent

According to the above analysis of the MOM^3 teleoperation system's characteristics and Agents' functions, designed the mixed architecture [9] of Agent as shown in Fig. 3. The architecture Agent can meet not only respond quickly to the demand, but also the demand for higher intelligence. Of which there are:

(1) Inductive Module: It is responsible for receiving the external environment (such as the operation orders, the state of the environment changes, and other information), and processing information into a knowledge-level expression.

(2) Reactive Module: It has the function of Reactive Agent. It receives the messages coming from Inductive Module and Communication Module, and classifies message in the basis of rules stored in Repository. Emergency or simple events are sent to the Execution Device and are implemented immediately, and the complicated events are processed further by Cooperative and Planning Module.

(3) Communication Module: It administers the information exchange between Agents. On the one hand, it receives the message of other Agents, and sends the message to Reactive Module for further processing. On the other hand, it sends the information of Reactive Module and Decision Module to other Agents.

(4) Database and Repository: They are used to store names, capacities, objectives, and other description information, and store rules, control knowledge, field knowledge and other correlative information.

(5) Cooperative and Planning Module: According to its own targets, it gives complex behavior of decomposition, planning, reasoning, solving with correlative knowledge, and the results will be sent to Decision Module. According to the Contract Net Protocol, it provides Agents with collaboration in rules.

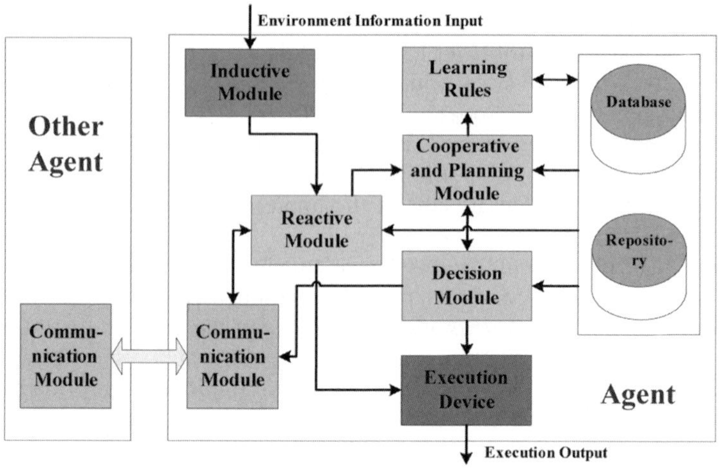

Fig. 3. Architecture of agent

(6) Learning Rules: According to the certain study rules, learns the planning and collaborative process, and uses acquired knowledge to update the Database.

(7) Decision Module: It receives the results outputted by Cooperative and Planning Module, and according to certain rules making conflict inspection and elimination. Then it sends the results to Execution Device or transmits the results to other Agents by Communication Module.

(8) Execution Device: It is the interactive tool of Agent and the environment. It brings actions to act on the environment (virtual scene, states of virtual robots) according to the information coming from Reactive Module or Decision Module.

4.2 Agent Implementation Example

Take Consistency Control Agent as an example to introduce the implementation method of the Agent.

Consistency control is the basis of VE teleoperation to work effectively. Consistency control of the system consists of two aspects: the consistency control of DVE model's state and the consistency control between virtual model and physical model. It only considers the consistency control between the virtual environments of two operators in the example, and uses Local Lag Based Consistency Maintaining Algorithm [10] to keep consistency of DVE. In order to facilitate the description, designed a typical communication structure of the Agents (two client as an example, not consider the robot side) is shown in Fig. 4.

Consistency Control Agent can be described by eight components : {*Inductive Module, Reactive Module, Database, Repository, Cooperative and Planning Module, Communication Module, Decision Module, Execution Device*}。 Components described as follows:

(1) Inductive Module: It gets operator's operational orders or the orders programmed by Operation Administration Agent, and processes orders into a knowledge-level expression, and then sent it to Reactive Module.

(2) Reactive Module: It completed two major tasks: *1)* Receives Inductive Module's messages, and puts the timestamps on the messages according to the lag time value which is stored in the Repository. Then it puts the messages in message queue of Agent, and executes tasks when the lag time is over to change the states of local VE. At the same time, Communication Module processes the messages into KQML format, and stores them in shared storage area (information-sharing pool of blackboard). Sub-system Administration Agent takes out the messages and sends them to the shared storage area of Client 2 by collaborating with Sub-system Administration Agent of the partner and use peer-to-peer communication mode with Contract Net Protocol. The Consistency Control Agent of Client 2 executes tasks explained by the messages to update the VE. *2)* Receives VE updating messages from Client 2 through Communication Module, and comparing the timestamp of the message with the local physical time. If it is not overtime, put the messages in the message queue to wait for implementation by Execution Device to update local VE. If it is overtime, the Cooperative and Planning Module will make a further processing on the messages.

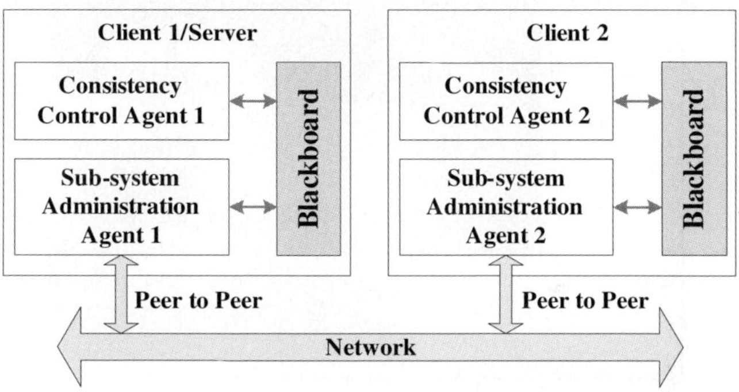

Fig. 4. Communication structure of Consistency Control Agent

(3) Database: It is used to store names, addresses, PRIs, capacities, targets, status (Invalid, Idle, Busy), and other information, of which fully describe the Consistency Control Agent. When Consistency Control Agent is activated, some of the information will be registered in the relevant Sub-system Administration Agent.

(4) Repository: It is used to store the rules of Local Lag Based Consistency Maintaining Algorithm, lag time value and the syntax of Time-Distorting State Repair Mechanism, and to store the implementation records of the system at specific time points.

(5) Cooperative and Planning Module: When it received information, the state of VE has been in a short period inconsistency (information transmission time is longer than local lag time). It uses the Time-Distorting State Repair Mechanism and the implementation records of the VE to make the repair orders for VE. The Decision Module makes the conflict check for the orders, and then sends them to Execution Device and to the Client 2 by Communication Module

(6) Communication Module: It is responsible for receiving the information of Reactive Module and Decision Module and processing the information into KQML format, and then put it in shared storage area. It processes the update information that stored in shared storage area and comes from Client 2 into a knowledge-level expression.

(7) Decision Module: It makes conflict inspection and elimination for the information of Cooperative and Planning Module, and sends the results to Execution Device to update local VE or to other Agent by the Communication Module.

(8) Execution Device: It is used to update the VE according to the information of Reactive Module and Decision Module.

4.3 Experiment

In order to verify the capability of the architecture of Agent, as is shown in Fig. 3, it takes achieved Consistency Control Agent as an example, considering only two clients' VE, establishes the experimental system shown in Fig. 4.

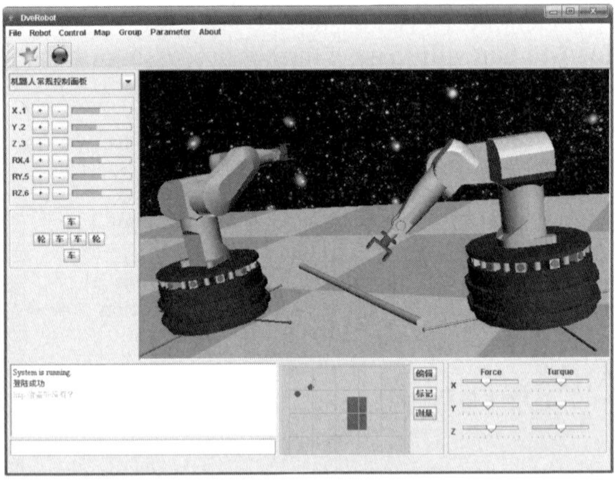

Fig. 5. Man-machine interactive VE

The experiment is carried out in the LAN, using delay simulator [11] to simulate random network latency, using Java / java 3D software create the virtual environment as shown in Fig. 5. When operators start their virtual environment software, each agent is activated. Two Sub-system Administration Agents communicate with each other by C / S mode to get the registration information of all the agents of other side. And then they exchange information by Contract Net Protocol.

Local lag time value is set to 200 ms, the range of latency time of delay simulator is set from 0 to 500 ms, and the probability of more than 200 ms delay is set up less than 5% (the probability of having a short period inconsistency is less than 5%). Firstly, two operators control the different virtual robots respectively, and then they operate the two virtual robots in turns in their own virtual environment, to achieve that, at the same time the two operators control the same virtual robot. Experimental results show that in the process of the operation, the state consistency of two virtual environments is all right, there are no halt and distortion in the process of operation, and Consistency Control Agent is steady.

5 Conclusion

Through the above study reached the following conclusions:

(1) Established sharing controlled and layerd architecture of MOM^3 teleoperation system, which is based on Multi-Agent technology, can distinctly describe the information interactive relationship between components of the system. So it can reduce the system's difficulties in controlling and implementation, and optimize intelligence distribution between human and robots. According to the characteristics of the MOM^3 teleoperation system, with the combination of the blackboard model and peer-to-peer model, a mixed-communication model that can optimize the communications between the Agents is proposed.

(2) The whole system is divided into several sub-systems in terms of their functions. The sub-systems in the basis of multi-Agent technology, having the characteristics of autonomy and coordination, can help to reduce the negative effects that are caused by communication delay on the system's part capability, to improve the stability of system and to enhance the system's ability to coordinate operation.

(3) A general architecture of Agent for MOM^3 teleoperation system is designed. Given by an example on the implementation of Agent, an experiment to verify the validity of the architecture is designed. It established the foundation for the realization of Multi-Agent-Based MOM^3 teleoperation system.

Acknowledgments

This work was sponsored by the National High Technology Research and Development Project (Grant No. 2006AA04Z245).

References

1. Suzuki, T., Fujii, T., Yokota, K., Asama, H., Kaetsu, H., Endo, I.: Teleoperation of Multiple Robots through Internet. In: IEEE International Workshop on Robot and Human Communication, Tsukuba, pp. 84–89 (1996)
2. Suzuki, T., Fujii, T., Yokota, K., Asama, H., Kaetsu, H., Endo, I.: A Multi-Robot Teleoperation System Utilizing the Internet. Advanced Robotics 11(8), 781–797 (1998)
3. Daniel, D.C.: Collaborating software blackboard and multi-agent systems & the future. In: Proceedings of the International Lisp Conference, New York (October 2003)
4. Zhang, L.X., Wu, L., Gao, H.M., Zhang, G.J.: Agent-based modeling and control of remote robotic welding system. In: RWIA 2006. Lecture Notes in Control and Information Sciences, pp. 2087–2094 (2006)
5. Liu, J.K., Er, L.J.: Overview of Application of Multiagent Technology. Contol and Decision 16(2), 133–140 (2001)
6. Sheridan, T.B.: Telerobotics, Automation, and Human Supervisory Control, pp. 1–12, 98–108. MIT Press, Cambridge (1992)
7. Smith, R.G., Davis, R.: Framework for Cooperation in Distributed Problem Solving. IEEE Transactions on Systems, Man and Cybernetics 11(1), 61–70 (1981)

8. Yan, J.H., Zhao, N., Zhao, J., Gao, S.: Research on adaptive virtual guide based telerobotics. Journal of Harbin Institute of Technology 39(1), 59–63 (2007)
9. Wooldridge, M., Jennings, N.: Intelligent. Agents: Theory and Practice. The Knowledge Engineering Review 10(2), 115–152 (1995)
10. Chen, L., Chen, G.C., Chen, C.: Local lag based consistency maintaining technology. Journal of Zhejiang University (Engineering Science) 38(2), 149–153 (2004)
11. Zhao, M.G., Zhao, J., Cui, Z., Cai, H.G.: An internet-based Telerobtics—Telerobot. Journal of Harbin Institute of Technology 33(1), 8–12 (2001)

Stable Multirate Control Algorithm for Haptic Dental Training System

Xiaowei Dai, Yuru Zhang, Yonggang Cao, and Dangxiao Wang

State Key Laboratory of Virtual Reality Technology and System, Beihang University
Beijing, P.R. China, 100083
daixw@me.buaa.edu.cn, yuru@buaa.edu.cn

Abstract. This paper proposes a multirate control algorithm to guarantee the stability of haptic dental training system. In terms of a high-frequency force interpolating model, a multirate system with two levels up-sampling is introduced. The first level up-sampling achieves the haptic rendering with 1K Hz and the second level achieves the interpolating algorithm with 10K Hz or higher. Due to the slow velocity of dental training system, the complex virtual tooth surface can be regarded as a series of consecutive virtual tangent planes, in which the interpolating algorithm is designed with virtual wall model. Theoretical analysis proves that the multirate control algorithm can enlarge the range of virtual stiffness and improve the stability. Numerical and experimental results of a three degree-of-freedom haptic device demonstrate the effectiveness of the proposed method.

Keywords: Haptic system, Stability, Multirate Control, Dental Training System.

1 Introduction

Stability is a prerequisite for a haptic dental training system. Unstable phenomena influence the trainee's haptic sensation for dental training. Wang et al. [1] developed haptic dental training systems with virtual spring model, in which the stability criterion can be defined as the range of virtual stiffness. The wider the range is, the more dental training applications the device can be applied to. For a haptic interaction system under the impedance control, several factors, both mechanical and control systems, affect the virtual stiffness.

The mechanical factors relate to the device damping, coulomb friction and transmission stiffness. J. Colgate et al [2] developed a theoretical model illustrating the impacts of device damping and sampling period on virtual stiffness and indicated that increasing the device damping or decreasing the sampling period can enlarge the range of the virtual stiffness. Y. Luo et al [3] concluded that the increase of transmission stiffness can enhance the virtual stiffness. N. Diolaiti et al [4] examined how the maximum achievable virtual stiffness interacts with the inertia, natural viscosity, and coulomb damping of a haptic device. M. Kawai et al [5] and J. Mehling et al [6] proposed two different methods to enlarge the system damping by adding mechanical damping and electronic damping to improve the stability. The control factors include

C. Xiong et al. (Eds.): ICIRA 2008, Part II, LNAI 5315, pp. 27–35, 2008.

sampling period, ZOH (zcro order holder), position and velocity resolution. J. Colgate et al [2] analyzed the effects of sampling period, sensor quantization and velocity filtering on virtual stiffness. J. Abbott [7] modeled the effects of position resolution and obtained a necessary and sufficient condition for passivity.

The above studies indicate that the sampling period is one of the major factors and it is possible to improve the stability by decreasing the sampling period. K. Akahane et al [9] introduced the 10K Hz high definition haptic rendering for both fidelity and stability. For the same purpose, J. Kim et al [10] proposed a multirate control framework with a slow rate for haptic rendering algorithm and a fast rate for low-level controller having energy bounding algorithm. In both of their papers, the stability analysis and condition about multirate control are not presented. K. Lee et al [11] applied multirate control to improve the stability. However, they did not take the computational time delay in the interpolating period into account.

Aiming at enhancing the virtual stiffness and improving the stability, this paper proposes a multirate control algorithm and presents the system stability condition under the multirate control. Section 2 describes the multirate control architecture. Section 3 introduces the multirate interpolating algorithm. Section 4 presents the stability condition under this algorithm. Section 5, in terms of the contrastive experiments, validates that the multirate control algorithm is efficient and feasible in improving stability. Section 6 is the conclusion.

2 Multirate Control Architecture

In haptic dental training system, PC is mainly responsible for virtual environment rendering and haptic rendering, the controller is mainly responsible to transfer the digital virtual force signal received from PC to analog signal, which is used to control the output torque of the driven motor. The controller updates the analog signal at the same frequency as PC updates the digital signal. The single control rate is the characteristic of the conventional impedance haptic control, which illustrated in Fig. 1. Where, $F_d(t)$ and $F_e(t)$ denote the output force of haptic device and the virtual force; $v(t)$ and $X(t)$ denote the velocity and displacement of haptic device.

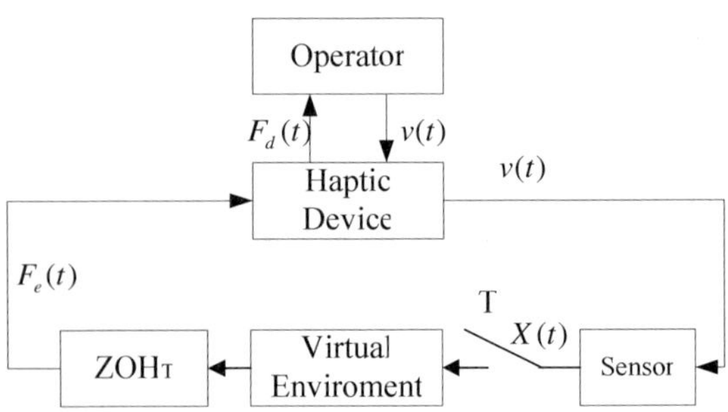

Fig. 1. Structure of conventional impedance control

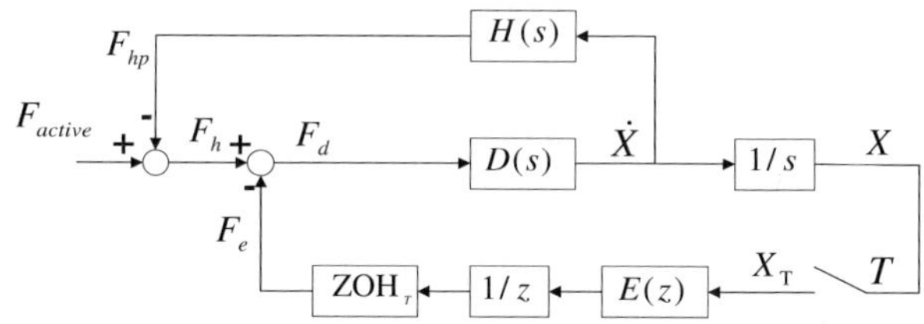

Fig. 2. System block diagram of single rate control

In Fig. 2, T, $1/z$, and ZOH_T respectively denote the sampling period, the computational time delay and the zero order holder with the sampling period T; $\dot{X}$, X and X_T denote the velocity, displacement and sampling displacement of the haptic device; F_{active}, F_{hp}, F_h denote the operator's active force, passive force and the composition of forces on the haptic device; F_e and F_d denote the force computed by virtual environment and the composition of forces imposed on the end of haptic device. The detailed expressions of $H(s)$, $D(s)$ and $E(z)$ are as follows:

$$H(s) = M_h s + B_h + \frac{K_h}{s} \tag{1}$$

$$D(s) = \frac{1}{M_d s + B_d} \tag{2}$$

$$E(z) = K_e X_T(z) \tag{3}$$

Therefore, the overall transfer function is,

$$\frac{\dot{X}(s)}{F_{active}(s)} = \frac{s}{(M_h + M_d + \frac{K_e T^2}{2})s^2 + (B_h + B_d - \frac{3K_e T}{2})s + K_h + K_e} \tag{4}$$

Consequently, the stability condition is as follows:

$$K_e < \frac{2}{3}\frac{B_h + B_d}{T} \tag{5}$$

Considering the stability condition, the decrease of sampling period can effectively enhance the virtual stiffness. This conclusion triggers the multirate control algorithm. The multirate control algorithm is implemented by high-frequency interpolating model, which samples the position and forecast the output force of the haptic device with 10K Hz or higher frequency. The system block diagram of multirate control algorithm is designed as shown in Fig. 3. The following part of this paper quantificationally analyzes the effect of multirate control on system stability.

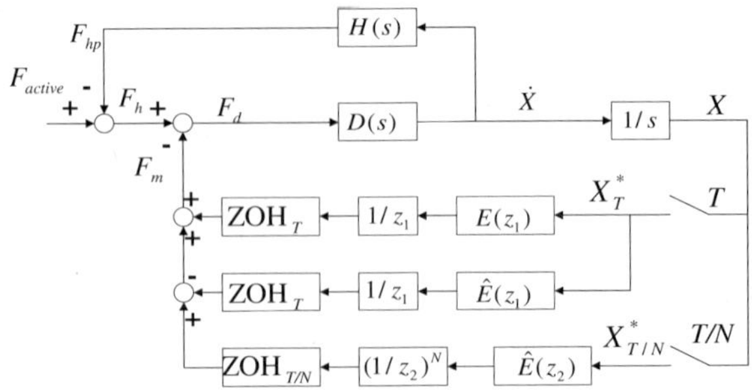

Fig. 3. System block diagram of the multirate control

Compared with Fig. 2, N denotes the proportion of interpolating frequency to the conventional update frequency; $\hat{E}(z_1)$ and $\hat{E}(z_2)$ denote the high-frequency interpolating model with different sampling periods T and T/N ; $1/z_1$ and ZOH_T denote the computational time delay and the zero order holder with the sampling period T ; $1/z_2$ and $\text{ZOH}_{T/N}$ denote the computational time delay and the zero order holder with the sampling period T/N .

3 High-Frequency Interpolating Model

The update period of force signals coming from PC is ΔT , however, the controller updates the motor torque signals in interval of $\Delta T/N$. The controller utilizes the information of the current device position and posture to compute the increment of output force on-line and interpolates the motor control force between the two consecutive force singals coming from PC. Fig. 4 illustrates the multirate interpolating algorithm with the virtual enviromen is virtual wall.

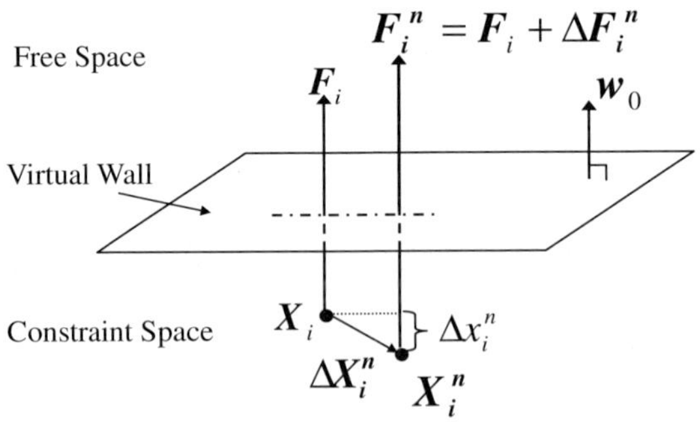

Fig. 4. The diagram of multirate interpolating algorithm

In Fig. 4, K_e denotes the stiffness of the virtual wall; $\boldsymbol{w}_0$ denotes the unit vector of the normal of virtual wall; $\boldsymbol{X}_i$, $\boldsymbol{F}_i$ denote the device displacement and virtual force at the initial time t_i; $\Delta\boldsymbol{X}_i^n$, $\Delta\boldsymbol{F}_i^n$ denote the increment of that at the interpolating time $t_i^n = t_i + n\times\Delta T/N$; $\boldsymbol{X}_i^n$, $\boldsymbol{F}_i^n$ respectively denote that at the interpolating time t_i^n; Δx_i^n denotes the projection of $\boldsymbol{X}_i^n$ in $\boldsymbol{w}_0$.

The detailed algorithm is as follows:

$$\Delta\theta_i^n = \theta_i^n - \theta_i \tag{6}$$

$$\Delta\boldsymbol{X}_i^n = J_i \cdot \Delta\theta_i^n \tag{7}$$

$$\Delta x_i^n = \Delta\boldsymbol{X}_i^n \cdot \boldsymbol{w}_0 \tag{8}$$

$$\Delta\boldsymbol{F}_i^n = K_e \Delta x_i^n \boldsymbol{w}_0 \tag{9}$$

$$\boldsymbol{F}_i^n = \boldsymbol{F}_i + \Delta\boldsymbol{F}_i^n \tag{10}$$

Where, θ_i is the motor angle at t_i; θ_i^n is the motor angle at t_i^n; J_i is the velocity Jacobian matrix at t_i.

In this algorithm, the high-frequency interpolating model is the same as the spring model with stiffness K_e, so

$$\hat{E}(z_1) = K_e X_T^*(z_1) \tag{11}$$

$$\hat{E}(z_2) = K_e X_{T/N}^*(z_2) \tag{12}$$

Fig. 5 demonstrates the model of tooth surface probing in the haptic dental training system. Although the surface curve of the tooth is complex, the point where the tool contacts the tooth can be considered as a virtual tangent plane during each update period because the velocity of the operator is relatively slow. Accordingly, the virtual wall model and the multirate interpolating algorithm can be used during the whole process, as shown in Fig. 6.

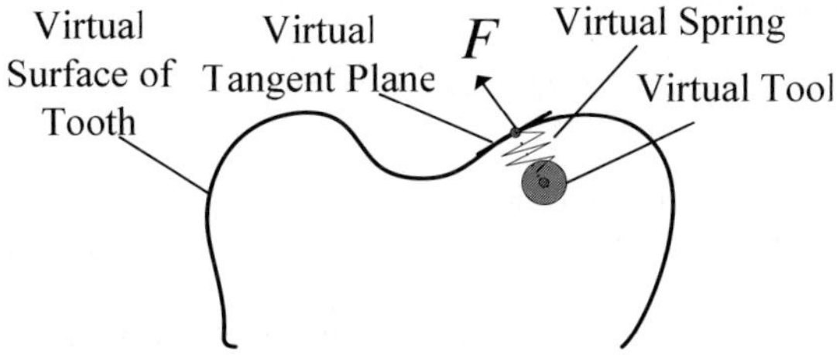

Fig. 5. Model of virtual tooth probing

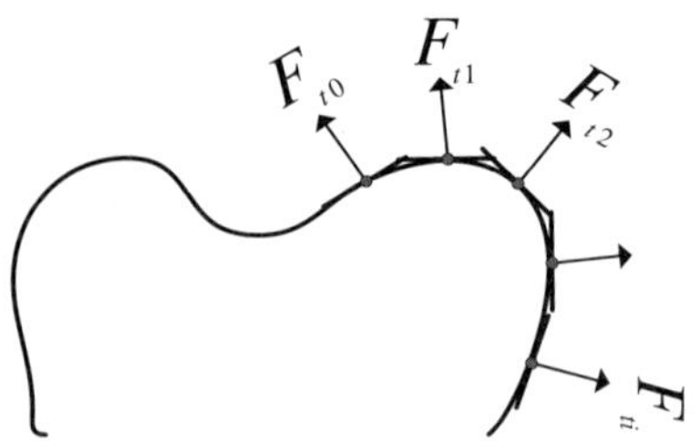

Fig. 6. Multi planes in virtual tooth probing

4 Stability Condition

The overall transfer function of the multirate control system, illustrated in Fig. 3, becomes,

$$\frac{\dot{X}(s)}{F_{active}(s)} = \frac{s}{(2N(M_h + m_d) + K_e T^2)s^2 + (2N(B_h + b_d) - (2N+1)K_e T)s + (2NK_h + K_e)} \tag{13}$$

The overall system is stable if and only if:

$$2N(M_h + m_d) + K_e T^2 > 0 \tag{14}$$

$$2NK_h + K_e > 0 \tag{15}$$

$$2N(B_h + b_d) - (2N+1)K_e T > 0 \tag{16}$$

The stability condition (14) and (15) are always satisfied, so the inequality (16) gives the system stability condition as follows:

$$K_e < \frac{2N}{2N+1} \frac{(B_h + b_d)}{T} \tag{17}$$

Considering the inequality (17), it can be inferred that if $N = 1$, the stability condition of multirate control is the same as that of single rate control (inequality (5)). Obviously, the range of the virtual stiffness is enlarged with the increase of N, and furthest it can increase to 150 percent.

5 Experiment

These experiments are conducted to derive the maximum virtual stiffness under single rate control and multirate control and to validate that multirate control can enhance the virtual stiffness. During following experiments, the virtual environment is a virtual wall with pure spring and the virtual wall exists at the origin of x axes. The virtual spring only exists in the constraint space where the x coordinate is negative. The operator operates the haptic device to contact the virtual wall from the free space.

PC updates the virtual force in 1K Hz frequency. However, the controller interpolates the control force imposed on the driven motor in 10K Hz under multirate control.

The 3DOF haptic device, as shown in Fig. 7, is usesd in the following experiments. The maximum force of the haptic device is 5N and the position resolution is 0.05mm.

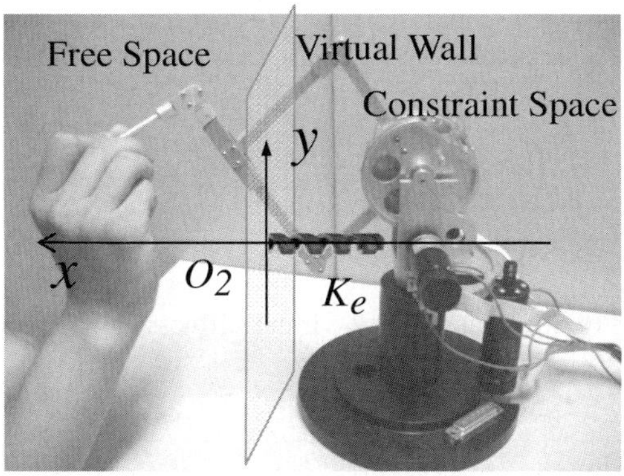

Fig. 7. 3DOF haptic device

In the experiments under single rate control, the operator can feel the haptic device vibrates violently when the haptic device contacts the virtual wall if the virtual stiffness reaches $3.0N/mm$. The similar vibration phenomenon doesn't take place if the virtual stiffness is no more than $2.8N/mm$. So the maximum achievable virtual stiffness is approximately $2.8N/mm$ under single rate control. The displacement and velocity of the haptic device are recorded, as shown in Fig. 8 and 9.

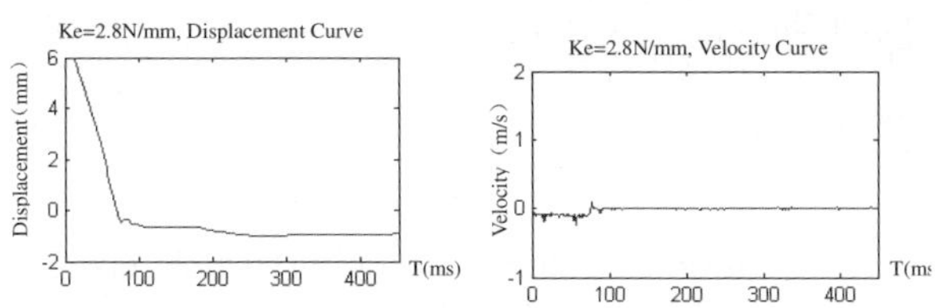

Fig. 8. Single rate control, virtual stiffness Ke=2.8N/mm

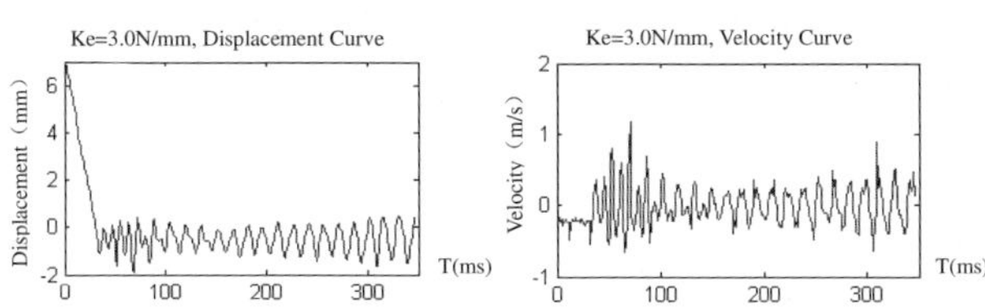

Fig. 9. Single rate control, virtual stiffness Ke=3.0N/mm

In the experiments under multirate control, the displacement and velocity of the haptic device are also recorded, as shown in Fig. 10 and 11. Compared with single rate control, the operator feels the violent vibration only if the virtual stiffness reaches $4.3N/mm$. Therefore, the maximum achievable virtual stiffness is approximately $4.1N/mm$ under multirate control.

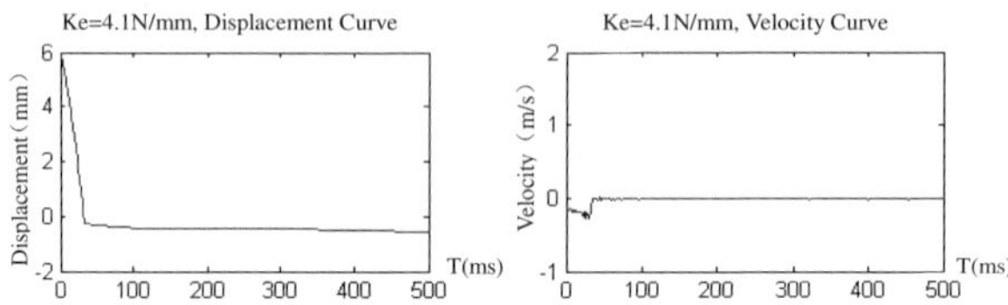

Fig. 10. Multirate control, virtual stiffness Ke=4.1N/mm

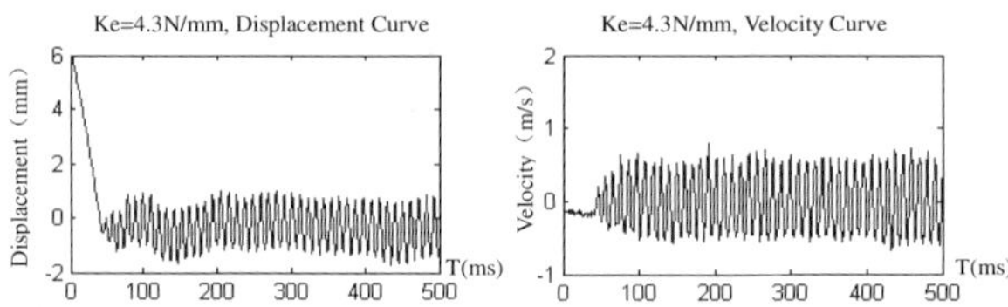

Fig. 11. Multirate control, virtual stiffness Ke=4.3N/mm

Comparing the numerical and experimental results, the multirate control increases the maximum virtual stiffness from $2.8N/mm$ to $4.1N/mm$, which is consistent with the theoretical result. These experiments prove the correctness and feasibility of the multirate control algorithm.

6 Conclusion

This paper proposes a multirate control algorithm which takes into account the computational time delay in the interpolating period. The stability condition under the multirate control is derived, which shows the working principle of the multirate control algorithm. Numerical and experimental results prove that the multirate control can enlarge the range of virtual stiffness and improve the stability of a haptic system compared with single rate control.

Acknowledgment

This work is supported by the National Natural Science Foundation of China under the grant No.50575011.

References

1. Wang, D., Zhang, Y., et al.: Cutting on Triangle Mesh Local Model Based Haptic Display for Dental Preparation Surgery Simulation. IEEE Transaction on Visualization and Computer Graphics 11(6), 671–683 (2005)
2. Edward Colgate, J., Michael Brown, J.: Factors affecting the Z-Width of a Haptic Display. In: Proceedings of the 1994 IEEE International Conference on Robotics and Automation, San Diego, vol. 4, pp. 3205–3210 (1994)
3. Luo, Y., Wang, D., Zhang, Y.: Modeling and Analysis of a Force Interaction System. Journal of Beijing University of Aeronautics and Astronautics 30(6), 539–542 (2004)
4. Diolaiti, N., Niemeyer, G., Barbagli, F., et al.: The Effect of Quantization and Coulomb Friction on the Stability. In: Proceedings of the First Joint Eurohaptics Conference and Symposium on Haptic Interfaces for Virtual Environment and Teleoperator Systems, pp. 237–246 (2005)
5. Kawai, M., Yoshikawa, T.: A New Haptic Interface Device Capable of Continuous-Time Impedance display within Sampling-Period: Application to Hard Surface Display. In: Proceedings of the 2001 IEEE International Conference on Robotics and Automation, vol. 1, pp. 880–885 (2001)
6. Mehling, J.S., Edward Colgate, J., Peshkin, M.A.: Increasing the Impedance Range of a Haptic Display by Adding Electrical Damping. In: Proceedings of the First Joint Eurohaptics Conference and Symposium on Haptic Interfaces for Virtual Environment and Teleoperator Systems, pp. 257–262 (2005)
7. Abbott, J.J., Okamura, A.M.: Effects of Position Quantization and Sampling Rate on Virtual-Wall Passivity. IEEE Transaction on Robotics 21(5), 952–964 (2005)
8. Lee, K., Lee, D.Y.: Multirate Control of Haptic Interface for Stability and High Fidelity. In: The 2004 IEEE International Conference on Systems, Man and Cybernetics, vol. 3, pp. 2542–2547 (2004)
9. Akahane, K., Hasegawa, S., Koike, Y., et al.: A Proposal of a Haptic Definition Haptic Rendering for Stability and Fidelity. In: The 16th International Conference on Artificial Reality and Telexistence–Workshops, pp. 162–167 (2006)
10. Kim, J.P., Seol, C., Ryu, J.: A Multirate Energy Bounding Algorithm for High Fidelity Stable Haptic Interaction Control. In: 2006 International Joint Conference, Busan, pp. 215–220 (2006)
11. Lee, M.H., Lee, D.Y.: Stability of Haptic Interface Using Nonlinear Virtual Coupling. In: The 2003 IEEE International Conference on Systems, Man and Cybernetics, vol. 4, pp. 3420–3424 (2003)

Ground Control Station Development for Autonomous UAV

Ye Hong, Jiancheng Fang, and Ye Tao

Key Laboratory of Fundamental Science for National Defense, Novel Inertial Instrument & Navigation System Technology, Beijing, 100191, China

Abstract. Unmanned Aerial Vehicle (UAV) has typically been used in civil and military field all over the world. Based on the UAV mission of autonomous flight, the ground control station (GCS) including hardware and software become important equipment to be developed. This paper emphasizes three parts to build a well functioning ground control station: a portable ground station hardware system, a virtual instrument panel for the attitude information and flight path showing, all kinds of error alert. Through the whole test on the ground and in the sky, GCS can show the remote sensing information precisely and send the control command in time. The system can be also used to assist in the function of autonomous cruise task for UAV.

Keywords: Unmanned Aerial Vehicle (UAV), ground control station, man machine interface, autonomous task.

1 Introduction

Autonomous Unmanned Aerial Vehicle (UAV) has the potential to act as low cost tools in variety of applications such as traffic monitoring, border patrol, search, rescue and surveillance. As the central Part of the UAV, GCS (ground control station) also have a continuous development [1-3]. It is also called for "planning and control station". Planning means to plan tasks of UAV during flying, and then to control actuating mechanism. GCS is often consisted of planning facility, display equipment, telemetry schedule, computer processor, data terminal on ground, communication equipment and protection device.

In 2002, the Air Force Technical School had developed onboard system and ground station for UAV [4]. The whole computer system is developed in the present study to include such tasks as data collection, analysis and computation, and control/monitor the UAV in flight, while the ground station monitors in real time the status of UAV and uplink commands or waypoints. All the flight information is archived either onboard the vehicle or downlink to the ground station.

A new design for an immersive ground control station is presented by Bryan E. Walter in Iowa State University. This ground station utilizes a virtual reality based visualization of the operational space and the graphical representation of multiple information streams to create a comprehensive immersive environment [5].

The unmanned airship has a capability of autonomous flight, navigation and guidance based on a telemetry command of the ground control station [6,7]. GSC is

C. Xiong et al. (Eds.): ICIRA 2008, Part II, LNAI 5315, pp. 36–44, 2008.

comprised of propulsion system, communication system, electrical system and other airship sensors were realized as a software-based program and do the same function of the real hardware system. The Ground Integration Test is performed to check the operation with engine running.

There are two ways to achieve the UAV flight: remote controlling the UAV via instrument data/real-time video and autonomous flight by UAV itself. The latter one is adopted in current study. To accomplish the goal, in this paper the ground control station provides attitude information and track showing, hands remote control and other function, such as sending control command to UAV, all kinds of error alert and building its database which can query flight information offline.

2 GCS Design Requirement

In order to make the program open, we use the modular structure to express the process design. The Basic process chart is shown in Figure1.

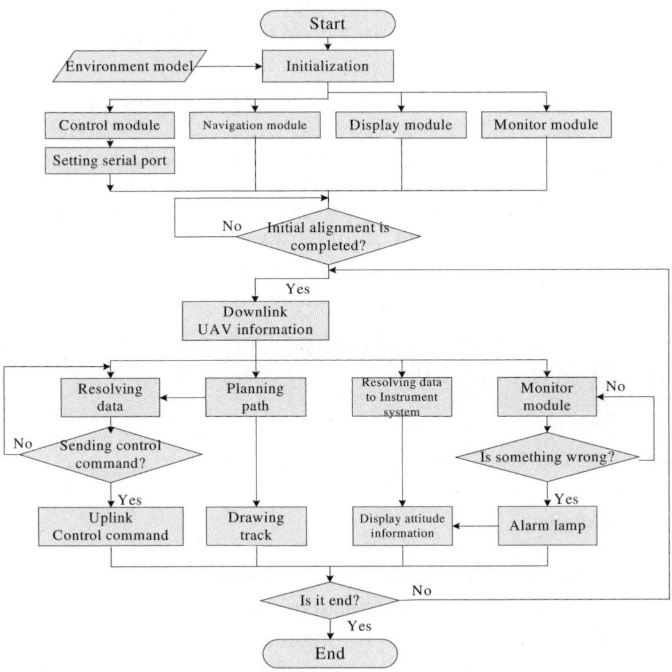

Fig. 1. Basic process chart

There are four modules to the whole system. Control modular is to resolve all information of UAV and send the control command to UAV. Navigation modular is to plan path before flight, and then draw the track. Display modular can show the attitude in the real time including the alarm lamps. Monitor modular is to take charge all kinds of error alert. The method has three merits: firstly, all modules have their own independence. We can add some new modules or bowdlerize old modules to complete other functions freely. Programming efficiency is high. Secondly, GCS should control any kinds of UAVs and can communicate any network. Finally, the software should be general for other user. The airborne system comprises an onboard system and a radio controlled aircraft. The GCS comprises a lab PC and a radio modern to communicate with onboard system. It can receive UAV flight information in real time, such as position, altitude, airspeed, heading, flight path, health condition of sensors and commands up-linking as well. On the other hand, it can send the control commands to on-board processor if necessary.

To achieve the basic communication link above all, the major design requirement of GCS should meet following function:

- planning the reasonable path according to current mission offline
- accepting down-link attitude information data from UAV
- carrying out the storage of the UAV data in time
- building up virtual instrument panel for the attitude information and tracking showing
- sending the up-link command data to UAV if necessary
- determining the position and the attitude with the data acquired from the navigation system
- monitoring the current status of systems and detecting the fault and failure on the platform
- coping with the emergency and performing all kinds of error alert

To be able to ensure a sufficient degree of confidence in performance during operations, both component and equipment of all hardware system should meet the physical and environmental conditions. Each part of systems of GCS must be able to withstand following temperature and humidity requirement:

- temperature : -20 to +50 degrees Celsius
- humidity : not greater than 85%

3 Ground Control Station System

3.1 Station Hardware

The on-board system of UAV consists of single-point GPS receiver, three single-degree of freedom silicon MEMS gyroscopes and two-degrees of freedom silicon MEMS accelerometer which installed orthogonally. The analog signals from above sensors plus air pressure sensor are converted to digital signals by an Analog-to-Digital Convert which is controlled by C8051 microprocessor. AT91RM9200 microprocessor is used as a navigation computer, receiving GPS data through serial port, completing navigation resolving and flight control algorithm, finally driving PWM (Pulse-Width Modulation) to steering engine for deflection and communicating with ground control station. The experiment system shows in fig. 2(a).

To permit manual flight of the vehicle during flying, a radio control (RC) receiver is built into the land system. The final control signals, whether generated from the control loops or manually from the RC receiver, are sent from the microcontroller to the servo actuators on the UAV. The user interface is from a ground terminal and radio control transmitter. The terminal is for preflight parameter modification in the flight code on the microcontroller. The RC transmitter is for manual flight of the vehicle. The flight control computer was chosen to be a programmable microcontroller. Ground control system interface was designed for a RS-232 serial link. To allow for autopilot flight, a changer lever system was also designed. Figure.2 (b) illustrates the flight control system on board and ground support hardware.

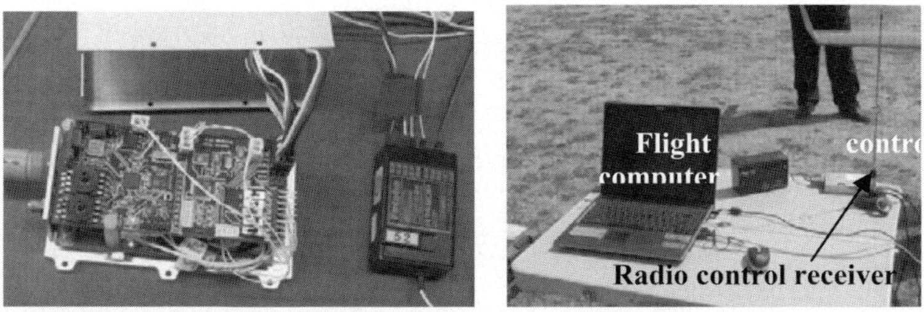

(a) On-board system (b) ground support hardware

Fig. 2. On-board system and ground support hardware

3.2 Station Software

The development of ground control station is mainly based on Microsoft Visual C++ 6.0 that is useful to show all data as soon as possible. The communication protocol between UAV and GCS should be known before the data transmission by quest. The frame is led by the strings of '@@@', and then 35 groups data is flowing, such as position, altitude and attitude. All data will be saved as a text file including the wrong data. After checking the remaining data, they will all be converted into different sets of information and displayed on the instrument panel on the screen. If there is something wrong of the data, the system will immediately give a warning with red light and beeping sound to notify us. Fig.3 displays the panel of the ground control station.

The main function of the panel is to show the information of UAV during the flight, such as position, altitude, attitude, airspeed, and heading. All of this data will be written down the edit frame on the right of the panel. Moreover, the tracking will be drawn with red lines in the center. These flight paths are all in the relative coordinate system. The cross point of axis is the initial position of UAV, and then the next point is recorded for the next location. There are three icons on the toolbar; they are view-out, view-in and view-move. When the flight path of UAV is overflowing the coordinate, we can click the view-out, and then the scale ratio is smaller in order to show the full tracking lines. We can also choose the button named "Mission point setup" to input the next expected mission point. When it is down, there is a cross iron on the screen that is the position of the cursor in the current. Moving the cross and clicking it at the suitable position, the message of the numerical value will be sent to UAV. All of the steps can be also operated in the flight control.

On the right-bottom of the panel, it is the instrument board. Three attitude director indicators will be shown, that is roll angle, pitch angle and yaw angle. All of them are

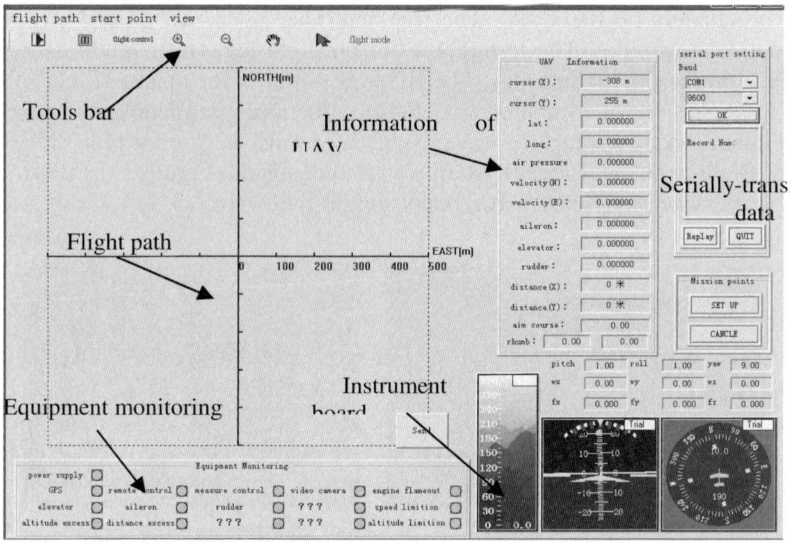

Fig. 3. Panel of the ground control station

refreshed with the downlink information 5 times a second. Height-position indicator is adjacent. We use the value of gas-pressure meter to remark the current height for UAV. All other important data will be written in the special edits.

For autonomous flight, the GCS interface also provides some flight states for users to choose, the entire function button is shown in the Fig.4. If you chose the "manual pilot", the UAV will be controlled by the steering handle on ground. When you knob down the button "autopilot", the UAV will run the autonomous mode. Other states will also be done, such as right-hover, climb, and slowdown. Now like a person UAV has its own decision making, but its information will be known by the instrument panel. It is also proved that the GCS is very important for early stage of autonomous flight.

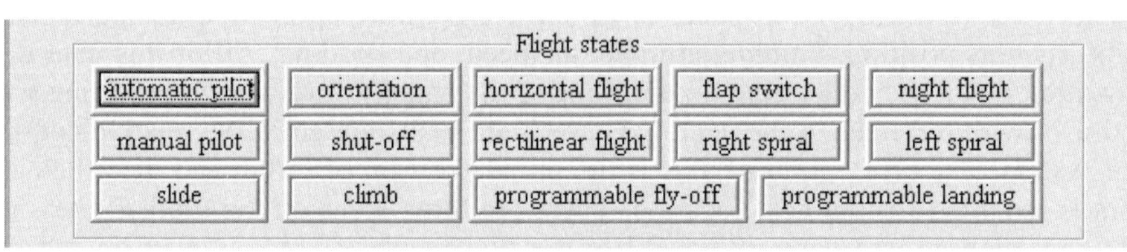

Fig. 4. Different flight states

During the program running, to accomplish sending the control command from GCS to UAV, three property pages named FLIGHT CONTROL is designed. Page one is to change the goal of the mission; the function can be realized in the program. Page two is to control actuator, and it is very important for sensitive adjustment of the steering engine. The order can be send to on-board system from radio-telegraphic transmitter wherever UAV on the ground or in the sky. Page three is the loops control. There are usually four loops to control and stabilize the attitude of UAV. Each loop has its own chain of command, but lateral direction and course have coupling. So the design of the loops must consider the relevance and dependence of each other. In this case, we use the PID method to stabilize and control the attitude angles and different state variables. To accomplish the attitude maintenance, constant height and turning control are the goal after all.

4 Test and Results

The overall system test can be divided into two important parts: ground phase and flight phase. UAV must be tested well on the ground before flight in the sky. The test on the ground is to detect the performance of the on-board system, and to test the liking of data. The integration test makes sure the entire system in regular status. The wireless data transmission test shows that the data delay in the ground station propagating with time increasing at the first beginning. The problem was solved soon, and the data can be synchronized both in airborne and ground system. The electromagnetic interference test is made to ensure that the electrical devices and wireless receiver do not influence with each other, and the communication between the onboard computer and the ground station will not be influenced by other factors. Finally, the dynamic ground test on a push car was implemented. Fig.5 is shown the flight path of the whole test.

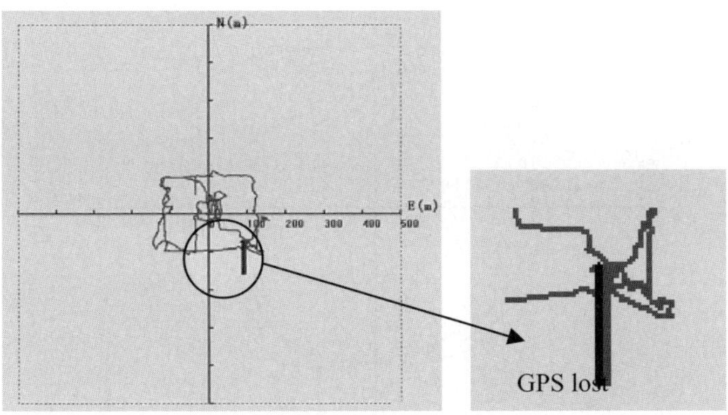

Fig. 5. Flight path of the whole test

Different from other ground control station, our system develops an algorithm to solve the problem of the global positioning system (GPS) lost. Some fight system only depends on the GPS receiver to get the position and attitude of UAV that is the system will be at a stand when GPS signal is lost. As the same with our system, it seems that the GPS lost track of signals for a while during the test in Fig.6. When the GPS receiver is wrong, the tracking of UAV will be disordered. In order to solve the problem, we develop a special compensation algorithm. The present navigation systems rely on Kalman filtering to fuse data from GPS and the inertial navigation system (INS). In general, INS/GPS integration provides reliable navigation solutions by overcoming each other shortcomings, including signal blockage for GPS and growth of position errors with time for INS.

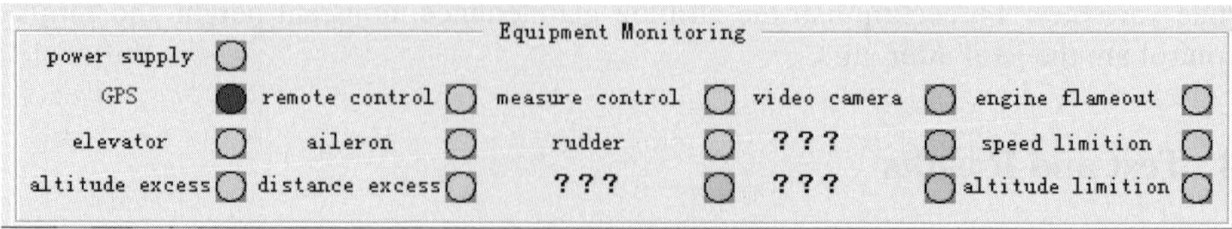

Fig. 6. Malfunction alarm panel

We can see in the right-bottom of the picture, there are some black-colored lines to express the no the GPS signal. Through the special compensation, the flight path looks like smooth. Fig.6 is shown that when the position data of the GPS receiver is wrong, there is the red light in the equipment monitoring. All other lights are green, and all of sensors are healthy. The malfunction alarm is finished, as soon as the GPS recuperate its heath.

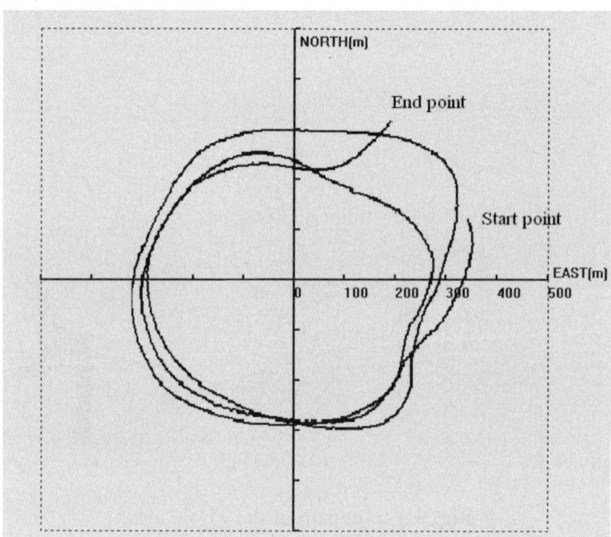

Fig. 7. The tracking of the cruise task

After the ground test, the flight test was put into practice. The major purpose is to validate the performance of the GCS above all, such as the real time data linking, the shown information of UAV and the function of equipment monitoring. After that, we also expect to accomplish the autopilot of UAV for an appointed task.

The whole fight test is 18 minutes long. The data of the ground control station is well displayed the condition during the flying for UAV in the sky including the manual flying and autopilot. To be assure the safe of the equipment on board, the cruise task command is sent up to UAV and then the autopilot system is run. UAV will enter the state to hover with 20m/s velocity. As shown as Fig.7, the purpose of the autonomous cruise task is to fly the circular area by a 300 meters radius. We can see the path tracking is smooth although the GPS signal is lost during 30 seconds. During the autonomous flight, the controller parameters are adjusted by UAV lateral controller to main the roll angle as constant. Fig.8 shows the roll angle and heading of the flight.

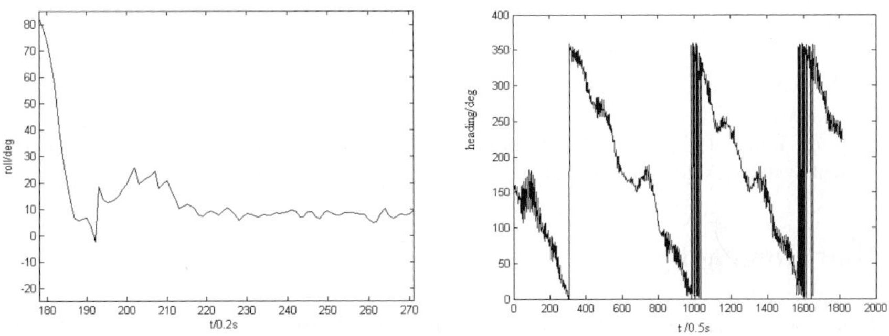

Fig. 8. Roll to level and heading track

5 Conclusion Remarks

The results of the tests show that the functions of the ground control station are verified in the both ground test and flight test. The ground control station has been developed successfully so that it can show data such as position, airspeed, altitude, heading, and health status for UAV. As the important function, the ground control station can send the autonomous control command to the system onboard. The information allows for implementation of basic ability for autonomous flight. But some significant problems can be conducted as following: Firstly, a portable graphical interface is not established. The electronic map can be used to display the position of UAV, and be moved and rotated to fix the position and heading of the UAV on the screen. It will be the next goal to realize in the future. Secondly, the power consumption is too large to maintain a long endurance flight. The method of power saving should to be given. Lastly, the complicated task can be designed for UAV to achieve the real autonomous flight.

Acknowledgments

This work was sponsored by a grant from Key Programs of National Natural Science Foundation of China (60736025); the work was sponsored by a grant from the Major Programs of China National Space Administration (D2120060013).

References

1. Cunningham, K., Foster, J.V., Shah, G.H., Stewart, E.C., Rivers, R.A., Wilborn, J.E., Gato, W.: Simulation Study of a Commer-cial Transport Airplane During Stall and Post-Stall Flight. In: 2004 SAE World Aviation Congress, vol. 113, pp. 1527–1537 (2004)
2. Taamallah, S., de Reus, A.J.C., Boer, J.-F.: Development of a Rotorcraft Mini-UAV System Demonstrator. In: The 24th Digital Avionics Systems Conference, vol. 2, pp. 11.A.2-1–11.A.2-15 (2005)
3. Lee, S.-J., Kim, S.-P.: Development of Autonomous Flight Control System for 50m Unmanned Airship. In: Intelligent Sensors, Sensor Networks and Information Processing Conference, pp. 457–461 (2004)
4. Kim, W.G.: The History of Airship and the New Concept Airship. Journal of the Korean Society for Aeronautical and Space Science 29(2), 152–155 (2001)
5. Ko, N.Y., Lee, B.H.: Avoid ability measure in moving obstacle avoidance problem and its use for robot motion planning. IEEE conference on Intelligent Robots and System 1(2), 1296–1303 (1996)
6. Tao, Y., Fang, J.C., Yang, C.: Design of low-cost-MEMS-based MUAV navigation and control system. Acta Aeronautica et Astronautica Sinica 29, 463–467 (2008)

Author Biography

Ye Hong was born in Heilongjiang Province, P. R. of China, in 1979. Now she is a postdoctoral candidate of Beihang University of Instrument Science & Optoelectronic Engineering in China. Her main research interests are related to the theory of autonomous control and the path planning for micro UAV.

Jiancheng Fang is professor and doctor tutor at school of Instrument Science and Optoelectronics Engineering in Beihang University. His main research area is at the technology of positioning and navigation, method of measurement and control, and theory of optimal estimation.

Ye Tao was born in Heilongjiang Province, P. R. of China, in 1979. Now he is a doctor candidate of Beihang University of Instrument Science & Optoelectronic Engineering in China. His main research interests are related to the theory of autonomous control for micro UAV.

Speech Emotion Recognition Using Spectral Entropy

Woo-Seok Lee, Yong-Wan Roh, Dong-Ju Kim, Jung-Hyun Kim,
and Kwang-Seok Hong

School of Information and Communication Engineering, Sungkyunkwan University, 300,
Chunchun-dong, Jangan-gu, Suwon, Kyungki-do, 440-746, Korea
grampus553@skku.edu, elec1004@skku.edu, raokdioguy@korea.com,
kjh0328@skku.edu, kshong@skku.ac.kr
http://hci.skku.ac.kr

Abstract. This paper proposes a Gaussian Mixture Model (GMM)–based speech emotion recognition methods using four feature parameters; 1) Fast Fourier Transform(FFT) spectral entropy, 2) delta FFT spectral entropy, 3) Mel-frequency Filter Bank (MFB) spectral entropy, 4) delta MFB spectral entropy. In addition, we use four emotions in a speech database including anger, sadness, happiness, and neutrality. We perform speech emotion recognition experiments using each pre-defined emotion and gender. The experimental results show that the proposed emotion recognition using FFT spectral-based entropy and MFB spectral-based entropy performs better than existing emotion recognition based on GMM using energy, Zero Crossing Rate (ZCR), Linear Prediction Coefficient (LPC), and pitch parameters.

1 Introduction

The ability to recognize, interpret and express emotions - commonly referred to as "Emotional Intelligence" [1] - plays a key role in human communication. Computers with emotion recognition and expression skills will allow a more natural and improved human computer interaction. An emotion-recognizing computer can "learn" during an interaction by associating emotional expressions (like pleasure or displeasure) with its own behavior, as a kind of reward and punishment [2]. In recent years, research that analyzed, human emotional information has been conducted, particularly in the fields of emotional speech, facial expressions, and body gestures etc. There are still few papers that address the problem of recognizing emotional states or human emotions contained in speech information, however and most of the papers are based on mathematical classification methods or pattern recognition techniques [3]. The most commonly analyzed aspects of emotion in speech are energy, tempo, duration, jitter, shimmer, LPC, Mel Frequency Cepstrum Coefficient (MFCC), pitch, and so on. The features that are most prominent in emotion recognition are pitch and energy [4], [5]. A probability model algorithm is used to classify speech and to derive the status of speaker's emotions. Generally, the emotion classifications are neutrality, anger, sadness, happiness, surprise and disgust [4].

This paper proposes to perform emotion recognition using speech information. Speech is able to deliver not only the meaning of speech but also information about

C. Xiong et al. (Eds.): ICIRA 2008, Part II, LNAI 5315, pp. 45–54, 2008.

emotions which is evident in aspects of speaker's speech that are able to be classified. The emotional speech database that is used in this paper consists of neutrality, anger, sadness, and happiness. The analytical methods for emotion recognition are FFT spectral entropy, delta FFT spectral entropy, MFB spectral entropy, delta MFB spectral entropy. We use a GMM algorithm as a pattern recognition algorithm for recognizing emotion in speech. The rest of this paper is organized as follows. Section 2 describes the previous variable emotion recognition methods. The proposed method is described in Section 3. Section 4 shows the experiment-based performance evaluation of the proposed method. Finally, conclusions are provided in Section 5.

2 Related Works

In this section, we describe work that has been done in emotion recognition. Kyung Hak Hyun [6] used non-zero-pitch for speech emotion recognition. Pitch information is quite useful in speech emotion recognition [6], and non-zero-pitch is the pitch contour that does not have a zero value. Because the zero value of the pitch causes some errors in the Gaussian distribution, it must be eliminated. Although the non-zero-pitch contour loses some information content such as unvoiced sounds, the emotion recognition result is improved. They have applied this concept to a Bayesian classifier and they obtained better results for emotion recognition than those obtained using the previous pitch contour.

Kwon et al. [7] used a CHMM (Continuous Hidden Markov Model) with a left-right topology and up to five states to model on the word level including a neutral style and three stress styles. Their paper showed an average emotion recognition rate of 70.1%, which was superior to the performance of a support vector machine (SVM) classifier that had a recognition rate of 67.1% [8]. For a second database containing short commands or greetings with several words using five basic emotions, an average recognition rate of 40.8% was achieved, but this time it was inferior to the SVM classifier's rate of 42.3%.

Jian Zhou [9] proposed a speech emotion recognition method based on rough set (RS) theory and SNM. Rough Set (RS) is a valid mathematical theory to deal with imprecise, uncertain, and vague information. They used energy, pitch contour, and the first, second, and third formants as features for speech emotion recognition. The mean emotion recognition rate is 74.75%.

3 A Proposal for Speech Emotion Recognition

In this paper, we used spectral entropy and MFB spectral entropy to analyze the features for emotion recognition. Spectral entropy calculates each frame, and uses a combination of delta spectral entropy. MFB spectral entropy uses 27 filter banks. In this section, we first describe the compilation flow and the block diagram of the emotion recognition analysis.

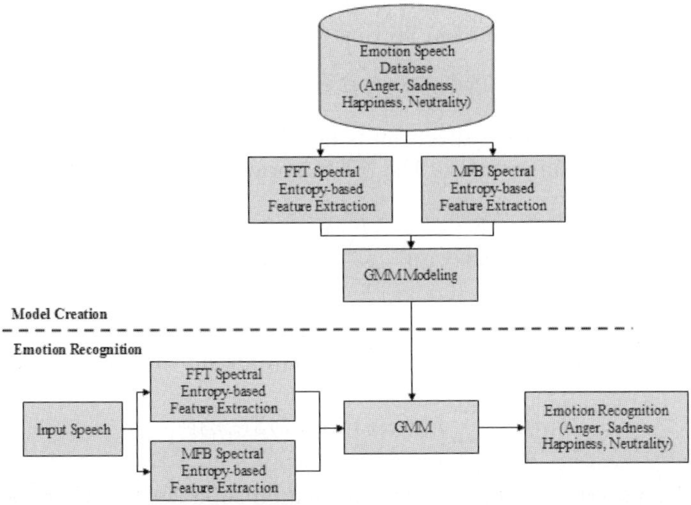

Fig. 1. Block Diagram of the Emotion Recognition Analysis

3.1 The Block Diagram of the Emotion Recognition Analysis

The emotion recognition system block diagram is shown in Fig. 1. In creating the model, we use the emotion speech database to perform FFT and MFB spectral entropy-based feature extraction using FFT spectral entropy, delta FFT spectral entropy, MFB spectral entropy, and delta MFB spectral entropy. The probabilistic model parameters are based on using the GMM. In recognizing emotions, we extract the FFT and MFB spectral entropy-based features and then the emotion recognition system compares the extracted parameters with the probabilistic models of the four emotions.

3.2 FFT Spectral Entropy

In this paper, we use FFT spectral entropy and delta FFT spectral entropy. Entropy is based on Shannon's information theory and it is the means of measuring the amount of information. In FFT spectral entropy, entropy theory is applied to speech emotion recognition.

The speech is first pre-emphasized using a pre-emphasis filter in order to spectrally flatten the signal, and then the pre-emphasized speech is separated into short segments called frames. This will significantly enhance the ability to identify the emotional aspects of speech in this paper. In order to reduce the familiar edge effects, a 512-point Hamming window is applied to each frame. The FFT of X(i,n) is given by equation (1).

$$X(i,n) = \sum_{m=1}^{M} x(m,n) e^{-j\frac{2\pi}{N}im} \tag{1}$$

Where X(i,n) is the nth frame and the ith frequency component. M denotes the number of points in the FFT. x(m,n) is the nth frame the mth sample. After the FFT block, the spectrum of each frame is filtered by a set of filters, and the power of each band is calculated. The power of each band S(i,n) is calculated using equation (2).

$$S(i,n) = |X(i,n)|^2 \tag{2}$$

The probability density of the spectrum is estimated by using a method that normalizes the frequency components. The FFT normalization P[S(i,n)] is defined in equation (3).

$$P[S(i,n)] = \frac{S(i,n)}{\sum_{m=1}^{M/2} S(m,n)} \tag{3}$$

The method of calculating the spectral entropy H(n) is shown in equation (4).

$$H(n) = -\sum_{i=1}^{M/2} P[S(i,n)] \log_2 P[S(i,n)] \tag{4}$$

The delta FFT power spectrum of each calculation subtracts the nth frame and the ith frequency component from the $n+1^{th}$ frame and the ith frequency component. The delta FFT power spectrum S´(i,n) is defined in equation (5).

$$S'(i,n) = S(i,n+1) - S(i,n) \tag{5}$$

We calculated the delta FFT power spectrum by taking the logarithm and the modulus, and then we calculated the spectrum normalization. P[S´(i,n)] is the delta FFT normalization, which is defined in equation (6). In addition, the proposed delta spectral entropy H´(n) is shown in equation (7).

$$P[S'(i,n)] = \frac{|S'(i,n)|}{\sum_{m=1}^{M/2} |S'(m,n)|} \tag{6}$$

$$H'(n) = -\sum_{i=1}^{M/2} P[S'(i,n)] \log P[S'(i,n)] \tag{7}$$

3.3 MFB Spectral Entropy

In this paper, we use MFB spectral entropy and delta MFB spectral entropy. The speech is first pre-emphasized using a pre-emphasis filter "$1\text{-}\alpha Z^{-1}$" in order to spectrally flatten the signal, where "α" is in the range 0.9 ~ 1. The default value of "α" is 0.97 [10]. Then the pre-emphasized speech is separated into short segments called frames. The frame length is set to 32ms (512 sample) to guarantee that the signal inside the frame is stationary. There is an 16ms (256 sample) overlap between two adjacent frames to ensure that the signals from one frame to the next are stationary. A frame can be seen as the result of multiplying the speech waveform by a rectangular pulse whose width is equal to the frame length. In order to reduce the edge effects, a 512-point Hamming window is applied to each frame. After the FFT block, the spectrum of each frame is filtered by a set of filters, and the power of each band is calculated. Each signal frame is processed through a Mel-scale filter bank resulting in a vector that contains 27 energy coefficients.

The MFB multiplies the FFT by the Mel-scale filter. The MFB describes M(b,n), which is shown in equation (8).

$$M(b,n) = \frac{\sum_{i=L_b}^{U_b} V_b(i) S(i,n)}{\sum_{i=L_b}^{U_b} V_b(i)} \tag{8}$$

where, M(b,n) is obtained by multiplying S(i,n) by the frequency response of the ith Mel-scale filter as$V_b(i)$. L_b and U_b are the start frequency and the end frequency of the ith Mel filter. The method of calculating the spectral entropy H(n) is shown in equation (9).

$$H_{MFB}(n) = -\sum_{b=1}^{B} P[M(b,n)] \log_2 P[M(b,n)] \tag{9}$$

The proposed delta MFB is M´(b,n), which is defined by subtracting the nth frame and the bth Mel-frequency filter bank by the n+1th frame and the bth Mel-frequency filter bank. The delta FFT power spectrum S´(i,n) is defined in equation (5). We calculated the delta MFB power spectrum by taking the logarithm and the modulus, and then we calculated the normalized delta MFB spectrum P[M´(b,n)] that is defined in equation (10).

$$P[M'(b,n)] = \frac{| M'(b,n) |}{\sum_{m=1}^{B} | M'(m,n) |} \tag{10}$$

where, b is the number of Mel-filters that is used in this paper. The proposed delta MFB spectral entropy is shown in equation (11).

$$H'_{MFB}(n) = -\sum_{b=1}^{B} P[M'(b,n)] \log P[M'(b,n)] \tag{11}$$

3.4 Emotion Recognition Using GMM

In this paper, we used a GMM to estimate the probability distribution instead of assuming that each class distribution is a normal distribution. A GMM uses various Gaussian distributions to model discrete probability distributions, so it can be optimized using the Expectation Maximization (EM) algorithm [11]. The modeled probability distribution using the GMM is defined in equation (12).

$$p(x | \lambda) = \sum_{i=1}^{M} p_i b_i(x) \tag{12}$$

where, b_i is the GPDF (Gaussian probability density function), and p_i is the mixture weight. We need u_i, Σ_i and p_i to express the Gaussian mixture density, where u_i is the mean vector and Σ_i is the covariance matrix. It is a set of three parameters that express the probability model for a Gaussian distribution of the speaker's emotion. This set is defined by the GMM, and shown in equation (13).

$$\lambda = \left\{ \rho_i,\ \mu_i,\ \sum_i \right\} \qquad i = 1,2,3,\ldots,M \tag{13}$$

All emotional features are modeled using the GMM with diagonal covariance matrices measured over all frames of a speech.

First, using all of the training data, a root GMM is trained with the EM(Expectation Maximization) algorithm with a maximum likelihood criterion, and then one GMM per class is adapted from the root model using the MAP(Maximum a Posteriori) criterion. MAP adaptation protects against overtraining and removes the need to optimize the number of Gaussians per class which may be necessary due to differences in the amount of available training data per class [12]. We use 32 Gaussians for spectral-based entropy and MFB spectral-based entropy.

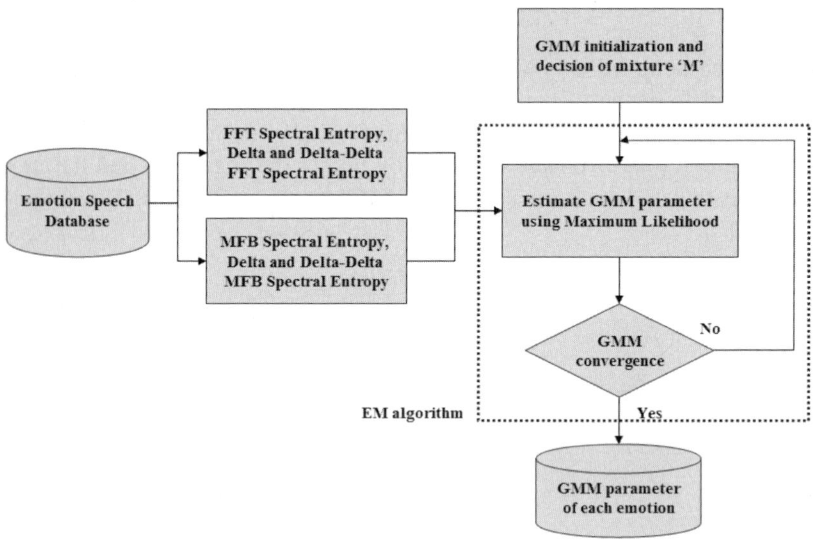

Fig. 2. Block diagram of the process of training the GMM parameters

Figure 2 shows emotion recognition using the GMM. In the training step, we estimate the GMM parameters including the maximum Gaussian in each emotional data set using EM algorithm.

4 Experiments and Results

4.1 Emotional Speech Databases

Given that in many languages the fundamental tendencies of sounds are expressed in similar ways, our results in recognizing the emotions of Korean language speakers can generally be applied to speakers of other languages. For this reason, we used a database produced by Professor C. Y. Lee from Media and the Communication Signal Processing Laboratory of Yonsei University in Korea with the support of the Korea Research Institute of Standards and Science. This data covers the four emotions of neutrality, happiness, sadness, and anger; and its principles are as follows [13]:

- easy pronunciation in anger, sadness, happiness and neutrality
- 45 dialogic sentences that express natural emotion

The original data is stored in the form of 16kHz. To use the data in MATLAB, we transformed the data for the training and simulation into a 16bit format through quantization with a pulse code modulation filter.

There are fifteen male and fifteen female emotional speech samples in the database. In this paper, 30 subjects listened to the utterances of one speaker played back in random order.

4.2 Speech Emotion Recognition Using the Existing Methods

The table 1 shows that the result of the emotion recognizing experiment using general features. The general features define energy, log-energy, ZCR, LPC, and pitch. The existing method use combination of general features. The judgment currently uses four emotions. The experiment used four classifications by dividing the group into men and women, and then dividing each of these groups according to whether or not the speaker participated in the training.

Table 1. Emotion recognition results: (a) General features; (b) General and delta general features

	Participate in training		Not participate in training	
	Male	Female	Male	Female
Anger	78.0%	79.3%	74.3%	76.3%
Sadness	71.3%	75.0%	61.6%	74.6%
Happiness	42.0%	58.6%	40.3%	54.0%
Neutrality	51.0%	60.3%	47.6%	52.3%
Average	60.6%	68.3%	55.9%	64.3%

(a)

	Participate in training		Not participate in training	
	Male	Female	Male	Female
Anger	80.3%	82.6%	74.3%	77.3%
Sadness	77.0%	78.0%	75.7%	76.3%
Happiness	53.3%	56.0%	50.3%	57.3%
Neutrality	51.6%	51.6%	46.0%	49.3%
Average	64.5%	67.1%	61.6%	65.1%

(b)

Table 1(a) is the result of the first experiment that used general features. Table 1(b) is the result of the second experiment that used general features and delta general features. In this experiment, the emotion recognition result using general features is 62.3%, and the emotion recognition result using general and delta general features is 64.6%. The experiment of emotion recognition using general feature showed a maximum recognize rate when using a combination of general features and delta general features.

4.3 Emotion Recognition Using the Proposed Method

In experimental environments, we used 12,600 sentences as training data, and we performed the context-independent speech emotion recognition using experimental data consisting of 3,600 sentences. The sentences used in the experiments were 200 randomly selected sentences for each emotion. The experiments consist of two methods of using FFTs for spectral entropy based emotion recognition. Table 2(a) shows the experimental results using the FFT spectral entropy based emotion recognition method. Table 2(b) shows the experimental results using the FFT spectral entropy method and the delta FFT spectral entropy based emotion recognition method. In the experimental results, the emotion recognition result using FFT spectral entropy is 65%, and the emotion recognition result using FFT spectral entropy and delta FFT spectral entropy is 72.75%. The experiment demonstrates that the emotion recognition using FFT spectral entropy, and delta FFT spectral entropy show the maximum recognize rate. The experiments consist of two parts for the MFB spectral entropy based emotion recognition methods.

Table 2. Emotion recognition results: (a) FFT spectral entropy; (b) FFT and delta FFT spectral entropy

	Participate in training		Not participate in training	
	Male	Female	Male	Female
Anger	78.0%	68.0%	72.0%	66.0%
Sadness	80.0%	74.0%	86.0%	78.0%
Happiness	52.0%	58..0%	46.0%	66.0%
Neutrality	60.0%	62.0%	52.0%	54.0%
Average	67.5%	65.5%	64.0%	66.0%

(a)

	Participate in training		Not participate in training	
	Male	Female	Male	Female
Anger	82.0%	84.0%	84.0%	78.0%
Sadness	78.0%	72.0%	44.0%	76.0%
Happiness	64.0%	52.0%	48.0%	54.0%
Neutrality	62.0%	58.0%	66.0%	50.0%
Average	71.5%	66.5%	60.5%	64.5%

(b)

Table 3. Emotion recognition results: (a) MFB spectral entropy; (b) MFB and delta MFB spectral entropy

	Participate in training		Not participate in training	
	Male	Female	Male	Female
Anger	78.0%	66.0%	74.0%	62.0%
Sadness	76.0%	84.0%	76.0%	86.0%
Happiness	54.0%	58..0%	42.0%	54.0%
Neutrality	68.0%	72.0%	72.0%	70.0%
Average	69.0%	70.0%	66.0%	68.0%

(a)

	Participate in training		Not participate in training	
	Male	Female	Male	Female
Anger	92.0%	80.0%	84.0%	78.0%
Sadness	72.0%	92.0%	72.0%	96.0%
Happiness	56.0%	58.0%	54.0%	52.0%
Neutrality	86.0%	74.0%	82.0%	74.0%
Average	76.5%	76.0%	73.0%	75.0%

(b)

Table 3(a) shows the experimental results using the MFB spectral entropy based emotion recognition method. Table 3(b) shows the experimental results using the MFB spectral entropy and delta MFB spectral entropy based emotion recognition method.

In the experimental results, the emotion recognition result using MFB spectral entropy is 68.25%, and the emotion recognition result using MFB spectral entropy and delta MFB spectral entropy is 75.13%. The experiment demonstrates that emotion recognition using MFB spectral entropy and delta MFB spectral entropy show the maximum recognize rate.

5 Conclusions

This paper proposed human emotion recognition using FFT and MFB spectral-based entropy. For emotion recognition, the GMM was used to design the emotion probabilistic model. An emotion speech database was used that consists of four emotions: anger, sadness, happiness and neutrality. We trained and tested the emotion recognition using the collected FFT and MFB spectral-based entropy from the emotion speech database. In experiments using the FFT spectral entropy-based method, we attained a maximum recognition rate of 65.8% when we used FFT spectral entropy and delta FFT spectral entropy. In experiments using the MFB spectral entropy-based method, we attained a maximum recognition rate of 75.1% when we used MFB spectral entropy and delta MFB spectral entropy. We also experimented using the existing method, and we experimented using the proposed emotion recognition method, and then we compared the results of the experiment using the existing method with the result of the experiment using the proposed method. We attained a maximum recognition rate of 64.6% using general features, such as energy, ZCR, LPC, and pitch and delta using these general features. From the experimental results, the proposed FFT spectral entropy-based method improves the recognizing rate 1.2%, and the proposed MFB spectral entropy-based method improves the recognizing rate 10.5% compared to the emotion recognition method that uses general features.

Acknowledgment

This research was supported by MKE, Korea under ITRC IITA-2008-(C1090-0801-0046) and the Korea Science and Engineering Foundation (KOSEF) grant funded by the Korea government (MEST)(No. R01-2008-000-10642-0).

References

1. Goleman, D.: Emotional Intelligence. Bantam Books, New York (1995)
2. Borchert, M., Dusterhoft, A.: Emotion in Speech-Experiments with Prosody and Quality Features in Speech for Use in Categorical and Dimensional Emotion Recognition Environments, Natural Language Processing and Knowledge Engineering. In: Proceedings of 2005 IEEE International Conference on IEEE NLP-KE 2005, 30 October-1 November (2005)
3. Kim, S.-i., Lee, S.-h., Shin, W.-j., Park, N.-c.: Recognition of Emotional states in Speech using Hidden Markov Model. In: Proceeding of KFIS Fall Conference, vol. 14(2) (2004)
4. Zhao, L., Cao, Y., Wang, Z., Zou, C.: Speech Emotional Recognition Using Global and Time Sequence Structure Features with MMD. In: Tao, J., Tan, T., Picard, R.W. (eds.) ACII 2005. LNCS, vol. 3784. Springer, Heidelberg (2005)
5. Schuller, B., Rigoll, G., Lang, M.: Hidden Markov Model-based speech emotion recognition. In: Proc. ICASSP, HongKong, China, pp. 401–404 (2003)
6. Hyun, K.H., Kim, E.H., Kwak, Y.K.: Improvement of Emotion Recognition by Bayesian Classifier Using Non-zero-pitch Cencept, Robot and Human Interactive Communication. In: IEEE International Workshop on ROMAN 2005, 13–15 August (2005)

7. Kwon, O.-W., Chan, K.-L., Hao, J., Lee, T.-W.: Emotion Recognition by Speech Signals. In: Eurospeech, Geneva, Switzerland (2003)
8. Wagner, J., Vogt, T., Andre, E.: A Systematic Comparison of Different HMM Design for Emotion Recognition from Acted and Spontaneous Speech. In: Paiva, A.C.R., Prada, R., Picard, R.W. (eds.) ACII 2007. LNCS, vol. 4738, pp. 114–125. Springer, Heidelberg (2007)
9. Zhou, J., Wang, G., Yang, Y., Chen, P.: Speech Emotion Recognition Based on Rough Set and SVM, Cognitive Informatics. In: 5th IEEE International Conference on ICCI 2006, July 17-19, 2006, vol. 1, pp. 53–61 (2006)
10. Young-Wan, R., Hong, K.-S.: Delta FBLC based Speech/Non-Speech Frame Decision in Real Car Environment. In: The 4th Conference on New Exploratory Technologies (Next 2007)
11. Hastie, T., Tibshirani, R., Friedman, J.: The elements of statistical learning - data mining, inference, and prediction. Springer, Heidelberg (2000)
12. Reynolds, D., Quatieri, T., Dunn., R.: Speaker verification using adapted Gaussian mixture models. Digital Signal Processing 10, 19–41 (2000)
13. Hyun, K.H., Kim, E.H., Kwak, Y.K.: Improvement of emotion recognition by Bayesian classifier using non-zero-pitch concept, Robot and Human Interactive Communication. In: IEEE International Workshop on ROMAN 2005, August 13-15, 2005, pp. 312–316 (2005)

Robot Auditory Search Realization Based on Virtual Reality

Xiaoling Lv and Minglu Zhang

School of Mechanical Engineering, Hebei University of Technology,
Tianjin 300130, China
lxl000418@163.com

Abstract. A novel robot auditory search system is proposed in this paper. The system consists of a robot which has a microphone array corresponding to human's ears and a virtual reality robot teleoperation system. Sound source localization is realized based on time delay of arrival (TDOA) estimation using microphone array. The sound source search is realized via virtual reality system. Virtual robot and virtual environment are set up according to the real scene. Virtual robot is the agent of the real robot. Data glove is used to operate the virtual robot to complete the control towards the real robot. It can make the operator control the real robot to find the sound source fast and conveniently. The system was tested in leaky chemistry container mending: robot could reach the leaky point successfully and accomplish the mending task smoothly. A great deal of experiments prove that this search system is reliable and efficient.

Keywords: Virtual reality, Sound source localization, Robot, Search.

1 Introduction

In recent years, with the rapid development of chemical technology, research on how to make robot work in dangerous and unknown surroundings has become a hot topic in the field of robotics.

Especially in mending leaky chemistry container, robot plays an important role. When accidents occur with a crash sounds, for example chemistry container leaks, the robot will be aware and localizes the sound source to find the leak point. The approach of using a moving microphone array to localize the sound source has been started recently as a challenging research topic of sound processing [1].There are a lot of advantages in using several microphones in any sound source direction estimation system that is applied to humanoid robot. Because the structure of the system is agile, the computational complexity is low.

But how to make the robot search the sound source includes a lot of complicated problems, such as path planning, collision detection and so on. So we propose a novel searching method by integrating robot audition and virtual reality.

This paper is organized as follows. In Section 2, we introduce robot auditory localization system and present the results of our initial localization experiments. Section 3 presents the virtual reality robot teleoperation system. Section 4 discusses the search realization based on integration of auditory and virtual reality. Section 5 presents our conclusions and plans for future work.

C. Xiong et al. (Eds.): ICIRA 2008, Part II, LNAI 5315, pp. 55–63, 2008.

2 Robot Auditory Localization System

There are several methods of sound source localization [2]. Considering for our localization system need real time realization, we adopt the localization method based on time delay of arrival (TDOA) [3].

The direction of a generated sound source can be estimated using the time difference between microphones and the characteristics of the sound. Most practical acoustic source localization schemes are based on time delay of arrival estimation for the following reasons: such systems are conceptually simple. They are reasonably effective in reverberant environment. Moreover, their low computational complexity makes them well-suited to real-time implementation with several sensors.

Time delay of arrival-based source localization is based on a two-step procedure：

(1)The TDOA between all pairs of microphones is estimated, typically by finding the peak in a cross-correlation or generalized cross-correlation function.

(2) For a given source location, the estimated TDOA and those geometry model could be used to evaluate the source location [4].

However, it is very difficult to create an estimation system using a computer and two microphones. Considering the microphone array would be fixed on the robot, it is also not appropriate to use a lot of microphones to localize the sound source. In this system we propose a novel sound source localization system. The squared microphone array in the proposed system consists of four microphones which are distributed on the front of the robot underpan. It is shown in Fig 1.

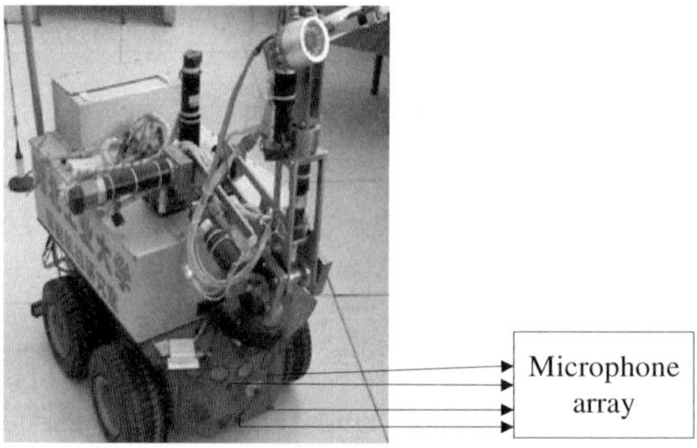

Fig. 1. Microphone array on robot

HEBUT-II robot consists of a mobile vehicle and a five-degree-of-freedom manipulator. The received signals of these four microphones are used to determine the position of the sound source.

Supposed there is a sound source in the working environment of robot. The position relationship between the microphone array and the sound source is shown in Fig 2. In the coordinate system, S denotes the sound source, M_1~M_4 represent microphones, R denotes radial distance, θ denotes azimuth angle, ϕ denotes zenith angle, and L denotes the side length of the squared microphone array.

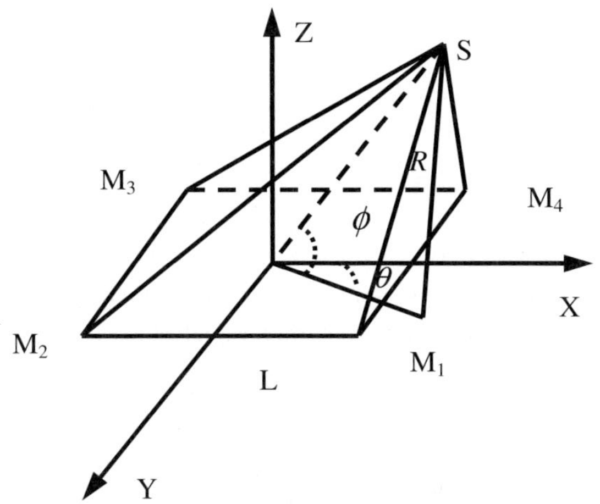

Fig. 2. Coordinate system of microphone array

We could get equations from coordinate system as follows:

$$\begin{cases} x^2+y^2+z^2=R^2 \\ (x-\frac{L}{2})^2+(y-\frac{L}{2})^2+z^2={R_1}^2 \\ (x+\frac{L}{2})^2+(y-\frac{L}{2})^2+z^2={R_2}^2 \\ (x+\frac{L}{2})^2+(y+\frac{L}{2})^2+z^2={R_3}^2 \\ (x-\frac{L}{2})^2+(y+\frac{L}{2})^2+z^2={R_4}^2 \end{cases} \tag{1}$$

$$\begin{cases} x=R\cos\theta\cos\phi \\ y=R\cos\theta\sin\phi \\ z=R\sin\theta \end{cases} \tag{2}$$

The position of the sound source can be determined by calculating the radial distance R , azimuth angle θ , and zenith angle ϕ from equations (1)-(2). The parameters could be calculated and expressed as equations (3)-(5). Where R1~R4 denote the distance between sound source and microphone array M1~M4 and C denotes the traveling velocity of sound wave.

$$tg\theta=\frac{\tau_{41}+\tau_{31}-\tau_{21}}{\tau_{21}+\tau_{31}-\tau_{41}} \tag{3}$$

$$cos\phi = \frac{C}{L}\sqrt{\frac{\tau^2{}_{31} + (\tau_{41} - \tau_{21})^2}{2}} \tag{4}$$

$$R = \frac{C \cdot \left[\tau_{31}^2 + (\tau_{41} - \tau_{21})^2\right]}{4 \cdot (\tau_{41} - \tau_{31} + \tau_{21})} \tag{5}$$

The time delay corresponds with the peak value of cross correlation function. If the cross correlation function of the signals received by microphone i and j is represented as $R_{ij}(\tau)$ .The time delay could calculated by equation (6).

$$\tau_{ij} = \arg\max(R_{ij}(\tau)) \tag{6}$$

Sound signal is time variable actually. We usually process sound signal in a very short time, for instance in 20ms, in short a time, it can be considered invariable, and this is the basic point of processing sound signals.

We make some experiments to test robot auditory localization system. The sound source is placed at 4m away from the microphone array. A multi-channels recording card is used to simultaneously record the sound signals from four microphones. Signals are band pass filtered at 250-16000 Hz to remove both high and low frequency background noise. This range was determined so as to retain as much useful information as possible. Sound signals received are divided into several frames, each of which has 512 samples. The noises involved in the sound would affect the accuracy on calculating time delays, there are 256 samples overlapped in the neighboring frames to avoid the blocking effect [5]. Sound endpoint detection which has simple calculation is adopted to detect sound signals, which can improve the performance of the system. When there is no sound, calculate Power Spectrum of the noise, and then reduce it from sound Power Spectrum. The time delay corresponds with the peak of cross correlation function. When the time delay of every microphone pair is got, we use the values to calculate the sound source position in the environment. The radial distance R , azimuth angle θ , and zenith angle ϕ could be got through equations (3)-(5). The localization simulation results are shown in Table 1.

From Table 1, we could see that noise greatly affects the localization results. So far, it is still one of the most difficult tasks to reduce the noise influence to sound source localization. In future, we'll find more effective means to solve this problem.

Table 1. Experiments results of the localization

	Parameter	θ	ϕ	R
L=0.2m	Theoretical values	70°	60°	4m
Quiet environment	Measured values	69.3°	63°	3.8m
	Deviations	0.7°	3°	0.2m
Noisy environment	Measured values	66°	70.5°	3.3m
	Deviations	4°	10.5°	0.7m

3 Virtual Reality Robot Teleoperation System

Virtual reality teleoperation is a natural and efficient human-computer interaction fashion [6-7]. The virtual reality robot teleoperation system is made up of data glove and stereoscopic glasses combine together with virtual reality software. The virtual robot is controlled by operator using data glove to complete task, the virtual robot is the agent of real robot, and thus the control to the remote true robot is carried out by controlling the virtual robot. Every movement of the virtual robot is transmitted to the real robot through WLAN, so that the virtual robot and the real robot always move synchronously. Meanwhile, real robot feedbacks information constantly for operator determine next task. It is a good human-computer interaction system.

The virtual reality teleoperation realization principle is shown in Fig 3.

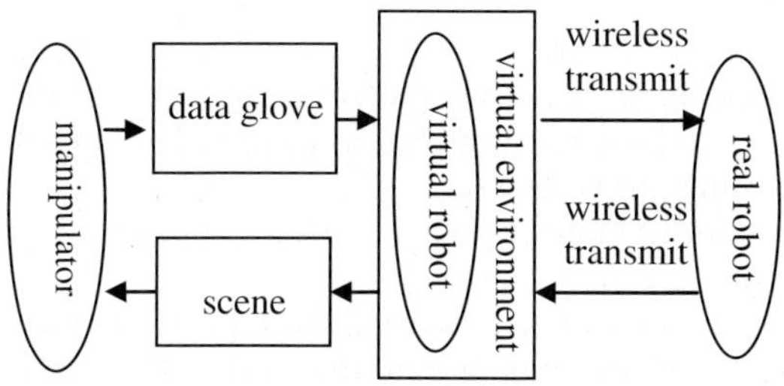

Fig. 3. Virtual reality teleoperation realization principle

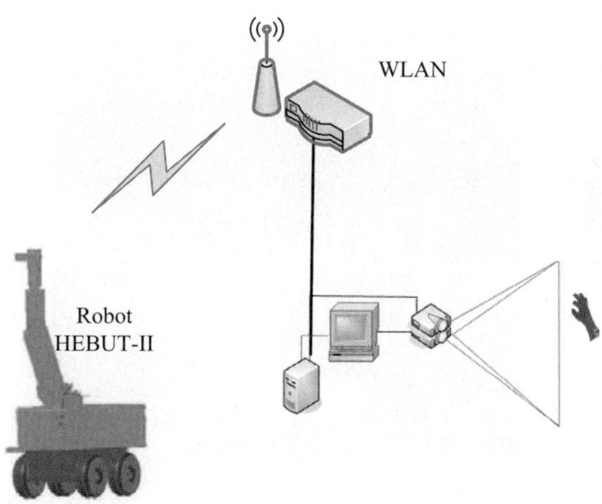

Fig. 4. Virtual reality robot teleoperation system

Operator in this system wears the data glove to send out instruction signals. That signals spread towards virtual robot. Virtual robot completes the corresponding action and feeds back to the operator. The virtual robot is the reflection to real robot, its move parameter of action and each joint can be passed to the remote real robot. The robot model in the virtual reality environment which acts as an agent to the real robot is the bridge of real robot contacting with operator. Virtual reality robot teleoperation system is shown in Fig 4.

In the whole operating process, the operator has to wear stereoscopic glasses, for our eyes could not see stereoscopic picture directly. The principle of producing a stereoscopic picture is light polarization. Two bunches of partial light are thrown to screen using two projectors. The operator then can see a stereoscopic picture using partial glasses. Data glove is used to operate target object in the virtual environment on the screen. The message is transmitted via WLAN between virtual environment and real environment. WLAN (Wireless LAN) has enough bandwidth; the bandwidth of this WLAN is 11Mbps, which is wide enough for our communication system.

The host computer is connected with two projectors, virtual environment can be thrown to projecting screen to produce stereoscopic picture. The data glove can operate stereoscopic picture directly. In the whole operating process, the operator has to wear stereoscopic glasses, for our eyes could not see stereoscopic picture directly. The principle of producing stereoscopic picture is light polarization. Two bunches of partial light are thrown to screen using two projectors. The operator only could see a stereoscopic picture using partial glasses.

Data glove which has 14 contact points is used to operate virtual robot in the virtual environment on the screen.

The robot model is set up using UG, for validating whether the module is similar to the real robot or not, we make simulation to the model. The experiment results prove that the model is very similar to the real robot. The environment scene is set up using 3dmax. The operation virtual environment based on EON is shown in Fig 5.

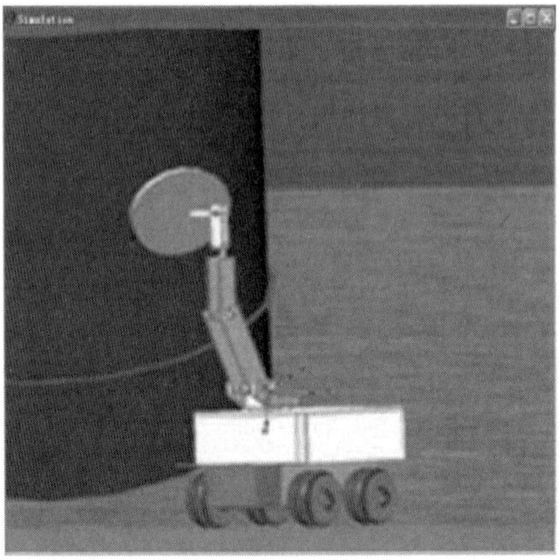

Fig. 5. Virtual environment based on EON

4 Search Realization Based on Robot Auditory and Virtual Reality

In the leaky chemical container mending task, when accidents occur with a crash sound, the robot will be aware and localize the leaky point. Sound source localization is realized by robot auditory localization system which is introduced in part 2. The leaky point position will be transmitted to the virtual environment via WLAN. The operator can use data glove to control the virtual robot to move in the virtual environment to the direction of leaky point, then the real robot also moves in the real environment to the leak point synchronously.

Because modeling error of the virtual environment and slide phenomena wheels exist inevitably, operators must use remote video guidance to eliminate these errors. The operator could judge whether position and pose of these two robots appear variance through observing remote videos and adjust them to keep consistent. The real environment inspecting interface is show in Fig 6. It can show videos from cameras on the robot and on the spot. The main window embedded in the interface display video from the camera on the spot, the other display video from camera of the manipulator. It is very effective for operator to manipulate the mending robot. The bandwidth of this WLAN is 11Mbps, which is wide enough for our communication system and video transmission. But we should avoid opening too many video windows at the same time considering for real time operation [8].

HEBUT-II robot consists of a mobile vehicle and a five-degree-of-freedom manipulator. The manipulator has five links which connected through rotary joints, so it is driven by five motors. Motors are controlled by PMAC (program multiple axis controller), and they occupy five of eight channels. Control signals of PMAC are sent to motor drivers, and then motors are driven by motor drivers to finish task. Because slide and slip phenomena exist inevitably, the real robot can hardly arrive at the leaky point accurately. With the operator's adjust; the robot can reach the leaky point successfully. When the vehicle arrives at the leaky point position and adjusts its posture, the leaky container can be repaired by constantly changing the postures of the manipulator.

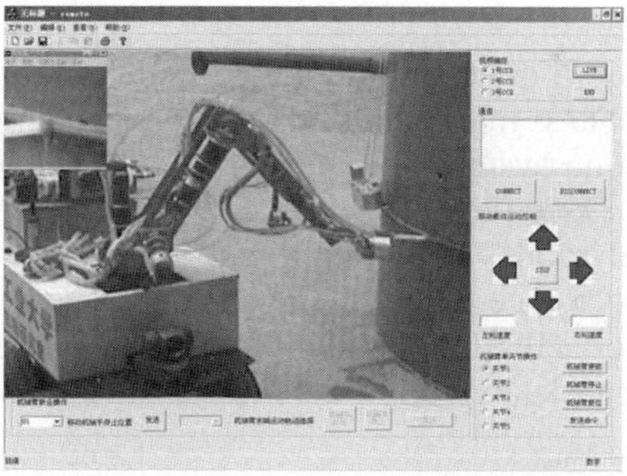

Fig. 6. Real environment inspecting interface

Operator's duty is to use data glove to control the real robot get to the leaky point position and to finish mending task. But this way may lead to collision between the robot and other objects because of operators' random operation. We install ultrasonic sensors on the real robot to protect the robot from danger. The robot should have the ability to avoid obstacle. Ultrasonic sensor is widely applied in obstacle voidance and navigation. In this system, ultrasonic sensors are used to form front and back sonar annulus which detecting obstacle in all directions. It is shown in Fig 7 and Fig 8. The characteristic of sensors layout is that they could provide a great deal of environment information.

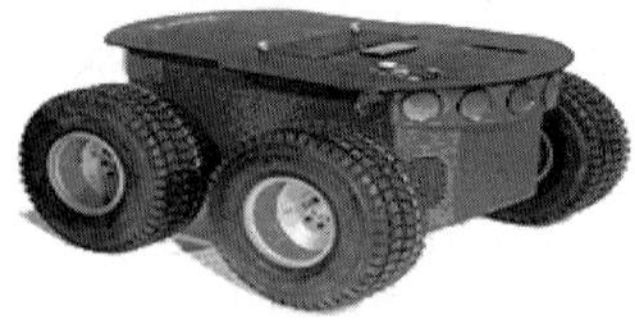

Fig. 7. Mobile noumenon sonar array

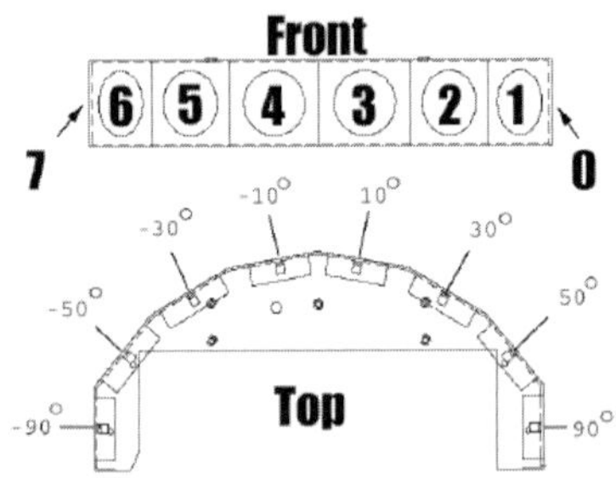

Fig. 8. Altrasonic sensors array

In the whole process, the mending robot can reach the leakage successfully and accomplish the mending task smoothly, no collisions happen. Experiments demonstrate that this method has good practicability and security.

5 Conclusion

In this paper, we propose a novel sound source search system. This system is composed of a robot which has a microphone array corresponding to human's ears and a virtual reality teleoperation system. The virtual robot is the agent of remote robot in the virtual environment. Data glove is used to operate the virtual robot to complete the control towards the real robot. The system can make the operator control the real robot to search the sound source fast and conveniently. The system is used in mending leaky chemical container; HEBUT-II robot can reach the leakage successfully and accomplish the mending task smoothly. It is proved to be practical and secure.

Acknowledgements

This work was supported by 863 (Grant No. 2006AA04Z221)□Tianjin Nature Science Fund (043601811).

References

1. Kulji, B., János, S., Tibor, S.: Mobile robot controlled by voice. In: International Symposium on Intelligent Systems and Informatics, pp. 189–192 (2007)
2. Peter, X., Liu, A.D.C., Chan, R., Chen, K., Wang, Y.: Voice Based Robot Control. In: International Conference on Information Acquisition, pp. 543–547 (2005)

3. Rahmadi Kurnia, M., Hossain, A., Nakamura, A., Kuno, Y.: Object Recognition through Human-Robot Interaction by Speech. In: International Workshop on Robot and Human Interactive Communication, pp. 619–624 (2004)
4. Zhizeng, L., Jingbing, Z.: Speech Recognition and Its Application in Voice-based Robot Control System. In: International Conference on Intelligent Mechatronics arid Automation, pp. 960–963 (2004)
5. Sakai, K., Asada, T.: Developing a Service Robot with Communication Abilities. In: International Workshop on Robots and Human Interactive Communication, pp. 91–96 (2005)
6. Youjun, X., Shiqi, L., Wentao, W.: Operating Technology Of Virtual Robot Based on Data Glove Drive[A]: Mechanical Science and Technology (23) (2004)
7. Mei, J., Lei, X.: Research on Virtual Object Manipulation Technology. Journal of System Simulation, 330–332 (2002)
8. Cui, F., Zhang, M., Mi, X.: A Semi-autonomous Teleoperation Method for Mending Robots Based on Virtual Reality and WLAN. In: International Conference on Mechatronics and Automation, pp. 1430–1435 (2006)

Application of Touch Sensing Technique Based on Magneto-Rheological Fluid in Constant Power Control of Coal Mining Machine

Can Zhao, Dan-dan Liu, and Chun-rui Tang

Heilongjiang Institute of Science and Technology, Harbin 150027, P.R. China
tcrldd@163.com

Abstract. In this paper, the power control method of coal mining machine of touch sensing technique based on magneto-rheological fluid is presented by analyzing to the performance of haulage and velocity modulation and the constant power control to coal mining machine in the real work. Controller outputs control signals which control touch sensing force-feedback devise base on magneto-rheological fluid by sampling current and rotate speed signals of cutting motor of coal mining machine. The manipulator adjusts haulage speed of coal mining machine to force the motors to operate approximately with rated power according as resistance touched by handle. The results of simulation and experiment indicate that the method can enhance obviously cutting efficiency of coal mining machine and void overload operating. The structure of the control method is simple and actualizes easily, so its outlook in application is good.

Keywords: Touch sensing force-feedback; magneto-rheological fluid; Coal mining machine; Power control.

1 Introduction

With energy industry rapid development, the power of coal mining machine increases from several dozens kilowatts to more than 2000 kilowatts presently. The growing of coal mining machine work efficiency enhancement is emphasized. At present, coal mining machines operate under the constant power through adjusting haulage speed. In the existing product, according to the related parameters and the experience, the manipulator adjusted the button of the manipulator to set haulage speed (limitation value). The machine actualizes automatic control and operation under full load of machines. In the practical application, because of the complex of the coal beds and the deficiency of manipulator's experience the coal mining machines is in frequently operating under under-loads, occasionally overloads. Operation under the long-term overload can accelerate its aging and increase the frequency of breakdowns, which cannot play its potency in application. Therefore, the more human-based operating mode is needed to settle the above questions radically.

The research of the ability of humanity acquisition information indicates that the sense of touch is the most important feeling except the sense of vision and hearing [1] [2] . Comparing with the visual feedback, the sense of touch not only can distinguish

C. Xiong et al. (Eds.): ICIRA 2008, Part II, LNAI 5315, pp. 64–72, 2008.

the size and the shape of the object, but also can distinguish hardness, quality of material, smooth degree and superficial mechanism, and so on. Magneto-rheological fluid provides a new direction for development of the sense of touch feedback system because of its unique flow-changing characteristics and good controllability [3] [4].

In order to achieve the precise and effective control to haulage speed of the coal mining machine and realize it and the power control to achieve the best efficiency, on the base of magneto-rheological valves which we develop independently, a kind of constant power control method of coal mining machine is designed based on touch sensing technique and magneto-rheological fluid, using special performance of magneto-rheological fluid – a new intelligent material.

2 The Sense of Touch Force-Feedback Device Based on Magneto-Rheological Fluid

When the hand of a man fetches an object, a moment is produced in the joint after the muscle of the fingers contracts; this moment causes the finger to produce a force. If this force affects on the surface of the object, the object produces a equal size, the opposite directional force to the finger, this force extrusion epidermis of the fingers, and stimulate sensory nerve cell, the stimulation signals are passed to human's cerebral cortex (nerve center). By analyzing these stimulation signals, the man hand can feel the force. This will form sensation of the force sense. During the conventional passive force-feedback devices working, when manipulator by remote control installment fetches an object, the force-feedback device produces a damping force to prevent the finger to do further grasp movement, according to the force signals transmitted by the long-distance manipulator. Here, the size and direction of this damping force have the same direction and the size of linear relation to the force produced by the real object to the fingers when a real object exists, which makes man feel that seems grasp the real object.

2.1 Working Models of Magneto-Rheological Fluid

Magneto-rheological fluid is the aerosol liquid which is formed by dispersing magnetic particles with the high saturation magnetic induction in nonmagnetic carrier liquid. Iron particles are magnetized when the role of the magnetic field, iron particles arranged along the direction of magnetic field. The mixture in seconds quickly turned into solid. Hundreds of KP magnitude shear stress can produce. It has better practical engineering value. The material phase change is not only rapid, but also reversible. Once the magnetic field completely removed, and the material restores fluid. What is more important is magneto-rheological material has controllability. The degree of phase change and size of interior shear stress can be controlled by the magnetic field. In the magnetic field, Magneto-rheological Fluid change Newtonian fluid of free flow into viscoplasticity body of certain yield shear strength, After removing the magnetic field, Magneto-rheological Fluid restore the free liquid state. This is Magneto-rheological effect. Magneto-rheological effect has the following characteristics: (1) Conversion is reversible; (2) Conversion is controllable; (3) control Conversion only controls the current signal strength of the magnetic induction; (4) control Conversion only response millisecond time; (5) energy of control Conversion is very low [3].

2.2 Designing of Magneto-Rheological Valve

Magneto-rheological valve is shown as Fig. 1. The valve body is made of nonmagnetic material. One end of it connects to working connection and another end to a piston cylinder body, which constitutes a seal connect cavity with magneto-rheological fluid in it. When magneto-rheological fluid valve work, the magneto-rheological fluid is flowing via magneto-rheological fluid entrance, magneto-rheological fluid bore, magneto-rheological fluid gap and magneto-rheological fluid channel. When excitation coil power turn-off, magneto-rheological fluid appear as favorable fluid without action of outer magnetic field. Magneto-rheological fluid valve open; when Excitation coil power turn-on, strong magnetic field is produced. Viscosity is enhanced two orders of magnitude within short time (millisecond level). Magneto-rheological fluid present similar solid mechanics character, its intensity is

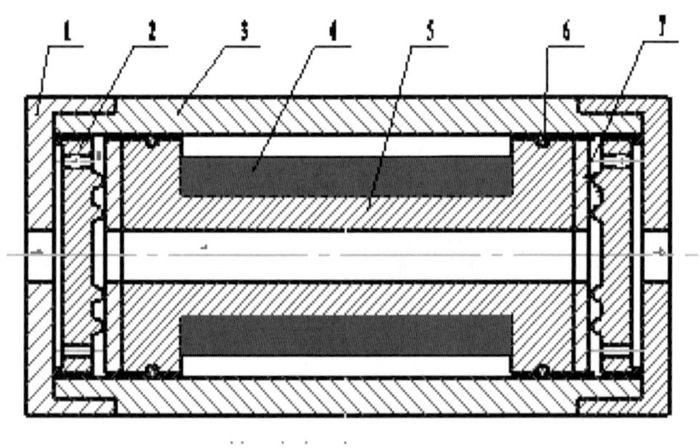

Fig. 1. Schematic diagram of magneto-rheological fluid valve(1. end cap 2. positioning block 3.valve body 4. excitation coil 5.bracket 6.seal ring 7.guide magnetism circle disc)

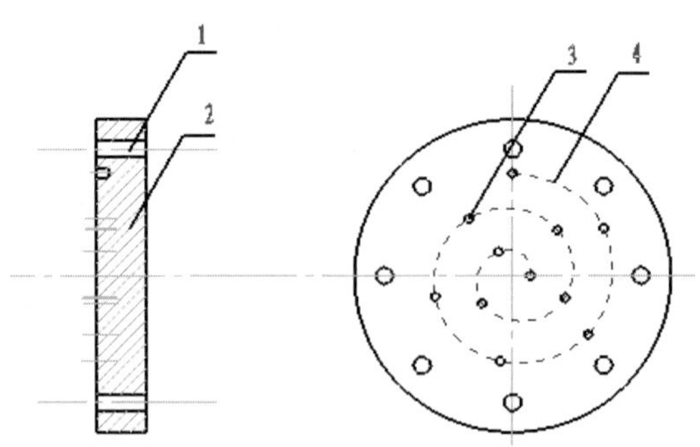

Fig. 2. Schematic diagram of magnetism gap space of magneto-rheological fluid valve(1.magnetizer 2.guide magnetic disc 3.non-flux sleeve 4.guide flow channel)

characterized by shearing yield stress, and that change of viscosity is consecutive and reversible. Magneto-rheological fluid valve are closed, and magnetic field is taken out, magneto-rheological fluid become fluid that is flowed.

In order to increase to adjust work voltage of magneto-rheological valve, schematic diagram of magnetism gap space of magneto-rheological fluid valve is shown in Fig 2. Magneto-rheological fluid flow magnetism gap space from entrance to non-line fluid flow channels, and last to exit of gap space.

2.3 Touch Sensing Force-Feedback Device Based on Magneto-Rheological Valve

Because this equipment will be installed in the manual manipulator, its structure should be simple and dexterous. The piston structure is advantageous to increase stability to the equipment, so the handle is connected to the piston by screw thread that is used as sensation of manipulator's touch in this design. The piston, steel body and magneto-rheological valve formed into a loop. Fig.3 is structure sketch of touch sensing force-feedback device based on magneto-rheological valve.

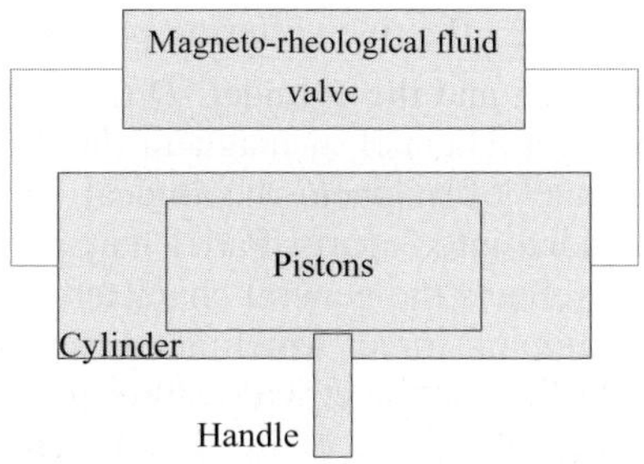

Fig. 3. Structure sketch of touch sensing force-feedback device based on magneto-rheological valve

With the handle driving piston, magneto-rheological fluid is impelled to flow into loop through the magnetic gap channel of magneto-rheological valve. In the condition of no magnetic field, magneto-rheological fluid is fluid feely as Newton free-flow, the piston motion is not affected by the resistance (only friction force of the system). When exert the magnetic field force on it, magneto-rheological fluid is transformed from the free-Newtonian flow to the viscous-plasticity body in several milliseconds. Magneto-rheological fluid is flowing in magnetic gap, it becomes the similar solid and the resistance to fluid increase. The constitutive relation of the similar solid may be described by the one of Bingham viscous-plasticity body [5].

$$\tau=\tau_y(B)+\eta\times(\frac{du}{dy}) \tag{1}$$

In formula (1), τ is the shear stress of magneto-rheological fluid; $\tau_y(B)$ is the shear yield stress; η is the kinetic viscosity of fluid; $\frac{du}{dy}$ is the velocity gradient; the first right item of formula 1 is called the Coulomb shear stress, the second right item is called the viscous shear stress; $\tau_y(B)$ is related to magnetic induction intensity, and is effected on the strength of the magnetic induction. So the shear yield stress can be controlled by magnetic field intensity.

To the shear flow, computational formula of the damping force is

$$F_B = L\pi D\tau = L\pi D\tau_y + \frac{L\pi D\eta}{h}u(t) \tag{2}$$

To the pressure-gradient flow, computational formula of the damping force is

$$F_P(\mathrm{t}) = \Delta P \times A_P = \frac{12\eta LA_P}{\pi Dh^3}A_P u(t) + \frac{3L\tau_Y}{h}A_P \tag{3}$$

Adding formula (1) to formula (2), considering the friction F_f of piston rod and bearing, computational formula of force-feedback dada gloves is gained, as following:

$$F(\mathrm{t}) = [\frac{12\eta LA_P^2}{\pi Dh^3} + \frac{L\pi D\eta}{h}]u(t) + [\frac{3LA_P}{h} + L\pi D]\tau_Y + F_f \tag{4}$$

In the formula (4), A_P is the effective suffering pressure area of the piston; $u(t)$ is the relative speed of the piston and the cylinder; D is the diameter of the piston; L is the length of the magnetic gap channel of magneto-rheological valve; h is the thickness of magnetic gap channel of magneto-rheological valve. From formula (4), the damping force may be divided into 3 parts. Part 1 may be called the viscosity damping force, which basically reflects the general characteristics of viscous fluid. Part 2 may be called Coulomb damping force, which is adjustable damping force of force-feedback device and reflects special electrical control performance of force-feedback device. Part 3 is the friction resistance of the piston rod and the bearing, which is treated as systemic error only to minimize, but not to be avoided.

3 The Coal Mining Machine Haulage Performance, Speed Regulation and Working Principle

Haulage performance of the coal mining machine reflects the relation among the haulage, haulage power, cutting power and haulage speed. Because the brittleness of coal crag, the flintiness f of coal bed, and the cutting impedance great range change, the haulage and the load power of electric motor great range change too and present the zigzag waveform stochastically. In the stability conditions, i.e. the change of f and *A* is small range, the haulage is given as formula (5), Cutting power as formula (6) by recursive computation according to experimental curve [6].

$$T = T_0 + Bv \tag{5}$$

$$N_t = N_0 + Cv \tag{6}$$

In the formula (5) and (6), T_0, N_0 are respectively the haulage and the no-load power of the cutting motor when the coal mining machine begins to operate (v=0). *B, C* is the constant. In given condition, it is related to the cutting impedance, the situation of clamping the gangue, the profile and the abrasion degree and the collocation of the cutting pick. The cutting impedance *A* is the main effect fact. The characteristic curve determined by the above two equations is Fig.4.

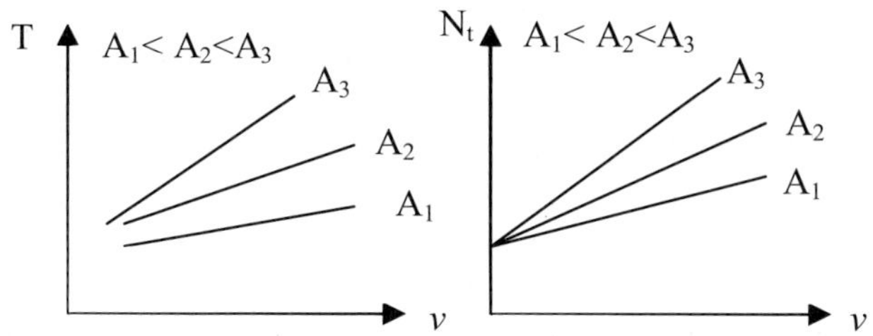

Fig. 4. The curve of haulage performance

The change of the cutting impedance is the input signal to cause the change of the parameters of the hauling part and the cutting part, through adjusting the hauling speed *v* to change the parameters. When *A* changes, keeping the power of the cutting motor constant, the change of its speed *v* is shown in Fig.5. To make the power of the cutting motor constant (working under full load), if *A* increases, v can be adjusted lowly from *v2* to *v3*. If the governor be used, the hauling speed can be regulated automatically with the change of *A* to keep the power of the cutting motor constant.

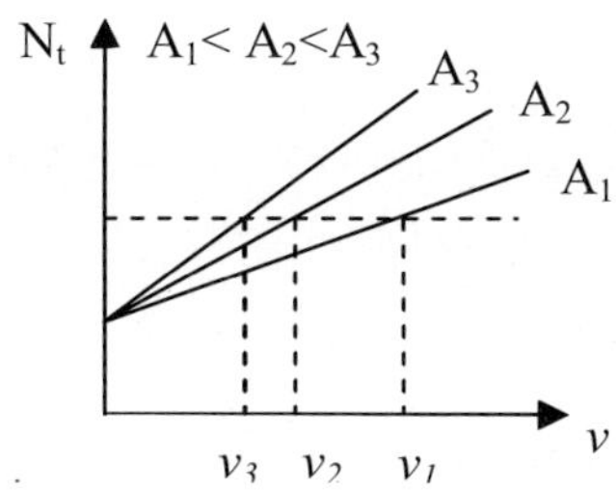

Fig. 5. The curve of speed regulation characteristic

4 Power Control of Coal Mining Machine of Touch Sensing Based on Magneto-Rheological Fluid

The cutting motor of the coal mining machine realizes basically the constant power control by force-feedback device based on magneto-rheological valve according to a certain control logics. The specific control flow is as following.

(1) Extracting the current and the rotate speed signals of the cutting motor of the coal mining machine by sensors such as instrument transformer.

(2) According to certain proportional relation, the controller output parallel codes by depending on the above signals. The current controller inputs control signals through the D-A conversion and outputs the current.

(3) Under the output current of the current controller of magneto-rheological valve, Magneto-rheological fluid flow through the magnetic valve flow channels that produces a certain resistance, the resistance to the piston changes along with it.

(4) The manipulator moves the piston by the slip handle and decides the movement direction by judging the resistance touched. The controller gets the displacement signal produced by the handle via the D-A conversion, and further to regulate the transducer to change the rotate speed of the haulage motor.

(5) The coal mining machine operates under new haulage speed, when it encounters different coal bed situations, the current and the rotate signals of the cutting motor of the coal mining machine corresponding change. The manipulator regulates the handle according to the new condition.

The control flow is given by Fig.6.

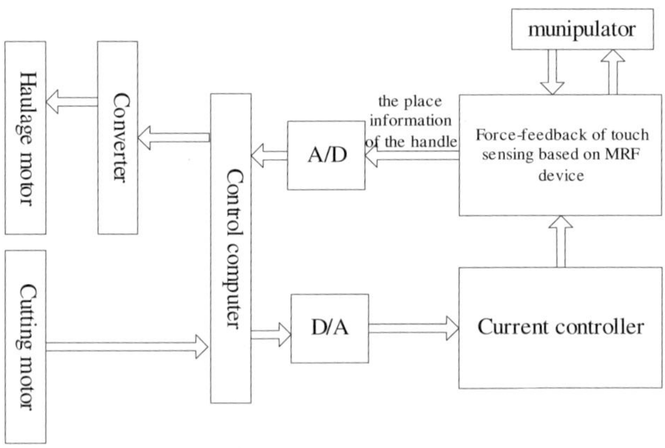

Fig. 6. Schematic diagram of power control of touch sensing based on magneto-rheological fluid of the coal mining machine

The handle will produce the resistance depending on the current and rotate signals of the cutting motor of the coal mining machine in this method. The manipulator moves the piston by the slip handle and decides the movement direction by judging the resistance touched. The controller gets the displacement signal produced by the handle by the D-A conversion, and further to regulate the transducer to change the rotate speed of the haulage motor. Comparing to the existent method to regulate haulage speed by the key, some questions such as the overload and under-load are settled and the reliability of the system are enhanced by the method in this paper. And the system can output the minimum power in the higher speed and reduce the noise when the coal mining machine is working under no-load. In this method, the definition and the responding speed of the system are advanced in largely extent, which is fit for working in the coal mine with bigger noise and lower visibility.

5 The Analyze to the Result of Simulation and Experiment

In the experiment, the mathematics model of a coal bed structure is established and stimulated by MALAB. The mathematics model, the electric control box of coal mining machine, the power control device of touch sensing based on magneto-rheological fluid, which constitutes the experimental condition. Compare the result of the stimulation with the speed got by the handle to regulate the electric control box, the experimental curve is given by Fig.7.

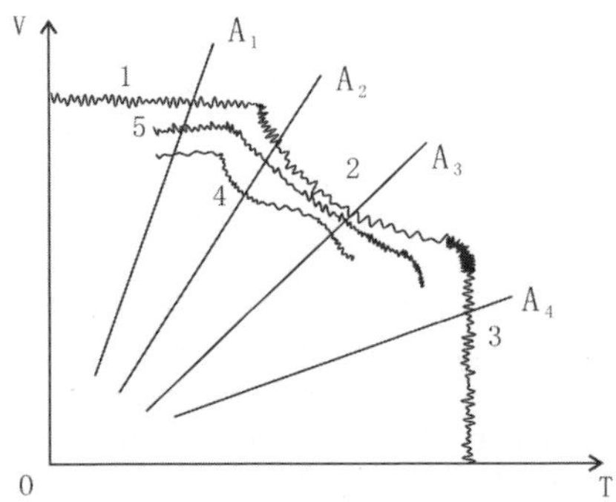

Fig. 7. The haulage speed curves produced by the different power output ways

The haulage speed course of coal mining machine is recorded in Figure 7, the horizontal axis denotes time, and the vertical axis denotes haulage speed. When the cutting motor adjusts the speed automatically by current signal to the constant power, the haulage speed curve should be closed within the region of the 1, 2, 3 curve and coordinate axis in Figure 7. This can ensure the cutting motor not to overload work. The operation curve of haulage speed of the actual manually by experience of a permit given is curve 4. In order to ensure the cutting part not to overload, the coal mining machine haves protective effect to overload decrease speed and overload stop by adjusting speed. This adjusting speed make that the cutting motor often work under less load or occasional overload conditions. The productivity of coal mining machine will not be very high. But control method of touch sensing technique based on magneto-rheological fluid in constant power control of coal mining machine in this paper takes full advantage of the operator of the tactile feel of the sensitive. The adjusting speed curve is curve 5. The power of cutting motor is closer to rated power than the experienced operatives power, the efficiency of the cutting motor has high improved.

6 Conclusion

In this paper, applying the force-feedback device of touch sensing based on magneto-rheological fluid to the control to the haulage speed of the coal mining machine, which regulates effectively the output power of the coal machine and enhances the work reliability and economizes energy consumption to reduce the cost of mining coal depending effectively on the definition and the responding speed of the hand touch of the manipulator. The algorithm is tested by the simulation based on the electric control box of coal mining machine and the power control device of touch sensing based on magneto-rheological fluid. After the function of the hardware is tested, this algorithm need be further tested in real machine to apply to the real mining coal.

References

1. Emst, M.O.: Humans integrate visual and haptic information in a statistically optimal fashion. J. Nature 415, 429–433 (2002)
2. Zhenglie, C., Matsunaga, K., Shidoji, K.: The effect of reaction force feedback on object-insert work in virtual reality environment. J. Research Reports on Information Science and Electrical Engineering of Kyushu University 7, 105–110 (2002)
3. Ynw, G., Anthony, M.R.: The development of variably compliant haptic systems using magneto-rheological fluids. In: Fortieth Annual Asilomar Conference on Signals, Systems and Computers, pp. 491–502. SPIE, San Diego (2005)
4. Ai-min, W., Jin-qiao, D.: A Passive Force Feedback Data Glove Based on a Smart Material. J. Measurement & Control Technology 26, 10–12 (2007) (in Chinese)
5. Changrong, L., Miao, Y., Weimin, C.: Study on design theory for magneto-rheological fluid damper using eyring constitutive relationship and experimental test. J. Chinese Journal of Mechanical Engineering. 14, 132–136 (2005) (in Chinese)
6. Dao-xing, A.: Analysis of Speed Regulation Principles and Hualage Properties of Electrical Shearer. J. Coal Mine Machinery 47, 47–48 (2005) (in Chinese)

Research on the Unmanned Air Vehicle Team Intelligence Control System Based on Multi-agent

Ning Guo, Junwei Lv, and Jihong Yu

Department of Control Engineering, NAEI, Yantai Shandong 264001, China

Abstract. Unmanned Air Vehicle is a kind of flying intelligence robot with real-time reaction ability. Using the multi-agent idea in the exploitation of the unmanned air vehicle team Intelligence control system (UAVTICS) will enhance its intelligence degree greatly. The article introduces the design idea of Cruise Missile Weapon Control System, build the multi-agent frame of UAVTICS, and design the architecture of the fly-control agent and single unmanned air vehicle agent with "human-machine integration approach". And the model of unmanned air vehicle team agent is also described.

Keywords: Unmanned Air Vehicle Team, Multi-Agent, Intelligence Control.

1 Introduction

With the development of the computer and information technology, great progress has been achieved on the researcher of UAV. Compared with manned air vehicle, UAV has many advantages as a flying intelligence robot, such as low cost, low risk, good flexibility. And it has been widely used in reconnaissance, surveillance, attacking the target, and so on. Whereas, because of the complexity of the aerial warfare circumstance, a single UAV is no longer adequate for the tasks such as mission re-project and new attacking decision-making. So we pay our attention to UAV team.

Multi-Agent Systems(MAS) is an important part of distributed artificial intelligence, its main idea is dividing a complex system into some smaller agents which can communicate and cooperate with each other, and the complex system can accomplish its function by the cooperation of these smaller agents. It will be easier to study the cooperation of the single UAV agents by using the multi-Agent technology, and will enhance the Intelligence degree of the system greatly. The article combines the artificial intelligence with the machine intelligence with the direction of "human-machine integration approach" (the idea has been used successfully in the design of the Cruise Missile Weapon Control System in USA), brings forward a design project of the UAVTICS faced to the multi-Agent, and shows a way to build its architecture.

2 The MAS Architecture of UAVTICS

Architecture is the first sect to develop the UAVTICS, so we begin with the Architecture design. The theory and practice of intelligence control shows us: it is not enough to depend on high-autonomic intelligence system excessively; human intelligence can

C. Xiong et al. (Eds.): ICIRA 2008, Part II, LNAI 5315, pp. 73–80, 2008.

not be exchangeable. The "battle-axe" Cruise Missile is representative. The system adopts the "man in loop" technique, whose essential is adding a human-machine interaction system in the control loop. The "battle-axe" Cruise Missile weapon control system(CMWCS) can communicates with the flying missile though the secondary planet date chain, gives a series of orders to the missile such as: going around for the attacking chance; re-aiming in the flying course; scouting the information that missile transmit; evaluating the attacking effect. The CMWCS has the power to control the missile launch and program the mission on the launch platform, it make the cooperation of the missile team comes true [1]. Considering the comparability of CMWCS and UAVTICS, the article introduces the design idea of CMWCS to develop the architecture of UAVTICS.

2.1 The Design Object of UAVTICS

The object of the UAVTICS is: Command center agent binds the mission date on the unmanned air vehicle team on the ground. When there is no suddenness happened, every unmanned air vehicle keeps the real-time connection with Command center agent, unmanned air vehicle team executes the date pre-bonded and keeps auto-aviating though the cooperation among single unmanned air vehicles. When changes have taken place in warfare circumstance, including weather condition, equipments' conking out, and enemy's attacking, unmanned air vehicle team agent should take responses as below: making judgments on the new circumstance, making real-time re-projection and decision, supervising the execution course on the mission projection. At the same time, UAVTA transmit the information to Command center agent through Communication Module. Having finished evaluating the condition, command center agent make new decisions and give the UAVTA new order.

2.2 The Design of MAS Architecture

According to the object, the article builds the UAVTICS model based on MAS as Fig.1:

The function of every unit is introduced as below:

- Launch Control Agent (LC-A).UAV launch unit, its function is mainly about binding tracking date, original setting, detecting the UAV before launch, UAV launch control.
- Command and Surveillance Center Agent (CS-A). which includes: ① Command／launch surveillance agent (LSC-A): its function is supervise and accredit LC-A, communicate with superior and neighbor unit in behalf of UAVTICS, coordinate the agent's work in the surveillance center agent; ② Fly Control Agent (FC-A): its function is supervise the flying state of UAVT, identify the target, evaluate the target damage degree and give new order to UAVT according to the battlefield situation. ③ Mission re-Projects Agent (MrP-A):this unit mainly in charge the work as below: receiving and checkout attack plan and track program from the superior, making launch project, re-project or amend the plan according to the mission changing, transmitting the

mission date; ④ Communication Management Agent(CM-A): its function is mainly about managing the information from the superior, neighbor unit.

- UAVT Agent (UT-A). The agent is composed of some single UAV agents. Every single agent communicates and cooperates with each other according to some stated rules, and keeps the real-time connection with Communication Management Agent. UT-A is the direct unit to carry out the mission, it carry out its work according to the pre-bonded date and make decisions accordingly. Its decision level is lower than MrP-A's in LSC-A.
- Communication Module Agent (CM-A). This unit is mainly composed of secondary planet and signal receiving station on the ground. Its job is the communication between CS-A and UT-A.

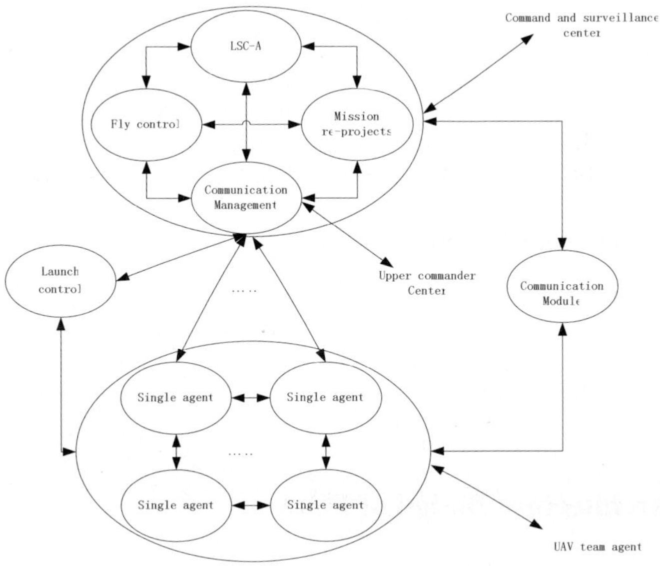

Fig. 1. The UAVTICS model based on MAS

3 The Communication and Cooperation Rule of UAVTICS

Excepting for the voice communication between the human-machine integration Agent, FIPA ACL format (an Agent communication language in intelligence physical fund organization) is used widely by the information transmitted in date form. The content and ontology of FIPA ACL message uses XML (eXtensible Markup Language) code. Communication among the Agents obeys FIPA communication [2]. The agent in CS-A communication though LAN; different kinds of wireless and lineate method is used among CS-A, LC-A and superior command system; CS-A connects with ground station of secondary planet and communicate with UAVT through the secondary planet date-line.

3.1 Cooperation Based on Organization Architecture

Organization architecture defines the rule, function and relationship of single agents. LSC-A plays a governor and controller role compared with LC-A, FC-A and UAVT. LSC-A, FC-A and MrP-A Cooperate equally with each other on the whole in the Command and surveillance center. Single UAV agents cooperate with each other though FC-A. The content of UAV cooperation includes time cooperation and attack direction cooperation, the method is composed of using attack project and track program planned before launch, plan regulation by LSC-A during the launch cause, remote control by FC-A to aero-UAV[3-4-5].

3.2 Cooperation Based on Promises

All agents promise to finish their conjunct work and obey the rules as below: ① Every Agent should keep the promise except for finding that the mission has been finished or the mission is impossible or unnecessary. ② When agents receive new order or the modificatory information of promised mission, they should execute new mission or actualize update as quickly as possible. ③ One agent must notify the other agents concerned when it has finished, abandoned or changed its promise…[2-3].

3.3 Cooperation Based on Shared Plan

All agents obey a shared plan to achieve dynamic combination and cooperation in the group. The plan contains all the detail and approach in the mission, single agent or agent group participate part of the plan. If the plan can not be abided, the surveillance center will take real-time adjustment to the shared plan and actualize control on it.

4 The Architecture Design of FC-A

FC-A is the core of UAVTICS on the ground and the key of system development. Considering FC-A's function is very complexity and the design idea of "battle-axe" Cruise Missile has been proved successfully, the article uses the idea for reference to enhance the intelligence degree of FC-A. Its main idea is "human-machine integration approach" [6]:it consider the agent as a whole consists of human, intelligence machine agent and common machine that help human acquire and transmit the information(such as telephone, fax). In the whole agent, human is the core, intelligence machine agent (IMA) is the assistant, they cooperate with each other to make decisions and carry out the mission. On the base of analysis to the mission feature, human characteristic and function demand, the key elements of the design includes: distribute the function of human and machine rationally; design the human-machine interface of IMA in order to best the human beings' ability to cognize the information and short the time that FC-A need to respond to the decision and action which might change with the situation [7]. The structure graph of FC-A was shown as Fig.2 [4-7]:

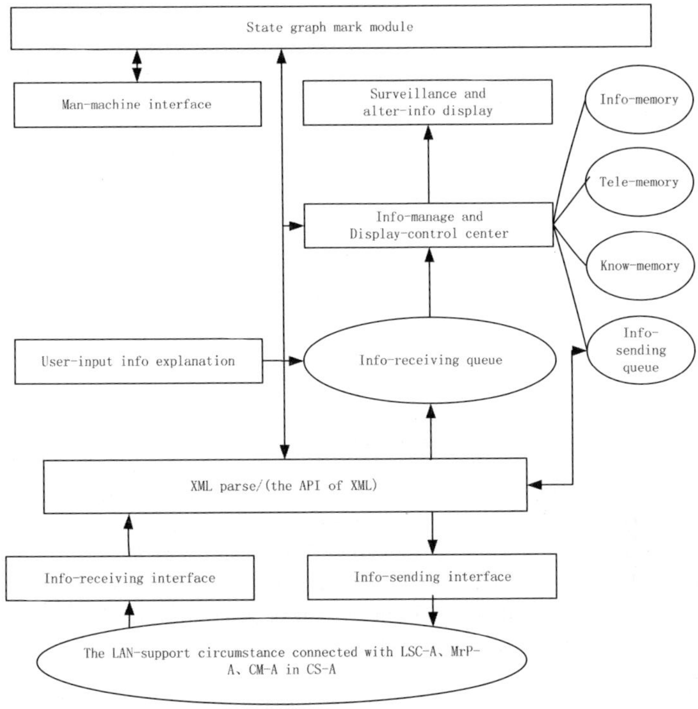

Fig. 2. The structure graph of FC-A

In Fig.2, the hardware of IMA consists of a workstation with a keyboard, a mouse and two link-monitors. Its main part includes:

(1) State graph mark module. It is consists of several parts: the army tab memory contains plot function which can create military standard; geography and map memory provides us date map and geography attribute of the battlefield; application program interface(API) contains the interface function provided for the display and operation of surveillance software; the program for the situation mark and control is in charge dealing with the information from human and API, read the date in database, command the bottom graph control program to mark on the map, store and manage map , turn human's operation into input affair to the command center then induce the corresponding action[7].

(2) Man-machine interface. this unit includes two parts: state graph surveillance machine and date surveillance machine. Their functions are both provide human with the information of the battlefield. We can conclude the difference between them, that is, the one shows graph and the other shows date.

(3) Info-manage and Display-control center. It is the intelligence core of IMA, its job is cognizing, responding to and disposing the information. In this way, IMA can communicate with human and other agents. XML parse machine analyses FIPA ACL message with XML code and puts the result in Info-receiving queue. Command center deals with the information according to the communication agreement, Info-memory

stores the date of faith aggregate for the display and decision; Tele-memory stores date and cyclostyle of Tele-message; Know-memory stores the preparative knowledge of IMA as arithmetic, consequence rules, communication knowledge. XML format is used in all the three above.

5 Structure Design of Unmanned Air Vehicle Team Agent

Because of the complexity of the aerial warfare circumstance, it is insufficient in actual combat with a single Unmanned Air Vehicle executing mission. Building an Unmanned Air Vehicle Team is essential. We construct a multi-agent system which can accomplish its mission by cooperating with every sub-agent. Firstly a single Unmanned Air Vehicle Agent's structure is given.

5.1 Structure Design of Single Unmanned Air Vehicle Agent

When we select method of Agent structure design, structure BDI was taken into account. Because structure BDI uses observe-think-act executing manner, which can obviously express Agent's Beliefs, Desires, Intentions and Programming. Furthermore structure BDI has perfect theory, flexibility and response. So we design the structure of single Unmanned Air Vehicle Agent based on the BDI.

The structure of single Agent was shown as Fig.3:

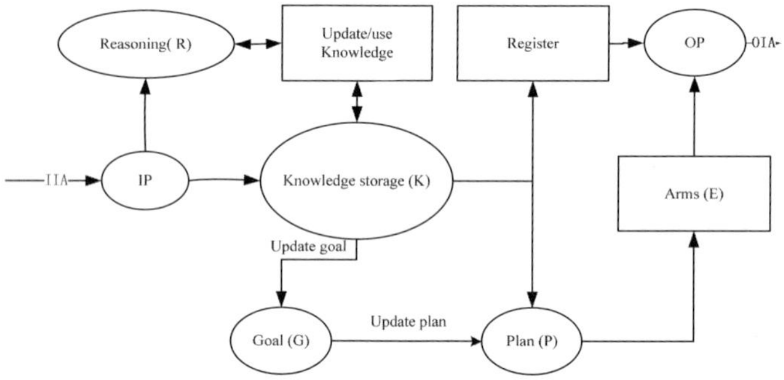

Fig. 3. The structure of single Agent

In the model BDI=(R,K,G,P,E,IP,OP,T,F,ILA,OLA,E).
Thereinto:

- R,K,G,P,E are abstract databases, they can be gauged by different mission.
- Reasoning(R) shows the reasoning and decision-making course of Unmanned Air Vehicle. During this course, Unmanned Air Vehicle makes decisions according to the information of its own, information offered by other Unmanned Air Vehicles and existing knowledge storage.
- Knowledge storage (K) is the finite set of database, which corresponds with the Beliefs of BDI. It shows the war field circumstance and the information of

other Unmanned Air Vehicle Agents (such as the number and position of goal and companion, the forecast of mobile intention).

- Goal (G) corresponds with the Desires of BDI, it shows Unmanned air vehicle Agent's motivation and final goals (such as air holding up, air convoy and air recovery), at last battle plan is set up on the battle intention.
- Plan (P) corresponds with the Intentions of BDI, it shows the action of Unmanned Air Vehicle Agent when it locks goal. Decision-making information which is set up by goal is input into corresponding control organization.
- Arms (E) is the implement organization of Unmanned Air Vehicle Agent, including flight control system, weapon control system and electro-war system [8].
- IP and OP are databases which contains input and output message.
- IIA and OIA show input and output interface of system model independently, they mainly describe communicating information and communicating behavior between agents and other sets. They are the service single UAV can get or provide, which can be exchanged with circumstance or other UAV. It is pivotal in the course of Multi-UAV agent cooperating with each other.
- Registration module shows that interrelated information must be registered or deleted when a new UAV joined in or exit the system.

When UAV agent firstly acquired war field situation by itself or accepted message from other agents, the message will be sent to the reasoning module(R) of agent, reasoning war field situation or mission on the base of knowledge storage, updating Agent's knowledge storage module (K), goal module (G) and programming module (P). If the similar message was accepted next time, it will be directly sent to knowledge storage, and agent will go ahead by former experience.

5.2 Cooperation Process among Unmanned Air Vehicle Team Agent

A lead plane agent, a wing plane agent and command center agent are included in a simple multi-UAV intelligent command control system structure model. UAV agent model can be gauged by Fig.3. In the process of aerial warfare, the attacking action of UAV Team is an action under the command of lead plane agent. UAV agents observe the war field situation by its sensors, and broadcast what it had to other UAV agents through communication module. Lead plane agent fuses the whole information based on the mission ordered by command center, information detected by itself and other wing planes, then makes out the whole aerial warfare situation, resets cooperating tactics, and redistributes wing plane agent mission. Under the lead plane agent's command, the wing plane agent makes an attack on goals according to programming and mobile tactics [9]. At last lead plane agent and wing plane agent transfer the actual state of mission to the command center agent by communications module. Having evaluated the attacking effect and our expenses, the command center agent reassigns lead plane agent by the existing troops.

6 Conclusions

The article introduces the multi-agent idea in the design of UAVICS, constructs the structure of MAS, and demonstrates its responsibility assignment, configuration, communications and cooperation. On the base of Cruise Missile Weapon Control System, we designed the control center—the architecture of the Fly-Control Agent and Single Unmanned Air vehicle Agent according to BDI model. And the cooperation process of Unmanned Air Vehicle Team Agent is also described. Reference [10] indicates that introducing the multi-agent idea to the design of UAVICS can exert high autonomy, response and intelligence of UAV. The article has just discussed the structure design of UAVICS, in the future we will research on the cooperating algorithms and project applications of Unmanned Air Vehicle Team Agent.

References

1. Besselman, J., logsdon, M., Whisnant, B.E.: The tactical tomahawk weapons control system.Interface design project, `http://www.sys.virginia.edu/hci/papers/capstonepaper5.doc`
2. Michael, W.A.: Introduction to MultiAgent Systems. Publishing House of Electronics Industry, Beijing (2003)
3. Zhang, W.M., Li, Y.: Intelligent and Cooperative Information Technology. Publishing House of Electronics Industry, Beijing (2002)
4. Zhang, O.Y., Tong, M.A.: Agent-Oriented Design of Cruise Missile Weapon Control System Architecture. Fire Control and Command Control 8, 33–36 (2007)
5. Huang, X.Y., Liu, W.H., Ma, X.X.: Mechanism of Human-Machine Cooperation Based on Agent and the Role of Human Being. Journal of Chongqing University Natural Science Edition 25, 32–35 (2002)
6. Robert, A.W.: Tactical Tomahawk Weapon Control System User Interface Analysis and Design. The School of Engineering and Applied Science University of Virginia (2001)
7. Zhu, N.Z., Zhu, D.C.: Command Automation System Engineering. Publishing House of Electronics Industry, Beijing (2001)
8. Liu, J.X., Tong, M.A.: Study on Models of Multi-Agent System Based Group Aircraft Cooperative Air Combat Command Control System. Electronics Optics & Control 31, 49–53 (2001)
9. Liu, J.X., Tong, M.A.: Cooperative Attack Action of Multi-UAV Team. Flight Dynamics 21, 16–19 (2003)
10. Tan, Y.Y., Zhao, R.C.: Intelligent Agent-Based Design and Implementation of Autonomous Task Manager for Small UAVS. Journal of Northwestern Polytechnical University 12, 757–759 (2006)

Transparency Oriented Virtual Coupling Design: New Approach and Application to a Novel Admittance Haptic Device

Yanhe Zhu[1,2], Jizhuang Fan[2], Qinxin Meng[1], Jie Zhao[2], and Hegao Cai[2]

[1] School of Mechanical and Electrical Engineering, Harbin Engineering University, Harbin 150001, China
[2] State Key Laboratory of Robotics and System , Harbin Institute of Technology, Harbin 150001, P.R. China
yhzhu@hit.edu.cn

Abstract. A novel admittance haptic device which has low inertia and high speed to guarantee the high force bandwidth for the haptic interaction system is presented. Friction wheel is used to implement a rapid adjustment of the velocity loop. According to the admittance character of the haptic interface, PI velocity feedback control is utilized in the haptic interaction system. By introducing the virtual coupling into the system, Llewellyn's stability criteria in circuit theory is used to derive the constraint conditions to guarantee the system's absolute stability. Furthermore the parameters of the virtual coupling are optimized oriented to high transparency of the system. Man-machine haptic interaction system is established with the novel admittance interface. The experimental results indicate that optimized virtual coupling guarantees the large range stability, as well as improving the transparency effectively.

Keywords: Admittance device; Two-port network; Virtual coupling; Stability; Transparency.

1 Introduction

As well as visual and audio capabilities, the sensation of force and touch is also the essential information passage for human being's perception of the external world. Human-machine haptic interface system is composed of operator, the haptic interface devices, and virtual environment. Stability and transparency of the system depend on the complicated interaction between each one of the three. In Virtual Reality and teleoperated system, the simulation and recreation of the sense of touch is the key way to strengthen the genuine feeling of the system, to create the effect of indulgence. Hence, the related research has already been focused on , and evolved into a completely new field for studying[1]. Since haptic interface devices can release energy, unstable state may result in not only the destruction of the hardware, but also the threat to the safety of the operator. Stability is prior to all the problems to be concerned when it comes to system-controller design. In general, stable state depends on many factors such as operator, hardware (Motors, sensors, controllers, etc), virtual environment and the complicated interaction between each individual of the

C. Xiong et al. (Eds.): ICIRA 2008, Part II, LNAI 5315, pp. 81–90, 2008.

previously mentioned three. Initial hard work to solve the problem proposed virtual coupling of the virtual environment and haptic device. Virtual Coupling is a kind of virtual mechanical system including combination of components which are connected in series or in parallel. These components between haptic interface and virtual environment can constrain the maximum or minimum impedance of the virtual environment, and guarantee the stability of the system. Firstly introduced by colgate[2] , the method was used to solve the problem of non-continuity in environment appearing in collision. Besides, Zilles and Salisbury[3] have promoted a similar approach called "god-object", which utilized a virtual spring damper between force-feedback device and virtual environment. Meanwhile, Adams and Hannaford have deduced the means of designing virtual coupling parameters using two-terminal network theory, concerning every combinations of the relationship of reason and result, which has less conservation than passive design.

In this paper, a novel 1-DOF admittance haptic device has been designed, and algorithm for controlling to ensure system stability and transparency through visual coupling optimization method has been studied, which has the assumption of passivity of virtual environment.

2 Novel 1-DOF Admittance Haptic Interface

The 1-DOF haptic interface is shown as Fig.1,made up of three parts: 1)power, including motor and digital RC motor, 2)transmission mechanism, including driving-wheel and directing-wheel, 3)sensors, including collinear displacement sensor and six-dimension force sensor.

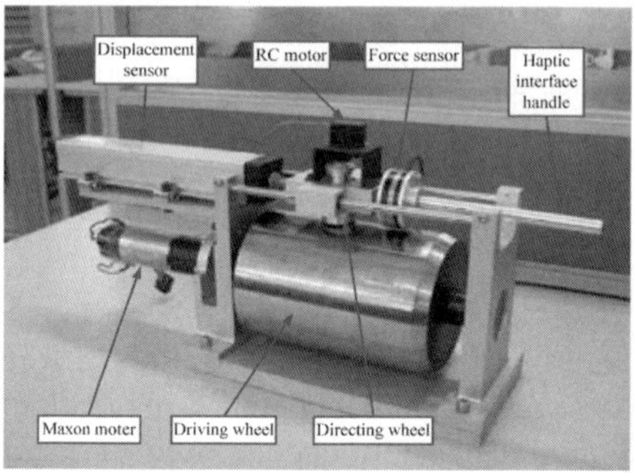

Fig. 1. The 1-DOF admittance haptic device

Two round surfaces have been used for transmission with the help of friction. Initially, the axis of the directing wheel is parallel to that of the driving wheel, which is obvious in Fig.2. At this time, there is no relative displacement between the two wheels. When the directing-wheel rotates along its axis Z1 for a certain degree θ, since the two axis are not parallel to each other, helical movement can be created, thus leading to linear movement. The advantage of such realization lies in rapid conversion of movement direction, for traditional transmission method makes sure that when moving part moves inversely, mostly motors will rotate in a different direction. In this way, processes for motor-speed deduction and increment have to be enhanced.

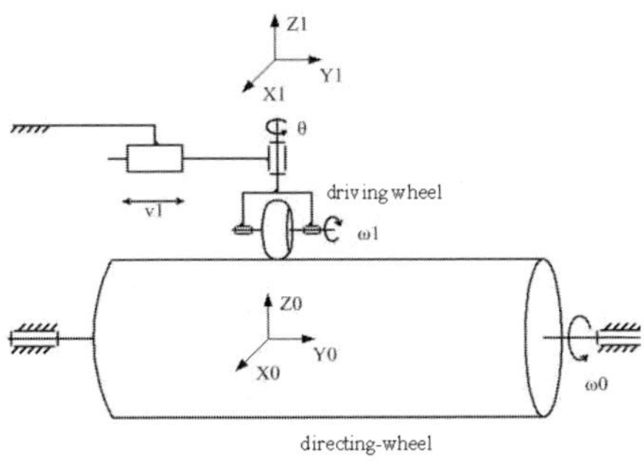

Fig. 2. Transmission diagram of the haptic device

3 Modeling of Admittance Haptic Interface System

3.1 Simplified Dynamic Model of the Haptic Device

Up to now modeling available for the operator comes in mainly two forms: 1)regarding the operator equivalently as passive impedance[4,5] 2)treating the operator as the equal linear combination of mass, spring, and damper[6,7,8], which is limited with particular operator and operating style concerned. In this paper the previous method will be used.

Taking 1-DOF haptic interface devices into consideration , corresponding dynamic model is depicted as Fig.3.

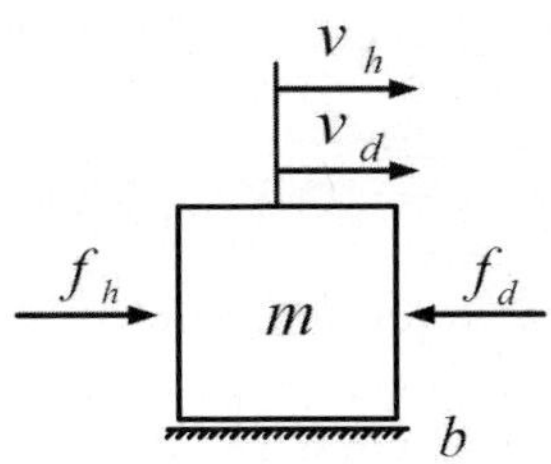

Fig. 3. Simplified dynamic model of the haptic deive

m is the total mass of the driving motor and the supplementary connecting parts, b is the damping of the device, f_h and v_h are the force and velocity of the driving point of the operator, f_d and v_d are the force and velocity of the driving point of the motor.

Dynamic equations of the device can be listed as follows:

$$\begin{cases} f_h - f_d = ms^2 x_d + bsx_d \\ x_h = x_d \end{cases} \tag{1}$$

For virtual environment, a reasonable dynamic model can be a combination of spring, damp and mass:

$$\begin{cases} f_e = m_e s^2 x_e + b_e s x_e + k_e x_e \\ f_h = f_e \end{cases} \tag{2}$$

In which f_e is the virtual force, m_e, b_e, k_e are virtual mass, virtual damping coefficient and virtual elastic factor, respectively.

3.2 Closed-Loop Control Model for the System

Haptic device discussed in this paper belongs to admittance type device. Its control model with speed closed-loop is shown in Fig.4.

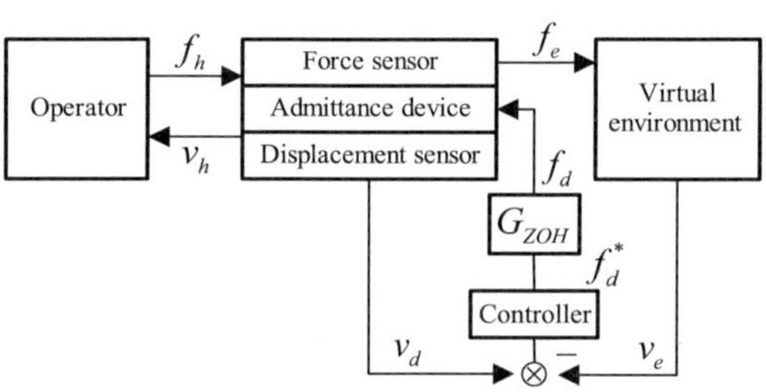

Fig. 4. The control model with speed closed-loop

A kind of internal speed closed-loop control strategy has been introduced, as Fig.4 illustrated, the control strategy is :

$$f_d^* = K_v(v_d - v_e) + K_p(x_d - x_e) \tag{3}$$

In which K_v is speed gain, K_p is position gain, v_e is the velocity in the virtual environment, the asterisk on the right upper position indicates discrete quantity. Velocity and position signals of the virtual environment are the inputs to the controller, considering phase-delay of the zero-order holder, obtained:

$$f_d = f_d^* G_{ZOH} \tag{4}$$

Based on the equivalent effect of mechanical system and electrical system, i.e. , force is equivalent to voltage, velocity is the counterpart to current, analysis of the relationship between force and velocity can be accomplished on the base of analyzing two-terminal network circuit. Equations (1)~(4) is converted to:

$$\begin{cases} f_h - f_d = msv_d + bv_d \\ v_h = v_d \end{cases} \tag{5}$$

$$\begin{cases} f_e = msv_e + bv_e + kv_e/s \\ f_h = f_e \end{cases} \tag{6}$$

$$f_d = [K_v(v_d - v_e) + K_p \frac{1}{s}(v_d - v_e)] \cdot G_{ZOH} \tag{7}$$

Utilizing equations (5)~(7),the following is got:

$$\begin{pmatrix} v_h(s) \\ f_e(s) \end{pmatrix} = \begin{pmatrix} G_{hh}(s) & -G_{he}(s) \\ 1 & 0 \end{pmatrix} \begin{pmatrix} f_h(s) \\ -v_e(s) \end{pmatrix} \tag{8}$$

In which

$$G_{ZOH} = 1 - e^{-sT}/s \approx 2/2 + Ts \tag{9}$$

$$G_{hh}(s) = 1/ms + b + (K_v + K_p/s) \cdot G_{ZOH} \tag{10}$$

$$G_{he}(s) = (K_v + \frac{K_p}{s}) \cdot G_{ZOH} \Big/ ms + b + (K_v + \frac{K_p}{s}) \cdot G_{ZOH} \tag{11}$$

4 Transparency Oriented Virtual Coupling Design

4.1 Stability Analysis for the Admittance Haptic System

For any two-terminal network system, the mapping relationship between input and output can be described by the admittance matrix $P_{2\times2}$ of the system, i.e. , y=Pu. According to Llewellyn's criterion, absolute stability of two-terminal network does exist on and only on the condition that:

$$\begin{aligned} &\mathrm{Re}(p_{11}) \geq 0 \,\&\, \mathrm{Re}(p_{22}) \geq 0 \\ &2\,\mathrm{Re}(p_{11})\mathrm{Re}(p_{22}) \geq | p_{12}p_{21} | + \mathrm{Re}(p_{12}p_{21}), \forall \omega \geq 0 \end{aligned} \tag{12}$$

Consulting to the research of Hogan[9], operator is passive. Meanwhile, virtual environment is assumed to be passive, thus the stability of the haptic interface system depends on the absolute stability of the haptic interface. Therefore, the mapping relationship between two-terminal network can be shown as equation (8), absolute stability rely on and only on:

$$\begin{aligned} &\mathrm{Re}(G_{hh}(s)) \geq 0 \\ &\mathrm{Re}(G_{he}(s)) \geq |G_{he}(s)|, \forall \omega \geq 0 \end{aligned} \tag{13}$$

In which the following can be easily found:

$$\frac{\mathrm{Re}(G_{he}(s))}{|G_{he}(s)|} = \cos(\angle G_{he}(s)) \geq 1 \tag{14}$$

For a system with sampling and holding, the lag or delay of phase ensures $\cos(\angle G_{he}(s)) < 1$, which means the haptic interface is not absolutely stable.

4.2 System Stability Conditions with Virtual Coupling Introduced

For such system, to guarantee that haptic interface is absolutely stable, the method preferred is to introduce the virtual coupling path, and for admittance-recreation approach, it means to add virtual mass-damping willingly unit between haptic interface and virtual environment. The two-terminal network is shown in Fig.5:

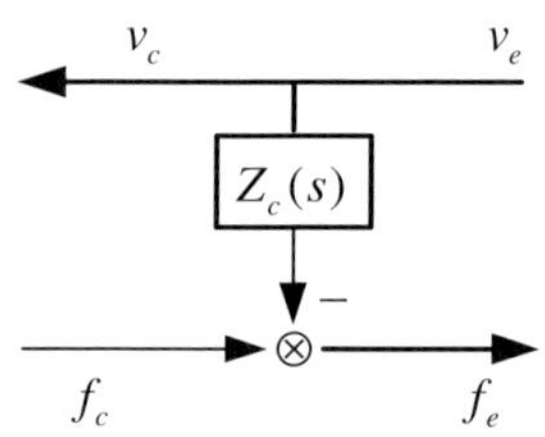

Fig. 5. Virtual coupling network composed of mass-damping

The relationship of the parameters in the virtual coupling is shown as following:

$$\begin{pmatrix} v_c(s) \\ f_e(s) \end{pmatrix} = \begin{pmatrix} 0 & -1 \\ 1 & Z_c \end{pmatrix} \begin{pmatrix} f_c(s) \\ -v_e(s) \end{pmatrix} \tag{15}$$

$$f_c = f_h \tag{16}$$

$$Z_c = \frac{b_c \cdot m_c s}{b_c + m_c s} \tag{17}$$

Substituting (15), (16), (17) into (8), we can obtain:

$$\begin{pmatrix} v_h(s) \\ f_e(s) \end{pmatrix} = \begin{pmatrix} G_{hh}(s) & -G_{he}(s) \\ 1 & Z_c(s) \end{pmatrix} \begin{pmatrix} f_h(s) \\ -v_e(s) \end{pmatrix} \tag{18}$$

Hence, for admittance-recreation approach, with virtual coupling path introduced, the stability of the system can be got through (12) :

$$\begin{aligned}&\mathrm{Re}(G_{hh}(s))\geq 0\ \&\ \mathrm{Re}(Z_c(s))\geq 0\\&\mathrm{Re}(Z_c(s))\geq\frac{|-G_{he}(s)|+\mathrm{Re}(-G_{he}(s))}{2\,\mathrm{Re}(G_{hh}(s))}\end{aligned}\tag{19}$$

From which we see that to make sure of the absolute stability of system, there are two steps: 1)choose appropriate speed closed-loop controller to get $G_{hh}(s)$ all positively real; 2)using the function of frequency to find proper virtual coupling path $Z_c(s)$ to ensure that the second description in equation (19) is true.

4.3 Transparency Oriented Virtual Coupling Optimization

Performance of the haptic interface system can be measured on the degree of transparency. For an ideal system, position of the main hand and force should be exactly corresponding to position and force in virtual environment. For the two-terminal network system we described, the mixture mapping matrix should satisfy:

$$\begin{pmatrix}v_h\\f_e\end{pmatrix}=\begin{pmatrix}0&-1\\1&0\end{pmatrix}\begin{pmatrix}f_h\\-v_e\end{pmatrix}\tag{20}$$

According to (20), to realize the thorough transparency in haptic interface system, the following should be satisfied:

$$\begin{aligned}&G_{hh}=\frac{1}{ms+b+(K_v+\frac{K_p}{s})\cdot G_{ZOH}}=0\\&G_{he}=\frac{(K_v+\frac{K_p}{s})\cdot G_{ZOH}}{ms+b+(K_v+\frac{K_p}{s})\cdot G_{ZOH}}=1\\&Z_c=\frac{b_c\cdot m_c s}{b_c+m_c s}=0\end{aligned}\tag{21}$$

To achieve the total transparency of the system, speed closed-loop gain should be increased as much as possible. At the same time, impedance of the virtual coupling path should be decreased as much as possible. However, the realization of the stability of haptic interface system should simultaneously satisfy the stability conditions listed by equation (19) , and this calls for us to find an equilibrium point between stability and transparency of the system. The is a multi-variable related, multi-goal, non-linear, complicated process.

The four parameters K_v, K_p, b_c, m_c in equation (21) can be used as design parameters for optimization, equation (19) can be used as constraint conditions for optimization, the three parameters G_{hh}, G_{he}, Z_c can be used as goal of optimization. Computation with the optimizing toolbox of MATLAB, utilizing linear search algorithm by Quasi-Newton, optimized velocity loop gain parameter and virtual coupling parameter can be achieved.

5 Experimental Research

Using the virtual coupling parameters obtained through optimization, the experiment of simulation and recreation of the virtual spring force and damping is done.

5.1 Spring Force Simulation

Assuming the stiffness of virtual environment is 200N/m, operator takes hold of the handle and move at a certain speed(approximately 10mm/s) along x-axis back and forth, the zero-force-position of the spring is at x=25mm,the tested result of the mapping relationship is illustrated in Fig.6.

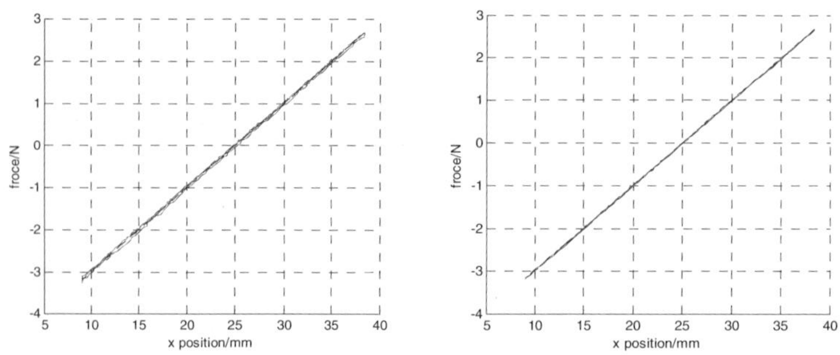

a) b)

Fig. 6. Experimental curve of the spring force simulation. a) with regular PID controller. b) with virtual coupling optimized controller.

It is obvious that force and displacement in Fig.6b) are related to each other in a more linear way than the one in Fig.6a), and during repetitive movement, the degree of non-overlapping of the loaded curve is less than 0.05N, indicating that optimized virtual coupling path has overcome the influenced caused by the damping and inertia of the hardware in a better way.

5.2 Damping-Force Simulation

Assuming the elastic coefficient of the virtual environment is 14N.s/m, and operator holds the handle, moving along the x-axis, the experiment result is shown in Fig.7:

In which the dashed line means the linear least square of the result point. As shown in Fig.7a), At approximately zero point, the working of the hardware transpose from static friction and dynamic friction, resulting in additional random interruption ,thus causing relatively larger force fluctuation at zero-speed area. In Fig.7b), it is easily seen that with the virtual coupling path under way, system keep stable, and the strengthening of transparency does good to the linear relationship of force and velocity.

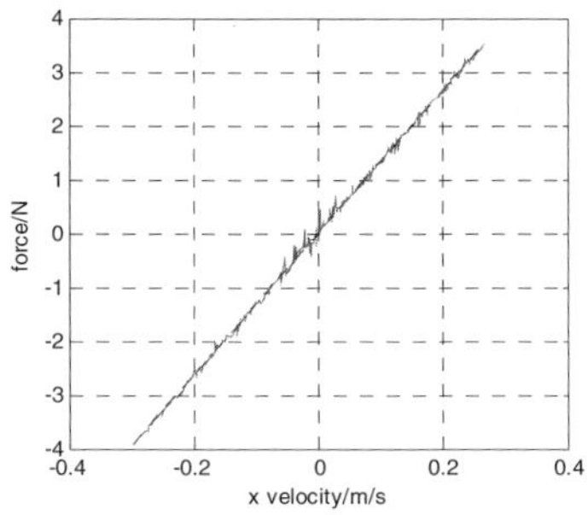

a)

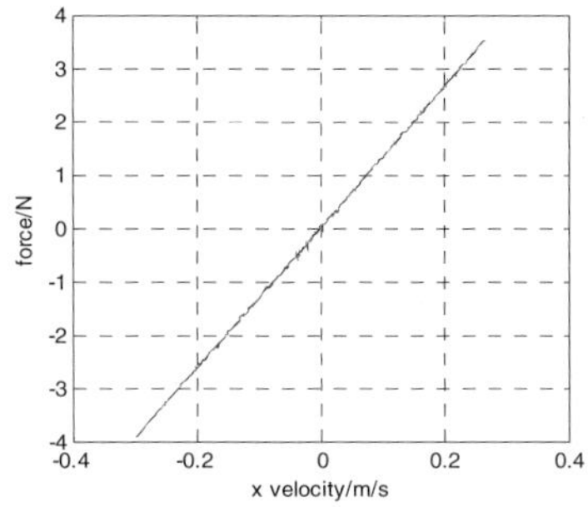

b)

Fig. 7. Experimental curve of the damping force simulation. a) with regular PID controller. b) with virtual coupling optimized controller.

6 Conclusion

A novel low-inertia, high bandwidth admittance haptic interface device is designed, the introduction of port network theory guarantees the absolute stability of new admittance haptic system. Moreover, through the optimization of the virtual coupling parameters and speed closed-loop gain parameters, higher transparency of the system is derived. By utilizing the new approach into the haptic system, experiments results have shown apparent improvement of transparency within the stable control domain. This paper has formed a basis for the transparency and stability oriented design and analysis for multi-degrees-of-freedom admittance haptic interface system.

Acknowledgement

The work reported in this paper is funded by the National High Technology Research and Development Program of China (Grant No. 2006AA04Z245).

References

1. Burdea, G., Coiffet, P.: Virtual Reality Technology, pp. 75–91. Wiley, New York (1994)
2. Colgate, J.E., Stanley, M.C., Brown, J.M.: Issues in the Haptic Display of Tool Use. In: Proc. of IEEE/RSJ Int. Conf. Intell. Robot. Syst., pp. 140–145. IEEE Press, Pittsburgh (1995)
3. Zilles, C.B., Salisbury, J.K.: A Constraint-Based God-Object Method for Haptic Display. In: Proc. of IEEE/RSJ Int. Conf. Intell. Robot. Syst., pp. 146–151. IEEE Press, Pittsburgh (1995)
4. Adams, R.J., Hannaford, B.: Stable Haptic Interaction with Virtual Environments. IEEE Trans. Robot. Automat. 15, 465–474 (1999)
5. Colgate, J.E., Schenkel, G.: Passivity of a Class of Sampled-Data Systems: Application to Haptic Interfaces. In: Proc. of the American Control Conference, Baltimore, Maryland, pp. 3236–3240 (1994)

6. Benali, A., Richard, P., Bidaud, P.: A Six D.O.F. Haptic Interface for Medical Virtual Reality Applications: Design, Control and Human Factors. In: IEEE International Conference on Virtual Reality, pp. 284–290. IEEE Press, New Brunswick (2000)
7. Youm, Y., Chung, W.K.: Human Kinematic Factor for Haptic Manipulation: The Wrist to Thumb Keehoon Kim. In: 10th Symposium on Haptic Interfaces for Virtual Environment and Teleoperator Systems, Orlando. Haptics Proceedings, pp. 319–326 (2002)
8. Daniel, R.W., McAree, P.R.: Fundamental Limits of Performance for Force Reflecting Teleoperation. International Journal of Robotics Research 17(8), 811–830 (1998)
9. Hogan, N.: Controlling Impedance at the Man/Machine Interface. In: Proc. of IEEE Int. Conf.on Robotics and Automation, pp. 1626–1631. IEEE Press, Scottsdale (1989)
10. Chen, W.K.: Modern Network Analysis, pp. 463–629. Post and Telecommunication Press, Beijing (1992)
11. Minsky, M., Ouh-Young, M., Steele, O., et al.: Feeling and Seeing Issues in Force Display. Computer Graphics 24(2), 235–243 (1990)
12. Adams, R.J., Hannaford, B.: Control Law Design for Haptic Interfaces to Virtual Reality. IEEE Transactions on Control Systems Technology 10(1), 3–13 (2002)

Self-collision Detection for Rigid Non-convex Multi-link Model

Shujuan Peng[1,*], Yuanxiang Li[1,2], and Hui Zeng[1]

[1] Department of Computer Science, Wuhan University, 430072, China
[2] State Key Lab. of Software Engineering, Wuhan University, 430072, China
shujuanpeng@gmail.com

Abstract. This paper presents an efficient algorithm to perform continuous self-collision detection for rigid non-convex multi-link model. Our algorithm precomputes the oriented bounding box (OBB) and the bounding volume hierarchy (BVH) of convex hulls for each link based on the surface convex decomposition and constructs the dynamic bounding volume hierarchies with axis-aligned bounding boxes (AABBs). Given two discrete configurations of the links, we use motion interpolation between two successive time steps and check the resulting trajectory for collisions. We employ the conservative advancement and temporal culling to calculate the potentially colliding links, and adopt spatial culling to reduce the conservative advancement iterations. If collision occurs, the algorithm reports the first time of contact as well as colliding features (vertex/ face or edge/edge contacts). We implement the algorithm on the avatar model consisting of many links and tens of thousands, the results demonstrate the algorithm is efficient to perform continuous self-collision detection between the rigid non-convex multi-link model.

Keywords: Self-collision detection, non-convex multi-link model, surface convex decomposition, conservative advancement, temporal culling.

1 Introduction

The goal of collision detection (CD) is to check the possible interferences between geometric models in the space. Collision detection is a crucial part to make objects look physically believable for the application simulating interaction impenetrable objects. Many collision detection algorithms have been presented to detect interfering objects in applications such as industrial applications (virtual prototype environments [1], virtual maintenance system [2]), assembly tests [3]), virtual museum [4], surgery simulation [5] and cloth simulation [6]. Depending on how collision detection algorithms handle the motion of objects, they

* Supported by the National Natural Science Foundation of China (60773009), the National High Technology Research and Development Program of China (863 Program)(2007AA01Z290) and Natural Science Foundation of Hubei Province of China (2007ABA009).

C. Xiong et al. (Eds.): ICIRA 2008, Part II, LNAI 5315, pp. 91–100, 2008.

can be usually split into two parts: discrete collision detection (DCD) and continuous collision detection (CCD). DCD algorithms sample fixed time intervals for the objects motions and detect objects interpenetrations. However, when objects are moving at a high speed or objects are thin, like cloth on virtual avatars [7], DCD algorithm can easily miss a collision between sampled time instances or the cause the penetration between two objects [8].

In order to overcome the limitations of DCD algorithms, CCD have been proposed that model the motion between successive time instances as a continuous path and check for collisions along these paths. Those research areas are mainly focused on complex geometrical models [9], the rigid and articulated bodies [10][11] and deformable objects [12][13][14] using different algorithms. Fedrowitz, C. H. [9] presented an efficient object-oriented collision detection engine for complex geometrical models defined constructively and for geometrical primitives which representation base on the widely used boundary representation geometric solid modeler ACIS. Redon [11] used line-skeletons with constant offsets and the virtual environment as a collection of polygonized objects to detect the continuous collision between a moving avatar and its surrounding virtual environment. The algorithm had been introduced the arbitrary in-between motion and swept volume (SV) to improve the efficiency. Govindaraju, N. K. [13] decomposed the problem into adjacent and non-adjacent collision detection, taking advantages of primitive connectivity information to perform efficient collision culling between bounding swept volumes to ensure no collision to miss between time steps. However, the use for CCD has been limited since it typically requires higher computational cost than discrete collision detection.

In this paper, we present an efficient continuous self-collision detection algorithm for rigid non-convex multi-link model in virtual environments using the arbitrary motion interpolation and temporal culling with dynamic volume hierarchy. Each link in the model is represented as the tight AABBs using OBBs. The algorithm can reduce the computational time cost through the conservative advancement (CA) and temporal culling. The paper is structured as follows. Section 2 is the key techniques for our algorithm. We present our multi-stages interactive self-collision detection algorithm in section 3 and describe the implementation results and analysis in section 4. Section 5 is the conclusion, limitations and the future work.

2 Overview

In this section, we give the key techniques in our algorithm. We first formulate the problem of CCD among general rigid non-convex links models; then briefly explain the basic idea of conservative advancement, surface convex decomposition and distance calculation our algorithm is based on.

2.1 Problem Formulation

Given an multi-link model A consisting of m rigid non-convex links A_1, ...,A_m with no closed loop, we use a directed acyclic graph to represent the link structure of A. We assume that many links may share the same parent link, but each individual link has only one parent (although the root link has no parent). For the sake of simplicity, we will assume that the index of the parent of link i is $i-1$. This notation can be easily modified when a parent has multiple children.

For a given link i, let i denote its associated reference frame, and let 0 represent the world reference frame. Let us further represent the orientation of i relative to j as ${}^{j}_{i}R$ on $SO(3)$ when $j < i$. Similarly, the relative transformation of i with respect to j at time t can be described by ${}^{j}_{i}\overline{M}(t)$ in SE(3). We will use $\overline{M}$ to distinguish a time-dependent, continuous transformation in $SE(3)$ from an instance M of $SE(3)$; we will also use ${}^{j}_{i}\overline{M}$ to represent ${}^{j}_{i}\overline{M}(t)$ if it is clear in the context. A similar notation is applied to $\overline{R}$ and $\overline{T}$. We use ${}^{j}L_i$ to denote the vector from the origin of j to that of i. Any point on link i can be represented by ${}^{j}_{i}r$ with respect to j.

As is the case with other continuous CD algorithms, one input to our algorithm must be the continuous motion of the models under consideration. In our algorithm, we use the motion interpolation [15] to synthesize the continuous motion, see fig.1. (a). Specifically, we only consider the initial and final configurations q^0 and q^1 for an articulated model, then synthesizes a continuous motion to interpolate q^0 and q^1 over the time interval $[0, 1]$. We can get the interpolating motion as follows:

$$ {}^{0}_{i}\overline{M}(t) = {}^{0}_{1}\overline{M}(t).{}^{1}_{2}\overline{M}(t)...{}^{i-1}_{i}\overline{M}(t) \tag{1} $$

$$ {}^{i-1}_{i}\overline{M}(t) = \begin{pmatrix} {}^{i-1}_{i}\overline{R}(t) & {}^{i-1}_{i}\overline{T}(t) \\ (0,0,0) & 1 \end{pmatrix} \tag{2} $$

where ${}^{i-1}_{i}\overline{R}(t)$, ${}^{i-1}_{i}\overline{T}(t)$ are the position and orientation of i with respect to $i-1$ at a given time t in $[0, 1]$.

Given two links A_i, B_i in multi-link bodies A , B with respective associated continuous motions ${}^{0}_{i}\overline{M}_A(t)$, ${}^{0}_{j}\overline{M}_B(t)$, we to know whether the following set is non-empty:

$$ \{t \in [0, 1] \,|{}^{0}_{i}\overline{M}_A(t)A_i \cap {}^{0}_{j}\overline{M}_B(t)B_j\} \tag{3} $$

In our algorithm, we consider the self-collision in the same model. So in the equation, we set $A = B$. For the equation, notice that when $A = B$ and $|i-j| > 1$, which means the self-collision between non-adjacent links. If the set is not empty, we want to determine the minimum value of t (called the TOC, τ) that that satisfies this equation, known as the time of contact, t_{TOC}. Here $\tau > 1$ means that there is no collision in the time interval [0,1].

2.2 Conservative Advancement

Conservative advancement (CA) is a simple technique to compute a lower bound on τ by repeatedly advancing a movable convex object A by $\triangle t$ toward another fixed convex object B while avoiding collision. Here, $\triangle t$ is calculated from the closest distance $d(A(t), B)$ between $A(t)$ and B, and the upper bound μ on the

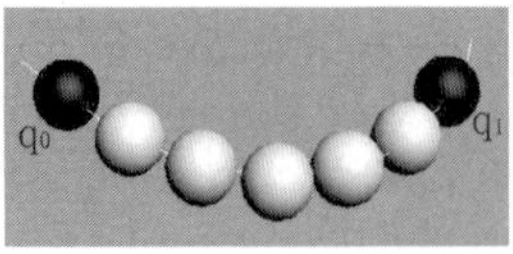

(a)

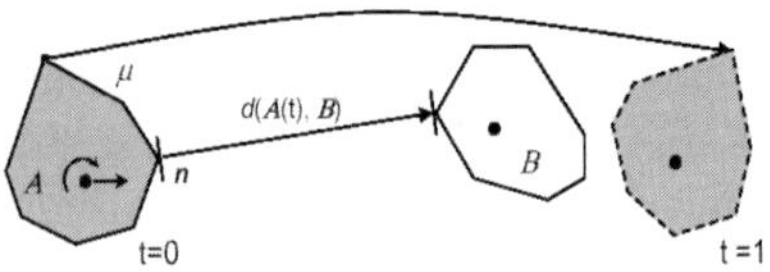

(b)

Fig. 1. Sub-figure. (a) is the motion interpolation for continuous motion, q_0, q_1 represents the initial and final motion respectively. Sub-figure. (b) is the conservative advancement.

motion along $d(A(t), B)$, traced at a rate of $A(t)$ over the time interval $[0, 1]$, as shown in Eq.(4)

$$\triangle t \leq \frac{d(A(t), B)}{\mu} \tag{4}$$

A can then safely advance from time t to time $t + \triangle t$ without collision (see fig.(1). (b)). The TOC, τ, is obtained by accumulating such time-steps $\Sigma\tau$ until $d(A(t), B)$ becomes less than some user specified distance threshold ε. Further, a tighter bound on μ can be obtained by projecting the motion of A on to the direction n corresponding to the shortest distance between A and B.

2.3 Surface Convex Decomposition

Collision detection is related to distance computation; two pieces are in collision if and only if the distance between the pieces is zero. To compute the distance between non-convex objects, we can break each object into convex pieces based on surface convex decomposition the and then use one of the above algorithms to determine the distance between pieces.

Convex decomposition can be divided into two class: the first one is based on solid model and the second one based on surface, which decompose the model surface into convex pieces: $boundary(A) = \bigcup_i c_i \forall i,\ j\ :\ i \neq j;\ c_i \cap^* c_j = \emptyset;\ c_i \subseteq boundary(C_i)$, where A represents the model, c_i^A the convex piece, $C_i = CH(c_i)$ which is the convex hull, and $boundary(A)$ the boundary for A. After the decomposition, we can get the surface decomposition position in which the union of C_i covers only the boundary of A; this is sufficient for distance calculation.

2.4 Distance Calculation

Starting from the root nodes of two convex hull trees, simultaneously traverses the two trees while performing Voronoi marching on the tree nodes and calculating their distance as well as their associated closest features. The recursive traversal continues until the closest distance cannot be further reduced. This tree traversal process can be also thought of as implicitly building a bounding volume traversal tree between two convex hull trees.

Given two convex pieces c_i^A, c_i^B, we need to construct the $BVHs$ (CHT_A, CHT_B) for c_i^A, c_i^B at given time t, starting from the root nodes of CHT_A, CHT_B. The algorithm is summarized as pseudo-code in the ***algorithm*** 2.1:

Algorithm 2.1. Closest distance calculation

Input: The BVH node h_i, h_j and the current distance $d_{current}$.
Output: The closest distance $d(\ h_i,\ h_j)$.
1. Creat a bounding volume traversal tree $h(i,j)$
2. perform Voronoi marching on h_i, h_j to find
   $d(h_i, h_j)$ and its closest vector $n(i,j)$
3. **if** $d(h_i, h_j) < d_{current}$, **then**
4.   **if** h_j is not a leaf node in CHT_B, **then**
5. $d_1 = BVTT(h_i, h_j .LeftChildTree)$
6. $d_2 = BVTT(h_i, h_j .RightChildTree)$
7.   **return** min (d_1, d_2)
8.   **else if** h_i is not a leaf node in CHT_A, **then**
9. $d_1 = BVTT(h_i .LeftChildTree, h_j)$
10. $d_2 = BVTT(h_i .RightChildTree, h_j)$
11.   **return** min (d_1, d_2)
12.   **else**
13.   Mark $h(i,j)$ as front and $n(i,j)$ is stored as it
14.   **return** $d(h_i, h_j)$
15.   **end if**
16. **else**
17.   Mark $h(i,j)$ as front and $n(i,j)$ is stored as it
18.   **return** d
19. **end if**

Specifically, when we consider the self-collision of the model, the two trees $CHT_A = CHT_B$. So, we can get the closest distance of links in the same model.

3 Interactive Continuous Self-collision Detection

In this section, we present our multi-stages interactive self-collision detection algorithm. We first describe the pre-processing phase followed by the runtime algorithm. The input of the algorithm is the multi rigid non-convex links, and output is the self-collision result, which is the first time of contact (TOC).

3.1 Preprocess

The main purpose of preprocess is to compute the oriented bounding box (OBB) and a BVH of convex hulls based on a surface convex decomposition for the m rigid non-convex links model. During the pre-process, decompose a given model A into convex pieces c_i^A and recursively builds a convex hull tree CHT_A where each node in the tree corresponds to a convex hull of its children nodes. We construct the OBB hierarchy using a standard top-down approach based on the convex pieces connectivity. The OBB hierarchy is constructed as a pre-process and is updated at run-time for the model.

3.2 Run-Time Algorithm

Algorithm 3.1. CCD algorithm for self-collision

Input: A list of PCLs.
Output: The first time of contact among PCLs
1. **for** each link pair PCL_i in PCLs **do**
2.   calculate its lower bound of TOC, τ_i^*
3. **end for**
4. sort PCL in the ascending order of τ_i^* into $\overrightarrow{PCL}$
5. $t_{min} = 1.0$
6. **for** each $\overrightarrow{PCL}_i$ in $\overrightarrow{PCL}$, **do**
7.   **if** $\tau_i^* > t_{min}$, **then**
8.   **return** $\tau = t_{min}$
9.   **else**
10.   advance the CA time of $\overrightarrow{PCL}_i$ to $\tau_i = \tau_i^*$
11.   Start of CA iterations
12.   **repeat**
13.   calculate the closest distance $d(\overrightarrow{PCL}_i)$ and direction **n**
14.   calculate the motion bounds μ
15. $\triangle t_i^j = \frac{d(\overrightarrow{PCL})}{\mu}$
16.   **if** $\tau_i + \triangle t_i^j > t_{min}$ **then**
17.   skip $\overrightarrow{PCL}_i$ and jump to **6**
18.   **else**
19. $\overrightarrow{PCL}_i$ to $\tau_i = \tau_i + \triangle t_i^j$
20.   **end if**
21.   **until** $d(\overrightarrow{PCL}) < \varepsilon$
22. $t_{min} = min(t_{min}, \tau_i)$
23.   **end if**
24. **end for**
25. **return** $\tau = t_{min}$

Our run-time algorithm consists of four stages:

Stage A: Construct the dynamic bounding volume hierarchies with AABBs. For each link in A, an AABB is first created to bound the extent of the motion of the associated link-level OBB under the interpolating motion. Meanwhile, computer the tight set of AABBs, here we use the Talor models, which is the generalization of interval arithmetic.

Stage B: Computer the tight upper bound on the motion. According to the given continuous motion of the model with constant angular and translational velocities for each link, we employ the conservative advancement to calculate the upper bound for the motion. The machinery of CA requires two basic components, the distance calculation and the determination of upper bound on the motion. Let ${}^0_ip$ be a point on a link A_i in the reference frame 0. As A_i undergoes ${}^0_i\overline{M}(t)$, ${}^0_ip$ will trace out a trajectory ${}^0_ip(t)$ in the 3D space. In order to calculate the μ,we need to derive the velocity ${}^0v_i = {}^0_i\dot{p}(t)$ in the world reference frame. So, the upper bound on the motion μ is: $\mu = \max_{{}^0_ip \in A_i} \int_0^1 |{}^0_i\dot{p}(t).\ n|\,dt = \max_{{}^0_ip \in A_i} \int_0^1 |{}^0v_i.\ n|\,dt$, where n is the direction vector that points at the closest other object in the environment.

Stage C: Calculate the potentially colliding links (PCLs). In order to judge whether the collision occurs between the links in the time interval $[t_0,\ t_1]$, we need to motion interpolation in the arbitrary interval, calculate the potentially colliding links. If an link A_i does not belong to the PCLs, it implies that A_i does not collide with any link of the model. Based on this property, we can prune the number of links pairs that need to be checked for exact collision.

Stage D: Return the mininum time of contact. A straightforward way of finding the time of contact τ of all potentially is to apply the CA algorithm to to each pair of potentially colliding links (PCLs) [16]that have survived the spatial culling, so that $\tau = \min(\tau_i)$, where τ_i is the collision time of the *ith* $PCL(PCL_i)$ and $\tau_i = \sum_{j=1}^{N_i} \triangle\, t_i^j$ where is the advancement time step determined as a result of the *jth* CA iteration for PCL_i, and N_i is the total number of CA iterations for PCL_i. When performing the CA iterations for all PCLs, we can get the total computation time $T = \sum_{j=1}^{N_1} T_1^j + \sum_{j=1}^{N_2} T_2^j + ... + \sum_{j=1}^{N_n} T_n^j$, where T_i^j is the time spent on the *jth* CA iteration for PCL_i. To reduce the computational cost of T, we need to either decrease the N_i or T_i^j. For N_i, the main approach is to simultaneously performing CA iterations for all pairs to determine pairs PCL_i. The algorithm is summarized as pseudo-code in the ***algorithm*** 3.1:

4 Results and Analysis

We have implemented our algorithm under Windows XP (Intel Core Duo 2.0GHz PC with 1GB main memory) using Visual C++, OpenGL API, proximity query library, SWIFT++, which is used for distance calculation and for the construction of a hierarchy using convex hulls. We use controlled threshold distance ε in the definition of τ is 0.001 throughout the algorithm.

The simulation experiment created a key-framed animation with self-collisions between links in a avatar model, which is the rigid non-convex multi-link model about 15 links and $20K$ triangles (about 4.8K convex pieces using the surface convex decomposition). The different sub-figure in fig. 2 is snapshot of the status for the model in different simulation frame steps with dynamic bounding box (OBB, AABB). Fig. 2. (a) is the initial state, fig. 2. (b-c)is the snapshot when

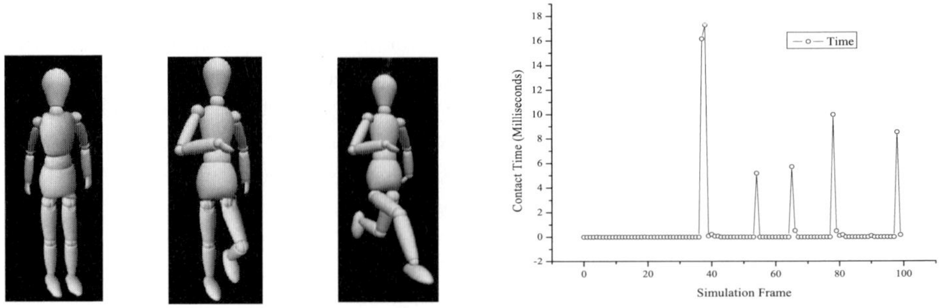

(a) (b) (c) (d)

Fig. 2. The different sub-figures (a-c) are the snapshot for the model in different simulation frame steps with dynamic bounding box (OBB, AABB). A avatar model consists of about 15 links and 20K triangles (4.8K convex pieces). (a)is the initial state, (b)(c)is the snapshot when self-collision occurs in different frames scenario. Sub-figure (d) is the time of contact for the self-collision from 0 to 100 frame, in which the average timing is $0.64ms$.

self-collision occurs in different frames scenario. Fig. 2.(d) is the time of contact for the self-collision from 0 to 100 frames. From the fig. 2. (d), it is clearly the algorithm detect the self-collision in the frame step 39, 40, 56,67, 80, 100, and costing time $16.1741ms$, $17.291ms$, $5.19376ms$, $5.71743ms$, $9.9925ms$, $8.52544ms$ respectively, noticing that the algorithm can get the collision result quickly when there is collision free.

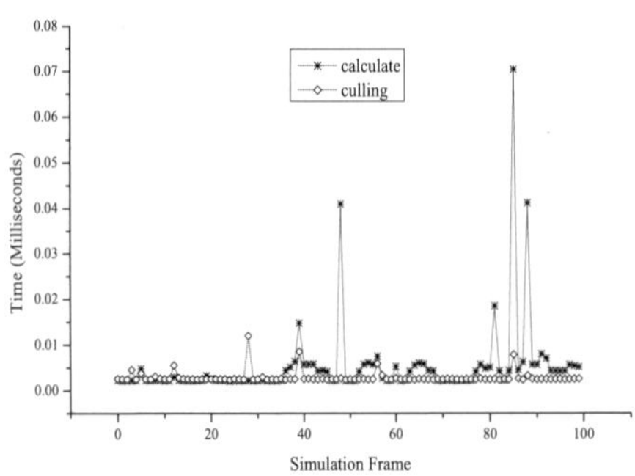

(a) AABBs calculating and culling

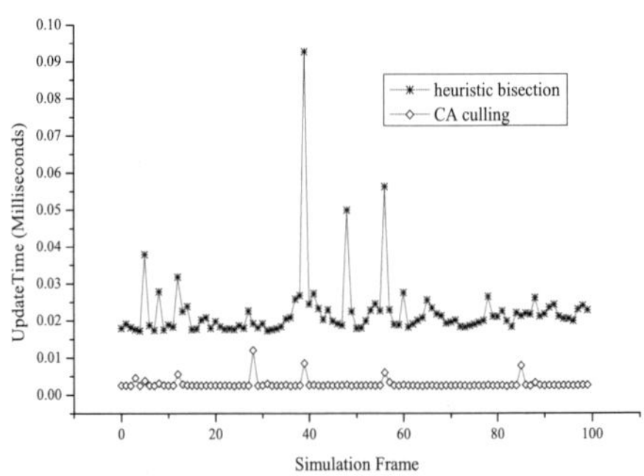

(b) Heuristic bisection search and CA culling

Fig. 3. Time comparison with frame steps.

Figure. 3. (b) is the time comparison for the AABBs calculating and culling. The number of links pairs for PCLs have been reduced due to tight dynamic BVH using Taylor models, so the time consume for culling is drastically reduced comparing to the AABBs calculating. In particular, for each pair of potentially colliding links, the CA advance the iteration time step adaptively to find τ, so the temporal culling algorithm performs very efficiently to improve the algorithm overall performance. Schwarzer [17] performs CCD in a similar way to our algorithm using motion bounds and distance calculations. However, the algorithm is based on on heuristic bisection search. For ours, we use motion projection for CA instead of the heuristic bisection search and can get quicker speed. Fig. 3. (b) is the comparison for the original (heuristic bisection search) and the changed culling (CA culling), the updated efficiency is greatly improved.

5 Conclusion and Future Work

We have presented an efficient continuous self-collision detection algorithm for rigid non-convex multi-link model in virtual environments. We decompose the model into several links, get the convex pieces in the preprocess stage using the surface convex composition, and construct the bounding-volume hierarchy construction with the AABBs and OBBs to get the dynamic BVH. When computing the AABBs, our algorithm takes advantages of the Taylor model to ensure the tight set. Then, calculate the potentially colliding links to prune the number of links pairs needed to be checked for exact collision. According to simultaneously perform CA iterations for all pairs to reduce the runtime time complexity, we have applied our algorithm to the avatar model consisting of multi-link with many thousands of triangles and got good results. But there also has some limitations for the algorithm: the implementation requires 2-manifold, the distance calculation based on convex decomposition needs much time complexity and not considering the avatar interaction with the environment. There are many avenues for the future work: use the motion capture data to drive movement of the avatar model, combine the graphics processors unit (GPU) to improve the collision detection speed and more complicated model to implement such as multi-avatar based on user and environment interaction.

References

1. Figueiredo, M.: Adjustable approach for collision detection in virtual prototype environments. In: Geometric Modeling and Imaging, GMAI 2007, pp. 44–47 (2007)
2. Su, Q.X., Liu, P.Y.: Research on collision detection in certain missile virtual maintenance system. In: Istm/2007: 7th International Symposium on Test and Measurement. Conference Proceedings, vol. 1-7, pp. 6103–6106 (2007)
3. Tamura, Y., Mizuguchi, N., Matsumoto, S., Ueki, H.A.U.H.: Construction of virtual assembly system with real-time collision detection. In: Mizuguchi, N. (ed.) 17th International Conference on Artificial Reality and Telexistence, pp. 284–285 (2007)
4. Sari, R.F., Muliawan: Interactive object and collision detection algorithm implementation on a virtual museum based on croquet. In: Muliawan (ed.) 4th International Conference on Innovations in Information Technology, pp. 685–689 (2007)
5. Yaacoub, F., Hamam, Y., Abche, A.: Collision detection in computer simulations for wrist arthroscopic surgery training. In: Hamam, Y. (ed.) EUROCON, 2007. The International Conference on Computer as a Tool, pp. 2088–2095 (2007)
6. Baciu, G., Wingo Sai-Keung, W.: Image-based collision detection for deformable cloth models. IEEE Transactions on Visualization and Computer Graphics 10, 649–663 (2004)

7. Vassilev, T., Spanlang, B., Chrysanthou, Y.: Fast cloth animation on walking avatars. Computer Graphics Forum 20, 260–267 (2001)
8. Redon, S., Kheddar, A., Coquillart, S.: Fast continuous collision detection between rigid bodies. Computer Graphics Forum 21, 279–287 (2002)
9. Fedrowitz, C.H., Duber, F.: An algebra for efficiently solving the continuous collision detection problem. In: Duber, F. (ed.) Proceedings IEEE/RSJ International Conference on Intelligent Robots and Systems, 1998, vol. 3, pp. 1628–1633 (1998)
10. Redon, S., Lin, M.C., Manocha, D., Kim, Y.J.: Fast continuous collision detection for articulated models. Journal of Computing and Information Science in Engineering 5, 126–137 (2005)
11. Redon, S., Kim, Y.J., Lin, M.C., Manocha, D.A.M.D., Templeman, J.A.T.J.: Interactive and continuous collision detection for avatars in virtual environments. In: Kim, Y.J. (ed.) Virtual Reality, 2004. Proceedings, pp. 117–283. IEEE, Los Alamitos (2004)
12. Larsson, T., Akenine-Mller, T.: Collision detection for continuously deforming bodies, pp. 325–333 (2001)
13. Govindaraju, N.K., Kabul, I., Lin, M.C., Manocha, D.: Fast continuous collision detection among deformable models using graphics processors. Computers & Graphics-Uk 31, 5–14 (2007)
14. Wong, W.S.K., Baciu, G.: Robust continuous collision detection for interactive deformable surfaces. Computer Animation and Virtual Worlds 18, 179–192 (2007)
15. Zhang, X.Y., Lee, M., Kim, Y.J.: Interactive continuous collision detection for non-convex polyhedra. Visual Computer 22, 749–760 (2006)
16. Zhang, X.Y., Redon, S., Lee, M.Y., Kim, Y.J.: Continuous collision detection for articulated models using taylor models and temporal culling. Acm Transactions on Graphics 26 (2007)
17. Schwarzer, F., Saha, M., Latombe, J.-C.: Exact collision checking of robot paths. Algorithmic Foundations of Robotics (2002)

Inter-enterprise Multi-processes Quality Dynamic Control Method Based on Processing Network

Yongtao Qin, Liping Zhao, Yiyong Yao, and Damin Xu

State Key Laboratory for Manufacturing Systems Engineering, Xi'an Jiao Tong University
School of Mechanical Engineering, Xi'an Jiao Tong University,Xi'an, China
qinyt23419@126.com

Abstract. During the course of inter-enterprise processing network quality control, for judging and analyzing the others process quality influence of the abnormal process quality, especially key process quality influence, and servicing whole the multi-processes quality control course, the inter-enterprise multi-processes quality control method based on processing network by means of inter-enterprise quality control model based on fractal network is proposed. In the method, multi-processes processing network is constructed by process mapping, the key process can be figured out based on the analysis of processing network sensitivity. To the key process, depending on multi-processes cost function based on cost influence coefficient among processes, the method can establish the comprehensive optimizing object function including cost and error propagation. Depending on the optimum solution of the object function solved by genetic algorithm, the key process can correct to regulate and distribute the control parameters to decrease accumulative error, to avoid false alarm and misstatements originated from the abnormal process. This application course of method could be applied with a multi-processes manufacturing example.

Keywords: Multi-Processes, Quality Control, Inter-Enterprise, Processing Network.

1 Introduction

To the complexity of product structure, the transformation of multi-processes quality control course from sample procedure to complex structure, and the degree of process relation among enterprises is more and more close, so that error propagation scope among processes extend from interior enterprise to exterior enterprise. The error propagation among processes should be created and will accumulated, especially some processes may be creating false alarm and misstatements owing to an abnormal process. Consequently, some measures should be adopted to assure the key process and others quality, decrease the error propagation among processes, and rationally distribute tolerance among processes be means of some rules to gain whole optimization in the quality and cost aspects.

In order to complete the quality dynamic control multi-processes, a lot of studiers had researched on the field at home and abroad. For example, Yang M. [1], Kano M. [2], Bayazita O.[3], and Lopez-ortega O.[4] researched inter-enterprise quality

C. Xiong et al. (Eds.): ICIRA 2008, Part II, LNAI 5315, pp. 101–110, 2008.

management system to gain product quality control. Liu D. [5], Sun H. [6] can adjust control parameters to dynamically control among processes. Dey S. [7], Wang H. [8], Choongyeun C. [9], and Loose J. [10] researched state space method to describe and solve error propagation. For dynamically adapting to the influence of the abnormal process, assuring the key process quality, and servicing for the whole multi-processes quality control course, depending on inter-enterprise quality control model based on fractal networks[11], the inter-enterprise multi-processes dynamically quality control method based on processing network is proposed. The method can build a multi-processes dynamically quality control processing network by means of process mapping. Based on the analysis of processing network performance to figure out the key process, and research the key process error influences propagated by the abnormal process. Depending on cost influence originated from among processes, the comprehensive optimizing object function including cost and error propagation can be established. Owing to the solution the object function, the key process can correct to regulate and distribute the control parameters to decrease accumulative error, to avoid false alarm and misstatements.

2 Multi-processes Dynamic Quality Control's Processing Network

2.1 The Construct of Multi-processes Processing Network

According to the fractal characteristic of inter-enterprise quality control function, based on fractal and complex networks theory, inter-enterprise quality control task execution units can be constructed as network nodes by the encapsulation of object-oriented technology. The constraint relationships among nodes are established based on hierarchical structure among enterprises and the relationship of product configuration. Based on network nodes and constraint relationships, combined with some quality control methods and supporting technologies, inter-enterprise quality control fractal networks model is established[11].

NR is constraint relation among nodes in the model.

$$NR = \left\{ \begin{matrix} MR \\ CR \end{matrix} \right\} \Bigg|_{k=0,1} = \left\{ \begin{matrix} 0 \\ 0,\ 1,\ 2 \end{matrix} \right\}_{k=0} = \left\{ \begin{matrix} 1, -1 \\ 0,\ 1,\ 2 \end{matrix} \right\}_{k=1} \tag{1}$$

where:

① MR is the management constraint of upper layer nodes to lower layer ones. $MR = 1$ represents there is management constraint between upper layer nodes and lower layer nodes. $MR = 0$ represents there isn't management constraint between upper layer nodes and lower layer nodes. $MR = -1$ represents lower layer nodes be used as backup selection or reference to upper layer nodes.

② CR is coordination constraint relation among nodes at the same layer. $CR = 0$ represents there is rejection coordination constraint relation, $CR = 1$ represents there is competition coordination constraint relation, $CR = 2$ represents there is necessity coordination constraint relation.

③ $k=0$ represents quality control function need no reconfiguration, $k=1$ represents quality control function need reconfiguration.

To the complex and dynamic multi-processes association relation, taking the product machining processes in the manufacturing cell nodes of the model as object, the network process nodes having autonomy and cooperation ability can be built by means of mapping. The constraint relation among manufacturing cell nodes is mapped as the association relations among processes. If S_t is association relations matrix among processes, there is $NR \to S_t$.

$$NR \to S_t = \begin{Bmatrix} 0, & 1, & -1 \\ 0, & 1, & 2 \end{Bmatrix}_{k=0,1} \to \begin{bmatrix} 1 & 0 & \dots & \lambda_1 & \lambda_1 \\ 0 & 1 & \dots & \lambda_1 & 0 \\ \dots & \dots & \dots & \dots & \\ \lambda_1 & \lambda_1 & \dots & 1 & 0 \\ \lambda_1 & 0 & \dots & 0 & 1 \end{bmatrix}_{N \times N} \tag{2}$$

where, λ_1 $(0 \le \lambda_1 \le 1)$ can express the connection relation dense degree(strong and weak) among processes nodes. The value of λ_1 can be determined by means of machining task, manufacturing resources, machining demand, cost factors, and so on. The range of λ_1 includes:

$$\lambda_1 = \begin{cases} 1, i=j,, \text{The self-connection relation among processes nodes(The maxmum degree).} \\ \lambda_1, \text{There is the direct connection relation among processes nodes} \\ \lambda_2, \text{There is the indirect connection relation among processes nodes.} \\ \lambda_3, \text{There is the bypassingconnection relation among processes nodes.} \\ 0, i \ne j, \text{There is't the connection relation among processes nodes(The minmum degree)} \end{cases} \tag{3}$$

Depending on the process nodes mapped by machining processes in the manufacturing cell nodes, and association relations among process nodes mapped by constraint relation among manufacturing cell nodes, The structure of inter-enterprise multi-processes processing network including machining process, process nodes, and equipment is established, and it can be described as Fig. 1.

In the structure, by the one-to-many mapping, the nodes of processing network could be mapped as manufacturing resources. That is the nodes of processing network can further correspond to equipment nodes in inter-enterprise quality control fractal networks model.

2.2 The Key Process Determination Based on the Sensitivity of Multi-processes Processing Network

The key process plays a key role in course of multi-processes quality control, so that it needs to be figured out and accurately control. In multi-processes quality dynamic control network, the sensitivity of multi-processes processing network can represent the key process and key machining path. The sensitivity of node represents the node's the influence degree to whole network operation. In multi-processes processing network, the sensitivity of process node can represent the process's the node is the key process to whole processing. Based on [12-13], the sensitivity of process node in multi-processes processing network S_k can be defined as followings:

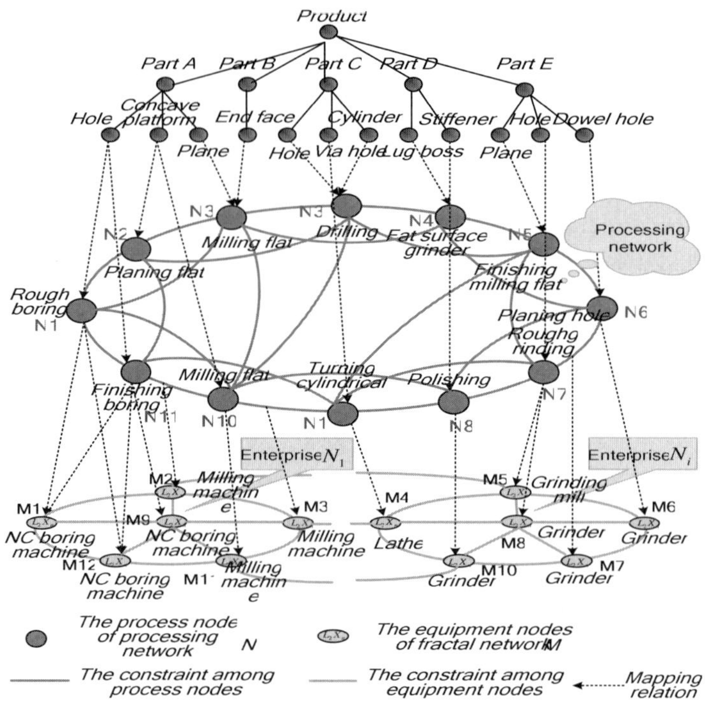

Fig. 1. The construct of inter-enterprise multi-processes processing network

$$S_k = \sup \frac{\left\| w\sigma^2{}_{out} \right\|_2}{\left\| \sigma^2{}_{in} \right\|} = \left\| w \cdot \left[\gamma^2(k) \right] \right\|_2 \tag{4}$$

where: w expresses the important degree of key quality's feature error, and it is weight coefficient. σ^2_{out} expresses the node key quality feature output. σ^2_{in} expresses the node key quality feature input. $\gamma^2(k)$ expresses relation matrix among nodes S_k can be defined as followings:

By the sensitivity of network path and process node, the key process and key machining path can be determined for multi-processes quality dynamic control.

2.3 The Cost Influence Coefficient among Processes

The key process figured out by the sensitivity of multi-processes processing network should decrease accumulative error, avoid false alarm and misstatements, optimize operation in quality and cost aspects, and has dynamic adaptation ability by means of the cost influence among processes[14-15]. Based on the quantitative analysis of among process nodes in multi-processes processing network, the cost influence coefficient among processes can be established for cost optimizing combined with cost function. There are some quantitative indexes to multi-processes measure cost influence, and they are as followings:

(1). Time influence coefficient among process nodes t_n

Time influence coefficient among process nodes t_n can be expressed in status waiting time among nodes, namely a interval time between a process node implement task time M_j and next node implement task time M_j. Time influence coefficient among process nodes t_n can be described as:

$$t_n = (M_j - M_i) \tag{5}$$

Because a node may be has many predecessor tasks, namely there are many processes, t_n can count the status waiting time to the node in every condition.

(2). The throughput influence coefficient among process nodes u_n

The throughput among process nodes can be expressed degree in processing network. To node u_i and node u_j, $\forall(u_i, u_j) \in u$, in stable status, the throughput influence coefficient among process nodes u_n:

$$u_n = u_i / u_j = P[M(S_i)] / P[M(S_j)] \tag{6}$$

where: $P[M(S_i)]$, $P[M(S_j)]$ expresses the probabilityof node u_i throughput $M(S_i)$ and the probability of node u_j throughput $M(S_j)$ respectively. u_n describes the influence degree of process task implement probability.

(3). Resource utilization influence coefficient among process nodes r_n

Resource utilization influence coefficient among process nodes r_n is probability ratio quality task implement among process nodes by resource utilization, and it expresses manufacturing resource supply and utilization influence degree in multi-processes. In any time, $\forall t \in T$, resource utilization influence coefficient among process nodes r_n is represented as followings:

$$r_n = P[H(S_i)] / P[H(S_j)] \tag{7}$$

where: $P[H(S_i)]$, $P[H(S_j)]$ expresses the probabilityof node u_i resource utilization $H(S_i)$ and the probability of node u_j resource utilization $H(S_j)$ respectively.

For describing to the cost influence coefficient among processes, combining with resource utilization influence coefficient r_n, throughput influence coefficient u_n, and time influence coefficient t_n, multi-processes cost influence coefficient c_n can be expressed as followings:

$$c_n = w_1 r_n + w_2 u_n + w_3 t_n \tag{8}$$

where: w_1, w_2, w_3 express weight value among influence coefficient, and their value can be determined by machining process, machining feature, material, manufacturing resource, and so on. There is $w_1 + w_2 + w_3 = 1$. Multi-processes cost influence coefficient c_n can be took as a part of cost object, and the error propagation equation of multi-processes based on state space method can be took as quality object, depending on the self-organization evolution law of multi-processes processing network, multi-processes can rationally distribute control parameter , such as tolerance, process redundancy, can decrease accumulative error, and avoid false alarm and misstatements created by abnormal process.

3 The Multi-processes Quality Dynamic Control's Implementation

In the multi-processes quality dynamic control cost function $TC = f(x_1, x_2, ...x_n)$, TC is whole product cost when manufacturing factors $(x_1, x_2, ...x_n)$ are inputted. $x_i (i = 1, 2, ...n)$ is i th manufacturing factor's input quantity[16-17]. When x_i 's cost coefficient is p_i, combining with multi-processes cost influence coefficient c_n, multi-processes quality dynamic control cost function is as followings:

$$TC = c_1 p_1 x_1 + c_2 p_2 x_2 + ...c_n p_n x_n = \sum_{i=1}^{n} c_i p_i x_i \quad (9)$$

For decreasing multi-processes manufacturing cost, combining with the minimum of error propagation.among processes, and completing cooperation and optimizing quality control, the comprehensive optimization object function is established as followings:

$$obj(f) = \min(y) + \min(TC) = \min(Cx_0 + v) + \min(\sum_{i=1}^{n} c_i p_i x_i) \quad (10)$$

$$\text{Constraint condition:} \quad TC = f(x_1, x_2, ...x_n) \quad (11)$$

$$\sum \delta_{id} \le \Delta X \quad (12)$$

$$\delta_{ij\min} \le \delta_{ij} \le \delta_{ij\max} \quad (13)$$

$$\delta_{ij} + \delta_{i,j-1} \le Z_{0j} - Z_{0j\min} \quad (14)$$

$$\delta_{id} = \delta_{im_i} \quad (15)$$

where: Formula(11) describes manufacturing cost constraint. Formula (12) describes tolerance constraint in the assembly process. i th part tolerance δ_{id} should less than assembly tolerance ΔX . Formula (13) describes the processing ability constraint among processes. ith part's j th process real tolerance should less than maximum allowable tolerance $\delta_{ij\max}$, and should more than minimum allowable tolerance $\delta_{ij\min}$. Formula (14) describes process redundancy constraint. δ_{ij}, $\delta_{i,j-1}$ are ith part's j th and $j-1$ th process tolerance. Z_{0j} is j th process nominal process redundancy. $Z_{0j\min}$ is j th process minimum allowable process redundancy. Formula (15) describes the last process tolerance δ_{in} should meet the demand of drawing regulations design tolerance δ_d .

Genetic algorithm has giant advantage to solving combined optimization problems in a large searching space[18-19]. Therefore, the multi-objective optimization genetic algorithm is adopted to realize comprehensive optimization object function among processes, depending on some constraint conditions. According to the result by means of genetic algorithm, key process' some control parameters can be obtained. The key process can correct to regulate and distribute the control parameters to decrease accumulative error, to avoid false alarm and misstatements from the abnormal process in controlled status for optimizing and dynamically control. The implementation of multi-processes quality control can be expressed in Fig. 2.

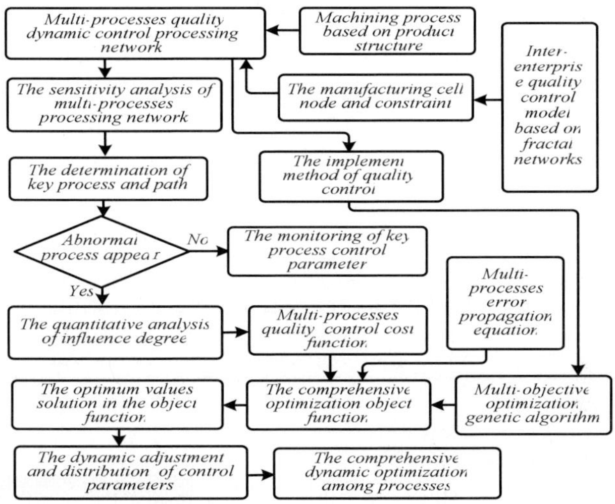

Fig. 2. The implementation procedure of multi-processes quality dynamic control

4 Example

The air-cylinder jacket is a critical part of engine, and it can be manufactured by more method and new material as high technology development. However, the processing course change more complex and involve more enterprise. The processing course can be expressed a network structure relation more than a flow structure relation. When the abnormal process is appeared in complex air-cylinder jackets machining correlation processes, other processes, especially key process, should decrease accumulative error, to avoid false alarm and misstatements, and carry out the quality and cost comprehensive optimization in controlled status. Taking Japan Daihatsu DL air-cylinder jackets processing quality dynamic control as example, the implementation of multi-processes quality dynamic control could be applied. Based on Japan Daihatsu DL air-cylinder jackets structure characteristics and commonprocessrule[20], assuming that rough boring inner hole is a abnormal process owing to some reasons such as machine wear or disoperation, depending on the process production technology of Tianxiang Electromechanical Industry General Corporation(Hengyang , China), the Japan daihatsu DL engine air-cylinder jackets's machining process and path can be established. The machining processes are described in Table 1.

Table 1. Japan Daihatsu DL engine air-cylinder jackets's machining processes[20]

NO.	*Process name*	*Type*	*Equipment*	*Fixture*	*Tool*
P1	centrifugal casting		centrifugal casting machine		
P2	cutting	QD-01	self-made trimming machine	three flap sleeve fixture	special cutter
P3	rough boring cylindrical	Ck620	self-made NC lathe	three flap sleeve fixture	cylindrical turning tool
P4	rough boring inner hole	TK716	vertical NC boring machine	jackets vertical fixture	rough boring tool
P5	rough turning cylindrical	Ck620	NC lathe	plasticssleeve fixture	cylindrical turning tool
P6	rouht turning reference	Ck618	self-made NC lathe	three flap sleeve fixture	cylindrical turning tool
P7	half refined reamers inner hole	TK716	vertical NC boring machine	jackets vertical fixture	half rough boring tool
P8	finish turning reference	CK762	multi-tools NC lathe	plasticssleeve fixture	gear turning tool
P9	refined reamers inner hole	T716	vertical NC boring machine	jackets vertical fixture	gold boring tool
P10	turning reference	Ck618	self-made NC lathe	three flap sleeve fixture	arcturning tool
P11	finish turning cylindrical	Ck620	NC lathe	plasticssleeve fixture	cylindrical turning tool
P12	finish boring inner hole	TK716	vertical NC boring machine	jackets vertical fixture	gold boring tool
P13	rough grinding inner hole	M4215	vertical grinding machine	three flap sleeve fixture	diamond whet-slate
P14	turning water sealing groove	CK620	NC lathe	three flap sleeve fixture	groove turning tool
P15	turning support shoulder	CK620	NC lathe	three flap sleeve fixture	end-face tool
P16	finish grinding inner hole	M4215	vertical grinding machine	four vertical post fixture	finish grinding whet-slate
P17	milling cylindrical	M131	cylindrical grinder	three flap sleeve fixture	whet-slate
P18	polishing inner hole	M4215	vertical grinding machine	four vertical post fixture	polishing grinding wheel

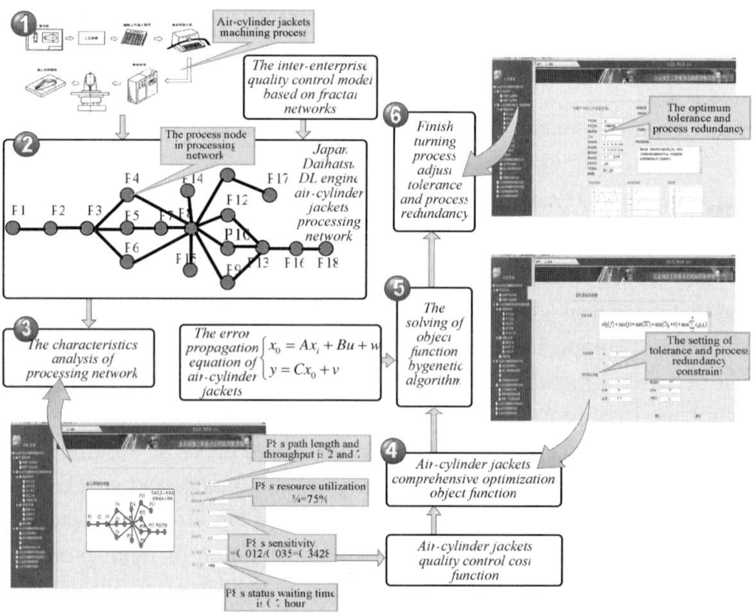

Fig. 3. The Daihatsu DL engine air-cylinder jackets quality dynamic control's implementation

The implementation procedure of Japan Daihatsu DL engine air-cylinder jackets quality dynamic control can be described in Fig. 3.

The implementation procedure includes: (1)Owing to the structural characteristics of the engine, machining path can be constructed assuming machining processes in Table 1. (2)Depending on air-cylinder jackets's machining processes and path, the air-cylinder jackets processing network can be established by mapping. (3). The finish turning reference process can be determined by the maximum sensitivity processing network. The air-cylinder jackets quality control cost function can be counted when cost influence coefficient among processes is combined. (4)The error propagation equation of air-cylinder jackets processing network can be built by means of state space method. The comprehensive optimization object function is established by error propagation equation and quality dynamic control cost function. (5)The object function can be counted by multi- objective optimization genetic algorithm. (6)The finish turning reference process can regulate tolerance and process redundancy depended on optimum tolerance and process redundancy.

5 Conclusion

The inter-enterprise multi-processes dynamically quality control method based on processing network can figure out the key process by means of the sensitivity of multi-processes processing network, can express the cost influence coefficient among processes. Depending on multi-processes quality dynamic control cost function by cost influence coefficient, and the error propagation of multi-processes by state space method, the comprehensive optimization object function is established. Owing to genetic algorithm, the optimum values in the object function can be obtained. Consequently, based on the optimum values, the key process can correct to regulate and distribute the control parameters to decrease accumulative error, to avoid false alarm and misstatements originated from the abnormal process, to implement the quality and cost comprehensive optimization, and to assure quality operation in controlled status for optimizing and dynamically control.

Acknowledgment

This work was supported by grant No. 2006AA04Z149 form the National High-Tech. R&D Program for Contemporary Manufacturing Integrated Technology, China.

References

1. Yang, M., Zhang, Y.: Intelligent Integrated Control Method in Manufacturing Process. In: IEEE International Conference on Automation and Logistics, August 2007, pp. 1640–1645 (2007)
2. Kano, M., Nakagawa, Y.: Data-based Process Monitoring, Process Control, and Quality Improvement: Recent Developments and Applications in Steel Industry. Computers & Chemical Engineering 32, 12–24 (2008)
3. Bayazita, O., Karpak, B.: An analytical Network Process-based Framework for Successful Total Quality Management (TQM): an Assessment of Turkish Manufacturing Industry Readiness. International Journal Production Economics 105, 79–96 (2007)
4. Lopez-ortega, O., Ramirezr, M.: A STEP-based Manufacturing Information System to Share Flexible Manufacturing Resources Data. Journal of Intelligent Manufacturing 16, 287–301 (2005)

5. Liu, D., Jiang, P.: E-quality Control Architecture for Multistage Machining Processes. Computer Integrated Manufacturing Systems 13, 782–790 (2007) (in Chinese)
6. Sun, H., Jiang, P.: Complex Weighted Networks-Based Analysis of Mobile Collaboration Space. Journal of Xi'an Jiaotong University 40, 573–576 (2006) (in Chinese)
7. Dey, S., Stori, J.A.: A Bayesian Network Approach to Root Cause Diagnosis of Process Variations. International Journal of Machine Tools & Manufacture 45, 75–91 (2005)
8. Wang, H., Pramanik, N., Roy, U., et al.: A Scheme for Mapping Tolerance Specifications to Generalized Deviation Space for Use in Tolerance Synthesis and Analysis. IEEE Transacion on Automation Science and Engineering 3, 81–91 (2006)
9. Choongyeun, C., Daeik, D.K., et al.: Decomposition and Analysis of Process Variability Using Constrained Principal Component Analysis. IEEE Transaction on Semiconductor Manufacturing 21, 55–61 (2008)
10. Loose, J., Zhou, S., Ceglarek, D.: Kinematic Analysis of Dimensional Variation Propagation for Multistage Machining Processes With General Fixture Layouts. IEEE Transacion on Automation Science and Engineering 4, 141–152 (2007)
11. Qin, Y., Zhao, L., Yao, Y., Xu, D.: A Study on Inter-enterprise Quality Control Function Self-organization Reconfiguration Based Fractal Networks. In: Proceedings of the 2007 IEEE International Conference on Robotics and Biomimetics, Sanya, China, December 2007, pp. 1733–1737 (2007)
12. Wang, L.: The Research on the Construction Method for the Quality Assurance System of the Manufacturing Network. Tianjin University, Tianjin China (2006) (in Chinese)
13. Zhang, M., Djurdjanovic, D., Ni, J.: Diagnosibility and Sensitivity Analysis for Multistation Machining Processes. International Journal of Machine Tools and Manufacture 47(3), 646–657 (2007)
14. Du, S., Xi, L., Ni, J., Ershun, P., Liu, R.: Product Lifecycle-Oriented Quality and Productivity Improvement Based on Stream of Variation Methodology. Computers in Industry 59, 180–192 (2008)
15. Lin, Y., He, L., et al.: Stochastic Physical Synthesis Considering Prerouting Interconnect Uncertainty and Process Variation for FPGAs. IEEE Transaction on Verylarge Scale Integration (VLSI) System 16, 141–152 (2008)
16. Du, S., Xi, L., Pan, E.: Modeling and Controlling of Dimensional Variation in Multi-Stage Manufacturing System. Journal of Shanghai Jiaotong University 40, 583–587 (2006) (in Chinese)
17. Zheng, L., Yang, X.M., Zhang, Z.H., Liu, T.I.: A Web-based Machining Parameter Selection System for Life Cycle Cost Reduction and Product Quality Enhancement. Computers in Industry 59, 254–261 (2008)
18. Mok, P.Y., Porter, B.: Evolutionary Optimization of Hedging Points for Unreliable Manufacturing Systems. International Journal of Advanced Manufacturing Technology 28, 205–214 (2006)
19. Gupta, S., Tiwari, R., Nair, S.: Multi-objective Design Optimization of Rolling Bearings Using Genetic Algorithms. Mechanism and Machine Theory 42, 1418–1443 (2007)
20. Gao, Z.: The Study and Development of the CAPP System of the Engine Air-cylinder Jackets. Central South University of Forestry and Technology, Changsha (2006) (in Chinese)

A Tele-operation System for Collaborative Works with Vision-Guided Autonomous Robot

Shiqi Li, Mingfu Li, Di Zhao, and Wenge Zhu

School of Mechanical Science and Engineering Huazhong Universty of Science and Technology, Wuhan, Hubei Province, China
sqli@mail.hust.edu.cn, Lmfwolmf2000@gmail.com,
vbscripzt@126.com, wgzhu2000@mail.hust.edu.cn

Abstract. Fully autonomous robot is limited by level of nowadays artificial intelligence. The research of interface between human and autonomous robot is a burgeoning area in robotics research. User Interface for dynamic autonomy is proposed in this paper for the sake of switch between different control modes to cope with dynamic verification in remote environment. Vision guided fully autonomous act as the basic function for the system. Shared autonomy based on natural image user interface and remote program act as default control mode to combine merits both of human and autonomous robot. The experiments show that the dynamic autonomy tele-operation system proposed in this paper is friendly for human operator and efficient.

Keywords: Dynamic autonomy; Human-robot interaction; User interface; Tele-operation.

1 Introduction

Remote environment often verify dynamically in tele-operation, timedelay is existed in the process as well. Traditional bilateral tele-operation can't handle with timedelay and dynamic verification at the same time. To cope with dynamic environment, telerobots required to be endowed with capability of local autonomy. However, fully autonomous robots are not yet competent for complex tasks operation in remote environment independently because nowadays autonomous systems are unapt at task definition and object recognition. Human operator is with stronger capability of task definition and object recognition than robot, but robot outshines human being in precision, and nowadays computer is not worse, even better than human being in task planning and path planning [1]. Therefore, the problem is expected to be solved by combining merits both of human being and autonomous robot to construct a collaborative tele-operation system.

However, the research of interface between human and autonomous (or semi-autonomous) robot is arisen only recently few years [2]. Researchers in CMU have the pioneer researches, Fong et al. [3] [4] present collaborative control which based on the interface of operator-robot ask, answer question and dialog, in the system humans and robots work as partners. Furthermore, human and autonomous robot exchange information and assist one another to achieve common goals. The researches

C. Xiong et al. (Eds.): ICIRA 2008, Part II, LNAI 5315, pp. 111–120, 2008.

revealed that interface of dialogue are valuable for tele-operation and significantly helped novices understand problems encountered by the robot.

Birk et al. [5] presented an adaptive human machine interface for rescue robots which supports adjustable autonomy by automatically changing its display and control functions based on relevant measures. Bruemmer et al. [6] developed a novel human-robot interaction concepts and interfaces for robust, mixed-initiative interaction between robots and humans. Those interfaces utilize simultaneous localization and mapping techniques that capture an abstracted representation of the robot's experience and exploit sensor-suites and fusion algorithms that enhance capabilities for sensing, interpreting, and "understanding" environmental features. These studies of interaction between humans and autonomous robots present a fascinating and crucial new area of research.

In this paper, user interface based on vision guided autonomous robot is developed to construct a dynamic autonomy tele-operation system. This paper is organized as follows. The framework and overview of the system is described in section 2. Fully autonomy mode of vision guided robotic tracking, reaching and grasping is presented in section 3. Section 4 discussed the natural image user interface and remote programming based shared autonomy tele-operation. Dynamic autonomy of switching between four control modes is discussed in section 5. Experiments of the system are presented in section 6. Conclusions and possible future directions are shown in section 7.

2 System Overview

Accessible and fluent interaction is vital for the sake of combining of human and autonomous robot to the same system. As dynamic verification in remote environment, relevant different control mode is proposed in this paper to suit different situation. Control mode of direct tele-operation, augmented reality and predictive display, shared autonomy and fully autonomy are developed in this paper. A controller clutch is presented to switch between these four control modes, feedback information filtrated according to selected control mode, and display by relevant channel for the operator. Remote robot is endowed with autonomous capability by vision guided reaching and grasping. The framework of multi-control-mode dynamic tele-operation as showed in Fig.1. The details of different modes will describe in following sections.

3 Fully Autonomous: Vision Guided Autonomous Robotic System

Fully autonomous is presented as a basic capability of telerobot in this paper. Telerobot can handle with certain tasks by close loop control, visual information which captured by vision sensors guide the robotic actuator execute expected tasks. The close loop control contains three aspects: object searching, visual tracking and vision guided reaching.

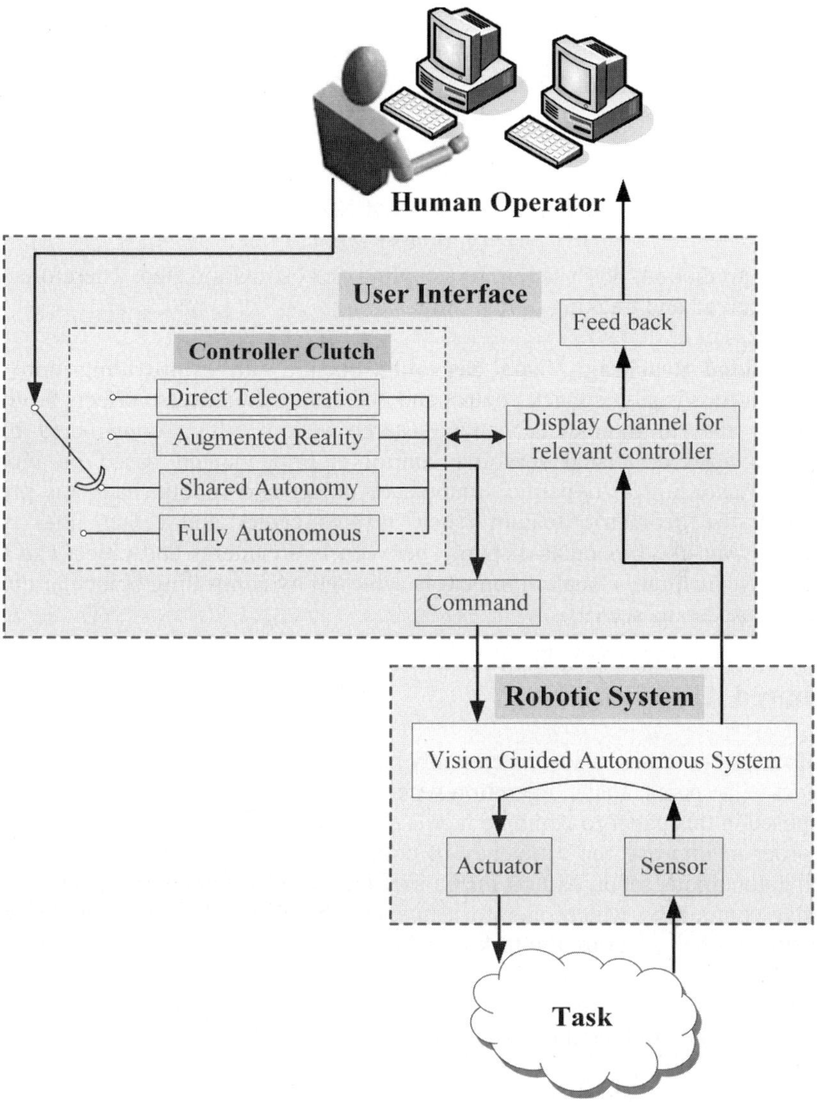

Fig. 1. System architecture of dynamic autonomy tele-operation system

Object Searching & Visual Tracking. A shape template can be constructed before hand by defining geometric parameter according to the method of template tracking [7]. And so, the position angle 'θ', distance from center to left-down point of image plane 'γ', width of object 'ω', length of object 'ι' and slope angle 'φ'. And so the position and status of object can be described by state vector 'S':

$$S=[\theta,\gamma,\omega,\iota,\varphi] \tag{1}$$

Contour is divided by J control points into J+1 segmented lines, visual tracking can be implemented by estimation of the observation likehood:

$$h(I_k|S_k) \equiv h(Z_k|S_k) = \prod_{i=1}^{I} h(z_{i,k}|s_{i,k}) \tag{2}$$

In Eq. (2), $h(z_{i,k} \mid s_{i,k}) \equiv \prod_{j=1}^{J} p(z_{j,i,k})$. CONDENSATION [8] tracking can be implemented by prediction, observation, re-sampling and estimation step. Therefore, object can be perceived and tracking in real time.

Vision Guided Reaching: Visual Servoing. For the sake of providing more visual information for visual feedback control and decreasing the adverse effects brought by contour overlay in monocular camera, stereo vision system constructed by two cameras is applied. Visual servoing control is implemented based on binocular disparity. According to dynamic contours of object and robotic hand (as previous described), the geometric feature (such as area center and center line) can be positioned. And the binocular disparity between two cameras and object can be got dynamically. Accurate visual alignment is achieved by controlling binocular disparity to zero (more details see [9]).

4 Shared Autonomy

Remote fully autonomous system can only handle with tasks which very specific such as object with special shape, operation with special flow and so on. Shared autonomy is proposed in this paper to combine merits of autonomous robot and human operator.

In order to improve the efficiency of communication between human and vision guided autonomous robot, natural image user interface is proposed in this paper based on active contour, by which operator can select the objects to be operated in natural video stream, then program the task based on shared autonomy remote program. The autonomous telerobot execute the tasks automatically which defined by remote program. In the process of tele-operation, human operator can intervene to cancel the current task, send command of exigency stop and override the commands at any moment.

4.1 Objects Pick-Up: Natural Image User Interface

On the one hand, natural image of video stream is directviewing for human operator to understand the situation in the remote environment. On the other hand, vision guide autonomous robot is constructed based on natural image feedback. Therefore, natural image can act as intermedium between human operator and telerobot for interacting and exchanging information each other.

One of the most important purposes of interaction between human operator and telerobot is to provide the objects to be operated. The objects are viewed as dynamic contour for telerobot, human operator pick-up contours in the natural image of feedback video stream by B-spline method. The position information of control points of

B-spline curve is sent to remote telerobot serve. Telerobot approximating and tracking the real contour by B-Snake [10].

According to B-spline, the curve $\boldsymbol{v(s)}$ ($\boldsymbol{r(s)}=(x(s),y(s))$) in the image plane can be defined by control points as follow:

$$\boldsymbol{v(s)}=\sum_{n=0}^{N-1} B_n(s)p_n \qquad 0\le s\le L \tag{3}$$

$B_n(s)$ are basis functions, p_n ($n=0,1,\cdots N-1$) are control points which picked by mouse or keyboard input, the initial curve $\boldsymbol{v}_0\boldsymbol{(s)}$ is got by applying B-Snake to approximating the real contour of the object. In order to track the contour at real time, the B-spline curve required plane affine transformation, affine space of $\boldsymbol{v}_0\boldsymbol{(s)}$ can be viewed as a set of linear transformation:

$$\boldsymbol{v(s)} = \boldsymbol{A}\boldsymbol{v}_0\boldsymbol{(s)} + \boldsymbol{C} \tag{4}$$

In which $\boldsymbol{A}=\begin{pmatrix} A_{11} & A_{12} \\ A_{21} & A_{22} \end{pmatrix}$, $\boldsymbol{C}=\begin{pmatrix} c_1 \\ c_2 \end{pmatrix}$, and so:

$$\begin{aligned}\boldsymbol{v(s)} - \boldsymbol{v}_0\boldsymbol{(s)} &= \boldsymbol{C} + (\boldsymbol{A} - \boldsymbol{I})\boldsymbol{v}_0\boldsymbol{(s)} \\ &= \begin{pmatrix} c_1 B^T(s) \\ c_2 B^T(s) \end{pmatrix} + (\boldsymbol{A} - \boldsymbol{I}) \begin{pmatrix} B^T(s) & 0 \\ 0 & B^T(s) \end{pmatrix} \begin{pmatrix} \boldsymbol{P}_0^x \\ \boldsymbol{P}_0^y \end{pmatrix}\end{aligned} \tag{5}$$

Let $\boldsymbol{\beta(s)}=\begin{pmatrix} B^T(s) & 0 \\ 0 & B^T(s) \end{pmatrix}$, then:

$$\begin{aligned}\boldsymbol{v(s)} - \boldsymbol{v}_0\boldsymbol{(s)} = {}& c_1\boldsymbol{\beta(s)}\begin{pmatrix} 1 \\ 0 \end{pmatrix} + c_2\boldsymbol{\beta(s)}\begin{pmatrix} 0 \\ 1 \end{pmatrix} + (A_{11} - 1)\boldsymbol{\beta(s)}\begin{pmatrix} \boldsymbol{P}_0^x \\ 0 \end{pmatrix} + \\ & A_{21}\boldsymbol{\beta(s)}\begin{pmatrix} 0 \\ \boldsymbol{P}_0^x \end{pmatrix} + A_{12}\boldsymbol{\beta(s)}\begin{pmatrix} \boldsymbol{P}_0^y \\ 0 \end{pmatrix} + (A_{22} - 1)\boldsymbol{\beta(s)}\begin{pmatrix} 0 \\ \boldsymbol{P}_0^y \end{pmatrix}\end{aligned} \tag{6}$$

Affine space of $\boldsymbol{v}_0\boldsymbol{(s)}$ can also defined by control points:

$$\boldsymbol{P}=\boldsymbol{W}\boldsymbol{X}+\boldsymbol{P}_0 \tag{7}$$

In which $\boldsymbol{W}=\begin{pmatrix} 1 & 0 & \boldsymbol{P}_0^x & 0 & \boldsymbol{P}_0^y & 0 \\ 0 & 1 & 0 & \boldsymbol{P}_0^x & 0 & \boldsymbol{P}_0^y \end{pmatrix}$ represent 6 DOF shape matrix, $\boldsymbol{P}_0 = \begin{pmatrix} \boldsymbol{P}_0^x \\ \boldsymbol{P}_0^y \end{pmatrix} = \begin{pmatrix} p_0^x, p_1^x, \cdots p_{N-1}^x \\ p_0^y, p_1^y, \cdots p_{N-1}^y \end{pmatrix}$ is initial curve, according to Eq.(6) and Eq.(7), the shape control vector X is:

$$\boldsymbol{X}=(c_1,c_2,A_{11}-1,A_{22}-1,A_{21},A_{12})^T \tag{8}$$

The real contour can be tracked at real time by control the parameter $c_1, c_2, A_{11} - 1, A_{22} - 1, A_{21}$ and A_{12}.

4.2 Remote Programming for Shared Autonomy

The objects contours can be picked in natural user interface based on B-spline curve, the objects have their index such as: object '1', object '2', …object 'N', user can name each object manually.

As the objects are defined by natural image interface, the operation task needs to determine by operator. As for tele-operation, the operation tasks include four parts: end effector or tool selection, operational action, status checking and speed setting. And the four parts constructs a tele-autonomy command to be sent to telerobot. Telerobot capture and track relevant objects, and execute the tasks according to program explain module.

Operator can programming in the user interface freely, for the users who unfamiliar with the system, the interface provide step by step textbox filling and generate tele-autonomy command finally. A shared autonomy command can be programmed as follow:

```
{Start:
 object enumeration (object '1',object '2',…object 'N')
////***For object 'n' (1•n•N) ***////////
object 'n':{
tool: (?dextrous hand  ?gripper  ?driller)
action:(?reaching  ?grasping  ?drilling  ?following
?releasing)
velocity: (?high  ? moderate  ?slow  ?following)
is action finished ? next object operation : repeat
current object operation
}
Wait: XXX(ms)
////***For object 'i' (1•i•N) ***////////
object 'i':{
 //include four parts: tool, action, speed and status
checking
 }
Is task finished? End: next object operation
}
```

5 Interface for Dynamic Autonomy

Dynamic autonomy is proposed for the sake of cope with dynamic verification in remote environment. Therefore, the interface must provide channel for smooth switching and convenient human intervention. Interface proposed in this paper contain a control mode clutch, fully autonomous mode, shared autonomy mode, augmented reality and predictive display mode and direct bilateral tele-operation.

Clutch for Control Mode Switching. A clutch is designed for control mode selection and switching. Operator can make switch from one control mode to another, furthermore, display channel also switch to suit relevant control mode. As show in Fig.1, the clutch also provide filter for information of feedback data and send out command to reduce human and robot error.

Fully Autonomy. Vision guided fully autonomy is basic capability of telerobot, however, as described in section 3, application of fully autonomous limited to special tasks and special object. Therefore, fully autonomous mode suggested to be selected in the situation of special tasks or special sub-task.

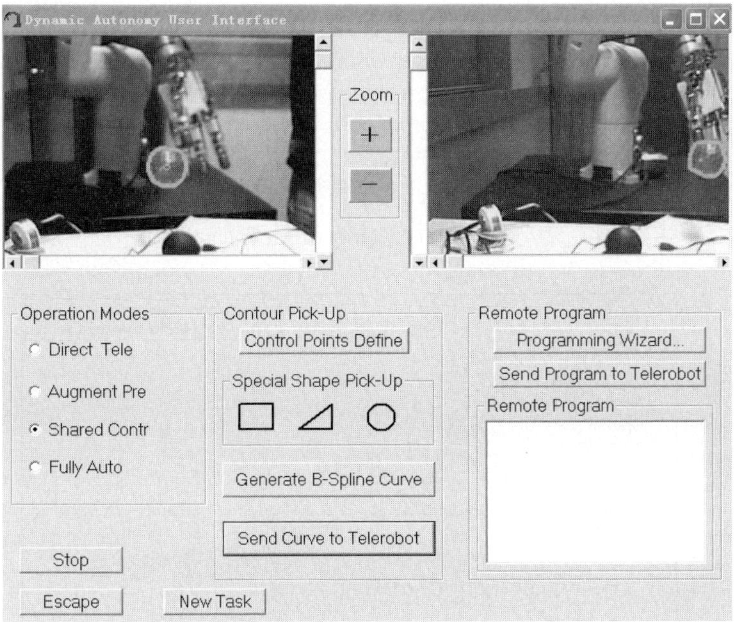

Fig. 2. Flow of shared autonomy remote programming

Augmented Reality Predictive Display. A virtual robot is registered to the real video image and becomes an interface between the operator and the telerobot, thus the time-delay is separated from interactive of the human-virtual robot (more details see [11]).

When shared autonomy encounter emergencies, by human operator intervene, this mode has the chance to be selected, especially when remote environment is unstructured.

Direct/bilateral Tele-operation. Direct bilateral tele-operation consists of transmitting video to local station. The operator can operate the telerobot by using control device such as space ball, data glove or joy stick. Since timedelay affect the quality of bilateral mode seriously, this mode only has the chance to be selected when without large timedelay.

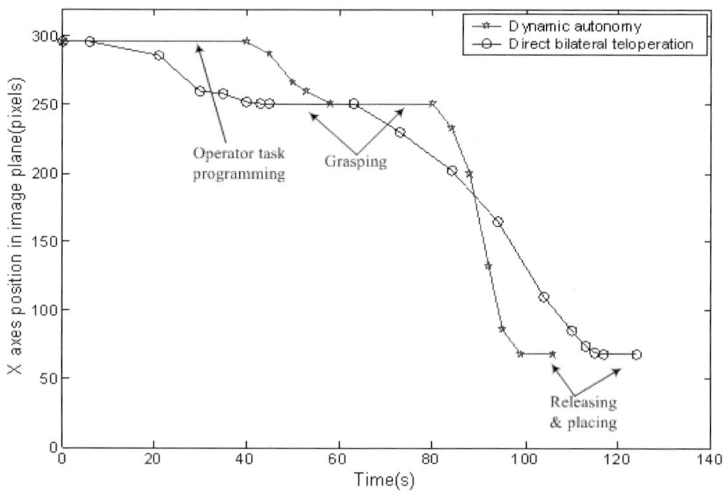

(a) Trajectory of X axes

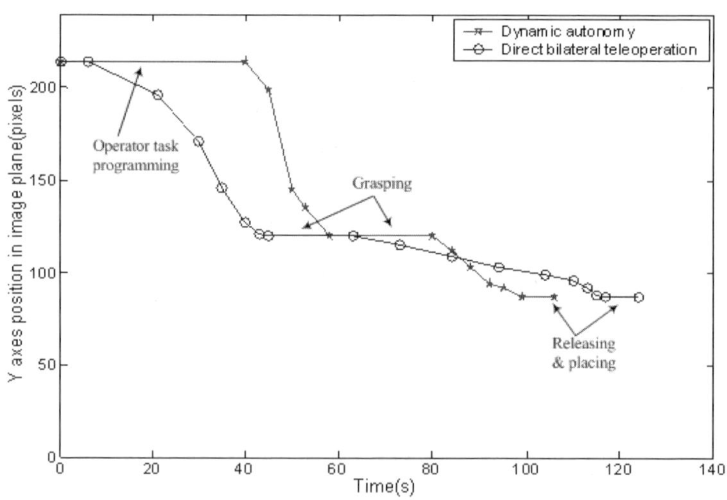

(b) Trajectory of Y axes

Fig. 3. Trajectory of robot finger by in the right camera image plane

6 Experiments

As described in section 5, shared autonomy is common use control mode while augmented reality predictive display is a standby control mode. Therefore, experiment of object tracking, reaching and grasping is implemented by the dynamic autonomy system include these two modes. The task of the experiment is to put a bottle into a bucket which both in remote environment. The dynamic autonomy tele-operation system is constructed by autonomous telerobot (Staubli RX40), robot server and local user interface. The experiment is take in local area network, in order to simulate the large time delay, fix manmade 6 seconds round trip time delay is added in the process. As a comparison, experiment of bilateral tele-operation also took under the same condition. In the dynamic autonomy tele-operation, when the contours of bottle and bucket are picked-up, the remote program set as described in section 4.2.

The experimental results as show in Fig.3, total time of dynamic autonomy tele-operation is shorter than fully bilateral tele-operation although task programming in dynamic autonomy could spend longer time. Furthermore, for the operator, dynamic autonomy is easier and lower pressure than bilateral tele-operation

7 Conclusions

User interface for dynamic autonomy tele-operation is proposed in this paper. The interface provide smooth switch between four control modes. As default and common use mode, shared autonomy tele-operation is friendly and easy for an operator who unfamiliar with tele-operation. Furthermore, shared autonomy tele-operation can cope with large time delay with high operational efficiency. The augmented reality predictive display mode and fully autonomous mode act as safe supporter for dynamic autonomy system. However, the deficiency to be improved is that the process of contour pick-up in natural user interface is not so easy for operator and could spend long time to do it.

Acknowledgments

The authors thank Dr. Ming Xie of Nanyang Technological University for providing useful insights contribution to this work.

References

1. Hauck, A., Sorg, M., Farber, G., Schenk, T.: A Biologically Motivated Model for the Control of Visually Guided Reach-To-Grasp Movements. In: Proceedings of the 1998 IEEE ISIC/CIRA/ISJ, Gaithersburg, pp. 295–300. IEEE Press, New York (1998)
2. Steinfeld, A.: Interface Lessons for Fully and Dynamic Autonomy Mobile Robots. In: IEEE International Conference on Robotics and Automation (ICRA).IEEE Press, New York (2004)
3. Fong, T., Thorpe, C., Baur, C.: Collaboration, Dialogue, and Human-Robot Interaction. In: Robotics Research: The 10th International Symposium, vol. 6, pp. 255–270 (2003)

4. Fong, T., Thorpe, C., Baur, C.: Collaboration, Robot, asker of questions. Robotics and Autonomous Systems 42, 235–243 (2003)
5. Birk, A., Pfingsthorn, M.: A HMI Supporting Adjustable Autonomy of Rescue Robots. In: Bredenfeld, A., Jacoff, A., Noda, I., Takahashi, Y. (eds.) RoboCup 2005. LNCS (LNAI), vol. 4020, pp. 255–266. Springer, Heidelberg (2006)
6. Bruemmer, D.J., Dudenhoeffer, D.D., McKay, M.D., Anderson, M.O.: Dynamic-Autonomy for Remote Robotic Sensor Deployment. In: Proc. Spectrum 2002, Reno (2002)
7. Masahide, S., Norikazu, I., Motonori, D.: Tracking of Fingers in Dynamic Image of Omni-direction Camera by CONDENSATION Algorithm. In: Proc ISCIE Int Symp. Stoch Syst. Theory Appl (Inst. Syst. Control Inf. Eng.), vol. 36, pp. 14–19 (2005)
8. Isard, M., Blake, A.: CONDENSATION – Conditional Density Propagation for Visual Tracking. Int. J. of Computer Vision 29(1), 5–28 (1998)
9. Li, M., Fu, Y., Li, S., Zhu, W., Zhao, D.: Robotic Hand-Eye Coordination Control Based on Binocular Disparity and Active Contour. Robot 30(3), 248–253 (2008)
10. Menet, S., Saint, M.P., Medioni, G.: B-Snakes: Implementation and application to stereo. In: DARPA Image Understanding Workshop, pp. 720–726 (1990)
11. Xiong, Y., Li, S., Xie, M.: Predictive display and interaction of telerobots based on augmented reality. Robotica 24(1), 447–453 (2005)

Occlusion Handling in Augmented Reality System for Human-Assisted Assembly Task

Chi Xu[1], Shiqi Li[1], Junfeng Wang[1], Tao Peng[1], and Ming Xie[2]

[1] School of Mechanical Science & Engineering, Huazhong University of Science & Technology, Wuhan, Hubei Province, 430074, China
[2] Nanyang Technological University, School of Mechanical & Aerospace Engineering, Block N3, Nanyang Avenue, 639798 Singapore
tomxu2008@yahoo.com.cn, sqli@mail.hust.edu.cn,
wangjf@mail.hust.edu.cn, pntao@smail.hust.edu.cn,
mmxie@ntu.edu.sg

Abstract. Augmented reality (AR) based human-machine interaction (HMI) provided a seamless interface between user and application environment, but occlusion handing remained as a tough problem in AR applications. Recently most AR occlusion handling algorithms aimed at general environment, more special research on AR occlusion handling for application in the context of industrial assembly, such as assembly training and assembly task guidance, is required. An occlusion handling method aimed at video see-through AR-based assembly system is presented based on the analysis of the occlusion between virtual part, visual assembly feature, navigation information, physical part and physical assembly environment in the context of virtual/physical assembly working space. The method was implemented in prototype AR-assembly system and was proved to be efficient in handling the virtual/physical occlusion in augmented assembly scene.

Keywords: Augmented reality; Human-machine Interaction; Virtual assembly; Occlusion; Depth image.

1 Introduction

In recent years, augmented reality (AR) and human-machine interaction (HMI) have been becoming more and more tightly interrelated, with the help of AR technology physical working space can be enhanced with various useful digital content [1]. In AR system for assembly task application, AR displays can enhance the user's perception of the physical assembly working space and assembly constraint feature between virtual/physical parts, providing access to information the user cannot directly perceive when unaided. AR can be used in a wide range of areas in the industrial assembly field, and potential applications can be concluded into following 5 aspects [2]: AR-based assembly feature design [3], AR-based assembly sequence evaluation [4], AR-based assembly training, AR-based assembly task guidance, and AR-based assembly inspection.

Two basic choices are available to accomplish the combining of virtual and physical scene: optical and video see-through HMD. Compare with optical see-through

C. Xiong et al. (Eds.): ICIRA 2008, Part II, LNAI 5315, pp. 121–130, 2008.

HMDs, video see-through HMD is widely used in AR applications because of its flexibility in combining strategies, easier to match the brightness of virtual and physical objects, and relatively cheaper. Video see-through HMD is used in Prototype AR system presented in this paper to achieve a virtual/physical mixed assembly environment (see **Fig. 8**).

Most of the AR application directly overlay the computer generated graphic of virtual parts on physical scene video captured by camera, therefore the image of physical parts is occluded by the graphic of virtual parts all the time (see **Fig. 1**). Many researches aimed at solving the incorrect occlusion problem: Fuhrmann [5] selected a portion of the physical scene and aligned 3d geometry models to them, and the 3d geometry information of models was used to manipulate occlusion. Yokoya [6] calculated depth information of physical objects by stereo vision theory, and the method cost large amount of calculation as it deals with the whole scene to calculate the depth information of physical environment, but stereo vision method can not be used in real-time AR system. Ohta [7] used client/server method to accelerate calculation speed, but vision field of client and server suffered from inconsistent problem. Lepetit [8] accelerated calculation speed by calculating approximate depth information of physical objects through their 2d contours in the video, however the method could not achieve the accurate depth information of complex 3d geometry object such as assembly part.

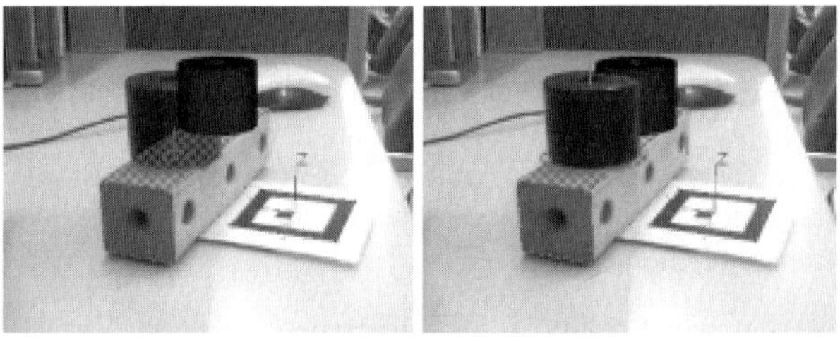

Fig. 1. Virtual/physical occlusion. (Left) Incorrect occlusion. (Right) correct occlusion.

Occlusion handling methods mentioned above are general methods, however there is seldom special research on occlusion between virtual/physical parts in the AR-based assembly applications. It is noted that accurate depth information of virtual and physical parts are required to manipulate occlusions by AR-based assembly system. However both accuracy and calculation speed of stereo vision theory based method need to be improved. It is considered that CAD model of physical assembly parts are always available in industrial assembly application, therefore occlusion handling method presented in this paper used 3d CAD model of physical parts to calculate depth information for virtual/physical occlusion handling.

2 Visual Elements in AR-based Assembly Scene

In the context of AR-based assembly application, visual elements can be classified into 2 categories: virtual and physical elements.

2.1 Virtual Elements

(1) Virtual Part. Virtual part does not exist in the physical assembly working space, and computer generates the graphic of virtual parts and overlays it on the video captured by camera mounted on the HMD. In the designing stage of an assembly project, AR system gets 3d geometry model of virtual parts from CAD software and merges it into virtual/physical environment to accomplish the pre-assembly procedure, and deficiency of the assembly design can be found and modified. In the training stage, virtual part was transformed to target place through defaulting path and then constrained in the computer driven mixed assembly scene, so that user can learn the assembly procedure intuitively.

(2) Visual Assembly Feature. Visual assembly feature means visual geometric elements representing assembly relations and constraints between assembly parts. AR-based assembly system help the user identify the constraints between assembly parts intuitively with visual assembly feature while manipulating the part to the target place. For instance, part A and part B have a face-mating relationship, AR system displays the faces to be mated on A and part B while part A approaching to part B, so that face-mating constraint of the parts can be augmented by visual assembly feature and be identified intuitively (see **Fig. 2**). Elements of assembly feature include:

- Line: including beeline, curve and circle, these assembly features are used to represent assembly constraints such as hole-shaft fitting, edge alignment and so on.
- Surface: including plane, curved and sphere surface, mainly used to represent constrains such as face-mating, face-parallel and face-alignment and so on.

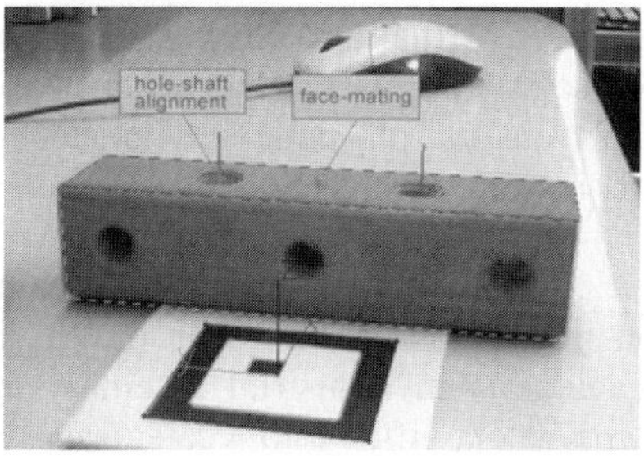

Fig. 2. Visual assembly feature with line and surface style

(3) Navigation Information. Navigation information includes product name, part name and id, guidance for assembly procedure in assembly handbook, prompt message (see **Fig. 2**), and also graphic elements such as line, rectangle, circle, arrow and so on, these elements are used to let the user pay attention to the assembly information such as active region, assembly direction, assembly path and so on (see **Fig. 7**).

2.2 Physical Elements

(1) Physical Part. Physical part means the assembly part exists in the physical assembly working space, and its feature is presented in the video capture by the camera mounted on the HMD.

It is possible that physical part's feature is not clear enough for user to identify in the physical scene video because of the insufficient light condition or out of focus, therefore physical part's outline contour need to be augmented. AR-based assembly system achieves 3d model data from CAD software, align the model to corresponding physical part's region in physical scene video captured by camera, and then enhanced the user's perception by overlaid physical part's location and geometry information.

(2) Physical Assembly Environment. Physical assembly environment means the physical working space in which assembly procedure takes place, including assembly platform, brace, clamp, and workshop etc. Physical assembly environment is dealt as background in the AR scene by default. Prototype AR-based assembly system presented in this paper dealt the physical assembly environment as bounding box and constrained assembly elements within certain range of physical space by collecting detection technology.

3 Occlusion between Virtual/Physical Elements

Virtual elements in the AR-based assembly scene include virtual part, visual assembly feature and navigation information; Physical elements include physical part and working environment. Occlusion between virtual and physical elements in AR assembly application is analyzed in this section.

3.1 Occlusion between Virtual Part and Physical Part

The most important portion in occlusion handling method in AR-based assembly application is occlusion between virtual and physical parts, because users always pay more attention to assembly relational region than other of the video image. Accurate depth information of both virtual and physical parts is needed for occlusion handling, for inaccurate depth information will lead to incorrect occlusion between virtual/physical parts when virtual part is attached to physical part through assembly constraint and tightly mated together. In this paper we calculate the accurate depth information of virtual and physical parts based on the 3d CAD model of assembly parts while it is always available in industrial assembly application. Occlusion of virtual and physical parts can be classified into 4 categories:

- Virtual occlude physical: When the location of virtual part is closer to the observer than physical part, system directly overlaid virtual graphic generated by computer up on the physical scene captured by camera mounted on the observer's head.
- Physical occlude virtual: On the other hand, if physical part's location is closer to the observer than virtual part, system remained the region of physical part in physical scene video unchanged and neglected virtual part's graphic in the same region.
- Virtual/physical mutual occlusion: In this case, virtual and physical parts occluded mutually (see Fig. 3) and we can not simply directly overlaid graphic of one part on to another. For the region of virtual part's graphic generated by computer and physical scene video captured from camera can be divided into pixels, and AR-based assembly system deals with virtual/physical occlusion region pixel by pixel to solve the mutual occlusion problem.

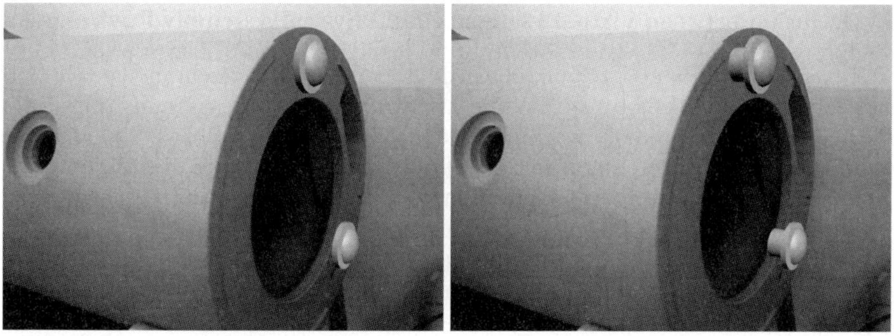

Fig. 3. (Left) mutual occlusion of virtual/physical parts: virtual part antenna is partial occluded by physical part shell, and physical part is also partial occluded by virtual part. (Right) Incorrect occlusion.

- Translucent occlusion: In this case, visual property of virtual part is translucent. In other words, physical part's feature behind the virtual part can be seen simultaneously by alpha channel blending method. In AR-based assembly application, if translucent occlusion mode is on, user could always perceive physical assembly part through video see-through HMD even when it is occluded by translucent virtual ones.

3.2 Occlusion between Visual Assembly Feature and Physical Part

Assembly constraints among assembly parts, such as face-mating, alignment, hole-shaft mating, can be augmented in the users' vision field intuitively by visual assembly feature in AR-based assembly system. Visual assembly feature is a kind of virtual 3d geometry object whose elements include line and surface as mentioned above. Similar to the virtual/physical parts' occlusion, the occlusion between visual assembly feature and physical part includes: virtual occlude physical, physical occlude virtual, virtual/physical mutual occlusion and translucent occlusion.

It is recommended that the property of surface element in visual assembly feature can be set to translucent style by defaulting, so the observer can always perceive the geometry and location of virtual and physical parts even when they are occluded by translucent assembly feature (see **Fig. 2**).

3.3 Occlusion between Navigation Information and Physical Part

2d navigation information is always visible and cannot be occluded by physical part or other visual elements, it occluded or translucently occluded other elements in mixed assembly environment. 3d navigation information such as arrow, rectangle region, and circle are virtual 3d geometry elements, Occlusion between 3d navigation information and physical part is similar to virtual and physical parts' occlusion described above, it includes: virtual occlude physical , physical occlude virtual , virtual/physical mutual occlusion and translucent occlusion.

3.4 Occlusion between Virtual Elements and Physical Assembly Environment

In AR-based assembly application, physical assembly environment includes assembly platform, brace, workshop, etc. While user is performing assembly task in virtual/physical mixed assembly working space, physical environment is shown as background in the scene, and computer generates virtual elements are directly overlaid on to the physical assembly environment in the video captured by camera, since physical environment was always further to the observer than virtual elements.

Bounding box is used to constrain virtual elements be in a certain region of working space and make sure that virtual elements to be always closer to observer than physical environment.

4 Occlusion Handling Method for AR-based Assembly Application

4.1 Placing Virtual Part in Contact with Physical Part in AR Assembly Scene

3d geometry models of virtual/physical parts are achieved from CAD software interface, they are placed in the AR assembly scene in contact with each other automatically by registration procedure. First parts' transform matrices from physical world coordinate to camera are estimated, and then parts' CAD models are transformed and projected onto image plane aligning with physical assembly scene. Great deal of researches can be found on this subject. Our registration method is similar to Kato's method, and the details can be found in [9] and [2].

It is noted that lens distortion of camera mounted on users' head would reduce precision of virtual/physical parts' alignment. The distortion can be approximated using the following expression:

$$P_d = (1 + k_1 r^2 + k_2 r^4 + k_3 r^6)\, P_n + dp. \tag{1}$$

where k1, k2, k3 are coefficients for radial distortion, dp is tangential distortion vector, and P_d is distorted position in image coordinate. Distortion of physical scene video is verified in our system by calibration procedure, details can be found in [2].

4.2 Virtual/Physical Depth Image

Virtual depth image records the depth information of virtual elements such as virtual part, visual assembly feature and navigation information within rending area, it is a gray scale image with the same size as computer generates graphic. The value of virtual depth image indicates the distance from observer to virtual element's surface being rendered at current pixel. Virtual depth image can be acquired from 3d graphic engine such as OpenGL and OpenInventor while rendering procedure.

Physical depth image records depth information of the video captured by camera mounted on observer's header pixel by pixel. AR system aligns physical part's CAD model to its corresponding region in physical scene video, by rending the physical model, its depth image can be easily achieved from rendering engine. The range of gray scale value in depth image is from 0 to 1, it is recommended that depth information of physical assembly environment be set to the maximal value 1, so that it will be directly overlaid by other elements in the mixed scene by default (see Fig. 4).

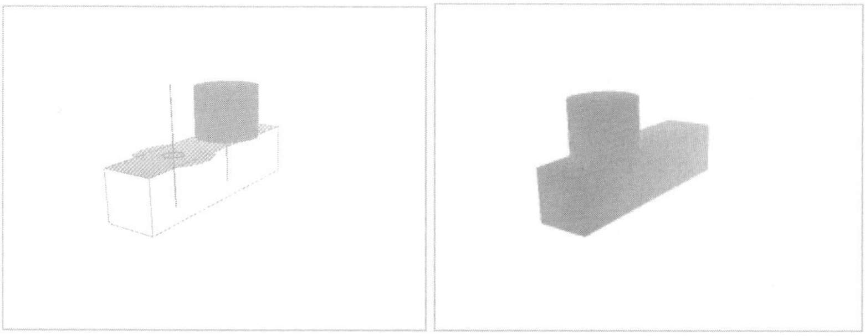

Fig. 4. (Left) depth image of virtual elements. (Right) depth image of physical elements.

4.3 Occlusion Handling Procedure

When virtual scene, virtual depth image, physical scene and physical image are available, system integrates the virtual/physical scene. Virtual scene is generated by computer, physical scene is captured by camera mounted on observer's head, and virtual/physical depth image are acquired from rendering engine mentioned above. While integrating, system compares the depth value of virtual scene with physical pixel by pixel: if physical depth value is less than virtual one, it means that virtual element's region at current pixel is further to observer and should be occluded by physical element, system fills current pixel with physical scene, and vise versa. Occlusion relation of 3d virtual elements and physical elements will be correctly dealt with through this procedure (see **Fig.5**).

After 3d geometry elements are integrated into one image, 2d navigation information will be overlaid on top of mixed video. It is noted that there are also occlusions between 2d navigation information, and the order of 2d information overlaying on the video is determined by their layer id. 2d information is drawn on the video from lest important to the most important for the sake that important information would not be occluded by less important ones. The whole procedure of occlusion handling method is illustrated below (see **Fig. 6**).

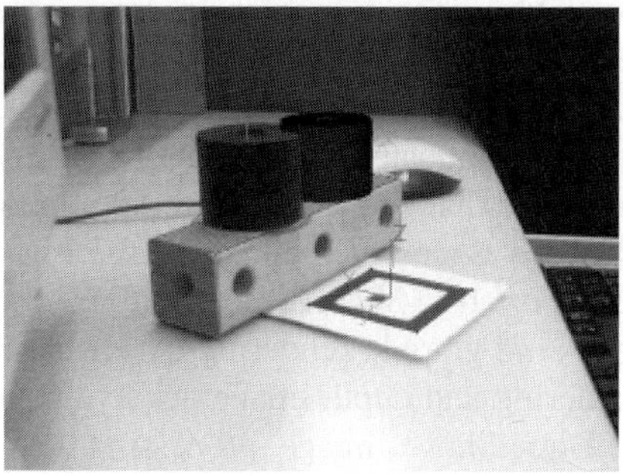

Fig. 5. Occlusion between virtual and physical 3d geometry elements

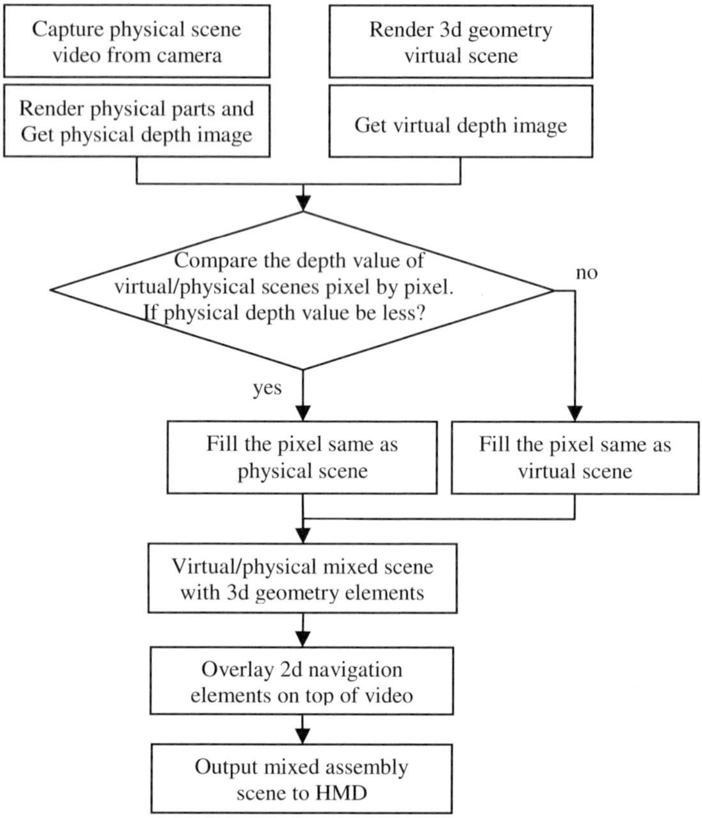

Fig. 6. Occlusion handling method

5 Prototype AR-based Assembly System

Prototype AR-based assembly system is a sub-system of smart assembly system which belongs to national defense "eleven five" foundational scientific research project committed by Huazhong university of science and technology. Prototype system presented in this paper was implicated in assembly task training for an aerospace product, and it has been proved that occlusion handling method can real-time manipulate the occlusion in AR-based assembly application (see **Fig. 7**).

Geometry model was exported to VRML file ".wrl" from CAD software pro/e; assembly scene management and graphic rendering by virtual reality SDK OpenInventor; assembly feature rendering and depth image achievement by OpenGL; capturing video from camera by DirectShow; image processing and occlusion handling by open-source library OpenCV. Development platform was Microsoft Visual C++ 6.0 and operation system was Microsoft windows XP.

Physical scene video was captured by camera mounted on the video see-through HMD "AR-vision-3D" (see **Fig. 8**), CMOS color sensor, resolution 640×480, maximal capture rate 48fps. Virtual scene is generated by pc with Intel Pentium 4 CPU 2.4G, GeForce MX 440 AGP8x 64M, memory 512M. Virtual/physical assembly scene was displayed on the HMD with solution 800×600 and rate 12fps.

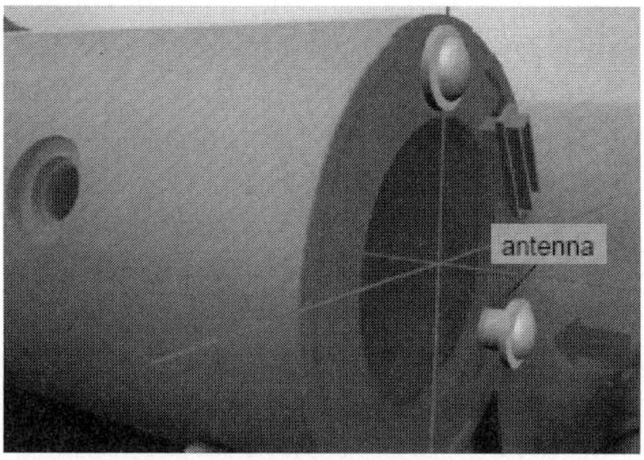

Fig. 7. Prototype AR-based assembly system

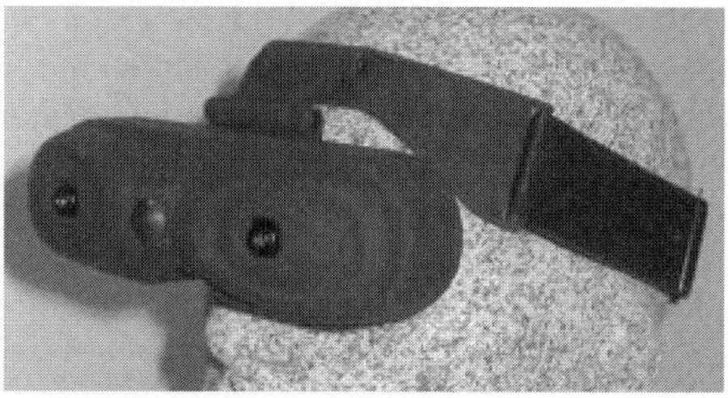

Fig. 8. Video see-through HMD "AR-vision-3D"

6 Conclusion

Augmented reality technology can be implicated in industrial assembly field to form a virtual/physical parts mixed assembly environment, and it can effectively improve the product quality, shorten period of development and reduce the cost of the product.

Virtual/physical occlusion handling is one of the main problems in AR technology, by now there is no special research that analyzed occlusion handling of virtual/physical elements in the industrial assembly field. In this paper occlusion among virtual part, visual assembly feature, navigation information, physical part and physical assembly environment is analyzed, and then occlusion handling method is presented for video see-through AR-based assembly application. The experiment of prototype AR system proved that occlusion handling method can solve the occlusion problem in industrial assembly application efficiently.

References

1. Azuma, R.T.: A survey of augmented reality. J. Presence: Teleoperators and Virtual Environments 6(4), 355–385 (1997)
2. Xu, C.: Research on the virtual/physical scene integration of augmented assembly system. M.Sc. Huazhong University of Science and Technology, WhuHan (2007)
3. Yan, P., Nee, A.Y.C., Soh Khim, O., Yuan, M., Youcef-Toumi, K.: Assembly feature design in an augmented reality environment. J. Assembly Automation 26(1), 34–43 (2006)
4. Klinker, G., Dutoit, A.H., Bauer, M., Bayer, J., Novak, V., Matzke, D.: Fata Morgana: a presentation system for product design. In: Proceedings of the IEEE and ACM International Symposium on Mixed and Augmented Reality, pp. 76–85. IEEE Comput. Soc., Darmstadt (2002)
5. Fuhrmann, A., Hesina, G., Faure, F., Gervautz, M.: Occlusion in collaborative augmented environments. J. Computers & Graphics 23(6), 809–819 (1999)
6. Okuma, T., Kiyokawa, K., Takemura, H., Yokoya, N.: An augmented reality system using a real-time vision based registration. In: Proceedings. Fourteenth International Conference on Pattern Recognition (Cat. No.98EX170), vol. 2, pp. 1226–1229. IEEE Comput. Soc., Brisbane (1998)
7. Ohta, Y., Sugaya, Y., Igarashi, H., Ohtsuki, T., Taguchi, K.: client/server depth sensing for see-through head-mounted displays. J. Presence: Teleoperators and Virtual Environments 11(2), 176–188 (2002)
8. Vacchetti, L., Lepetit, V., Fua, P.: Combining edge and texture information for real-time accurate 3D camera tracking. In: Third IEEE and ACM International Symposium on Mixed and Augmented Reality, pp. 48–56. IEEE Comput. Soc., Arlington (2004)
9. Kato, H., Billinghurst, M.: Marker tracking and HMD calibration for a video-based augmented reality conferencing system. In: Proceedings 2nd IEEE and ACM International Workshop on Augmented Reality (IWAR 1999), pp. 85–94. IEEE Comput. Soc., San Francisco (1999)

Research on the Wave-Variable Based Tele-operation with Force-Feedback

Di Zhao, Shiqi Li, Mingfu Li, and Wenge Zhu

School of Mechanical Science and Engineering Huazhong University of Science and Technology, Wuhan, Hubei Province, China
vbscript@gmail.com, sqli@mail.hust.edu.cn,
Lmfwolmf2000@gmail.com, wgzhu2000@mail.hust.edu.cn

Abstract. In this paper, we describe a wave variable based tele-operation system with force feedback. The wave variable is imported to the system, and the stabilization is discussed with passive theory. We calculated virtual force in VR environment and extrapolated it to achieve smooth force feedback to the human operator. The immersion is provided as well to help the operator finish the tele-operation task. At the end of the paper, an experiment was introduced.

Keywords: Tele-operation, wave-variable, force-feedback.

1 Introduction

The tele-operation system can drive the telerobot working under a dangerous environment or a place unreachable to human being. The working environments lead to distribution of the master-slave parts are in distance. And the time delay is also an important problem. The experiments indicate that when the time delay is larger than 0.25s, it will sharply decrease the system stability and affect the judgment of the operator in common bilateral control tele-operation system with force feedback. This will reduces efficiency and safety of tele-operation. Scientists suggested a lot to reduce the efficiency such as transparency, caused by time delay, such as tele-program, predictive control and event based supervisory control. Traditional method to reduce that efficiency is using VR based predictive display to simulate the working environment [1], [2], [3]. The operator interacted with the virtual reality environment continually, and the results can be showed in VR environment, then the telerobot would act as the one in the VR environment by time delay [4].

The network propagation delay can not be ignored when there is long distance between the master and slave .For example, the propagation delay between ground station and on-orbit telerobot reach 3~6s [5]. When only traditional methods are used in the tele-operation system, the system will become instability because of the time delay. Sometimes, the remote environment is changed by outside influence factors while the local VR environment is not updated in time, so working only with the graphic simulation in VR will limit the ability of the tele-operation system to deal with the external contingency. The force & video feed-back is delayed far behind the VR environment. It is not dependable to make real-time judgment only by the feed-back

C. Xiong et al. (Eds.): ICIRA 2008, Part II, LNAI 5315, pp. 131–140, 2008.

sensors, the tele-operation system will work as "move-wait" way. In this paper, virtual force is calculated in the VR environment to instead the real force feedback which is getting from the remote side to the operator. This will help the operator making real-time judgment. The delayed remote force sensor information is used to revise the virtual force. This will improve the immersion and the interaction and the transparency of tele-operation system. CyberGrasp is used as force feed-back equipment in this case.

Tele-operation is widely used in the maintenance of airspace equipment. German Aerospace Center (DLR) first operated the ROTEX(Robotic Technology Experiment) on "Columbia" (Space Shuttle) using tele-operation on the ground in 1993. Japan tele-operated the robot on ETS-VII (Engineering Test Satellite VII) to finish two extravehicular operation experiments, rendezvous of two on satellite robot systems and remote tele-operation in 1999.

Based on passive theory, focus on the energy transmission, a wave variable based technique is developed by Niemeyer and Slotine in 1991 [6]. And passive control arithmetic is developed. After that, wave variable becomes an important method to stable the tele-operation system under variable time-delay.

In this paper, we study a ground research system, which is used to simulate the ground-space tele-operation system. This system includes VR based tele-operation system with force-feedback and wave variable is used to make sure the system is stable. In chapter 3, stable analysis of the wave variable based tele-operation system is discussed. In chapter 4, force feed-back and the virtual force extrapolation is studied. The experiment set up and result analysis is in chapter 5.

2 System Descriptions

The structure of a tele-operation system is shown as fig.1:

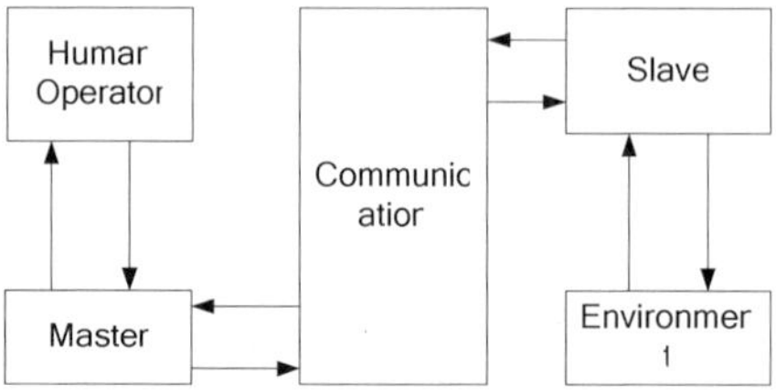

Fig. 1. A structure of tele-operation system

In a master-slave tele-operation system, the operator interacts with the master side. The master side sends the command to the slave side by the communication block. The tele-robot in slave side interacts with the environment, and sensor feedback is send back to the master side through the communication block. The time-delay of the tele-operation is mainly in the transmission process, which is in communication block.

In this paper, wave variable is imported in the transmission process of the tele-operation systems to make system stable under a time-vary delay. Wave variable based tele-operation is a method based on passive theory. It is considered in passive theory that the robustness control theory can be designed in a passive system, while a non-passive system can be converted to a passive system in a way.

The transmission block of a tele-operation system can be treated as a two port network [7-9] in fig2:

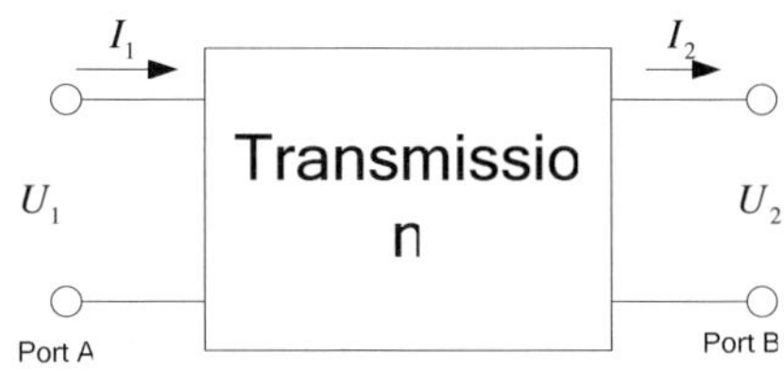

Fig. 2. Two port transmission network

The force F and the velocity v in tele-operation system is mapped with the voltage V and the current I in the circuit, that is $F \rightleftarrows V$, $v \rightleftarrows I$. The transmission delay T in the tele-operation system is mapped with l/v_0 in two port network. So a tele-operation system can be mapped as a two port network. And circuit theory can be used to analyze tele-operation system. It is considered that the transmission process should be passive to stabilize a system; otherwise there is no need to transmit energy from port A to port B.

3 Stabilization Analysis of a Wave Variable Based Tele-operation System

An ideal non-dissipation transmission system is shown in fig 3. The operator is non-passive in a tele-operation system, but operator is adaptable with the system. So the operator is able to adapt the passive system.

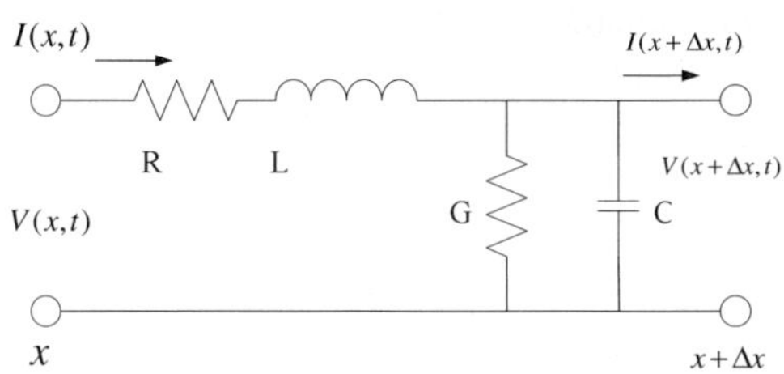

Fig. 3. An ideal non-dissipation transmission circuit

There are typical inductances and capacitors in the circuit. The voltage is referred as V, the current is referred as I, the capacitor is referred as C and the inductance is referred as L.

$$\frac{\partial V(x,t)}{\partial x} = -L\frac{\partial I(x,t)}{\partial t}$$
$$\frac{\partial I(x,t)}{\partial x} = -C\frac{\partial V(x,t)}{\partial t} \tag{1}$$

After Laplace transform, using impedance matrix to separate the voltage V and the current I.

$$\begin{bmatrix} V_1(s) \\ V_2(s) \end{bmatrix} = \begin{bmatrix} Z_0 \coth \frac{sl}{v_0} & Z_0 \operatorname{cosech} \frac{sl}{v_0} \\ Z_0 \operatorname{cosech} \frac{sl}{v_0} & Z_0 \coth \frac{sl}{v_0} \end{bmatrix} \begin{bmatrix} I_1(s) \\ -I_2(s) \end{bmatrix} \tag{2}$$

Z_0 is impedance characteristic of transmission process, v_0 is transmission velocity, the lower mark 1&2 is referred as master & slave side.

Because of the time-delay:

$$V_1(t) = V_2(t-T)$$
$$I_2(t) = I_1(t-T) \tag{3}$$

In tele-operation system it means :

$$F_1(t) = F_2(t-T)$$
$$\dot{x}_2(t) = \dot{x}\ (t-T) \tag{4}$$

Consider about the pure time-delay statement, at time t, force at the master side equals to the force at the slave side but T delay ago, while the velocity at the slave side equals to the one at master side but T delay ago.

Import wave variables U, V:

$$u_l = \frac{b\dot{x}_l + F_l}{\sqrt{2b}}, w_l = \frac{b\dot{x}_l - F_l}{\sqrt{2b}} \tag{5}$$

The two port network is changed as shown in fig 4:

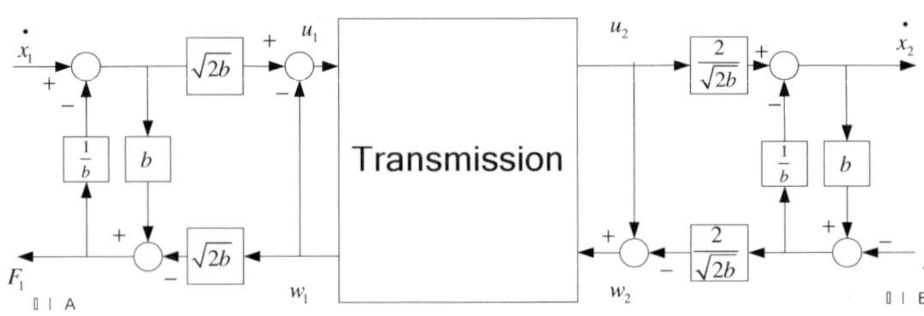

Fig. 4. The framework of the transmission process imported with the wave variable

By calculating the energy flow of the two port network, it can be proved that energy flow into the network is larger than the flow out, which means the network is passive, so that the system is stable.

The proof is as follow (assume there is no energy in the network at first):

$$\underline{F} = \begin{bmatrix} F_1 \\ F_2 \end{bmatrix}, \quad \underline{\dot{x}} = \begin{bmatrix} \dot{x}_1 \\ -\dot{x}_2 \end{bmatrix} \tag{6}$$

At time t, the energy in the transmission process is:

$$E_{net}(t) = \int_0^t \left(\underline{F}^T \underline{\dot{x}} \right) d\tau = \int_0^t \left(F_1 \dot{x}_1 - F_2 \dot{x}_2 \right) d\tau \tag{7}$$

If the network is passive, the flow in energy is larger than the flow out. Means:

$$\int_0^\infty \left(F_1 \dot{x}_1 - F_2 \dot{x}_2 \right) d\tau \geq 0 \tag{8}$$

Using the scatter operator S

$$S(s) = \begin{bmatrix} -\tanh(sT) & \sec h(sT) \\ \sec h(sT) & \tanh(sT) \end{bmatrix} \tag{9}$$

$$\underline{F}(s) - \underline{\dot{x}}(s) = S(s) \left[\underline{F}(s) + \underline{\dot{x}}(s) \right] \tag{10}$$

$$\left\| \underline{F}(s) + \underline{\dot{x}}(s) \right\|^2 - \left\| \underline{F}(s) - \underline{\dot{x}}(s) \right\|^2 \geq 0 \tag{11}$$

$$\int_0^\infty \left[\left(\underline{F} + \underline{\dot{x}} \right)^T \left(\underline{F} + \underline{\dot{x}} \right) - \left(\underline{F} - \underline{\dot{x}} \right)^T \left(\underline{F} - \underline{\dot{x}} \right) \right] d\tau = 4 \int_0^\infty \left(\underline{F}^T \underline{\dot{x}} \right) d\tau \geq 0 \tag{12}$$

Means the energy flow into the two port network is larger than the flow out, the transmission network is passive, and the tele-operation system is stable.

4 Tele-operation System with Force Feedback

According to the research, force feedback can enhance the immersion of the tele-operation system, and improve the efficiency and veracity of the operation. If people operate the master side only depends on the VR graphic simulation without force feedback, the modeling error will lead to the failure. And it is not safe and reliable. Force feedback provides huge agility and high efficiency to the tele-operation system [10]. Some scientists studied on the master-slave tele-operation system with and without force feedback, the research indicate that force feedback can reduce 40% time to accomplish the task.

Human can feel force variations about 300~1000HZ. The lower frequency will lead intermission to human's haptic feelings. Direct sensor force feedback frequency from remote is low. The force feedback depends on the calculating speed of the virtual force. In this paper, two methods are combined to calculate the virtual force in VR environment, and feedback to the human operator in time.

Based on the mapping relationship of the robot hand and the VR environment, using the angle displacement of fingers on robot hand to instead of the move of the robot hand, and calculate the virtual force by Hooke's law. Then update the force feedback to the operator.

Use the insert-value method to extrapolate the virtual force based on time sequence, disperse the force value which is gotten in experiment and save to a database. Calculate the virtual force in VR environment as a symbol, and query from the database to extrapolate and feedback to the human operator. This will achieve smooth force feedback and conquer the impulse of the force feedback.

The force changes because of the move of the robot hand which made the distortion of face-contacted of the object. Considered the characteristics of the robot hand, the angle displacement of fingers R is referred to the position changes P of the fingers. While the angle displacement is easier to get than the position change, the angle displacement is used to instead the distortion of the face-contacted in virtual force calculation. This approximation will reduce the calculation of virtual force. The t time virtual force $F(t)$ changes from

$$F(t) = \begin{cases} f(P_n) & t = n \\ f(a_{n+i}) & n < t < n+1 \end{cases} \tag{13}$$

$$F(t) = \begin{cases} f(R_n) & t = n \\ f(a_{n+i}) & n < t < n+1 \end{cases} \tag{14}$$

Function f is referred to the mapping of the angle displacement and it can be query in the database, P_n referred to the position of the finger, R_n referred to the angle displacement of the finger, $f(a_{n+i})$ referred to the extrapolation of the virtual force.

4.1 Virtual Force Extrapolation Based on Material Characteristics

Calculating speed of the virtual force is not fast enough to catch up human operator's feeling. An extrapolation of virtual force based on material characteristics by testing in experiment is studied in this paper. The approaches are:

1. Operate the HIT/DLR robot hand to grasp object and save the force value and draw a curve.
2. Disperse the force value and save to the database
3. Using the calculated virtual force in the VR environment as a symbol, extrapolate the virtual force.

An angle displacement R_n is gotten in every refresh of the VR environment. The virtual force is calculated by function $F(t) = f(R_n)$. Query the most near force value $f(a_n)$ in database, feedback $f(a_n) \dots f(a_{n+i})$ to human operator until next update of VR. The calculation should judge the grasp and release action to decide the orientation of the extrapolation. The extrapolation of $F(t_n)$ is

$$F(t) = \begin{cases} F(t_n) & t = t_n \\ F(a_{n+i}) & t_n < t < t_{n+1} \\ F(t_{n+1}) & t = t_{n+1} \end{cases} \tag{15}$$

The process is shown as fig5

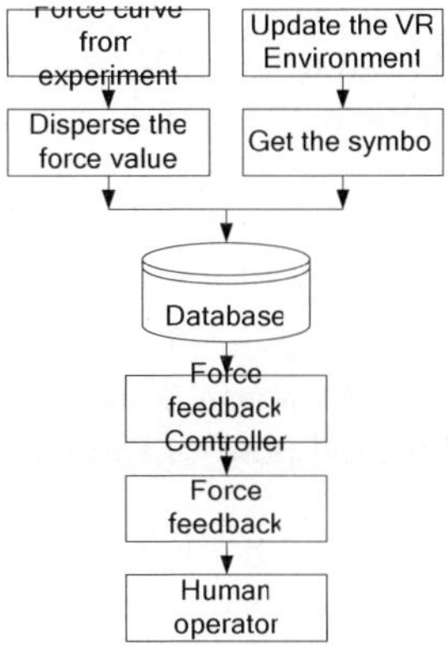

Fig. 5. The approach of virtual force extrapolate

This extrapolation of virtual force is based on material characteristics, so the extrapolation is very close to the real force feedback. The next update and re-query will avoid the accumulative errors.

5 Experiment Setup

The operator interacts with the virtual slave in the master side. The virtual slave provides VR environment to simulate the real slave side and graphic feedback to the operator. The tele-operation commands are examined in virtual slave to be inerrant before send to the robot in slave side by transmission network. At the same time, the slave side feedback remote sensor to master side. The master side updates the VR environment of virtual slave and provides force feedback to the operator by CyberGrasp equipment. Operator makes decision by those feedback information and step on the next operation (fig7).

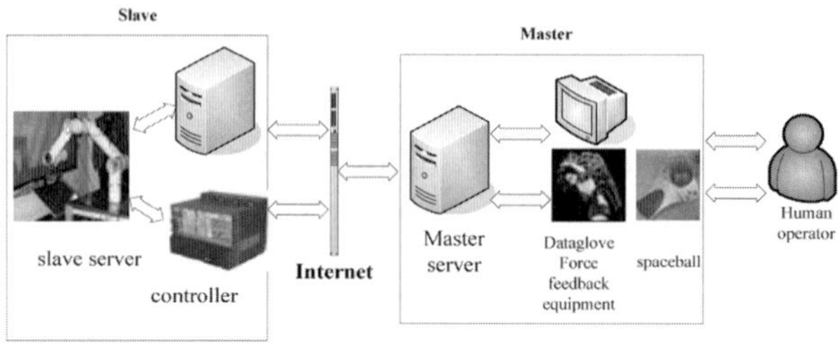

Fig. 6. Force feedback tele-operation based on VR

A 4DOF robot arm and a 4-finger robot hand (13DOF) are used as the slave robot system in this tele-operation experiment. Spaceball 5000 (6DOF) is used as a input equipment to operate the robot arm and CyberGlove dataglove is used to operate the robot hand, while CyberGrasp is used as the force feedback equipment. Through the internet, a tele-operation experiment between Wuhan and Harbin was held to push to unfolding the invalid sun panels and to wipe the polluted camera lens on the satellite. A time-vary delay was added in the transmission network to simulate the maintenance on the of airspace equipment.

When the tele-operation started, the contact was established between the master & slave side, initialized by the remote sensor feedback.

- With the help of local VR environment, the operator use the Spaceball to move remote robot system (including robot arm & hand) to approach the sun panel
- When reaches the panel, adjust the pose of robot arm and initialize the robot hand to grasp
- Grasp the handle on the sun panel with robot hand by using CyberGlove dataglove, the force feedback is provided by Cybergrasp equipment so that the operator could confirm a stable grasp to the handle
- Program a path and push the sun panel to a correct position
- Release the handle and take back the robot system in the slave side

Wave variable method is used in tele-operation system to reduce the impact of time-delay. The experiment shows that the force feedback becomes smooth by extrapolating virtual force (fig7).

Obviously, the force feedback is smoother when virtual force extrapolation is used. The disadvantage of this method is the material characteristics should be tested beforehand.

Because of the transmission delay, the force sensor and the position statement information are delayed in the master side. The impact of time delay is reduced by importing wave variable. The command from the master side and the sensor feedback from slave side of the robot's first joint are shown in fig8.

The tele-operation system is stable during the experiment.

(a) (b)

Fig. 7. The Force-feedback results with & without virtual force extrapolate, (a) is virtual force feedback without extrapolation, (b) is virtual force feedback with extrapolation

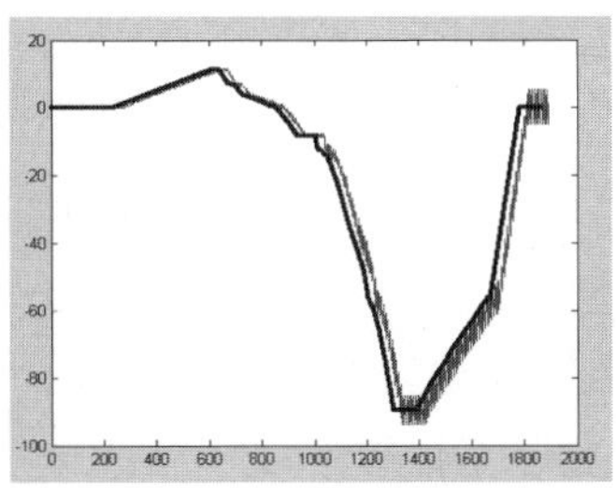

Fig. 8. The command from the master side and the sensor feedback. The blue curve is the command and the red curve is the sensor feedback.

6 Conclusion and Future Work

A wave variable based tele-operation system with force feedback is analyzed in this paper. The stabilization of the tele-operation system imported wave variable is discussed by using passive theory. By calculating virtual force and extrapolation, a smooth force feedback is provided to human operator, and an immersion is provided as well. In future, the stabilization of tele-operation system needed to be studied under time-vary delay. A new virtual force algorithm is required to reduce the reliance to the material characteristics.

Acknowledgments

The research works are generously funded by CAST foundation of China. And the authors thank Dr. Ming Xie of Nanyang Technological University for providing useful insights contributing to this work.

References

1. Kim, W.S.: Computer Vision Assisted Virtual Reality Calibration. IEEE Transactions On Robotics And Automation 15(4), 450–464 (1999)
2. Hirzinger, G., Brunner, B.: ROTEX— The First Remotely Controlled Robot in Space. In: IEEE International Conference on Robotics and Automation, pp. 2604–2611 (1994)
3. Oda, M., Kibe, K., Yamagata, F.: ETS-VII, Space Robot In-Orbit Example Satellite. In: IEEE International Conference on Robotics and Automations, pp. 739–744 (1996)

4. Jun, Z., Ping, Q., Zengqi, S.: Distributed telerobotic system with large time delay. Journal of Tsinghua University 40(1), 80–83 (2000) (in Chinese)
5. Sheridan, T.B.: Space tele-operation through time delay: review and prognosis. IEEE Trans on Robotic and Automation 9(5), 593–606 (1993)
6. Niemeyer, G.: Using Wave Variables in Time Delayed Force Reflecting Tele-operation [M]. PhD thesis, MIT, Cambridge, MA (September 1996)
7. Lawrence, D.A.: Stability and transparency in bilateral tele-operation. IEEE trans. Robotics and Automation 9(5), 624–637 (1993)
8. Hashtrudi-Zaad, K., Salcudean, S.E.: Transparency in time-delayed systems and the effect of local force feedback for transparent tele-operation. IEEE trans. Robotics and Automation 18(1), 108–114 (2002)
9. Adams, R.J., Hannaford, B.: Stable haptic interaction with virtual environments. IEEE transaction on Robotics and Automation 15(3), 465–474 (1999)
10. Xiong, Y., Li, S., Xie, M.: Predictive display and interaction of telerobots based on augmented reality. Robotica 24(1), 447–453 (2005)

On-Line Simulation for Shop Floor Control in Manufacturing Execution System

Yunqing Rao, Fei He, Xinyu Shao, and Chaoyong Zhang

State Key Laboratory of Digital Manufacturing Equipment and Technology, Huazhong University of Science and Technology, Wuhan, Hubei Province, China
Mackintosh_Storm@163.com

Abstract. This paper presents and discusses the structure and components of a novel on-line simulation system for real-time shop floor control in manufacturing execution system (MES). The framework of the simulation system is constructed in association with a MES. The on-line simulation system can collect data from physical shop floor and communicate with a scheduling controller through the MES. Furthermore, MES can provide much of the dynamic information required by the simulation model, and can also execute the shop floor control strategy which is solved by the simulation system. A multi-pass simulation method is introduced and applied to control the shop floor.

Keywords: On-Line Simulation; Shop floor control; Manufacturing Execution System.

1 Introduction

Increasing economic pressure has steadily driven manufactures toward partial or complete automation of their production facilities, and the manufacturing companies are always investing large sums of money in advanced production facilities such as computer hardware and software, robotics, automated material handling, machine tools and so on. However, the result of better quality, less direct labor and faster throughput which are expected by the use of the facilities have not been reached in many cases. One of the primary reasons for this is the difficulty involved in scheduling and controlling manufacturing activities in a dynamic environment on the shop floor [1]. Therefore the manufacturing planning, scheduling and control systems should be able to be dynamically adapted to the changing requirements and unforeseen situations in the shop floor.

This paper presents and develops a real-time shop floor decision making system which is based on the simulation technology. Simulation is commonly used to gain insight into manufacturing systems, and is based on a logical model of how a series of processes interact combined with statistical and deterministic information about the individual process.

Traditionally, simulation has been applied to the long-term planning, design and analysis of manufacturing systems. These models have been termed as "throw away models" because they are seldom used after the initial plans or designs are finalized [2]. In recent years, as opposed to the traditional use of simulation, there has been an

C. Xiong et al. (Eds.): ICIRA 2008, Part II, LNAI 5315, pp. 141–150, 2008.

increasing trend towards integrating the simulation model with the shop floor control system. Simulation can be used as a tool for real-time evaluation in manufacturing systems [3].

Although recent researchers have examined the responsibilities and underlying function of the on-line simulation, but they always view the simulation software as a "black box" and seldom examine its interaction with other system components [1]. Thus the research of the framework for on-line simulation system and its interaction with other system components is still needed.

Actually, the manufacturing execution system (MES), which can collect real-time production information and execute optimized task to increase manufacturing efficiency, is one of the typical shop floor control system [4]. Most of components such as data collection devices, control mechanism, and process planning functions in the MES can support the implementation of the on-line simulation.

Some researchers have mentioned the information transfer between the on-line simulation and MES. For example, Kouiss and Najid presented a combination of a MES and an on-line simulation model for controlling a flexible manufacturing system . Lee and Chan developed an object-oriented simulation for MES [5]. But none of these researchers has discussed the relationship between them, and the framework which integrate the on-line simulation and MES has not been constructed. These issues will discussed and solved all of these problems.

The structure of the remainder of the paper is as follows. After a brief review of the on-line simulation, the relationship between MES and on-line simulation is firstly analyzed, and then a general framework for the on-line simulation is constructed in section 4. The workflow how the on-line simulation can control the shop floor is shown in section 5, and the implementation of the on-line simulation is described in section 6. Finally, the conclusions are drawn.

2 A Review of On-Line Simulation

2.1 The Concept and Utilization of On-Line Simulation

The on-line discrete event simulation is a promising technology to support real-time decision makings on shop floor. Manivannan and Banks define on-line discrete event simulation as "a computerized system capable of performing both deterministic and stochastic simulation in real-time or quasi real-time, to monitor, control, and schedule parts and resources in a discrete part manufacturing environment" [6]. If the on-line simulation integrates with the information system, it can reach two powerful features: 1) the ability to reliably predict the future behavior of the shop floor, and 2) the ability to emulate and/or dictate the control logic of a manufacturing system.

Figure 1 shows the general information relationship between the on-line simulation and external software components. According to this architecture, the summarized utilization of on-line simulation can be described as follows, the first three of which are closely related to MES.

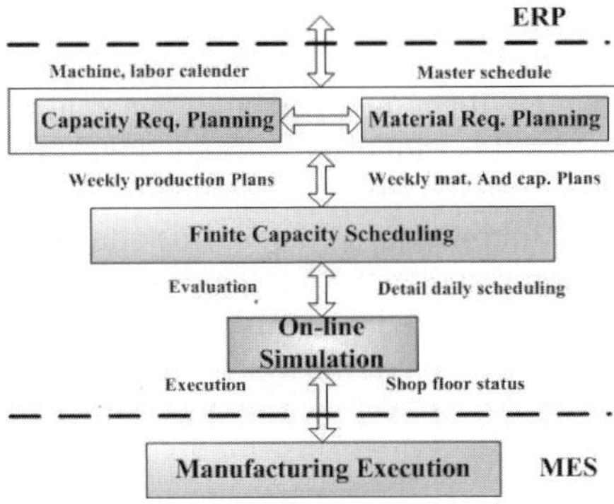

Fig. 1. General use of on-line simulation

Firstly, simulation can help capacity planners determine order lot sizes, release dates, and work calendars for resources by incorporating simulated scheduling constraints in their decision making [7].

Secondly, the simulation model can be initialized to the current state of the shop floor and a human scheduler can use it to predict the performance of alternative decision options to help make the most appropriate choice.

Thirdly, once the desired operational strategy and part mix have been determined, simulation can interact in real-time with shop floor management. Work lists can be generated and distributed to shop floor execution or dispatched on line in a task-by-task manner. Running parallel to the actual system in real-time allows the simulation system to keep track of current status and send feedback to the scheduling function on the current schedule's performance.

Fourthly, the simulation model would be to allow personnel to use it to predict order completion time for customers on-line. This application would ensure that promises made to customers were based on valid estimates of completion times.

Finally, the simulation system must interact with engineering for the necessary data to perform valid analysis. Simulation output can give feedback to the engineering function on the performance of a current design.

2.2 The Classification of On-Line Simulation

Generally, the on-line simulation based shop floor control approach can be classified into four categories: 1) general SRDM (Simulation-Based Real-time Decision-Making) approaches; 2) artificial intelligence-based approaches; 3) distributed system approaches; and 4) virtual manufacturing and/or virtual factory approach [8].

The general on-line simulation is always employed to evaluate a set of alternative scheduling algorithms such as heuristic and dispatching rules, and then to select the one with the best performance. For instance, Kim and Kim presented a simulation-based on-line scheduling mechanism for flexible manufacturing systems [9]. The simulation mechanism executes a series of simulation runs to evaluate a set of dispatching rules, and then the selected dispatching rule is applied to the shop floor.

Applications of artificial intelligence techniques for on-line simulation can conquer some drawbacks for the SRDM approach. For example, the performance highly depends on the quality of the candidate heuristic and dispatching rules. In recent years, most of the researches in this area have been focusing on knowledge-based approaches.

The distribution approach introduced to the on-line simulation can provide two important benefits. Firstly, they provide flexible environment for collaboration among components. Secondly, the distributed systems approach is adequate to model and simulate large-scale complex manufacturing systems.

In this paper, we focus on the SRDM approach as well as its communication with MES.

3 Relationship between On-Line Simulation and MES

As an integrated shop floor control system, MES can support manufacturing across a wide range of functions, including plant management and engineering, quality management, real-time supervisory control and monitoring. In order to implement the real-time process control, an on-line decision support system may be adapted to and integrated with the requirements of MES functions [10]. Then the on-line simulation which is one of the most important on-line decision tools can be combined with optimization tools for decision making and evaluation.

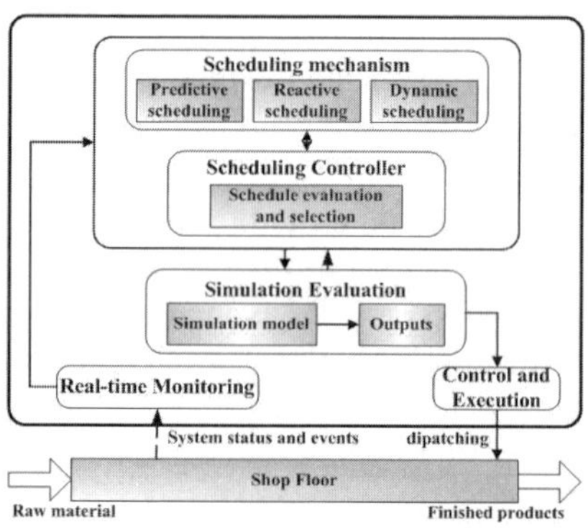

Fig. 2. The structure of a general on-line simulation system

In Figure 1, both the MES and ERP communicate with on-line simulation, but how the on-line simulation can control the shop floor has not been described more exactly. A more detailed control mechanism which the on-line simulation performs is shown in Figure 2.

A general on-line simulation system is composed of four components: a real-time monitoring system for collecting data from the physical shop floor; a simulator for generating simulation models, running simulations and analyzing simulation results; a decision-making system for generating decisions such as schedule components which contain scheduling mechanism and scheduling controller; and an execution system for controlling the shop floor [8].

The ***monitoring component*** receives events from the shop floor, and periodically monitors the performance of the shop floor. According to the information, the ***scheduling controller*** selects the better scheduling approaches for further simulation evaluation based on actual manufacturing conditions, and subsequently selects the best approach to be used on the shop floor.

The component of ***simulation evaluation*** includes a simulation model constructed based on the physical shop floor status from the factory database. When the scheduling controller passes control to simulation evaluation, a series of simulation runs are initialized with the generated schedules under the same stochastic conditions. The ***control and execution component*** sends all scheduling control information to the shop floor and dispatches jobs to the machines accordingly.

Actually, except the simulator, all the other components are also the functions of MES. For example, the scheduling module is one of the most important components to control the production process and WIP in MES.

According to MESA (Manufacturing Execution System Association International), the full functions of MES include: 1) resource allocation and status; 2) operation and detailed scheduling; 3) dispatching production units; 4) document control; 5) data collection and acquisition; 6) labor management; 7) quality management; 8) process management; 9) maintenance management; 10) product tracking and genealogy; 11) performance analysis.

By this classification, the components numbered by 1, 5 and 10 can be seen as the monitoring component. The first and fifth components can provide the most static information to support the simulator generate simulation models, "Product Tracking and Genealogy" can collect the dynamic process information especially the disturbance information to direct the on-line decision making.

The second and third components can be regarded as the scheduling controller component. "Operations and Detailed Scheduling" is used for medium-term or short-term schedule control, which can provide sequencing based on priorities, attributes, characteristics, and/or recipes associated with specific production units. "Dispatching Production Units" can manage flow of production units in the form of jobs, orders, batches, lots, and work orders.

"Process Management" can monitor production and provide decision support to operators for correcting and improving in-process activities. These activities may be intra-operational and focus specifically on machines or equipment being monitored and controlled as well as inter-operational, which is tracking the process from one operation to the next. "Process Management" can provide more powerful function than control and execution component in the simulation system.

Moreover, other components in the MES can also provide important information to on-line simulation and make some decisions. For example, "Labor Management" can provide status of personnel in and up-to-the-minute time frame. By the information, the on-line simulation can evaluate the prior production calendar and rank a better one. "Quality Management" and "Maintenance Management" can also provide the processing information and equipment information to ensure the schedule controller to make a better scheduling scheme to adapt the physical shop floor environment.

According to these analyses, it can be conclude that there exist a sophisticate relationship between on-line simulation and MES. MES can provide more reality and exactly real-time information to the simulator which can ensure the simulator to solve the most correct production plan. Meanwhile, the best scheduling results can be delivered to the physical shop floor more rapidly by the MES.

4 General Framework

As analyzed in section 3, on-line simulation can be regarded as one component of MES. Figure 3 shows a general software infrastructure of MES which incorporates the simulation function.

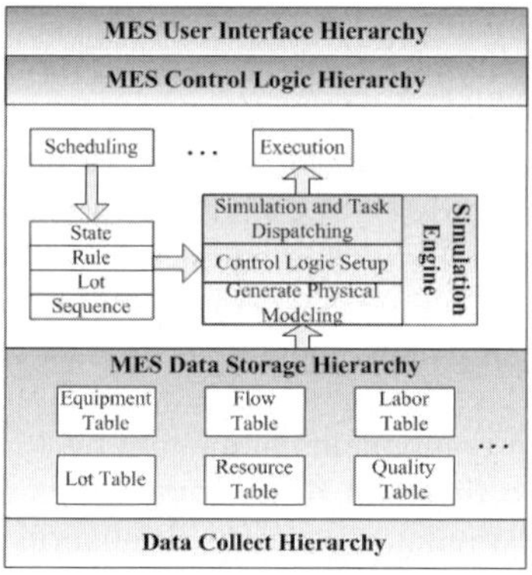

Fig. 3. General software infrastructure of MES include simulation function

Traditionally, the software infrastructure of MES can be classified as three hierarchies which are user interface hierarchy, control logic hierarchy and data storage hierarchy. The simulation component which is integrated with MES can also be structured by this three hierarchy format.

User interface hierarchy is used to show the simulation modeling, simulation process and simulation results, and it can alternate information between users and software system.

Control logic hierarchy includes three functional elements of the simulation which are physical model generation, control logic setup, simulation and task dispatching. Physical model generation is the definition of machines, people, tooling, transporters, and storage areas in the facility, as well as layout and decision points of the manufacturing process. Control logic setup is to integrate the operation rules, simulation run-time parameters, and exception handling into the physical model. Task dispatching is the simulator's I/O link with external components for task dispatching and the protocol of these messages. In Figure 3, the simulation engine contains these three elements and exchange information with other components.

Data storage hierarchy supports the input and output of the simulation. Simulation inputs contain the product definitions, product demand, work calendars and so on. Simulation outputs contain start- and end-times for tasks in the system. These times may include additional "tag" information such as task codes, affected products, or utilized resources.

In order to describe the relationship between the MES components and on-line simulation, Figure 4 is introduced and showing a complete modeling and emulates process.

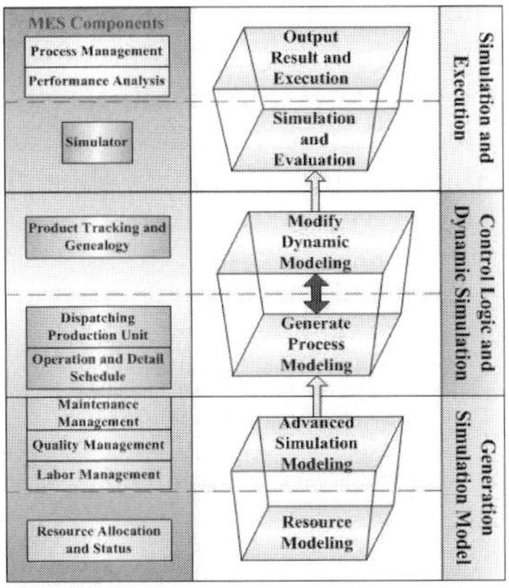

Fig. 4. Modeling and simulation process in MES

Firstly, by communicating with the "Resource Allocation and Status" component, resource modeling can be constructed. This model just considers the number and types of physical facilities in the workshop such as machines, tooling, transporters, buffers and the layout of these facilities. Advanced simulation modeling is conducted by using the date obtained from "maintenance management", "quality management" and "labor management" to modify and expand the resource modeling. By this advanced model, a more detailed and exact simulation experiment can be carried out, and the results may match the physical shop floor environment more exactly.

The process modeling is used to define how the resources are used to test the product. In a typical back-end operation the same devices may be processed using different steps due to the fact that one device corresponds to multiple products. In addition a proportion of products have alternative operation routes. All of these process routes can be provided by the "Operation and Detail Schedule". By "Production Tracking and Genealogy", the current status can be used to modify the simulation modeling and feedback to the scheduling component to generate a new schedule strategy.

After the simulation experiments, the alternative results are compared and the best one can be executed by the "Process Management" component.

5 Shop Floor Control by On-Line Simulation

Traditionally, simulation is always associated with scheduler to control the shop floor. By emulating the alternative schedule strategies, the best scheme can be executed in the physical shop floor. But this method can not deal with some various unexpected events more rapidly. In order to solve these problems, Young J.S. has proposed a multi-pass simulation method [1]. The multi-pass simulation is composed of two simulations – a real time simulation and a preview simulation.

In this paper, the multi-pass simulation concept is employed, but the workflow is changed in order to adapt the software infrastructure of MES. In our approach, the preview simulation is used to evaluate the prior schedule scheme and the real-time simulation acts as a real-time shop floor controller. The workflow of the simulation is shown in Figure 5, and the approach is composed of four steps as described bellow.

Step 1: Initial schedule development: Various scheduling algorithms, rules, Petri nets, are used for off-line initial scheduling. The output of this step is several schedule schemes which is fed to the preview simulation, through a dynamic database, for implementation. This dynamic database includes: part arrival time, part processing time, setup time, parts completion time, resources allocation time, transfer time, and breakdown time.

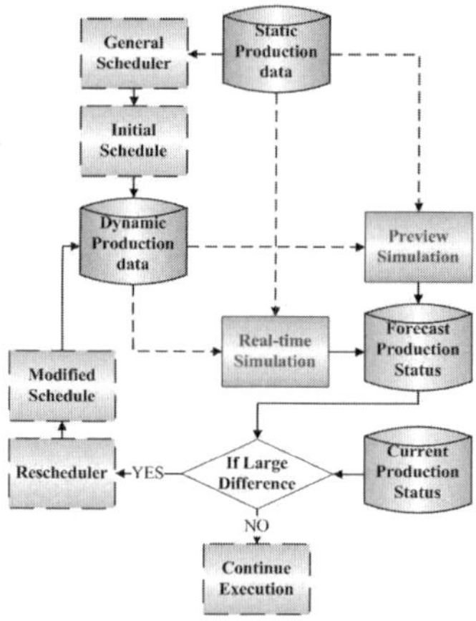

Fig. 5. Workflow of simulation process to control the shop floor

Step 2: **Preview simulation model implementation.** A preview simulation model of the manufacturing system is first implemented according to the input data obtained from the current actual manufacturing system and the dynamic date given by step 1, and then the best simulation result is executed.

Step 3: **Compare execution results.** By the collection of current production status through the MES, the physical production condition and simulation results can be compared. If the difference is remarkable, it means that the preview simulation result can not be executed continuously, so a new schedule and simulation must be implemented, and the simulation process can skip to step 4. If the different is slight, the simulation result can be executed continuously

Step 4: **Rescheduling.** According to the current status of the manufacturing system, rescheduling algorithms are invoked to revise the original schedule. The modified schedule is then updated into the simulation model. The results of the on-line simulation execution are stored in a database and then be executed in the physical shop floor.

By selecting the best simulation result, the shop floor can be controlled more rapidly and exactly. But the method has a disadvantage that is difficult to decide the best point when the rescheduling and real-time simulation can be executed. Generally, the value of this point is always given according to the experience, but the value may not be exact. And more research on this problem must be carried out in the future.

6 Implementation

In this paper, Plant Simulation^{TM} is applied as the target simulation software. Plant Simulation defines the standard for object-oriented, graphical and integrated modeling, simulation and animation of systems and business processes. It contains three important functions to support the implementation of on-line simulation integrate with MES.

Firstly, the socket component supports real-time shop operation coordination via TCP/IP communication capability. A socket object is provided in the Plant Simulation class library, where the connection to the other application is defined.

Secondly, the Plant Simulation ODBC is the interface for bidirectional communication between Plant Simulation and diverse ODBC servers.

Thirdly, the integrated language Sim Talk can create the simulation model graphically and interactively. However, it can also automatically create a model based on the parameters entered from external software system.

According to these three functions, the simulation system can get the static information from the database easily and obtain the real-time information from physical shop floor immediately. The result solved by the simulation model can also be saved and executed. Otherwise, the simulation model can be generated and changed immediately no matter when the simulation system is off-line or being executed. Figure 6 shows the main window of simulation model.

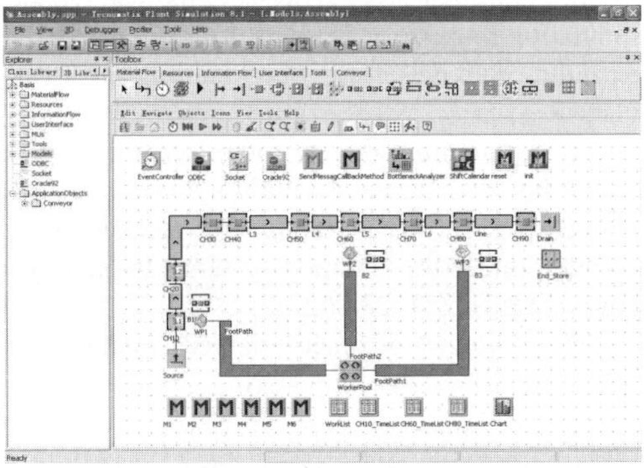

Fig. 6. The main window of simulation model

The major structure of MES software is developed by the JAVA techniques, using ORACLE as DBMS, and adopting the three hierarchies of B/S model to actualize the scenario of shop floor control with the on-line simulation. The simulation engine is triggered by MES, and the control program is written in operation logistic hierarchy.

7 Conclusion

In this paper, a novel on-line simulation system integrated with the MES is presented. The simulation system can improve the production efficiency through the information interaction with the physical shop floor and schedule control system.

Firstly, the relationship between on-line simulation and MES is discussed. The analysis shows that the simulation has a sophisticate relationship with MES, and it can be regarded as one important component in the MES. Through associating with the components of MES, the integrated simulation can reach more capability than a single simulation system. Secondly, a general framework is constructed, in which some components of MES are integrated with the process of simulation modeling. Then a mutli-pass simulation method is presented, where the four steps for controlling shop floor are demonstrated. Finally, the Plant Simulation^{TM} is employed to implement the on-line simulation.

Acknowledgement

This research work is partially supported by the National High Technology Research and Development Program of China (863 Program) under Grant #2007AA04Z186 and #2007AA04Z107, National Natural Science Foundation of China under Grant No. 50775089.

References

1. Son, Y., Rodriguez-Rivera, H., Wysk, R.A.: A multi-pass simulation-based, real-time scheduling and shop floor control system. Transactions: The Quarterly Journal of the Society for Computer Simulation International 16(4), 159–172 (1999)
2. Thomson, M.B.: Expanding Simulation Beyond Planning and Design. Industrial Engineering 26(10), 65–67 (1994)
3. Rogers, P., Gordon, R.j.: Simulation for real-time decision making in manufacturing systems. In: Proceedings of the 1993 Winter Simulation Conference, pp. 866–874 (1993)
4. Choi Byoung, K., Kim Byung, H.: MES (manufacturing execution system) architecture for FMS compatible to ERP (enterprise planning system). International Journal of Computer Integrated Manufacturing 15(3), 274–284 (2002)
5. Lee, A., Chan, H.: A Development of objec-oriented simulator for manufacturing execution systems. Computers and Industrial Engineering 37, 239–242 (1999)
6. Manivannan, S., Banks, J.: Design of a knowledge-based on-line simulation system to control a manufacturing shop floor. IIE Transactions 24, 72–83 (1992)
7. Drake, G.R., Smith, J.S.: Simulation system for real-time planning, scheduling, and control. In: Proceedings of the 28th conference on winter simulation, pp. 1083–1089 (1996)
8. Yoon, H.J., Shen, W.: Simulation-based real-time decision making for manufacturing automation systems: a review. International Journal of Manufacturing Technology and Management. 8, 188–202 (2006)
9. Kim, M.K., Kim, Y.D.: Simulation-based real-time scheduling in a flexible manufacturing system. Journal of Manufacturing Systems 13, 83–85 (1994)
10. Iassinovski, S., Artiba, A., Fagnart, C.: A generic production rules-based system for on-line simulation decision making and discrete process control. International Journal of Production Economics 112(1), 62–76 (2008)

Realization of the Synchronization Mechanism of Step and Scan Projection Lithography

Liangliang Yang[1], Yunfei Zhou[1], Haihong Pan[2], and Wei Teng[1]

[1] Huazhong University of Science and Technology, Wuhan, China
[2] GuangXi University, Nanning, China
yigaoyang319@tom.com

Abstract. Analyze the synchronous motion process of the step and scan projection lithography. Classify the subsystems of the machine into synchronous master subsystems and synchronous slave subsystems; realize the state broadcasting of synchronous master subsystem by synchronous serial bus; analyze the communication among subsystems and their data-collection systems and realize the communication using high speed serial hotlink. In order to validate the synchronization mechanism, a synchronous experimental platform is established. The experimental result shows the system is stable, reliable and satisfied with the requirements of synchronization and engineering.

Keywords: Step and scan projection lithography; synchronization control; state synchronization; high speed high precision motion control.

1 Introduction

With size of DRAM、ASIC becoming larger and larger, the IC manufacturers are required to decrease the exposure times of silicon chip to enhance the efficiency and reduce the cost of lithography by increasing Numerical Aperture(NA) and enlarging the exposure field. Considering the trade-off between high exposure resolution and Depth of focus, the fabrication of lens with large exposure field and NA has reached the physical limit and become a bottleneck to block the improvement of IC manufacturing industry. Under this tough condition, Step and Scan Projection lithography become the key equipment in IC manufacturing industry. It utilizes the constant speed and linear scan motion of regular narrow image field to realize the exposure of large exposure field projecting on the silicon chip. Differed from the traditional step lithography, the quality of image exposed by the step and scan projection lithography depended on not only the optical system but also the dynamic position precision and dynamically synchronous tracking precision between reticle stage and wafer stage. As three most important criterions to evaluate the performance of lithography: exposure precision、overlay precision and efficiency, it is required that the lithography should reach position precision、motion precision and synchronization precision of nanometer level. For example, A commercialized wafer stepper, PAS5500, the step and scan projection lithography of ASML, the reticle stage speed, wafer stage speed and acceleration of which reach 1000mm/s, 250mm/s, 10g respectively with the position error below 10nm and standard position error below 6nm.

C. Xiong et al. (Eds.): ICIRA 2008, Part II, LNAI 5315, pp. 151–161, 2008.

The Synchronization Mechanism is one of the most key technologies of the Step and Scan Projection Lithography. During process of the silicon exposure, cooperation is needed among different subsystems, In case synchronous timing requirements are not met with, the synchronous error will be produced and nanometer level precision of the motion control is unable to achieve, which leads to silicon exposure failure. For example, if the synchronous timing error of 10ns is existed between the wafer stage and reticle stage, 2.5nm of the synchronous displacement error will be produced on the exposure field during exposure process. Therefore, how to coordinate the timing between various subsystems which involved in the working process efficiently to achieve the synchronization required by actual application becomes a key issue to be discussed.

Synchronization mechanism involved in various subsystems was seldom discussed in current literatures. Reference [1] put forward a method using uniform clock with high frequency produced by RF monofier to realize synchronization between short pulse laser and synchronous accelerated radiator. Reference [2] proposed a method applied in laser intelligent manufacturing system to realize synchronization. However, the above proposed synchronization method could not be directly applied to the step and scan projection lithography due to the different characteristics among control targets. Though reference [3] proposed a synchronous control algorithm applied to the step and san projection lithography, it only discussed about the control algorithm not about the realization of the clock synchronization of the hardware layer. Aimed at solving the above mentioned questions, this paper classifies the subsystems of step and scan projection lithography involved in synchronous motion into two categories: synchronous master subsystems and synchronous slave subsystems and suggests the following questions should be taken into account through analyzing working principle and motion characteristics of the machine: First of all, the classification of various subsystems; Second of all, the states and state-jumping diagram of master and slave respectively; The third, the state synchronization between master and slave; The last one, sampling synchronously among all subsystem. And this paper is organized as follow: the first paragraph discusses the working process of the step and scan projection lithography. The second paragraph analyzes the synchronous motion of the step and scan projection lithography and the timing of every subsystem involved in synchronization. The third paragraph classifies the subsystems involved in synchronization into master subsystems and slave subsystems and discusses how to realize the state synchronization between two categories of subsystems. The forth paragraph discusses the synchronously sampling among all subsystems and how to realize it. The fifth and the last paragraphs establish an experimental platform to verify the synchronization mechanism of the step and scan projection lithography and the experimental data and diagrams are demonstrated to show that feasibility and reliability of the proposed synchronization mechanism.

2 The Working Principle of Step and Scan Projection Lithography

The structure of step and scan projection lithography is demonstrated in the figure 1, the reticle stage is used to place mask with schematics and the wafer stage is used to place the wafer on which the schematics is projected and exposed field by field through alignment scan, leveling and focus scan and exposure scan using short pulse laser and shrunken lens with big NA. the step and scan projection lithography consisted of the following subsystems: step stage and wafer stage motion control subsystem, shutter motion control subsystem, alignment and leveling and focus subsystem, projection and lens control subsystem, laser position measure subsystem and a global control system. The process of exposure comprised with a series of step-scan motions which is explained as follow:

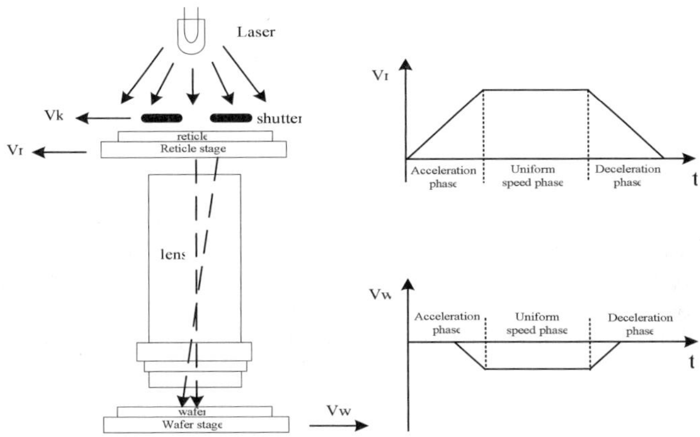

Fig. 1. Working principle of step and scan projection lithography

During the process of current step-scan, the global control system obtains the minimum prepare time and scan time of all subsystems associated with the synchronous motion by negotiations with them and plans the time sequence, which is a sequence pair of state-time. Then, the global control system respectively writes the planed sequence pair of state-time into the state FIFO and duration FIFO located in the reticle stage and wafer stage motion control subsystem before accomplishment of current step-scan. After the beginning of the next step-scan, the state-time sequence pairs jump from the state FIFO and duration FIFO pair by pair and is broadcasted to all subsystem through synchronous bus before synchronous machine clock comes which means the synchronous time point then the new state lasts for the time of state-time pair. At that time, all other subsystems keep monitoring the state broadcasted on the synchronous bus and receiving the state in their own buffer, once synchronous machine clock comes and the state in the buffer is the one interested by the subsystem, a pre-set time sequence of the subsystems will be carried out. After the time of state-time pair expires, the new state-time sequence pair jumps from the FIFOs again. The whole wafer will be exposed though repetition of the process mentioned above. A whole process of exposure consisted of placing, aligning, leveling and focusing, exposing, fetching. And the scan stages comprised with reticle stage and wafer stage are the mainly moving part of step and scan projection lithography with the characteristic of point-to-point path. Namely, the path is divided into three phases: acceleration phase, constant speed phase and deceleration phase. There may not be constant speed phase existing in the point-to-point path planning in other applications according to the limit of speed, acceleration and distance but in the application of step and scan projection lithography there must be a constant speed phase. Because when the shutter opens, only a part of the schematics is projected on the wafer due to the limitation of the lens. Therefore, having a constant speed phase is the characteristics of step and scan projection lithograph.

3 Synchronous Motion Analyzing of Step and Scan Projection Lithography

There are three kinds of step-scan motion used by the step and scan projection lithography. They are exposure scan, leveling and focus scan, alignment scan, all paths of which are point-to-point. All of the three motions are different in functions but are similar to their algorithm of path planning.

Every mechanical system has a limited control bandwidth; hence, a step input can not be tracked accurately because of its infinite bandwidth. In order to avoid an undesired output response, a third-order position S-profile with a limited input bandwidth is used in the mechanical system so that the output position can track the reference command accurately. Equation (1) governs the third-order S-profile generation.

$$\begin{cases} \dfrac{da(t)}{dt} = \{J_{\max}, 0, -J_{\max}\} \\ v(t) = \int a(t)dt \\ s(t) = \int v(t)dt \end{cases} \tag{1}$$

where $a(t)$, $v(t)$, and $s(t)$ are acceleration, velocity, and position of the S-profile respectively, while $J_{\max}$ is a preset jerk constant. For our motion control system of retical stage and wafer stage, two typical point to point position profiles derived from a pick-and-place automation machine need to be tracked. The frequently tracked short-distance position profile is shown in A of figure 2. Another long-distance position profile to be tracked is depicted in B of figure 2.

Based on the above mentioned algorithm of path planning, one of the synchronous motion processes of reticle stage and wafer stage, exposure scan, is indicated as below:

As figure 3 shows, the dot line is a speed curve of wafer stage and the solid line is reticle's. reticle stage starts to move at t0, the wafer stage starts to move towards the opposite direction at t1. They achieve their synchronous scan speed of v0 and v1 respectively at t2 after acceleration for a while and they come into the constant speed scan motion at t4 simultaneously after their respective settling time. Shutter NO.1 starts to move at t3 and has to open the narrow slot at t4 and stops moving at t5. The projection system begins to project the schematics evenly on the wafer by laser. After keep moving for an exposing time the wafer stage and reticle stage stop scan-move and enter into the deceleration motion at t7 simultaneously. The projection system also shuts down the laser at t7 immediately. And Shutter No.2 starts to move to close the narrow slot. Wafer stage stops moving at t9 and reticle stage stops moving at t10. An exposure of an exposure field is finished until then. And then reticle stage and wafer stage enter into the next exposure scan for next exposure field. The laser position measure system keeps locking and sampling the position data during exposure scan process.

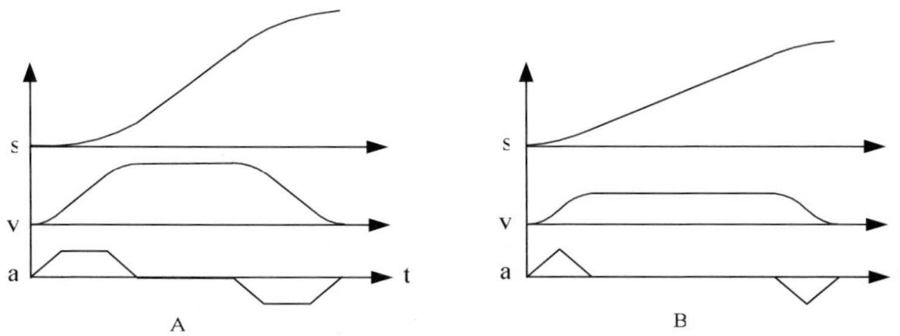

Fig. 2. Two frequently position profile

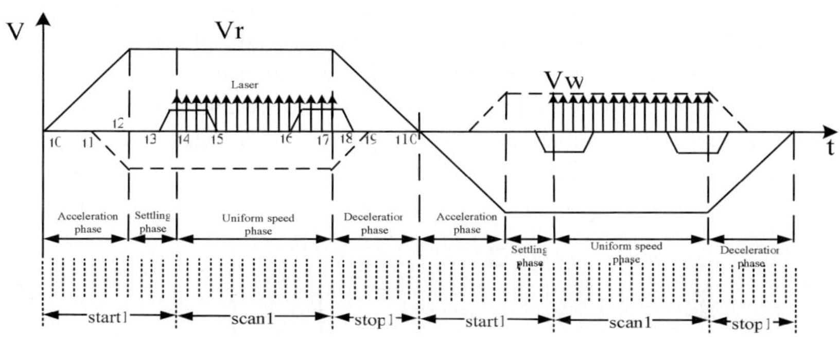

Fig. 3. Two synchronous exposure process of step and scan projection lithography

From the analyzing above, an exposure scan can be divided into three obvious phases: start phase which includes acceleration phase and the settling phase, scan phase which includes constant speed phase and stop phase which includes deceleration phase. In start phase, wafer stage and reticle stage are controlled to reach synchronous scan speed and settle for some time. And then, the two stages come into the constant speed scan phase and perform constant speed scan for a while, and then, the two stages come into the stop phase simultaneously. Therefore, the exposure scan can be divided into three states of start, scan, stop plus two states of end and error (entering into the error state when detecting an error). The duration time of each state is integer times of the servo interval obtained by negotiation. leveling and focus scan and alignment scan are also divided into these five states.

In the practical application, the algorithm of path planning and process of state jumping are realized in the digital signal processor according to the servo interrupt with frequency of 5 KHz. Therefore, they should be discretized before application. After discretization, the discrete expression of equation (1) is described in expression (2) and path planning corresponded to the state jump is illustrated in figure 3, the interval between two vertical dot lines in the figure 3 denotes a servo interval. Therefore the state of start of the exposure scan No.1 is composed of 12 servo intervals, the state of scan 14 servo intervals and state of stop 8 servo intervals respectively. The exposure scan No.2 is similar to No.1.

$$\begin{cases} a(k) = a(k-1) \\ v(k) = v(k-1) + a(k-1) \\ s(k) = s(k-1) + v(k-1) \end{cases} \qquad k = k+1 \tag{2}$$

4 The State Synchronization between Synchronous Master Systems and Synchronous Slave Systems

It is educed that the reticle stage and wafer stage motion control subsystem can be divided into five states of stop, start, scan, end and error from the analyzing of synchronous motion process and the duration time of each state is integer times of the servo interval. Other subsystems keep monitoring the state of the reticle stage and wafer stage motion control subsystem and run its own internal time sequence. Therefore the reticle stage and wafer stage motion control subsystem can be categorized as synchronous master subsystems and the other subsystems needed to be synchronized as synchronous slave subsystems.

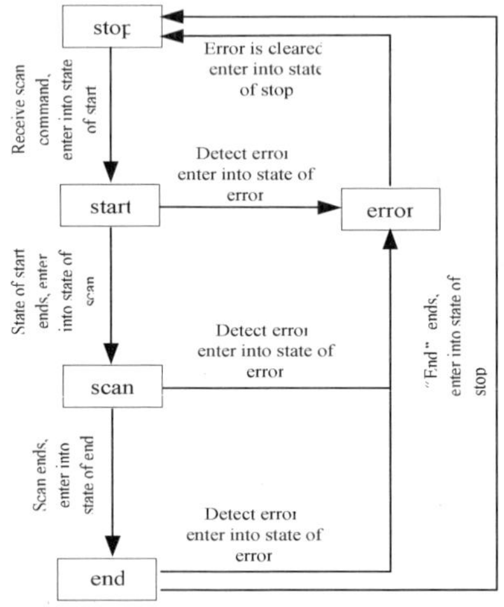

Fig. 4. State-jump diagram of step and scan projection lithography

The state jump diagram of synchronous master that is similar to the state jump diagram of step and scan projection lithography is demonstrated in the figure 4. Path is planed according to the permitted maxim velocity, maxim acceleration and interval of point-to-point through negotiations. The obtained sequence pairs of state-time after negotiations are written into the synchronous master. after receiving the "start" command the synchronous master starts to read the state-time pair by pair and sends the state of the pair though high speed serial synchronous bus.

The state jump diagram of synchronous slave is demonstrated in the figure 5.. There are two registers in every synchronous slave subsystem. One is trigger state register which is responsible for storing the state to be triggered. And the other is delay register which is responsible for time delay. When the two registers is set, the synchronous slaves are monitoring the high speed serial synchronous bus and keep comparing the new coming state with the trigger state in the state register at the synchronous time point. When the new coming state is same to the trigger state, the synchronous slave delay for the set time in the delay register and run the internal time sequence automatically after finishing time delay.

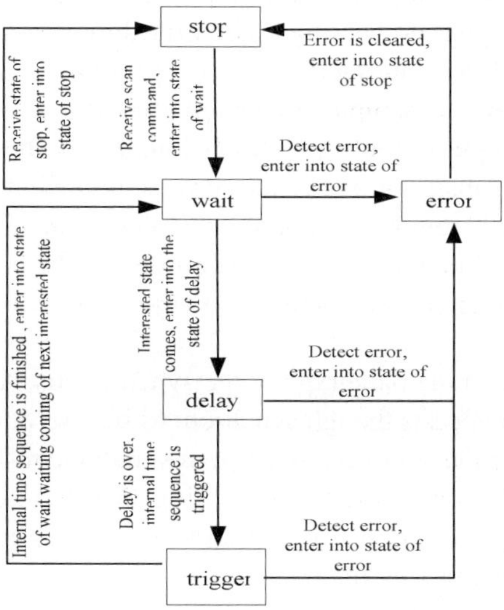

Fig. 5. State-jump diagram of synchronous slave subsystems

The synchronous state communicated between synchronous master systems and synchronous slave systems are broadcasting through high speed serial synchronous bus which is demonstrated in figure 6. The synchronous bus is composed of three serial lines, one is clock line, another is input line and the third is output line. The synchronous master system uses the output line to send the 4 bits synchronous state and 1 bit checkout code serially to the synchronous slave system and uses the input line to receive the 2 bits state and 1 bit checkout code from the synchronous slave system as one of the judgments for state-jump. In order to avoid the noise from other electric devices the synchronous bus use differential signal to transfer state and use odd to avoid transfer error.

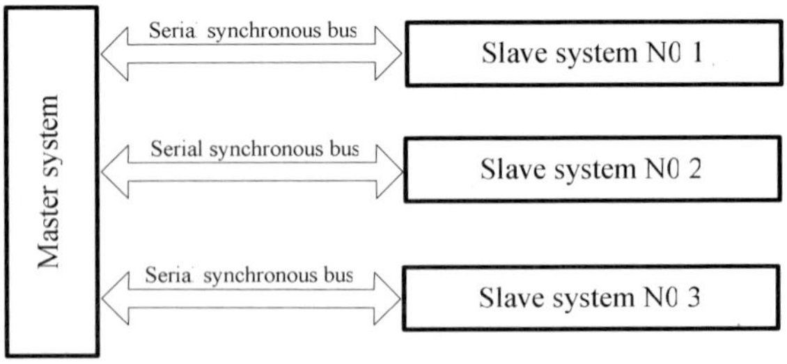

Fig. 6. The connective diagram between master system and slave system

5 The Synchronous Communication between Subsystems and Their Remote Input-Output Module

Every subsystem of step and scan projection lithography has its own digital signal processing boards. For example, reticle stage and wafer stage motion control subsystem has 7 digital signal processing boards for digital signal processing and there are two high speed fiber interfaces on every digital signal processing board to communicate with remote sample or actuator boards called remote input-output module. All remote input-output modules belonging to the reticle stage and wafer stage motion control subsystem are required to sample simultaneously and the time difference between two remote input-output modules should be less than 0.5us. In order to meet the real-time requirement, the burden of the communication should be low and the communication delay should be adjustable with precision of microsecond level.

From the analyzing in the paragraph 3, the synchronous state of step and scan projection lithography broadcasts though synchronous bus, so does the sample command. Synchronous bus controller of every subsystem simultaneously broadcasts the sample command to its entire digital signal processing boards after receiving the sample command and the command is sent to the remote input-output module by fiber interface on the digital signal processing board.

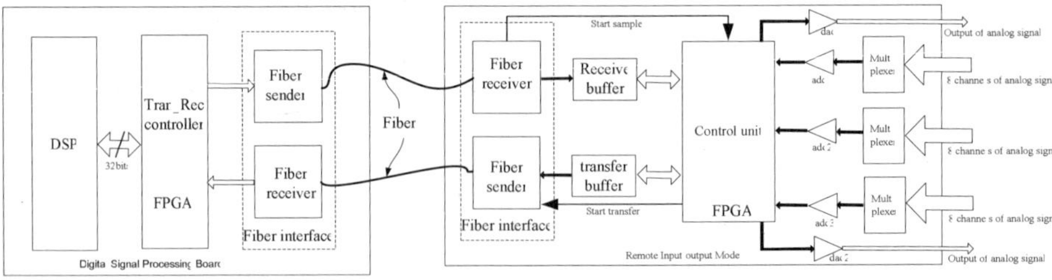

Fig. 7. The structure of the remote input-output module and the connection diagram

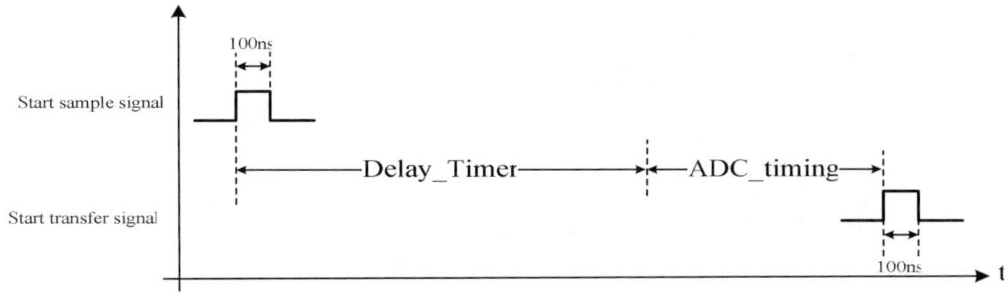

Fig. 8. The working timing of remote input-output module

Considering the great characteristics of FPGA (field programmable gate array), such as high density, high clock frequency, precise time sequence control and flexibility of programming, the fiber interface and the control part of the remote input-output module are realized by FPGA. When the remote input-output module receives the sample command (RX_TRIGGER) coming from the fiber interface, the remote input-output module enters into the wait state waiting for an preset time (TX_TIMER).when the preset time is over, controller module in FPGA generates a trigger signal to sample 24 ADC channels serially. When the samples of all channels are over, a "start transfer" signal is generated by the controller module in FPGA to the fiber interface on the remote input-output module for transferring the sampling data to the digital signal processing board. The structure of the remote input-output module and the connection between it and digital signal processing board is demonstrated in figure 7. And the remote input-output module working timing is demonstrated in figure 8.

6 Experiment and Result

An experimental platform demonstrated in figure 9 is established to prove the feasibility of the principles discussed above. The circuit boards in the figure are self-made. The synchronous bus controller and one of 7 digital signal processing board are placed in the same VME rack. The digital signal processing board and two remote input-output modules are connected by fibers. Based on this experimental platform, the synchronous state transfer between synchronous master system and synchronous slave system and synchronous data sampling between digital signal processing boards and the remote input-output module synchronous slave are proved feasible.

In the experiment, a logical analyzer built in the synchronous bus controller is used to monitor and trace the process of the communication between synchronous master system and synchronous slave systems which is demonstrated in figure 10. The servo interval is 200us and the machine state is read from the synchronous state register and sent to all subsystems every servo interval through synchronous serial bus. (Showed in ellipses in the figure 10).

Also, a logical analyzer built in the remote input-output module is used to monitor and trace the communication process between subsystems and remote input-output module, which is demonstrated in figure 11. when remote input-output module receives the sample command from fiber, a trigger is generated immediately and then three ADC triggers are generated to start sampling real-time data serially after delay of preset time. The timing of two signals, serial_clk and serial_datain used as communicating line between FPGA and ADC are demonstrated in figure 11.

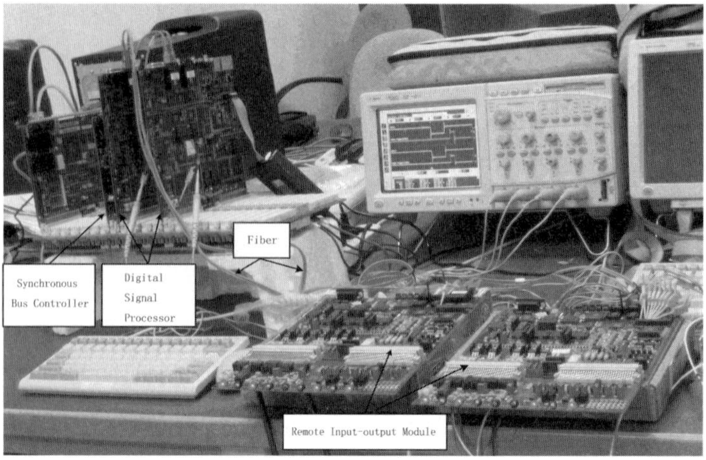

Fig. 9. The experimental platform of synchronization mechanism

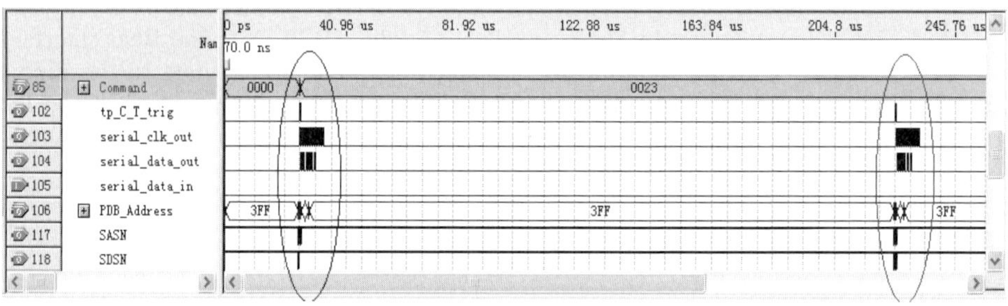

Fig. 10. The broadcast of states of synchronous master system

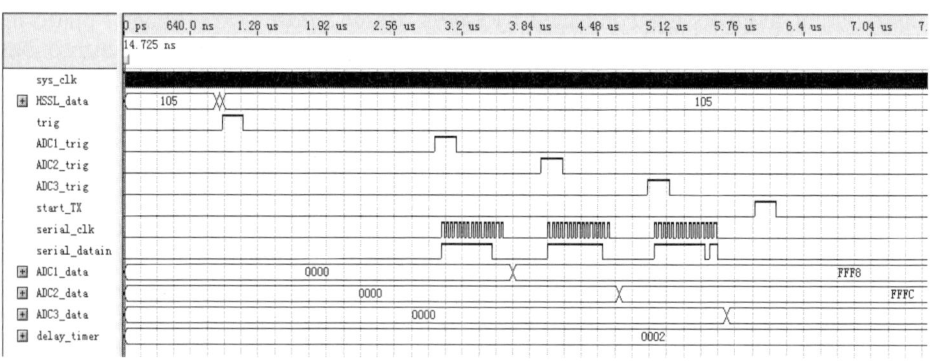

Fig. 11. Synchronously sampling of synchronous slave systems

7 Conclusion

Step and scan projection lithography is one of the most important machines applied in the IC manufacturing industry. Many technologies, such as field bus technology, programmable logical control, digital signal processes are used in the actual application to meet the requirement of high precision in the synchronous motion. Meanwhile, with the high precise synchronous control algorithm, the above synchronous hardware structure is applied to the actual application of step and scans projection lithography and has gained a good performance with nanometer level motion precision.

Acknowledgements

The authors acknowledge the financial supports from National Natural Science Foundation of China (No. 507775088). The authors also wish to thank Shanghai Nanpre Mechanics Co. Ltd. which provided valuable suggestions and experimental assistance.

References

1. Yosibito, T.: Synchronization of picosecond laser pulses to the target X-ray pulses at spring-8. J. Nuclear Instruments and Methods in Physics Research A 467, 1451–1454 (2001)
2. He, X.J., Hu, G.: Realization of synchronous control in laser intelligent manufacturing system. J. Chinese Journal of Mechanical Engineering 40, 126–130 (2004)
3. Hu, X.X., Tai, X.Q., Yang, K.J.: Study on the synchronizing Control and Wafer Deformation Error Compensation Technology for Step Scanning Photoetching Machine. J. Chinese Journal of Mechanical Engineering 15, 192–195 (2004)
4. Pahk, H.J., Lee, D.S., Park, J.H.: Ultra Precision Positioning System for Servomotor-piezo Actuator Using the Dual Servo Loop and Digital Filter Implementation. J. Machine Tools & Manufacture 41, 51–63 (2001)
5. Tong, D., Veldhuis, S.C., Elbestawi, M.A.: Control of a dual stage magnetostrictive actuator and linear motor feed drive system. J. Int. J. Adv. Manuf. Technol. 33, 379–388 (2007)
6. Alter, D.M., Tsao, T.: Stability of turning process with actively controlled linear motor feed drives. Trans. ASME 116, 298–306 (1994)
7. Natale, C., Velardi, F., Visone, C.: Modeling and compensation of hysteresis for magnetostrictive actuators. In: Proc IEEE/ASME International Conference on Advanced Intelligent Mechatronics, pp. 744–749 (2001)

A Thin-Type Traveling Wave Ultrasonic Motor and Phenomenon Analysis of Experiment with Single-Phase Voltage

Hui Guo[1] and Chun-Sheng Zhao[2]

[1] School of Mechatronics Engineering, University of Electronic Science and Technology of China, Chengdu 610054, China
[2] Research Center of Ultrasonic Motors, Nanjing University of Aeronautics & Astronautics, Nanjing 210016, China

Abstract. A thin-type traveling wave ultrasonic motor has been designed and fabricated, and the major properties of traveling wave in the stator of the annular ultrasonic motor have been analyzed. It has pointed out that part areas of the annular stator inner circumference surface have the power to drive the rotor. Moreover, the performance test of the stator and the operating experiment of the motor have been accomplished. In the experiment it has been found that the motor can operate normally even with single-phase voltage. To above mentioned phenomenon, the paper discusses the tooth motion of the inner surface on the annular stator in bend mode and distinguishes the different effects of normal motion and radial motion of the tooth and analyzes the drive action of the six teeth of the stator inner surface to the rotor during one period. On the basis of the analysis, a thin-type standing wave ultrasonic motor can be designed and made further

Keywords: Ultrasonic motor stator tooth displacement drive with single-phase voltage.

1 Introduction

At present, some researchers have done a lot of significant work into developing the annular ultrasonic motor, and recently they have focused on the new drive mechanism of annular motors. In the published papers, with a view to innovating polarization sub area manner of piezoelectric ceramics, reference 1 put forward the scheme of 32 sections, and developed a kind of traveling wave motor driven by bend mode of B08. In reference 2, the stator was designed to the shape of cymbal--a musical instrument, and a new kind of annular standing wave ultrasonic motor was fabricated. Also a new thought was brought forward in reference 3, in which two lines of waves that excited separately were used to drive the motor in the stator and the rotor. So apparently reference 2 and 3 emphasized particularly on the innovation in drive mechanism. The new drive mechanism is beneficial to realization of the properties of this kind of motor and miniature further the size of the motor, so as to adapt for the development trend of high precision minimization and miniature mechatronics system.

C. Xiong et al. (Eds.): ICIRA 2008, Part II, LNAI 5315, pp. 162–169, 2008.

Mostly, the annular piezoelectric ultrasonic motor utilizes the bend mode of the stators to drive the rotor, so the interface between the stator and the rotor are annular surface. This kind of motor can be made easily with stable properties and bigger output torque. But the thickness of the motors is limited by the contact structure of the stator and rotor of the motor along axial direction. Reference 4 studied another kind of annular piezoelectric ultrasonic motor which utilizes inner surface mode of the annular stator, it is non axisymmetric mode. The interface of the stator and the rotor turns into inner or outer circumference side face instead of the annular surface. This kind of motor can minimize the motor thickness and miniaturize the motor. In this paper the motor structure adopts inner face mode, uses the inner or out circumference side face to drive the rotor, that is bend mode of the stator. Thus the paper analyzes the motions of the stator particles in traveling wave. The stator scanning experiment and running test of the motor have done for the sample motor and the experiment results have been obtained. In the experiment, the motor can be run normally only with single-phase voltage and the mechanism of this phenomenon is analyzed. A new thin-type standing wave ultrasonic motor has been fabricated based on this mechanism analysis.

2 Motor Structure Character

Fig.1 shows the structure of the thin-type ultrasonic motor. The motor consists of annular stator, two pieces of semicircle lamella rotor and strings. The two pieces of semicircle lamella rotor are installed on inside track of the stator, and the strings are installed inside the lamella rotor. Therefore, through the spring pressure the external circumference side of the rotor and the internal circumference side of stator contact each other.

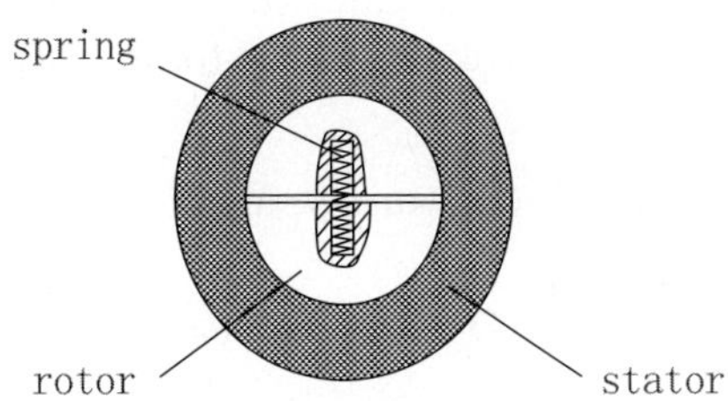

Fig. 1. Structure of ultrasonic motor

The stator is made of annular steel chips and piezoelectric ceramic chips, which are felted together. The middle layer is annular steel chip, whose front face felt. The annular steel chip is between the piezoelectric ceramic chips and its front face and back face felt piezoelectric ceramics chips. Rectangle teeth are distributed uniformly in the inner circumference side of the annular steel chip which was made into a structure of circular truncated cone face on the two ends and a cylindrical surface in the middle. Accordingly one end of the rotor also has the same taper surface in order to contact perfectly with the stator, therefore the contact surface of the stator and the rotor is the combination of cylindrical surface and circular truncated cone face rather than simple one of the both styles. In this structure contact surface of the stator and the rotor is along the stator's internal circumference side instead of the annular end side. In addition, the pre-tight between the stator and the rotor exerts along the radial direction of the stator ring in order to avoid motor thickness increasing occurred by pre-tight.

3 Mechanism Theory Analysis of Two Excitation Means

Concerning the theory of mechanism in motor when adapting two-phase excitation, the paper make the analysis from the displacement character of surface particles of the stator excited with two-phase voltage. Firstly, set up a column coordinate system, make the annular stator axes as z-axis, and make the below annular surface of the stator as x-y plane. Excite piezoelectric ceramics chips of the stator with two-phase of sine and cosine voltages, research all the particles' displacements of entire circumference whose radius is one set value in the annular stator in any moment. So the whole circumference outspread is a wave curve, figure 2 shows the mode B(0,7) of the annular.

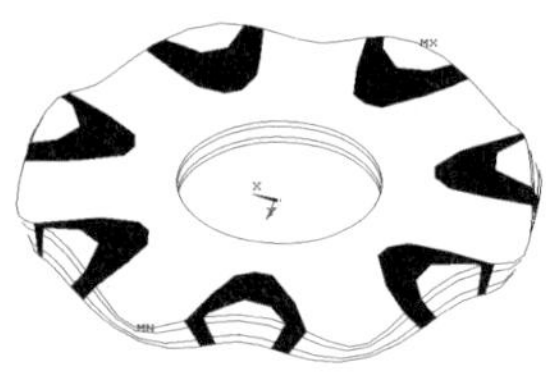

Fig. 2. Mode B(0,7) of annular lamella

On the other hand, a list of bending traveling wave is excited in the annular stator of the motor when the stator is excited with two-phase voltages. The motion of any particle on the annular stator can be expressed as formula (3) which is the composition of (1) and (2).

$$S_2 = AJ_m(kr)\sin m\varphi \sin \omega t \tag{1}$$

$$S_2 = AJ_m(kr)\sin m\varphi \sin \omega t \tag{2}$$

$$S_z = S_1 + S_2 = AJ_m(kr)\cos(m\varphi - \omega t) \tag{3}$$

where J_m is the Bessel functions of m order, m is wave number, ω is circular frequency and r is the pole radius ordinate of the particle. Expression (3) shows that at any time the amplitude of the annular stator particles is related to the traveling wave transmit direction, namely, the ordinate φ of the circle direction as well as its pole radical ordinate r. The section graph at the wave peak as figure 3 of the annular plate shows that the particle amplitude increases with the pole radical ordinate r. Point A in the section graph shows that the replacement of the particles on the annular plate has an additional radical component S_r, besides the vertical component, and the relation of the vertical component to the radical ordinate r and z coordinate can be expressed as following:

$$S_r = R(r, z)\cos(m\varphi - \omega t) \tag{4}$$

where R is the particle maximal displacement along the radical direction.

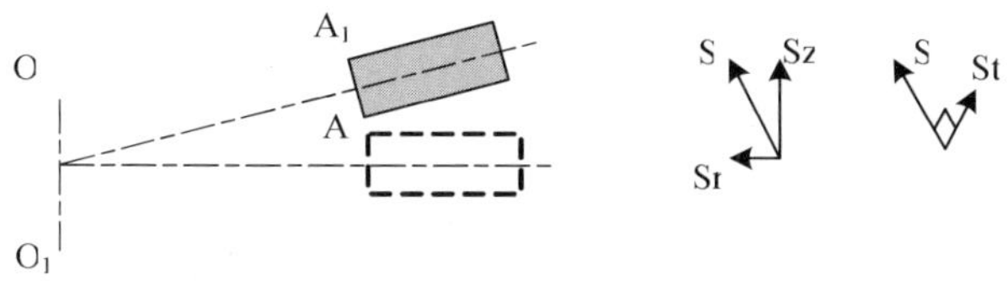

Fig. 3. Particle displacement in the direction of radius of annular stator

The radial component S_r makes the elliptical motion of the stator particles tilt. Then the two symmetry axes of the elliptical motion of the particles are axial displacement S and tangential direction S_t respectively. When the additional component S_r points towards annular plate axes, the plane of the elliptic motion of particles on the stator will tilt to the axes of annular plate axes. This tilt results in each narrow cylindrical side face on inner column side upper end and lower end of stator cirque. The elliptical motion of the stator particles on the narrow column side face can rotate the rotor. Utilizing the elliptical motions of the particles in the above narrow column side and the end face of the annular stator makes the motor have bigger output power. Therefore, in structure the stator inner side is the combination of the two circular truncated cone faces and one cylindrical surface. In the running experiment, the motor can operate normally even with one-phase voltage. The mechanism is analyzed as following: Fig.4 and Fig.5 show the structure of the motor stator and the Electrode arrangement of piezoelectric ceramic chip respectively. The piezoelectric ceramic chip is divided equally into 12 sections that are circularly arranged according to two-positive and two-negative order and connected with wires by one-positive and one-negative order so as to form two-phase input of the motor. A list of traveling wave excited with two-phase input can drive the rotor, which has been analyzed in the paper. A list of standing wave is excited with single-phase voltage, which has three wave crests and three wave troughs along the circumference, namely, one B(0,3) mode. As set forth, when standing wave is excited in motor stator, the stator annular outspread graph is one wave plane (see fig.2). This makes the teeth on the inner circumference surface swing correspondingly with the wave plane.

Expression (1) indicates that the displacement along z direction of the stator is changed with its pole radius, and the particle has one radical component which makes the stator and the rotor contact each other only at the crest and troughs of the wave, no longer along the whole circumference surface. The displacements along above two directions had the six teeth most near the crest and troughs, which drive the rotor. Suppose the vibration period of the mode B(0,3) is T, time is t, outspread the inner circumference surface of the stator.

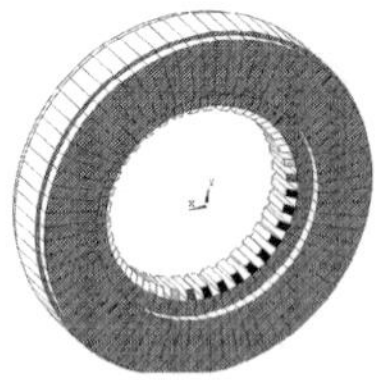

Fig. 4. Stator structure of motor

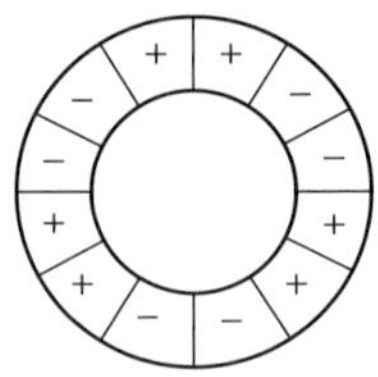

Fig. 5. Electrode arrangement of PZT

Fig.6 shows that when t=0, both the tangential displacements and the radical displacements of the 6 teeth were zero. When 0<t<T/4, the wave plane of the annular stator begin to form along circumference surface, the teeth 1, 2, 3, 4, 5, 6 wave with the plane. The teeth 1, 3, 5 move anticlockwise, and teeth 2, 4, 6 move clockwise. Also, because of the displacement change of the stator along the radical direction, the displacements of up ends of the teeth 1, 3, 5 point to axes, so up ends of the teeth contact with the rotor and the incremental elasticity can drive the rotor. While the displacements of down ends of the teeth 1, 3, 5 leave axes, so up ends of the teeth cannot contact with the rotor, can not drive the rotor.

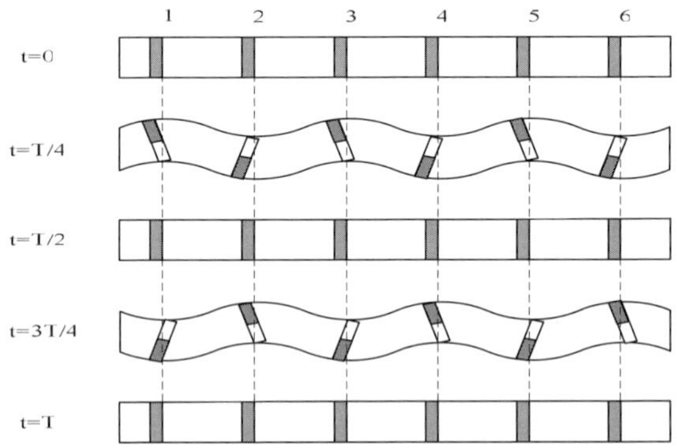

Fig. 6. Drive mechanism of the motor excited with single-phase voltage

On the contrary, the displacements of down ends of the teeth 2, 4. 6 point to axes, so down ends of the teeth contact with the rotor and the incremental elasticity can drive the rotor. While the displacements of up ends of the teeth 2, 4. 6 leave axes, so down ends of the teeth cannot contact with the rotor, can not drive the rotor. Fig.6 shows the contact status of the up ends and down ends with the rotor. In the figure, the black parts stand for the contact between the teeth and the rotor. When t=T/4, the teeth 1, 3, 5 turn anticlockwise to the biggest displacement along the tangential direction. In the meantime, the up ends of the teeth 1,3,5 produce the biggest displacement which point to the axis, and the down parts conduct the biggest displacement which is apart from the axis. The teeth 2, 4, 6 turn clockwise to the biggest displacements in the tangent direction. In the meantime, the teeth 2, 4, 6 up produce the biggest displacement which is apart from the axis, and the down part conduct the biggest displacement which point to the axis. From above analyze, The six teeth were excited with single-phase voltage, the up part of teeth 1,3,5 and the down part of teeth 2,4,6 produce the displacements towards the axis and contact with the rotor, and their tangential displacements were consistent, so these parts can rotate the rotor. While, because the radial displacements leave the axis, the other parts can not rotate the rotor.

When $T/4<t<T/2$, the teeth 1,3,5 move clockwise, and the teeth 2,4,6 move anti-clockwise. The radical changes of the stator displacements make the up parts of the teeth 1,3,5 produce displacements which is apart from the axis, the up parts of the teeth deviate from the rotor, cannot drive the rotor. While the displacements of down ends of the teeth 1, 3, 5 point to axes, begin to contact with the rotor, can drive the rotor. On the contrary, the down ends of the teeth produce displacements which point to the axis, begin to contact with the rotor and drive the rotor. While the up ends of the teeth produce the displacements which is apart from axes, deviate the rotor, so can not drive the rotor.. When $t=T/2$, the 6 teeth return to the status when $t=0$.

According to the same principle, when $T/2<t<t3T/4$, the down ends of the teeth 1,3,5 contact with the rotor, the elasticity of them increase, and the rotor is driven. The up ends of the teeth 1,3,5 produce displacements which is apart from the axis, and deviate from the rotor, so they cannot drive the rotor. While the up ends of the teeth 2, 4, 6 produce the displacement which point to the axis, begin to contact with the rotor and drive the rotor.When $3T/4<t<T$, the down ends of the teeth 1,3,5 gradually deviate from the motor, and the down ends contact with the rotor. While the up ends of the teeth 2,4,6 gradually deviate from the motor, and the up ends contact with the rotor. When $t=T$, the six teeth return to the status when $t=0$ again.

From above movement analyses of the six teeth on inner annular surface of the stator during one period, it is known that with single-phase voltage, by dint of their tangential and radial displacements the stator can rotate the rotor along the fixed direction, and change the drive voltage phase, the motor can reverse.

4 Experiment Result

Frequency characteristics experiment has been done for the stator of the motor with the instrument of HP3562 to verify the excitation results of the motor. Fig.7 shows the scanning result. In the experiment, the piezoelectric ceramic chip was felted with steel chips, and the stator was excited with single-phase voltage without the rotor. The result shows that in the frequency range from 20kHz to 50kHz, a formant comes at the spot 29.45kHz for the motor stator. The model motor was fabricated and excited with two-phase voltage. Fig.8 showed the speed-frequency relation with no load. The scatter points were the experimental datum. Apparently the max speed of the motor is gained at the frequency range of 29.2kHz~29.3kHz. This is accordant with the resonance frequency of 29.45kHz in Fig.7. The result has proved that the design of the prototype motor is practical. In the above drive experiment it has turned out that the motor has bigger torque, and the torque is bigger when the axial load is put on.

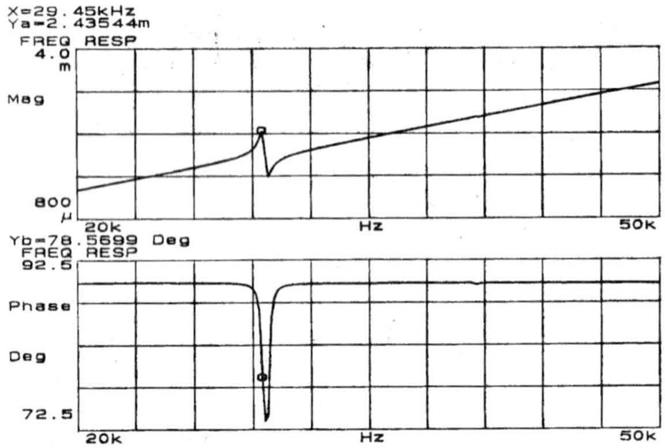

Fig. 7. Frequency characteristics of stator

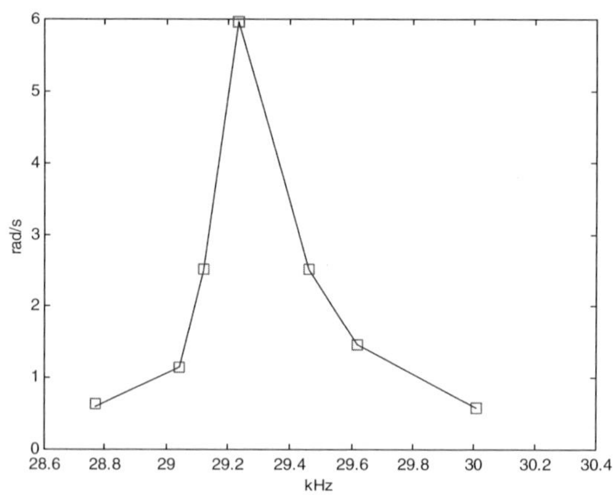

Fig. 8. Speed-frequency characteristics with no load

5 Conclusion

This paper put forward a thin-type traveling ultrasonic motor and the model motor is fabricated. The running experiment result turns out that the scheme is practical. To the phenomenon that the motor can operate normally with single-phase voltage, the paper analyzes the characteristics of normal motion and radial motion of the particles on inner surface of annular stator in bend mode and the drive action of the six teeth of the stator inner surface to the rotor in one period. According to the analysis, a thin-type standing wave ultrasonic motor can be designed.

In practical design of this thin-type motor, the following aspects should be taken into account:

1. Determining the optimal obliquity of the circular truncated cone face for the contact surface of the stator and the rotor.

2. Determining the height of the circular truncated cone face for the contact surface of the stator and the rotor.

References

1. Rayner, P.J., Whatmore, R.W.: Traveling Wave Ultrasonic Motor Using the B08 Flexural Mode of a Circular Membrane. IEEE Transactions on Ultrasonics Ferroelectrics and Frequency Control 48, 683–690 (2001)
2. Leinvuo, J.T., Wilson, S.A., Whatmore, R.N.: Flextensional Ultrasonic Motor Using the Contour Mode of a Square Piezoelectric Plate. IEEE Transactions on Ultrasonics Ferroelectrics and Frequency Control 51, 929–936 (2004)
3. Bai, D., Ishii, T., Nakamura, K., Ueha, S., Yonezawa, T., Takahashi, T.: An Ultrasonic Motor Driven by the Phase-Velocity Difference between Two Traveling Waves. IEEE Transactions on Ultrasonics Ferroelectrics and Frequency Control 51, 680–685 (2004)
4. Lebrun, L., Petit, L., Gonnard, P.: Piezoelectric Motor Using a (1,1) Non-Axisymmetric Mode. Ultrasonics 34, 251–255 (1996)

A Vertical Sidewall Surface Piezoresistor Technology Based on DRIE and Its Typical Application in Micro xy-Stages

Jiachou Wang[1,2], Lining Sun[1], Weibin Rong[1], and Xinxin Li[1]

[1] State Key Laboratory of Robotics and System, Harbin Institute of Technology, Harbin, 150001, Heilongjiang Province, China

[2] State Key Laboratory of Transducer Technology, Shanghai Institute of Microsystem and Information Technology, Chinese Academy of Sciences, Shanghai 20050, China

jiatao_wang@163.com

Abstract. A vertical sidewall surface piezoresistor technology is developed for single-wafer-processed MEMS of in-plane lateral piezoresistors configuration. The technology based on the deep reactive ion etching (DRIE) and the ion implantation technology can be used to integrate piezoresistive sensor on the vertical sidewall of trench or beam easily. The developed technology has been successfully applied to a nano-positioning micro xy-stage integrated with displacement sensor based on the piezo-resistance effect, in which the piezoresistor has been fabricated on the vertical sidewall surface of the detecting beam to improve the displacement sensitivity and resolution of sensor. Besides satisfactory electric principles of the piezoresistors obtained, the experimental results also verify the sensitivity of the fabricated piezoresistive sensors is better than 0.903mV/μm without amplification, the linearity is better than 0.814%, which are well with design.

Keywords: MEMS, DRIE, Vertical sidewall piezoresistor, micro xy-stage.

1 Introduction

With the development of the surface micromachining and bulk micromachining, varieties of formation fabricated piezoresistor technology based on inductively coupled plasma (ICP) deep reactive ion etching (DRIE) process have been developed for single-wafer-processed MEMS of in-plane lateral piezoresistor configuration, such as oblique ion implantation technology[1][2][3] and the trench-sidewall single-wafer-MEMS technology[4][5]. In the former process, the piezoresistors are formed by ion implantation technology, so the trenches have to be widely opened enough for oblique implantation which may make difficulties in squeeze-film damping and electrostatic actuating designed, besides, this process has the disadvantage of integration incompatibility. For the latter process, the piezoresistors are formed by ion diffusion technology, so it is not limited by the width of the trench, but this process is more complicated and the piezoresistive region is more difficult to be controlled. New technology featuring improved integration capability, low cost and high yield is in demand. A vertical sidewall surface piezoresistor technology based on DRIE and ion

C. Xiong et al. (Eds.): ICIRA 2008, Part II, LNAI 5315, pp. 170–177, 2008.

implantation technique is proposed in this paper. With this process, the piezoresistor can be integrated on the trench or beam sidewall easily. The technical details of the proposed vertical sidewall surface piezoresistor and the typical application will be described in following sections.

2 Processes of the Vertical Sidewall Piezoresistor

The fabrication process of the vertical sidewall surface piezoresistor is mainly based on DRIE technology and ion implantation technology. The process includes four patterning and one DRIE etching step. The fabrication process for sidewall piezoresistor is depicted in fig. 1 and described as follows.

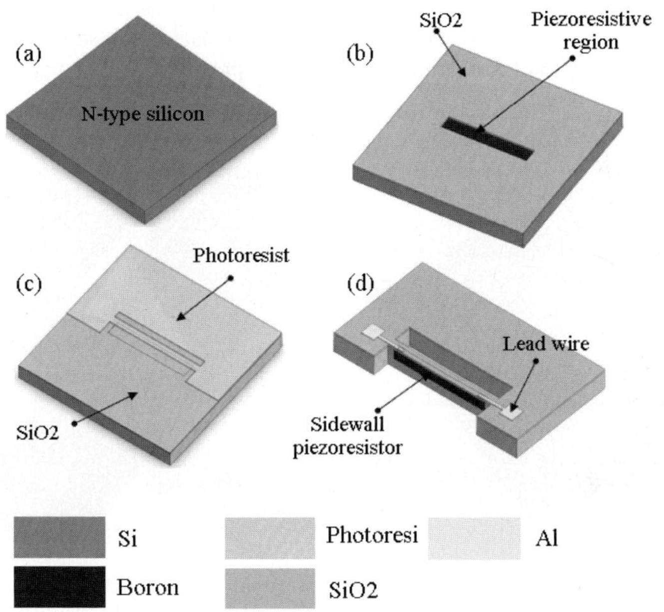

Fig. 1. Fabrication process of the vertical sidewall piezoresistor

(1) Starting from double polished n-type (100)-oriented 4 inch ordinary silicon wafers with a resistivity of 1～10 Ω·cm;

(2) The SiO_2 layer is grown on both side of the silicon wafers by the thermally oxidation process; The SiO2 layer thickness is controlled to be approximately 0.5μm and then the first time photolithography is conducted on the front side of the wafer to pattern the resistor region, then buffer HF acid is used to etch SiO_2 with photoresist as the etching mask;

(3) The surface piezoresistors are formed by boron ion implantation process. In order to reduce the temperature sensitivity of piezoresistors and form better ohmic contact in the next step, the impurity concentration on the wafer surface is controlled at about 10^{19} atoms/cm^{-3};

(4) After the second time photolithography, the contact hole is formed by buffer HF acid etching, and then aluminum is sputtered and patterned with the third time photolithography, metallization process is performed for interconnection. Finally, the fourth photolithography is used to shape the detecting beam and the sidewall piezoresistor based on the formed surface piezoresistor, the inductive coupled plasma (ICP) deep RIE is performed to release detecting beam and form veridical sidewall piezoresistors, synchronously, the protective layer on the surface of the sidewall piezoresistor is form with the polymer by the protective gas of C_4F_8 during the DRIE.

3 Experiments and Typical Application

For evaluating the capability of the vertical sidewall surface piezoresistors technique, a nano-positioning micro xy-stage integrating displacement sensor based on the piezo-resistance effect is fabricated by the process proposed in this paper, as shown in fig.2.

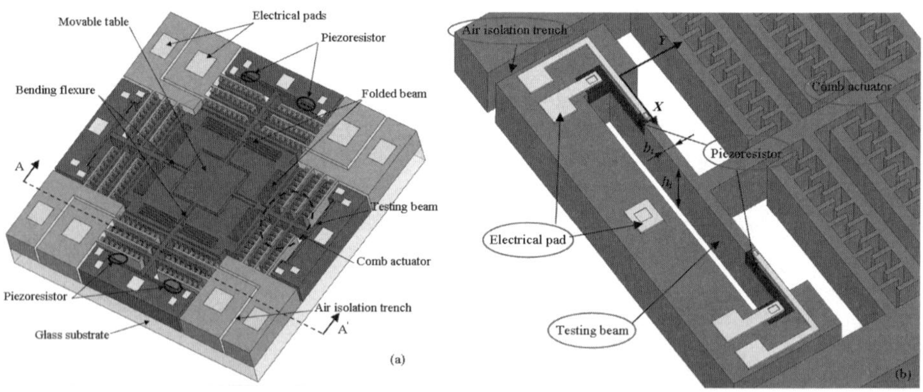

Fig. 2. (a) Schematic of the micro xy-stage and (b) a 3D sketch of the testing beam and piezoresistors

Fig. 2(b) shows a 3D schematic of the detecting beam and the sensor configuration. The sensing direction of the displacement sensor base on piezoresistor is in the wafer plane. The transversely deflecting clamped-clamped beam (detecting beam) is designed to measure the lateral displacement of the movable stage. The aspect ratio of the detecting beam cross section is designed as 1:3.75 to decrease the cross-sensitivity of orthogonal direction. Two vertical sidewall surface piezoresistors have been fabricated on the outboard surface of the both end of the detecting beam respectively, and there are two detecting beams with the identical construction located at the both side of the movable stage. At the middle of which are connected to the movable stage. Fig. 3 shows a simplified mechanism of the fabricated micro xy-stage. When the movable stage moves along the *x*-direction, the detecting beams deflect along the *x*-direction

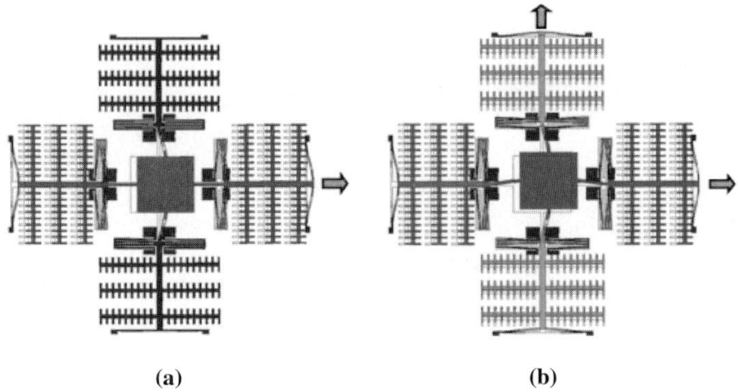

Fig. 3. The driving mechanism of the micro xy-stage :(a) x-actuation; (b) x-and y-actuation

too, Two resistors increase their resistance, whereas, the others decrease. So the four piezoresistors can be used to form a full Wheatstone bridge (see fig.2 (a)).

Fig.4 shows a brief process flow of the micro xy-stage as a cross-sectional process at the dash-dotted line A-A' in fig.2 (a). Fig. 5(a) and (b) show the top-view CCD micrograph of the piezoresistor. In figure 5(a) shows the surface piezoresistor before forming the vertical sidewall surface piezoresistor by using DRIE, and (b) shows the fabricated vertical sidewall surface piezoresistor after being released by the DRIE. The fig. 5(c) shows the close-up views of the end of the detecting beam, on the vertical sidewall surface of which there is a fabricated piezoresistor and fig. 5(d) shows the SEM photo of the fabricated micro xy-stage chip.

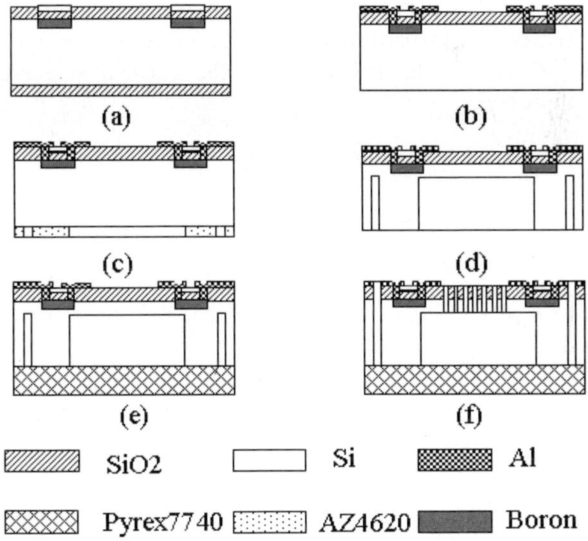

Fig. 4. Cross-sectional process flow of the xy-stage at the dash-dotted line A-A' in fig.2 (a)

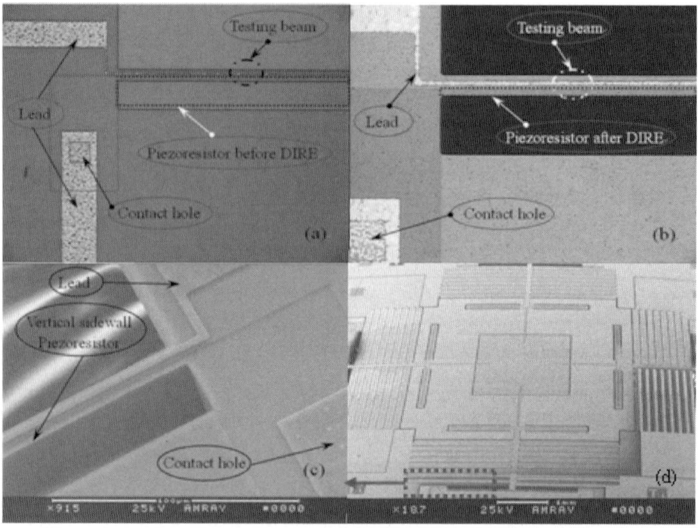

Fig. 5. The photograph of piezoresistor during the fabricating process, the fabricated micro xy-stage and the close-up view of the fabricated testing beam and piezoresistors

Using the fabricated micro xy-stage structure, the vertical sidewall piezoresistor technique can be evaluated by electric principle characterization. Fig. 6(a) shows measured *I-V* principle of a sidewall piezoresistors. About 5.4kΩ sidewall-piezoresistance with sheet resistance of about 95Ω/□ is also measured. Fig. 6(b) shows the measured breakdown voltage of two adjacent piezoresistors. Higher than 45V breakdown voltage is measured this is enough for the sensor operation. From the measured electric principles, the feasibility of the vertical sidewall piezoresistors technique can be approved.

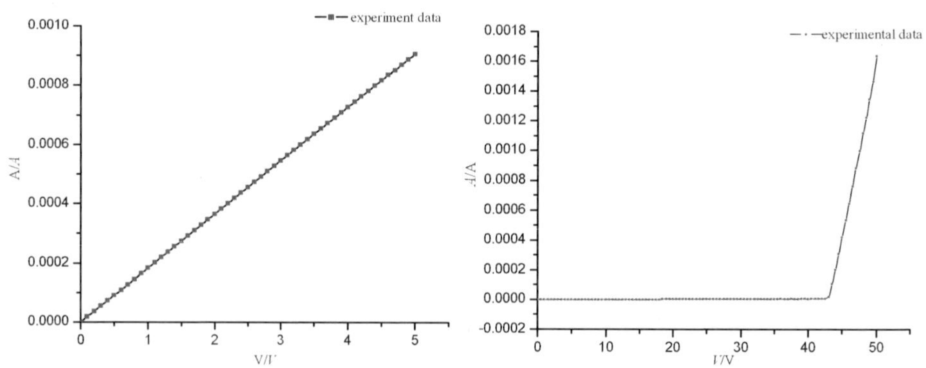

(a) (b)

Fig. 6. Measure sidewall piezoresistors electric principles. (a) Linear *I-V* principle of a sidewall piezoresistor with sheet resistance of about 95Ω, and (b) Higher than 45V breakdown voltage is measured between two adjacent piezoresistors.

Fig. 7 shows the curve relationship between the displacement and the measured voltage of the displacement sensor without amplification. The experimental data are estimated by the method of least squares. After the fitting, the relationship between the displacement of stage and the measured voltage can be, respectively, expressed as:

$$\begin{aligned} y &= -0.00177x + 0.37519, \quad in+x\ direction \\ y &= +0.00129x + 0.36308, \quad in-x\ direction \\ y &= +0.00117x + 0.23696, \quad in+y\ direction \\ y &= -0.00090x + 0.23963, \quad in-y\ direction \end{aligned} \qquad (1)$$

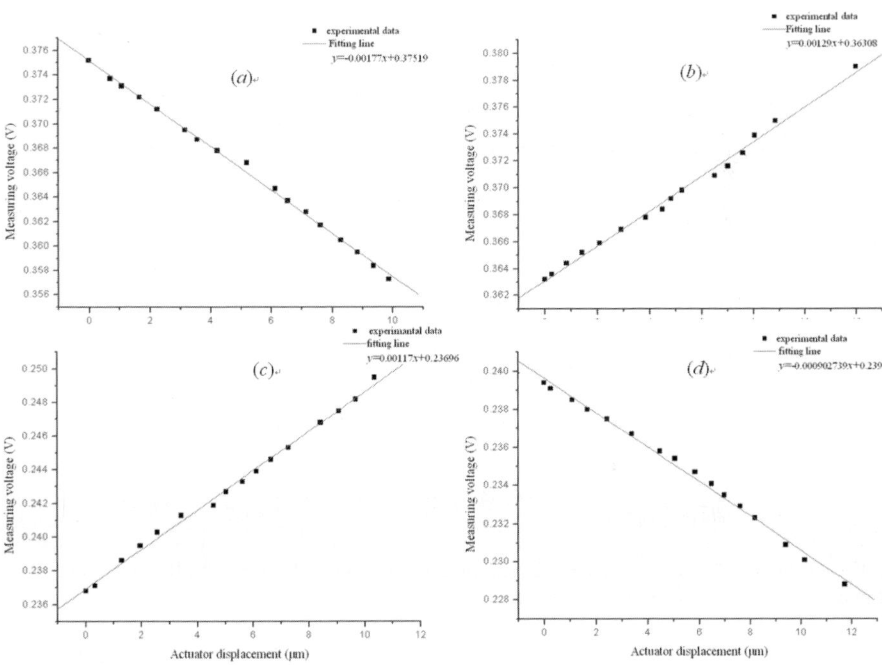

Fig. 7. Curve between the displacement and measured voltage. (a) relationship between displacement and measured voltage in +x direction; (b) relationship between displacement and measured voltage in -x direction; (c) relationship between displacement and measured voltage in +y direction and (d) relationship between displacement and measured voltage in -y direction.

Table 1. The sensitivity and linearity of displacement sensor

Actuator(direction)	+x	-x	+y	-y
Sensitivity(mV/μm)	-1.77	1.29	1.17	-0.903
Linearity (%)	0.814%	0.510%	0.429%	0.346%

The sensitivity of response to the displacement of the xy-stage and linearity of the piezoresistive sensor are listed in Table 1. If taking fabrication imperfections into consideration, the measured results agree well with design.

Using the displacement sensor composed of sidewall piezoresistors, the dynamic behavior (natural frequency) of the stage is also obtained experimentally. Fig. 8 is a bode plot. The measured first resonant frequency is found at 983Hz as shown in fig. 8. It is 15.9% lower than the simulated first undamped natural frequency, 1169Hz. The discrepancy that is observed may arise from fabrication imperfections and the since the stiffness of the flexures is sensitive to their dimensions. Further, approximations made in the finite element modeling and the effect of the damping condition is not to be taken into account during the experiment all may also contribute to this discrepancy. So the measured results also agree well with design.

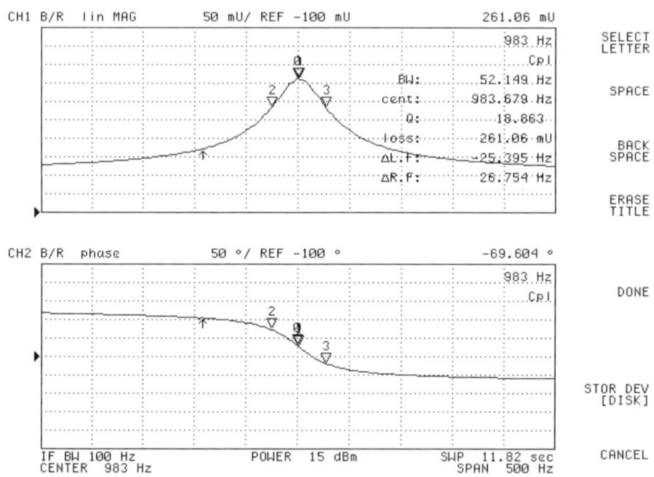

Fig. 8. Measured frequency response of the in-plane component, both amplitude (upper traces) and phases (lower traces). Response curves yielded values o f0=983Hz, Q=18.86.

4 Conclusions

From the results of the micro xy-stage integrated with the sidewall piezoresistive sensor, the capability of the vertical sidewall surface piezoresistors technique is verified. As a standard process for single wafer integration of in-plane MEMS configuration, the proposed technology is promising to be widely used.

Acknowledgments

The authors gratefully acknowledge the High Technology Research and Development Programme of China through Grant Number 2007AA04Z315 and the Program for Changjiang Scholars and Innovative Research Team in University (PCSIRT).

References

1. Partridge, A., Reynolds, J.K., Chui, B.W., et al.: A High-Performance Planar Piezoresistive Accelerometer. J. Microelectromech. Syst. 9, 58–66 (2000)
2. Chui, B.W., Kenny, T.W., Mamin, H.J., Terris, B.D., Rugar, D.: Independent detection of vertical and lateral forces with a sidewall-implanted dual-axis piezoresistive cantilever. Appl. Phys. Lett. 72, 1388–1390 (1998)
3. Chui, B.W., Mamin, H.J., Terris, B.D., Rugar, D., Kenny, T.W.: Sidewall-implanted dual-axis piezoresistive cantilever for AFM data storage readback and tracking. In: MEMS 1998, pp. 12–17 (1998)
4. Li, X.X., Cheng, B.L., Wang, Y.L., Gu, L., et al.: A Trench-sidewall single-wafer-MEMS technology and its typical application in High-performance accelerometers. In: IEDM 2004, pp. 43–45 (2004)
5. Gu, L., Li, X.X., Bao, H.F., et al.: Single-wafer-processed nano-positioning XY-stages with trench-sidewall micromachining technology. J. Micromech. Microeng. 16, 1349–1357

Three-Dimensional Tracking at Micro-scale Using a Single Optical Microscope

Liguo Chen, Zhiliang Yang, and Lining Sun

State Key Laboratory of Robotics and System, Robotics Institute, Harbin Institute of Technology, Harbin 150080, China
{clg,yangzhiliang,lnsun}@hit.edu.cn

Abstract. 3D tracking is of fundamental importance to the development of practical visual applications to micromanipulation and microassembly. In this paper, a new 3D tracking method based on CAMSHIFT and Depth-from-Defocus is developed for micromanipulation and microassembly task. CAMSHIFT algorithm is used to find the size and location of moving object even the micro-objects is highly blurred. And Depth-from-defocus method is used to recover the depth information of the object from a measure of the level of defocus. The experimental results of blurring tracking and depth recovery of micro gear validate the feasibility of the proposed 3D tracking method.

Keywords: 3D tracking, autofocus, microscope, micromanipulation, microassembly.

1 Introduction

Visual tracking of microscopic images is of fundamental importance to micromanipulation and microassembly in providing noncontact dynamic measurement of poses of the objects of interest and their spatial relations. It also increases the flexibility of micromanipulation and microassembly by reducing the dependence on precise calibration. In a typical 3D microassembly situation, the micro object should be tracked in the 3D space in real time, while general optical microscope can not get the depth information for its limited depth of field. Confocal laser scanning microscopy is much too slow for real time tracking. The limited optical working distance between a microscope lens and a device to be manipulated indicates that stereo vision is not feasible. Therefore, how to get the depth information in 3D tracking has become a major roadblock to the development of practical visual applications to micromanipulation and microassembly.

In prior research efforts, many methods were attempted to accomplish the 3D tracking using a single optical microscope. However, most work employs 2-D recognition methods [1-5] sometimes in combination with an auto-focusing system, which ensures that the object to be recognized always stays in focus [6][7]. So the object can just be tracked but can not obtain 3D trajectories which are essential to visual servoing. Geometric Hashing and the Bounded Hough Transform have been used to recognise with up to 4 degrees-of-freedom for micromanipulation and microassembly[8-10]. However, as both recognition and tracking are purely combinatorial

C. Xiong et al. (Eds.): ICIRA 2008, Part II, LNAI 5315, pp. 178–187, 2008.

approaches, the memory requirements for the algorithms are high and image features can not be extracted when the level of defocus is significant. Because of the unique properties of microscope optics, microscopic computer vision differs significantly from macroscale computer vision. The small depth-of-field of microscope optics is a fundamental constraint that must be considered in developing microscopic computer vision techniques for micromanipulation and microassembly. Small amount of displacement error of working distance causes significantly blurred of target object in sight. Therefore, how to track the blurred object and get the 3D trajectories is totally important. Using a quantitative defocusing method to obtain 3D trajectories of cells using a fluorescent microscope successfully [11][12].

In this paper, a novel imaging technique that tracks (x,y,z,t)coordinates of micro-object for micromanipulation and microassembly using a single optical microscope is proposed. A widely used macroscale 2D track method called camshaft is used for microscopy images to track defocusing miro-object. And a depth from defocus based method is used to obtain the depth information in z direction. The integration of these two techniques is implemented successfully for obtaining 3D trajectories of micro-object.

The paper is organized as follows. Section II briefly introduces the 3D tracking technique based on CAMSHIFT and DFD and gives the corresponding theoritical analysis which is feasible for microscopy images. In section Ⅲ, Experiments are performed to test the effect of this tracking method. Conclusions and future work are discussed in Section Ⅳ.

2 3D Tracking Technique for Microscopy Image

2.1 CAMSHIFT Based Blurred Image Tracking for Microscopy Images

CAMSHIFT algorithm is widely used in face tracking about apperceiving user interface now [12-16]. It makes use of color information in region to track object and adopts a non-parameter technique and searches moving target by clustering method.

The CAMSHIFT algorithm is a modification of the meanshift algorithm which is a robust statistical method of finding the mode (top) of a probability distribution. Typically the probability distribution is derived from color via a histogram, although it could be produced from correlation, recognition scores or bolstered by frame differencing or motion detection schemes, or joint probabilities of different colors/motions etc. To be brief, CAMSHIFT algorithm applies target's hue character to find the size and location of the moving object in video image. Initial value of search window is set as current position and size before search [13]. In the next frame video image, search window is initialized by current position and size of moving object. The process is repeated to realize continuous object tracking. The theoretical analysis can be found in [14-16].

In this application, we use only the most simplistic approach: A 1-D Hue histogram is sampled from the object in an HSV color space version of the image. In our experiments we find that even the micro-objects is highly blurred, the color information is still reserved which is shown in Fig.1. It indicates that CAMSHIFT method can also be used to track burred micro-objects.

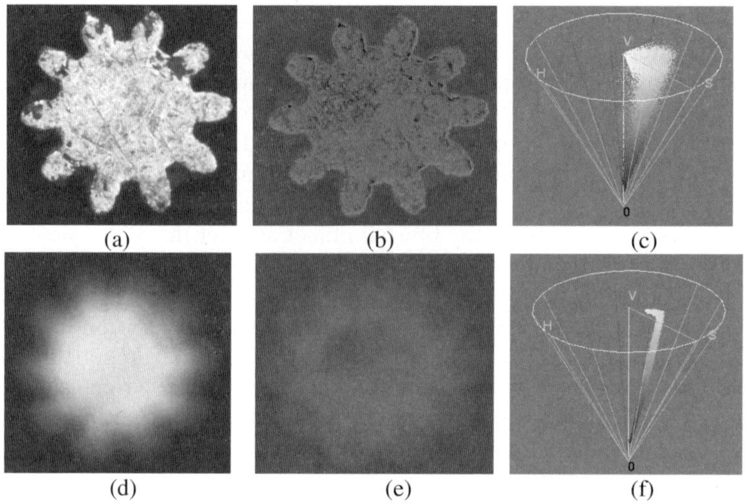

Fig. 1. Color information of focus image and blurred image of a micro gear: (a) Focus RGB image , (b)Focus HSVimage , (c) focus HSV model; (d)blurred RGB image (e) blurred HSVimage, (e) blurred HSV model

2.2 Depth Tracking Based on Depth from Defocus

Depth from defocus (DFD) was proposed by Pentland [16], it directly estimates the depth information from a measure of the level of defocus, which makes it suitable for real-time depth tracking. Blur is modeled as a point spread function (PSF). The sigma parameter of the PSF is proportional to the level of defocus and the depth information is related to the level of defocus, therefore, the depth information is obtained finally.

A spatial-domain Convolution/Deconvolution Transform (*S* Transform) has been developed for images and n-dimensional signals for the case of arbitrary order polynomials [13] [14]. If *f*(x, y) is an image that is a two-dimensional cubic polynomial defined by:

$$f(x,y)=\sum_{m=0}^{3}\sum_{n=0}^{3-m}a_{mn}x^m y^n \tag{1}$$

where a_{mn} is the polynomial coefficient; *m, n* are orders of the polynomial.

The restriction on the order of *f(x, y)* is made to valid by applying a polynomial fitting least square smoothing filter to the image. The blurred or defocused image *g(x, y)* can be described as the result of convolving the focused image *f(x, y)* with the point spread function (PSF) *h(x, y)*:

$$g(x,y)=h(x,y)*f(x,y) \tag{2}$$

For any circularly symmetric PSF h(x, y), the spread parameter δ is defined:

$$\delta^2=\int_{+\infty}^{-\infty}\int_{+\infty}^{-\infty}(x^2+y^2)h(x,y)dxdy \tag{3}$$

According to Equation (1), Equation (2) and Equation (3) can be rewritten as:

$$f(x,y)=g(x,y)-\frac{\delta^2}{4}\nabla^2 g(x,y) \tag{4}$$

And obtain the following relations.

$$\delta^2 = \frac{4\iint_A (g(x,y) - f(x,y)dxdy}{\iint_A \nabla^2 g\ (x,y)dxdy} \tag{5}$$

where ∇^2 is the Laplacian operator.

Equation (5) is a very useful deconvolution formula and it provides a spatial-domain method to get the spread parameter.

As the depth information has direct relation with the spread parameter, the depth of the object can be gain through calculation of the spread parameter of a defocus image. A look-up table based calculation method is adopted in this paper to get the depth of the object in images. And the look-up table itself is obtained through calibration as follow.

(1) First an object is placed in the center of field-of-view. The light microscope is moved to the focus location and a focused image *f*(x, y) is obtained.

(2) The light microscope is then moved to another position and the distance between this position and the focused position are recorded. Then a defocused image was gain and the corresponding spread parameter was calculated through Equation (5).

(3) Repeat the process of step (2), and a look-up table was gain which links the distance between the defocus image position and the focused image position through spread parameter.

Therefore, when a blurred image of the object is recorded, the corresponding spread parameter is calculated and its depth information can be gain through the look-up table. The depth tracking process can be shown in Fig.2.

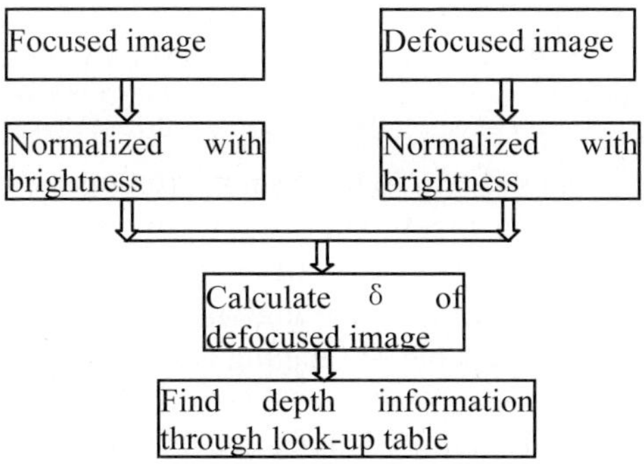

Fig. 2. Depth tracking process based on DFD method

2.3 3D Tracking Integrate CAMSHIFT and DFD Technique

As described above, the CAMSHIFT method can be used to track the X-Y position of the moving object, and the depth tracking can be realized based on DFD technique, therefore, the 3D tracking of moving object under microscope can be realized through integration of CAMSHIFT and DFD tracking method. The process of 3D tracking is shown in Fig.3.

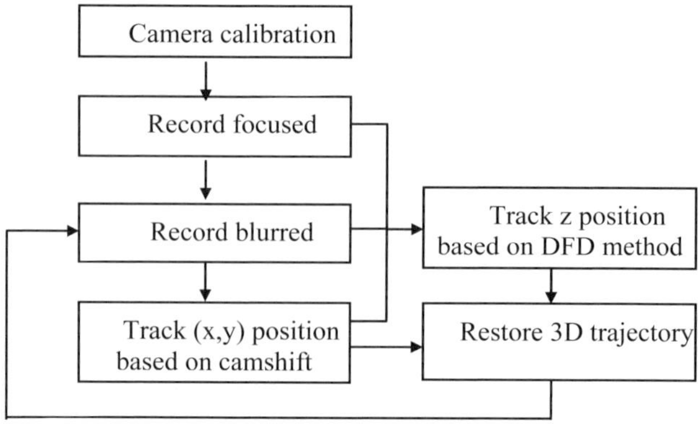

Fig. 3. 3D tracking process based on integration of CAMSHIFT and DFD

Firstly, the microscope system should be calibrated and a focused image is gain through autofocusing adjustment. Then, the object of interest is moved to a random position and a blurred image was recorded. The current (x,y) position of the object can be tracked through CAMSHIFT method. Accordingly, the calculation region in focused image and blurred image is obtained. Thirdly, the z position of the blurred object can be gain through look-up table calibrated beforehand based on DFD method. Finally, the 3D trajectory of the moving object can be gain by calculation at each position.

3 Experiment and Results

3.1 Microscope System

Experiment system is composed of a light zoom microscope, a CMOS camera and an auto focusing motor shown in Fig.4. The magnification of the microscope can be changed between 0.25×—1.8×. Because of the unique properties of zoom microscope, the depth-of-field is a little larger than the traditional microscope in the same magnification. The CMOS camera is capable of imaging a total of 800x600 pixels with each pixel 2.33μm.

The light microscope can be adjusted along the Z direction driven by a step motor. The positioning precision of the Z direction motor is about 0.05μm which corresponds to one step number of the motor. The speed of the step motor is 2000 steps per second which corresponds to 10μm per second. The 3D tracking algorithms can be programmed and executed on the computer.

3.2 Tracking Blurred Object

CAMSHIFT method has been proved to be effective for tracking an object in focus. This experiment aims to test its tracking character when an object is blurring under

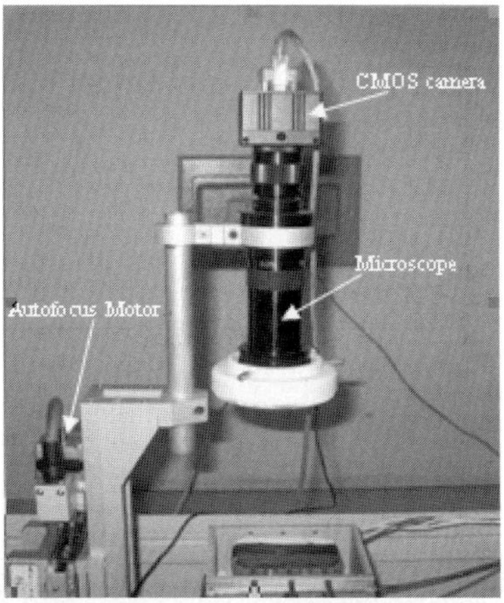

Fig. 4. Microscopic System

microscope. A micro gear with 1mm diameter was used to perform the tracking experiment. Firstly, the micro gear is positioned at the center of field of view of microscope, and the microscope is adjusted to gain in focus image of micro gear and the initials position of micro gear is recorded as (390,328) in pixels. Then, the microscope was adjust along Z direction with step of 100μm, and the defocus level of the current position is described with the distance between current position and the focus position. Finally, the center of micro gear was tracking with CAMSHIFT method, and the tracking error of this position was calculated. The tracking result was shown in Table 1, and the tracking error was shown in Fig.5, each pixel is 4.76μm.

Experiment results show that when the defocus level is less than 600μm, the average tracking error is under 10μm. Further increasing of the level of defocus will gradually increase in its tracking error, but do not exceed 50μm which is still acceptable to micromanipulation and microassembly. Therefore CAMSHIFT method gives a good result to track blurred microscopy images. Fig.6 shows the in focus image and a blur image of micro gear.

Table 1. Tracking result based on CAMSHIFT method

defocus Level (μm)	100	200	300	400	500	600	700	800	900	1000
X center (pixels)	390.0	390.0	389.5	389.5	389.5	389.5	387.5	386.5	385.5	384
Y Center (pixels)	327.0	327.0	328.0	327.5	327.0	327.5	327.0	327.0	327.0	327.5
Tracking error(μm)	4.76	4.76	2.38	3.37	5.32	3.37	8.58	12.82	17.33	28.66

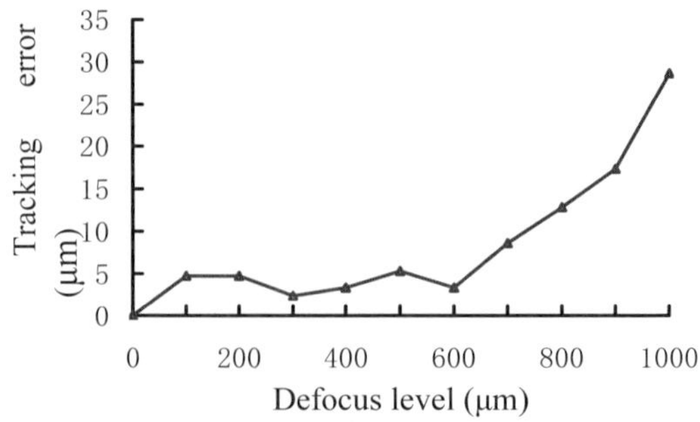

Fig. 5. Tracking error

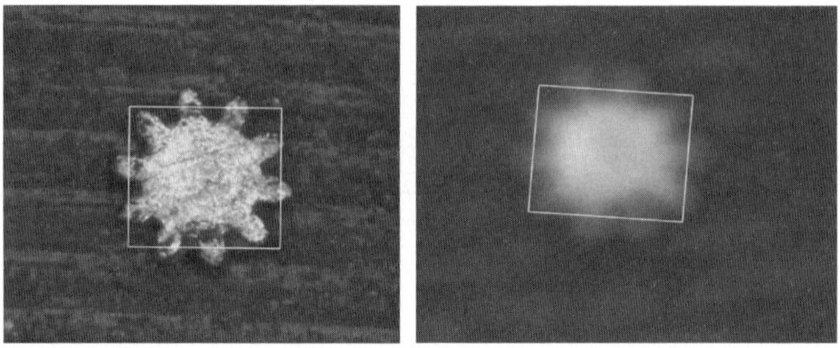

(a) (b)

Fig. 6. Images of micro gear in different position during tracking based on camshift (a) In focus image; (b) a blur image of micro gear

3.3 Depth Recovery

As described in Section II, depth information of a defocused object can be gain through look-up table. Therefore, the look-up table must be calibrated beforehand.

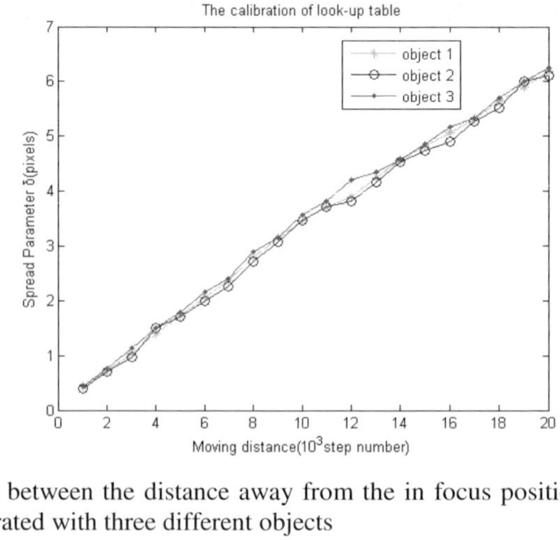

Fig. 7. Relationship between the distance away from the in focus position and the spread parameter which calibrated with three different objects

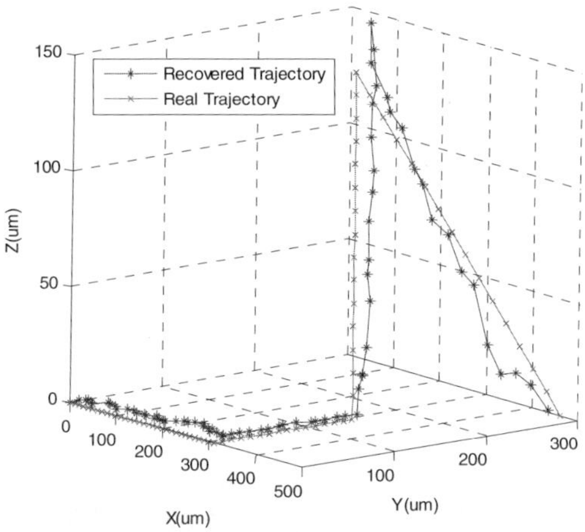

Fig. 8. Recovered 3D trajectory of micro gear in X, Y, Z direction

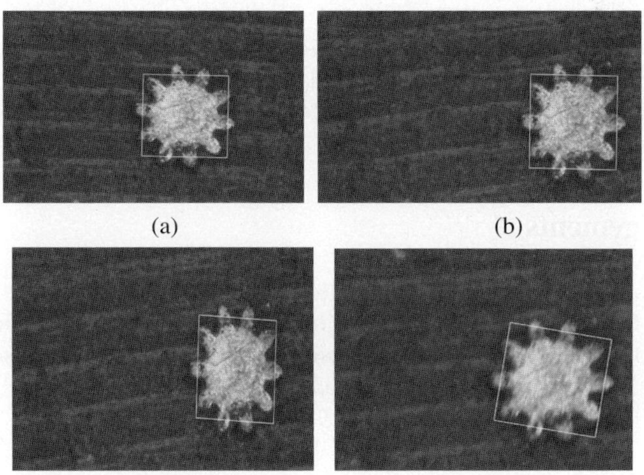

(a) (b)

(c) (d)

Fig. 9. Images in different tracking stages (a) Initial position; (b) Moving along X axis; (c) Moving along Y axis; (d) Moving in three direction at the same time

In this paper, three different objects are used to calibrate the look-up table. The calibrated result is given in Fig.7. As for the large depth of field of zoom microscope, the distance away from the in focus position and the spread parameter is approximate linear relationship. At the same time, the relationship is indispensable to the content of image.

Then a micro gear depth tracking experiment is performed, and the tracking error is about 8μm.

3.4 Trajectory Recovery

In this section, a 3D trajectory of micro-gear is recovered through integration of CAMSHIFT and DFD method. The micro gear is moved respectively along X axis, Y axis and Z axis, and then move in three direction at the same time, the travel line is shown in Fig.8 with red line. The recovered trajectory of the micro gear is shown with blue line. The tracking images at each stage are shown in Fig.9.

4 Conclusion

In this paper, a new 3D tracking method based on CAMSHIFT and DFD using a single camera is constructed. The CAMSHIFT based tracking method is proved to be effective even when the tracking object is blurring under microscope. Depth-from-defocus method based on look-up table is used to recover the depth information of an object in different focus plane. Through integrating the two methods, three dimensional information of micro object can be gain. The tracking experiments of micro gear under zoom microscope are performed and the experimental result validates the effectiveness of proposed tracking method.

Zoom microscope based vision system is usually used in micromanipulation and microassembly system, the tracking method presented in this paper is experimentally demonstrated to be efficient and effective for common optical microscope to micromanipulation and microassembly.

Acknowledgements

The authors would like to thank the National High Technology and Research and Development Program of China through Grant Number 2006AA04Z256 for the support to this work. And the project is also supported by the scientific research foundation of Harbin Institute of technology (HIT.2003.25).

References

1. Yang, G.: Scale-based integrated microscopic computer vision techniques for micromanipulation and microassembly. Ph.D. dissertation,Mech. Eng. Dept., Univ. Minnesota Twin Cities, Minneapolis, MN (2004)
2. Blasko, G., Fua, P.: Real-time 3d object recognition for automatic tracker initialization. In: Fourth international symposium on augmented reality, New York, pp. 175–176 (2001)
3. Greenspan, M., Shang, L., Jasiobedzki, P.: Efficient tracking with the bounded hough transform. In: CVPR 2004: Computer Vision and Pattern Recognition (2004)
4. Ashbrook, A., Thacker, N., Rockett, P., Brown, C.: Robust recognition of scaled shapes using pairwise geometric histograms. In: Proceedings of the BMVC, vol. 2, pp. 503–512 (1995)
5. Meikle, S., Amavasai, B.P., Caparrelli, F.: Towards real-time object recognition using pairs of lines Real-Time Imaging 11(1), 31–43 (2005)

6. Surya, G., Subbarao, M.: Continuous focusing of moving objects using image defocus. In: Proceedings of SPIE's international symposium, Machine Vision Applications, Architectures, and Systems Integration III, October 1994, vol. 2347 (1994)
7. Wei, T., Subbarao, M.: Continuous Focusing of Moving Objects using DFD1F. In: Proceedings of SPIE IS Symposium on Electronic Imaging Science and Technology, San Francisco (February 1994)
8. Lamdan, Y., Wolfson, H.J.: Geometric hashing: A general and efficient model-based recognition scheme. In: Second International Conference on Computer Vision, December 5-8, 1988, pp. 238–249. IEEE, New York (1988)
9. Shan, Y., Matei, B., Sawhney, H.S., Kumar, R., Huber, D., Hebert, M.: Linear model hashing and batch ransac for rapid and accurate object recognition. In: Proceedings of the 2004 IEEE Computer Society Conference on Computer Vision and Pattern Recognition, vol. 2, pp. 121–128 (2004)
10. Wedekind, J., Boissenin, M., Amavasai, B.P., Caparrelli, F.: J. Travis Object Recognition and Real-Time Tracking in Microscope Imaging
11. Wu, M., Roberts, J.W., Buckley, M.: Three-dimensional fluorescent particle tracking at micron-scale using a single camera. Exp. Fluids 38, 461–465 (2005)
12. Speidel, M., Jonas, A., Florin, E.-L.: Three-dimensional tracking of fluorescent nanoparticles with subnanometer precision by use of off-focus imaging. Opt. Lett. 28, 69–71 (2003)
13. Chu, H.Y., Guo, S., Qingchang Liu, X.: Object Tracking Algorithm Based on CAMSHIFT Algorithm Combinating with Difference in Frame. In: IEEE International Conference on Automation and Logistics, August 18-21, 2007, pp. 51–55 (2007)
14. Bradski, G.R.: Computer vision face tracking for use in a perceptual user interface. Intel. Technol. J. 2(2), 1–15 (1998)
15. Intel. Open Computer Vision library (2005), `http://www.intel.com/research/mrl/research/opencv/` [Open source library]. Retrieved, from the World Wide Web, `http://www.intel.com/research/mrl/research/opencv/.N`
16. Zhu, Q., Cheng, K.-T., Wu, C.-T., Wu, Y.-L.: Adaptive learning of an accurate skin-color model. In: The Proc. 6th IEEE Internat. Conf. on Automatic Face and Gesture Recognition (2004)

Bionic Flying Robot: Design, Fabrication and Experiment

Yu Hou and Jianyi Kong

School of Mechanical Automation, Wuhan University of Science and Technology, Wuhan, 430081, China
fly_houyu@163.com

Abstract. Bionic flying robots are new conceptual air vehicles that mimic the flying modes of birds and insects. They have the advantages of small sizes, light weights, low costs, good stealth abilities and high maneuverability, and widely used in the fields of military and civil applications. Based on statistics and analysis of structural parameters, kinematical parameters and dynamic parameters of 68 types of different birds, the bionic formulas was brought forth and original flying robot design was carried out. According to the bionic results, the flapping mechanism and the flexible wing of flapping-wing flying robot were designed. The aerodynamic characteristics of the flapping wing movement were analyzed emphatically. According to the status and function of each part, the system configuration of flying robot can be divided into five child systems. The robot prototype is driven by micro DC motor and polymer lithium battery, and made of carbon fiber fuselage and polyester membrane wing. The total weight of the robot is about 16.5g, wingspan is 200mm, and beat frequency is 12~15Hz. The wind tunnel experiments results indicated that the aerodynamic forces increased by the increase of flapping frequency, wind velocity and attack angle of the wing. Flying test and experiments verified the effectivity and feasibility of the design. The results of research are helpful to the design, fabrication and application of bionic flying robot.

Keywords: Bionic flying robot; Bionic design; flapping mechanism; wind tunnel experiment.

1 Introduction

Bionic flying robots are new conceptual air vehicles that mimic the flying modes of birds and insects. Compared with fixed wing air vehicle and rotary wing air vehicle, the bionic flapping wing air vehicle integrated lifting, thrusting and hanging function into a flapping wing system, and has the ability to cruise a long distance without energy supply, at the same time bionic flying robot has high maneuverability and flexibility. The flapping wing mode of flying creatures in nature gives us edification that flapping wing mode is superior to fixed wing and rotary wing modes when the wingspan is less than 15cm, and the results of bionics and aerodynamics prove it [1].

Now most researches about flapping-wing flying robot concentrated on theory study [2-4], but not on overall design method. According to bionics, aerodynamics, mechanism kinematics and dynamics, an engineering design method that is proper to bionic flying robot was proposed in this paper, and the total design order is: bionic

C. Xiong et al. (Eds.): ICIRA 2008, Part II, LNAI 5315, pp. 188–196, 2008.

primary design, flapping mechanism design and aerodynamic analysis, flexible wing design, system configuration design, and robot prototype fabrication and experiments.

2 Bionic Design of Flying Robot

After ten million years evolution, birds and insects have excellent flying ability, and their flying mode and theory can be the primitive inspiration when designing flapping-wing flying robot.

On the premise of geometry comparability, different flying parameters can be related by dimension analysis. According literature [5], when level flying, the weight *W*, lift *L* and mass *M* of a bird can be expressed as following formula by character length l :

$$W = L = mg \propto l^3 \tag{1}$$

Similarly, wing area *S* can be expressed as

$$S \propto l^2 \tag{2}$$

Wing load *W/S* is

$$W / S \propto l \tag{3}$$

If take wing span *b* as character length, we can get the relationship between wing span *b* and mass *m* from (1)

$$b \propto m^{1/3} = m^{0.33} \tag{4}$$

By the same principle, according to the physical meanings, the flying parameters such as wing area, wing beating frequency, etc., can be expressed as following approximate formula.

$$C = am^b \tag{5}$$

Take logarithm for both side of (5), we can get

$$\ln C = \ln a + b \ln m \tag{6}$$

If define $y = \ln C$, $a_0 = \ln a$, $a_1 = b$, $x = \ln m$, then (6) transfer to a linear expression:

$$y = a_0 + a_1 x \tag{7}$$

Where a_0 and a_1 are objective parameters.

Based on statistics and analysis of structural parameters, kinematical parameters and dynamic parameters of 68 types of different birds, from the smallest goldcrest, which mass is 0.006kg, wingspan is 0.155m, to the largest wondering albatross, which mass is 8.5kg, wingspan is 3.4m, a_0 and a_1 are acquired and the bionic formulas are brought forth by the least two multiplication method.

$$\begin{aligned}
&\text{wingspan} \quad b = 1.237m^{0.368} \\
&\text{wing area} \quad S = 0.164m^{0.667} \\
&\text{aspect ratio} \quad AR = 9.339m^{0.069} \\
&\text{beating frequecy} \quad f = 3.991m^{-0.202} \\
&\text{drag coefficient} \quad C_d = 0.027m^{-0.034} \\
&\text{minimum power velocity} \quad V_{\min p} = 8.704m^{0.158} \\
&\text{minimum drag velocity} \quad V_{\min d} = 11.591m^{0.158} \\
&\text{flying power output} \quad P_{fly} = 45.211m^{0.728} \\
&\text{maximum power output} \quad P_{\max} = 84.388m^{0.734}
\end{aligned} \tag{8}$$

These bionic formulas are approximate formulas with statistics meaning, and don't coincide with actual birds completely, they are used to acquire the approximate scale of every flying parameter.

According to flying bionic formulas, the mass m of flying robot is the fundamental variable of other flying variables. Commonly, m should contain the mass of fuselage, wing, transmission mechanism, power, etc., and the available load including sensor, control, and communication. In theory, we hope the self mass of flying robot to be smallest, but in fact, the mass is restricted by the actual design, technics, materials, and energy power. Considering the factual situation, the smallest mass of the flying robot is about 16g, in which micro motor is 5.3g, battery is 3.2g, transmission mechanism is 3.5g, fuselage is 1.5g, wing is 1.5g, and empennage is 1.0g.

After calculation, the initial flying parameters of the flapping-wing flying robot is acquired: whole wingspan $b = 0.27\text{m}$, wing area $S = 1.04 \times 10^{-2}\text{m}^2$, aspect ratio $AR = 7.02$, beating frequency $f = 9.2\text{Hz}$, minimum power velocity $V_{\min p} = 4.53\text{m/s}$.

3 Design and Analysis of Flapping Mechanism

Based on the initial design results, the flapping wing form, transmission layout, power scheme, and total structure of the flying robot can be designed. Figure 1 is the 3D design model of flying robot.

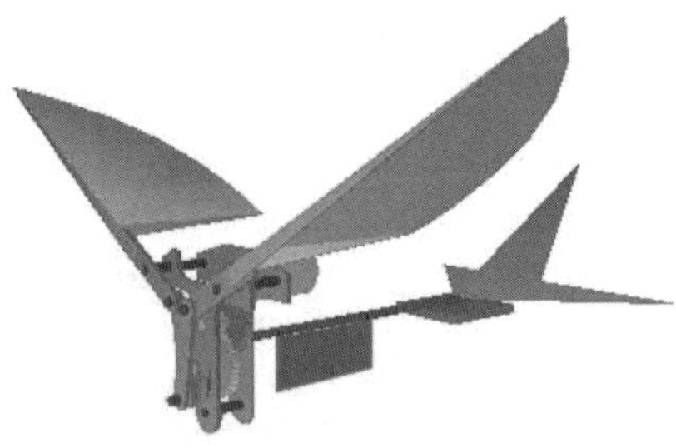

Fig. 1. Design model of flying robot

The characteristics of flapping wing mode lie in the lift and thrust is produced by downstroke and upstroke of the wings, so the design of efficient and reliable flapping mechanism is more important. For flying robot, the design, fabrication and study of dynamic characteristics of micro flapping mechanism are key questions. The transmission scheme is from micro DC motor to two grade gear speed-down, then to crank rocker mechanism, then to flapping wing. Figure 2 is the sketch of flapping mechanism. The advantages of the mechanism include simple and compact structure, high efficient and reliable transmission, and light weight.

The specified parameters of the flapping mechanism such as gear ratio, rod length of the linkage mechanism, wingspan, wing area, can be choose according to former result of bionic design. Meanwhile, the property of the motor should be considered in design.

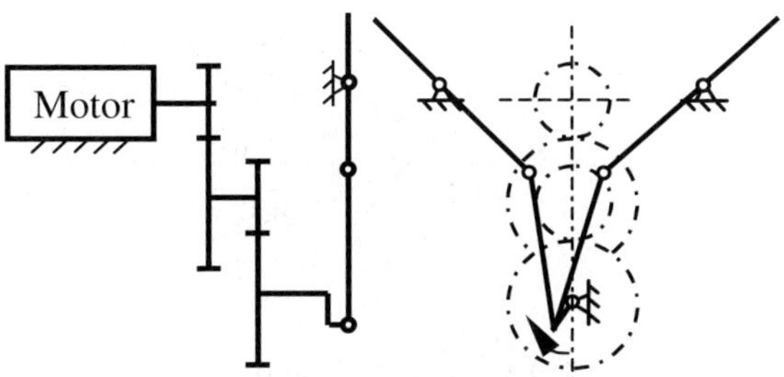

Fig. 2. Flapping mechanism

Based on the design of flapping mechanism, the aerodynamic analysis should be carried on to calculate the lift and thrust during the course of actual flying.

Up to now, there is not a complete and accurate analysis method about flapping-wing flying aerodynamic in low Re number. On account of involving nonstable aerodynamics, shape deformation of flexible wing, rapid adaptive system, it is more complicated for the sturdy of flapping wing flying than fixed wing flying. On the premise of satisfying engineering application, the approximate analytical method is adopted to study the aerodynamic characteristic of flapping wing flight.

Based on bionic analysis, the aerodynamics simplified model of flapping-wing flying robot can be set up as figure 5. OXYZ is the absolute coordinate system fixed on the ground, $O_1X_1Y_1Z_1$ is the movement coordinates fixed on the mass centre O_1 of flying robot, its axes are always parallel to the axes of absolute coordinate system. Axis X_2 is coincident with the flap axis of flapping-wing robot, and the angle is γ between axis X_1 and axis X_2. The flap plane which is made up of the linkage lines of airfoil section aerodynamic centres is vertical to the flap axis.

The wing is divided into many wing elements along the wingspan direction, and its airfoil section is illustrated in figure 6. When considering the bending and torsional deformation, the flap angle around flap axis and the torsional angle around revolving axis of the wing element which distance is r from wing root are as follows:

$$\begin{cases} \phi(r,t) = \phi_0 + \phi_1(r)\sin(\omega_\phi t + \beta_\phi) \\ \psi(r,t) = \psi_0 + \psi_1(r)\sin(\omega_\psi t + \beta_\psi) \end{cases} \tag{9}$$

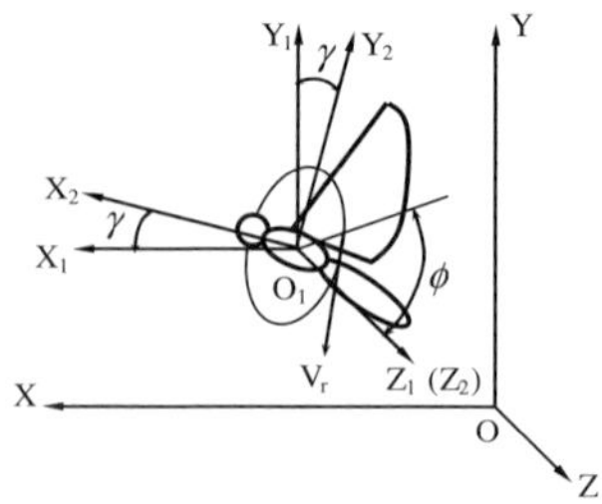

Fig. 3. Coordinate system of flying robot model

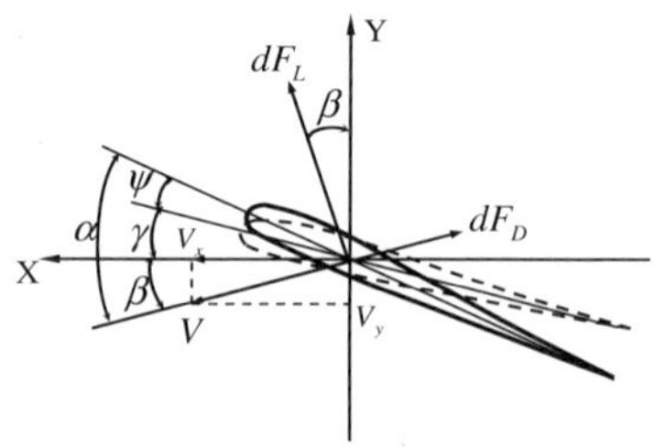

Fig. 4. Airfoil section

According to the flapping-wing movement rule, the velocity V_r of the airfoil aerodynamic center which distance is r from wing root is

$$V_r(r,t) = r\frac{\partial\phi}{\partial t} = r\phi_1(r)\omega_\phi \cos(\omega_\phi t + \beta_\phi) \tag{10}$$

V_{rx}, V_{ry} and V_{rz}, the projection, of V_r on axis XYZ, are as follows:

$$\begin{aligned} V_{rx} &= V_r \cos\phi \sin\gamma \\ V_{ry} &= -V_r \cos\phi \cos\gamma \\ V_{rz} &= V_r \sin\phi \end{aligned} \tag{11}$$

The components of flying velocity of robot mass center along axis X and Y are $\dot{x}$ and $\dot{y}$, respectively. So the absolute velocity V of wing aerodynamic center and the angle between V and axis X are as follows:

$$\begin{aligned} V &= \sqrt{V_x^2 + V_y^2} \\ \beta &= \arctan(V_y / V_x) \end{aligned} \tag{12}$$

V_x and V_y are components of V along axis X and Y.

$$\begin{aligned} V_x &= \dot{x} + V_{rx} \\ V_y &= \dot{y} + V_{ry} \end{aligned} \tag{13}$$

From Figure 6, if the torsion angle of airfoil section at a certain moment is ψ (as shown in dotted line for the initial location, and solid lines for the torsional position), at this time, the attack angle α of airfoil on aerodynamic center is

$$\alpha = \gamma + \psi + \beta \tag{14}$$

Due to the flap of wing, the aerodynamic forces on wing element is

$$\begin{aligned} dF_L(t,r) &= \frac{1}{2} C_L(\alpha(t))\rho c(r) V^2(t,r) dr \\ dF_D(t,r) &= \frac{1}{2} C_D(\alpha(t))\rho c(r) V^2(t,r) dr \end{aligned} \tag{15}$$

In (16), dF_L and dF_D are lift and drag on wing element, ρ is density of air, c is chord length of wing. V is velocity of wing relative to airflow, C_L and C_D are dimensionless lift and drag coefficients, which can be expressed as functions of attack angle α. Here according to the literature [2], the empirical calculation formula of lift and drag coefficient can be obtained from the test results.

$$\begin{aligned} C_L &= 0.225 + 1.58\sin(2.13\alpha - 7.20) \\ C_D &= 1.92 - 1.55\cos(2.04\alpha - 9.82) \end{aligned} \tag{16}$$

The aerodynamic force imposed on wing element due to the action of rotation cycle is

$$dF_N(t,r) = C_{rot}\rho c(r)^2 V(t,r)\omega dr \tag{17}$$

$C_{rot} = \pi(3/4 - x_0)$ is the revolving force coefficient, and is independent of attack angle. x_0 is the dimensionless length from the revolving axis to the leading edge of wing. ω is the angular velocity of wing relative to revolving shaft. The force is a pure normal force and its action direction is vertical to airfoil profile.

If project dF_L, dF_D and dF_N on axis X and Y, respectively, and calculate the integral of these forces along wing length. According to the superposition principle, the total lift L and drag D are as follows.

$$\begin{aligned} L(t) &= \int_0^{b/2} \{dF_L(t,r)\cos\beta + dF_D(t,r)\sin\beta + dF_N(t,r)\cos(\gamma+\psi)\} \\ D(t) &= \int_0^{b/2} \{dF_L(t,r)\sin\beta - dF_D(t,r)\cos\beta - dF_N(t,r)\sin(\gamma+\psi)\} \end{aligned} \tag{18}$$

Similarly, the resultant force of each wing element is multiplied by the distance r from the wing root, and the integral along the wingspan direction is calculated, so the instantaneous aerodynamic resistance moment M_{aero} on the wing can be obtained.

There is a need to explain that it is fast and easy to estimate flapping aerodynamic force, and set design scale to use approximate analytical method, but calculation accuracy is relatively low. It is accurate but time-consuming using the numerical simulation method of computational fluid dynamics (CFD). The actual design can use analytical method for rapid estimation, and then use numerical method for certification.

4 Flexible Wing Design of the Flying Robot

The wing structure of birds are sophisticated and complex, it is very difficult to mimic totally. Simply the pursuit of complexity and precision make the design become an ideal design drawings and never practical. On the basis of grasping the main features of birds' wings, we should seek to the aim that the design and process are simple and feasible.

The flapping wing design of flying robot includes wing structural design, airfoil design, size parameters design, and so on. Two typical wings structure are as follows.

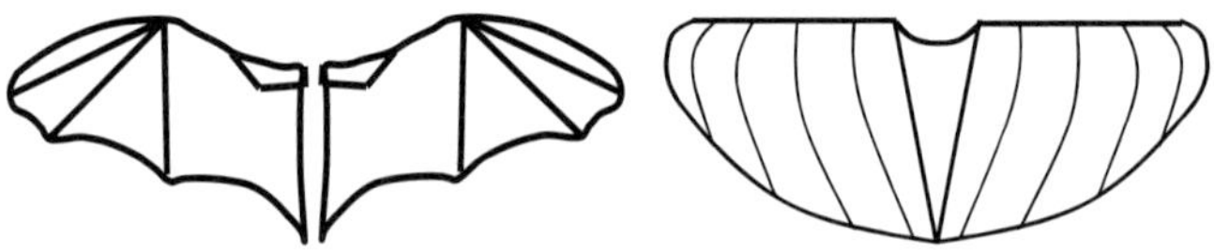

(a) bat-like wing (b) arc surface wing

Fig. 5. Wing structure

It should be noted that the common characteristics of various wings is that the diameter and thickness of the main skeleton reduce from wing base to wing tip gradually. It is a kind of variable stiffness structure. This design imitates the feature of birds, and its advantage is to reduce the energy consumption and skeleton stress.

5 System Configuration and Prototype Fabrication

According to the status and function of each part, the system configuration of flying robot can be divided into five child systems: energy and power system, fuselage and flapping wing system, flying control system, sensors system and communication system.

Total configuration is improved continually based on theory analysis and repeated experiments. The fix attack angle of flapping wing, the stance angle of stabilizer, center of gravity of the flying robot, position of aerodynamic center are adjusted in order to make the flying robot have fine flying stability and maneuverability.

The layout sketch of flying robot is shown as figure 6. The main structure include: 1. flapping wing; 2.transmission and drive mechanism; 3. micro motor; 4. micro switch; 5. radio receiver; 6. polymer lithium cell; 7. rudder motor; 8. vertical empennage; 9. stabilizer; 10. elevator; 11.rudder; 12.support rod; 13.fuselage keel.

Based on the bionic design, dynamic analysis, and total system design, the bionic flying robot prototype is fabricated shown as Figure 7. The flying robot use polymer lithium battery as power and is driven by micro DC motor. The fuselage is made of carbon fibre, and the flexible wing is made of polyester membrane. Total weight of the flying robot is about 16.5g, the wingspan is 200mm, and the flapping frequency is 12~15Hz. The flying robot is controlled by remote radio, and can fly 3~4 minutes.

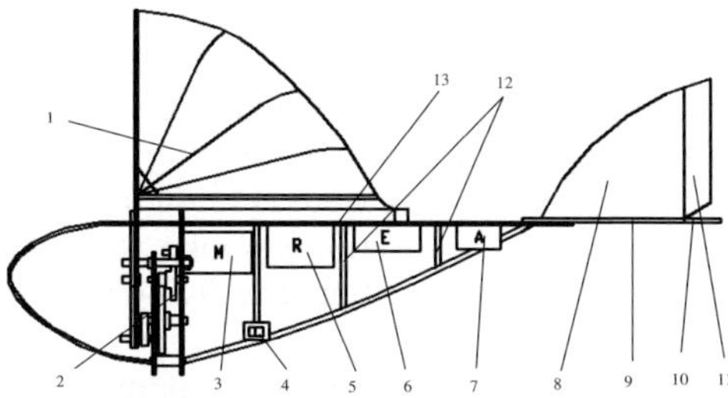

(a) Side view

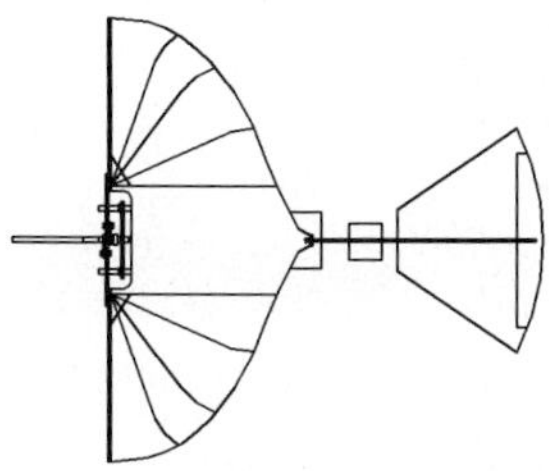

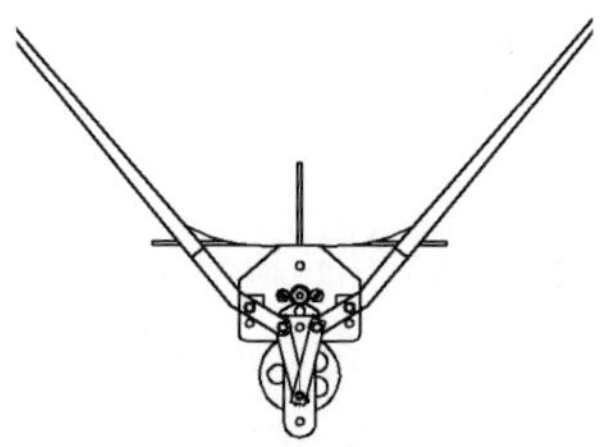

(b) Planform view (c) Former view

Fig. 6. Layout sketch of flying robot

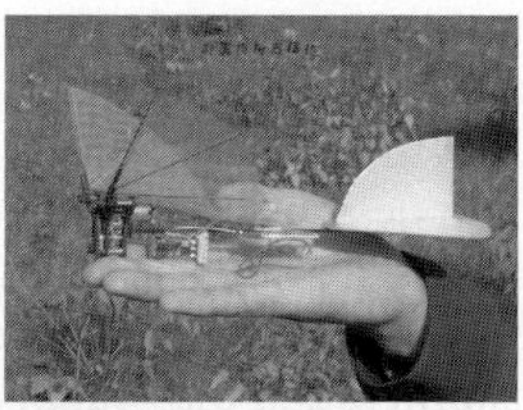

Fig. 7. Flying robot prototype

6 Wind Tunnel Experiments

The flying robot prototype is tested in the low turbulence wind tunnel, in which the wind speed is 2m/s~10m/s, Reynolds number is about 2,625 (wind speed 5m/s).

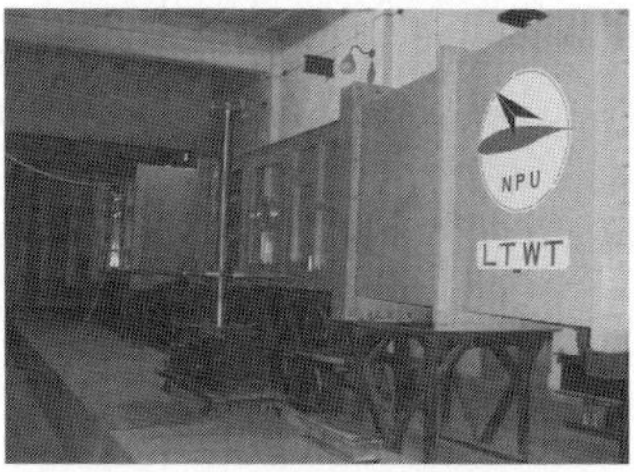

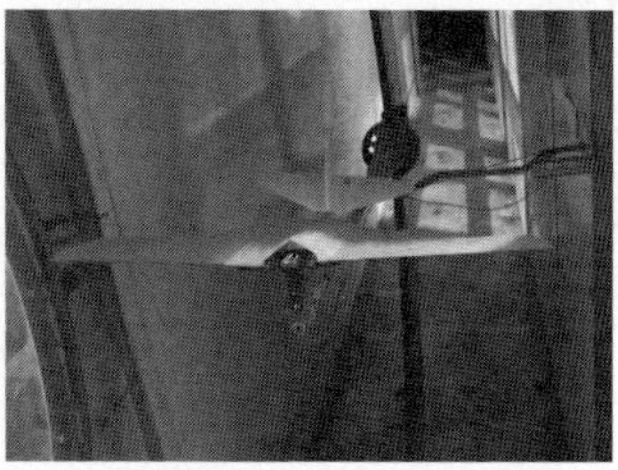

(a) Low turbulence wind tunnel (b) Inner view of wind tunnel

Fig. 8. Smoke wind tunnel experiment

The experiments results indicated that the aerodynamic forces increased by the increase of flapping frequency, wind velocity and attack angle of the wing.

The results also showed that the flapping frequency and lift was smaller than the calculated results. It was analyzed that the errors were caused probably because the contour drag and induced drag of the wing were ignored in calculation.

Furthermore, the flow field test is made in a smoke wind tunnel. The disturbance situation of flow field during the course of flapping flying is shown in Figure 9.

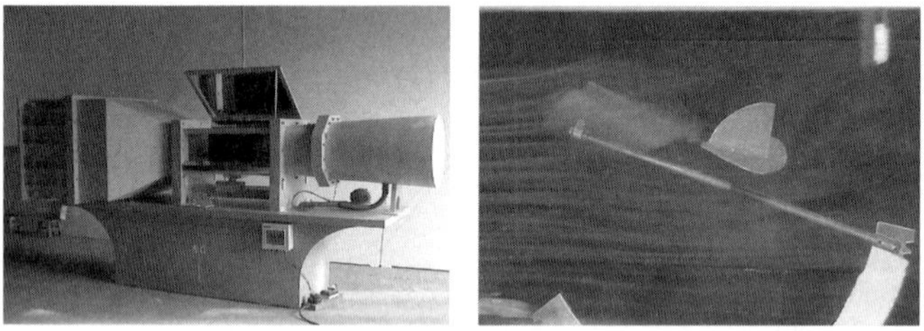

(a) Smoke wind tunnel (b) Flying robot in wind tunnel

Fig. 9. Smoke wind tunnel experiment

7 Conclusion

Bionic flapping-wing flying robots are new conceptual air vehicles. They surpass the research fields of traditional airplane design and aerodynamics, and initiate a new multidisciplinary research field. A new method is proposed in this paper to design flapping-wing flying robot and the design course include bionic primary design, total structure design, aerodynamic analysis, system configuration, and fabrication and test of robot prototype. The theoretical calculations and experimental results show that this method is effective and feasibility, and thus supply an overall engineering design method for flapping-wing flying robot.

Acknowledgments

This paper is supported by the Hubei Key Laboratory of Mechanical Transmission and Manufacturing Engineering.

References

1. Dickonson, M.H.: Wing Rotation and the Aerodynamic Basis of Insect Flight. Science 284, 1954–1960 (1999)
2. Delaurier, J.D.: An Aerodynamic Model for Flapping-wing Flight. Aeronautical Jorunal 10, 125–130 (1993)
3. Charsles, P.E., Coen, B.: Leading-edge Vortices in Insect Flight. Nature 384(12), 19–26 (1996)
4. Graham, K.T.: Mechanics and Aerodynamics of Insect Fight Control. Biol. Rev. 76, 449–471 (2001)
5. Wei, S., Mats, B., Daniel, L.: Flapping and Flexible Wings for Biological and Micro Air Vehicles. Progress in Aerospace Sciences 35, 455–505 (1999)

Fuzzy Logic Control for Vehicle Suspension Systems

Chuanyin Tang[1], Lijie Yue[2], Lixin Guo[1], Shuwen Zhou[1], Wei Zhou[3], and Zhaowen Wang[4]

[1] School of Mechanical Engineering and Automation, North Eastern University, Shenyang, China
[2] School of Material Science and Engineering, Shandong University of Science and Technology, Qingdao,China
[3] China Ministry of Communications Research Institute of Highway, Beingjing, China
[4] School of Materials and Metallurgy ,North Eastern University, Shenyang, China
monsigor@yahoo.com.cn

Abstract. An active suspension system for vehicles using fuzzy logic controls is presented in this paper. The model is described by a linear system with six degrees of freedom, subject to irregular excitations from the road surface. Based on control theory, the fuzzy control system of the active suspension is proposed. With the aid of software Matlab/simulink, a lot of simulation process is done. Simulation results indicate that the proposed active suspension system proves to be effective in the vibration isolation of the suspension system. What's more, a mechanical dynamic animation of six-degree-of -freedom half body of vehicle suspension system is obtained, with the aid of software ADAMS and media player. The animation demonstrates the mechanism principle of suspension system more vividly and visually.

Keywords: suspension system; fuzzy control; Matlab/simulink; simulation; animation.

1 Introduction

The major purpose of suspension system is to provide passenger with ride comfort while maintaining the vehicle to be safe and stable .Passive suspension system can only offer a compromise between these two conflicting criteria by providing spring and damping coefficients with fixed rates. Active suspension control system can produce corresponding control force according to running status and road oscillations to maintain the suspension system to be the optimal status.

A variety of research projects and publications deal with different types of active suspension systems have been discussed in [1], [2] and [3], .Different vehicle dynamic models have been adopted according to different study purposes during research. A two degree-of -freedom quarter body of vehicle suspension system model has been widely applied in vehicle suspension control research, while it can only indicate the vehicle body vertical movement ,not include the pitching movement of the vehicle body. Although a seven degree-of -freedom whole-body of vehicle

C. Xiong et al. (Eds.): ICIRA 2008, Part II, LNAI 5315, pp. 197–206, 2008.

suspension system model can describe not only the vertical movement of the four wheels and the body center of gravity , but also present the pitching and lateral movement, the model is too complicated to be widely applied [4]. A four degree-of -freedom half body of vehicle suspension system model can describe both the vertical movement of the body center of gravity ,and the pitching movement, which got widely used in suspension dynamic model. In our research, a six-degree-of -freedom half body of vehicle suspension system model is obtained, which has the advantages of six degree-of -freedom model, what's more, it can demonstrate the effect of seat and passenger, which makes it to be an ideal model for suspension dynamic description.

The purpose of this paper is to propose an active suspension system for vehicles, using the fuzzy-logic controller. The model is described by a linear system, subject to irregular excitation from the road surface. In particular, a mechanical dynamic animation of six degree-of -freedom half body of vehicle suspension system is obtained, with the aid of software ADAMS and media player. Finally, some concluding remarks are given.

2 Modelling

2.1 Six Degree-of -Freedom Model

The model of half-body system is shown in Figure1. The half-body suspension system is represented as a linearized six degree-of-freedom system. It consists of a single sprung mass connected to two unsprung masses ,the seat mass and the passenger mass. The sprung is free to heave and pitch while the unsprung masses and the seat and the passenger mass are free to bounce vertically with respect to the sprung mass. The suspensions between the sprung and unsprung masses are modeled as linear viscous dampers and spring elements, while the tires are modeled as simple linear springs without damping. For simplicity, all pitch angles are assumed to be small.

After applying a force- balance analysis to the model in Fig.1.,the equations of motion are given as

$$\begin{aligned}
m_1\ddot{z}_1 &= k_{21}(z_1' - z_1) + c_1(\dot{z}_1' - \dot{z}_1) - k_{11}(z_1 - r_1) - u_1 \\
m_2\ddot{z}_2 &= k_{22}(z_2' - z_2) + c_2(\dot{z}_2' - \dot{z}_2) - k_{12}(z_2 - r_2) - u_2 \\
m_p\ddot{z}_p &= -k_p\left(z_p - z_c\right) - c_p\left(\dot{z}_p - \dot{z}_c\right) \\
m_c\ddot{z}_c &= k_p\left(z_p - z_c\right) + c_p\left(\dot{z}_p - \dot{z}_c\right) - k_c\left(z_c - z_3 + \theta e\right) - c_c\left(\dot{z}_c - \dot{z}_3 + \theta e\right) \\
m_3\ddot{z}_3 &= -k_{21}(z_1' - z_1) - c_1(\dot{z}_1' - \dot{z}_1) - k_{22}(z_2' - z_2) - c_2(\dot{z}_2' - \dot{z}_2) + k_c\left[z_c - (z_3 - \theta e)\right] \\
&\quad + c_c\left[\dot{z}_c - \left(\dot{z}_3 - \dot{\theta} e\right)\right] + u_1 + u_2 \\
J\ddot{\theta} &= a[k_{21}(z_1' - z_1) + c_1(\dot{z}_1' - \dot{z}_1) - u_1] - b[k_{22}(z_2' - z_2) + c_2(\dot{z}_2' - \dot{z}_2) - u_2] \\
&\quad - e\left\{k_c\left[z_c - (z_3 - \theta e)\right] + c_c\left[\dot{z}_c - \left(\dot{z}_3 - \dot{\theta} e\right)\right]\right\}
\end{aligned} \tag{1}$$

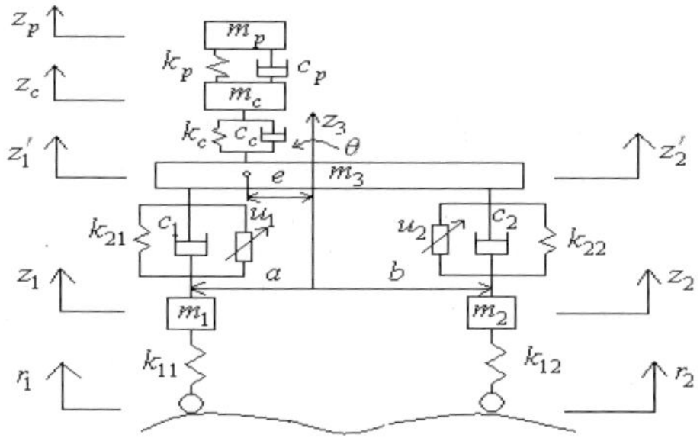

Fig. 1. Model of half body six degree-of -freedom of suspension

The system states are assigned as

$x_1 = z_1$ front wheel unsprung mass height
$x_2 = z_2$ rear wheel unsprung mass height
$x_3 = z_3$ heave position
$x_4 = \theta$ pitch angle
$x_5 = \dot{z}_1$ front wheel unsprung mass velocity
$x_6 = \dot{z}_2$ rear wheel unsprung mass velocity
$x_7 = \dot{z}_3$ heave velocity
$x_8 = \dot{\theta}$ pitch angular velocity
$x_9 = z_c$ seat heave height
$x_{10} = \dot{z}_c$ seat heave velocity
$x_{11} = z_p$ passenger heave height
$x_{12} = \dot{z}_p$ passenger heave velocity

This results in the system state equations below:

$$X = (x_{1,} x_{2,} x_3 ......x_{12})^T \tag{2}$$

And

$$x_1 = z_1, x_2 = z_2, x_3 = z_3, x_4 = \theta, x_5 = \dot{z}_1, x_6 = \dot{z}_2$$
$$x_7 = \dot{z}_3, x_8 = \dot{\theta}, x_9 = z_c, x_{10} = \dot{z}_c, x_{11} = z_p, x_{12} = \dot{z}_p \tag{3}$$

The state space equations in matrix are given by

$$\dot{X} = AX + BR + CU \tag{4}$$

With the control input defined as the force generated at the front, rear suspensions respectively as $U = [u_1 \quad u_2]^T$, and the disturbance input defined as $R = [r_1 \quad r_2]^T$. Signals z_1, z_2, z_3, z_c and z_p are the heave height at the front wheel , rear wheel ,vehicle body, seat and passenger ,respectively.

The model parameters selected for this study are given in Table 1.

Table 1. Parameters of system model

model parameters	value	model parameters	value
font wheel mass m_1/kg	40	rear wheel massm_2/kg	36
Sprung mass m_3/kg	730	front tire spring stiffness k_{11}/ N/m/ N/m	17500
rear tire spring stiffness k_{12}/ N/m	17500	front suspension spring stiffness k_{21}/ N/m	19960
rear suspension spring stiffness k_{22}/ N/m	17500	front suspension damping c_1 /N.s/m	1290
rear suspension damping c_2/ N.s/m	1290	pitch axis moment of inertia/ kg.m^2	1230
Passenger mass m_p/ kg	60	Seat spring equivalent stiffness k_c / N/m	2400
seat mass m_c /kg		Cushion equivalent damping c_p N.s/m	152.8
seat equivalent damping c_c N.s/m	875	Cushion equivalent stiffness k_p / N/m	8228.7
distance between front of vehicle and center of gravity of sprung mass a/ m			1.0
distance between rear of vehicle and center of gravity of sprung mass b/ m			1.8
distance between the passenger-seat system action point and the center of gravity of vehicle body **e**/ m			0.1

2.2 Road Input Modelling

The road irregularity formula is defined as

$$\dot{x} = -2\pi f_0 x + 2\pi\sqrt{G_0 v}\omega(t) \tag{5}$$

Using Grade B road surface, which is the common road ,gives the irregular road coefficients as $G_0 = 64\times10^{-6}\ \mathrm{m}^2/\mathrm{m}^{-1}$ and velocity v is $20\mathrm{m/s}$.

3 Control System Design

The fuzzy logic control is one of the most attractive parts where fuzzy theory can be effectively applied. The fuzzy logic translates the mathematical control strategy into the linguistic control strategy. The fuzzy logic controller is usually based on the operator's knowledge, fuzzy modelling of the operator's control actions and fuzzy modelling of the process.

The fuzzy logic controller consists of three steps. The first step is the fuzzification, the second step is the reasoning using the fuzzy rule base, the last step is the defuzzification.

In the paper, the fuzzy logic controller is used to adjust the vehicle's body acceleration errors[5].

Figure 2 shows the block diagram of the vehicle body acceleration used. The error block is the difference between the actual body acceleration and the reference body acceleration.The fuzzy logic controller is designed to reduce the acceleration errors.

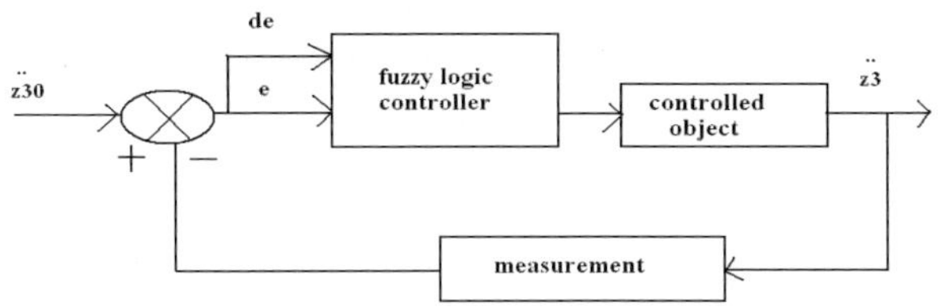

Fig. 2. Block diagram of the acceleration control system

3.1 Fuzzification

The first step in making a fuzzy logic controller is to take the inputs and determine the degree to which the inputs belong to each of the appropriate fuzzy sets via fuzzy membership function. The input is always a numerical value and must be fuzzified. The fuzzification of the input becomes a membership function to be evaluated. The fuzzy membership function can be described as follows:

$$K = \{(x, u_k(x)) \mid x \in K, u_k(x) \in [0,1]\} \tag{6}$$

where $u_k(x)$ is the membership function specifying the grade of degree for any element in K which belongs to the fuzzy set K . The lager values of $u_k(x)$ indicate the higher degrees of membership.

The trimf membership is selected. It has seven grades; negative big (NB), negative medium (NM) ,negative small (NS) ,zero (ZE), positive small (PS), positive medium (PM), and positive big (PB).

3.2 Fuzzy Rule Base

The Mamdani fuzzy logic type is used. The fuzzy control rules are designed by a collection of if-then rules. In general, the input to an if-then rule is the current value for the input variable and the output is an entire fuzzy set. This set will later be defuzzified, assigning one value to the output.

In the paper, the fuzzy controller controls the multi-input-single-output system and the fuzzy rule is described as follows:

$$Ri: IF\ x\ is\ A_i ..., AND\ y\ is\ B_i ..., THEN\ z = C_i, D_i, E_i, F_i$$

A total of seven grades are used for the control force in the paper: negative big(NB),negative medium (NM), negative small (NS),zero (ZE), positive small (PS), positive medium (PM), and positive big (PB).The fuzzy rule table shown in Table 2 is developed based on these if-then rules.

3.3 Defuzzification

The defuzzification is a mapping from a space of the fuzzy control action into a space of the non-fuzzy control action. This process is necessary because the action is required to actuate the controller in many practical applications. In most cases , the

Table 2. The rules of fuzzy control

u		*de*						
		NB	NM	NS	ZE	PS	PM	PB
e	NB	NM	NS	NS	NS	ZE	PS	PM
	NM	NM	NM	NM	NS	PS	PM	PM
	NS	NB	NM	NM	NS	PM	PB	PB
	ZE	NB	NB	NM	ZE	PM	PB	PB
	PS	NB	NB	NM	PS	PM	PM	PB
	PM	NM	NM	NS	PS	PM	PM	PM
	PB	NM	NS	ZE	PS	PS	PS	PM

input for the defuzzification process is a fuzzy set and the output is a single number. The famous defuzzification method is the centroid calculation, which returns to the centre of the area under the curve.

In this paper, the defuzzification using the centre of area method is used and the defuzzification outputs are the controlled force. This method yields

$$Z^* = \sum_{j=1}^{n} \mu_c(z_j) z_j \Big/ \sum_{j=1}^{n} \mu_c(z_j) \tag{7}$$

where n is the number of quantization levels of the output, z_j is the amount of control output at the quantization level j, $\mu_c(z_j)$ represents its membership value in the fuzzy output set.

The fuzzy inference system compiler and membership function complier are showed in figure 3 and figure 4.

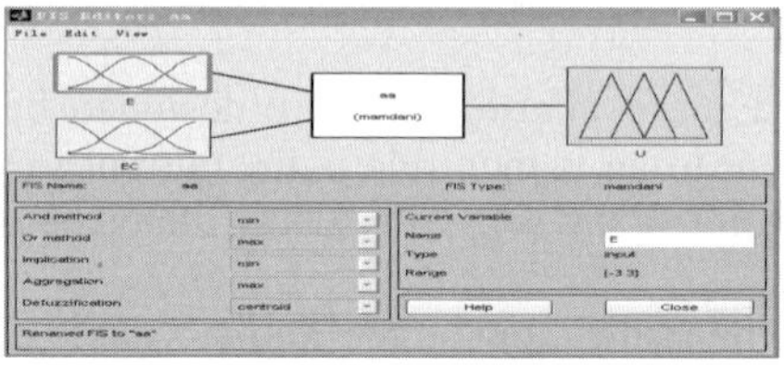

Fig. 3. Fuzzy inference system complier

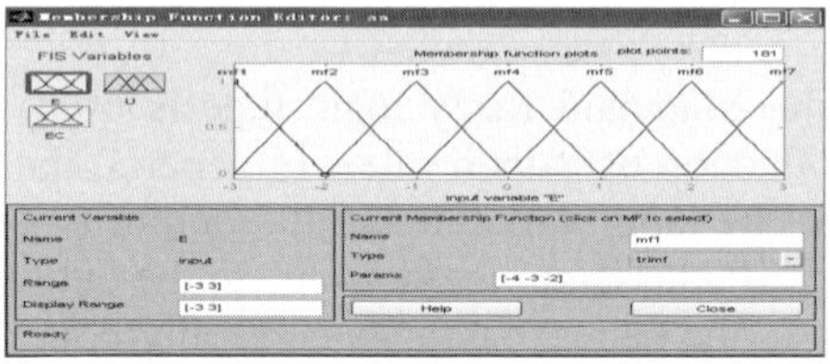

Fig. 4. Membership function complier

4 Results and Discussion

The established dynamic vehicle model and the fuzzy logic controller are used to improve the vehicle comfort using Matlab/Simulink.

Figure 5shows the corresponding Simulink block diagram of six degree-of - freedom half-body of vehicle suspension system.This Simulink block calculates the vehicle body acceleration, velocity, displacement, pitch acceleration, front and rear suspension displacement ,tire travel, seat movement and passenger movement as well. The E(acceleration error) and dE (variation acceleration error) are the input of the fuzzy logic controller. The control forces are the output of the fuzzy controller.

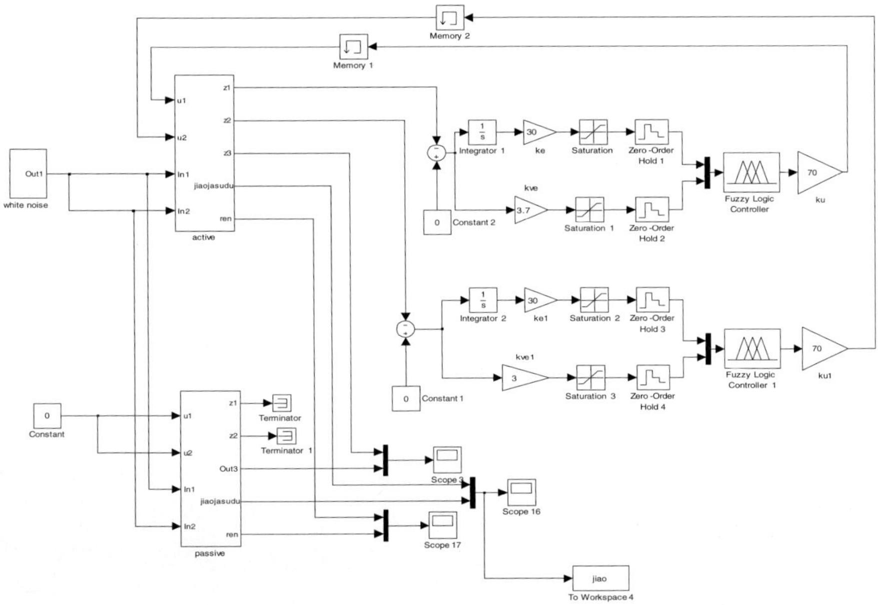

Fig. 5. Simulink block diagram of suspension system

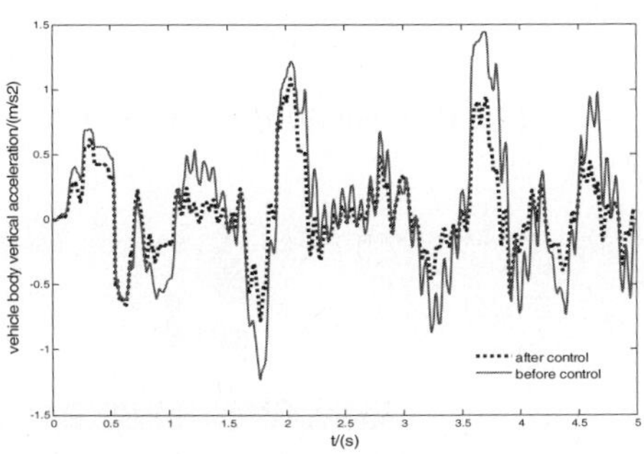

Fig. 6. Vehicle body vertical acceleration

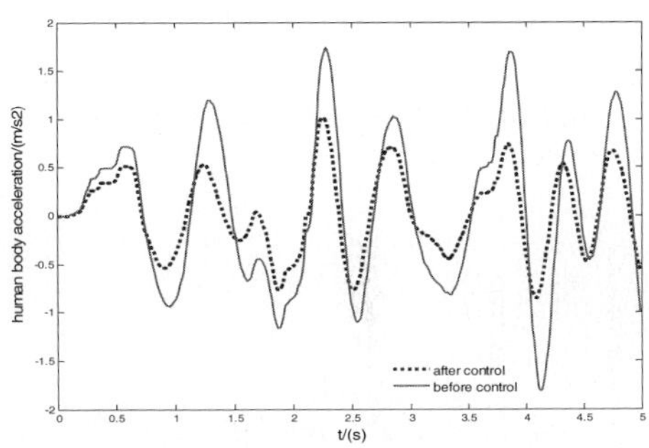

Fig. 7. Human body vertical acceleration

Figure 6 shows the controlled body acceleration response and the passive system body acceleration response. For compare, they are out in one figure. The solid line indicates the passive system, the dash line presents the controlled system. Figure 7 shows the controlled acceleration response and the passive system acceleration response of passenger. Figure 8. shows the controlled pitching angular acceleration response and the passive system pitch angular acceleration response. Figure 9and Figure 10 show the front suspension displacement and rear suspension displacement response, respectively. Figure 11and Figure 12 show the front tire dynamic load and rear tire dynamic load response, respectively.

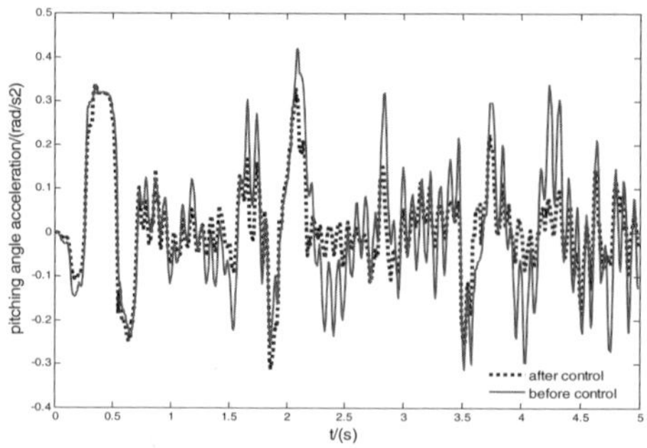

Fig. 8. Pitching angular acceleration

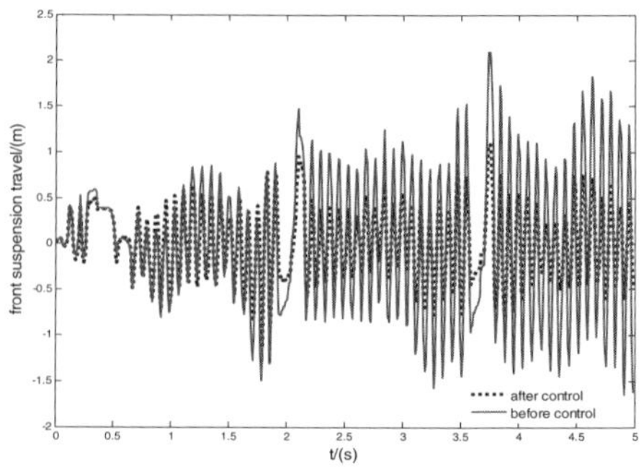

Fig. 9. Front suspension displacement

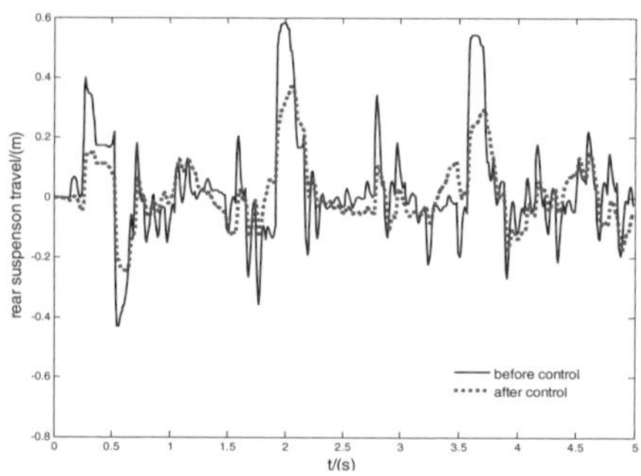

Fig. 10. Rear suspension displacement

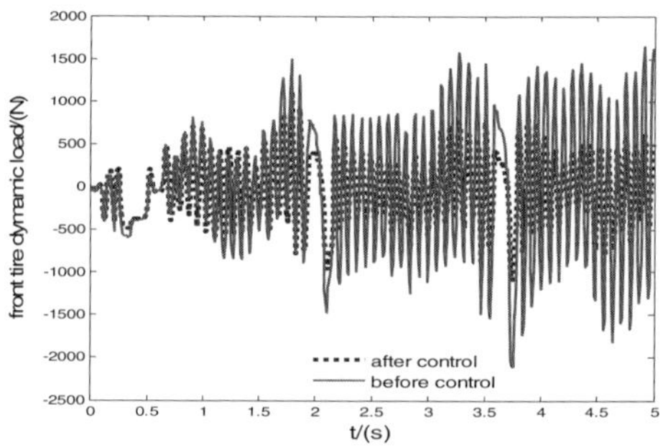

Fig. 11. Front tire dynamic load

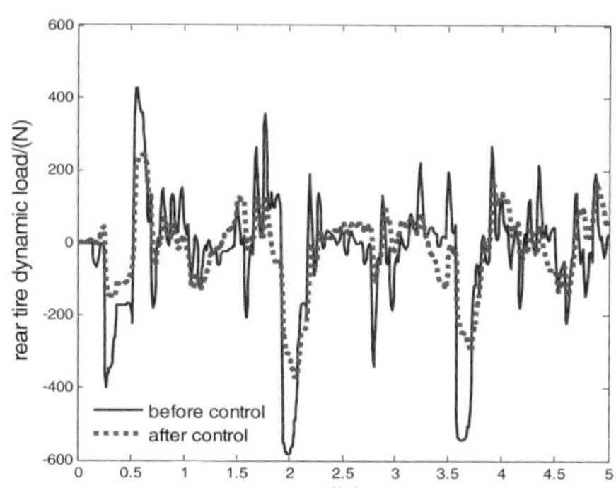

Fig. 12. Rear tire dynamic load

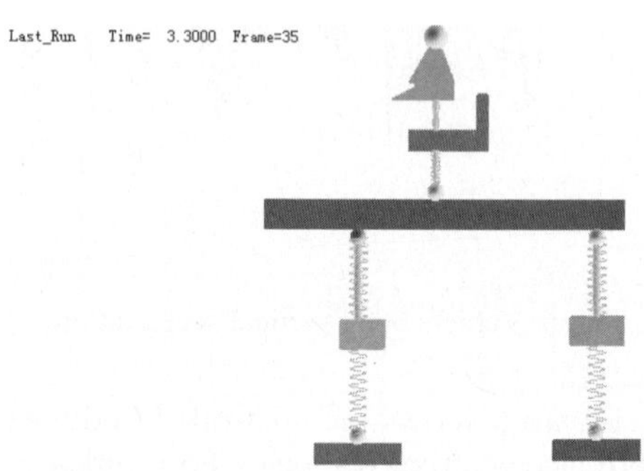

Fig. 13. Mechanical dynamic animation

Table 3 includes the performance analysis of the system. The body acceleration and pitching angular acceleration is greatly decreased, and the passenger acceleration is reduced dramatically ,which indicates that the fuzzy controller is effective in improving the system riding comfortability [6]. The compare of tire dynamic loads show that the system holding ability is meliorated.

Table 3. Performance analysis

	Body acceleration (m/ s^2)	Pitching angular acceleration (rad/s^2)	Passenger Acceleration (m/ s^2)	Front suspension displacement (m)
passive	0.4722	0.1760	0.2205	0.7503
controller	0.2679	0.1212	0.1126	0.3947
Performance melioration	43.3%	31.1%	49%	47.4%
	Rear suspension displacement (m)	Front tire dynamic load (N)	Rear tire dynamic load (N)	
passive	0.1756	750.36	175.18	
controller	0.1124	394.7	111.98	
Performance melioration	35.9%	47.9%	36.6%	

5 Animation Demonstration

First, using the software ADAMS ,the mechanical model of six degree-of-freedom half body suspension system is established, then with the aid of software media player ,a mechanical dynamic animation of six degree-of -freedom half body of vehicle suspension system is obtained, as demonstrated in figure 13. The animation illustrates the mechanism principle of suspension system more vividly and visually.

6 Conclusions

In this paper an active suspension control approach combining a fuzzy control scheme was proposed for a six degree-of-freedom half body suspension system in order to reduce heave, pitch acceleration and improve ride comfortability of the vehicle. The percentage improvement for the ride comfort compared with a passive suspension averages around 40%. It was shown that the proposed fuzzy controller proves to be effective in the vibration isolation of the suspension system. Performance of the suspension system was demonstrated in simulations.

Acknowledgement

Thanks for the fund supported by National Basic Research Program of China(973 Program)(Number: 2007CB210305) & Western Communications Construction Project ,Research Institute of Highway (Number:2005031822322). And thanks for Northeastern university for providing us with the resources.

References

1. Lin, Y.J., Lu, T.Q., Padovan, J.: Fuzzy Logic Control of Vehicle Suspension Systems. Int. J. Vehicle Design 14, 457–470 (1993)
2. Liu, H., Nonami, K., Hagiwara, T.: Active Following Fuzzy Output Feedback Sliding Mode Control of Real-Vehicle Semi-active Suspensions. Journal of Sound and Vibration 314, 39–52 (2008)

3. Sung, K.G., Han, Y.M., Cho, J.W., Choi, S.B.: Vibration Control of Vehicle ER Suspension System Using Fuzzy Moving Sliding Mode Controller. Journal of Sound and Vibration 311, 1004–1019 (2008)
4. Chen, S.A., Liu, H.G., Lu, S.L., He, R., et al.: Fuzzy Control System for Automobile Active Suspension with Four Dimensions. Automobiles Engineering 23, 375–380 (2001)
5. Chen yang.:Active Suspension System of Automobile Based on Fuzzy Control, Northeastern University (2007)
6. Yu, Z.s.: The Theory of Automobiles. The Press of Industrial Mechanics (2000)

A Sidewall Piezoresistive Force Sensor Used in a MEMS Gripper

Tao Chen[1], Liguo Chen[1], Lining Sun[1], Jiachou Wang[1], and Xinxin Li[2]

[1] State Key Laboratory of Robotics and System, Robotics Institute, Harbin Institute of Technology, Harbin 150080, China
{Tao Chen,cht22}@sina.com, {Liguo Chen,clg}@hit.edu.cn, {Lining Sun,lnsun}@hit.edu.cn, {Jiachou Wang,jiatao_wang}@163.com

[2] State Key Lab of Transducer Technology, Shanghai Institute of Microsystem and Information Technology, Chinese Academy of Sciences, Shanghai 200050, China
{Xinxin Li,xxli}@mail.sim.ac.cn

Abstract. This work reports the design and development of a MEMS based, piezoresistive sensor for micro-force measurement. Surface and bulk micromachining technology is employed to fabricate the force sensor from single crystal silicon wafer (i.e., no silicon on insulator wafer is used). Boron diffusion process combined with deep reactive ionic etching (DRIE) technique is used to form the side direction force sensors. The force sensor is integrated in a four arms structure MEMS gripper to experimentally verify the performance of the sensor. The resolution of the force sensor is in the micronewton range and, therefore, provides feedback of the forces that dominate the micromanipulation processes. Testing results show that the sensitivity of the piezoresistive sensors is better than 72V/N and the resolution is better than 3μN. Experimental show that it can successfully provide force sensing and play a main role in preventing damage of microparts in micromanipulation and microassembly tasks.

Keywords: MEMS, Microgripper, Sidewall piezoresistive sensor.

1 Introduction

With the development of micromanipulation and microassembly and the miniaturization of the objects to manipulate, particularly efficient, reliable and precise handling strategie are required. Microobjects are hard to manipulate because their different behavior. In order to handle small objects effectively and efficiently under uncertain environment, feedback-sensor is critical in the process of manipulation, and they allow for the controllable actuation with a range and resolution of force and displacement matching the required size scale. Micromanipulation of those objects requires the use of miniaturized tools with end-effectors on the size-scale of the manipulated objects. So the integration of the force sensor in the manipulation tools is a difficult and key technique. MEMS technology allows for the fabrication of such devices that meet these requirements.

C. Xiong et al. (Eds.): ICIRA 2008, Part II, LNAI 5315, pp. 207–216, 2008.

Grippers or tools integrated with piezoresistive force sensors or semiconductor strain-guage sensors have been reported in recent years. Arai F [1] fabricated the micropyramids and the integrated piezoresistive force sensor on the micro end-effector to reduce and control the adhesive force in microgripping tasks. Hybrid gripper designs have been demonstrated in [2] having integrated piezoresisitve force sensors. In [3] a micro-gripper is designed and fabricated to manipulate the small object like a cell. On the gripper a piezoresistive sensor is integrated for sensing the gripping force. A prototype miniature robotic instrument consisting of a microfabricated microgripper, instrumented with semiconductor strain-gauges as force sensors is described in [4]. A magnetically actuated gripper with piezoelectric force sensing has been reported in [5], and an optical method for force measurement is presented in [6]. These designs provide a reasonable sensitivity and resolution, but complicated and expensive assembly processes are required to build the grippers. In [7], an electro-thermally actuated microgripper with integrated force sensor is presented. It is fabricated on the wafer level using a simple fabrication process. Unfortunately, the sensitivity is much lower compared to hybrid designs, making it impossible to measure the small forces dominating micromanipulation processes. The gripper proposed by Y.Sun [8] was actuated by electrostatic force and include a capacitive force sensor measuring the gripping force, while measuring the small capacity change is also a difficult work.

Piezoresistive sensing is mostly employed because of its compatibility with operation in solutions and the simple fabrication process. This paper presents a new design for piezoresistive force sensing integrated in a gripper to sensing the gripping force. This sensorized microgripper can be successfully used in microassembly system for force-controlled micro gripping.

2 Design of the Force Sensor

Now the most general semi-conductor pressure sensor is the PN junction type pressure sensor that made by distribution process. Main advantage of the piezoresistive sensor is the simple process, low cost. In this paper the vertical sidewall surface piezoresistor can be deep-reactive ionic etching (DRIE) form at the outboard surface of the both root of the testing cantilever.

Fig. 1(*a*) shows the configuration of this piezoresistive force sensor and the position in the MEMS gripper. This sensor has been designed to measuring rang from 5μN to 500μN. The end-effector of the gripper is a four arms structure. Two arms both sides are fixed as the force sensor cantilevers. The intermediate two arms are moveable which are actuated by electrostatic comb. It means that there are two tweezers in one gripper and the gripping force can be sensed. Two force sensor cantilevers are along <110> crystal orientation. The piezoresistors are located at the outboard surface of the both end of the cantilevers.

To pick up an object, the moveable arms are pushed to close with the fixed arms. This generates a gripping force that deflects the fixed arms shown in Fig. 1(*b*). This deflection is measured by the piezoresistor for force sensing on the end of the fixed cantilevers. The deflection of the arm is proportional to the gripping force and is independent of the size or the mechanical properties of the object which is gripped.

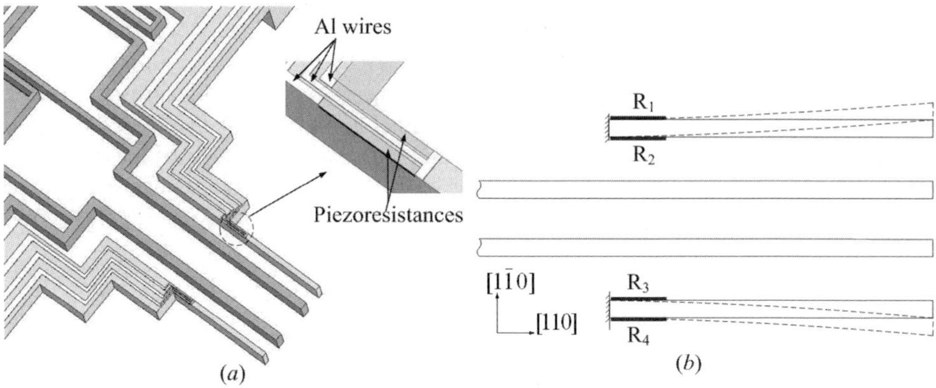

Fig. 1. Sketch of the force sensor

How to get the reasonable maximal stress is key point. It determines the measuring range and the resolution of the sensor. And the maximum stress of the cantilever must be lower than the yield strength. Based on the Material Mechanics and Finite Element Analyze, stress in the position A is maximal in Fig. 2:

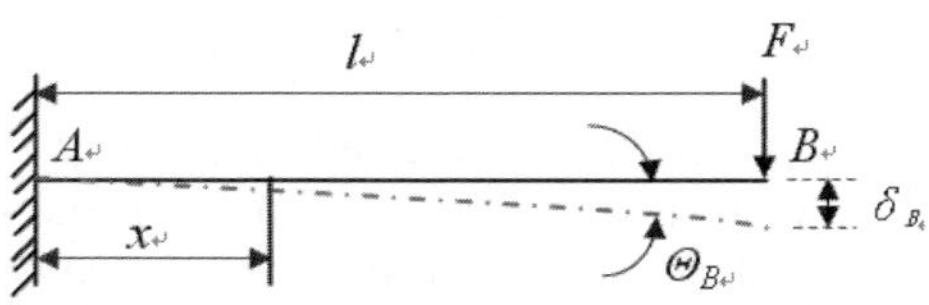

Fig. 2. Sketch of the deflection of the force sensor cantilever

Measuring band width of the sensor is limited by the resonance frequency of the cantilever. In general, the measuring band width is expected to less than half of the resonance frequency. Moreover, the cantilever with low resonance frequency is easily influenced by the environment. So the analyze of the frequency is necessary. The FEA results are shown in Table 1. The first-order is most important in the using of this sensor. And Modal analysis shows that it is 183524Hz which can satisfy the frequency influence completely in gripping relative to the frequency of the environment and the driven voltage.

Table 1. Modal analysis

Exponent number	1	2	3	4
Frequency(Hz)	183524	408075	1138982	2403305

The piezoresistive sensor uses the change of the electrical resistivity due to the strain variation according to the applied force. The resistance change is expressed as the summation of multiplication of the resistivity and the stress in the longitudinal and transverse direction. The resistance change due to the mechanical stress is given by [9]:

$$\Delta R / R = (\pi_l \sigma_l + \pi_t \sigma_t) . \tag{1}$$

Where $\Delta R / R$ is the relative change of resistance in a conventional piezoresistor due to the longitudinal stress, π_l and π_t are the longitudinal and the transverse piezoresistance coefficients, σ_l and σ_t are the longitudinal and the transverse stresses, respectively. The σ_t can be neglected in the bending cantilever so the equation (1) can be reduced to:

$$\Delta R / R = \pi_l \sigma_l . \tag{2}$$

The longitudinal piezoresistance coefficients are given by:

$$\pi_{l,110} = (\pi_{11} + \pi_{12} + \pi_{44}) / 2 . \tag{3}$$

Where π_{11}, π_{12}, π_{44} are three independent coefficients of the first order piezoresistive tensor. The values are given in Table 2. Relative to π_{44}, π_{11} and π_{12} can be neglected.

Table 2. Resistivity according to the Material Type

Type	$\pi_{11}/(10^{-11}\text{m}^2/\text{N})$	$\pi_{12}/(10^{-11}\text{m}^2/\text{N})$	$\pi_{44}/(10^{-11}\text{m}^2/\text{N})$
P-type	+6.6	-1.1	+138.1

Two piezoresistors are placed and connected at the end of the beams so as to maximize the sensitivities to various components of force and moment. The piezoresistive effect of conventional single crystalline piezoresistors can be expressed as below:

$$S = \Delta R / R = \left(\int_0^l \frac{1}{2} \pi_{44} \sigma_l (x) dx \right) / l . \tag{4}$$

In the measuring system, two resistances form is designed in a Half Wheatstone bridge. The resistances of two sensing resistors change in opposite direction if a lateral force is applied. The bridge configuration of the resistors compensates for the signals caused by the deflection. When a lateral load is applied to the tip of the cantilever, the differential change of resistance occurs on two resistors R_{s1} and R_{s2}. The other piezoresistors R_1, R_2 are the compensation resistors.

When the piezoresistor value is changed byΔR, the lateral output signal is given by:

$$\Delta V = \Delta R \cdot V_{power} / 2R = \pi_{44} \sigma_{l,\max} V_{power} / 4 . \tag{5}$$

Where V_{power} is the supply voltage and R is the resistance of the non-stressed piezoresistor. The V-I characteristic curve of piezoresistor is shown in Fig. 3.

The main process of piezoresistor is boron ion implantation. Implantation is along z direction, and forms the resistance areas 100μm×4μm in x-y coordinate surface as shown in Fig. 4.

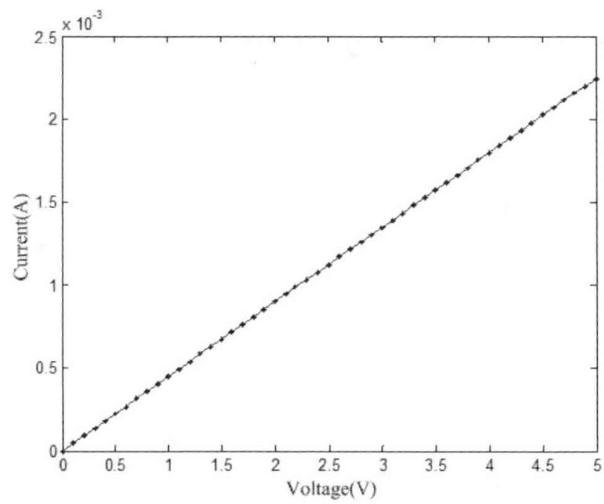

Fig. 3. V-I characteristic curve of piezoresistor

But in this paper, the force F is lateral direction along y direction and the bend of the cantilever is in x-y coordinate surface. Then the boron ion implantation is utilized to form the piezoresistor on y-z surface. 1μm -1.2μm depth PN junction is formed in this paper. Therefore the area of the piezoresistor to measure the gripping force F is about 100μm×(1μm -1.2μm), and depth is 4μm. Two piezoresistors are located at the bilateral root of the cantilever.

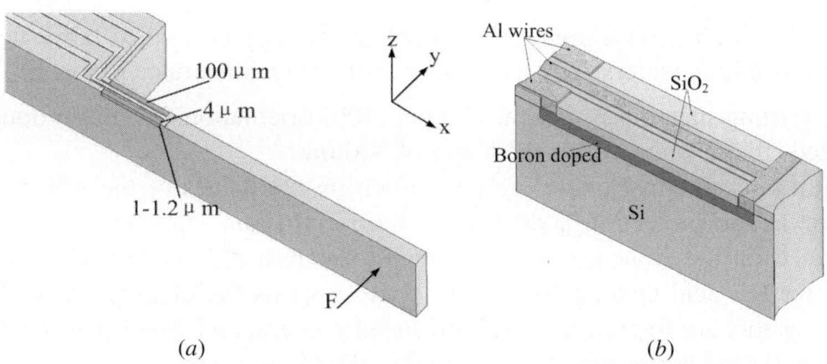

Fig. 4. (*a*) The sketch of piezoresistor cantilever. (*b*) The close-up view of the piezoresistor. The Al wires and Si are electrically isolated by the previously formed SiO_2.

For the special structure of the sidewall piezoresistor, the shape is only designed to be rectangular. The value of the resistance can be given:

$$R = R_s L / W \,. \tag{6}$$

Where R_s——sheet resistance;
L——length of the piezoresistor;
W——width of the piezoresistor

According to the standard process of the piezoresistor and the dimension of the testing cantilever, the sheet resistance is about 80Ω/□, width of the piezoresistor is 4μm. From the equation (6), the length of the piezoresistor can be given as 100μm. The dimensions of the sensor are 100μm×20μm×1.2μm.

The resolution of testing cantilever is limited by the four intrinsic noises in semiconductors, which include Johnson noise, shot noise, generation-recombination noise and Hooge noise. In all of which, frequency-independent Johnson noise and low-frequency Hooge noise are two dominant noise sources. The voltage noise power can be expressed as

$$V_n = \sqrt{\left(\alpha V_{power}^2 / N_p W t b_p\right) \ln\left(f_{\max} / f_{\min}\right) + 4 k_B T R \left(f_{\max} - f_{\min}\right)} \,. \tag{7}$$

Where α is parameter independent of dimensions, which dependent on anneal for implant resistors, N_p is the impurity concentration (4.5×10^{15}/cm^3), W is the piezoresistor width and t is the piezoresistor thickness. k_B is the Boltzmann's constant, f_{max} and f_{min} are, respectively, the upper limit and the lower limit of the bandwidth and T is the temperature in Kelvin.

It is evident that the resolution is determined by more parameters, besides the dimensions of the testing cantilever, the parameters of the doped piezoresistors also play more important role in the displacement resolution.

3 Fabrication of the Force Sensors

Surface and bulk micromachining fabrication technology is used to fabricate micro-grippers from silicon wafers. The fabrication sequence is illustrated in Fig. 5.

a) The starting material is 4-inch, N-type, (100) orientation, 1-10Ωcm double polished silicon wafer with a thickness of 300μm.
b) 0.5μm thick thermal oxide layer is grown on both sides of the wafer which is used as the protection layer for the boron infusion. Photolithography is conducted on the front side of the wafer to pattern the piezoresistors, and then buffer HF acid etching SiO2 with photoresist as the etching mask. The piezoresistors are formed by boron diffusion process, and then drive-in process is done to send boron ions deeper into the silicon substrate.
c) The contact holes are patterned by photolithography and opened by wet etching in buffered HF solution.
d) 1 μm-thick aluminum wires and bonding pads are formed by vacuum evaporation, photolithography, and etching processes. The aluminum thin film is photoetched for interconnection, and stripped by plasma etching.
e) The testing cantilever structure and the vertical sidewall surface piezoresistors on the testing cantilever are patterned photoresist and SiO_2 as the etching mask.
f) DRIE is used to form the testing structure and the piezoresistors synchronously. In order to ensure the identical dimension of the each piezoresistor. the parameters of the DRIE should be controlled strictly.

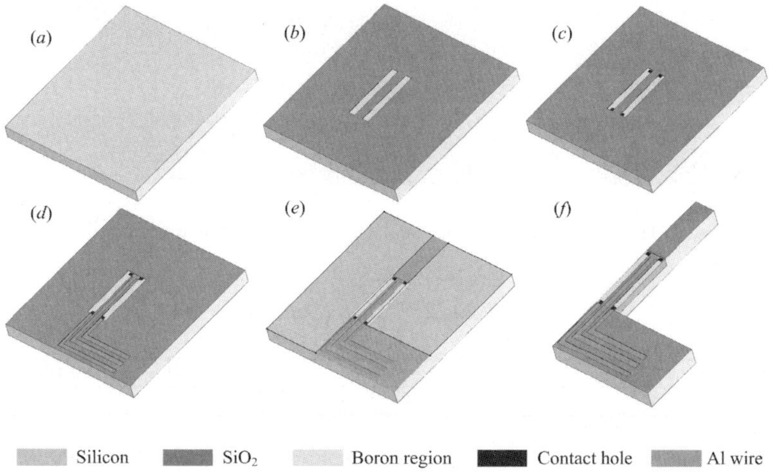

Fig. 5. Process flow schematic of piezoresistor fabrication. *(a)* The double polished N-type (100)-oriented silicon wafer; *(b)* the SiO_2 mask and boron ion implantation; *(c)* The contact holes etching; *(d)* The vacuum evaporation and stripping of aluminum lead; *(e)* Photoresist coating and patterning; *(f)* DRIE of the structure.

4 Testing and Discussion

Fig. 6 shows SEM images of the end effector of the gripper and the piezoresistor.

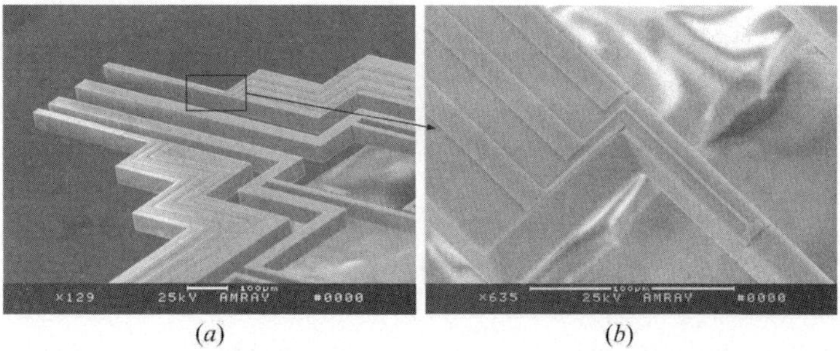

Fig. 6. SEM images. *(a)* The end effector of the gripper. *(b)* The piezoresistor and the Al wires.

The microscope photographs of the local view of the piezoresistive cantilever are shown in Fig. 7.

For calibrating the piezorisistance sensor, an electronic scale and a precision voltage meter are used. The resolution of the piezoresistor sensor is 3μN given by the calibration. The relationship curve of the gripping force and the sensor voltage output is linear shown in Fig. 8. The sensitivity 72V/ N can be received from the curve. Considering the influence of the actual process, the dimensions of the cantilevers and the result of the doped piezoresistor are different with theoretical calculation. The sensitivity 72V/ N satisfies the request of the manipulation.

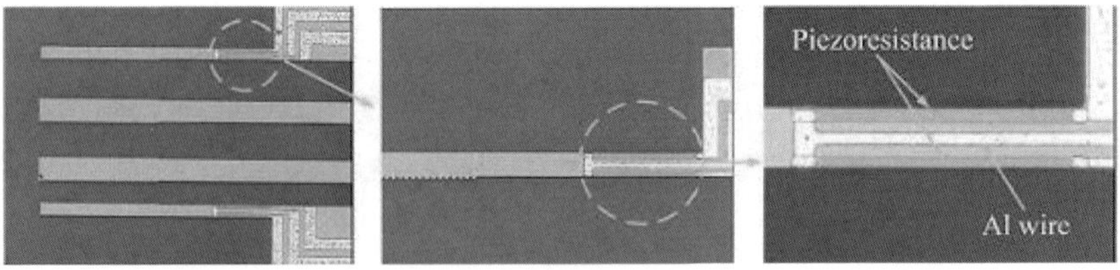

Fig. 7. The photographs of the local view of the piezoresistor cantilever

Table 2. Testing results

Force measuring range	Sensor Resolution	Breakdown voltage of Piezoresistor
5-500μN	3μN	32V

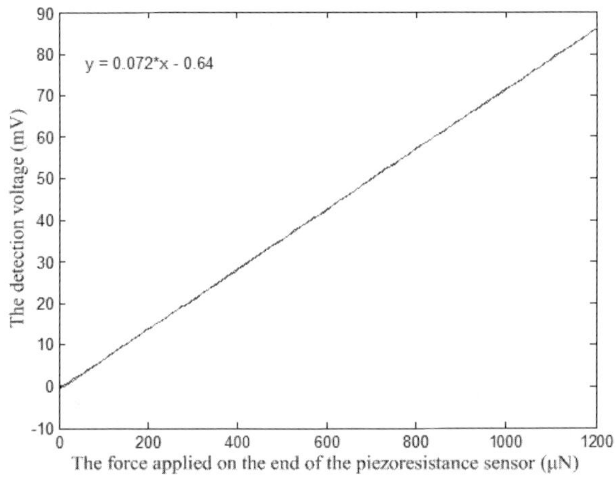

Fig. 8. The relationship of the force applied on the sensor and the detection voltage. The range from 0-400μN is commonly used in the manipulation.

The testing results of the force sensor are stated in Table 3.

An experiment of grasping polystyrene microsphere with different sizes is performed with the gripper shown in Fig. 9. Different voltages are applied during pick-and-release manipulations, and the signal output of the force sensor is shown in Fig. 10. By closing and opening the gripper arm, the signal has a step up and down. The voltage corresponds with the negative gripping force. The values of the voltages reflect different gripping force.

It is found that this fabrication technology and the microgripper configuration are reliable by experiment.

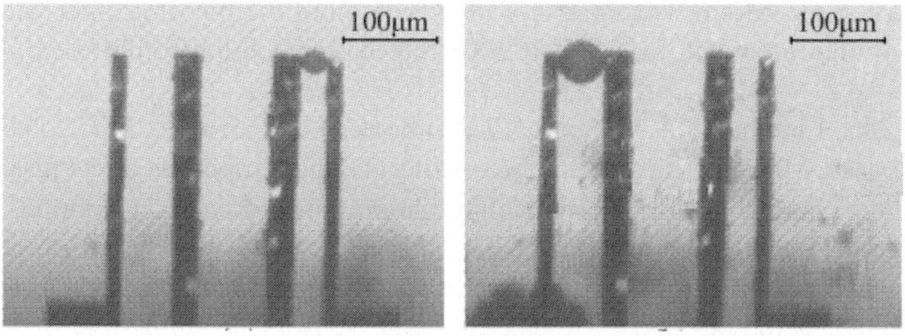

Fig. 9. Grasping the polystyrene microspheres in the gripper

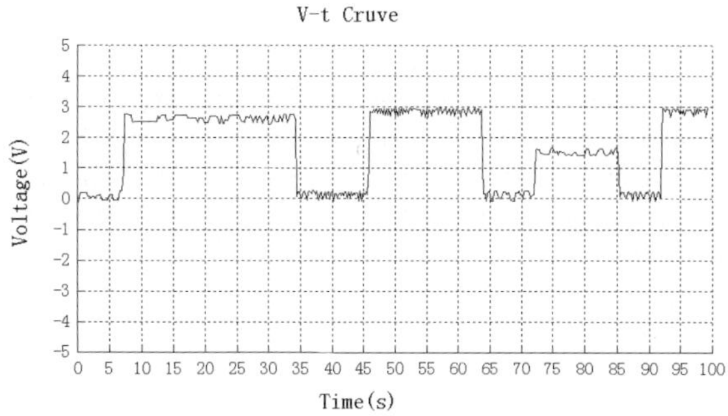

Fig. 10. The signal output of the force sensor. The step up means the picking operation and the step down means the placing operation. Different driving voltages generate the different amplitudes.

5 Conclusion

A novel vertical sidewall surface piezoresistor technique based on bulk-micromachining technologies is proposed in this paper. We combine Boron diffusion process with DRIE technique to form the side direction force sensors. The design and fabrication of the force sensor is presented based on the process and the characteristic of the MEMS gripper. The piezoresistors are integrated in the MEMS gripper ingeniously to measuring the gripping force. Which is High-yield low-cost fabrication technology, with the process, the piezoresistor of random dimension can be located on the vertical sidewall surface easily. Testing results verify the vertical sidewall surface piezoresistor technique, the sensitivity of the fabricated Piezoresistive sensors is better than 72V/N and the resolution is better than 3μN. Experimental show that it can successfully provide real-time force feedback with a high sensitivity sensing and play a main role in preventing damage of microparts in micromanipulation and microassembly tasks.

References

1. Arai, F., Lee, G.U., Colton, R.J.: Integrated microendeffector for micromanipulation. IEEE/ASME Transac. Mechatronics 3(1), 17–23 (1998)
2. Park, J., Moon, W.: A hybrid-type micro-gripper with an integrated force sensor. Microsystem Technol. Micro. Nanosyst. Inf. Storage Process. Syst. 9(8), 511–519 (2003)

3. Han, K., Lee, S.H., Moon, W., Park, J.-s.: Fabrication of the micro-gripper with a force sensor for manipulating a cell. In: SICE-ICASE International Joint Conference, pp. 5833–5836 (2006)
4. Menciassi, A., Eisinberg, A., Scalari, G., Anticoli, C., Carrozza, M.C., Dario, P.: Force Feedback-based Microinstrument for Measuring Tissue Properties and Pulse in Microsurgery. In: Proceedings of the 2001 IEEE, International Conference on Robotics and Automation, pp. 626–631 (2001)
5. Kim, D.H., Lee, M.G., Kim, B., Sun, Y.: A superelastic alloy microgripper with embedded electromagnetic actuators and piezoelectric force sensors: A numerical and experimental study. Smart Mater. Struct. 15, 1265–1272 (2005)
6. Zhou, Y., Nelson, B.J.: Adhesion force modeling and measurement for micromanipulation. In: Proc. SPIE Int. Symp. Intell. Syst. Adv. Manufact., vol. 3519, pp. 169–180 (1998)
7. Molhave, K., Hansen, O.: Electro-thermally actuated microgrippers with integrated force-feedback. J. Micromech. Microeng. 15(6), 1265–1270 (2005)
8. Beyeler, F., Bell, D.J., Nelson, B.J., Sun, Y.: Design of a Micro-Gripper and an Ultrasonic Manipulator for Handling Micron Sized Objects. In: Proceedings of the 2006 IEEE/RSJ, International Conference on Intelligent Robots and Systems, pp. 772–777 (2006)
9. Stephen, D.: Microsystem design. In: Senturia, ch. 18, pp. 469–495. Kluwer Acedamic Publishers, Dordrecht (2001)

Estimation of the Cell Deformation

Mingli Han, Yanliang Zhang, Cheng Yap Shee, and Wei Tech Ang

School of Mechanical and Aerospace Engineering
Nanyang Technological University, Singapore
hanm0005@ntu.edu.sg

Abstract. Biomembranes can withstand the external forces by changing the cell shapes. Shape changes of the biomembrane produce evolution to the organism. To introduce desired chemistries to the cell by changing its shapes, the model to describe the mechanical property of the cell is necessary to be characterized. Estimation of the cells deformation is the major part for the characterization of mechanical properties. A novel method is proposed in this paper to quantify the strain for deformed biomembranes. The method estimates the global change of the deformed biomembranes which is induced by the injection pipette. The experimental results show that the estimation of the cells deformation is reasonable and quantifiable to model the mechanical property of cells.

Keywords: Biomembrane, boundary extraction, least square.

1 Introduction

Cells, to some extent, are the basic units of life. They perform all essential vital functions: extracting energy and producing materials from their environment, constructing, repairing and cleaning up themselves, regulating their own internal operations, and reproducing themselves periodically.

Biologists are devoted to figure out the underlying mechanisms and their relationship to the environment that enable cells to perform these functions. Their researches are normally conducted by aborative operations with high accuracy and reproducibility. As recent advances in the biological field, operations in the scale of micro are highly required. Micromanipulation is the technique to handle cells on a microscope stage, performing micro procedures via microtools. Conventionally, micromanipulation is conducted manually by operators. It usually takes months or one year to train operators to be professional. However, low success rates, poor reproducibility due to fatigue and unexpected contamination from human involvement all appeal for an automatic system to perform the micromanipulation task without or eliminating the direct human involvement to samples. In recent years, many researches are conducted to develop automatic micromanipulation systems ([1], [2], [3], [4]). Studies for individual cells can be proceeded into the micro level by using these developed automatic micromanipulation systems.

Although there are a number of kinds of cells, they display common architecture and reflect similar basic functions. All cells have a semi-permeable boundary, i.e. biomembrane, which selectively separate the cells contents from their environment.

C. Xiong et al. (Eds.): ICIRA 2008, Part II, LNAI 5315, pp. 217–223, 2008.

Biomembranes not only have the ability of preventing the cells contents from water but also can repair themselves when it is necessary. The flexible biomembranes can help cells changing the shape to respond to the changing environment. However, from the biological perspective, molecular filaments are the reinforcing elements to strengthen the thin biomembrane of the cell, like the roles of the ropes and masts played in the construction of boats. Biomembranes can be compressed or tensed is because of the networks built by filaments. The network can sustain the whole cell, and the exterior membrane is just the cladding. Usually, thick filaments appear stiff while the thin filaments are more convoluted. In other words, the cell accommodates the pressure it suffers by reinforcing its biomembrane with a network of filaments. When forces are acted on the cell, it faces the problem of explosion because of the higher interior pressure of the cell than its surroundings [9].

Functions performed by the cell can be looked upon from different aspects. Chemical functions of the cell introduce the internally chemical changes in the cell, like production of energy, manufacturing of proteins. Functions of information processing are more related with relationships of cells and how does the cell recognize other cells as friend or foe. Cell mechanics is investigated the cell from the physical perspective. There have been few studies to investigate the mechanical property changes of the cell ([5], [6], [7], [8]). An analytical biomembrane elastic model is constructed to describe biomembrane mechanical properties in [5]. However, the biomembrane deformation brought by the external force is estimated by the local dimple geometry change only without considering the global geometry change of the deformed biomembrane. Young's modulus is also calibrated in [6] by using an elastic microfabricated PDMS (polydimethylsiloxane) device. It takes time to fabricate this micro device and the following image processing work is very complicated to deal with the shadow area caused by devices deflection. Mechanical property of a single tomato suspension cell is also measured by compressing a cell between two parallel flat surfaces [7]. But the deformation is detected by two cameras through two objectives on the microscope. In this paper, the biomembrane refers to the structures around cells which look like the sheet.

With the exclusion of nucleus, all the materials inside the cell are defined as cytoplasm for animal and plant cells. Various filaments create a variety of cytoskeletons which are organized to form networks and produce different mechanical properties of biomembranes. Biomembranes can withstand the external forces by changing the cell shapes. When the cells shape changes, the deformation it creates also produces evolution to the organism. If the deformation of the cell is controllable, we can introduce desired chemistries by changing the cell shape to a proper extant. During the controller development, the estimation of the biomembrane deformation is the most important factor which directly influences the performance of the controller.

2 Estimation of Cell Deformation

Normally, the deformation of the biomembrane is expected to be a dimple as shown in Fig. 1. Then the strain is modeled by analyzing the indentation of biomembranes. The estimation of cell deformation is rigorous in this way if only the local geometry change exist. But the change of cells outline is so obvious, as shown in Fig. 1, that it should not be ignored when calculate the cells deformation.

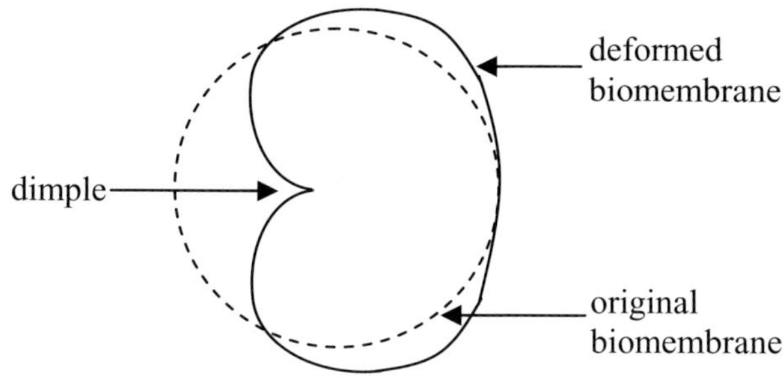

Fig. 1. Comparing the deformed biomembrane with the original biomembrane

2.1 Extraction of the Boundary

To measure the outline of deformed cells, the boundary is extracted from the image first. The extraction of the boundary is to detect the contour of the biomembrane based on the gray level difference. Images are converted to binary images for there are only one object is going to be analyzed except the background. The object of injection pipette is not the research interest for this application.

The extraction of biomembrane contour begins from a starting point which is a nonzero pixel. The position of the starting pixel is set by the experimental experience. Then, the boundary of the biomembrane is traced from the starting point and the specified search direction along the 8-connected neighborhood [10]. Pixels with gray level of *1* are set to be the object, i.e. the deformed biomembrane, and pixels with gray level of *0* are background. The boundary is stopped detecting when the specified number of pixels are identified. A set of points, *(x, y)*, which are represented the boundary of the deformed biomembrane, are used to estimate the global geometry change of cells outline.

2.2 Estimation of the Boundary

In estimating the boundary, first consider the geometry shape which is suitable to approximate the outline of the cell. In this paper, ellipse is proposed to approximate the boundary of deformed biomembranes. Comparing with the parabola and hyperbola, the shape of ellipse is closer to the real profile of the boundary, as shown in Fig. 1. Comparison between different deformations is also easier to proceed by using parameters of ellipses than using of multiple curves of parabola. However, there is an alternative of approximating the boundary by combining multiple parabolas, which consumes more computations time.

In the Cartesian plane, ellipse is defined by the equation of form

$$ax^2 + bxy + cy^2 + dx + ey + f = 0 \tag{1}$$

where all of the coefficients are real and $b^2 < 4ac$. The equation (1) can also be written in the form of

$$P(A) = uA = -f \tag{2}$$

where $u = (x^2, xy, y^2, x, y)$, $A = (a,b,c,d,e)^t$ is the vector of coefficients to be estimated. The aim is that the ellipse should follow the real boundary points and, at the same time, the error for doing so should be minimized. The objective function is then defined to be

$$J(A) = (P_m + F)'(P_m + F) \tag{3}$$

where $P_m(A) = UA$ is the vector function of all the boundary points *(x, y)*, *F* is the column vector with elements of *-f*, *N* is the number of boundary points. Then (3) becomes

$$J(A) = (UA + F)'(UA + F) = A'U'UA + 2F'UA + NF^2 \tag{4}$$

The estimated ellipse is derived by finding the parameters which minimize the objective function. This reduces to a least square problem and the solution can be obtained by using the Least Square method. Deviation of the objective function with respect to the vector of parameters *A* is

$$\frac{\partial J}{\partial A} = A'U'U + F'U = 0 \tag{5}$$

rearrange equation (5) and normalized it by $-F$ becomes

$$A = \frac{U}{U'U} \tag{6}$$

then, the center and the axis, semi major axis *sa* and semi minor axis *sb*, of the ellipse are calculated by using the square completion method

$$\begin{aligned} x_0 &= -\frac{d}{2a}, \; y = -\frac{e}{2c} \\ sa &= \sqrt{abs(\frac{-f + d^2/4a + e^2/4c}{a})} \\ sb &= \sqrt{abs(\frac{-f + d^2/4a + e^2/4c}{c})} \end{aligned} \tag{7}$$

throughout the fitting of ellipse by using extracted boundary points *(x, y)*, it is assumed that the ellipse is non-tilted to avoid the unnecessary rotation of the fitted ellipse caused by noisy points from *(x, y)*.

3 Experiment Design and Results

The automatic micromanipulation system used in this application is composed of an injection unit and a vision unit. A three degree of freedom motorized translation stage and a micromanipulator are the main parts for the injection unit. The motorized translation stages have a travel range of *50×50×50* mm, with a resolution of 1.25 *u*m. Two phase stepping motors mounted on the stages have 200 steps per revolution. The micromanipulator is mounted on the vertical stage. The injection pipette, with diameter of 100 um, is installed on the micromanipulator. Control the position of translation stage drives the micromanipulator approaching the sample.

The vision unit consists of an upright microscope, a CMOS camera and a host computer. 4 times magnification is used for the upright microscope (EclipseFN1 of Nikon), since zebrafish egg is the sample in the experiment. Normally, diameter of zebrafish eggs is *700-1000* um which is a relative large sample for microscopes. The camera (Basler exA640-180m) mounted on the rear port of the microscope has a maximum frame rate of 176 frames per second. During the experiment, a set of images are saved while the translation stage is controlled by the host computer. Every image corresponds to a certain position of the translation stage. Images are then processed off-line on the host computer.

Fig. 2 shows a raw image of a deformed cell. The shadow surrounding the cell is the solution. The original cell is considered to be round.

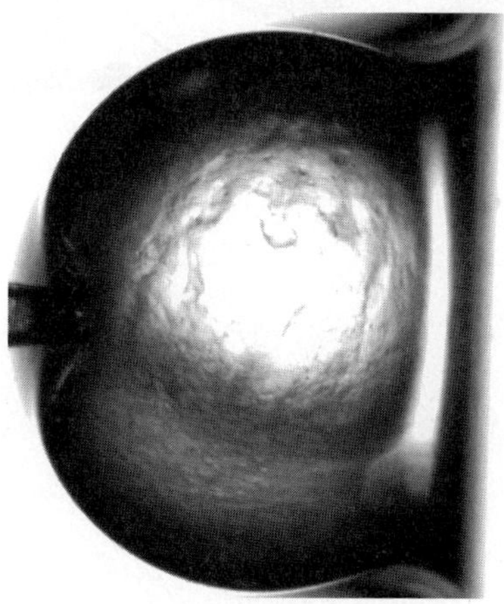

Fig. 2. A deformed cell caused by the manipulator

To reduce the variability of the gray values at each pixel position, 10 images are captured at each manipulator position. The image $\overline{I}(x, y)$ is formed by averaging 10 different noisy raw images,

$$\overline{I}(x, y) = \frac{1}{N}\sum_{i=1}^{N} I_i(x, y), \qquad N = 10 \tag{8}$$

After processing the image, $\overline{I}(x, y)$, by the method proposed in the section 2, boundary and the estimated ellipse are obtained, as shown in Fig. 3. The outline of the deformed biomembrane is estimated by the fitted ellipse quite well. Although the error is up to 20 pixels in some part of the biomembrane, the overall outline changes of the biomembrane are still provided by the fitted ellipse. By combining the global and local, i.e. the dimple, changes, deformations of the biomembrane caused by the external force can be estimated more accurately. The image is converted to a binary image and the two axis of the ellipse are plotted by the dotted lines in Fig. 3.

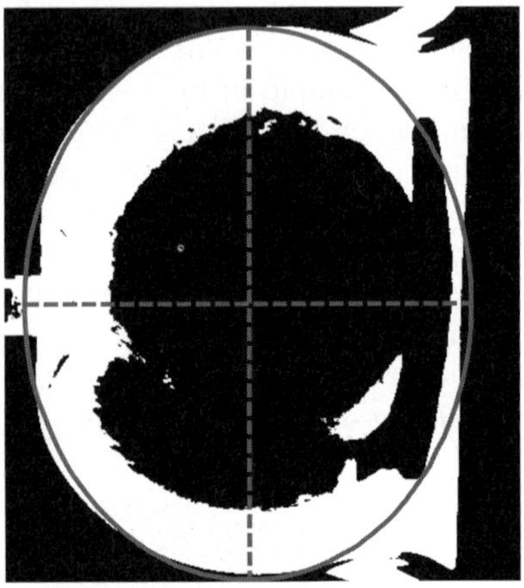

Fig. 3. Estimate the deformed cell by the ellipse

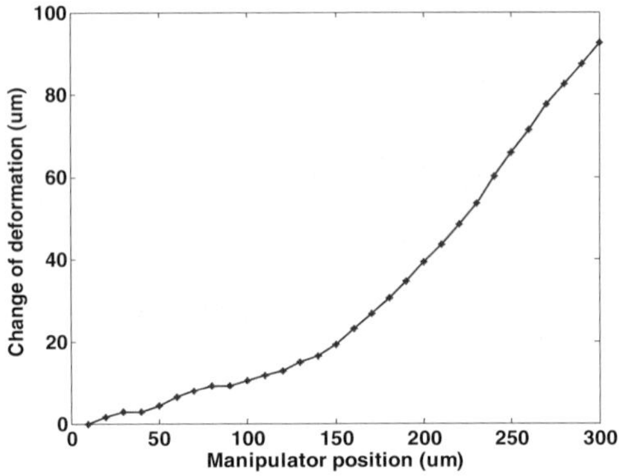

Fig. 4. Change of deformation $|\Delta sa| + |\Delta sb|$ vs the position of the manipulator

Parameters of estimated ellipses are compared with the undeformed cell. The change of the deformation is defined to be $|\Delta sa| + |\Delta sb|$. Fig. 4 shows that the change of deformation is consistently increasing as the manipulator penetrates into the cell.

4 Conclusion

The ellipse is proposed to estimate the global geometry changes of deformed biomembranes in this paper. Based on the image processing algorithm, the boundary of the biomembrane is extracted. Parameters of the fitted ellipse are computed by the least square method. An automatic micromanipulation system is implemented to investigate changes of biomembranes deformation. By combining the dimple estimation and the outline estimation presented in this paper, a more accurate model could be developed to describe the mechanical property for cells.

References

1. Sun, Y., Nelson, B.J.: Biological Cell Injection Using an Autonomous MicroRobotic System. International Journal of Robotics Research 21, 861–868 (2002)
2. Shim, J.H., Cho, S.Y., Cha, D.H.: Vision-guided micromanipulation System for Biomedical Application. In: Proceedings of SPIE, vol. 5604, pp. 98–107 (2002)
3. Lu, Z., Chen, P.C.Y., Nam, J., Ge, R.W., Lin, W.: A Micromanipulation System with Dynamic Force-feedback for Automatic Batch Microinjection. Journal of Micromechanics and Microengineering 17, 314–321 (2007)
4. Huang, H., Sun, D., Mills, J.K., Li, W.J.: Visual-based Impedance Force Control of Three-dimensional Cell Injection System. In: IEEE International Conference on Robotics and Automation, vol. 10, pp. 4196–4201 (2007)
5. Sun, Y., Wan, K.T., Roberts, K.P., Bischof, J.C., Nelson, B.J.: Mechanical Property Characterization of Mouse Zona Pellucida. IEEE Transactions on Nanobioscience 2(4), 279–286 (2003)
6. Liu, X.Y., Sun, Y., Wang, W.H., Lansdorp, B.M.: Vision-based Cellular Force Measurement using an Elastic Microfabricted Device. Journal of Micromechanics and Microengineering 17, 1281–1288 (2007)
7. Blewett, J., Burrows, K., Thomas, C.: A Micromanipulation Method to Measure the Mechanical Properties of Single Tomato Suspension Cells. Biotechnology Letters 22, 1877–1883 (2000)
8. Wang, C.X., Wang, L., Thomas, C.R.: Modeling the Mechanical Properties of Single Suspension-Cultured Tomato Cells. Annals of Botany 93, 443–453 (2004)
9. Boal, D.: Mechanics of the Cell. Cambridge University Press, Cambridge (2002)
10. Gonzalez, Woods: Digital Image Processing. Prentice Hall, Englewood Cliffs (2002)

Optimizing Mechanism for a Polymorphic Tracked Robot

Jia Xu, Qingsheng Luo, Ningjun Fan, and Jiwei Yang

School of Aerospace Science and Engineering,
Beijing Institute of Technology, Beijing, China
mailxujia@gmail.com

Abstract. A new type shape-shifting mechanism of the polymorphic tracked robot has been designed and optimized. A virtual prototype has been established under Adams. We analyzed the sensitivity of design parameters and optimized the design variables using the Design Evaluation Tools of Adams. In order to find the optimized result, sequential quadratic programming has been selected to running the iterative simulation. The optimized mechanism can control the track configuration neither too loose nor too tight, which achieved the tension requirement of the crawling mechanism. The driving mode of the shape-shifting mechanism has also been optimized to improve transforming process of the track configuration.

Keywords: polymorphic tracked robot, shape-shifting mechanism, design variable, changing rate of the track perimeter.

1 Introduction

With its excellent climbing obstacle capability, tracked robot counts for crucial role among the ground mobile robots. By combining variable poses and changing the approach angle of multiple tracks (Fig.1 shows an example), the polymorphic tracked robot further enhances the adaptability to terrain [1].

Since the position of its front idler is changeable in vertical direction, polymorphic tracked robot mentioned in this paper shares both the abilities of passing through the low gaps and stepping across the high obstacles [2]. The key point in its mechanical design, among this kind of robots, lies in the method how to keep the tracks moderate tense as its configuration is changing and thus protecting the tracks from loose or fracture. Usually, there are mainly two methods adopted in design: 1) by using the special elastic tension devices 2) keeping the perimeter of a polygon constituted by bracing gear trains constant or oscillatory within a small area.

Reference [3] designed a variable configuration tracked robot. It keep the tracks real-time tense as its configuration is changing by applying a theorem that the perimeter of a triangle which originated from an arbitrary point and two focus points of the same elliptic is const and a series of transmission mechanisms. However, this kind of robots is usually complex and huge (Fig.2 shows an example), and hard to miniaturize. Therefore it's necessary for us to further develop a new shape-shifting mechanism, which could satisfy the practical needs for the miniaturization of robots.

C. Xiong et al. (Eds.): ICIRA 2008, Part II, LNAI 5315, pp. 224–231, 2008.

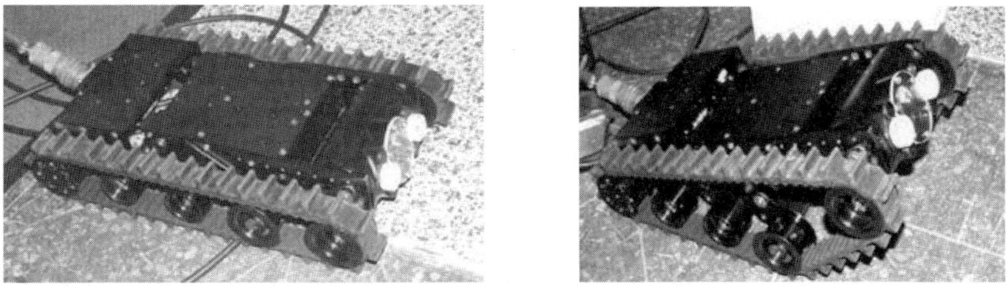

Fig. 1. Polymorphic tracked robot in its down position (left), partly raised position (right)

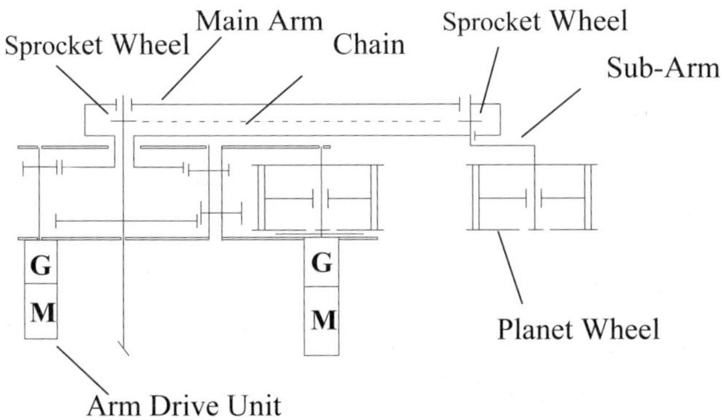

Fig. 2. Arm transmission mechanisms of the robot in reference [3], the mechanism is so complex that is difficult to miniaturize

2 Analyze on Characteristics of the Shape-Shifting Mechanism

First of all we make analyze on the shape-shifting mechanism which is without tension device. As Fig. 3 shows, the radius of road wheels and front idler are both R; the length of the main arm is A; the distance between the road wheels is L and the angle of main arm is α. The shaft of the main arm locates on the connect centre between the two road wheels.

When $0° \leq \alpha \leq 90°$

The perimeter C can be shown as follows:

$$C = L + 2\pi R + \sqrt{A^2 + (L/2)^2 - 2AL\cos(\alpha)} + \sqrt{A^2 + (L/2)^2 + 2AL\cos(\alpha)} \quad (1)$$

In order to facilitate the analyze toward C, and simultaneously make sure that polymorphic tracked robot has rational mechanism, we presume that: A= （160, 180, 200, 220, 240）; L=200; R=20.

As figure 4 shows, C is varying with α and monotone increasing; when A varies from 150 to 240, the difference between the maximum and minimum is monotone decreasing:

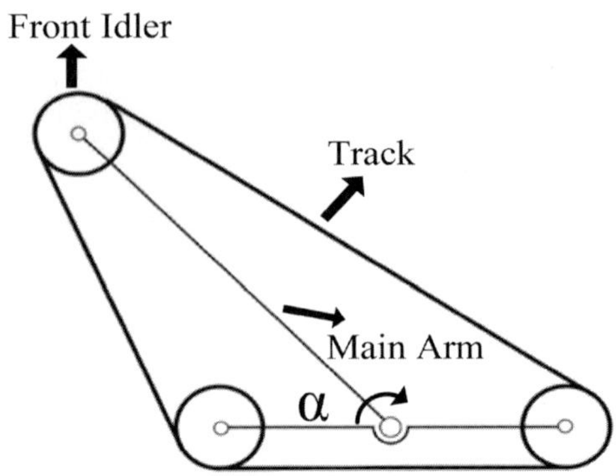

Fig. 3. Sketch map of shape-shifting mechanism without tension device

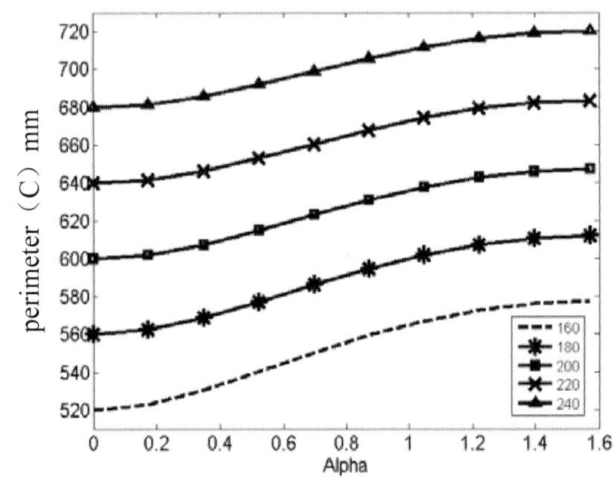

Fig. 4. Variety of the tracks perimeter as the length of main arm is changing

$$\Delta C = C_{max} - C_{min} \tag{2}$$

$$\eta = \Delta C / C \tag{3}$$

However, its rate of change remains above 5%. When the main arm is raised up, the tense tracks begin to fall off. When the main arm is brought down, the tense tracks will fracture, which is unacceptable for the tracked vehicle.

Aiming at these problems, we adopt the diamond pantograph mechanism [4] (see figure 5) instead of rigid linkage between the road wheels, and connect the revolute joint M on main arm and on pantograph mechanism with linkage. When the main arm is raised up around the revolute joint O, the diamond pantograph mechanism is accordingly shortened, which means decreasing L, thus minishing the change range of perimeter C as much as possible.

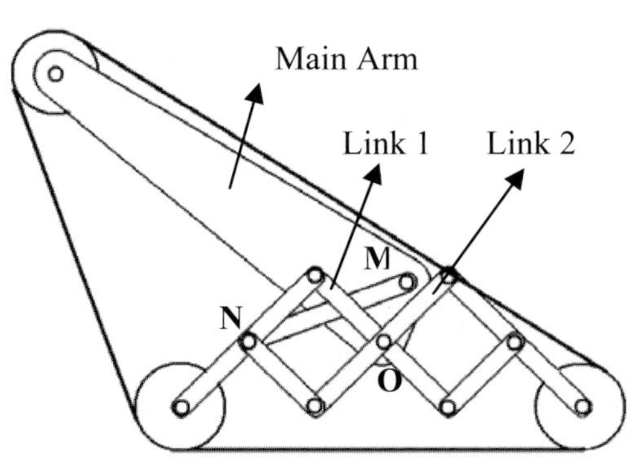

Fig. 5. Diamond pantograph mechanism for shape shifting

3 The Establishment of Optimal Design Model

Aiming at the shape-shifting mechanism as figure 5 shows, we establish parametric model in Adams to study its characteristics both in dynamics and kinematics. Since the main focus in optimal design is to control the variety extent of perimeter C, we set the minimum of η

The mechanical design parameters in this model are mainly including: $X = [x_1, x_2, x_3, x_4]^T$, where x_1 denotes the distance between the shaft of main arm and front guide wheel axle; x_2 denotes the length of links in diamond pantograph mechanism; x_3 denotes the horizontal coordinate of revolute joint M in main arm coordinate system, while x_4 denotes its vertical coordinate(see Fig. 6).

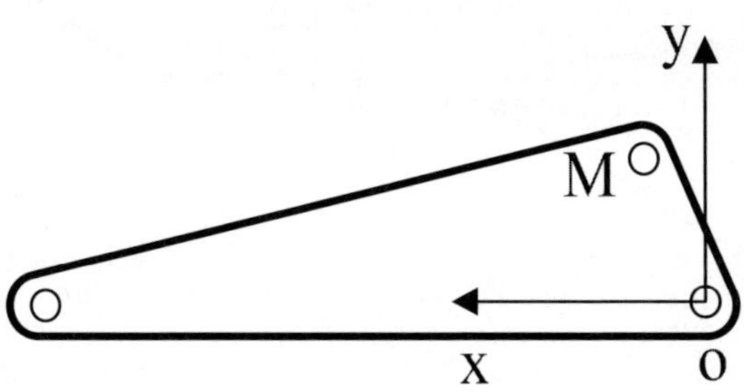

Fig. 6. Coordinate system of main arm

4 Optimal Design for Shape- Shifting Mechanism

4.1 Sensitivity Analyze on Design Parameter

Before optimization, we are obliged to discuss the sensitivity of the four parameter mentioned above, and then pick up the greater one to optimize, thus enhancing the efficiency [5].

We can have an intuitive analyze on the sensitivity of mechanism parameter by freely use of 'Design Evaluation tool in Adams simulation environment. We first define all the parameters as variables, and give their value range and initiate value. Then we define a new 'design study', where we select the design variables we need. Subsequently Adams will work out the kinematics simulation of model automatically, and draw up variation curves of track perimeter according to different value of design parameters.

Fig. 7 shows the different cases for the track perimeter when these parameters change. It is obviously seen that the rate of change η is more sensitive to x_3 and x_4, which clearly indicates that the position of revolute joint M on the main arm is one of the main influential factors for the change of the track perimeter.

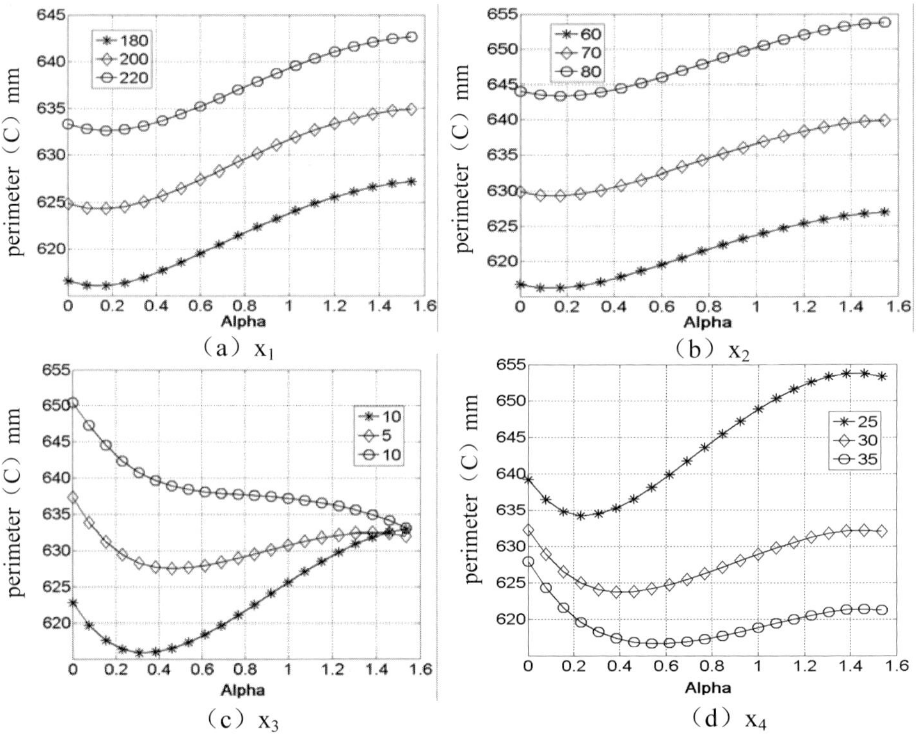

Fig. 7. Sensitivity analyze on design parameter

Up to this point, the mechanism optimal model of polymorphic tracked robot can be described as follows [6]:

Get a value of $X = [x_3, x_4]^T$, then let:

$$\eta(x) \rightarrow \min \tag{4}$$

Such that:

$$x_{\min} \le x_i \le x_{\max} \qquad i = 3,4 \tag{5}$$

$$0^\circ \le \alpha \le 90^\circ \tag{6}$$

$$\overline{MN} \le x_2 \tag{7}$$

Where $x_{\max}, x_{\min}$ is the upper and lower limit of design parameter; α is the angle of main arm; $\overline{MN} \le x_2$ is the length of link MN

4.2 The Optimal Design Result of Shape-Shifting Mechanism

According to the optimal model established in 4.1, we adopt sequential quadratic programming [7] to optimize the two parameters x_3 and x_4. Fig. 8 shows the iterative process, and Fig. 9 shows the final result. When x_3 equals to 43.83 and x_4 equals to

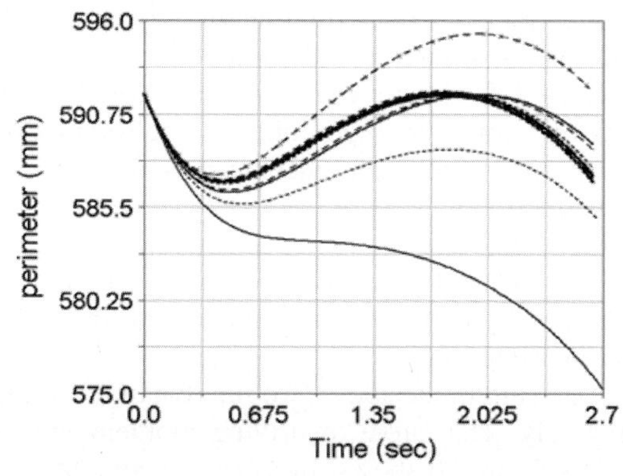

Fig. 8. Iterative process of the optimization

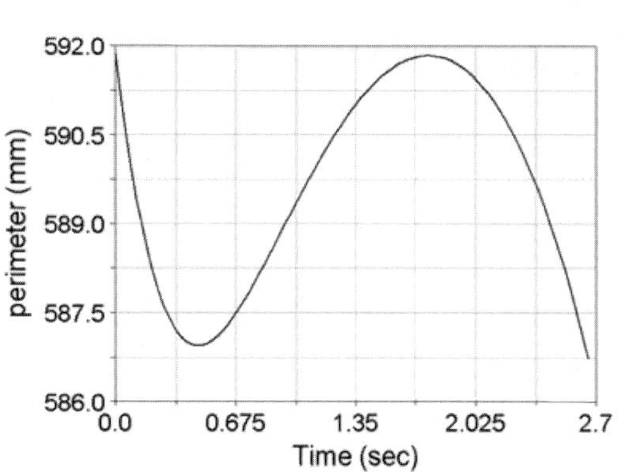

Fig. 9. Final result of the optimized track perimeter

86.15, the change of the length of track in the shape shifting process ΔC is 4.91, which means η is 0.67%. As for the tracked vehicle, the tracks are moderate tense when the change of perimeter is restrained by suspension and support devices within 1%, and the tracked vehicle can run normally , without falling off or fracture.

5 Optimal Driving Mode for Shape-Shifting Mechanism

With the size optimization above, we achieve the optimal mechanism size for polymorphic tracked robot. Based on this, we are necessary to discuss the driving mode of shape-shifting mechanism from the point view of power, then select a driving mode with low energy consumption.

As Figure 5 shows, when the main arm is rotating, the two links between the main arm and diamond pantograph mechanism rotates around revolute joint M. Here, we call link 1 to the link whose rotating direction is the same to the main arm's and link 2 to the link rotating in the opposite direction. The shape-shifting mechanism driving mode can be summarized as the following three:

Scheme 1: direct drive main arm, the rotation directly works on the main arm, with the driving main arm rotating around revolute joint O;

Scheme 2: direct drive link 1, the rotation directly works on the drive link 1, with its driving device rotating around revolute joint O. The rotation of link 1 is passed to main arm, through diamond pantograph mechanism and link MN, and then drive the main arm in the same direction;

Scheme 3: direct drive link 2, the rotation directly works on the drive link 2, with its driving device rotating around revolute joint O. The rotation of link 2 is passed to main arm, through diamond pantograph mechanism and link MN, and then drive the main arm in the opposite direction.

Aiming at the three driving mode above, we run dynamic simulation on Adams virtual prototype respectively. The curve of driving moment varied with the angle of main arm is achieved as figure 10 shows. In scheme 1, the driving moment gradually decrease as the main arm is raised, ultimately approaching to 0; in scheme 2 and 3, the driving moment keeps staying above 200mmN, and suddenly increasing when the

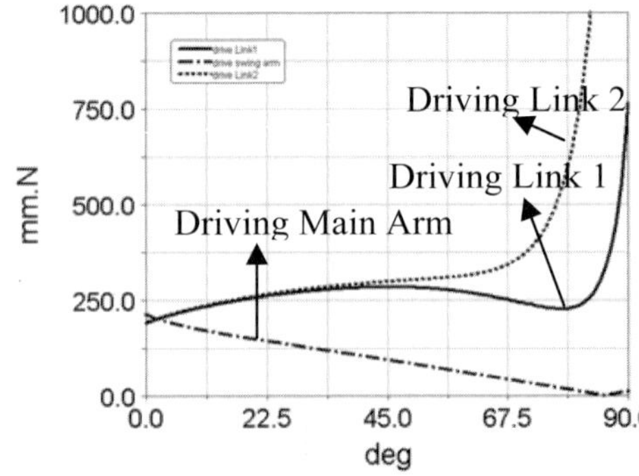

Fig. 10. The curve of driving moment varied with the angle of main arm

angle of main arm is approaching to 90° due to self-locking of mechanism when link MN and O-M are overlapped. Above all, scheme 1 requires little about the output of driving device, which can be selected as the best scheme for the shape-shifting mechanism.

6 Conclusions

This paper introduces a kind of shape-shifting mechanism for micro polymorphic tracked robot, and build parametric virtual prototype in the Adams simulation environment. After accomplishing the optimal design of shape-shifting mechanism and optimal the driving mode, we achieve these following conclusions:

1) Adams can be freely used to make sensitivity analyze on each design parameter. The result intuitively reflects the influence of design parameter to optimal target, which simplifies the variable and enhances the design efficiency.
2) The final result is achieved through the optimization towards design variables by using Design Evaluation tool and iterative simulation towards variables by applying sequential quadratic programming algorithm. In this method, the optimal result is quickly achieved and intuitively reflected on virtual prototype without encountering great work of modeling the complex mechanism.
3) The final result guarantees that the change rate of tracks perimeter is no higher than 1% during the shape shifting process, which meets design requirement that the tracked vehicle should be always tension.
4) Comparing three schemes for the driving mode of shape-shifting mechanism, we conclude that the direct drive main arm scheme requires low about the output of driving device, and is considered as first choice for the shape-shifting mechanism.

References

1. Drury, J.L., Yanco, H.A.: Changing Shape: Improving Situation Awareness for a Polymorphic Robot. In: Proceedings of HRI 2006, Salt Lake City, Utah, USA (2006)
2. Murphy, R.R.: Marsupial and shape shifting robots for urban search and rescue. J. IEEE Intelligent Systems, 14–19 (2000)
3. Iwamoto, T., Yamamoto, H.: Mechanical Design of Variable Configuration Tracked Vehicle. J. Journal of Mechanical Design. 112, 289–294 (1990)
4. Xia, D., Liu, J.: Optimization design of loading disc of precision centrifuge based on sensitivity analysis. J. Mechanical Design 23, 7–9 (2006)
5. Qizheng, L., Li, D.: Mechanisms for scaling Planar Graphs. J. Chinese Journal of Mechanical Engineering 147, 140–143 (2005)
6. Sun, J., Liang, Y.: Mechanical Design and Optimize. China Machine Press, Beijing (2007)
7. Qian, L., Zhong, W., Cheng, G., Sui, Y.: Sequential Quadratic Programming Approach Engineering Structural Optimization. J. Chinese Journal of Solid Mechanics 4, 469–480 (1983)

Design on the Driving Mode of MEMS Vibratory Gyroscope

Ranran Yi, Bangcheng Han, and Wei Sheng

Key Laboratory of Fundamental Science for National Defense, Novel Inertial Instrument & Navigation System Technology, Beijing, 100191, China

Abstract. Driving mode of MEMS (Micro-Electro-Mechanical Systems) Vibratory Gyroscope is discussed in the paper. We analyze the closed-loop circuit of MEMS gyroscope from two aspects of amplitude fixed and frequency locking. In the amplitude fixed circuit, Automatic Gain Control (AGC) circuit is employed to update the amplitude of the driving force, together with a PI controller to improve the accuracy and stability of the system. In the frequency locking circuit, two ways of PLL (Phase Locked Loop) and self-oscillation are used to improve the reliability of the system. Different levels of simulation and circuit implementation are made using the working mode and parameter of the dual-tuner output-quality pieces of silicon MEMS gyroscope which is designed by our own laboratory.

Keywords: MEMS, PLL, self-oscillation, Multisim, fixed amplitude.

1 Introduction

Since the 1980s, MEMS (Micro-Electro-Mechanical Systems) gyroscope has been developed with the development of silicon surface micro-machining technology. MEMS gyroscope is used in various fields for its advantages of small size, light weight, low cost and high reliability. The difference between MEMS gyroscope and gyroscope before is the MEMS gyroscope uses Principle of Coriolis force. It is a low cost inertial measurement of rotation angular velocity by sensing the Coriolis force, which changes the Coriolis force into electrical volume in the following circuit and gets the rotation angular velocity by calculation the electrical volume. A whole MEMS gyroscope system includes the mechanical system and the detecting circuit which make the oscillation of the gyroscope stable and resolve the micro-displacement of the mechanical system [1]. It must be kept the stability of the velocity of the oscillation mass if we want to resolve the rotation angular velocity exactly, because the Coriolis force yielding in the rotated mass is the coupling of the rotation angular velocity and oscillation velocity. Along with the increasing of accuracy requirements of MEMS gyroscope increasing, the position of the driving circuit is more and more important because it plays a key role in the course of keeping the stability of the oscillation as the entrance of the MEMS gyroscope.

This paper designs various driving circuits based on the simulation of Simulink and Multisim with the operation mode and parameter of the double-mass resonant output MEMS gyroscope which is designed by our own laboratory; and experimental analysis and comparison have been conducted preliminarily.

C. Xiong et al. (Eds.): ICIRA 2008, Part II, LNAI 5315, pp. 232–239, 2008.

2 The Principle

2.1 The Principle of the Double-Mass Resonant Output Gyroscope

The structure of the double-mass resonant output gyroscope is shown in Fig.1. The principle of driving mass is the same as tuning fork gyroscope; the difference between them is detecting mass of the double-mass resonant output gyroscope uses resonator, which overcomes the small displacement of the capacitance in C-V detecting approach because it uses the change of the resonator as the detecting value. The proof mass is driven relative to the outer frame using embedded lateral comb drive actuators. Specialized combs can be employed for self-test and for quadrature error cancellation. If an external rotation is applied to the chip about the z-axis, the Coriolis force acting on the driving mass is transmitted to the outer frame. A lever mechanism amplifies this force prior to being communicated axially onto two double-ended tuning fork (DETF) resonators placed on either side of the outer frame to provide for a differential output. The two tines of each tuning fork vibrate anti-phase to each other and parallel to the direction of motion of the inner driving mass. The periodic compression and tension of the tuning fork tines causing by the Coriolis force at the driving mass drive frequency modulates the resonant frequency of these force sensors. Each force sensor comprises of the tuning fork mechanical structure embedded in the feedback loop of an oscillator circuit. Thus, the rotation rate applied to the device can be estimated by demodulating the oscillator output frequency.

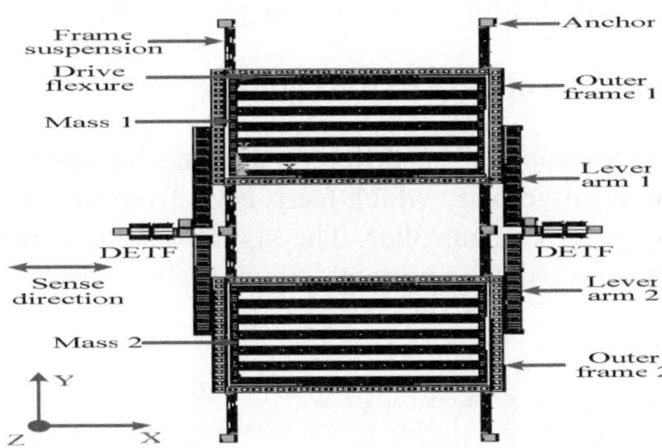

Fig. 1. The schematic of the mechanical structure illustrating the principle of operation

2.2 The Principle of the Driving Mass

The mechanical system of MEMS gyroscope is composed by the two parts of driving mass and detecting mass. The driving mass of the double-mass resonant output gyroscope in this paper is composed with both fixed comb and movable comb, and the detecting mass is composed with a resonant. The interface of the circuit part and mechanical system of the whole close-loop driving circuit includes two parts: The interface that the electrostatic force which comes from driving voltage is applied to the driving mass; The interface that the electrical volume outputs, which yields in the course of sensing the rotation outside. That means the whole close-loop driving circuit includes two conversion processes between the electrical volume and the dynamic volume. The key point in these processes is the electrostatic force that yields in the course of the oscillating mass sensing rotation angular velocity outside.

According to the following equation:

$$F = 2m\Omega \times v \tag{1}$$

where m is the driving mass, Ω is the angular velocity outside, v is the oscillation velocity of the driving mass, and $\times$ denotes the vector product, the oscillation velocity of the driving mass must be constant to make sure the Coriolis force expresses the angular velocity outside actually. The simple open-driving circuit can make the driving mass vibrate only, but it can't feedback the vibration of the driving mass. So it can't control the amplitude of the vibration. Therefore, we must use the closed-loop driving circuit and add the use of the driving detection to feedback the vibration [2] and [3].

3 Design and Realization of the Closed-Loop Driving Circuit

As said above, the stability of amplitude of the vibration is the key element which confines the accuracy of the MEMS gyroscope, so we must control the amplitude to improve the measurement accuracy at the same time optimizes the structure of the gyroscope. It means that the first goal of any driving circuit is to keep the stability of the amplitude. That is the control of the fixed amplitude [4] and [5].

3.1 Closed-Loop Control of the Fixed Amplitude

This design uses PI controller. The differential value between reference signal and amplitude of the vibration velocity which feeds back from the driving detecting comb yields a correction by the PI controller. The signal outside drives the MEMS gyroscope by the driving mass [6]. The principle block is shown in Fig.2.

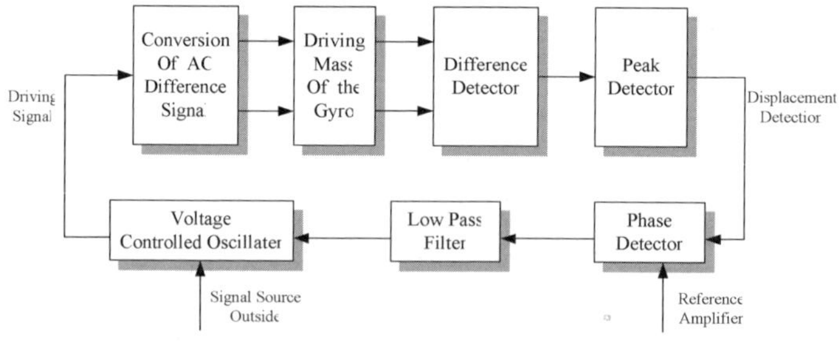

Fig. 2. The schematic block of the closed-loop control of the fixed amplitude

If we set the parameters combining with the actual parameters and make the oscillating frequency of the signal source outside in the natural frequency of the machine structural and the reference amplitude 1.25v, we will get the vibration displacement in Fig.3.

We will see that the amplitude of the gyro's final output is fixed in 1.25v. This circuit gets the goals of the amplitude fixed.

Fig.4 shows the change of the output of the vibration velocity and driving force as the natural frequency changes. The first figure shows the change of the driving force and the second figure shows the change of the vibration velocity. We will see that, though the amplitude of the vibration velocity will reduce when the frequency of the driving force is drift from the natural frequency, it returns to the reference amplitude quickly because of the adjustment of the closed-loop circuit.

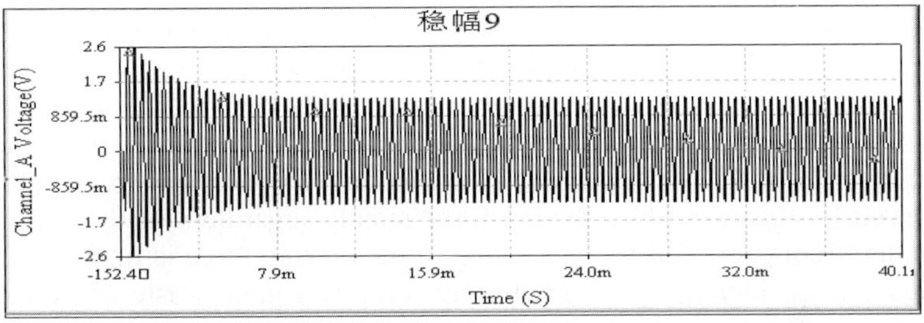

Fig. 3. The vibration displacement of the driving mass

Table 1. This table analyses the data of Fig.3, gives us the time when the system reaches the stabilization and the stability of displacement

Time of stability	Stable amplitude	Expectable amplitude	Relative error of amplitude
10ms	1.252v	1.25v	1.25v

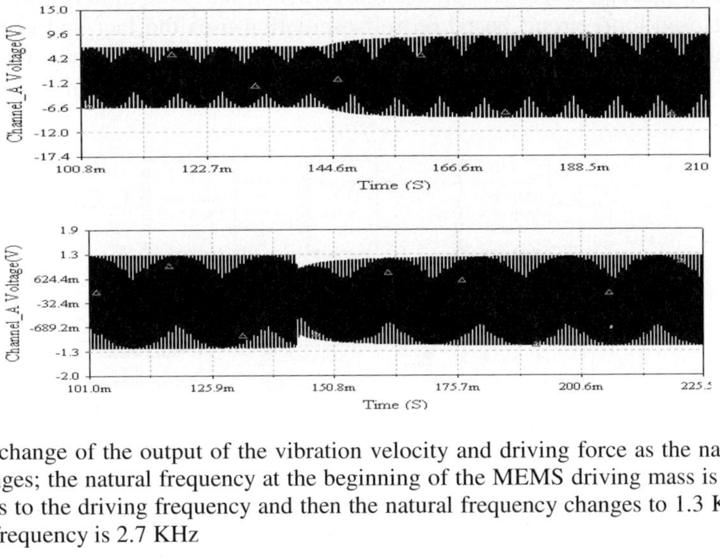

Fig. 4. The change of the output of the vibration velocity and driving force as the natural frequency changes; the natural frequency at the beginning of the MEMS driving mass is 2.7 KHz which equals to the driving frequency and then the natural frequency changes to 1.3 KHz, also the driving frequency is 2.7 KHz

Table 2. This table analyses the data of Fig.4, gives us the amplitude when the system operates on its natural frequency and the amplitude when the system doesn't operates on its natural frequency. Also it gives us the comparation.

Amplitude on the natural frequency	Amplitude on any frequency(1.3k)	Relative error on the natural frequency	Relative error on any frequency
1.252v	1.231v	0.16%	1.5%

3.2 Closed-Loop Control of the Frequency Locking

It is the basic requirement and goal to get the control of fixed amplitude. We must get the control of the driving-force frequency if we want to improve the performance of the gyro better. As known by the character of the MEMS gyro, the amplitude of the driving mass will reduce greatly if the frequency of the driving force is unequal to the natural frequency of the driving mass. It is available theoretically to keep the amplitude constant by increasing the driving force simply regardless of the change of the gyro's nature frequency. But the increasing of the driving force is limited by the analog device and the increasing of the driving force is a great waste of power. So the track of the natural frequency based on the fixed amplitude is needed in the driving circuit. Now, there are two approaches to realize the track of the frequency which one is based on PLL (Phase Locked Loop) and another is based on self-oscillation. We will discuss the approaches of self-oscillation in this paper [7].

Closed-loop circuit based on self-oscillation

Though the closed-loop circuit based on self-oscillation can make the oscillating frequency changed followed with the natural frequency of the gyro, extra circuit will be designed to satisfy the requirement of fixed amplitude, which increases the complexity of the circuit. So self-oscillation circuit which can realize the goal of amplitude fixed and frequency locking using a single circuit at the same time is proved.

The closed-loop circuit based on self-oscillation uses the fact that oscillation will be produced in the positive feedback circuit if there is little noise existing. The condition of the positive feedback is made up to make the whole circuit oscillate without

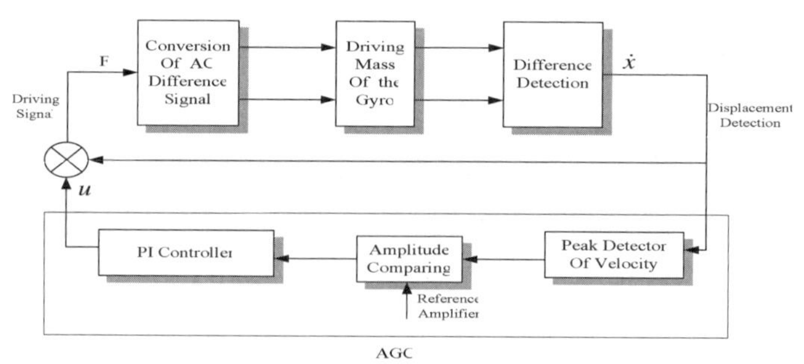

Fig. 5. The schematic block of the closed-loop circuit based on self-oscillation

motivation outside. The mechanical structure of gyro is the part of frequency selection which makes the system of self-oscillation oscillates with its natural frequency. The amplitude of the vibration is adjusted to the reference value by the AGC circuit. Fig.5 shows the schematic block of the closed-loop circuit based on self-oscillation [8].

The transfer function between the force applied to the driving mass and the vibration velocity can be expressed as follows [9] and [10]:

$$P(s) = \frac{1}{m}\frac{s}{s^2 + \frac{\omega_x}{Q}s + \omega_x^2} \tag{2}$$

where m is the proof mass, ω_x is the natural frequency of the proof mass, Q is the quality factor.

$$\frac{\dot{x}}{F} = \frac{1}{u} = P(s) \tag{3}$$

where x is the proof mass displacement, F is the driving force, u is the variable gain.

$$\frac{x}{usx} = \frac{1}{m}\frac{1}{s^2 + \frac{\omega_x}{Q}s + \omega_x^2} \tag{4}$$

Set the initial condition as 0, make Laplace inverse transform:

$$\ddot{x} + \frac{\omega_x}{Q}\dot{x} + \omega_x^2 x = \frac{u\dot{x}}{m} \tag{5}$$

$$\ddot{x} + \left(\frac{\omega_x}{Q} - \frac{u}{m}\right)\dot{x} + \omega_x^2 x = 0 \tag{6}$$

Make the damping term as 0 by changing the value of u. The system oscillates without damp, $\ddot{x} + \omega_x^2 x = 0$ and $x = B\sin(\omega_x t + \varphi)$ .The displacement of the vibration is a sine signal whose frequency is the natural frequency of the gyro. The control of oscillation frequency is realized.

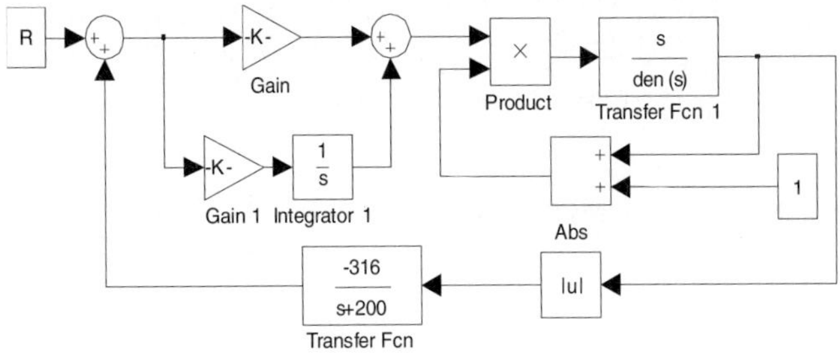

Fig. 6. The emulation block of closed-loop circuit based on self-oscillation

If we set the reference amplitude as 1.25v and make the Simulink emulation of self-oscillation driving using the parameter of the gyro designed by our own lab. Fig.6 shows the emulation block. The detection of the velocity amplitude uses the approach of rectifying and filtering. A constant deviation is applied to the circuit because the data is perfect in the environment of emulation.

Fig.7 shows the result of vibrating velocity of the driving mass.

Because the Q-factor is a little small, longer time is needed to make the system oscillating. Limiting circuit must be designed to overcome the large amplitude at the beginning actual circuit designs. Fig.8 shows the partial result.

As shown in Fig.8, amplitude of the vibrating output can be stabilized in the reference value by the control of the self-oscillation circuit.

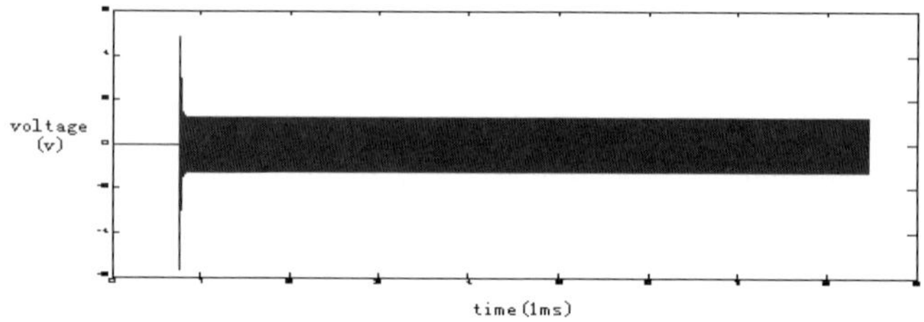

Fig. 7. The result of the vibrating velocity of the driving mass

Table 3. This table analyses the data of Fig.8, gives us the time when the system reaches the stabilization and the stability of displacement

Time of stability	Stable amplitude	Expectable amplitude	Relative error of amplitude
50ms	1.243	1.25	0.56%

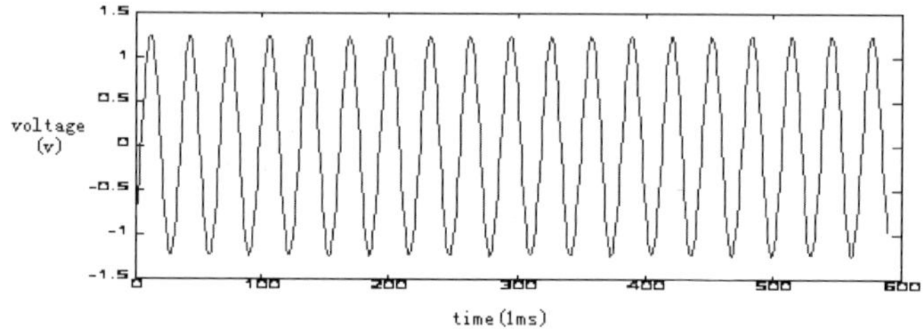

Fig. 8. The partial result of the vibrating velocity of the driving mass

4 Conclusion

This paper has designed closed-loop driving circuits according to the amplitude and frequency requirement of the MEMS vibrating gyro. It has formulated from simple to complex. Different levels of simulation and circuit implementation are made using the operation mode and parameter of the double-mass resonant output gyroscope which is designed by our own laboratory. The approaches improve the practicability and the correction and lay the fundament for the working following.

Acknowledgments

The work was sponsored by a grant from Key Programs of National Natural Science Foundation of China (60736025); the work was sponsored by a grant from the Major Programs of China National Space Administration (D2120060013).

References

1. Robert, P.L., Lipkin, Y., Highsmith, A.: Adaptive Oscillator Control for a Vibrational Gyroscope. In: Proceedings of the American Control Conference Denver, pp. 3347–3352. IEEE Press, Colorado (2003)
2. Park, S., Horowitz, R.: New Adaptive Mode of Operation for MEMS Gyroscopes. Transactions of the ASME 126, 800–810 (2004)
3. Chao, W.G., Yan, S., Rong, W.S.: Research on Self-Excited Driving of the Silicon Micromachined Vibratory Gyroscope Driver. Chinese Journal of Sensors and Actuators 19, 364–366 (2006)
4. Robert, P.L.: Adaptive Control of a MEMS Gyroscope Using Lyapunov Methods. IEEE Transactions on Control Systems Technology 14, 278–283 (2006)
5. Dong, J.K., Robert, T.M.: A Systematic Method for Tuning the Dynamics of Electrostatically Actuated Vibratory Gyros. In: IEEE Transactions on Control Technology, vol. 14, pp. 69–81 (2006)
6. Ming, L.J.: Research on High Signal-Noise Ratio of Capacitive Micromechanical gyroscope. [D], North University of China (2005)
7. Marc, S.W., Anthony, K.: Error Sources in In-Plane Silicon Tuning-Fork MEMS Gyroscopes. Journal of Microelectromechanical Systems 15, 479–491 (2006)
8. M'Closkey, R.T., Vakakis, A., Gutierrez, R.: Mode Localization Induced by a Nonlinear Control Loop. In: Nonlinear Dynamics, pp. 221–236 (2001)
9. Oboe, R., Antonello, R., Lasalandra, E., Durante, G.S., Prandi, L.: Control of a Z-Axis MEMS Vibrational Gyroscope. IEEE/ASME Transactions on Mechatronics 10(4) (2005)
10. Yen, C.C., R.T. M'Closkey, Tuan, A.T.: A Control and Signal Processing Integrated Circuit for the JPL-Boeing Micromachined Gyroscopes. In: IEEE Transactions on Control System Technology, vol. 13, pp. 286–300 (2005)

Investigation on the Key Technologies of Micro Machine Tool and Prototype Development

Jiashun Shi[1], Jintai Mi[1], Jinsheng Wang[1,2], Kui Chen[1], Wanshan Wang[1], and Guangqi Cai[1]

[1] Laboratory of Advanced Manufacturing and Automation, Northeastern University, Shenyang, China

[2] Laboratoire de Génie Industriel et de Production Mécanique, Université de Metz, Metz, France

jshshi@mail.neu.edu.cn, jswang@neu.com.cn

Abstract. In this work, the key technologies of Micro Machine Tool (MMT) are discussed in detail. A three-axis MMT prototype is developed. It is driven by ultra precision linear motors with high resolution linear encoders as feedback. It is equipped with a high speed electro-spindle and an CCD stereo microscope as a monitoring device. Meanwhile, the entire machine is controlled with an open numerical control system based on motion controller. The Human-Machine Interface (HMI) software is developed with G code compatibility. At last, the evaluation tests have been done on the MMT, and the results are very satisfactory and show its excellent performances.

Keywords: Machine tool design; Micro machine tool; Motion control system; Human-machine interface; Positioning accuracy; Micromilling.

1 Introduction

Nowadays, with the emergency requirements in many industry fields for micro parts, such as aerospace, biomedical, electro communication and so on [1,2], various related manufacturing techniques emerges one after another, such as etching, LIGA, laser and plastic micro-injection etc. [3]. Compared with other micromachining methods, micromilling is specialized in machining 3D micro parts in large range of workpiece materials from the metal alloy to other machinable nonmetallic materials such as polymer, plastic, ceramics etc. [4]. Meanwhile, it is cheaper and more flexible than other techniques and it can be monitored and controlled in process [5].

Due to the specialities of micro machining, the demands to the machine tool include the long stroke, micro feed, high positioning accuracy, excellent dynamic performances. Two types of machines are adopted to achieve the micromachining either in the industry or laboratory level. The first one is the traditional precision machine tool [6]. The second one is the micro machine tool (MMT). Compared with the traditional precision machine tool, the MMT is cost-effective due to the less materials requirement, and it is easy to achieve good thermal balance

C. Xiong et al. (Eds.): ICIRA 2008, Part II, LNAI 5315, pp. 240–249, 2008.

and environmental isolation. And due to its lower mass, its natural frequency is higher and the vibration amplitude is lower. Hence, Since the introduction of Japans Mechanical Engineering Lab microfactory concept is put forward in 1998 [7], more and more researchers resorted to develop several MMTs.

Subrahmanian and Ehmann [8] developed a three-axis meso-scale machine with $15 \times 15 \times 15mm^3$ workspace, $0.5\mu m$ encoder resolution, and $200,000RPM$ spindle. In University of Illinois at Urbana-Champaign (UIUC), after Vogler et al. [9] developed the first generation MMT, Honegger et al. [10] has beed developed the seconde prototype. Both of them are 3-axis and actuated by voice-coil motors. The second one is equipped with $160,000RPM$ air-turbine, $0.1mm$ encoder and reaches $25 \times 25 \times 25mm^3$ workspace. Ni and his group [11] has developed a 3-axis micro/meso machine tool, which is driven by a miniaturized piezoelectric linear stage with $13mm$ stroke and $0.25\mu m$ encoder resolution in each direction, as well as an air-turbine spindle with $120,000RPM$ maximal speed. Some other MMTs development includes the contribution from Bang et al [12], Ashida and Okazaki [13].

In this work, the key technologies of MMT are discussed in detail. A self-developedvthree-axis MMT prototype is introduced. At last, the evaluation tests have been done on the MMT, and the results are satisfactory and show its excellent performances.

2 Key Technologies of MMT

The entire MMT system is composed by some key components, and frequently they can be categorized as follows. How to develop these high quality components is critical to the MMT performance.

2.1 Feeding System

Because the feeding system of MMT must satisfy the demands of large feed, precision position, fast respond etc, the high quality feeding system is very important to the MMT performances. Some approaches which are primarily adopted to achieve the requirements will be discussed as follows.

Linear Driving System. The prismatic DoF is frequently adopted in the machine tool configuration, and the linear driving system can be used without the transferring chain in order to achieve the direct driving (DD). With the rapid development of the linear driving system, it has been applied in the machine tool industry more and more widely. The voice-coil motor, linear motors, and some similar types are included in this category. These motors can supply outstanding dynamic response as much as 5G acceleration, fast-speed positioning, high stiffness and good control ability [9]. Hence they are widely used in the MMT equipment [14,15].

Rotatory Driving Unit + Ball Screw System. This combination is commonly used in the traditional machine tool system. The rotatory driving unit, primarily rotatory motor, outputs the moment. Through the coupling unit, the ball screw system leads the stage movement. Compared with the linear driving system, they are less-cost, but the main problems are backslash and creeping phenomena in the ball screw system. So the error compensation devices or algorithms must be developed in order to improve its performances.

Non-motor Driving System. The non-motor driving system includes the piezo-electric actuator (PA), shape memory alloy (SMA), etc. They are well-known for their nano positioning precision, and widely used in the fields as MEMS/NEMS, micro manipulation, sensors, actuators and others. Some researchers adopted them into the MMT systems. Rusnaldy [16] used the PA to drive a three-axis MMT. Malukhin and Ehmann [17] have developed a 2D micro stage by SMA for thin wall structure fabrication. But the stroke of PA and SMA is relative small, the normal value is less than $1mm$. And their dynamic response is lower, so the displacement amplifier should be adopted when the machining feed rate is higher.

Micro Parallel Stage. In recent years, the theory of parallel robot have been developed rapidly and realized in many fields. And some researchers have developed the micro parallel stage for micromaching. Their DoFs range from 2 to 6 with higher stiffness. Furutani et al. [18] adopted the stacked piezo-electric actuators to form a Stewart parallel platform, which is used for nanometer cutting research. However, the workspace of the parallel mechanism is smaller and it is expensive to setup a high precision parallel stage.

2.2 Spindle System

Due to the tool tip diameter of the micromill is always smaller than $1mm$, the cutting speed is much smaller than the common sense. In order to improve the cutting speed to prolong the tool life and enhance the surface quality, the high speed spindle ($\geqslant 10,000RPM$) must be integrated into the MMT system. It can be categorized as bellows [19].

Electro Spindle. Today, the electro spindles are the brushless DC motors. Their speed can achieve as high as $200,000RPM$, and it is easy to be controlled by the digital signal from inverter. However, they are larger dimensions, heaver mass and the additional cooling system is necessary to decrease the temperature due to the inner heat generation.

Air Turbine. The speed of air turbine ranges from $50,000RPM$ to $200,000RPM$. But the size of them are relative larger, about $45mm$ diameter. Due to the driving source is the air flow, they can be cooled by themselves.

2.3 Sensing System

Because the functions of MMT are in the microscale, the sensors in conventional range are not capable to detect the signals for MMT. Many special sensors have been developed to improve the MMT performances. The linear encoder system can reach nanometer resolution in long stroke. The precision dynamometer with $2mN$ resolution and $40KHz$ sampling frequency are already widely used in the laboratory level. Other novel type sensors, such as laser sensor, acoustic emission senor et al, are integrated in the advanced MMTs.

2.4 Control System

Nowadays about 90% MMTs utilize the hierarchical control system. The PC/IPC is in the top level, and the motion controller is in the middle level. The controller compiles and sends the commands to the motor drivers in the machine language format. The feeding system moves according to the command and the sensors feedback form a closed-loop control system. Most researchers work under the controller software environment. Some investigators resorted to develop the interface software between the motion controller and the operator to achieve the operation directly. In order to be compatible with the G-code programming, the numerical control (NC) systems for the micromachining are developed. Hence the MMT can fulfill complex surface fabrication.

2.5 Monitor System

Due to the tiny tool size, the tool wear and breakage issues are really important to the micromilling operation [20]. Meanwhile, according to some tool catalogs, the tool life of micromill is only a few hours. Therefore, monitoring the machining process online is very useful to check the tool condition. In microscale machining process, the CCD stereo microscope is capable to supply large field-of-view and accepted depth-of-view. And the cutting force and acoustic emission sensors are also available.

3 Prototype Development

In this paper, the three-axis micromilling machine prototype is composed by a electro high speed spindle, three ultra precision linear motor, three linear encoders, open numerical control system, 3-component precision cutting force dynamometer, CCD stereo microscope with $40\times \sim 240\times$ magnification, HMI with G-code programming function, vibration-isolation system and spindle-cooling system. The entire prototype is shown in Fig.1. The dimension of the prototype is $400 \times 320 \times 100mm^3$ with $50 \times 50 \times 50mm^3$ workspace.

3.1 Feeding System

In order to realize the requirements of the machine motion, three micro feeding units are adopted. Each unit is composed by a Parker permanent magnet servo linear motor with $4G$ acceleration and $50mm$ stroke and a Reinshaw linear encoder with $10nm$ resolution. This configuration forms a closed-loop control system to improve the performance of the micromilling process.

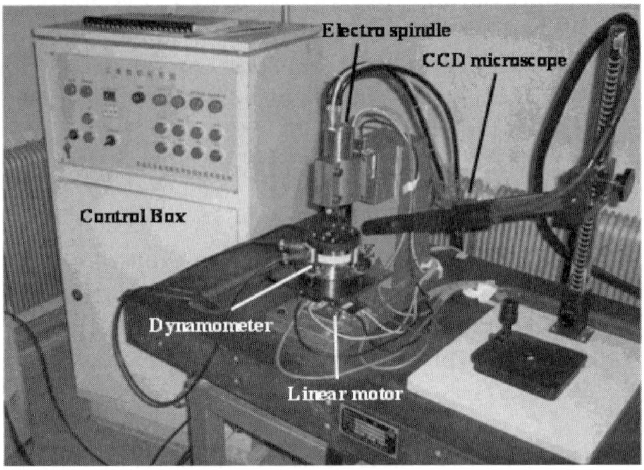

Fig. 1. Three-axis MMT system

3.2 Spindle System

A high speed electro spindle is integrated into the MMT system and moving in Z direction. The maximal rotating speed is $60,000RPM$. The run-out in radial and axial directions are $3\mu m$, which is satisfactory with the requirements of micromilling operation.

3.3 Control System

This control system structure is PC + 6K multi-axis motion controller + VIX linear motion driver, shown in Fig.2. The PC communicates with the 6K motion controller either by ethernet or serial port. The controller drives three linear motor drivers in each direction. With the feedback of linear encoders, the PID control is used to improve the motion performance and the motor conditions are monitored in real-time.

3.4 Human Machine Interface (HMI)

Because 6K motion controller couldn't provide the interface for numerical control of the micromilling process with G-code compatibility, a specialized HMI software is developed. It includes 4 function module, communication setting, parameters setting, manual manipulation and auto manipulation. The software can replace the programming environment of the 6K controller, and the G-code is interpreted into the corresponding commands to the motion controller. Fig.3 is the interface that the auto manipulation module is working with G-code.

3.5 Other Components

A CCD stereo microscope with $40\times \sim 240\times$ magnification is used to monitor the micromilling process and to do the online measurement. A three component

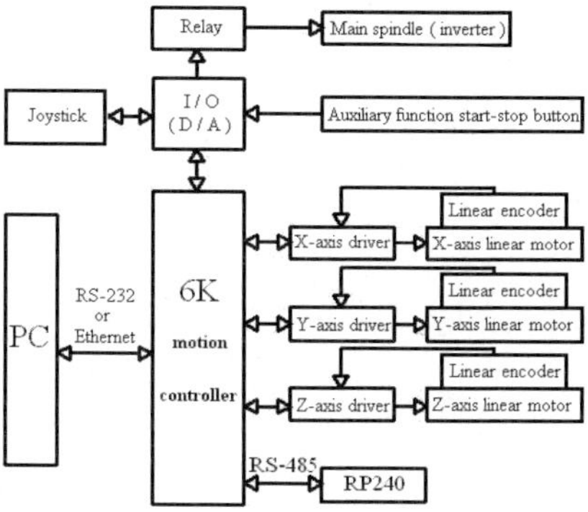

Fig. 2. MMT control system

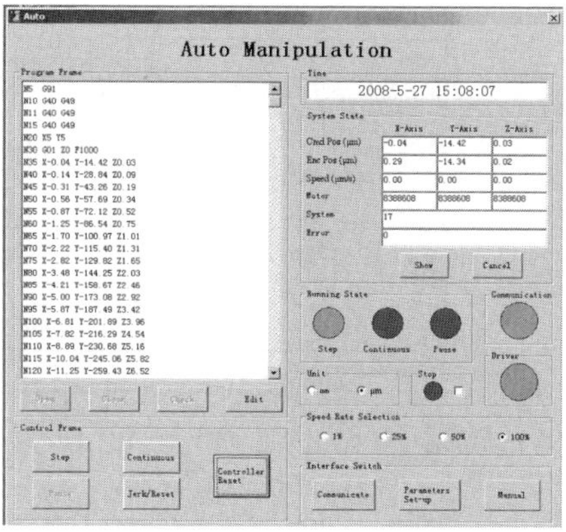

Fig. 3. HMI of MMT prototype

precision dynamometer SDC-CJ3SAS is assembled on the X-Y stage, with $10mN$ threshold and $250N$ maximum. The marble platform is used for the machine tool base in order to isolate the environmental vibration. The cooling system is used for decreasing the spindle temperature.

4 MMT Prototype Test

In order to evaluate the MMT prototype performances, the positional accuracy test and the machining test have been conducted on it.

4.1 Positional Accuracy Test

The evaluation criteria of the machine tool positional accuracy includes bi-directional positional accuracy, bi-directional repeatability and reversal value. According to the ISO-230-2:1997 standard, the positional accuracy tests of the motion platform used bidirectional evaluation method and linear circulation measurement. The target location points number $n = 10$, sequential numbered by $j = 1, 2, ..., n$, and the target measurement interval $t = L/n = 5mm$, with the cycle number $m = 5$.

The motion stage in each direction stopped steadily after it arrived the target point, the actual position from the linear encoder was fed back to the PC and displayed in the HMI. The Z axis test data were shown in Fig.4. And the X and Y directions were tested in the same way.

In Fig.4, $\uparrow$ and $\downarrow$ represented the test data were obtained from the positive and negative directions respectively, for example $X_{ij} \uparrow$ and $X_{ij} \downarrow$. Based on the evaluation data, the positional accuracy of the MMT was listed in Table.1. The test results showed the bi-directional positional accuracy and the bi-directional repeatability of the prototype is in sub-micron level, which is satisfactory to the requirements of micromilling operation.

Point j	1		2		3		4		5	
P_j (mm)	0		5.510		10.025		14.953		20.042	
Direction	↑	↓	↑	↓	↑	↓	↑	↓	↑	↓
Position Error X_{ij} (um) i	-0.38	-0.36	-0.46	-0.48	-0.38	-0.54	-0.55	-0.55	-0.33	-0.32
	-0.54	-0.44	-0.44	-0.41	-0.36	-0.40	-0.35	-0.32	-0.42	-0.43
	-0.44	-0.36	-0.38	-0.36	-0.38	-0.36	-0.37	-0.40	-0.50	-0.42
	-0.38	-0.46	-0.52	-0.42	-0.36	-0.56	-0.38	-0.36	-0.38	-0.39
	-0.54	-0.52	-0.42	-0.51	-0.48	-0.36	-0.57	-0.57	-0.37	-0.38
Point j	6		7		8		9		10	
P_j (mm)	25.051		30.066		34.879		40.027		45.048	
Direction	↑	↓	↑	↓	↑	↓	↑	↓	↑	↓
Position Error X_{ij} (um) i	-0.53	-0.54	-0.43	-0.36	-0.51	-0.52	-0.49	-0.49	-0.44	-0.42
	-0.37	-0.38	-0.42	-0.43	-0.37	-0.38	-0.41	-0.42	-0.52	-0.51
	-0.43	-0.39	-0.33	-0.37	-0.43	-0.43	-0.38	-0.46	-0.39	-0.38
	-0.53	-0.42	-0.45	-0.45	-0.42	-0.43	-0.36	-0.36	-0.41	-0.41
	-0.42	-0.46	-0.46	-0.45	-0.43	-0.42	-0.41	-0.42	-0.44	-0.42

Fig. 4. Positional accuracy test data for Z axis

Table 1. The positional accuracy of the MMT prototype

Dir.	Bi-dir. positional accuracy	Bi-dir. repeatability	Reversal value
X	$0.2734\mu m$	$0.2682\mu m$	$0.04627\mu m$
Y	$0.2800\mu m$	$0.2618\mu m$	$0.0347\mu m$
Z	$0.4534\mu m$	$0.4510\mu m$	$0.0520\mu m$

4.2 Micromilling Experimental Test

Some micromilling tests were done by the prototype. One 4-flute carbide micromill with $0.4mm$ diameter was chosen for the test. The workpiece was a specialized Mg-Zn-Y alloy for biomedical application [21]. Here, the slab and thin wall micromilling tests are given.

Slab Micromilling Experiment. In this test, the spindle speed was $30,000RPM$, the feed rate per tooth $3\mu m$, and the axial depth was $15\mu m$. Three slabs with $3 \times 2mm^2$ dimension were fabricated. The surface quality was measured by optical profiler and the average roughness value was $S_a = 0.123 \pm 0.0181\mu m$. The 2D and 3D surface figures from the profiler of one sample are shown in Fig.5. Obviously, the MMT prototype is able to produce the surface with high quality.

Thin Wall Milling Experiment. The parameters setting was $30,000RPM$ spindle speed, $1.5\mu m$ feed rate per tooth and $20\mu m$ axial depth in each step.

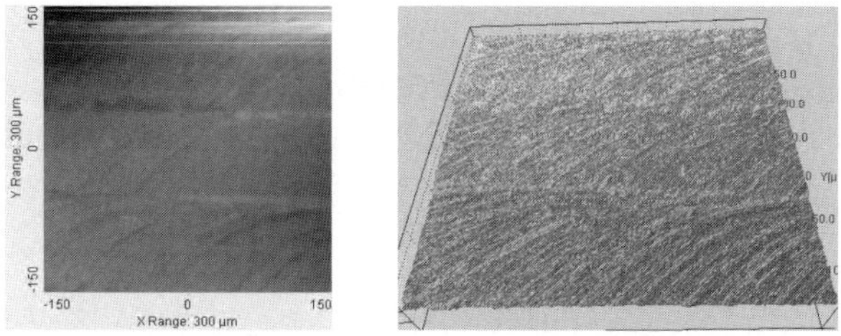

(a) 2D view (b) 3D view

Fig. 5. The micro slab surface figures

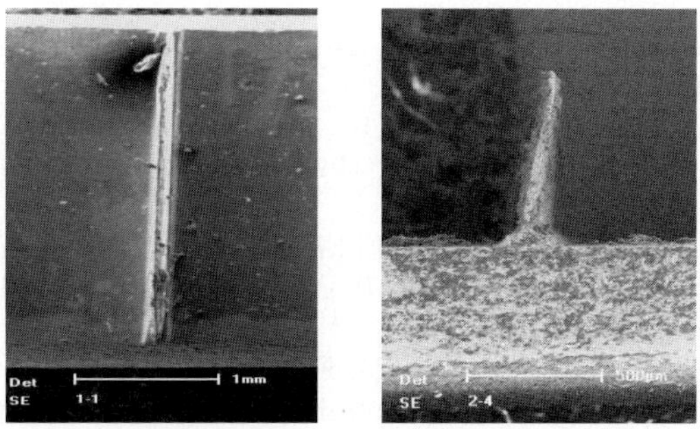

(a) Top view (b) Front view

Fig. 6. The thin wall structure

The desired section dimensions of the thin wall were $70\mu m$ in thickness and $780\mu m$ in height. The actual dimensions of it were about $65.5\mu m$ in average width, $778.7\mu m$ in height and $3.43mm$ in length, with high aspect ratio near 12 as shown in Fig.6. In this test, the axial machining error was acceptable. But from the front view, the wall bottom thickness was greater than the one in the wall top, because the tool vibration and deflection influences as discussed by Gong et al. [22].

5 Conclusions

In this work, the critical technologies of MMT are discussed in detail. A 3-axis MMT prototype is developed with large workspace and precision resolution. Through the positional accuracy test of the motion stage, the prototype expressed the excellent performances. In the machining test, the MMT prototype is able to produce high quality surface with suitable machining parameters setting. Meanwhile, it is capable to create high aspect ratio as thin wall structure.

Acknowledgements

This work was supported by Chinese 985-II foundation, Northeastern University PhD foundation 200705, French Research Ministry, and Lorraine Region Council.

References

1. Dornfeld, D., Min, S., Takeuchi, Y.: Recent advances in mechanical micromachining. Annals of CIRP 55(2), 745–768 (2006)
2. Filiz, S., Xie, L., Weiss, L., Ozdoganlar, O.: Micromilling of microbarbs for medical implants. International Journal of Machine Tools & Manufacture 48, 459–472 (2008)
3. Alting, L., Kimura, F., Hansen, H., Bissacco, G.: Micro engineering. Annals of CIRP 52(2) (2003); STC–O
4. Wang, J., Gong, Y., Abba, G., Chen, K., Shi, J., Cai, G.: Surface generation analysis in micro end-milling considering the influences of grain. Microsystem Technologies 14(7), 937–942 (2008)
5. Wang, J., Gong, Y., Abba, G., Cao, J., Shi, J., Cai, G.: Micro milling technologies for mems. In: Proceeding of 3rd MEMSTECH, Lviv-Polyana, Ukraine, May 2007, pp. 86–95 (2007)
6. Luo, X., Cheng, K., Webb, D., Wardle, F.: Design of ultraprecision machine tools with applications to manufacture of miniature and micro components. Journal of Materials Processing Technology 167, 515–528 (2005)
7. Furuta, K., Ishikawa, Y., Mikuriya, Y., Takahashi, Y.: The microfactory system in national r&d project of miti. In: Proceedings of the International Workshop on Microfactories, Tsukuba, Japan, December 1998, pp. 193–196 (1998)
8. Subrahmanian, R., Ehmann, K.F.: Development of a meso-scale machine tool (mmt) for micro-machining. In: Proceeding of Japan-USA Symposium on Flexible Automation, Hiroshima, Japan, July 2002, vol. 1, pp. 163–169 (2002)
9. Vogler, M., Liu, X., Kapoor, S., DeVor, R., Ehmann, K.: Development of meso-scale machine tool (mmt) systems. Transactions of North American Manufacturing Research Institution 30, 1–9 (2002)
10. Honegger, A., Kapoor, S., DeVor, R.: A hybrid methodology for kinematic calibration of micro/meso-scale machine tools (mts). ASME Journal of Manufacturing Science and Engineering 128, 513–522 (2006)
11. Lee, S.W., Mayor, R., Ni, J.: Dynamic analysis of a mesoscale machine tool. ASME Journal of Manufacturing Science and Engineering 128, 194–203 (2006)
12. Bang, Y., Lee, K., Oh, S.: 5-axis micro milling machine for machining micro parts. International Journal of Advanced Manufacturing Technology 25, 888–894 (2005)
13. Okazaki, Y., Mishima, N., Ashida, K.: Microfactory-concept, history, and developments. ASME Journal of Manufacturing Science and Engineering 126, 837–844 (2004)
14. Wang, J., Shi, J., Gong, Y., Abba, G., Cai, G.: A micro milling model considering metal phases and minimum chip thickness. Key Engineering Materials 375-376, 505–509 (2008)
15. Zhang, L., Zhao, D., Zhang, J., Sun, X., Pang, C.: Development of miniaturized numerical control milling machine tool used in micro cutting. Journal of Southeast University (Natural Science Edition) 137(1), 26–29 (2007)

16. Rusnaldy, T.J.K., Kim, H.S.: An experimental study on microcutting of silicon using a micromilling machine. International Journal of Advanced Manufacturing Technology (2008), doi:10.1007/s00170–007–1211–9
17. Malukhin, K., Ehmann, K.: Identification of direct metal deposition (dmd) process parameters for manufacturing thin wall structures from shape memory alloy (niti) powder. Transactions of the North American Manufacturing Research Institution of SME 35, 481–488 (2007)
18. Furutani, K., Suzuki, M., Kudoh, R.: Nanometer-cutting machine using stewart-platform parallel mechanism. Measurement Science and Technology 15(2), 467–474 (2004)
19. Kapoor, S.: Current state of micro-scale machine tool systems and machining research. In: Workshop on micromanufacturing, natural science foundation, University of Illinois at Urbana-Champaign (2004)
20. Tansel, I., Arkan, T., Bao, W., Mahendrakar, N., Shisler, B., Smith, D., McCool, M.: Tool wear estimation in micro-machining. part 1: tool usage ccutting force relationship. International Journal of Machine Tools & Manufacture 40, 599–608 (2000)
21. Zhang, E.L., He, W.W., Du, H., Yang, K.: Microstructure, mechanical properties and corrosion properties of mg-zn-y alloys with low zn content. Materials Science and Engineering: A 488(1-2), 102–111 (2008)
22. Gong, Y., Wang, J., Abba, G., Antoine, J., Shi, J.: Tool tip trajectories investigation and its influences in micromilling operation. IEEE Review on Advances in Micro, Nano and molecular Systems (in press)

Forward Kinematics and Solution Methodologies for a Flexure-Based Micro-manipulator

Yanling Tian[1,2], Bijan Shirinzadeh[1], Dawei Zhang[2], and Gursel Alici[3]

[1] Robotics and Mechatronics Research Laboratory, Department of Mechanical and Aerospace Engineering, Monash University, Clayton, VIC 3800, Australia
[2] School of Mechanical Engineering, Tianjin University, Tianjin 300072, China
[3] School of Mechanical, Materials and Mechatronic Engineering, University of Wollongong, NSW 2522, Australia
{yanling.tian,bijan.shirinzadeh}@eng.monash.edu.au, medzhang@tju.edu.cn, gursel@uow.edu.au

Abstract. This paper presents the forward kinematics of a five-bar compliant micro-manipulator, where lever mechanisms are used to enlarge the working range in Cartesian space. Based on the configuration of the proposed flexure-based micro-manipulator, the entire system has been divided into a five-bar mechanism and two four-bar amplification mechanisms. The amplification factor of the lever mechanism is derived based on the analytical solution of the four-bar linkage. For the five-bar mechanism, the closed-form forward kinematics is obtained according to the established geometric relationship. The velocity of the end-effector is also obtained by differentiating the forward position kinematic equation. Based on the simplified methodologies such as linearising the trigonometric functions and constant Jacobian matrix, numerical simulations have been carried out to investigate the performance of the five-bar compliant manipulator. The comparisons between the exact solution and the simplified methodologies are carried out. It is noted that the linearising trigonometric simplification has a higher accuracy and is more suitable for the kinematic calculation of the micro-manipulator, but the constant Jacobian matrix method can efficiently calculate the forward kinematics of the micro-manipulator with the acceptable accuracy.

Keywords: micro-manipulator, flexure hinge, forward kinematics.

1 Introduction

Micro/nano manipulation is one of the key techniques for the nanotechnology applications such as x-ray lithography, micro-manufacturing, biomedicine, micro-surgery, and nano- metrology [1-4]. In these engineering fields, the required motion and positioning precision is generally within the order of magnitude of nanometer. It is well known that the positioning precision and resolution of the micro-manipulators mainly depend on the topology and mechanical structure, actuator and transducer, sensing and measurement, and control methodologies [5]. It is impossible to make the conventional manipulator to fulfill the requirements of the micro/nano manipulation tasks. The main reasons that prevent the conventional manipulator from improvement

C. Xiong et al. (Eds.): ICIRA 2008, Part II, LNAI 5315, pp. 250–259, 2008.

of the positioning accuracy are mainly due to the backlash and stiction of the revolute joints and the geometric and dimensional errors of the components of the manipulator [6]. Therefore, different manipulators must be developed that can overcome these problems. One of the best choices to overcome the problems is using flexure-based compliant mechanism, where the conventional kinematic pairs are replaced by the flexure hinges. These types of the joints have a number of advantages including no backlash, zero friction, and negligible hysteresis [7-10]. In addition, such a flexure-based micro-manipulator can be monolithically manufactured, and thus reduce assembly errors and guarantee the machining accuracy [11]. Furthermore, the flexure-based micro-manipulator can be combined with the conventional macro-positioning manipulators to form the dual positioning system. Thus, the large range of precision positioning can be achieved [12, 13]. Research efforts have focused on the development of many aspects of the micro-manipulators for conducting nano-scale tasks beyond the limits of human manipulation and patience [14-17]. The development of these design methodologies for the flexure hinge, novel micro-actuators, and adaptive robust control strategies for precision positioning will help facilitate the micro-manipulator with high dynamic performance and resolution [18-21]. It is known that the piezoelectric parallel-actuated closed-loop mechanisms made up of flexure hinges have demonstrated a considerable potential for the applications in the micro-manipulation tasks [22]. The forward kinematics is one of the important research areas in the applications of the parallel micro-manipulator.

This paper presents the closed-form forward kinematics for the Cartesian displacement and velocity of a flexure-based micro-manipulator with lever mechanism. The amplification factor of the lever mechanism is achieved by considering the amplification mechanism as a special four-bar linkage. The velocity of the end-effector of the five-bar mechanism is obtained by differentiating the forward position kinematic equation. Based on the simplified methodologies such as linearising trigonometric functions and constant Jacobian matrix, numerical simulations have been carried out and calculation precision of the simplified methodologies is presented.

2 Kinematic Modeling

The 3D model of the five-bar compliant micro-manipulator with lever mechanisms is shown in Fig.1. The main components of the compliant mechanism include the rectangular links and flexure hinges. Compared with other types of flexure hinges, circular flexure hinge with rectangular cross-section has high precision for rotational accuracy and is the optimal choice as the revolute joint for precision mechanism design and construction. A stationary frame is used to support the compliant mechanism and connect with other equipment.

From the kinematic point of view, a rectangular circular flexure hinge can be simplified as a revolute joint. This indicates that the drift of the center of rotation during the motion of the relative links is not taken into consideration. Thus, the kinematic model of the five-bar mechanism is obtained and shown in Fig.2, where *OA* and *DB* are the active links, *AP* and *BP* are the passive links, and *PM* is the extended part of the passive link *AP*. The active links *OA* and *DB* have the initial angular positions of θ_1 and θ_2 from the positive direction of the x axis. The length of the links is

r_i (i=0, 1, ···, 5), and the angle α is the angle of link *PM* separating from link *AP*. Based on the geometric and motion relationships, the following equations can be given:

$$\boldsymbol{r}_1 = r_1 \cos\theta_1 i + r_1 \sin\theta_1 j \tag{1}$$

$$\boldsymbol{r}_6 = (r_0 + r_5 \cos\theta_2) i + r_5 \sin\theta_2 j \tag{2}$$

$$\boldsymbol{q} = \boldsymbol{r}_6 - \boldsymbol{r}_1 = Ci + Dj \tag{3}$$

where $C = r_0 + r_5 \cos\theta_2 - r_1 \cos\theta_1$, $D = r_5 \sin\theta_2 - r_1 \sin\theta_1$.

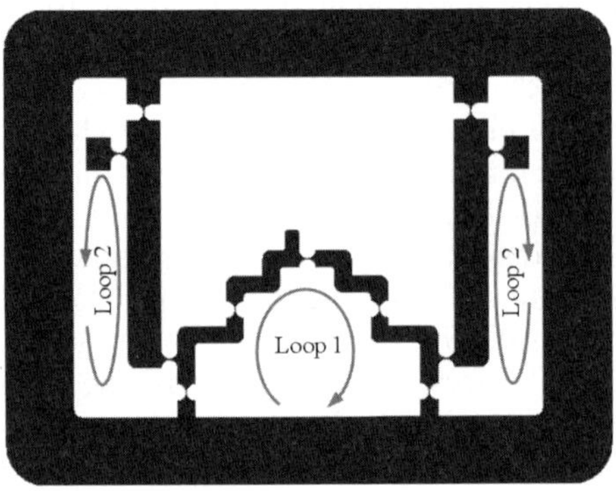

Fig. 1. 3D model of the five-bar micro-manipulator

The coordinates of the point *P* can be determined by the intersection of two circles whose centers locate at the points *A* and *B*, and the radii of the two circles are r_2 and r_4, respectively. It must be mentioned that the locations of the points *A* and *B* are the functions of the input angles θ_1 and θ_2. The two intersections are the possible solution for the point *P*. Based on the specified link lengths and driving angles, the coordinates of points $P_1(x, y)$ and $P_2(x, y)$ are given as follows:

$$\begin{cases} x_{P1} = r_1 \cos\theta_1 + r_2 (QC - DE) \\ y_{P1} = r_1 \sin\theta_1 + r_2 (QD + CE) \end{cases} \tag{4}$$

and

$$\begin{cases} x_{P2} = r_1 \cos\theta_1 + r_2 (QC + DE) \\ y_{P2} = r_1 \sin\theta_1 + r_2 (QD - CE) \end{cases} \tag{5}$$

where $Q = \dfrac{r_2^2 + q^2 - r_4^2}{2r_2 q^2}$, $E = \sqrt{1/q^2 - Q^2}$.

Thus, the possible locations of point $M(x, y)$ can be given as follows:

$$\begin{cases} x_{M1} = x_{P1} + r_3 \cos\alpha (QC - DE) - r_3 \sin\alpha (QD + CE) \\ y_{M1} = y_{P1} + r_3 \cos\alpha (QD + CE) + r_3 \sin\alpha (QC - DE) \end{cases} \tag{6}$$

and

$$\begin{cases} x_{M2}=x_{P2}+r_3\cos\alpha(QC+DE)-r_3\sin\alpha(QD-CE) \\ y_{M2}=y_{P2}+r_3\cos\alpha(QD-CE)+r_3\sin\alpha(QC+DE) \end{cases} \tag{7}$$

Based on the geometric relationship, Eq. (6) is chosen as the forward kinematics of the five-bar mechanism.

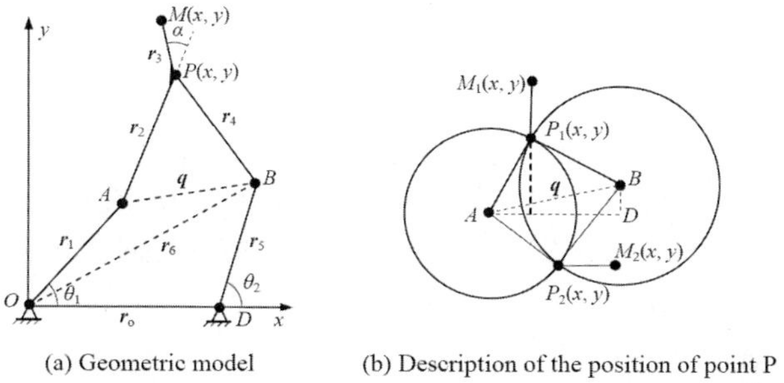

Fig. 2. Kinematic model of the five-bar mechanism

Assume that the links OA = DB, AP = BP, respectively, -i.e. r_1=r_5 and r_2=r_4. For the brevity and without loss of generality, two vectors $\boldsymbol{\Gamma}=(x_M, y_M)^{\mathrm{T}}$ and $\boldsymbol{\Theta}=(\theta_1,\theta_2)^{\mathrm{T}}$ are introduced.

By differentiating Eq. (6) with respect to time, the following relationship is given:

$$\dot{\boldsymbol{\Gamma}}=\begin{bmatrix} \dfrac{\partial x_M}{\partial(\theta_1,\theta_2)} \\ \dfrac{\partial y_M}{\partial(\theta_1,\theta_2)} \end{bmatrix}\dot{\boldsymbol{\Theta}}=\boldsymbol{J}\dot{\boldsymbol{\Theta}} \tag{8}$$

where $\boldsymbol{J}=\begin{bmatrix} J_{11} & J_{12} \\ J_{21} & J_{22} \end{bmatrix}$ is the Jacobian matrix and defined by:

$$J_{11}=-r_1\sin\theta_1+r_1(r_2+r_3\cos\alpha)\left[\frac{\sin\theta_1}{2r_2}+E\cos\theta_1+\frac{D}{q^4E}(C\sin\theta_1-D\cos\theta_1)\right]$$

$$-r_1r_3\sin\alpha\left[-\frac{\cos\theta_1}{2r_2}+E\sin\theta_1-\frac{C}{q^4E}(C\sin\theta_1-D\cos\theta_1)\right]$$

$$J_{12}=r_1(r_2+r_3\cos\alpha)\left[-\frac{\sin\theta_2}{2r_2}-E\cos\theta_2+\frac{D}{q^4E}(-C\sin\theta_2+D\cos\theta_2)\right]$$

$$-r_1r_3\sin\alpha\left[\frac{\cos\theta_2}{2r_2}-E\sin\theta_2-\frac{C}{q^4E}(-C\sin\theta_2+D\cos\theta_2)\right]$$

$$J_{21} = r_1\cos\theta_1 + r_1(r_2 + r_3\cos\alpha)\left[-\frac{\cos\theta_1}{2r_2} + E\sin\theta_1 - \frac{C}{q^4E}(C\sin\theta_1 - D\cos\theta_1)\right]$$
$$+ r_1r_3\sin\alpha\left[\frac{\sin\theta_1}{2r_2} + E\cos\theta_1 + \frac{D}{q^4E}(C\sin\theta_1 - D\cos\theta_1)\right]$$
$$J_{22} = r_1(r_2 + r_3\cos\alpha)\left[\frac{\cos\theta_2}{2r_2} - E\sin\theta_2 - \frac{C}{q^4E}(-C\sin\theta_2 + D\cos\theta_2)\right]$$
$$+ r_1r_3\sin\alpha\left[-\frac{\sin\theta_2}{2r_2} - E\cos\theta_2 + \frac{D}{q^4E}(-C\sin\theta_2 + D\cos\theta_2)\right]$$

The lever mechanism (loop 2 shown in Fig.1) can be considered as a four-bar mechanism and illustrated in Fig.3, where the length of the links is l_i (i=0, 1, 2, 3), and θ_i (i=3, 4, 5) is the angle of the links with respect to the positive direction of x' axis.

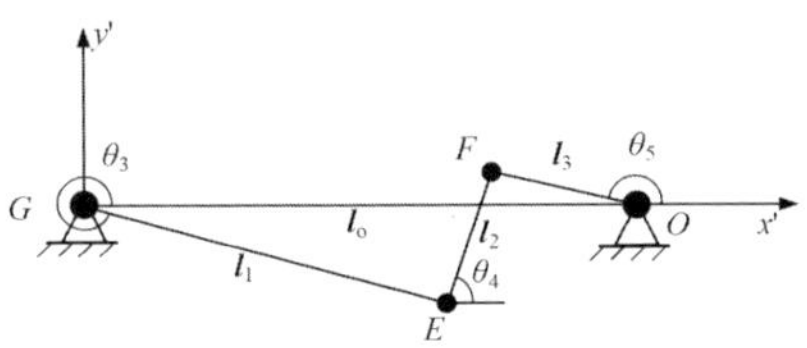

Fig. 3. Kinematic model of the lever mechanism

Thus, the four links form a closed-loop equation and the projection on x' and y' axes are given, respectively:

$$l_1\cos\theta_3 + l_2\cos\theta_4 - l_3\cos\theta_5 - l_0 = 0 \tag{9}$$

$$l_1\sin\theta_3 + l_2\sin\theta_4 - l_3\sin\theta_5 = 0 \tag{10}$$

Substituting Eq. (9) into Eq. (10), and eliminating θ_4, yields:

$$f = (l_1\cos\theta_3 - l_3\cos\theta_5 - l_0)^2 + (l_1\sin\theta_3 - l_3\sin\theta_5)^2 - l_2^2 = 0 \tag{11}$$

Thus, the relation between θ_3 and θ_5 can be derived as follows:

$$\frac{d\theta_5}{d\theta_3} = -\frac{\partial f/\partial\theta_3}{\partial f/\partial\theta_5} = -\frac{l_1(l_3\sin(\theta_3 - \theta_5) + l_0\sin\theta_3)}{l_3(l_1\sin(\theta_5 - \theta_3) - l_0\sin\theta_5)} \tag{12}$$

When link l_1 is parallel to link l_3, - i.e. $\theta_3 - \theta_5 = \pi$, Eq. (12) can be simplified and rewritten as:

$$d\theta_5 = -\frac{l_1}{l_3}d\theta_3 \tag{13}$$

It is noted that the amplification factor of the lever mechanism is proportional to the ratio of the links l_1 and l_3, when the mechanism moves within a small range. In addition, the link l_2 should be perpendicular to the links l_1 and l_3, in order to obtain a large transmission angle.

The exact solution of the forward kinematics of the five-bar mechanism can be carried out based on the Eq. (6). In order to improve calculation efficiency, the solution of the forward position problem has been implemented by two simplified methods: (a) linearising the trigonometric functions for small displacement in Eq. (6), and (b) approximating the velocity equation, in Eq. (8), for small displacement equation in the actuation and Cartesian spaces. Thus, the small displacement mapping between the actuation and Cartesian spaces can be given as follows:

$$\begin{bmatrix} \delta x \\ \delta y \end{bmatrix} = \boldsymbol{J} \begin{bmatrix} \delta\theta_1 \\ \delta\theta_2 \end{bmatrix} \tag{14}$$

where δx and δy are the small displacement of the end-effector in the Cartesian space, $\delta\theta_1$ and $\delta\theta_2$ are the small displacement of the active links in the actuation space.

The similar method can be used to determine the velocity of the five-bar manipulator in Cartesian space. The first approach is based on the linearising all the trigonometric functions in Eq. (8). The second method uses a constant Jacobian matrix through the range of motion while evaluating the Cartesian velocity vector.

3 Numerical Results and Discussion

Under the special configuration of the lever mechanism, -i.e. the active link l1 is parallel with the link l_3 of the five-bar mechanism as shown in Fig.3, the amplification factor of the lever mechanism is constant and equal to the length ratio of the two corresponding links. Thus, the kinematic and dynamic characteristics of the compliant mechanism are determined by the configuration of the five-bar mechanism. Assuming that the link lengths for the five-bar mechanism are r_0=145 mm, r_1=r_5=60 mm, r_2=r_4=55 mm, and r_3=10, α=π/6 rad, and the initial position of the active links are chosen as θ_1= π/3 rad and θ_2= 2π/3 rad. The strokes of the active links are set as $\delta\theta_1$= $\delta\theta_2$= ±20×10-6 rad with a step s=0.5×10^{-6} rad. The angular velocities of the active links are chosen as $\dot{\theta}_1 = \dot{\theta}_2 = 1\times10^{-4}$ rad/s. Thus, the position and velocity of the points P and M are determined using the developed forward kinematic formulations and the simplified methodologies described in the previous section. The position errors of the points P and M in x and y directions corresponding to four different simplified forward kinematic solutions are provided in Figs. 4 and 5, respectively. The linearised function plots (Figs. 4a and 5a) show the position errors between the exact position solutions and the simplified solutions with linearised sine and cosine functions in the forward kinematic equations. It is noted that the error contours are the lines with almost the same slope, and the position errors are negligibly small. The position errors of the point P in the x and y direction are within the bands of $\delta x \approx 1.3\times10^{-11}$ m and $\delta y \approx 1.5\times10^{-11}$ m, and those of the point M in the x and y directions are located in the ranges of $\delta x \approx 1.7\times10^{-11}$ m and $\delta y \approx 1.8\times 10^{-11}$ m. In addition, the error contours of the point P are symmetric and those of point M are asymmetric. When Eq. (14) is used to evaluate the position of the end-effector, the position errors of the point P (Fig. 4b) in x and y directions increase to the ranges of $\delta x \approx 3.0\times10^{-11}$ m and $\delta y \approx 5.5\times10^{-11}$ m, and those of the point M (Fig. 5b) reach up to the bands of $\delta x \approx 3.4\times10^{-11}$ m and $\delta y \approx 6.2\times10^{-11}$ m in the x and y directions, respectively. Furthermore, the position errors in

y direction of the points P and M become asymmetric. When the trigonometric functions of the Jacobian matrix are linearised, the error contours of the points P and M (Figs. 4c and 5c) are the same as the solutions based on the exact Jacobian matrix. When the constant Jacobian matrix for the configuration of $\theta_1 = \pi/3$ rad and $\theta_2 = 2\pi/3$ rad are utilized to calculate the forward position of the five-bar compliant mechanism (Figs. 4d and 5d), the magnitude of values of position errors for the points P and M, are similar to those of exact or linearised Jacobian matrix, but the signs of the errors are opposite. From the computational results, it can be concluded that the linearising trigonometric functions in forward kinematic equation obtains the higher order of the magnitude precision for position prediction. The forward kinematic solution using simplified methods such as linearised and constant Jacobian matrix can be obtained with the similar precision for forward position prediction. Those simplified methods have the same order of magnitude for the precision of prediction. In addition, the constant Jacobian matrix corresponding to any configuration of the manipulator within the specified ranges of θ_1 and θ_2 can be used to calculate the forward kinematic position prediction, and the error ranges will not change significantly. This conclusion is in agreement with the research results, and it is important and useful for the forward kinematic calculation of the parallel micro-manipulators. It is also noted that the simplified methods can induce larger position errors at the point M. Thus, the point M should be chosen as close as possible to the point P. This conclusion is similar to that drawn from the local mobility index consideration.

The velocity errors in x and y directions of the points P and M are shown in Figs. 6 and 7. It is noted that the error contours are also the lines with almost the same slope, during the angles of the active links change within the ranges of $\theta_1+\delta\theta_1$ and $\theta_2+\delta\theta_2$.

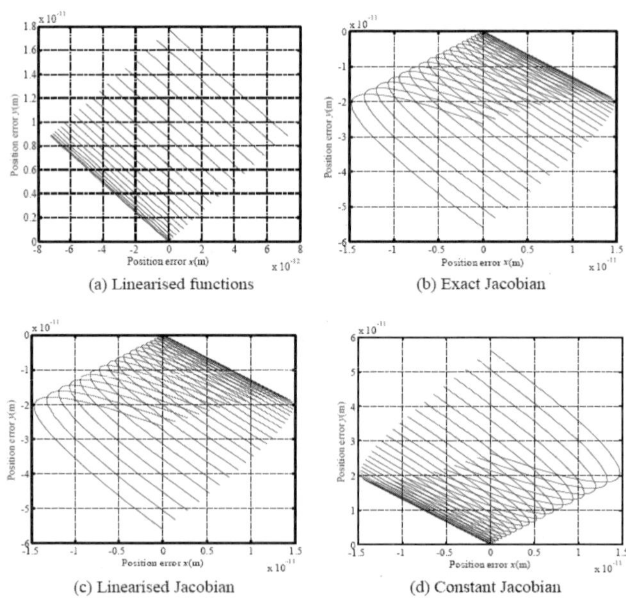

Fig. 4. Position errors of the point P in x and y directions

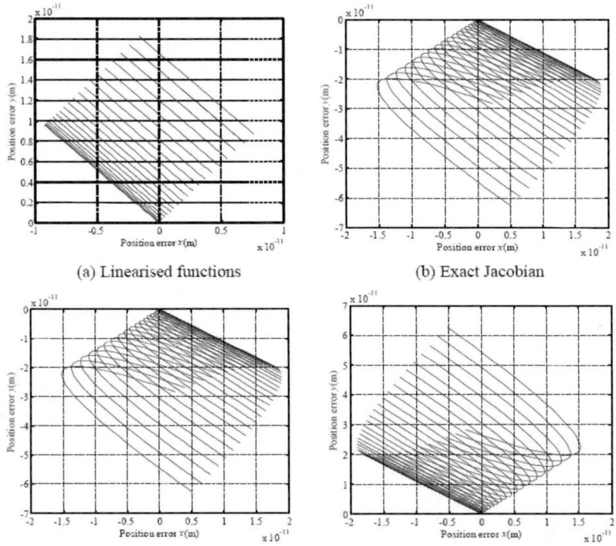

(a) Linearised functions

(b) Exact Jacobian

(c) Linearised Jacobian

(d) Constant Jacobian

Fig. 5. Position errors of the point *M* in *x* and *y* directions

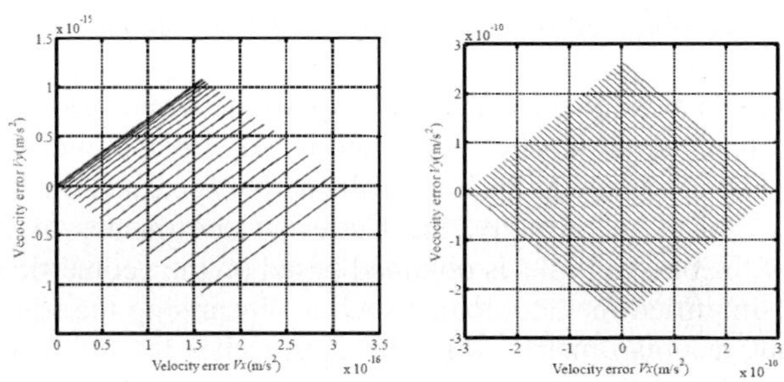

(a) Linearised Jacobian

(b) Constant Jacobian

Fig. 6. Velocity errors of the point *P* in *x* and *y* directions

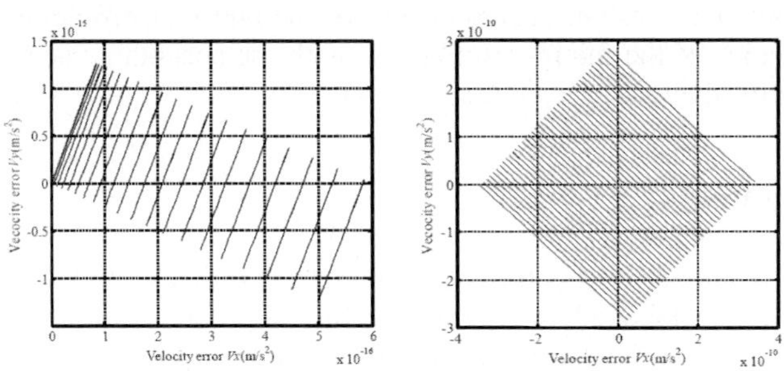

(a) Linearised Jacobian

(b) Constant Jacobian

Fig. 7. Velocity errors of the point *M* in *x* and *y* directions

When the trigonometric functions of Jacobian matrix are linearised to calculate the Cartesian velocity of the end-effector, the velocity errors of the point *P* in the *x* and *y* directions locate within the ranges of $\delta\dot{x} \approx 3.2\times10^{-16}$ m/s and $\delta\dot{y} \approx 2.2\times10^{-15}$ m/s, respectively. Similarly, the velocity errors of the point *M* in the *x* and *y* directions stay within the ranges of $\delta\dot{x} \approx 5.8\times10^{-16}$ m/s and $\delta\dot{y} \approx 2.5\times10^{-15}$ m/s, respectively. When the constant Jacobian matrix is utilized to calculate the velocity of the end-effector, the velocity errors of the point *P* dramatically increase to the ranges of $\delta\dot{x} \approx 6.0\times10^{-10}$ m/s and $\delta\dot{y} \approx 5.0\times10^{-10}$ m/s. The velocity errors of the point *M* will reach up to the ranges of $\delta\dot{x} \approx 6.8\times10^{-10}$ m/s and $\delta\dot{y} \approx 5.6\times10^{-10}$ m/s. Although the constant Jacobian matrix can induce larger prediction errors than the linearised Jacobian matrix, the computational errors are very smaller compared to the absolute velocity of the end effector. Thus, the constant Jacobian matrix can be used to calculate the velocity of the end-effector with an acceptable precision and high computational efficiency, and this is important for the realization of real-time control algorithm.

4 Conclusions

A five-bar compliant mechanism with lever mechanisms has been described. From the kinematic point of view, the entire compliant micro-manipulator has been divided into a five-bar mechanism and two four-bar amplification mechanisms. The amplification factor has been obtained by considering the lever mechanism as a special four-bar linkage.

The forward kinematics for the Cartesian displacement and velocity of the five-bar compliant micro-manipulator has been obtained by solving the intersection of the two circles with the centers located at the end of the active links and the radii equal to the length of passive links. Accordingly, the Cartesian coordinates of the end-effector attached to one of the passive links is obtained based on the geometric relationship.

Based on the simplified methodologies such as linearising the trigonometric functions and constant Jacobian matrix, different approaches for the forward kinematics have been proposed and the performance of the five-bar compliant manipulator is investigated. The comparisons between the exact solutions and simplified methods were carried out. It is noted that the linearization of trigonometric functions has a higher accuracy and is more suitable for the kinematic calculation of the micro-manipulator, but the constant Jacobian matrix method can efficiently calculate the forward kinematics of the micro-manipulator with the acceptable accuracy and is the optimal choice for the real-time control system.

Acknowledgments

This research is supported by the Australian Research Council (ARC) Discovery under Grant No. DP 0668052, ARC Linkage Infrastructure, Equipment and Facilities under Grant No. LE 0668508, National Natural Science Foundation of China under Grant No. 50705064, and Natural Science Foundation of Tianjin under Grant No. 08JCYBJC01400.

References

1. Yao, Q., Dong, J., Ferreira, P.M.: Design, analysis, fabrication and testing of a parallel-kinematic micropositioning XY stage. Int. J. Mach. Tool Manu. 47, 946–961 (2007)
2. Smith, S.T., Chetwynd, D.G., Bowen, D.K.: Design and assessment of monolithic high precision translation mechanisms. J. Phys. E: Sci. Instrum. 20, 977–983 (1987)
3. Miller, J.A., Hocken, R., Smith, S.T., Harb, S.: X-ray calibrated tunneling system utilizing a dimensionally stable nanometer positioner. Precis. Eng. 18, 95–102 (1996)
4. Choi, K.B., Lee, J.J.: Passive compliant wafer stage for single-step nano-imprint lithography. Rev. Sci. Instrum. 76, 075106 (2005)
5. Alici, G., Shirinzadeh, B.: Kinematics and stiffness analysis of a flexure-jointed planar micromanipulation system for a decoupled compliant motion. In: Proceedings of 2003 IEEE International Conference on Intelligent Robotics and Systems, pp. 3282–3287. IEEE Press, Las Vegas (2003)
6. Craig, J.J.: Introduction to Robotics: Mechanics and Control, 3rd edn. Pearson, Upper Saddle River (2005)
7. Paros, J.M., Weisbord, L.: How to design flexure hinges. Mach. Design. 37, 151–156 (1965)
8. Zhang, D., Chetwynd, D.G., Liu, X., Tian, Y.: Investigation of a 3-DOF micro-positioning table for surface grinding. Int. J. Mech. Sci. 48, 1401–1408 (2006)
9. Lobontiu, N., Paine, J.S.N.: Design of circular cross-section corner-filleted flexure hinges for three-dimensional compliant. J. Mech. Design-T ASME 124, 479–484 (2002)
10. Smith, S.T., Badami, V.G., Dale, J.S., Xu, Y.: Elliptical flexure hinges. Rev. Sci. Instrum. 68, 1474–1483 (1997)
11. Elfizy, A.T., Bone, G.M., Elbestawi, M.A.: Design and control of a dual-stage feed drive. Int. J. Mach. Tool Manu. 45, 153–165 (2005)
12. Gao, Y., Zhang, D.W., Yu, C.W.: Dynamic modeling of a novel workpiece table for active surface grinding control. Int. J. Mach. Tool Manu. 41, 609–624 (2001)
13. Stephen, J.L., David, A.C., Joseph, A.C.: Design of a rotary fast tool servo for ophthalmic lens fabrication. Precis. Eng. 23, 253–259 (1999)
14. Speich, J., Goldfarb, M.: A compliant mechanism based three degree of freedom manipulator for small-scale manipulation. Robotica 18, 95–104 (2000)
15. Culpepper, M.L., Anderson, G.: Design of a low-cost nano-manipulator which utilizes a monolithic, spatial compliant mechanism. Precis. Eng. 28, 469–489 (2004)
16. Gao, P., Swei, S.M.: A six-degree-of-freedom micro-manipulator based on piezoelectric translators. Nanotechnology 10, 447–452 (1999)
17. Dollar, A.M., Howe, R.D.: A robust compliant grasper via shape deposition manufacturing. IEEE-ASME T. Mech. 11, 154–161 (2006)
18. Li, Y.M., Xu, Q.S.: A novel design and analysis of a 2-DOF compliant parallel micromanipulator for nanomanipulation. IEEE T. Autom. Sci. Eng. 3, 248–254 (2006)
19. Liaw, H.C., Shirinzadeh, B., Smith, J.: Enhanced sliding mode motion tracking control of actuators. Sensor. Actuat A-Phys. 138, 194–202 (2007)
20. Tseytlin, Y.M.: Notch flexure hinges: An effective theory. Rev. Sci. Instrum. 73, 3363–3368 (2002)
21. Lobontiu, N., Paine, J.S.N., O'Malley, E., Samuelson, M.: Parabolic and hyperbolic flexure hinges: flexibility, motion precision and stress characterization based on compliance closed-form equations. Precis. Eng. 26, 183–192 (2002)
22. Liaw, H.C., Shirinzadeh, B., Smith, J.: Robust motion tracking control of piezo-driven flexure-based four-bar mechanism for micro/ nano manipulation. Mechatronics 18, 111–120 (2008)

Approximate Numerical Solution of Hydrodynamic Gas Journal Bearings*

Haijun Zhang[1,2], Changsheng Zhu[1], and Qin Yang[2]

[1] College of Electrical Engineering, Zhejiang University, Hangzhou, Zhejiang Province, China
[2] College of Mechanical-Electrical Engineering, Jiaxing University, Jiaxing, Zhejiang Province, China
zhjzszs_537@hotmail.com

Abstract. Considering small pressure change in the gas film of hydrodynamic gas-lubricated journal bearings, the corresponding nonlinear Reynolds equation is linearized through appropriate approximation and approximate Reynolds equation is derived and solved by means of finite difference method (FDM). The gas film pressure distribution of hydrodynamic gas-lubricated journal bearing is attained and load capacity is calculated. The approximate numerical solution shows better agreement with experimental data than direct numerical solution and demands less computer time. It is of interest to note the eccentricity ratio ε at which approximate numerical solution is better agreement with experimental data is different when bearing number is changing. The approximate numerical solution is slightly larger when the eccentricity ratio is smaller, and becomes slightly smaller when the eccentricity ratio is larger.

Keywords: hydrodynamic gas-lubricated journal bearings; Reynolds equation; nonlinearity; finite difference method (FDM).

1 Introduction

Gas bearings operate with the pressure generated for lubricating film. Because gas bearings have such characteristics as low fiction, high precision and low pollution, they have been successfully used in many commercial applications, such as navigation systems, computer disk drives, high-precision instruments and sensors, dental drills, machine tools, and turbo-compressors [1]. There had been a research boom of gas bearings in the 60-70 of 20th century. In recent years study on gas bearings has been paid much attention to with the advent of MEMS research [2, 3].

Reynolds equation is the fundamental equation with which the performance of hydrodynamic gas-lubricated bearing is investigated. Duo to gaseous compressibility, Reynolds equation is nonlinear and its analytical solution usually is difficult to obtain. Therefore numerical method is an effective means to study gas-lubricated journal bearings. All numerical methods used will be treated in two classes: analytical-numerical and direct-numerical [4]. In the former class either some features of the particular bearing

* This work is supported by National Science Foundation of China (10472101).

C. Xiong et al. (Eds.): ICIRA 2008, Part II, LNAI 5315, pp. 260–268, 2008.

under study are taken advantage of or some approximations are made in order to partially solve the problem by analytical means. Harrison first presented solutions for infinitely long gas-lubricated slider and journal bearings [5]. His work on the infinite journal bearing was improved upon by Katta and Soda [6] who gave an approximate analytical solution. Ausman [7] published the linearized ph solution for small motion of journal bearing of finite length. Methods of the latter class approach the problem immediately with numerical approximations, the accuracy of which is often easier to control. Elrod and Burgdorfer [8] presented solutions for the infinite journal bearings, i.e., length-to-diameter ratio is infinite ($L/D=\infty$). Ramondi [9] obtained solutions for full journal bearings with L/D ratio of 2, 1, and 0.5. Qi [10] transformed Reynolds equation into standard elliptic partial differential equation form and gained solutions using Matlab's PDE solver.

Because increased amount of time is spent on solving the non-linear Reynolds equation with direct numerical approaches, it is essential to find a simple and convenient method for the problem. Considering small pressure change in the gas film of hydrodynamic gas-lubricated journal bearing, the corresponding nonlinear Reynolds equation is linearized through appropriate approximation. Approximate Reynolds equation is derived and solved by means of finite difference method (FDM). The gas film pressure distribution of hydrodynamic gas-lubricated journal bearing is attained and load capacity is calculated. Finally the approximate numerical solution shows better agreement with experimental data than direct numerical solution, which proves its validity.

2 Reynolds Equation for Hydrodynamic Gas Journal Bearings

Reynolds equation, which determines pressure distribution of the bearings, can be derived from the motion equation, continuity equation and energy equation for gas. The gas-lubricated journal bearing model, composed of two plates, is shown in Fig.1, in which the upper plate is stationary and the lower one is moving at the velocity u_0.

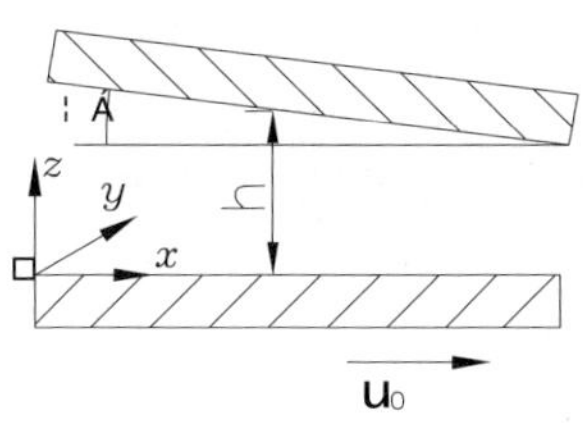

Fig. 1. Gas-lubricated journal bearing model

By assuming steady conditions and neglecting the inertial terms, body forces, x-direction and y-direction components of viscosity force induced by flow gradient, as shown in Fig.1, Reynolds equation is derived

$$\frac{\partial}{\partial x}\left(\frac{\rho h^3}{\mu}\frac{\partial p}{\partial x}\right)+\frac{\partial}{\partial y}\left(\frac{\rho h^3}{\mu}\frac{\partial p}{\partial y}\right)=6u_0\frac{\partial(\rho h)}{\partial x}+12\frac{\partial(\rho h)}{\partial t} \tag{1}$$

where ρ is gas density, μ gas absolute viscosity, h is gas film thickness, p is gas film pressure, u_0 is x-direction component of gas velocity, t is time variable.

Reynolds equation relating pressure, density, surface velocity, and film thickness is a 2-dimension elliptic differential one, which is fundamental in gas-lubricated journal bearing field. The solution to the Reynolds equation provides the pressure distribution throughout the film, given the geometry, property, and state parameters. Once the pressure distribution is known, the other properties of the gas film are readily determined.

Gas-lubricated film obeys a polytropic relation [1],

$$p\rho^{-n}=\text{constant} \tag{2}$$

where n is the polytropic gas-expansion exponent, whose value lies between 1 and γ. When flow is adiabatic, i.e., there is no transferred heat and the change in internal energy equals the compression work, (2) with $n=\gamma=c_p/c_v$ follows directly from the equation of state and the energy equation. When flow is isothermal, (2) with $n=1$ derives from the equation of state. c_p is the specific heat per unit weight for constant pressure and c_v is the specific heat per unit weight for constant volume.

The viscosities of common gases increase with temperature but are comparatively insensitive to moderate temperature and pressure changes. Within a gas lubricating film, temperature and pressure changes are normally small, and viscosity is considered to be constant.

Therefore, by assuming constant temperature, (1) becomes

$$\frac{\partial}{\partial x}\left(p h^3\frac{\partial p}{\partial x}\right)+\frac{\partial}{\partial y}\left(p h^3\frac{\partial p}{\partial y}\right)=6\mu u_0\frac{\partial(p h)}{\partial x} \tag{3}$$

For hydrodynamic gas-lubricated journal bearings shown in Fig. 2, (3) becomes

$$\frac{\partial}{\partial \theta}\left(ph^3\frac{\partial p}{\partial \theta}\right)+r^2\frac{\partial}{\partial y}\left(ph^3\frac{\partial p}{\partial y}\right)=6\mu u_0 r\frac{\partial(ph)}{\partial \theta} \tag{4}$$

The non-dimensional form for (4) is

$$\frac{\partial}{\partial \theta}\left(PH^3\frac{\partial P}{\partial \theta}\right)+\frac{\partial}{\partial \zeta}\left(PH^3\frac{\partial P}{\partial \zeta}\right)=\Lambda\frac{\partial}{\partial \theta}(PH) \tag{5}$$

where

$$x=r\theta, y=r\zeta, u_0=r\omega, P=p/p_a, \Lambda=\frac{6\mu\omega}{p_a}\left(\frac{r}{c_0}\right)^2, h=c_0\cdot(1+\varepsilon\cos\theta)=c_0 H$$

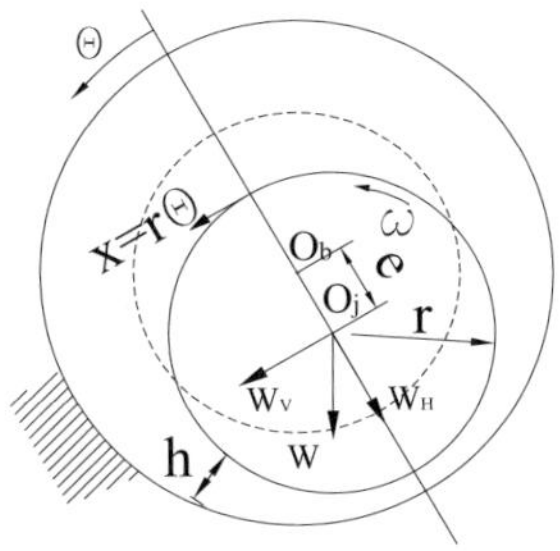

Fig. 2. Schematic diagram of hydrodynamic gas-lubricated journal bearing

where θ,ζ is the non-dimensional circumferential coordinate and axial coordinate respectively, H,P is the non-dimensional gas film thickness and gas film pressure, r is journal radius, ω is journal angular velocity, p_a is ambient pressure, ε is eccentricity ratio and c_0 is radial clearance.

The boundary conditions for (5) are

$$\begin{aligned} &P\left(\theta,\pm\frac{L}{2r}\right)=1 \\ &P(0,\zeta)=P(2\pi,\zeta) \\ &P(\theta,\zeta)=P(\theta,-\zeta) \end{aligned} \tag{6}$$

where $\theta\in[0,2\pi]$, $\zeta\in\left[-\frac{L}{2r},\frac{L}{2r}\right]$

Equation (5), a non-linear partial differential equation with respect to non-dimensional pressure P, can be solved directly by the finite difference method (FDM). However, as mentioned above, the disadvantages of direct-numerical method are: increased amount of computer time, the need for an efficient computer system and instability in the convergence of iteration process.

3 Reynolds Equation Approximation

Because Reynolds equation is a non-linear partial differential one, the calculation method of direct-numerical solution is more complex and occupies much more computer time. In order to simplify calculation, Reynolds equation is linearized as follows. First (5) becomes

$$\begin{aligned} &H^3\left(\frac{\partial^2 P}{\partial\theta^2}+\frac{\partial^2 P}{\partial\zeta^2}\right)+3H^2\frac{\partial H}{\partial\theta}\frac{\partial P}{\partial\theta}-\Lambda\frac{dH}{d\theta}= \\ &-\frac{H^3}{P}\left[\left(\frac{\partial P}{\partial\theta}\right)^2+\left(\frac{\partial P}{\partial\zeta}\right)^2\right]+\Lambda\frac{H}{P}\frac{\partial P}{\partial\theta} \end{aligned} \tag{7}$$

Considering the compressibility, small viscosity and small pressure of gas-lubricated journal bearings, $\left(\frac{\partial P}{\partial \theta}\right)^2, \left(\frac{\partial P}{\partial \zeta}\right)^2$ are considered to be small. The pressure gradient of gas film, $\frac{\partial P}{\partial \theta}, \frac{\partial P}{\partial \zeta}$, have the same trend as eccentricity ratio ε, i.e., $\frac{\partial P}{\partial \theta}, \frac{\partial P}{\partial \zeta}$ increase with ε increasing. Therefore it is appropriate to make the following approximation,

$$\left(\frac{\partial P}{\partial \theta}\right)^2 + \left(\frac{\partial P}{\partial \zeta}\right)^2 \approx \varepsilon \frac{\partial P}{\partial \theta} + \varepsilon \frac{\partial P}{\partial \zeta} \tag{8}$$

Harrison [5], Katto and Soda [6] substituted $p_a c$ for ph in deriving linearized ph solution of Reynolds equation, and the same approximation is adopted here. Therefore, the non-dimensional pressure P in the denominator of right hand in (7) is replaced by $\frac{P_0}{1+\varepsilon \cos\theta} = \frac{1}{H}$, (7) becomes

$$\begin{aligned} &H^3\left(\frac{\partial^2 P}{\partial \theta^2} + \frac{\partial^2 P}{\partial \zeta^2}\right) + 3H^2 \frac{\partial H}{\partial \theta}\frac{\partial P}{\partial \theta} - \Lambda \frac{dH}{d\theta} + \\ &H^2\left(\varepsilon \frac{\partial P}{\partial \theta} + \varepsilon \frac{\partial P}{\partial \zeta}\right) - \Lambda \frac{\partial P}{\partial \theta} = 0 \end{aligned} \tag{9}$$

As soon as (9) is solved by the means of FDM, the characteristics of gas bearings, such as pressure distribution, load capacity, etc., are obtained.

Load capacity of hydrodynamic gas-lubricated journal bearings is constituted by two parts: one is W_H in the direction of center-line, and the other is W_V normal to the direction of center-line, as shown in Fig.2.

$$\begin{cases} W = \sqrt{W_H^2 + W_V^2} \\ W_H = 2\int_0^{L/2}\int_0^{2\pi} p\cos\theta r d\theta dy \\ W_V = 2\int_0^{L/2}\int_0^{2\pi} p\sin\theta r d\theta dy \end{cases} \tag{10}$$

After discretization of solution region, (10) becomes

$$\begin{cases} W_H = p_a \cdot 2\pi r L \sum_{i=1}^{n-1}\sum_{j=1}^{m-1} P_{i,j} \cos\theta_i \Delta\theta\Delta\zeta \\ W_V = p_a \cdot 2\pi r L \sum_{i=1}^{n-1}\sum_{j=1}^{m-1} P_{i,j} \sin\theta_i \Delta\theta\Delta\zeta \end{cases} \tag{11}$$

where n, m are the circumferential and axial nodes of gas-lubricated journal bearings.

4 Load Capacity Calculation and Comparison

To demonstrate the validity of approximation numerical solution, numerical results are compared with experimental data in the literature. The parameters for gas-lubricated journal bearings have the same value as that in the literature [11], as shown in Table 1.

Table 1. Gas-lubricated journal bearings parameters

Parameters	Value
Journal radius r (mm)	25.4
Radial clearance c_0 (mm)	12.7×10^{-3}
Bearing width L (mm)	76.2
lubricant	Argon
Absolute viscosity μ ($N\cdot s/m^2$)	2.29×10^{-5}
Ambient pressure p_a (N/m^2)	1.033×10^5

Fig.3 demonstrates the pressure distribution of hydrodynamic gas-lubricated journal bearings. It can be seen that pressure distribution for gas bearings is different from that for oil bearings because of gas compressibility. (1) There is large pressure peak value in the convergent region while small pressure peak value in the divergent region, i.e., the magnitude of pressure in the convergent region is larger than that in the divergent region. (2) The pressure in the convergent region ascends smoothly while that in the divergent region descends quickly. (3) Contrary to oil bearings, the magnitude of pressure change is small, which explains smaller load capacity of gas bearings.

Comparing with direct numerical solution, approximate numerical solution demands less amount of computer time. When the geometry parameters of journal bearings and computation nodes are the same and the bearing number is different, the computation efficiency of the two methods in solving bearings' pressure distribution can be compared from CPU time data of Table2.

Table 2. CPU times for the approximate numerical solution and direct numerical solution

Bearing number Λ	Direct numerical solution (s)	Approximate numerical solution (s)
3	124.5156	105.0313
5	128.2500	81.7813
10	110.4531	46.9219
20	85.9531	17.9844

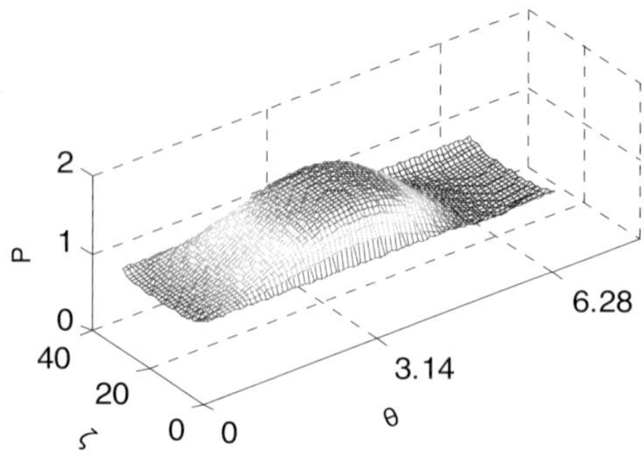

Fig. 3. The non-dimensional pressure distribution of hydrodynamic gas-lubricated journal bearings

It is of interest to compare the calculated values with experimental data. The comparisons of load capacity versus eccentricity ratio ε among direct-numerical solution, approximation numerical solution and experimental data for different bearing number Λ are shown in Fig.4, 5, 6.

It can be seen that load capacity for hydrodynamic gas-lubricated journal bearings increases with increasing eccentricity ratio ε. For the same bearing number Λ, both the value of direct numerical solution and that of approximation numerical solution are larger than experimental data. The difference between approximation numerical solution and experimental data is smaller than that between direct numerical solution and experimental data. Especially when the bearing number Λ increases, the consistency between approximation numerical solution and experimental data is better.

In addition, the eccentricity ratio ε at which approximating numerical solution is better agreement with experimental data is different when bearing number is changing. The approximating numerical solution is slightly larger when the eccentricity ratio is smaller, and becomes slightly smaller when the eccentricity ratio is larger.

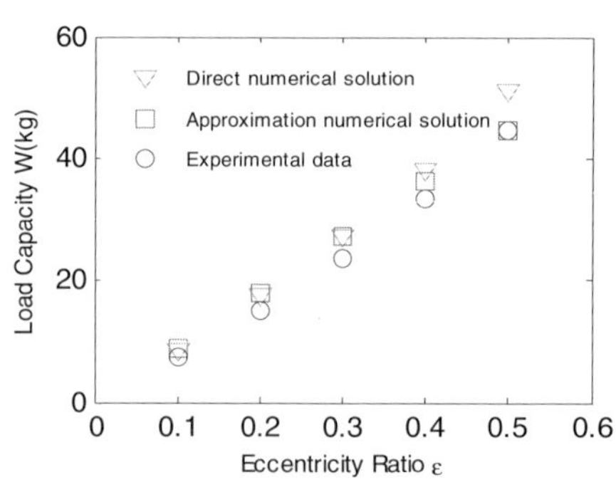

Fig. 4. Comparison when the bearing number Λ is 1.63

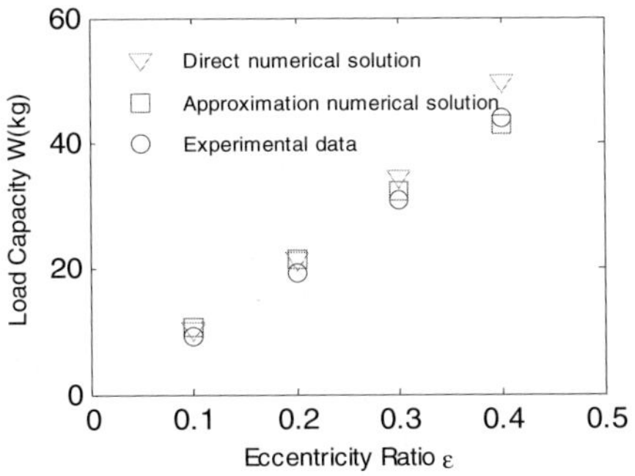

Fig. 5. Comparison when the bearing number Λ is 3.26

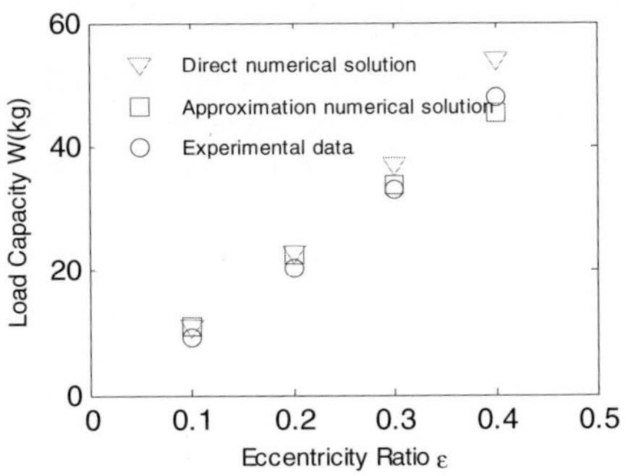

Fig. 6. Comparison when the bearing number Λ is 4.89

5 Conclusion

As a non-linear partial differential equation, Reynolds equation for hydrodynamic gas-lubricated journal bearing is difficult to obtain exact analytical solution. It is simple and convenient to transform Reynolds equation into linear partial differential one through proper approximation and attain numerical solution by the means of FDM. The study demonstrates that the approximating numerical solution shows better agreement with experimental data than direct numerical solution and demands less computer time, from which we think it superior to the direct numerical solution. It is of interest to note the eccentricity ratio ε at which approximating numerical solution is better agreement with experimental data is different when bearing number Λ is changing. The approximating numerical solution is slightly larger when the eccentricity ratio ε is smaller, and becomes slightly smaller when the eccentricity ratio ε is larger.

References

1. Gross, W.A., et al.: Fluid Film Lubrication. John Wiley & Sons, New York (1980)
2. Epstein, A.H., Senturia, S.D.: Microengineering: macro power from micro machinery. Science 276(5316), 1211 (1997)

3. Gad-el-Hak, M.: The Fluid Mechanics of Microdevices—The Freeman Scholar Lecture. Journal of Fluid Engineering 121(1), 5–33 (1999)
4. Castelli, V., Pirvics, J.: Review of numerical methods in gas bearing film analysis. Journal of Lubrication Technology 90(4), 777–792 (1968)
5. Harrison, W.J.: The dydrodynamical theory of lubrication with special reference to air as a lubricant. Trans. Cambridge Philosophical Society 22, 34–54 (1913)
6. Katto, Y., Soda, N.: Theory of lubrication by compressible fluid with special reference to air bearing. In: 2nd Japan National Congress for Applied Mechanics Tokyo, pp. 267–270 (1952)
7. Ausman, J.S.: An improved analytical solution for self-acting, gas-lubricated journal bearings of finite length. Journal of Basic Engineering 83, 188–194 (1961)
8. Elrod, H.G., Burgdorfer, A.: Refinement of the theory of gas-lubricated journal bearings of infinite length. In: 1st International Symposium on Gas Lubricated bearings, Washington, D.C (1959)
9. Raimondi, A.A.: A numerical solution for the gas lubricated full journal bearing of finite length. Trans. ASLE 4, 131–155 (1961)
10. Qi, S.M., Geng, H.P., Yu, L.: New method for the calculation of the characteristics of aerodynamic bearings. Journal of Mechanical Strength 28(3), 369–373 (2006) (in Chinese)
11. Whitley, S., Betts, C.: Study of Gas-Lubricated, Hydrodynamic, Full Journal Bearing. British Journal of Applied Physics 10, 455–463 (1959)

Modeling and Control of Macro-micro Dual-Drive High Acceleration and High Precision Positioning Stage Using for IC Packaging

Yanjie Liu, Teng Li, and Lining Sun

State Key Laboratory of Robotics and System, Harbin Institute of Technology, Harbin, China
yjliu@hit.edu.cn

Abstract. Macro-micro dual-drive positioning stage has particularly good potential application in high acceleration and high precision positioning stage using for IC packaging. In this paper, the positioning stage which is composed by VCM (voice coil motor) as macro driver and PZT as micro driver is used. Coupling characters of the stage are discussed by analyzing dynamic model firstly, then models of macro drive positioning stage and micro drive positioning stage are built separately which both contain mechanism and driver part. Finally, a control structure, micro drive positioning stage dynamic compensate the positioning error produced by macro drive positioning stage, is proposed, in this control structure, LQG control method is used to control macro drive positioning stage, and PID control method is used to control the micro drive positioning stage. Detailed designs are conducted for the proposed approach, and the simulation results demonstrate the good performance of the proposed controller.

Keywords: macro-micro dual-drive, positioning stage, motion couple, modeling, LQG.

1 Introduction

IC (integrated circuit) manufacturing technique is developed rapidly, the integrated level of IC chip is improving and its volume is reducing with the increasing I/O leg wires' density. So high machine accuracy and high productivity are urgently required for package equipment.

Positioning stage with high acceleration and high precision, as a central component in the package equipment, plays a key role. In package process, the positioning stage is required to run and stop frequently with high acceleration, such that the system must have high bandwidth, so many structures have been proposed to solve the problem. Presently, macro-micro dual-drive technique, which is proved an effective method to achieve long stroke, high acceleration and high precision, is presented by some institutes and scholars [1, 2]. This structure uses two independent mechanisms for a single degree of freedom motion, it can widen the bandwidth of system and reduce the effective inertia of end effectors [3, 4], but the motion coupling of the two positioning stages effects the performance of the whole positioning stage, and

C. Xiong et al. (Eds.): ICIRA 2008, Part II, LNAI 5315, pp. 269–278, 2008.

performance of this system may vary depending on the control method employed. So, in this paper, system's coupling characters are analyzed firstly, according to the results, the system can be treated as two separate positioning stage and models can be built separately. Based on the model, macro positioning stage has vibration, so PID controller in forward path plus LQG controller in the feedback loop is proposed to satisfy the track following performance and restrain vibration simultaneously.

This paper is organized as follows: in section 2, structure of the dual-drive positioning stage is displayed and in section 3, motion coupling between two positioning stage is analyzed by dynamic equation, in section 4, whole models for two positioning stage are built, which contain driver and mechanism part, then the control structure is constructed and controllers are designed in section 5, and the simulation results are shown, finally, in section 6, conclusions are drawn.

2 Structure of Macro-micro Dual-Drive Positioning Stage

Usually, the positioning stage for IC packaging has two degrees-of-freedom, and each has the same structure and characters, so here we use a single axis as an example to discuss. Fig.1 shows the structure of single axis macro-micro dual-drive positioning stage. VCM together with the PZT are adopted to drive the macro positioning stage and micro positioning stage, high resolution grating scale is integrated into the close-loop feedback of macro drive positioning stage and capacitance micrometer is used to measure the displacement of micro drive positioning stage.

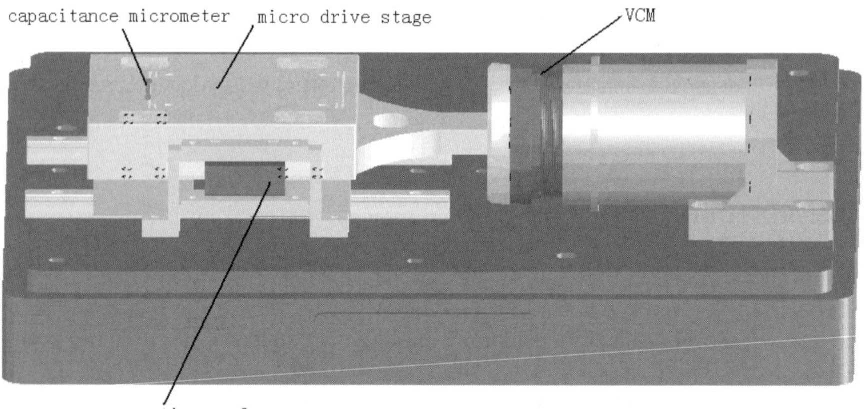

Fig. 1. Structure of macro-micro dual-drive positioning stage

The micro drive positioning stage is working at a nanometer level resolution and positioning accuracy via the double layer elastic hinges driven by PZT. The simplified structure of the micro drive positioning stage is shown in Fig.2.

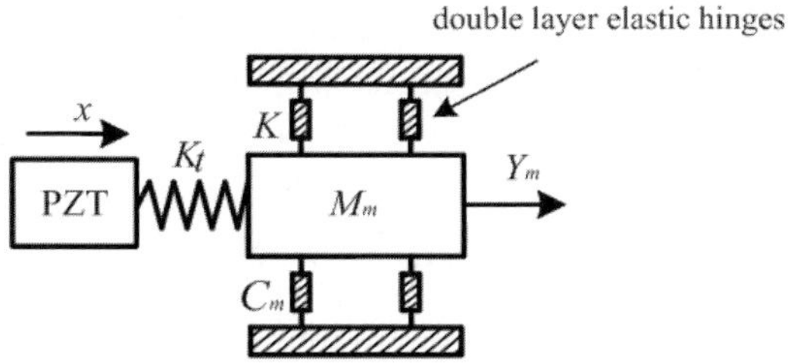

Fig. 2. The structure of micro positioning stage

Where, K_t is the stiffness of transmit part, K is the stiffness of double layer elastic hinges, M_m is the inertia of motion part in the micro stage, C_m is the damping ratio of micro stage, x is the input displacement by PZT, Y_m is output displacement. In our system, $M_m = 0.43kg$, $K = 2.0\times10^7 N/m$, $K_t = 12.0\times10^7 N/m$, and $C_m = 0.02Ns/m$.

3 Motion Coupling of Macro-micro Dual-Drive Positioning Stage

Since the micro drive positioning stage place on the macro drive positioning stage, there is force act on micro drive positioning stage when the macro dive positioning stage is moving, and vice versa, so the motion coupling should be discussed firstly as the guidance of modeling and controller design of the stage. In this paper, the motion coupling is discussed by analyzing dynamic model of the dual-drive stage.

The mechanism parts, as a kind of finite rigid body, have certain flexibility which causes remnant vibration in high-acceleration motion, reduces accuracy of the stage and prolongs the settling time. Therefore, the flexibility of the micro drive positioning stage and guiding plates should be considered. On the basis of the rigid-flexible dynamic analysis of mechanical system, the system can be simplified to a mass-damping system, as shown in Fig.3.

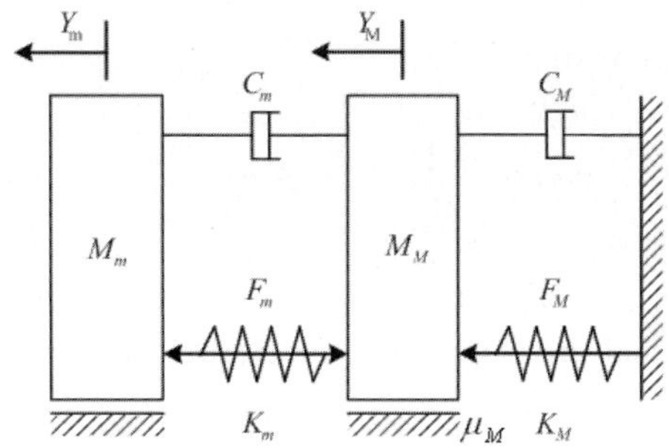

Fig. 3. The rigid-flexible model of dual-drive positioning stage

where, K_M , C_M ,and M_M are the stiffness, damping ration and inertia of stage driven by VCM, K_m ($K_m = K + K_t$), C_m and M_m are the stiffness, damping ration and inertia of stage driven by PZT , μ_M is the coefficient of friction of the linear guide, F_M , F_m are the drive force of VCM and PZT separately, Y_M, Y_m are the corresponding displacements. According to Newton's second law, dynamic differential equation of the macro-micro dual-drive positioning stage can de derived:

$$\begin{cases} M_m \ddot{Y}_m = F_m + K_m(Y_M - Y_m) + C_m(\dot{Y}_M - \dot{Y}_m) \\ M_M \ddot{Y}_M = F_M - F_m - K_M Y_M - K_m(Y_M - Y_m) - C_M \dot{Y}_M - C_m(\dot{Y}_M - \dot{Y}_m) - \mu_M \dot{Y}_M \end{cases} \tag{1}$$

Written in the form of matrix:

$$[M]\{\ddot{Y}\} + [C]\{\dot{Y}\} + [K]\{Y\} = [A]\{F\} \tag{2}$$

where, output vector: $\{Y\} = \begin{Bmatrix} Y_m \\ Y_M \end{Bmatrix}$, input vector: $\{U\} = \begin{Bmatrix} F_m \\ F_M \end{Bmatrix}$, $[M] = \begin{bmatrix} M_m & 0 \\ 0 & M_M \end{bmatrix}$, $[C] = \begin{bmatrix} C_m & -C_m \\ -C_m & C_M + C_m + \mu_M \end{bmatrix}$, $[K] = \begin{bmatrix} K_m & -K_m \\ -K_m & K_M + K_m \end{bmatrix}$, $[A] = \begin{bmatrix} 1 & 0 \\ -1 & 1 \end{bmatrix}$. In our system, $M_M = 1.92kg$, $K_M = 6.5\times 10^7\, N/m$, $C_M = 0.05Ns/m$, $\mu_M = 0.03Ns/m$.

Rewrite the above equation after do the Laplace transform on both side of it, the transfer function matrix can be obtained:

$$\begin{bmatrix} Y_m \\ Y_M \end{bmatrix} = \begin{bmatrix} \dfrac{1}{M_m s^2 + C_m s + K_m} & 0 \\ \dfrac{1}{C_m s + K_m} & \dfrac{1}{M_M s^2 + (C_M + C_m + \mu_M)s + K_M + K_m} \end{bmatrix} \begin{bmatrix} F_m \\ F_M \end{bmatrix} \tag{3}$$

Form (3) the motion coupling of macro drive positioning stage and micro drive positioning stage is:

$$Y_M = \frac{1}{C_m s + K_m} F_m \tag{4}$$

Do the inverse Laplace transform of it:

$$Y_M(t) = \frac{1}{C_m} e^{-\frac{K_m}{C_m} t} F_m(t) \tag{5}$$

K_m is far greater than C_m, so $Y_M(t) \approx 0$, that is, the motion coupling of the two stage can be neglected, the dual-drive stage can be treated as two single-drive positioning stages.

4 Modeling of Macro-micro Dual-Drive Positioning Stage

In this section, models of macro drive positioning stage and micro drive positioning stage are constructed. The model includes the mechanism part and the driver part.

4.1 Modeling of Macro Drive Positioning Stage

From electrical equivalent model of VCM and Kirchhoff law, the voltage balance equation can be written:

$$U = U_R + U_L + U_B \tag{6}$$

where, U is the overall voltage in coil, $U_R = Ri$ is the voltage in resistance, the induction voltage is $U_L = L(di/dt)$, the back electromotive force by coil's motion is $U_B = K_B V$, i is circuit current, V is motion speed, K_B is the back electromotive force constant. So we have:

$$U = Ri + L(di/dt) + K_B V \tag{7}$$

The force balance equation is:

$$F_M = M\ddot{Y}_M + (C_M + \mu_M)\dot{Y}_M + K_M Y_M \tag{8}$$

where, $F_M = K_F i$, K_F is force sensitivity of VCM, $M = M_M + M_m$, that is, micro drive stage is treated as one of the loads of macro drive stage.

According above two equations, the block diagram transfer function of macro drive stage is shown in Fig.4.

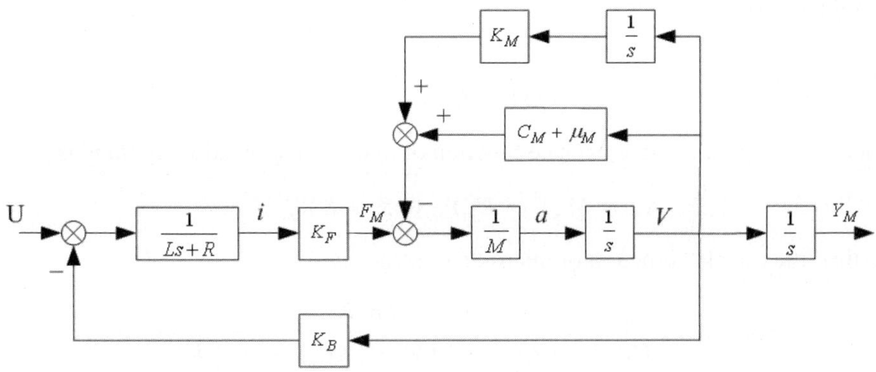

Fig. 4. Block diagram transfer function of macro drive positioning stage

So the transfer function of macro drive stage is:

$$G_M(s) = \frac{Y_M(s)}{U(s)} = \frac{K_F}{LMS^3 + (LC_M + L\mu_M + RM)s^2 + (K_M L + RC_M + R\mu_M + K_F K_B)s + RK_M} \tag{9}$$

In our system, $L = 2.5mH$, $R = 2.4\Omega$, $K_F = 21.35N/A$, $K_B = 21.36V/m/s$.

4.2 Modeling of Micro Drive Positioning Stage

The equivalent circuit of PZT is shown in Fig.5, R_i is the inner resistance of PZT power supply, R_p and C_p is the resistance and capacitance of PZT, and $R_i << R_p$, U_i is the input voltage of PZT power supply and U_p is the voltage act on PZT.

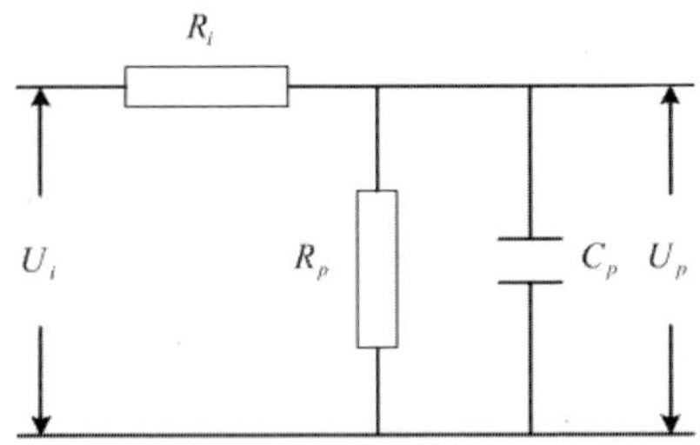

Fig. 5. The equivalent circuit of PZT

So the transfer function can be written as:

$$\frac{U_p(s)}{U_i(s)} = \frac{1}{R_i C_p s + 1} \tag{10}$$

According to the electric displacement character of PZT, and ignoring the nonlinearity of PZT, the displacement of PZT is proportional to the U_p, that is:

$$x = aU_p \tag{11}$$

a is the ratio coefficient, so

$$\frac{X(s)}{U_i(s)} = \frac{a}{R_i C_p s + 1} \tag{12}$$

Then from Fig.2 the force balance function of micro drive positioning stage is:

$$K_t x = M_m \ddot{Y}_m + C_m \dot{Y}_m + (K_t + K)Y_m \tag{13}$$

So that, the transfer function of micro drive stage is:

$$G_m(s) = K_p \frac{Y_m(s)}{U_i(s)} = \frac{aK_t K_p}{(R_i C_p s + 1)(M_m s^2 + C_m s + (K + K_t))} \tag{14}$$

K_p is the magnification of PZT power supply. In our system, $a = 0.267 \times 10^{-6} m/V$, $K_p = 15$, $R_i = 11\Omega$, $C_p = 14.5\mu F$.

5 Control of Macro-micro Dual-Drive Positioning Stage

The classic method using for control macro drive stage is PID, but for our system, from the transfer function above we know that the damping ratio is small, so the system will vibrate seriously while motion. The design of vibration damping controller is formulated as a standard LQG problem [5, 6]. In this paper, we design LQG controller as the feedback part to restrain vibration, and PID controller in forward path to ensure the track following character. The controller structure is shown in Fig.6.

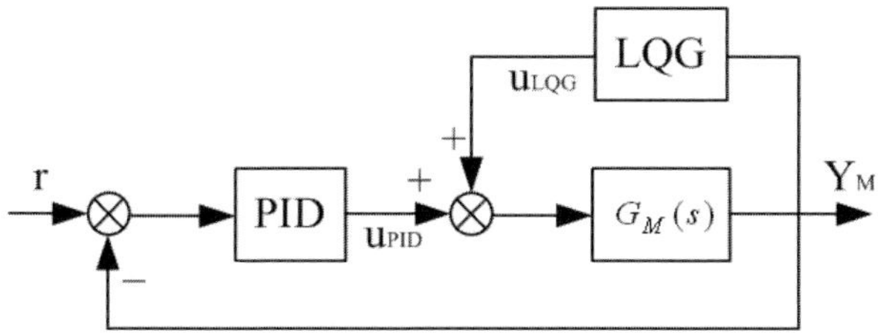

Fig. 6. Control structure of macro drive positioning stage

First, the state space model of macro drive stage is written:

$$\begin{pmatrix} \dot{x}_1(t) \\ \dot{x}_2(t) \\ \dot{x}_3(t) \end{pmatrix} = \begin{bmatrix} -\dfrac{LC_M + L\mu_M + RM}{LM} & -\dfrac{LK_M + RC_M + R\mu_M + K_F K_B}{LM} & -\dfrac{RK_M}{LM} \\ 1 & 0 & 0 \\ 0 & 1 & 0 \end{bmatrix} \begin{pmatrix} x_1(t) \\ x_2(t) \\ x_3(t) \end{pmatrix} + \begin{pmatrix} \dfrac{K_F}{LM} \\ 0 \\ 0 \end{pmatrix} u(t) \tag{15}$$

$$y(t) = x_3(t)$$

where state vector $\begin{pmatrix} x_1(t) \\ x_2(t) \\ x_3(t) \end{pmatrix} = \begin{pmatrix} \ddot{Y}_M(t) \\ \dot{Y}_M(t) \\ Y_M(t) \end{pmatrix}$.

The covariance of disturbance in state equation and measurement noise in observation equation for Kalman filter model are 1 and 0.01.

The cost function for this LQ design is:

$$J = \int_0^t (Y_M^2(t) + u_{LQG}^2(t))dt \tag{16}$$

Fig.7 and Fig.8 show the step response of system under PID controller and PID plus LQG controller. From the figure we can see that the system has a certain following ability under PID controller, but vibration is obvious, by adding the LQG feedback controller, the vibration is restrained assuredly.

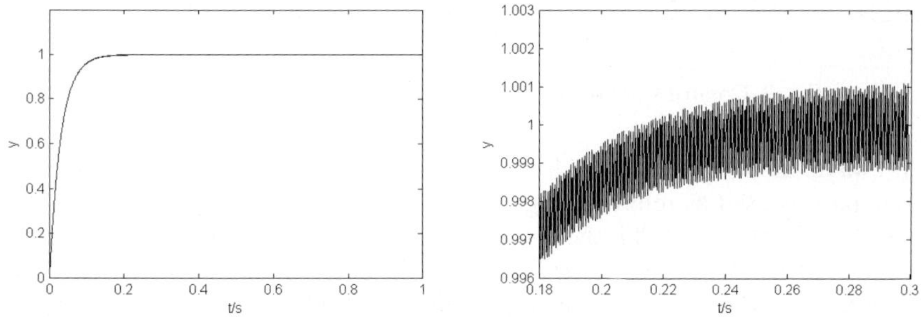

Fig. 7. Step response of macro drive positioning stage under PID controller

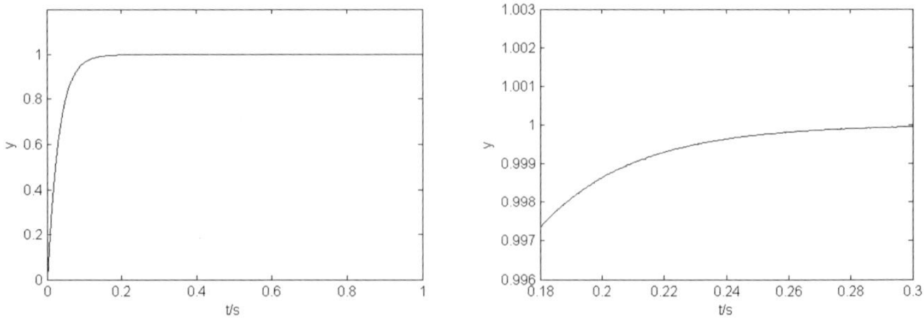

Fig. 8. Step response of macro drive positioning stage under PID plus LQG controller

For the PZT drive positioning stage, though the output displacement of PZT is proportional to input voltage, because of the nonlinear character of PZT, using the open-loop controller would not obtain good performance, so with the capacitance micrometer the micro drive positioning stage can form closed-loop control structure in our system.

Fig.9 shows the proposed controller structure for macro-micro dual-drive positioning stage. r_M is the reference input which is a periodic signal for IC packaging application, r_m is the reference input of micro stage, which is the error signal of macro drive positioning stage. In this structure, micro drive positioning stage dynamic compensate the positioning error of macro drive positioning stage, so the positioning error of the whole system is reduced by adding micro drive stage.

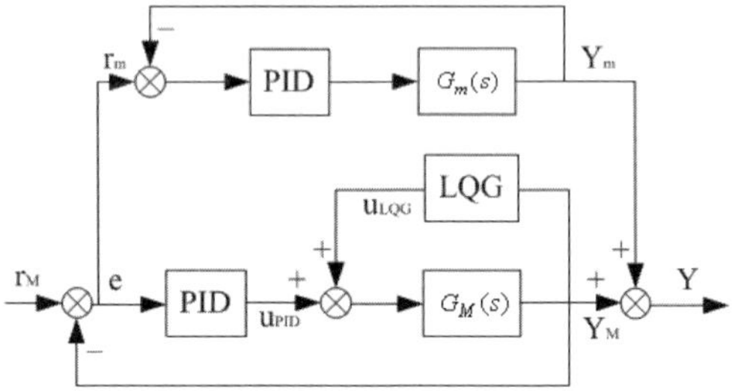

Fig. 9. Control structure of macro-micro dual-drive positioning stage

Sine wave, amplitude is 2mm, frequency is 10rad/s, and use absolute value of the negative part, is used as reference signal, which is similar to the periodic signal in IC packaging. Fig.10 and Fig.11 show the response curve of the system without micro drive stage. From these two figures, we can see that by adding micro drive stage, the positioning precision is an order of magnitude greater than the positioning stage driving only by macro driver.

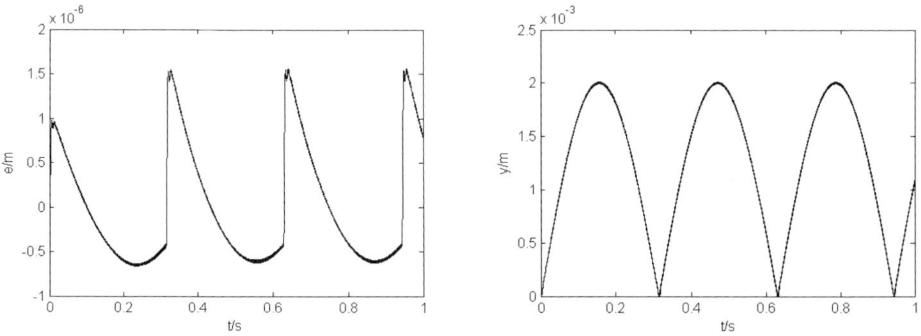

Fig. 10. Response of macro-micro dual-drive positioning stage to sine wave, the left figure is error curve of the whole positioning stage, the right figure is the response curve. In the right figure, the solid line is the reference input, and the dashed line is the response curve.

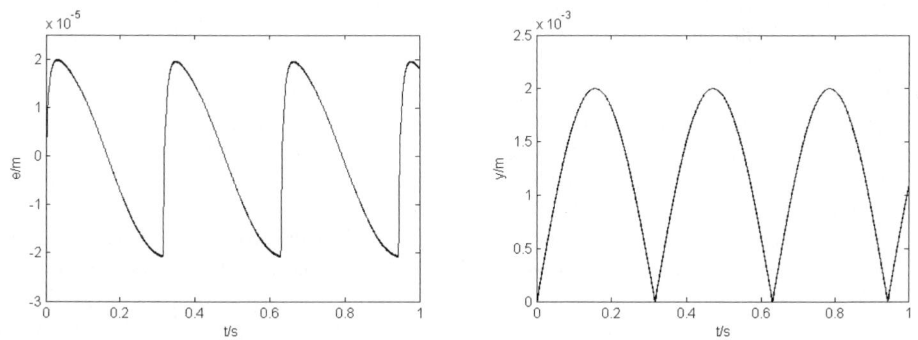

Fig. 11. Response of macro drive positioning stage to sine wave, meaning of figures are similar with Fig.10

6 Conclusions

In this paper, model building and controller design of macro-micro dual-drive positioning stage are discussed. Mechanism structure that this paper studied is composed by a VCM and a PZT, and both of them have displacement sensors. By analyzing dynamic model of the whole system, motion coupling of the two positioning stage is discussed, which conclude that the coupling action of two positioning is so small that can be neglected. Basing on the result, models of two positioning stage are built, both including mechanism part and driver part. From the model of macro positioning stage, we known that vibration is an important character of it, so we proposed a controller contain PID and LQG to satisfy the tracking following performance and improve vibration damping ability, simulation results verify the proposed controller. For the dual-drive positioning stage, we proposed a control structure that micro drive positioning stage dynamic compensate the positioning error produced by macro drive positioning stage, the simulation results also shows the good performance of it.

Acknowledgment

This paper is supported by the Cheung Kong scholars creative team plan IRT0423, the National Natural Science Foundation of China under Grant 50705027 and the National High Technology Research and Development Program of China (863 Program) under Grant 2007AA04Z315.

References

1. Sangjoo, K., Wan, K.C., Youngil, Y.: On the Coarse/Fine Dual-stage Manipulators with Perturbation Compensator. In: The 2001 IEEE International Conference on Robotics & Automation, Seoul, Korea, pp. 121–126 (2001)
2. Heui, J.P., Dong, S.L., Jong, H.P.: Ultra Precision Positioning System for Servo Motor-piezo Actuator Using the Dual Loop and Digital Filter Implementation. International Journal of Machine Tool & Manufacture 41, 51–63 (2001)
3. Sharon, A.: The Macro/Micro Manipulator: An Improved Architecture for Robot Control. Degree of Doctor of Philosophy, Thesis, Mechanical Engineering Department, Massachusetts Institute of Technology (1988)
4. Khatib, O.: Reduced effective inertia in macro-mini Manipulator Systems. In: Fifth Int. Symp. on Robotics Research, pp. 279–284 (1990)
5. Li, Y., Marcassa, F., Horowitz, R., Oboe, R.: Track following control with active vibration damping of a PZT actuated suspension dual-stage servo system. In: Proc. Am. Control Conf., pp. 2553–2559 (2003)
6. Huang, X., Horowitz, R., Li, Y.: Track-following control with active vibration damping and compensation of a dual-stage servo system. Microsyst. Technol. 11, 1276–1286 (2005)

Conceptual Design Modeling for Microcomponent Based on FES

Xiangtong Yan[1] and Pingyu Jiang[2]

[1] School of Mechanical Engineering, Xi'an University of Science and Technology, Xi'an 710054, China
[2] CAD/CAM Institute, School of Mechanical Engineering, Xi'an Jiaotong University, Xi'an 710049, China

Abstract. Conceptual design method and modeling technology for microcomponent are introduced. Concerning the important meaning of conceptual design in the product development, a modeling framework for the microcomponent conceptual design is studied. FES (Function- Effect-Solution) model is put forward. The function modeling, effect modeling and solution modeling of microcomponent are described respectively. The relationship of function, effect and solution is analyzed, and a case is used to illuminate the conceptual design process of microcomponent. Effective design information is provided by the conceptual design model for later design phases.

Keywords: conceptual design modeling; microcomponent; FES.

1 Introduction

A decision in an early stage of design may cause a great impact in the rest of design processes. Conceptual design is therefore the most important stages for innovation in the design process. For MEMS product development, typical concept to product development and release cycle has been 15 years. One reason for this is the lack of a comprehensive and effective MEMS design model or methodologies that cover conceptual design through detail design of MEMS product development process [1]. For MEMS conceptual design is not well practiced. Since MEMS design is strongly restricted by the manufacturing technology today, there is not much chance to think about alternatives for the same function [2]. Therefore the conceptual design of MEMS is an important and complex task.

Conceptual design modeling is the key technology of conceptual design and also is the foundation of solving conceptual design problem and building knowledge base. To address the conceptual design problem of microcomponent, this paper proposes a FES (Function-Effect-Solution) framework model to support conceptual design of microcomponent. The model can help user to finish functional decomposition and physical embodiment.

2 Function-Effect-Solution Framework of Microcomponent

Based on the idea of hierarchical modeling, the different phases in conceptual design can be represented by different layers. Layers map each other by carriers, and inter

C. Xiong et al. (Eds.): ICIRA 2008, Part II, LNAI 5315, pp. 279–288, 2008.

link between layers are established. According to this a modeling framework for microcomponent conceptual design is established, namely Function-Effect-Solution framework. The modeling framework consists of three layers, namely function layer, effect layer and solution layer. The function layer defines the main design task and requirements. The effect layer describes the underlying principles of the main functions and sub-functions and working principles embody effects. The solution layer describes the physical carrier to finish functions and topology structures. Figure 1 shows the FES modeling framework.

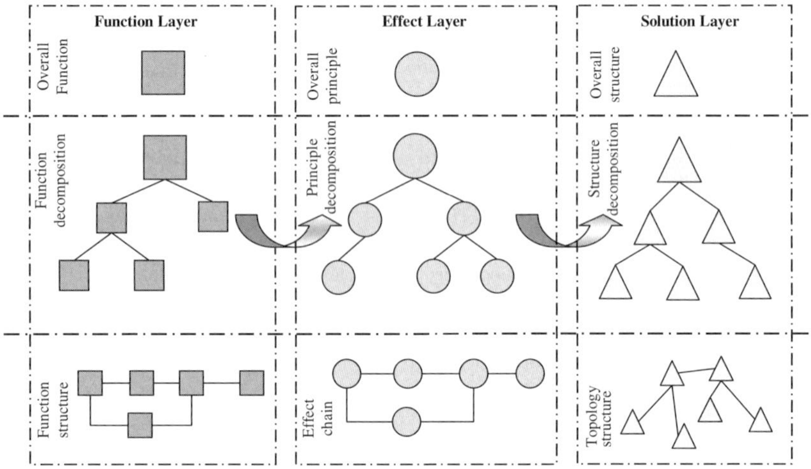

Fig. 1. The FES modeling framework of microcomponent

By the mapping relations between function, effect and solution, transitions are fulfilled between the required function, the effect and principle realizing the function and structure realizing the principle. All the composing parts in the framework are discussed in details in the following subsections.

3 Function Modeling of Microcomponent

Conceptual design is a process of step-wise refinement, namely the process of function evolution. Function understanding is the foundation of all conceptual design related research. Function-based modeling is useful for capturing engineering design intent at an abstract level.

3.1 Function Definition of Microcomponent

For modeling the function of microcomponent, the function concept should be defined clearly. Function is a statement to describe the transformation of input and output flows, aiming to achieve the designer's purpose. Recently many researchers at home and abroad have studied the definition of function, but there is not a universally accepted concept of function. Some researchers define function as a description of action and effect according to design requirement and change of system external environment, namely what to do something [3, 4]. The definition is similar to functional understanding and description of product, usually expressed in natural language. In this paper this definition is used.

3.2 Function Representation of Microcomponent

Function representation is an abstract behavior of function expressing and the foundation of function modeling. According to former literatures the representation methods of function mostly have three kinds: verb-noun form, input-output flow form and input-output state change form [5].

Based on analyzing input and output flow model and function definition, the function representation of microcomponent consists of several parts: Function Name, Function description and attribute value and so on. Verb-noun pair is used to describe the function and attribute value pair is used to describe the functional attribute, as shown in Fig.2. Correspondingly the function adverbials supply the engineer with additional description about the required functions. The part of Function description is expressed as "(adverb) +verb+ (adjective) +noun".

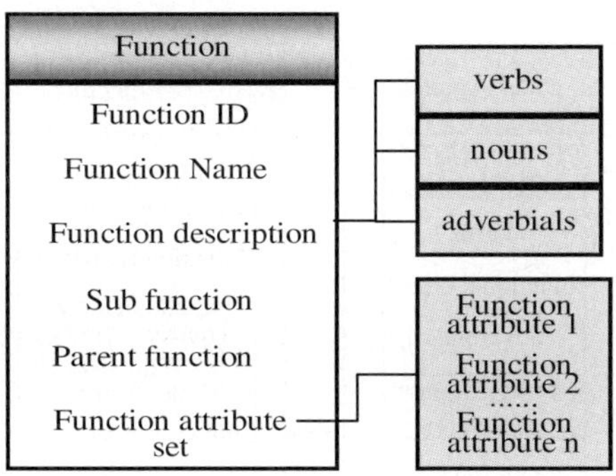

Fig. 2. Function description of microcomponent

3.3 Function Model of Microcomponent

According to the basic function of microcomponent in microsystem, microcomponent can be divided into three classes, namely microsensor, microactuator and microlink. For each big class, it can in turn be subdivided according to different action object and action principle. For microsensor, according to the kinds of conducting energy it can be classified into mechanical sensor, electric sensor and chemical sensor etc. Microcomponent works usually occured with transformation each other of different energy form. Therefore in analyzing the function of microcomponent energy mostly acts as object.

Based on combining kinds of microcomponent functions with funciton definition and classification in macro machinery, microcomponent functions can be devided into

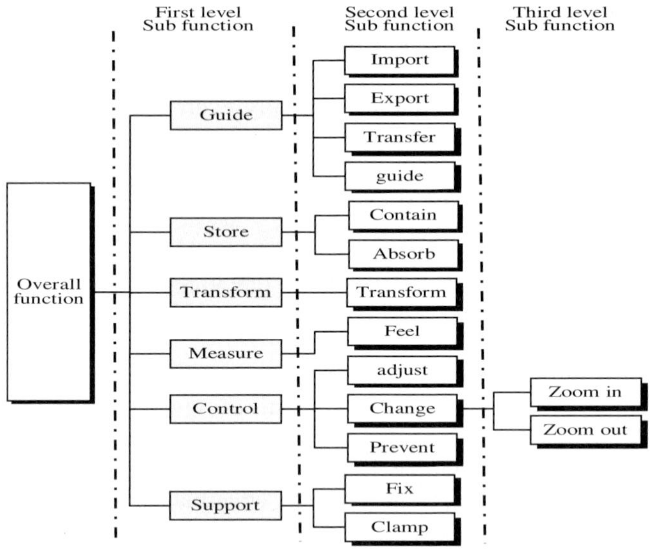

Fig. 3. The function classifying of microcomponent

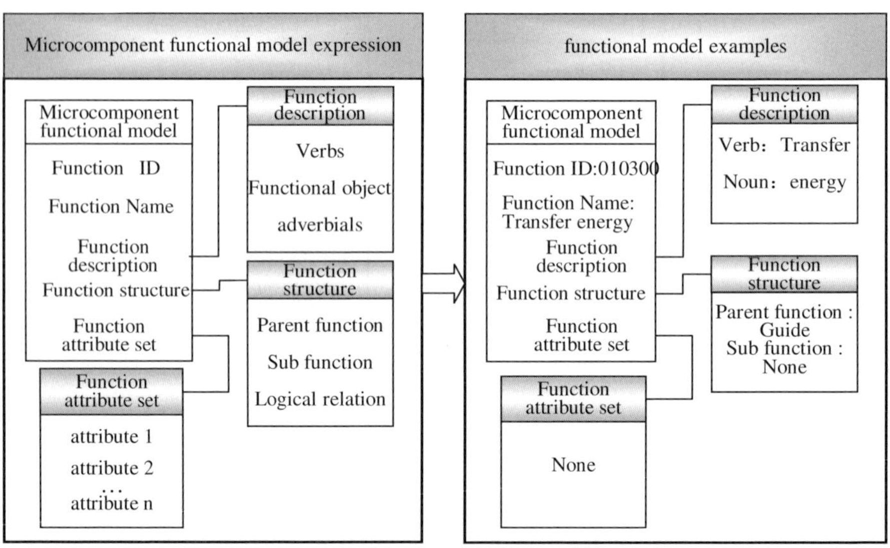

Fig. 4. The function model of microcomponent

several classes, as shown in Fig.3. The six general function verbs described: guide (import, export, transfer, guide), store, transform, control, measure and support.

Based on the analysis of above description, the function model of microcomponent can be represented by five part information, as shown in Fig.4.

a. Function ID: to identify the function of microcomponent, and also be the index of design catalogue and case base of microcomponent;
b. Function Name: to describe the function generally;
c. Function description information: detailed description of function by verb-noun pair form, including verb part, function object and function modificatory word;
d. Function structure relationship: to describe the parent function, sub-function and logical relation of these functions;
e. Function attributes set: to describe the attribute parameters of the function.

4 Effect-Principle Modeling of Microcomponent

4.1 Basic Concepts

In order to understand the principle and modeling process of effect modeling, the definitions of effect and relevant concepts are defined as follow [6]:

a. Effect: An Effects is an input and output relationship that combines the laws of science including physics, mathematics, chemistry and geometry, and their corresponding engineering applications. According to the included information effects can be divided into physical, chemical, geometric effects, etc. According to realizing modes effect is divided into single effect mode, combined effect mode and control effect mode [7].
b. Principle: is the working principle of microcomponent realization. Working principle includes all kinds of effects to realize a function and geometrical and material characteristics. Even if an effect is used to realize the same function, there are different working principles due to different geometrical and material characteristics.

4.2 Effect Analysis of Microcomponent

In the design and realization process of MEMS, all kinds of devices need apply different forms of principle and effect to optimize the function. In conceptual design process of microcomponent effects need to be analyzed in details and the map relationship between function and effect principle need to be established in order to search directly effect and effect chain to realize this function. The effects chains model fulfilling functions is set up by the studies of relations between effect and function.

MEMS is a coupled research field including multi-discipline. Effect plays an important role in microsystem. The combination of different effects can produce different principles and that form different function device to finish different function. According to different information including in the effect, effect can be divided as physical effect, chemical effect, biological effect and geometrical effect and so on. Through analyzing and refining the working principle of variety of devices and considering the classes of microcomponents, an effect tree of microcomponent is established, as shown in Fig.5.

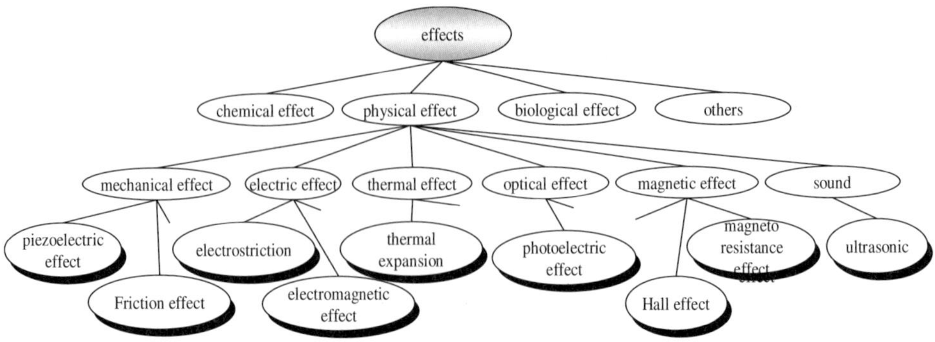

Fig. 5. Effect tree of microcomponent

4.3 Formal Description of Microcomponent Effects

The parameters given below can be used to represent the transition relationship between input and output quantity in effect. The effects and examples are categorized by function and the effects database with delaminated structure based on FES model is set up. The effect database cannot only realize the rapid search but also improve the function, and it is the effective way to solve problem by using effect.

Effect ID: is the only identification of effect;
Effect Name: is the general description of effect;
Effect Description: is the detailed specification of effect;
Formula And Parameters: the basic formula and parameters of effect;
Precondition: the precondition of applying an effect;
Inputs: the input quantities of an effect;
Outputs: the output quantities of an effect;
Remark: some information about source and references of effect;
Example: examples of applying the effect.

4.4 Effect Model of Microcomponent

Based on the analysis of above description, the effect model of microcomponent can be represented by three part information such as effect index information, the basic description of effect, effect constraint and remark, as shown in Fig.6.

a. Effect index information: identify the effect by effect ID and effect Name, and confirm the distinguish between effects and index feature.
b. Effect description: the basic physical, chemical and biology laws and principles of the effect are described by information such as basic formula, schematic and parameters .
c. Effect constraint and remark: describe the precondition, references and application examples of the effect.

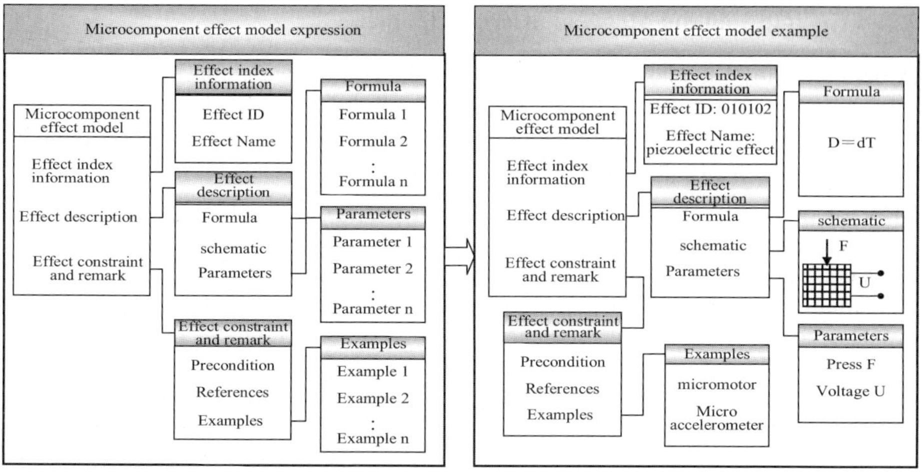

Fig. 6. The effect model of microcomponent

5 Principle Solution Modeling of Microcomponent

In conceptual design phase the principle solution modeling is to abstractly describe the basic physical structure of function, and schematic is usually used to describe the model. Principle solution model is the foundation of detailed design.

5.1 Establishment of Parameterized Microcomponent Libraries

In MEMS component is the basic composing unit. Component can make up of MEMS device and can also be a part of microsystem by itself at the same time. Kinds of component libraries and IP modular play an important role in IC design. In MEMS design parameterized microcomponent and microdevice libraries can be established to improve design efficiency.

The construction of microcomponent and microdevice libraries can be finished through two hierarchies. First according to the basic function of microcomponent in microsystem, microcomponent can be divided into three classes, namely microsensor, microactuator and microlink. For each big class, it can in turn be subdivided according to different action object and action principle. For microsensor, according to the kinds of conducting energy it can be classified into mechanical sensor, electric sensor and chemical sensor etc. Microactuator consists of micro motor, micropump, micro electromagnet, bimetallic film etc. Microlinks are basic micro components, including kinds of micro electronic component and mciromechanical component, for example inductance coil, variable capacity, micro gear, mass, static gap.

The second hierarchy is to establish parameterized model of these components. The parameterized model is described by parameter array. These parameters include geometry, material, performance parameter and dimension parameter.

5.2 Principle Solution Model of Microcomponent

Principle solution model of microcomponent is a solution for function and also response the action results of effects. The model can be represented by four part information such as function information, effect principle information, description of structure components and constraint and remark.

a. Function information: describe the basic function of the solution, including function ID and function Name;
b. Effect and principle information: describe effects and working principles of the solution including effect ID, effect Name, and basic formula etc.
c. Description of structural components: specify the structural components of realizing the solution, including component Name, schematic and parameters .
d. Constraint and remark: describe the constraint condition and application examples of the solution.

6 Case Study

We illustrate our approach by a case study of an actual MEMS component- micropump. In contrast to other MEMS-devices, micropumps are one of the components with a largest variety of operating principles. Many different types of micropumps have been designed to handle small, precise volumes for chemical, medical and biomedical applications.

6.1 Function Analysis

A design can be broken up using a technique based on the flow of signals, energy, and materials. First, the overall function of micropump is abstracted according to the design requirement. In the micropump design input material is fluid and output material is high energy fluid. From the point of energy view, through black-box the kinetic energy, potential energy or pressure energy of fluid increase. Signals flow mainly realizes the control and feedback function of information. So, the overall function of micropump is to “Convey fluid”.

Then the overall function may be decomposed again. For the muti-disciplinary characteristic of microcomponent the technology principles of sub-functions have more choices. According to the corresponding principle or effect of the function we can confirm when to stop decomposition. The function decomposition of micropump is depicted in Figure 7 below.

6.2 Choice of Effects

Each sub-function is associated with physical effects. After finishing function decomposition potential effects or action principles can be find according to the mapping relationship between function and effect principle. The designer of micropump can choose appropriate effect principle on the basis of their own experiences. For example, the function “transfer energy” can be realized by piezoelectric effect, electrostatic effect, thermal drive or ultrasonic drive. The model of function-effect mapping of sub-function of micropump “transfer energy” is shown as Figure 8.

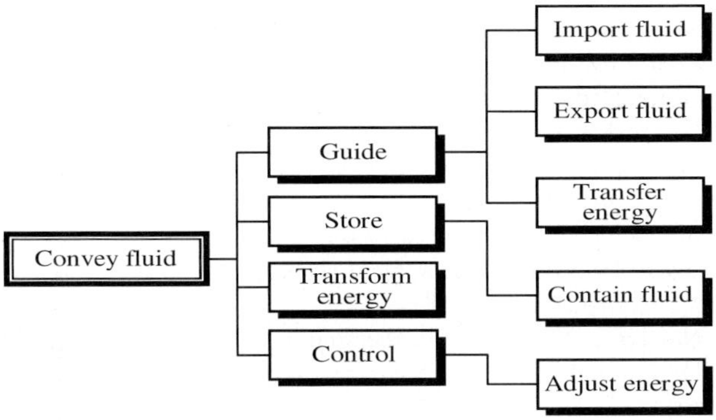

Fig. 7. The function decomposition of micropump

6.3 Determination of Principle Solution

Through the mapping from effect to principle solution, selective physical entity both realizes corresponding effect and realizes required function. In this case, function of "import fluid" is carried out by microchannel and microvalve; function of "transfer energy" can be realized by piezoelectric effect and a structure component is piezoelectric actuator, or electrostatic effect and electrostatic actuator.

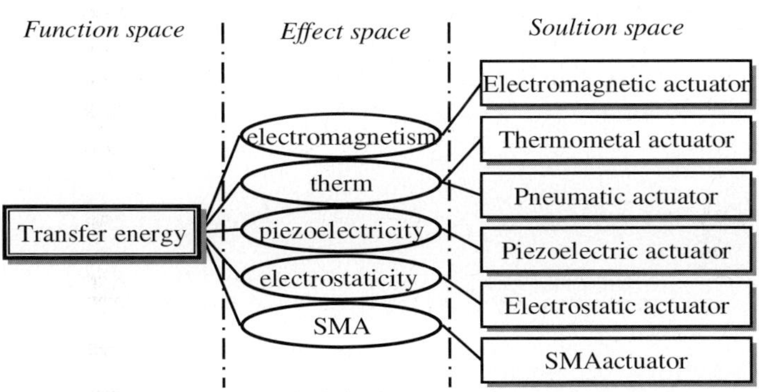

Fig. 8. The function-effect mapping of sub-function of micropump

7 Conclusions

This paper proposes a modeling framework of microcomponent to support the conceptual design of microcomponent. Based on FES (Function-Effect-Solution) model, the function modeling, effect modeling and solution modeling of microcomponent are described respectively. The relationship of function, effect and solution is analyzed. A design example of a micropump is presented to demonstrate the proposed conceptual design methodology and prove that the model is feasible.

Our next work will be integrating the proposed conceptual design framework with the existing downstream design activities, so as to achieve seamless transformation between MEMS conceptual design and detailed design.

References

1. da Silva, M.G.: MEMS design for manufacturability (DFM) (2002), http://www.coventor.com/dfm/
2. Kiriyama, T., Nakajima, N., et al.: A conceptual design environment for Micromechanisms. In: European Design and Test Conference and Exhibition, pp. 448–453. IEEE Press, Los Alamitos (1996)
3. Deng, Y.-M., Tor, S.B., Britton, G.A.: A computerized design environment for functional modeling of mechanical products. In: 5th ACM Symposium on Solid Modeling, pp. 1–12. ACM, New York (1999)
4. Tomiyama, T., Umeda, Y., Yoshikawa, H.: A CAD for Functional Design. Annals of the CIRP 42(1), 143–146 (1993)
5. Ren, G., Liu, Y., Zhang, Y.: Conceptual design and its representation of function for mechanical products. Machinery 29(4), 1–4 (2002)
6. Cao, G.: Study on Effect Based on Triz and its Software Development. CMFD, Beijing (2003)
7. Cao, G., Tan, R., Zhang, R., Jiang, P.: Study on Conceptual Design Process Model Based on Effects. China Mechanical Engineering 16(9), 823–827 (2005)

Clamping Modeling - State-of-the-Art and Future Trends

Jürgen Leopold

Am Bahrehang 95,
09114 Chemnitz, Germany
Info.leo@web.de

Abstract. Automated assembly is generally confined to mass production environments such as the manufacture of cars and white goods. Even in this environment high-level automated assembly is restricted to the OEMs where production volumes are high and flexibility and the ability to quickly reconfigure systems are not major drivers. In the aerospace industry the problem is further complicated by the move to thin walled monolithic parts and the increasing use of composite structures. Monolithic structures have been introduced to reduce the costs of assembling large numbers of components. Although the benefit of using monolithic parts is a large reduction in overall manufacturing costs the downside is a more difficult component to handle and assemble. In addition, there are thin walled components with sometimes-internal stresses and in our case made of nickel based alloys, which only can be cut with difficulties. Machining the flexible structure and maintaining close tolerance is difficult, transferring to assemble is difficult as well. Machining fixtures are used to locate and constrain a workpiece during a machining operation. To ensure that the workpiece is manufactured according to specified dimensions and tolerances, it must be appropriately located and clamped. Minimizing workpiece and fixture tooling deflections due to clamping and cutting forces in machining is critical to machining accuracy. An ideal fixture design maximizes locating accuracy and workpiece stability, while minimizing displacements. In this paper, a review of the state of the art approaches of Clamping modeling is provided. The current drawbacks of the existing approaches and the research areas to focus on in the near future are also identified.

Keywords: Clamping, Fixing, Modeling, Simulation, FE-Analysis, Multiphysics.

1 Introduction

A fixture is a mechanism used in manufacturing to hold a workpiece, position it correctly with respect to a machine tool and a cutting tool, and support it during machining. Typically, fixture design involves the identification of clamp, locator, and support points, and the selection of corresponding fixture elements for their respective functions. The automation of fixture design activities in manufacturing is an important research area, which must be addressed to achieve the integration of design and manufacturing. Fixture design is a complex task, which is as a critical design–manufacturing link, especially in a modern computer integrated manufacturing environment [1,2,3,4]. The computer- based automation of the fixture design activities is

C. Xiong et al. (Eds.): ICIRA 2008, Part II, LNAI 5315, pp. 289–300, 2008.

commonly referred to as computer - automated or computer - aided fixture design (CAFD).

The quality of a fixture design is defined through the requirements from design and manufacturing engineers. The main four commonly required areas are:

- Locating Performance Analysis. Studies workpiece DOFs (degree of freedom) constrained by locators, workpiece constrained status, locating performance index, and locator layout optimization.
- Tolerance Analysis. Studies machining accuracy provided by the fixture and locator tolerance assignment based on machining surface tolerances.
- Stability Analysis. Studies workpiece stability and minimal clamping forces.
- Accessibility Analysis. Studies point and surface accessibility.

To measure the quality defined above, two models – one geometric and one kinetic – will ne normally created to describe the fixture and workpiece relationship (Kang, 2001). The geometric model describes the relationship between workpiece displacement and locator displacements, and it is based on the Jacobian Matrix. The properties of the Jacobian Matrix can be used in finding locating performance and locating accuracy. The Jacobian Matrix is generally used to formulate the relationship between a 3D object and its locators, and it is also used in robotic hand grasping problems [5].

1.1 Initial Fixture Design

There have been many published papers in the area of fixture design. Attempts to automate the fixture design process are not new. In the initial work of Markus [6] and Miller [7], the locator and clamp positions were not determined automatically. The approach adopted was interactive where the user specified the clamping, locating, and support points, and then selected the appropriate fixturing components in the desired positions. In [8], the primary locating surface and its related locator positions are assumed as a given, and the problem was reduced to determining the secondary and tertiary planes with their respective locator positions. The work of Chou [9] focused on the clamping aspects of fixture design. A fixture clamping procedure was developed based on the twin criteria of workpiece stability and total restraint requirement. The total restraint requirement was ensured by restricting the degree of freedom of a given workpiece using clamps and balancing the cutting forces.

1.2 Expert Systems

Researchers have long recognised the importance of developing computer-automated fixture design (CAFD) approaches, in which the clamp, support, and locator design attributes are generated automatically for varying part designs. The use of artificial intelligence (AI) approaches, as well as expert system applications in fixture design, has also been reported. An expert system approach was adopted by Nee et al. [10] to perform the fixture design task where a heuristic rule base was used to generate a list of fixing recommendations including the locating and base elements for the fixture. A CAD model of a given product design was used as an input to the fixture design task. A heuristic rule base was used to generate a list of fixing recommendations including the locating and base elements for the fixture. In [11], a rule-based expert system is described, which identified the locating and clamping faces for rotational parts. Gandhi et al. [12] discussed an expert system architecture to perform fixture design using modular fixture components. Other expert-system oriented fixture-design methods include AIFIX [13] in which the fixing problem is solved as sub problems leading to the final workholding goal. Wright and Hayes [14] described the development of Machining Planner, which is an expert system for the set-up planning of rectangular parts in parallel-sided vices on a three-axis milling machine; later, an automated toe-clamp fixture was also used as a clamping device. Based on this study, the relationships between the force of the vice and the cutting forces were proposed. Markus [6] developed an expert system which configures clamps about a part using design specifications and rules related to geometrical constraints; Asada and By [15] implemented conformable clamps for assembly operations using magnetic tables, locators, and a robot. NIST has designed and implemented a programmable vice including a variable-depth jaw, to hold varying part shapes and sizes using controlled pressure [16]; fluidised beds have been reported [17] to hold parts of unusual shapes. Case-based reasoning has also been used to aid in automated fixture design activities [10,18].

1.3 Recent Approaches to CAFD

In [19], a semi-automated system is described where (when fixture points and planes are selected) modular components are automatically identified and assembled. However, the identification of the clamp, locator, and support (CLS) points is not determined within the system (they are provided as inputs to the system). In a related paper [20], the focus is on geometric analysis, which uses analysis of the geometric relationships between the CLS components and the workpiece, the initial conditions for fixture assembly are developed automatically. Dai et al. [21] described a modular element database creation method, which can be used effectively for integrating with a CAD system and for modelling fixture subassemblies. In [22], an innovative approach to fixture design based on genetic algorithms (GA) and neural networks (NN) is described. The GA searches among a population of fixtures, and each feasible fixture chromosome is evaluated using a defined objective or fitness function; the major drawback of this approach is that the design space (or search space) is very large even for fixture problems corresponding to simple part designs. In [23], fixing surfaces and points are automatically determined based on fixture surface accessibility, stability and feature accuracy. In addition to this, some investigations has been directed to tolerance analysis of locators, source errors analysis and fixture loading techniques [24, 25].

1.4 Summarized Methods Applied to Clamping Optimization

Although numerous CAFD techniques have been proposed and implemented, fixture design still continues to be a major bottleneck in the integration of CAD and CAM activities. One reason for this is that fixture design approaches being developed are not fully integrated with other product and process design activities. Future fixture design approaches must focus on methods which not only serve as a bridge between CAD and CAM, but, more importantly, seek to support cross-functional participation and concurrent engineering approaches. In today's virtual enterprise oriented manufacturing environment, the planning and process design resources may be physically distributed around the globe. There is a need to develop fixture design methods for this changing international manufacturing landscape.

The main activities of Clamping optimization are summarized in Figure 1.

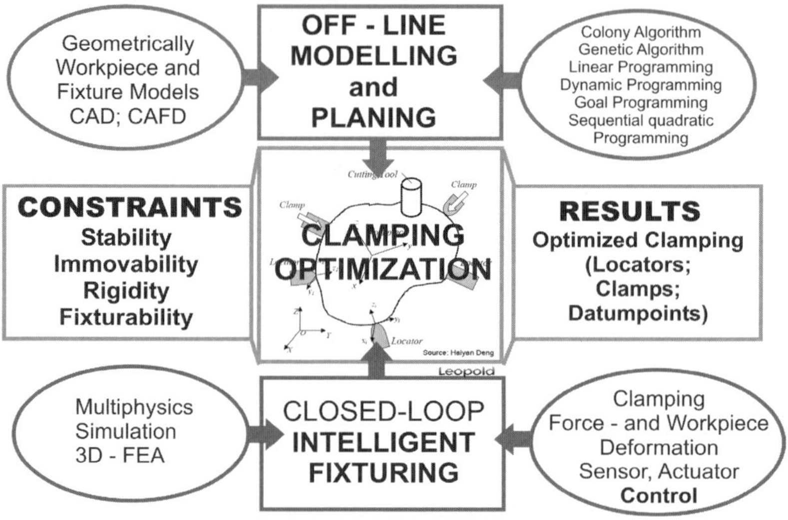

Fig. 1. Methods applied to clamping optimization

2 Modular and Intelligent Fixing Systems

Other computer-automated fixture design work includes Sakurai [26], Boerma and Kals [27], and Rong and Zhu [28]. In [26], the development of a system is described to automate set-up planning and fixture design. Both algorithmic and heuristic methods were developed to generate and analyse the set-up plan and fixture configurations. A solid model of the component (part) is used as the input for the fixture design task. The requirements for set-up planning and fixture design included accurate location of the workpiece, total restraint of the workpiece during machining and interference aspects between the cutting tool, workpiece, and fixture components. Another related aspect studied was the deformation of the workpiece during machining. Features occurring in part design have also been used by other researchers to develop fixture designs [29]. In [30], a mathematical model is used to determine the fixture locator and clamps; kinematic analysis based fixture design is described in several publications, including [8,11,31]. Other researchers, including DeVor et al. [32,33], have analysed the cutting forces and built mechanistic models for drilling, and other metal cutting processes, which can be used to determine clamping requirements. In [34], assembly constraints are defined to model spatial relationships between modular fixture elements. Modular fixture design elements are described in detail in [35]; the use of standardised fixtures or modular fixture components is intended to eliminate the need for single-purpose fixtures. It is an alternative to custom-built fixtures, which are more expensive. A predetermined grid of holes and components such as studs, clamps, etc. can be used to build a fixture. Several researchers have employed modular fixing principles to generate fixture designs [1,3,12,28]. Fixing is process-specific. At some positions along the tool path, small forces may be adequate, but large forces may be required at others. The minimum clamping forces to secure a workpiece are different as the cutter moves along its intended tool path. Hence, our attention is focused on the force distribution. We attempt to design an Intelligent Fixing System such that the fixture elements can be manipulated to provide dynamic clamping forces during the entire machining and fixing process. For the Intelligent Fixing, the clamping forces are adaptively adjusted to optimal values according to the cutter position and the cutting forces during machining with the objective of minimizing workpiece distortion while ensuring that it is adequately secured. Since adaptive clamping forces appropriate to the dynamic machining environment are provided, the proposed IFS offers higher quality of machined parts and greater robustness to disturbances. The developed Intelligent Fixing System [37] is characterized by on-line monitoring, dynamic clamping forces, and real-time fixing process control (Fig. 2).

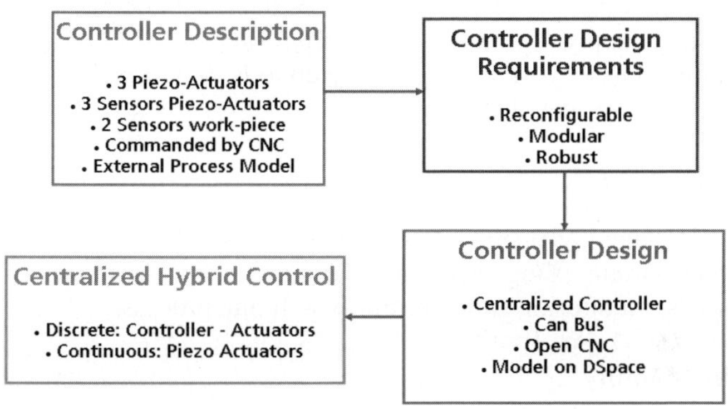

Fig. 2. Requirements for Intelligent Fixing Systems (IFS) [37]

2.1 Design Requirements

The general design requirements pertinent to ordinary fixtures also apply to the intelligent fixing system. The functional requirements of a fixture include total restraint, positive location, repeatability and rigidity. Since the IFS still needs to adjust the clamping forces at different cutting tool positions and the magnitude of the cutting forces vary during machining, sensor feedback, clamping control and programmability are required to realize its functions.

2.2 Open- and Closed-Loop

In an open-loop IFS, the optimal clamping forces with respect to the different cutting tool positions are pre-computed before machining. During machining, the control unit of the IFS adjusts the clamping system – based on a database - according to the deformation of the workpiece. In a closed-loop IFS, the optimal clamping forces with respect to the different cutting tool positions are calculated in real-time during machining. Cutting forces acting on the workpiece are obtained from sensors in the system and optimal clamping forces are then deduced and applied. Unlike the mechanism of open-loop IFS, the optimal clamping forces provided by the closed-loop IFS are continually adjusted by monitoring and measuring forces on the workpiece. To ensure that the controller has a sufficiently short response time, the models and algorithms should be as simple as possible.

2.3 Sensor Feedback

Sensor feedback is most important for the design of an intelligent system. Sensors allow real-time information to be transferred between the fixing system and its controller. In [APT] piezoelectric sensors are mounted on the locators to monitor and easure the reaction forces during machining.

2.4 Clamping Control

Clamping devices are designed to apply variable clamping forces to the workpiece during the machining process. Through a remote interface circuit, a CPU controls the clamping system to apply the required clamping forces as the cutting tool moves to different locations on the workpiece. The objective is to minimize the deformation of the workpiece caused by the clamping forces.

2.5 Programmability

The sensing and clamping operations of the IFS are controlled by a CPU through a remote interface circuit using customized programs for the processing of the input/output signals, monitoring and control of the fixing process.

2.6 Fixturing Stability

A stable fixturing system must hold a workpiece stable in place during machining. Positive reaction forces at the locators ensure that the workpiece maintains contact with all the locators from the beginning of the cutting operation up to the end. A negative reaction force at the locator must be avoided. If one or more of the reaction forces should go to zero, this indicates that the workpiece is no longer in contact with the corresponding locators and the fixing system is considered unstable. Hence, a fixing stability criterion is considered here and it states that all the reaction forces at the locators must be positive during the entire machining process.

2.7 Initial and Optimized Clamping Force

The optimal clamping forces are defined here as the minimum clamping forces necessary to keep the workpiece in static equilibrium throughout the entire machining process, but on the other hand, some thin-walled workpieces can be deformed due to the clamping forces. So, in addition to the initial clamping forces, process depending clamping forces should be used.

2.8 Control-Clamp at Datum Points

The control-clamp of a locator refers to the clamp that has the greatest influence on the reaction forces at the locator. All the clamps in a given fixing system are labeled as the control-clamps of a certain locator. If a reaction force at a locator is near or equal to zero during machining, its control-clamps will be adjusted to increase the clamping forces so that the reaction force will not reach the critical state.

2.9 Intelligent Controller

A model-based control scheme is proposed for the IFS - as illustrated in Fig. 3. Three different models are employed: fixture–workpiece model, stability monitoring model and process model. At the start of the machining process, the reaction forces are measured through the sensors embedded in the locators. According to the fixture–workpiece model, the cutting forces are estimated, and from the estimated cutting forces and the optimization model, the required optimal clamping forces are predicted. The predicted optimal clamping forces are then applied in real-time to the workpiece using the specially designed clamping system. Once unstable phenomena are detected, the stability monitoring model issues a command to the clamping system to increase the appropriate control-clamp until stability is restored. These processes are repeated until the completion of the machining process. In this way, reaction forces at the locators are monitored and serve as feedback information as the clamping forces are varied automatically throughout the entire machining process. The computation times of the fixture–workpiece and optimization models must be fast enough for real-time control.

3 Fixture - Workpiece Model and Simulation

For the Application of Intelligent Fixing Systems it is important to distinguish three families of workpieces – machine tool – cutting tool - clamping systems (Fig. 4)

a.) stable workpiece – unstable cutting tool
b.) unstable workpiece – stable cutting tool
c.) flexible sheet metal parts with internal stress situation (spring back)

A fixture–workpiece model aims to relate the interaction between the fixture and the workpiece during the machining operation. Several kinds of fixture–workpiece models have been developed in the past decades [38-43]. Different forms of fixture–workpiece model have been derived in order to make its application more convenient for the subjects under study. Many thin-walled structure components widely used in aero industries not only have complex structure and large size, but also need high machining accuracy. However, because of their poor rigidity, it is easy to bring machining deformation caused by the existence of the initial residual stresses, the fixing stresses, cutting forces and cutting heat. The difficulty in ensuring their machining accuracy becomes a big problem, so that how to effectively predict and control the machining deformation has become an important subject in the development and production of aero parts [44,45].

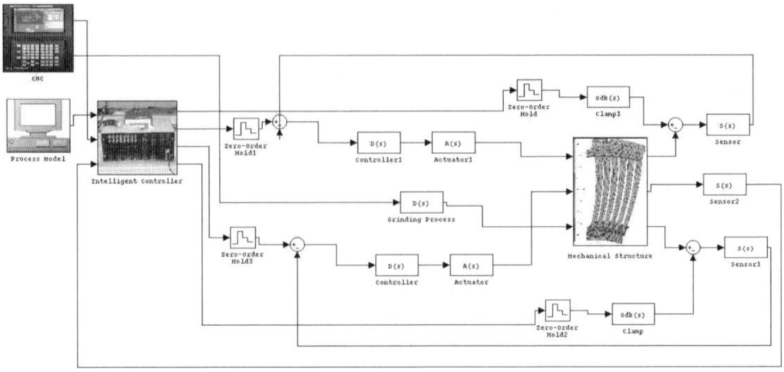

Fig. 3. Intelligent Controller for a Clamping System of Nozzle-Guide-Vans [37]

The FEM is most suitable to analyze the elastic deformation of a workpiece-fixture system in the presence of clamping and cutting forces. The finite element model built in this work includes contact stiffness, element stiffness, spring-damping properties and frictional force as well as grinding forces.

To realize the proposed Intelligent Fixing System Principle, a multiphysical simulation has been developed [ ]:

To realize the proposed Intelligent Fixing System Principle, a multiphysical simulation has been developed [ ]:

1. The Workpiece Model (material properties; friction conditions; boundary conditions for fixing)
2. The Machine Tool and the Cutting Tool Model – including instability charts
3. The process model for the applied machining operation (milling, drilling, grinding) – machining simulation based on FEA; cutting force predicition by simulation or predictive modelling
4. Sensor – Actor – Models - based on hybrid mechanical-thermal-electrical simulation

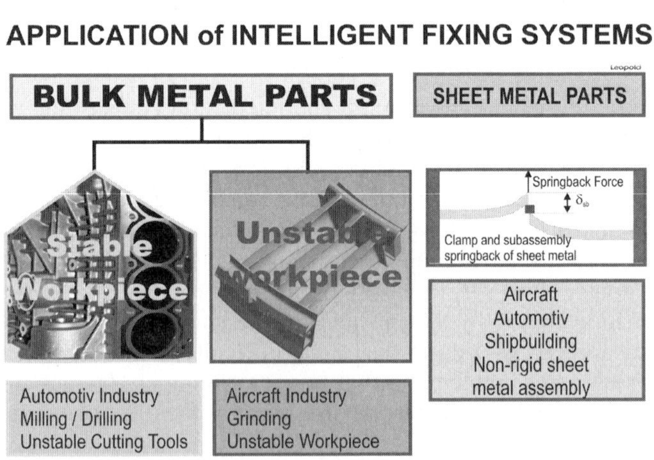

Fig. 4. Intelligent Fixing Systems for three different industrial applications

To realize a near real-time simulation, the proposed model for the Intelligent Fixing System is based on a reduced mechanical model, started with a full FE-Model, a parametric model up to an analytical model [37].

For the mechanical modelling, the following conditions must determine.

3.1 Cutting Forces

The thermo-mechanical phenomena of machining are so complex with so many elements involved that even for single-point cutting it is not simple to estimate the cutting forces accurately. A number of validated models have been reported in the literature for milling, drilling, and grinding.

3.2 Friction

It is well known that the frictional force between two objects is indeterminate until slippage occurs. Due to such uncertainty, the analysis of friction in a fixing system is difficult. Coulomb friction force between the workpiece surfaces and the fixture elements are usually assumed. This is considered to be the simplest and effective way to deal with friction. For some machining fixtures, unlike the problem of robot grasping, frictional forces are not relied on or necessary to hold the workpiece because the cutting forces can be very large and are inherently dynamic. Friction shows no significant influence on the fixturing system. Other machining fixtures, such as vises, chucks or strap clamps, rely mainly upon friction to maintain the fixturing stability. The friction coefficient is depending on the working environment, such as the use of cutting fluid. Since the objective is to obtain the minimum clamping forces, the critical situation of slippage should is assumed.

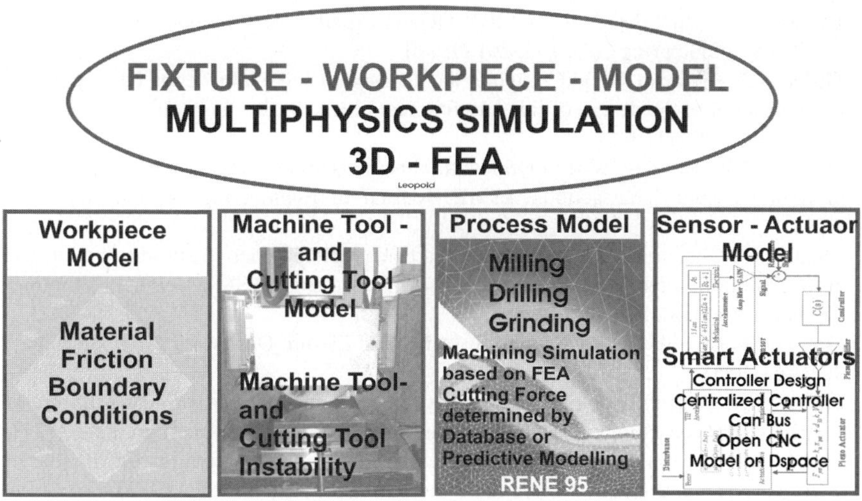

Fig. 5. Multiphysics approach to investigate intelligent fixing systems

3.3 Spring-Damping Properties

In order to produce a more accurate model for predicting the behaviour of the fixture–workpiece system, the FEM model must includes fixture stiffness [46, 47], which past models have assumed as rigid bodies. The spring-damping properties of the clamping devices have a strong influence on the dynamically behaviour of the intelligent fixing system [48].

Acknowledgments

Special thanks to my colleagues and students Anke Poppitz, Matthias Klärner, Anne-Kathrin Schmidt and Jens Berger for their assistance throughout the last year's research. Additional thanks to Professor Caihua Xiong for some fruitful discussions.

References

1. Cecil, J.A.: Fixture design in a CIM environment, PhD dissertation, Texas A& M University, Department of Industrial Engineering, College Station (1995)
2. Kumar, A.S., Nee, A.Y.C., Prombanpong, S.: Expert fixture design system for an automated manufacturing environment. J. of Computer Aided Design 24, 316–326 (1992)
3. Nee, A.Y.C., Tao, Z.J., Kumar, A.S.: An Advanced Treatise on Fixture Design and Planning. Series on Manufacturing Systems and Technology, vol. 1 (2004)
4. Kang, Y.: Computer-Aided Fixture Design Verification, PhD-Thesis Worchester Polytechnic Institute (2001)
5. Xiong, C., Li, Y., Xiong, Y., Ding, H., Huang, Q.: Grasp Capability Analysis of Multifingered Robot Hands. Robotics and Autonomous Systems 27, 211–224 (1999)
6. Markus, A.: Fixture design using PROLOG: an expert system. Robotics and Computer Integrated Manufacturing 1(2), 195–201 (1984)
7. Miller, A.S., Hannam, R.G.: Computer aided design using a knowledge base approach and its application to the design of jigs and fixtures. Proceedings – Institute of Mechanical Engineering 199(B4) (1985)
8. Menassa, R.J., Devries, W.R.: Optimization methods applied to selecting support positions in fixture design. Transactions ASME, Journal of Engineering for Industry, 412–418 (1991)
9. Chou, Y.C., Chandru, V., Barash, B.: A mathematical approach to automatic configuration of machining fixtures: analysis and synthesis. Transactions ASME, Journal of Engineering for Industry 111(4), 299–306 (1989)
10. Nee, A.Y.C., Whybrew, K., Kumar, S.: Advanced Fixture Design for FMS. Springer, Heidelberg (1995)
11. Bausch, J.J., Youcef-Toumi, K.: Computer planning methods for automated fixture layout synthesis. In: Proceedings of Manufacturing International 1990, vol. 1, pp. 225–232 (1990)
12. Gandhi, M.V., Thompson, B.S.: Automated design of modular fixtures for flexible manufacturing systems. Journal of Manufacturing Systems 5(4), 243–252 (1987)
13. Ferreira, P.M., Liu, C.R.: Generation of workpiece orientations for machining using a rule based system. Robotics and Computer Integrated Manufacturing 4(3/4), 545–555 (1988)
14. Wright, K., Hayes, C.C.: Automated planning in the machining domain, Knowledge Based Expert Systems for Manufacturing. ASME PED-24, 221–232 (1986)

15. Asada, H., By, A.: Kinematic analysis of workpart fixturing for flexible assembly with automatically reconfigurable fixtures. IEEE Journal of Robotics and Automation 2, 86–93 (1984)
16. Slocum, A.H., Peris, J., Donmez, A.: Development of a flexible automated fixturing system, Progress Report: US National Bureau of Standards, Automated Production Technology Division (1985)
17. Thompson, B.S., Gandhi, M.V.: A literature survey of fixture design automation. International Journal of Advanced Manufacturing Technology, 240–255 (1985)
18. Sun, S.H., Chen, J.L.: Modular fixture design system based on case based reasoning. International Journal of Production Research 34, 3487–3497 (1995)
19. Wu, Y., Rong, Y., Ma, W.: Automated modular fixture planning: geometric analysis. Robotics and Computer Integrated Manufacturing 14, 1–15 (1998)
20. Wu, Y., Rong, Y., Ma, W.: Automated modular fixture planning: accuracy, clamping, and accessibility analysis. Robotics and Computer Integrated Manufacturing 14, 17–26 (1998)
21. Dai, J., Nee, A.Y.C., Fuh, J.Y.H.: An approach to automating modular fixture designand assembly. Proceedings of the Institution of Mechanical Engineers, Part B, Journal of Engineering Manufacture 211, 509–521 (1997)
22. Kumar, A.S., Subramaniam, V., Seow, K.C.: Conceptual design of fixtures using genetic algorithms. International Journal of Manufacturing Technology 15(2), 79–84 (1999)
23. Ma, W., Li, J., Rong, Y.: Development of automated fixture planning systems. International Journal of Advanced Manufacturing Technology 15(3), 171–181 (1999)
24. Cai, W., Hu, S.J., Yuan, J.X.: A variational method of robust fixture configuration design for 3D workpieces. Journal of Manufacturing Science and Engineering 119, 593–602 (1997)
25. Choudhuri, S., De-Meter, E.C.: Tolerance analysis of machining fixture locators. Journal of Manufacturing Science and Engineering 121, 273–281 (1999)
26. Sakurai, H.: Automatic setup planning and fixture design for machining. Journal of Manufacturing Systems 11(1) (1990)
27. Boerma, J.R., Kals, H.J.J.: Fixture design with FIXES. Annals CIRP 38, 399–402 (1988)
28. Rong, Y., Zhu, J.: Fixturing feature analysis for computer aided fixture design. Intelligent Design and Manufacturing, ASME WAM, 267–271 (1993)
29. Dong, X., Gilman, C., Wozny, M.: Feature-based fixture design and set-up planning artificial intelligence in optimal design and manufacturing. Prentice-Hall, Englewood Cliffs
30. Cecil, J.A.: Impact of information technology on manufacturing practices, Virtual Enterprise Engineering Laboratory (VEEL) Report, Utah State University (July 2000)
31. Kang, Y., Rong, Y., Sun, M.: Constraint based modular fixture assembly modelling and automated design. Proceedings of the ASME Manufacturing Science and Engineering Division 8, 901–908 (1998)
32. Hoffman, E.G.: Jig and Fixture Design, Delmar, Albany, NY (1985)
33. Xiong, C., Ding, H., Xiong, Y.: Fundamentals of Robotic Grasping and Fixturing. Series on Manufacturing Systems and Technology, vol. 3. World Scientific, Singapore (2008)
34. Leopold, J., Poppitz, A., Klärner, M., Clauß, D., Bandoli, M., Merlo, A., Giménez, M., Larranaga, J.: Investigations to New Fixturing Principles for Aerospace Structures. In: Proceedings of the International Conference on Applied Production Technology, Bremen, September 17-19, 2007, pp. 173–189 (2007); ISBN 978-3-933762-21-4
35. Mittal, R.O., Cohen, P.H., Gilmore, B.J.: Dynamic modeling of the fixture–workpiece system. Robotics and Computer- Integrated Manufacturing 8(4), 201–217 (1991)
36. Fuh, J.Y.H., Nee, A.Y.C.: Verification and optimization of workholding schemes for fixture design. Journal of Design and Manufacturing 4, 307–318 (1994)

37. Shawki, G.S.A., Abdel-Aal, M.M.: Effect of fixture rigidity and wear on dimensional accuracy. International Journal of Machine Tool Design and Research 5, 183–202 (1965)
38. Chou, Y.C., Chandru, V., Barash, M.: A mathematical approach to automatic configuration for machining fixtures: analysis and synthesis. Journal of Engineering for Industry, Transaction of the ASME 103, 725–735 (1981)
39. DeMeter, E.C.: Min–max load model for optimizing machining fixture performance. Journal of Engineering for Industry, Transaction of the ASME 117, 186–193 (1995)
40. Wu, N.H., Chan, K.C., Leong, S.S.: Fixturing verification based on the analysis of multidiscipline frictional contacts. Manufacturing Science and Engineering, ASME MH3–1, 735–745 (1995)
41. Guo, H., Zuo, D.W., Wang, S.H., Xu, L.L., Wang, M., Hu, J.: The application of FEM technology on the deformation analysis of the aero thin-walled frame shape workpiece. Key Engineering Materials 315-316, 174–179 (2006)
42. Shaogang, L., Zheng, L., Zhang, Z.H., Wen, D.H.: Optimal fixture design in peripheral milling of thin-walled workpiece. Int. J. Adv. Manuf. Technol. 28, 653–658 (2006)
43. Tan, E.Y.T., Kumar, A.S., Fuh, J.Y.H., Nee, A.Y.C.: Modeling, Analysis, and Verification of Optimal Fixturing Design. IEEE Transactions on Automation Science and Engineering 1(2) (October 2004)
44. Zheng, Y.: Finite Element Analysis for Fixture Stiffness Ph.D. Dissertation, Worchester Polytechnic Institute (2005)
45. Leopold, J., Poppitz, A., Klärner, M., Schmidt, A.-K., Berger., J.: Interaction between machining and new fixturing principles for aerospace structures. International Journal of Material Forming (2008); ISSN 1960-6206 or ISSN 1960-6214

A Feasibility Study of the Design and Calculation of Fully Hydraulic Paper Cutting Machine System

Xinxiang Wang[1], Guoqing Hu[2], and Haifeng Zhou[1]

[1] Marine Engineering Institute, Jimei University, Xiamen 361021, China
[2] School of Mechanical and Automotive Engineering, South China University of Technology, Guangzhou, 510641, China
gqhu@scut.edu.cn

Abstract. As sort of traditional paper process machinery equipments, paper cutting machines are developing rapidly in hydraulic, digital display and computer control machines. But a great number of products of the paper cutting machines in the market are that the pressing paper units are controlled by hydraulic drive and cutting paper units still adopt mechanical driven by worm wheel and worm. These kinds of paper cutting machines have many disadvantages, such as: complex structure, low driven efficiency and low availability factor of hydraulic system and so on. One type of the paper cutting machine with fully hydraulic system both in pressing paper and cutting paper units is studied in detail. The hydraulic system element circuit are delivered and analyzed in detail. The loading and working condition of hydraulic system are also analyzes and calculated; the main parameters of performing elements including the power of motor are confirmed as well.

Keywords: Paper cutting machine; fully hydraulic control; design and calculation; hydraulic circuit; Motor.

1 Introduction

Paper cutting machine is a sort of paper machinery equipments. It is extensively used for paper making industry, paper carton, leather, plastic and food industry. With the developing of these industries, technical level of paper cutting machine becomes higher and higher. It's developing from mechanical machine to hydraulic, digital display and computer control machine. With the width use of hydraulic products, hydraulic control is adopted in the paper pressing unit of paper cutting machine. Because this pressing paper unit driven by hydraulic system has many advantages, such as: smooth working, high precision, heavy cutting force, broader pressure adjusting range [1], and so on. Nowadays, most products in inland and all products in developed countries adopt pressing paper unit driven by hydraulic system. But, at the same time, a great number of them still adopt traditional cutting paper unit driven by worm wheel and worm. The paper cutting machine having adopted this kind of cutting paper unit has advantage of low cost, but availability factor of its hydraulic system is low, and this cutting paper unit driven by worm wheel and worm has many disadvantages, for example: this type of cutting paper unit has complex structure and low driven

C. Xiong et al. (Eds.): ICIRA 2008, Part II, LNAI 5315, pp. 301–310, 2008.

efficiency. The cogwheels engaged between worm wheel and worm are easily worn; For the reason that break tray has remaining magnetism, it makes the electromagnetic clutch action more slowly and makes break capability reduce, safety decline. If gear wheel skids for a long time, the friction would produce heat, make gear wheel wear rapidly; the solenoid of electromagnetic clutch heat easily, voltage fluctuation is heavy, interference strong; the gear driven system has disadvantage of heavy noise; small and fixed cutting force, so the output torque is changing and the instability cutting paper quantity[2]~[4].

If cutting paper unit can adopt hydraulic control as pressing paper unit does, it markedly improves the availability factor of hydraulic system; and because the hydraulic system has characteristics of rapidly response and adjustable pressure, it commendably settle the matter of fixed cutting force and badly break capability. As the worm wheel and worm driving unit and electromagnetic clutch is removed, the problems caused by them will be settled, such as, serious wear and tear, heavy noise, high heating, unstable torque output and so on. In this paper, the authors major study in detail in the design and calculation of one type of fully hydraulic system of the paper cutting machine.

2 The Analysis of Pressing Paper Unit System and Cutting Paper Unit

The cutting paper part of the paper cutting machine are composed of pressing paper and cutting paper units, which controlled by fully hydraulic system.

Pressing paper unit [4] is shown in figure 1. When the piston of hydraulic cylinder moves upward, the lever construction makes the pressing paper machinery move downward. In order to ensure the quantity of paper, the pressure of the pressing paper machinery can be adjusted and kept stability, the gauge pressure should modulated within 4~10 *MPa* and not allow to exceed 15 *MPa* [5].

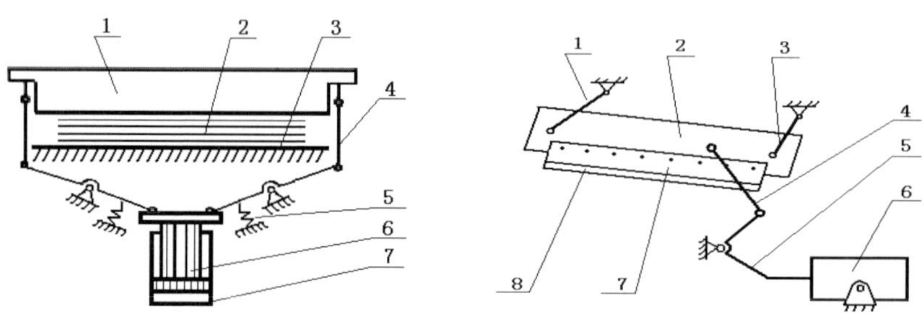

1. pressing paper machinery; 2. paper pack
3. working table; 4. pull rod; 5. spring
6. piston; 7. pressing paper hydraulic cylinder

1. swinging arm *a*; 2. guillotine knife;
3. swinging arm *b*; 4. pull rod;
5. crank; 6.cutting paper hydraulic cylinder;
7. cutting knife; 8. knife blade

Fig. 1. (a) pressing paper unit (b) cutting paper unit

Cutting paper unit [6] is shown in figure 2. The cutting knife moving along with the complex curve locus is realized, when the advanced technology has been used in the paper cutting machine. The characteristic of this oblique blade style is: When the piston of hydraulic cylinder moves towards the left, pulls paper cutting machinery downward, the cutting knife making an angle of α with paper. Cutting knife has a minuteness turning when it's moving. When knife blade touches the paper, only cuts a part of paper. As the descending of the knife blade; the knife blade touches the cutter blade slips gradually and the angle α decreases gradually to 0, both sides of papers separate gradually along with the width direction of paper pack in succession, so the cutting force is lesser than other cutting styles, and it approximates to a constant. The advantage of this oblique blade is reducing the cutting resistance of stuff and the shock force of the knife blade, improves cutting quantity. This oblique blade style is divided into two kinds of way according to the angle blade slope: $\alpha > \arctan(h/l)$ and $\alpha < \arctan(h/l)$. The way of $\alpha > \arctan(h/l)$ is almost impossible, because the structure of paper cutting machine is limited. Therefore, there are a lot of products are adopted the way of $\alpha < \arctan(h/l)$, the authors selected the way for further study. $\alpha < \arctan(h/l)$ cutting way is shown in figure 3.

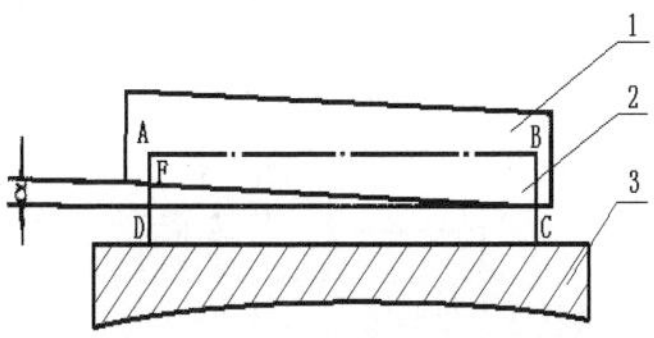

1. cutter knife; 2.paper pack
3. working table

Fig. 1. The oblique blade style of

The four corners of the paper are named as A, B, C, and D. When the knife blade moves to the corner C, cutting force increases to the maximum value, the corner A has already been cut off at this time. The cutting area having been cut off is a trapezoid, the equation to calculate cutting force [4] is:

$$F_{ic} = S_{afcb}\tau = \left[(h - L\tan\alpha) + h\right]L\tau \div 2 = Lh\tau - 0.5L^2\tau\tan\alpha \tag{1}$$

where: F_{ic}: The cutting force of the oblique blade (N); L: The width of the paper (m); h: The thickness of the paper (m); τ: The paper's anti-break strength. The white cardboard paper is 2.156×10^5 (N/m^2); α: cutting angle of the knife

3 The Design of Hydraulic Circuit

The hydraulic system is shown in figure 4. At first, hydraulic system downloads pressure through 2/2 way electromagnetic directional valve. When hydraulic system begins to work, the electromagnetic YA5 is on and the systemic pressure is established.

When worker pedals machine, the electromagnetic YA2 is on. The mineral oil passes through 3/4-way electromagnetic directional valve to the right chamber, pilot operated check valve, and modulation speed valve to the down-chamber of the pressing paper hydraulic cylinder. The pressing paper machinery decreases, the pressure of down-chamber increases quickly after the machinery has touched on the paper pack. When pressure increases to the target maximum value, pressure sensor sends a signal to electromagnetic YA2 and makes it off. 3/4-way electromagnetic directional valve works in middle position. The mineral flows into the down-chamber of hydraulic cylinder keeps pressure in stability by pilot operated check valve. When pressure decreases to target minimum value, pressure sensor sends signal to electromagnetic YA2 and makes it on, at the same time, YA1 is off. The system can be realized the mineral oil in the hydraulic system automatic compensation and pressure automatic stability. When the electromagnetic YA1 is on, 3/4-way electromagnetic directional valve works in the left position, the pressing paper machinery moves upwards.

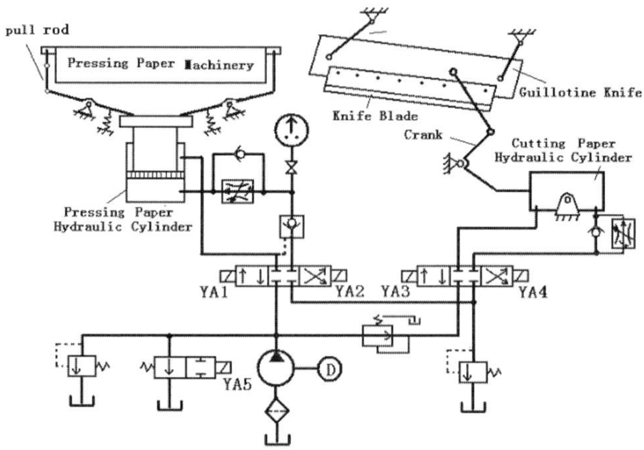

Fig. 2. Hydraulic system

If the pressure of down-chamber increases to the setup maximum value, the electromagnetic dowel is on. The dowel is magnetized from the knife-hole and then the electromagnetic YA4 is on, the cutting knife declines. When knife touches the downside and switch is on, the electromagnetic YA4 is off and YA3 is on, at the same time, the knife returns till touches the upside and switch is on, then electromagnetic YA3 is off, the electromagnetic dowel is off and return to knife-hole under the effect of spring. These measures can avoid the cutting knife declining itself.

The electromagnetic acting order is shown in table 1

Table 1. The electromagnetic acting order

Electromagnetic / Action	YA1	YA2	YA3	YA4	YA5	YA6
stop	-	-	-	-	-	-
Start	-	-	-	-	+	-
Pressing paper machinery decrease	-	+	-	-	+	-
Pull out the dowel	-	+	-	-	+	+
Paper cutting machinery decrease	-	+	-	+	+	+
Paper cutting machinery and Pressing paper machinery returns	+	-	+	-	+	+
Insert the dowel	-	-	-	-	+	-
Start	-	-	-	-	+	-

4 The Design and Calculation of the Hydraulic System

The height of the paper pack is set 100*mm*. this is because, the more higher the paper pack is, the more higher cutting resistance of the paper pack is, the more higher pressure the pressing paper machinery need thus, enlarges the deflections and distortion of the paper pack, the paper pack having been cut off, it maybe appear the case of up long and next short. So the best height of paper pack is below 100*mm*. the different height of paper pack is adjusted from the different thickness the paper[6]. The width of the paper pack is set 920*mm*. The cutting angle of the cutting knife is set 1.5º.

4.1 Design the Parameter of Cutting Paper Hydraulic Cylinder

4.1.1 Calculating the Speed of the Cutting Knife

For Most hydraulic control or programmable control paper cutting machine, cutting frequency is about 40 times/ *min*, thereout, so, the period of the cutting knife is following:

$$T=1min/40=60s/40=1.5s$$

To ensure the requirement of the period of 1.5*s*, the circulating period can be separated as following in detail: descending is 1*s*, rising is 0.5*s*; the distance of rising and descending is 12*mm*. So the average speed v_1 and v_2 of descendent and rising for cutting knife can be calculated, respectively. Here: $v_1=0.12m/s$; $v2=0.24m/s$.

4.1.2 The Maximum Cutting Force of Cutting Knife

According to the calculation equation of oblique blade style [2]: Substitute parameters into equation (1), got $F_{ic}=17445.96(N)$.

Assume the ratio of tension arm compares with heavy tension arm is 1 to 1.

In consideration of the whole loss in the transmission mechanics, and the gravity of guillotine knife, when computes the maximum pushing force of cutting hydraulic cylinder, need remain 20% amount. if the maximum pushing force F_{max} is 21807.45(*N*).

4.1.3 Working Pressure and Back Pressure of Cutting Paper Hydraulic Cylinder

According to the working pressure under different load conditions is shown in table 2.

Table 2. The working pressure under different load conditions [10]

Load F (*N*)	Working pressure ofhydraulic cylinder (*MPa*)
<5000	<0.8~1
5000~10000	1.5~2
10000~20000	2.5~3
20000~30000	3~4
30000~50000	4~5
>50000	≥5~7

Primary assume the working pressure of cutting paper hydraulic cylinder as 4 *MPa*.

According to the experience data of back pressure in hydraulic system [10] is shown in table 3

Table 3. The experience data of back pressure

Character of circuit	Back pressureP_2(*Pa*)
Meter-in inlet	$(1\sim2)\times10^5$
Meter-in inlet and back pressure valve is set in return circuit	$(2\sim5)\times10^5$
Meter-out outlet	$(6\sim15)\times10^5$
Close circuit with affixes pump	$(10\sim15)\times10^5$
Working pressure exceed 25MPa	0
Use inner-curve hydraulic motor	$(7\sim12)\times10^5$

If the back pressure of the circuit is 0.5 *MPa*.

4.1.4 The Parameter of Cutting Paper Hydraulic Cylinder

Because the chamber without pole is the work chamber, according to the simultaneous equations (2) and (3) [11]:

$$P_1A_1 - P_2A_2 = \frac{F_{\max}}{\eta_{cm}} \tag{2}$$

$$\frac{v_2}{v_1} = \frac{D_1}{(D_1 - d_1)} \tag{3}$$

P_1, P_2 : the pressure of working chamber and returning chamber of hydraulic cylinder, respectively (*Pa*); A_1, A_2: the effective area of rodless chamber and rod chamber of hydraulic cylinder, respectively (m^2); $F_{\max}$,: the maximum load force in hydraulic cylinder (*N*); η_{cm}: the mechanical efficiency (0.9~ 0.97); v_1, v_2: the speed which guillotine knife descend and ascend, respectively, (*m*/*s*); D_1, d_1: the diameter of hydraulic cylinder and diameter of piston, respectively (*m*)

Substitute all parameters into equations (2) and (3), get D_1 =89.8m*m*, d_1=44.9*mm*

If pressure of the cutting hydraulic cylinder increased appropriately, cutting will be easy. Therefore, the authors got the standard diameter of cylinder is smaller than that of calculating. From the regular of GB/ T 2348-1993 and GB/※7933-1987[12], the diameter of standard cylinder and piston are 80*mm* and 50*mm*, respectively.

Thereout, the working area and working pressures of cutting paper hydraulic cylinder are as following:

Rodless chamber area $A_1 = \pi D_1^2/4 = 5.02\times10^{-3}$ (m^2)

Rod chamber area $A_2 = \pi(D_1^2 - d_1^2)/4 = 3.06\times10^{-3}$ (m^2)

Substitute the parameters F=21807.45*N*, $\eta_{cm} = 0.95$, , P_2, A_1 , A_2 , got working pressure $P_1 = (F/\eta_{cm} + P_2A_2)/A_1 = 4.88$(*Mpa*)

The maximum flow $q_{\max}$ can be given:

$$q_{\max} = A\ v_{\max} \tag{4}$$

A_1 or A_2: the area of hydraulic cylinder (m^2), respectively, $v_{\max}$: the maximum speed of hydraulic cylinder (*m/s*).

Substitute all parameters into equation (4), and got $q_{\max}$ is 0.734×10^{-3} (m^3/s).

4.1.5 Check Strength and Stability of Cutting Paper Hydraulic Cylinder

1) The thickness of cutting paper hydraulic cylinder

If low-pressure system or $\delta/D\leq 0.08$, the thickness of hydraulic cylinder is consideration as thin wall.[13,14]

$$\delta \geq \frac{P_{max} D}{2[\sigma]} \tag{5}$$

$$[\sigma] = \frac{\sigma_s}{n_s} \tag{6}$$

δ: the thickness of hydraulic cylinder (m); P_{max}: the maximum allowable pressure. (MPa); When working pressure $P\leq 16MPa$, $P_{max}=1.5P$; D: the diameter of hydraulic cylinder (m); $[\sigma]$: Allowable stress of cylinder's material (MPa); σ_s: Material's bow limit, $\sigma_s=355MPa$; n_s- Safety coefficient n_s=1.5~2.5, here is 2.55 commonly.

Substitute all parameters into equations (5) and (6), and got $\delta \geq 2.06\times 10^{-3}(m)$.

So the outside diameter of the cylinder is D_2 is $84.12\times 10^{-3}(m)$

For the regular the standard [14], the outside diameter is $D_2=0.095m$, nominal pressure $P_N=16MPa$.

2) The strength of piston [13]

$$d \geq \sqrt{\frac{4F}{\pi[\sigma]}} \tag{7}$$

$$[\sigma] = \frac{\sigma_s}{n_s} \tag{8}$$

D: The diameter of piston. (mm); F- Load applies on the piston(N); $[\sigma]$: Allowable stress of piston's material.(MPa); σ_s: Material's bow limit, $\sigma_s=355MPa$; n_s=2~4.

Substitute all parameters into Eq. (7) and (8), and got $d \geq 17.69$ *and* $[\sigma]=88.75$

So, the diameter of piston is chosen as 50mm, satisfied the requirement of the strength.

4.2 The Parameter of Pressing Paper Hydraulic Cylinder

4.2.1 Working and Back Pressure of Pressing Paper Hydraulic Cylinder

From the regulation of paper enterprising, the value of pressure gauge in pressing progress should maintain the scope of 4~10 MPa, not over 15 MPa[6]. Therefore, the working pressure P_1 of pressing paper hydraulic cylinder is chosen as 11 MPa. From table 3, the back pressure of the hydraulic system is chosen as 0.5 MPa

4.2.2 The Maximum Push Force of Pressing Paper Hydraulic Cylinder

The pressure of the pressing paper machinery i.e. the force on the stuff prepare cutting, its value equals to the pressure resistance and its direction contrary. The maximum pressing force is one of the main performances of paper cutting machine[5]. The type of 920 Litong paper cutting machine's maximum pressing force is 35000N, other types of 920 paper cutting machines are about 30000N. Therefore, the maximum pressing force of paper cutting machine is chosen as 35000 N.

So, the results of the load of pressing paper hydraulic cylinder in different working condition are as follows:

When pressing paper machinery falls, but still not touch the paper pack, considers load as 0. After having touched the paper pack, the pressure of pressing paper hydraulic cylinder is loading. When pressure loading process is over, load is equal to the maximum pressing force. Meanwhile, the pushing force of pressing paper hydraulic cylinder is up to maximum.

While pressing paper machinery returns back, considers load as 0.

4.2.3 The Speed of Pressing Paper Machinery

As the pressing paper machinery descends to touch paper pack, pressing paper hydraulic cylinder enter to pressure loading process. In this process, the paper is pressed solidly. Because the different kinds of paper need different pressing force, the pressure of pressing paper hydraulic cylinder should be controlled between 4~10 *MPa*[6]. The pressing time of pressing paper machinery is corresponded to vary between 0.5*s*~ 5*s* [9]. The softer the texture of paper which needs to cut is, the bigger the pressing force adopts and the longer pressing time is.

Therefore, for calculating the moving speed of pressing paper machinery, supposition as follows.

The moving time of the pressing paper machinery from starting to contact the paper pack is 0.2*s*, the distance is 20*mm*; From touching the paper pack to pressure loading over, spend 5s, the distance is also 20 *mm*. The return speed of pressing paper machinery is 0.0024*m/s*.

The average falling speed of pressing paper machinery v_1=0.1(*m/s*);

The average falling speed of pressure loading process: v_2=0.004*m/s;* the average returning speed, v_3=0.24*m/s*

4.2.4 The Parameter of the Pressing Paper Hydraulic Cylinder

If the chamber with rodless is the working, in term of the simultaneous equations (2) and (3) [11]: Substitute all data into equations (2) and (3), got: D_1 =0.0663(*m*); d_1=0.0386(*m*)

To be ensure that the pressing paper hydraulic cylinder could maintain pressure over 10MPa after having been designed. The serial standard diameter of cylinder is smaller than calculated.

In term of the regular standard GB/ T 2348-1993 and GB/※7933-1987[12], the standard diameter of cylinder and piston are 63*mm and* 45*mm,* respectively.

Thereout, the working area and working pressures of pressing paper hydraulic cylinder are as following:

Rodless chamber area $A_1 = \pi D_1^2/4 = 3.12\times10^{-3}\ m^2$

Rod chamber area $A_2 = \pi(D_1^2 - d_1^2)/4 = 1.53\times10^{-3}\ m^2$

Working pressure $P_1 = (F/\eta_{cm} + P_2A_2)/A_1 = 12.05 Mpa$

Substitute data into equation (4), calculate the max. flow $q_{\max} = 0.367\times10^{-3}\ (m^3/s)$.

4.2.5 Check Strength and Stability of Pressing Paper Hydraulic Cylinder.

(1) Checking the thickness of pressing paper hydraulic cylinder.

Substitute all data into equations (5) and (6), got $\delta \geq 4\times10^{-3} m$

Because $\delta/D = 0.063 \leq 0.08$, the thin wall equations (5) and (6) are not suit for computing the thickness, the thickness of hydraulic cylinder is consideration as medium wall equations for checking. The medium equations [13] (6) and (9):

$$\delta \geq \frac{P_{\max} D}{2.3[\sigma]-3P_{\max}} \tag{9}$$

δ: the thickness of hydraulic cylinder. (*m*); $P_{max:}$ the maximum allowable pressure. *MPa*; when working pressure $P \leq 16MPa$, $P_{max}=1.5P$; *D*: the diameter of hydraulic cylinder (*m*); [σ]: Allowable stress of cylinder's material (*MPa*); $\sigma_{s:}$ Material's bow limit, $\sigma_s=355MPa$. n_s: Safety coefficient n_s=1.5~2.5 commonly.

Substitute all data into equations (6) and (9), got δ ≥4.18*mm;* and the outside diameter $D_2=D+2\delta=71.36$ *mm*

The outside diameter is[14], $D_2=78mm$, nominal pressure $P_N=25MPa$.

(2) The strength of piston [13].

Substitute all data into equations (7) and (8), got d≥22.41*mm;* So the diameter of piston is chosen as 45*mm*, satisfied the requirement of the strength.

5 Design Hydraulic Pump

5.1 The Working Pressure of Hydraulic Hump

$$P_p = P_l + \Sigma\Delta P_l \tag{10}$$

P_p: the maximum pressure of the pump (Mpa); P_l: the maximum pressure of the components (MPa); $\Sigma\Delta P_l$: the total pressure loss of the inlet circuits in the same working condition (MPa); $\Sigma\Delta P_l$ is an experiment data: the throttle speed control system or simple system, $\Sigma\Delta P_l$ = 0.2~0.5 *MPa*, Meter-in inlet or complicated system, $\Sigma\Delta P_l$=0.5~1.5 *MPa,* here: $\Sigma\Delta P_l$=0.5

Substitute P_l =12.05*Mpa* and $\Sigma\Delta P_l$=0.5 *Mpa* into equation (10), got P_p =12.55*Mpa*

5.2 The Flow of Hydraulic Pump

$$Q_p \geq K\,(\Sigma Q_i)_{max}, \tag{11}$$

Here: Q_p: the flow of hydraulic pump; *K*: the leakage coefficient of circuit; ΣQ_i: the total flow of all components

To throttle flow speed control system, the total flow of the system is the maximum flow of the flow control system and the minimum flow of the relief valve (5×10^{-5} m^3/s). Substitute all data into equation (11), got $Q_p \geq 8.8\times10^{-4}$ m^3/s

The gear pump of type CB-F_c31.5 is chosen here, it has character as follows and is satisfied the requirement.

And confirm the power of motor is 11.16*KW*

Table 4. The parameters of the type CB-F_c31.5

type	Theoretic displacement ($ml\cdot r^{-1}$)	Rated pressure (MPa)	Maximum pressure (MPa)	Rated rotate speed ($r\cdot min^{-1}$)
CB-$_c$31.5	32.02	16	20	2000

6 Conclusions

The hydraulic system draft of the fully hydraulic paper cutting machine was got; the control system process was studied in detail in the paper. In term of the structure and cutting method of the paper cutting machine, the different kinds of the loads and speeds of the cutting and pressing paper hydraulic cylinders are calculated. From above results, the diameter of the cutting paper hydraulic cylinder is 80mm, the diameter of the piston is 50 mm; the diameter of the pressing paper hydraulic cylinder is 63mm, the diameter of the piston is 45mm. The strength of the hydraulic cylinder was checked. From the analysis, the parameters of gear pump are: the displacement is 32.02 ml/r, nominal pressure is 16MPa, Nominal rotation is 2000rpm. The power of the motor is over 11.16KW.

References

1. Li, Y., et al.: The Research of Fuzzy Control on Hydraulic of Paper Cutting Machines. China Academic J. Equipment and Instrument (add) 24(4) (2003)
2. The Paper Cutter Gearing in Paper Cutting Machine, China patent No: 02266637.0
3. The Hydraulic Cutting Mechanism of Paper Cutting Machine, China patent No: 2005200002589.5
4. The Electromagnetic Clutch in Gearing of Paper Cutting Machine, China patent No:200420021858.8
5. Zhang, X.S.: A Research for Tests on the Pressure Resistance of Main Loading of Slitters. J. Beijing Institute of Printing 6(2), 14–20 (1998)
6. The Analysis of the main Mechanical Factor which Influences Cutting Quantity, http://www.hc360.com
7. Zhang, X.S.: The Research of Tests on the Main Cutting Resistance of Loading of Slitters. J. Beijing Institute of Printing 5(2), 17–23 (1997)
8. Chen, Y.W.: Analysis and Calculation of Guillotine Level Blade and Oblique Blade Cutting Force. J. Packing and Food Machine 23(5), 27–28 (2005)
9. Hu, Y.K.: The Application of C200H Programmable Controller in QZX1300 Paper Cutter. J. Changzhou Institute of Technology 14(4) (2001)
10. Jia, M.X.: Hydraulic Transmission and Control (ver.2). Defense Industry Publisher (2001)
11. Zhang, L.P.: Hydraulic Transmission System and Designs. Chemistry Industry Publisher (2000)
12. Cai, C.H.: M.E.H Design Handbook. Machine Industry Press, Northeast Univ. press (1997)
13. Dong, F.L.: Hydraulic and Pneumatic Drive. Chemistry Industry publisher (2006)
14. Cheng, D.X.: Mechanical Design Handbook. Chemistry Industry Publisher (2004)

Towards a Network Video Conference System Based-On Group Cooperation Mode for Multidisciplinary Collaborative Product Design

Pengfei Zeng[1,2], Yongping Hao[1], Weiping Shao[1], and Yongxian Liu[2]

[1] R&D Center of CAD/CAM Technology, Shenyang Ligong University
Shenyang, Liaoning Province 110168, China
[2] School of Mechanical Engineering & Automation, Northeastern University
Shenyang, Liaoning Province 110004, China
pfzeng@163.com

Abstract. To meet the needs of multidisciplinary collaborative design process in Web environment, a pure software network video conference system was developed. The system architecture adopts a similarity Browser/Server (B/S) structure. Java Media Framework (JMF) and streaming media transmission and control technology were introduced to system development. System framework and function design were achieved. Interactive processes management and multimedia control mechanism was implemented among media streams of clients' browsers. It was integrated with previous developed Product Data Management (PDM) system. The system provides a real-time multimedia application environment for knowledge communion, information sharing, and conflict resolution, in multidisciplinary collaborative product design process.

Keyword: Multidisciplinary collaborative design, network video conference, group cooperation mode, similarity B/S structure, JMF.

1 Introduction

With the growth of information and computer network technology, computer aided product design are available by means of group cooperation mode. It is mainly developing tendencies of academic research and engineering development in multiple disciplinary domains [1]. Mechanical product development is comprehensive system engineering in modern social. It is difficult to realize product development if we solely rely on knowledge or designers from one particular disciplinary field. Collaborative works of multiple disciplinary experts have become inevitable [2]. In distributed multidisciplinary design process, the information exchange and sharing ways have been extended from E-mail, telephone and white-board to real-time multimedia application environments. Via real-time multimedia interactive environment, the exchange and sharing of knowledge and information is effectively improved, design conflicts are resolved, design cycle is shortened, and the quality of group cooperation is enhanced in the collaborative process.

At present, the existing video conference systems have mostly been realized based on the special network video mode or hardware-based video conference solutions

C. Xiong et al. (Eds.): ICIRA 2008, Part II, LNAI 5315, pp. 311–320, 2008.

[3~7]. The investment costs of hardware or software are expensive, the network environment of system configuration and running requirements are fairly strict, and man-machine operations are complicated to system users. These factors also seriously restrict the usage of traditional video chat tools [8, 9]. They are difficult to meet rarely requirement of video conference for real time, light-weight, quickly response, security, portability, cross platform and scalability, in the collaborative design process.

Extensibility is on the solution to achieve the best effect of the meeting for adapting different conferencing environments by modifying some values and parameters. Up to now, most researches in this respect focus on adaptability of the system for different network surroundings [10]. Three queue models for speech mixing are put forward and analyzed to optimize the program structure and codes for a video-conferencing system [11], which is useful to strengthen the extensibility of the video-conferencing system with the function of real-time speech mixing. One of the goals for system design is to provide efficient solutions for adaptive multimedia transmission over different access networks in all-IP environment [12].

Reference [13] introduces a video-audio meeting system (VAMS) based on H.263 compress method and UDP, design principle and realize process of meeting room was generalized. The difficult problem is explained particularly, for instance, the create process of meeting room, command analysis, synchronization of Audio play and Video display, stereo process of audio data, the transmission of agent server. Reference [14] presents a video conference solution with high ration of performance to price, which based on hardware and ISDN networks. According to the ITU-T Recommendation H.323 Draft 4, the author designed and implemented a multipoint video conference system in [15], which is based on the TCP/IP network and Client/Server structure and running in centralized mode. Reference [16] describes a software development tool-GridON, aimed to provide a video transcodification service using Grid architecture and user controlled lightpaths (UCLP) software for the communication of the participants in an international high-bandwidth network. In reference [17], real-time multimedia applications are integrated into a Web-based robotic telecare system.

In this paper, a video conference system is developed with streaming media technology and JMF [18] for multidisciplinary product collaborative design in Web-based network environment. One of the goals of system design is to provide efficient solutions for adaptive scalability multimedia video conference over different access networks in all-IP network and across Internet environment. System development makes use of Java Bean, Servlet and Applet programming technology. Java Applets detect, capture, acquire, encode and compress multimedia data stream in the client browser side, and form RTP packets and send to the server side. Servlet program modules of server-side are realized to real-time monitor, receive, maintain and transport the video-audio media stream from client browser. Finally, the multimedia data stream is transmitted to others Applet processors, on the demand of participants, it is decoded and playbacked in others client.

The rest of the paper is organized as follows. Section 2 gives an overview of group cooperation and multidisciplinary product collaborative design. Section 3 analysis system development key technologies. Section 4 describes the system architecture design, software functions realization, and PDM system integration. Finally, Section 5 summarizes the conclusions and presents ongoing research and work.

2 Group Cooperation Mode and Multidisciplinary Product Design

A group is composed of some staffs that jointly undertook and completed a job or activity. Virtually, group work consists of a set of group activities and includes personal work and group collaborative work. The emergence of computer supported collaborative work (CSCW) [19] makes the computer not only support individual work, but also support group cooperation together. Consequently, it can give support to multidisciplinary collaborative design work. Multidisciplinary collaborative product design has some characteristics, e.g., distributed, real-time, heterogeneous, complex and parallelism, and so on. The key goals of system realization are to design a video conference system, to adapt for computer supported group cooperation mode, to resolve challenges to distributed-heterogeneous and real-time features of conference processes.

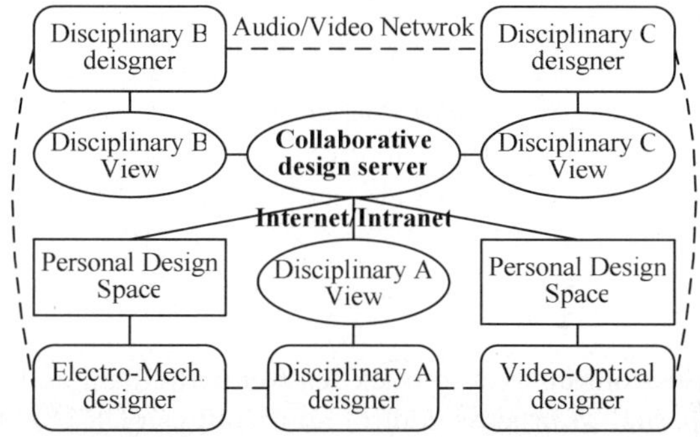

Fig. 1. Integrated multidisciplinary collaborative design in group cooperation mode

In the group cooperation mode, integrated multidisciplinary collaborative product design environment is composed of some model that distributed and multiple disciplinary application tools designed. The environment refers integration and convergence of multiple disciplinary and technology domains, integrates engineering design and analysis technology, modeling and simulation technology, virtual reality technology, et al. Moreover, complex collaborative management of different data, model, engineer, design and activity process are included in the environment. Through network interconnection, group collaborative environment that includes disciplinary designers, engineers, design views and personal design spaces, is established based on the design server. Multimedia interactive environment of audio and video is implemented for each design branch point. The user can distributed and collaborative complete design job or activity. The multidisciplinary collaborative design for group cooperation mode is showed in Fig.1.

3 JMF Media Framework Technology

3.1 JMF

JMF is a series of class set that display and capture multimedia data in Java applications and Applets. JMF API defines an infrastructure, which can capture, transport and play media stream, and the message processing mechanisms and programming design interface. It enables programmers to cross-platform and equipment-independent access audio and video media facility, and provides real-time media playback technology in distributed application environment. It also defines a series of API Plug-ins that enable advanced developers to mort easily customize and extend functionality, and supports media capture and addresses the needs of application developers who want additional control over media processing and rendering. Its high-level architecture is depicted by Figure 2. The application program interface is extended to provide for media processing and multimedia conferencing in JMF 2.1.1e version, which fully supports RTP/RTCP protocols.

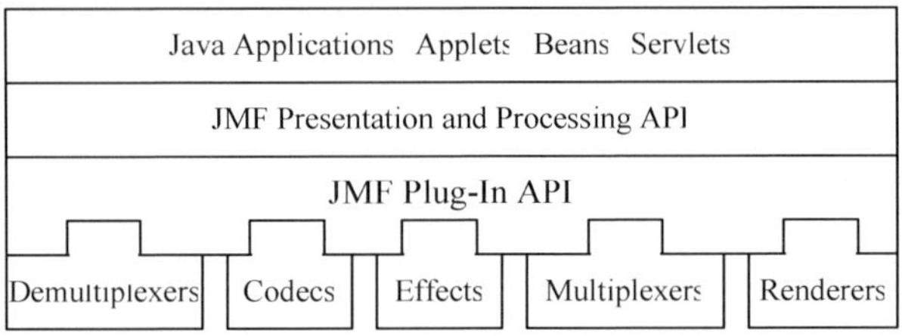

Fig. 2. JMF high-level architecture

JMF RTP uses SessionManager to track session participant and to monitor state of transmission stream, and to process control notifications of RTCP for the sender and the receiver. SessionManager maintains a single RTPStream object for each RTP data packet of session participant. The RTPStream object is divided into send stream object and reception stream object, which separately processes send stream and reception stream. When the SessionManager detects a new RTP datasource, it automatically calls createSendStream to create a send stream object. RTP event are responsible for reporting state of session and media stream.

3.2 Streaming Media Transport and Control

Streaming media is a rising network transmit technology, it can real-time orderly transmit and play audio/video multimedia content of continuous time-based data flows on Internet. Streaming media technology includes capture of media data, encode and decode, store, transmission and playback of video/audio stream. Streaming media control technologies include controllable streaming technology and double-grade buffer technology. The former, streaming media transmission was effected by play rate, bandwidth and client buffer sizes, system dynamically monitors and adjusts these parameters' change to ensure media stream coherent and coordinative. The latter technology that buffer zone is set up in the client end and server side both with a certain redundancy, which makes system may adapt to uncertainty of network transmission and operating system I/O delay, and ensures steady streaming media play over complex network conditions.

RTCP is adopted to enable received-side to synchronize multiple RTP streams. It requests the sender-side send unique marked datasource canonical name for each transmission. Although different media streams have different synchronization source from single datasource, they have the same canonical name, also the received-side knew which streams were relative. While the information contained in the sender-side report packets, can be used to coordinate timestamp values between media streams by the received-side. An absolute time value that expressed network time protocol (NTP) format was included in send-side report packets. That time produced absolute time value, namely the same time engendered TimeStamp field in RTP grouping packets. Since the same absolute time were used by all sent flows and reports from the send-side, the receiver can compare the absolute time of two flows from the same datasource, and conform how timestamp value of one stream can map to another.

RTCP inspects performance and quality of data streams, dynamically controls audio and video flows. Control packet of RTCP manages and controls the creation process of media transmission, according to the control process, transmits local presentation information to other remote nods that provide same multicast address, receives remote presentation information from these nods, establishes elementary link state table, and maintains the link table on the basis of nodes status of withdraw or accession. Consequently, current state of node link is reflected in time, group list of cooperative members is managed and maintained. Each destination nod adjusts the data encode format based on feedback information, checks and locates network faults, controls status of network transmission, drives video/audio encoder to response these changes, raises or lowers production rate of data stream.

4 System Development and PDM Integration

4.1 The Similarity B/S Structure Design

Web-based system has become a platform people acquire information and share knowledge. Distributed application of B/S structure may remarkably shorten costs of enterprises. However, all computing work focus on server-side, which makes server load increase and client-side computing resource fail to full usage. Combining C/S with B/S mode, computing resource is well balanced, cross-platform application is available, and system management and maintain is convenient. In our project, we integrate merits of B/S and C/S structure and adopt the similarity B/S architecture to realize the conference system. The similarity B/S architecture is shown in Figure 3. In the framework, client browsers are accessed to server, security Java Applets are embedded in browser. According to given parameters, Applets can realize different operations, make use of client computing resources to carry out media devices detection, and audio/video capture, encode and compress, reception and transport, decode and display, et, al. Server-side Servlet modules that resemble line concentrator are mainly

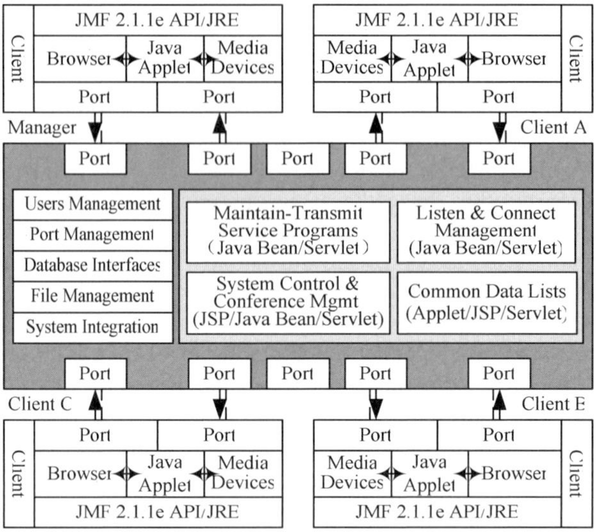

Fig. 3. The group network video conference system architecture

responsible for maintain, transmission, management and control media streams from the client browser, and complete system control and conference data management.

The similarity B/S structure is light-weight, lower costs and higher efficiency. Computing workload is accomplished in client. Server burthen is greatly reduced. The structure makes the users numbers that simultaneously access the system enormously enhance. The conference system is composed of server and client browser. The server-side mainly consists of streaming media server, web server, file/database management server, and programs of JSP, Java Bean/Servlet. Client-end merely needs browser and JMF and JRE. Client operating system may be alternative. Since development program is designed with Java language, which enables the system to run in different platforms, to expediently been transplanted to other servers, and to contribute to cross-platform application integration.

The Web server provide operating platform for JSP, Java Bean/Servlet programs. They answer for interception, analysis and response client browser requests. Programs server-side running is the hard core of the video conference system. Their functions include detection, reception and transmission media streams that are sent to server-side by clients. The port is an important flag to distinguish different media streams. In the system, the same IP address may send different streaming media. It cannot distinguish from different media streams that just using IP address. Therefore, it is very indispensable for each streaming media to set a specific port. Java Applets provide resolutions for browser to employ client computing resources. Login and authentication of system users are realized via client browser. Authorized users can enter the video conference system. In the kind of system framework, HTTP links are fulfilled over JSP pages. Java Applets carry out capture, transmission and display of streaming media in the pages.

4.2 Server Modules and Client Browser Design

The core of the conference system design is centralization-maintain and transmission-on-demand. User makes browsers' Java Applet to detect, compress and pack local media flow, and send it to video server. The maintain modules of server's Java Bean hold media flows from client browser, register its IP address and media stream Port into the common data area, and wait for other clients to request the media stream. If conference user needs to view other clients' media stream, he must send request to the server. Then, the server will search the requested media stream within the maintain array of the common data list. If existing requested clients' media stream, the server will start transmission module and copy media packets from the corresponding port in time, and send it to the user. The system functions design is depicted by Figure 4.

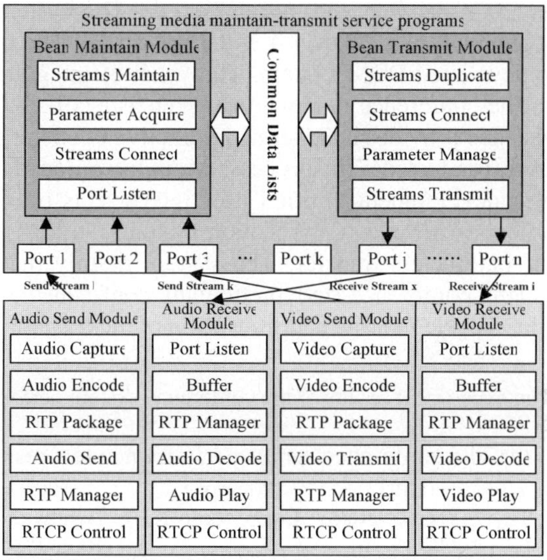

Fig. 4. Network video conference system function design

Via JSP establishing video conference, at the same time, receive Bean and transmit Bean are both instantiated and wait for user operations. When Java Bean receives parameters from client-end, relative operational modules are activated to response user request. The server sets up Java Bean parameters by using the attribute of set and get in JSP pages. The procedure may realize server passive interception. According to these parameters, server turns up listen thread. Servers programs mainly include maintain and transmit services module, interception and connect management, system control and data management, and the common data area. Maintain module is composed of streaming media maintain, parameter acquire, connect management and port interception. The functions of transmit module are divided into media stream replication, connect management, parameter management and transmit function.

Contrast to server, the client browser correspondingly uses the design idea of transmit-request. The process user joins the video conference, mainly includes system login, media send and reception, and so on. Detection Applet module completes media device detection work in login page. When user succeeds in entering the conference room, he can choose to send the local media stream to conference or request other users' media streams. JSP pages access browser parameters. The Applet captures media devices and compresses media streams and sends it to the server. When user requests media content, applet sends request parameters to server, and server transmits the requested stream to client browser Applet, which constructs a media manager to manage it and the process of decompression and playback in time. If user chooses to logout, the server withdraws user information and releases user media stream manager, and aborts transmission of media stream.

4.3 System Realization and PDM Integration

We choose Windows 2000 Server to develop the conference system, adopt Apache 2.0.59 and Tomcat 5.0.30 as web and system server. The system software running environment is implemented with JDK 1.4 and JMF 2.1.1e. The project is integrated into the previously developed PDM system. The work of integration with PDM was accomplished [20]. The conference modules are taken as a collaborative workspace in the PDM. The workspace provides a real-time interactive cooperative environment for network collaborative product design process. Modularization design technology is introduced to system development, unified user interface is provided, which predigests integration process with others application systems. In fact, the system integration is a process of parameters transfer. The system mainly includes two kinds of functions, management conference and participant conference. Audio/video detect module, sent module, receive module and transmit module are embedded in the PDM.

Table 1. The experiment results of the conference system performance test

(a) The conference server performance test results

User Counts	CPU Usage Ratio (%)	Memory Usage Ratio(KB)	100M Bandwidth Usage Ratio (%)
1	2.4	10045	1.2
2	8.1	10530	4.5
3	17.9	15105	8.3
4	28.4	23780	17.9
5	36.9	32195	22.3

(b) The video browser-end performance test results

User Counts	CPU Usage Ratio (%)	Memory Usage Ratio(KB)	100M Bandwidth Usage Ratio (%)
1	9.8	10345	1.2
2	14.7	12015	2.3
3	17.1	15470	3.5
4	25.3	20185	4.8
5	35.4	31680	6.2

The adopted client browser is Microsoft Internet Explorer, which version was 6.0. In our experimental setting, the conference management server is used with a Pentium IV CPU 2.0 GHZ processor, 512MB over the Internet with global IPv4 address; the client browser side is an Intel Pentium III 733 MHZ processor, 256MB in Windows 2000 Professional OS, which select a Logitech QuickCam Pro 4000 Webcam with USB connector as video camera, and a 100M LAN network card. The experimental results of system performance test are listed in Table 1. Table 1(a) is the result of server performance test in which user counts change from1 to 5, and Table 1(b) is the experimental result of client browser terminal in the conference process.

5 Conclusions

Aimed at integrated multidisciplinary collaborative product design process in group cooperation mode, the pure software network video conference system is developed. It is Web-based similarity B/S structure. The system makes full use of multimedia technology and JMF architecture technology. RTP programming mechanisms and RTCP streaming media control and synchronize mechanisms are come true. System framework, functions and interactive processes control design are achieved. Computer codes are compiled, and integration with PDM system is realized. Through JMF and relative technologies of multimedia data process, the network conference is achieved for remote distributed group collaborative product design.

Modularized design is convenient for integrating with others legacy systems. As a result of introducing to Java language, transplantable of cross-platform is well guaranteed. Via application and proof, the system performance is comparatively stabile, and has preferably compatibility, extendibility and reliability. The conference system supplies a real-time, lower cost, higher effective and agile, and friendly interface multimedia applications environment for network multidisciplinary collaborative design process. However, system usage was affected by other factors, for instances, client computer performance, and network connection speed and concurrency users' numbers. The next step will lucubrate to improve the system quality of services (QoS) of media streams.

Reference

1. Lei, Y.: Study of Common Integrated Framework Supporting Group Work. Doctor dissertation. Institute of Computing Technology, Chinese Academy of Sciences (2001)
2. Liang, C., Guodong, J.: Research on Product Multi-disciplinary Collaborative Design Based on Multiple Views Model. China Mech. Eng. 23 15, 2092–2097 (2004)
3. Qinghua, F., Zhenghong, D., Wei, Z.: Design and Realization of Distributed Video Meeting System in WAN. Computer Engineering. 17 30, 157–159 (2004)
4. Ling, S., Yan, C.: Research and Implement of a Software Videoconferencing System Based on H.323. Computer Engineering and Applications. 19 42, 208–211 (2006)
5. Chuanjian, Y., Zhe, C., Yonglin, Z.: IP Multicast Desktop Video Conferencing System in IE Browser. Computer Engineering and Design. 19 27, 3568–3570 (2006)
6. Civanlar, M.R., Özkasap, Ö., Çelebi, T.: Peer-to-Peer Multipoint Video Conferencing on the Internet. Signal Processing: Image Communication. 8 20, 743–754 (2005)

7. Wang, C., Griebel, S., Brandstein, M.: Robust Automatic Video Conferencing with Multiple Cameras and Microphones. In: IEEE Int. Conf. on Multimedia and Expo, ICME 2000, New York, NY, USA, vol. 3, pp. 1585–1588 (2000)
8. Xu, G., Subin, S., Guanqun, G.: Design and Implemention of a Network Video Tool for Video Conferencing over Internet. Computer Applications. 8 20, 11–13 (2000)
9. Guifang, Z., Guiming, F.: Design and Implementation of Platform Independent Video on Demand System Based on JMF. Application Research of Computers. 4 24, 235–238 (2007)
10. Strobel, N., Spors, S., Rabenstein, R.: Joint Audio-Video Object Localization Using a Recursive Multi-state Multi-sensor Estimator. In: IEEE Int. Conf. on Acoustics, Speech and Signal Processing, ICASSP 2000, vol. 6, pp. 5–9 (2000)
11. Yang, S., Ma, B.: Study on the Extensibility of Video Conferencing with Speech Mixing. Computer Communications. 11 29, 2026–2033 (2006)
12. Huusko, J., Vehkaperä, J., Amon, P., et al.: Cross-Layer Architecture for Scalable Video Transmission in Wireless Network. Signal Processing: Image Communication. 3 22, 317–330 (2007)
13. Xining, L., Yushan, Z.: Research and Design of VAMS Based on H.263 Compress Method and UDP. Computer Engineering and Design. 7 28, 1578–1580 (2007)
14. Xiaochun, C., Zhen, Y., Jianhua, L.: A Solution of Video Conference with High Ratio of Performance to Price. Computer Engineering. 11 26, 136–137 (2000)
15. Yong, C., De, X.: Design and Implementation of a Video Conference System over Internet. Computer Engineering and Applications. 13 41, 221–223 (2005)
16. Grasa, E., Figuerola, S., Recio, J., et al.: Video Transcoding in a Grid Network with User Controlled Lightpaths. Future Generation Computer Systems. 8 22, 920–928 (2006)
17. Hou, C., Jia, S., Takase, K.: Real-Time Multimedia Applications in a Web-based Robotic Telecare System. Journal of Intelligent and Robotic Systems 38, 135–153 (2003)
18. JMF-Reference, `http://java.sun.com/products/java-media/jmf/reference/index.html`
19. He, F., Han, S.: A Method and Tool for Human-Human Interaction and Instant Collaboration in CSCW-based CAD. Computers in Industry. 57, 740–751 (2006)
20. Pengfei, Z., Yongping, H., Chonghai, W., et al.: The research of Technology for Product Data Management with Web. Manufacturing Information Engineering of China. 11, 75–77 (2004)

Straightening Model and Prediction of Straightening Stroke of Precision Linear Guide Rail

Hong Lu[1], Xiao Zhang[1], Juergen Leopold[2], He Ling[1], and Changqiao Guo[1]

[1] School of Mechanical and Electronic Engineering, Wuhan University of Technology, Wuhan, China
[2] Fraunhofer Institute for Machine Tools and Forming Technology, Chemnitz, Germany
{Hong Lu,landzh}@whut.edu.cn

Abstract. In order to improve the straightening precision of flexible automatic straightening machine, a new way of establishing straightening model and predicting straightening stroke is proposed based on bending experiment. In this paper, aiming at the LG series linear guide rails, the mathematical load-stroke model of press straightening process is established based on elastic-plastic theory. The stroke-deflection model can be obtained by simulating the bending process of guide rails based on loading-unloading FEA analysis. And then the precision straightening model of predicting straightening stroke, which is describe as a simplicity formula, can be fit out based on establishing compensation knowledge base achieved from bending experiment and experimental data processing. The experimental results verify this method's feasibility. It will be helpful to the development of automatic straightening machine's control system.

Keywords: Straightening; Load-stroke model; Linear guide rail.

1 Introduction

Because of the external or internal force and temperature variation in work processing and transporting, metal bar may be bending or being distortion deformed easily. In order to obtain the high precision product, it should be straightened. The press straightening method, having big straightening force, best flexibility and high controllability and precision, could be applied to various degrees contraflexure of metal bar extensively.

With the appearance of automatic straightening machine, the theory of straighten process have gradually becoming the focus of current precision straightening controlling research. However, improving the precision of straightening theoretical model is still difficult. Reference [1] and [2] propose a way of establishing straighten theoretical model by controlling stroke, which is key factor of the straighten stroke accuracy calculation. Generally, the straighten stroke can be calculated according to the theory of elastic-plastic, FEM or empirical formula. But all of them have their limitation. At present, most studies focus on shaft and tubular bar, seldom on the irregular sectional. Besides, the straightening models rely overly on theory and have large calculation difficulty and lack practicability.

C. Xiong et al. (Eds.): ICIRA 2008, Part II, LNAI 5315, pp. 321–328, 2008.

The purpose of this paper is to establish precision straighten model and predict the straightening stroke which aiming at the LG series linear guide rails of irregular section. Firstly, the load-stroke model can be established by different conventional methods. Then the most important is the precision straightening model of predicting straightening stroke which is describe as a simplicity and precision formula can be fit out based on establishing compensation knowledge achieved from bending experiment and experimental data processing. Comparing these models, the precision straightening model will also verify and modified the former. It will be helpful to the development of automatic straightening machine's control system.

2 The Straightening Model Based on Elastic-Plastic Theory

2.1 Press Straightening Process of 3-Points Reverse Bending

In the process of press straightening, linear guide rail can be divided into a number of single-arcs to do multi-step straightening. Take single-arc for example, straightening process is comprised of reverse bending phase and elastic springback phase.Fig.1. shows the load-stroke (F-δ) curve model of straightening process[2]. In this figure, the loading process includes elastic deformation stage AB and elastic-plastic deformation stage BC, according to the simple law of unloading , the stage CD is considered elastic springback stage, so the line of AB and CD have the same slope K, point B is the yield point of elastic stage. If we have measured the initial deflection of guide δ_0, the location of point D will be defined, and then the location of point C which determines the corresponding straightening stroke δ_c and straightening load F_c can be known.

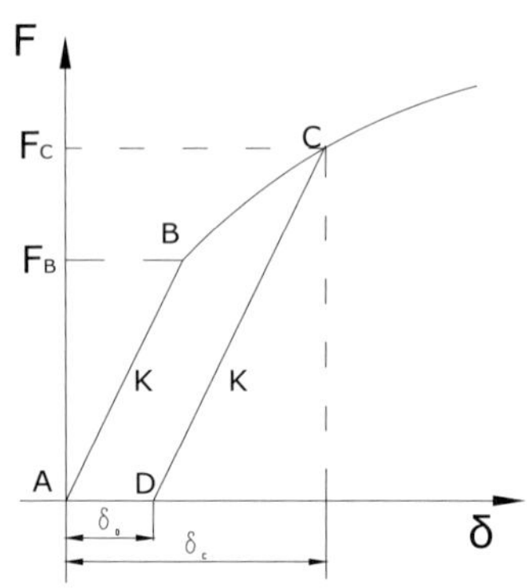

Fig. 1. The Load-Stroke Model

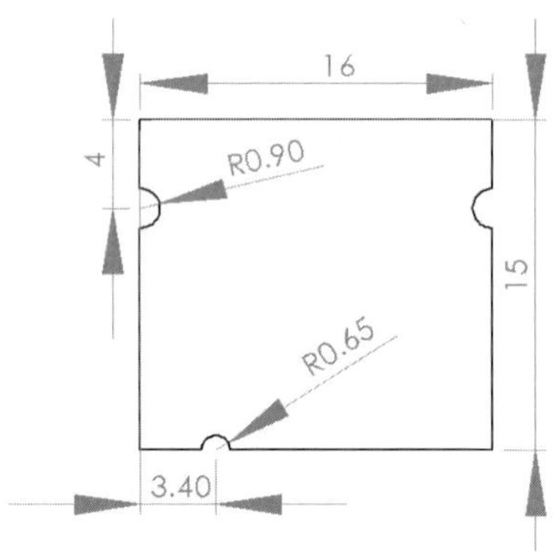

Fig. 2. The Cross-Section of Linear Guide Rail

2.2 The Mathematical Model of Straightening Process

We do analysis of straightening process on the basis of plane assumption and ignoring the impact of Bauschinger effect due to the deformation of bending is relatively so small for span. Fig.2 Shows the cross-section diagram of LG series linear guide rail. The material of rails is GCr15 bearing steel, so the stress-strain model was assumed to be an ideal model for elastic-plastic materials. As this cross-section is similar to rectangle, we analysis it according to the theory of rectangular section while the actual sectional moment of inertia (I) should be calculated. According to Fig.1, the mathematical model of each stage had been established.

2.2.1 The Elastic Loading and Unloading Stages

In Fig.2, the Load-Stroke relationship in elastic loading stage (AB segment) is:

$$F = \frac{6EI}{l^3}\delta \qquad (0 < F \le F_B) \tag{1}$$

The Load-Stroke relationship in elastic unloading stage (CD segment) is:

$$F = \frac{6EI}{l^3}(\delta - \delta_0) \qquad (0 < F \le F_C) \tag{2}$$

Where F is the value of load, δ is the value of stroke, δ_0 is the value of initial deflection, E is elastic modulus for the material, I is sectional moment of inertia, l is half of span. F_b is the limit load for elastic; F_c is the limit load for elastic-plastic.

2.2.2 The Elastic-Plastic Loading Stage[3]

On the elastic-plastic loading stage, according to the bending stress-strain relationship of the guide rail and the material property, and by analyzing the relationship between deflection and curvature in the elastic-plastic deformation, the pushdown stroke (δ) at the middle point of the guide rail can be expressed as[3]

$$\begin{cases} \delta = \dfrac{M_t}{3EI}\dfrac{l^2}{\overline{M}^2}[5-(3+\overline{M})\sqrt{3-2\overline{M}}\,] \\ F = \dfrac{2M_t}{l}\overline{M} \end{cases} \qquad (\overline{M} \in [1,1.5]) \tag{3}$$

where $\overline{M}$ is plastic-bending ratio, M_t is the elastic ultimate moment.

2.2.3 The Straightening Load-Stroke Model

Aiming at the LG series guide rail, the property of material and parameters as following: the elastic modulus E=190089MPa, yield stress σ_t =382Mpa, span 2l=200(mm). So the straightening load-stroke model of linear guide rail can be calculated through mathematic model. (As Fig.3.)

Programming in MATLAB software based on this model and mathematical model, it will be convenient to get the straightening stroke when the initial deflection has been measured. From this Fig, each time the max straightening stroke is 3(mm), or the guide rail may be break down. So the guide rail can be straightened by muti-step.

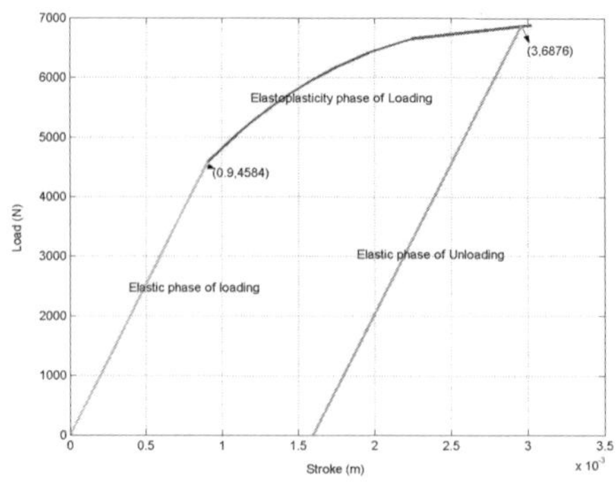

Fig. 3. The Straightening Load-Stroke Model based on Theory

3 The Straightening Model Based on FEM Simulation

3.1 The Process of Simulation Analysis

Analyze the press straightening process of 3-points reverse bending of LG guide rail by using finite element analysis software ANSYS. It is a process for Material Nonlinear analysis. Firstly, the finite element model of the LG guide rail has been established. The guide rail is 220 mm long while the span is 200 mm and the initial deflection is 0. Some parameters of material property which gained from the bending experiment of the sample are all the same with the former while Poisson's ratio P= 0.28. We adopt 3-dimensional solid element (SOLID185) which can give accurate result to do this simulating. The model is constituted of 7898 elements and 9453 nodes.

The rail has been defined the boundary conditions by actual load case, that is constraining both ends of the span and loading at the mid-span position. The simulation process includes loading and unloading steps. Then we can use the APDL language to program the whole process. Thus the corresponding pushdown stroke and residual deflection can be received in postprocess when apply a group of pressures or strokes.

3.2 Results and the Stroke-Deflection Model

Fig.4 shows the displacement contoured map of Y direction when loads 1000(N) pressure at the mid-span of guide rail while Fig.5 shows the map when unload the pressure to 0. The max stroke is 0.173 mm in loading stage (AS Fig.4) while the residual deflection is 0.218e-8 mm after unloading (as Fig.5). It can be seen the guide rail is at fully elastic stage from this. So the load–stroke model (as Fig.6) can be established from the data of load, stroke and residual deflection during the whole process. It is similar to the model established by elastic-plastic theory (as Fig.3) that proves the validity of the theoretical model. According to the model, the stroke-deflection models which can predict the straightening stroke of guide rail by only know the initial deflection can be established as fig.7.

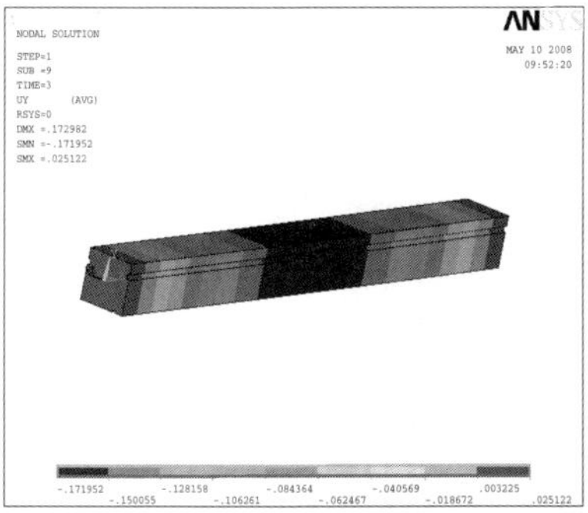

Fig. 4. The displacement contoured map by load1000N

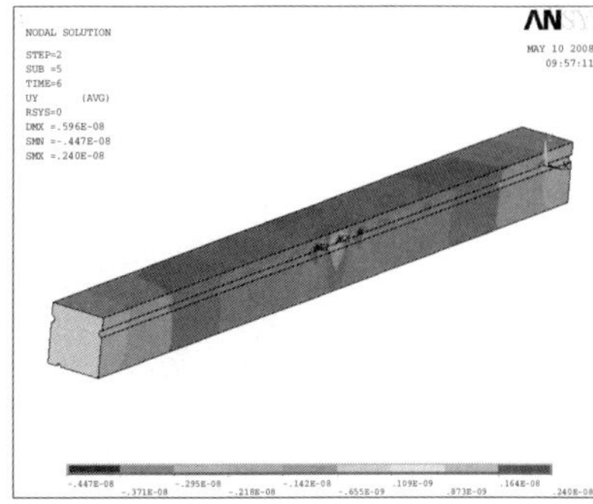

Fig. 5. The displacement contoured map after unload

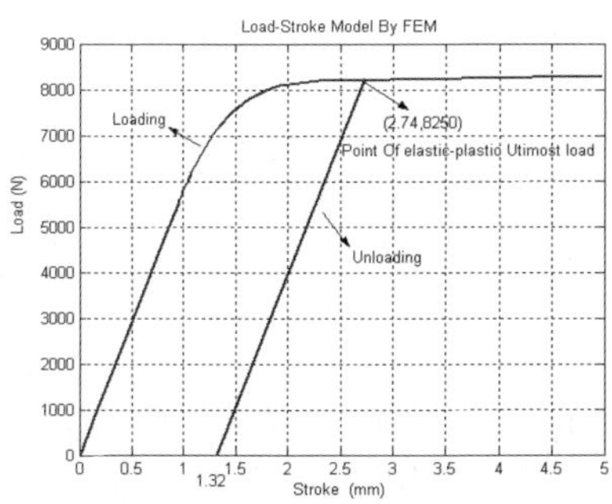

Fig. 6. The load-Stroke Model by FEM

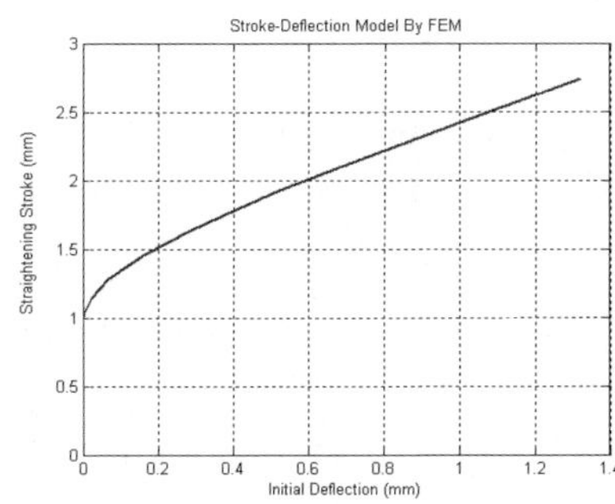

Fig. 7. The Stroke-deflection Model by FEM

4 Experiment

3-points bending experiment has been adopt to research the law of structure deformation in response to the load in the mid-span of this guide rail due to the press straightening process is really a 3-points reverse bending process. The load–stroke model can be established by the experiment data and consist of the compensation knowledge base of straightening model. It will be standard model to verify and modify the model which established by other methods .The straightening stroke also can be accurately predict from it.

4.1 Experiment Scheme

The bending experiment was carried out by the Instron1341 electro-hydraulic servo material testing machine, which has relative error of load precision less than 0.5%.The displacement and load data are exported through corresponding sensor .The whole working process are operated through software.

Fig.8 shows the bending experiment apparatus .The material and the experiment conditions are all the same of the simulation conditions. The bending process has been divided into three steps: pressure control loading, stroke control loading and unloading step, which in order to measure the accurate value of stroke and position of guide rail because of the experiment equipment restriction.

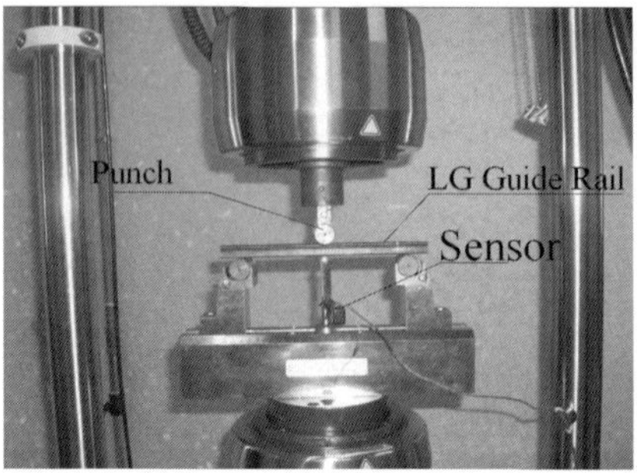

Fig. 8. The Bending Experiment Apparatus of the Guide Rail

The first step of bending process is controlled by loading 1000N pressure, which located in fully elastic stage. When loading out of 1000N, it comes to the second step, which is loading by displacement control and the displacement can be set in rang of limit stroke. When the guide rail arrive the designated position, it comes to the third step that is unloading completely. Do this experiment by different value of pushdown stroke, then a lot of real-time data of position and pressure in the mid-span of rail can be obtained from the computer. Therefore we have to obtain the stroke and corresponding residual deflection which used to established straightening model by data processing.

4.2 Experimental Data Processing

The recorded experimental data are real-time absolute position and pressure of the mid-span of rail. The initial position of mid-span of the rail can be got from each curve model by this data. The material stage of guide rail also can be seen from them. The initial position in the first experiment is 29.203mm, which is set to be the relative coordinate 0 and the pushdown direction is set to be the positive direction for the purpose of conveniently dealing with the data. Table 1 shows the stroke and load data after data processing.

Table 1. The Load-Stroke Data of Experiments

Experimental sequence number	Stroke(mm)	Relative position before loading(mm)	Relative position after unloading(mm)	springback (mm)	Load (N)
1	0.612	0	0	0.612	3252.78
2	0.714	0	0.00346	0.71054	3434.6
3	0.811	0.00346	0.0036	0.81086	4773.92
…	…	…	…	…	…
29	3.221	2.54816	3.90416	1.865	7983.5
30	3.722	3.90416	5.6416	1.98456	8450

4.3 Experimental Results

The straightening load-stroke model can be reverse established from the bending experiment data in table 1 as show in Fig.9.The model is one component of the straightening model compensation knowledge base which can verify and modify the form models.

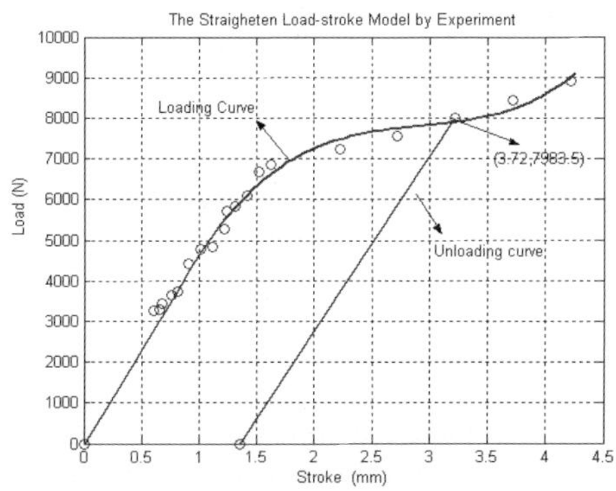

Fig. 9. The Straightening Load-Stroke Model based on Experiment

4.4 The Precision Straightening Model and Prediction Formula of Straightening Stroke of LG Guide Rail

Fig.10 is the contrast diagram of Straightening load-stroke model of LG Guide Rail which established by three different methods. It can be seen there are similar on the whole such as the distribution of three stages in press straightening process and the max deflection can be straightened at a time. However, the ultimate stroke in elastic-plastic stage and the corresponding pressure has large difference. It may be caused by the stress-strain model which was assumed to be an ideal model for elastic-plastic materials while the model is more complicated in fact.

By comparison, the straightening load-stroke model established by experiment data can be regarded as the precision straightening model. (As Fig.9 shows).From this model and the experiment data, the precision straightening stroke-deflection model can be fit as Fig.11. The simplicity formula for Predicting the Straightening Stroke ,which will be more useful to automatic straightening machine's control system ,can be fit to polynomial by using the least square method in MATLAB software. It is expressed as:

$$\begin{aligned} &S = -0.1398D^3 - 0.1268D^2 + 2.369D + 0.9066 \\ &D \in (0,1.4) \end{aligned} \tag{4}$$

Where S is the straightening stroke, D is the initial deflection.

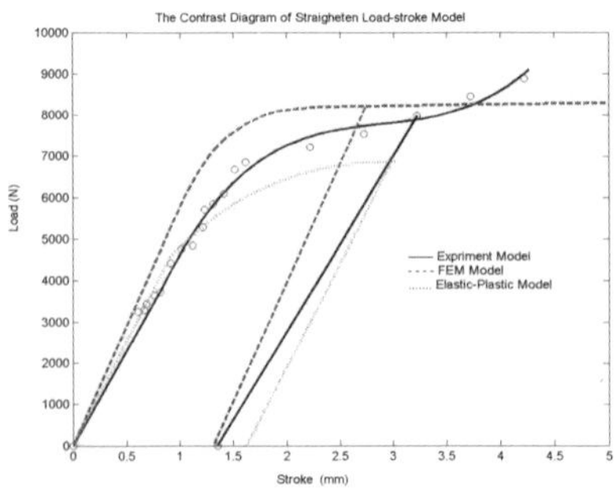

Fig. 10. The Contrast Diagram of Straightening Load-stroke Model

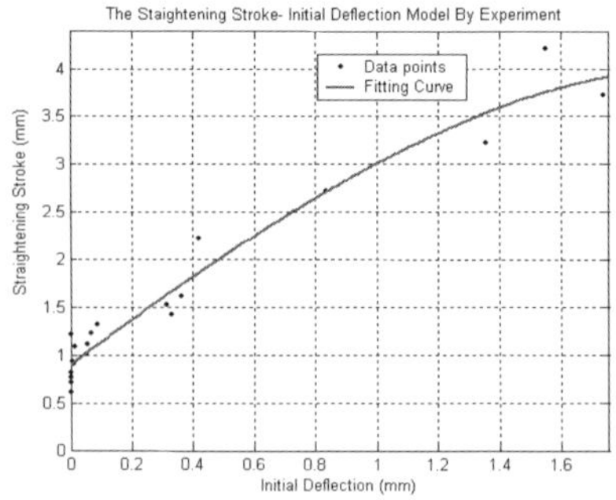

Fig. 11. The Precision Straightening Stroke-deflection Model

5 Conclusion

In the above, the straightening model compensation knowledge base of LG series linear guide rail has been established by experimental method.It has been compared with the straightening load-stroke model established by elastic-plastic theory and the straightening load-stroke model established by FEM simulation. Thus the precision straightening model has been defined and the simplicity of simplicity formula for predicting the Straightening Stroke can be fit based on the stroke-deflection model. The model obtained by this way has higher precision, and the stroke prediction formula can be applied to automatic straightening machine conveniently.However, certain limitations exist in this way ,such as the cost of experimental is high, the experimental method is suited to the parts which should be straightened in mass and the part is muti-deflection bending. Therefore, the theory of multi-point and multi-step straightening control is the emphasis of research in next step.

References

1. Qin, M.H., Ke, Z.Z., Jiang, S.R., et al.: Study On Straightening Technical Theory of Shaft-kind in Exact Straightening Press. Journal of Mechanical Engineering 33(2), 48–53 (1997) (in Chinese)
2. Li, J.: Research On Theoretical Model of Press Straightening Process and Its Experiment. Journal of Mechanical Strength 27(5), 636–639 (2005) (in Chinese)
3. Pu, C.: Straightening Theory and Parameters Calculation. Mechanical Industry Press, Beijing (1994) (in Chinese)
4. Li, J., Xiong, G.L., Zhou, H.J.: Process Modeling and Stroke Calculation for Shaft Straightening. J. Heave Machine 6, 41–44 (2004) (in Chinese)
5. Das Talukder, N.K., Singh, A.N.: Mechanics of bar straigtening. Part 1: General Analysis of Straightening Process. Journal of Engineering for Industry 113(2), 224–227 (1991)
6. Katoh, T., Urata, E.: Measurement and Control of a Straightening Process for Seamless Pipes. Journal of Engineering for Industry 115(3), 347–351 (1993)

Finite Element Modeling of Part Distortion

T.D. Marusich, S. Usui, and K. J. Marusich

Third Wave Systems, Inc, 7900 West 78th St. Suite 300, Minneapolis, MN 55439

Abstract. Airframe designs for modern commercial and military aircraft contain hundreds of monolithic metal structural components machined from solid plate or forgings of aluminum and titanium. The start-to-finish weight ratio for these components is easily 20:1 and greater, meaning that more than 95% of the initial material is machined away. The resulting thin-walled structure often distorts due to the removal of bulk material stresses and the application of machining-induced stresses. To alleviate the distortion, current practices rely on taking small depths of cut and flipping the part several times. This results in long cycle times, high cost and under utilization of large machining equipment. A finite element model has been developed specifically to predict and control these distortions. The model takes into consideration the machining induced residual stresses as well as the bulk stresses in the material from the manufacturer. It is the combination of these two residual stress components coupled with the geometry of the part and type of material that allows us to accurately predict, manage and control the shape and magnitude of deformation in large thin walled structures. The model can be used to determine the ideal cutting conditions for the process as well as determine the best location within the stock plate to machine the part from. Multiple machining tests have been done in order to validate the accuracy of the model.

1 Introduction

Residual stresses in the part have a significant quality and cost impact in many machining operations. This is particularly true for large airframe and similar components, since strains induced by residual stresses may lead to significant distortion. This can lead to a high scrap rate for some components, and to extended machining times if material is removed in multiple light passes to control distortion.

Residual stresses in machined parts result from two sources. Prior to machining, bulk stresses from primary processes such as rolling or forging may be present in the workpiece. Superimposed on these are residual stresses induced by the machining process, which result from differential plastic deformation and surface temperature gradients [1]. Significant distortions can arise from both sources, particularly in thin-walled parts.

There has been considerable research on predicting machining-induced residual stresses, most recently using finite elements methods [2-7]. Predictions of the most advanced models are qualitatively accurate (with respect to the shape of the subsurface stress distribution and the influence of major input variables); given the difficulty of repeatably measuring residual stresses, model predictions are as reliable as

C. Xiong et al. (Eds.): ICIRA 2008, Part II, LNAI 5315, pp. 329–338, 2008.

measurements in many cases. There has been little work, however, on predicting distortion in a machined structure due to bulk residual stresses from a primary process, although as noted above distortions from this source are often significant in thin-walled structures.

This paper describes an integrated approach to predicting distortions in machined structures due to both bulk and machining-induced residual stresses. Previously reported work on predicting machining-induced residual stresses through finite element modeling is briefly reviewed in Section 2. In Section 3, the integration of theses stresses into a toolpath analysis program which also takes into account bulk stresses to predict distortions is described. Preliminary comparison of analytical predictions with measurements for airframe components are reviewed in Section 4. Section 5 summarizes conclusions and areas for further research.

2 Finite Element Calculation of Machining Induced Residual Stresses

For this research, machining residual stresses were calculated using AdvantEdge™, an explicit dynamic, thermo-mechanically coupled finite element model specialized for metal cutting. Features necessary to model metal cutting accurately include adaptive remeshing capabilities for resolution of multiple length scales such as cutting edge radius, secondary shear zone and chip load; multiple body deformable contact for tool-workpiece interaction, and transient thermal analysis. A comprehensive discussion on the numerical techniques and validation examples are available in the literature [8,9].

In order to model chip formation, constitutive modeling for metal cutting requires determination of material properties at high strain rates, large strains, and short heating times and is quintessential for prediction of segmented chips due to shear-localization [10,11]. Specific details of the constitutive model used are outlined in [8]. The model contains deformation hardening, thermal softening and rate sensitivity tightly coupled with a transient heat conduction analysis appropriate for finite deformations.

Machining-induced residual stresses are computed by thermo-mechanically relaxing the workpiece after machining. After the tool passes, thermo-mechanical computations are continued until transient thermal gradients in the machined surface dissipate and the work sample comes an equilibrium configuration with a resultant residual stress distribution.

3 Integrating Bulk and Machining Induced Residual Stresses

To determine the effects of both machining induced and bulk residual stresses on distortion of a machined structure, an approach combining FEA results with toolpath-level analysis is required. Fig. 1 show the approach used in this research. The Tool Path Analysis component, adapted from the AdvantEdge Production Module, a commercially available mechanistic model for 5-axis end milling [12], reads in the initial workpiece geometry, tool path, workpiece material properties, and generates the final geometry of the workpiece. The Distortion Prediction component generates a mesh of the final geometry of the workpiece, builds a finite element model, imposes bulk stresses and residual stresses from machining onto the model and performs an equilibrium analysis. Results of predicted workpiece distortions are displayed through a visualization tool.

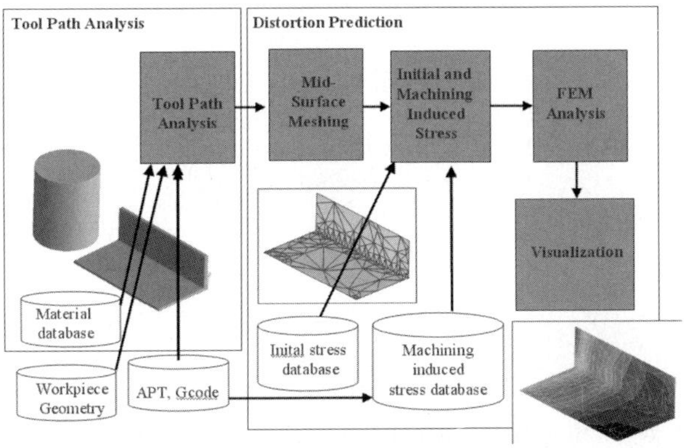

Fig. 1. Approach to modeling distortion

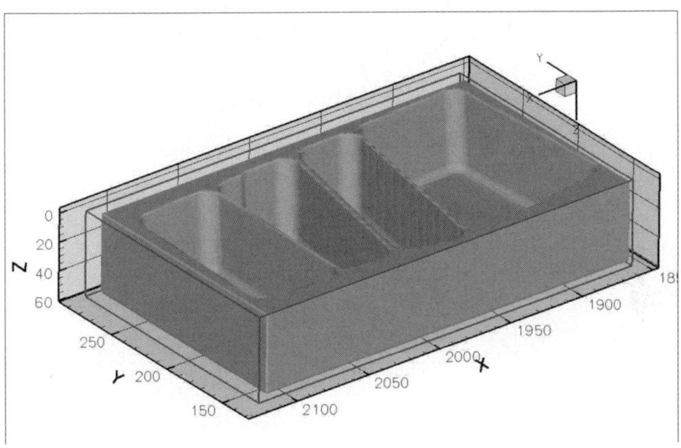

Fig. 2. Solid model of four pocket part

The Toolpath Analysis component is based on well known mechanistic modeling approaches and will not be described. The modules that make up the Distortion Prediction component are described in the following.

Workpiece Meshing

Using existing methods for toolpath generation and Boolean subtraction of workpiece material along toolpath, the final geometry of the thin-walled workpiece is generated. From the final geometry, a shell mesh is generated.

A typical part for illustrating this procedure is shown in Fig. 2. In this part all ribs are perpendicular to the XY plane, but can taper in the Z-direction.

The thin-walled workpieces are modeled by a mesh of triangular shell elements. The solution is obtained by implicit methods.

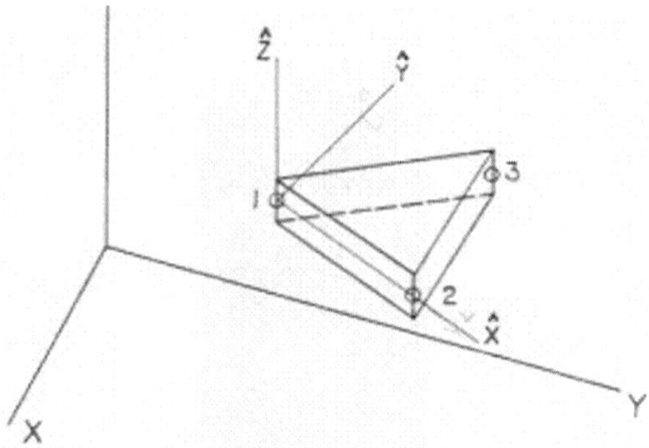

Fig. 3. Local and global coordinate systems

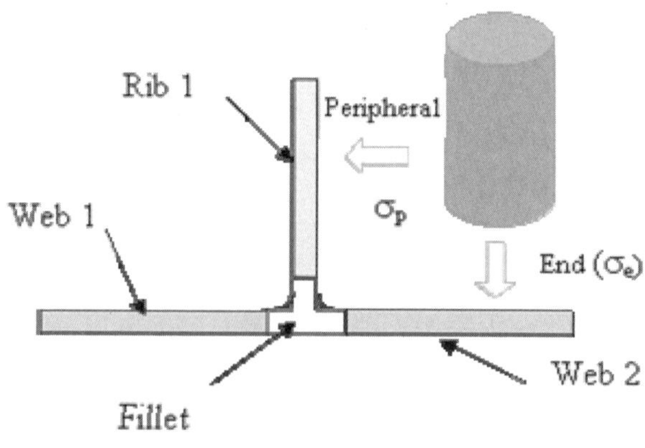

Fig. 4. Typical thin-walled section

Explicit stiffness matrix expressions for plate element are used where all stiffness matrix computations are done in a local coordinate system defined for each element. With reference to Fig. 3, the origin of the local coordinate system is located at node 1. The local X-axis is defined by the unit vector ($\mathbf{e}_{12}$) along a line connecting node 1 to node 2.

The unit vector along local Z axis ($\mathbf{e}_z$) is obtained by taking the cross product of $\mathbf{e}_{12}$ and $\mathbf{e}_{13}$, where $\mathbf{e}_{13}$ is the unit vector along a line connecting node 1 to node 3. Finally, unit vector along local Y axis ($\mathbf{e}_y$) is obtained by taking the cross product of $\mathbf{e}_z$ and $\mathbf{e}_{12}$.

The rearranged stiffness matrix is transformed to global coordinate system and assembled into the global stiffness matrix.

Fig. 4 shows a section of typical thin-walled components to be analyzed. The geometry consists of ribs (walls), webs (flanges) and fillets. Ribs are subjected to machining induced stresses from side cutting whereas webs are subjected to machining induced stresses from end milling. In general, the fillet region is small compared to the cross-section of the component. As a first approximation, it may be assumed that stress in the fillet regions do not contribute significantly to the overall distortion of the part. With this, the mapping task simplifies to determining procedures for wall and rib mapping.

Machining induced stresses for different process conditions, computed through finite element calculations as discussed above, are stored in a machining induced stress database. The database consists of machining induced stress profiles (Fig. 5) as function of the cutting speed, feed rate, depth of cut, tool nose radius, and radial and axial rake angles.

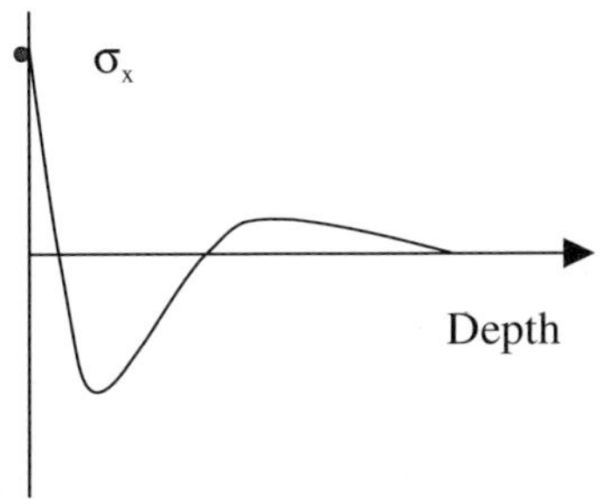

Fig. 5. Typical machining induced stress profile

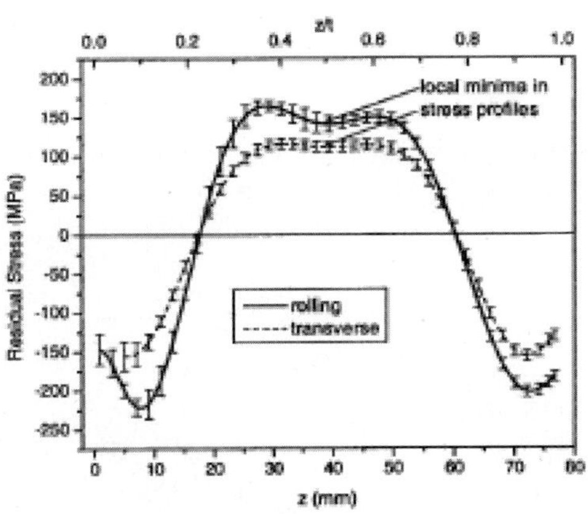

Fig. 6. Residual stresses in 80 mm thick 7050 T74 Al plate [13]

Fully three-dimensional stress profiles on the machined surface can be stored.

The toolpath is used to obtain the solid model of the final geometry of the workpiece. The machining induced stress mapping is performed on the surface of the thin-walled workpiece. Residual stresses are determined from the database with process parameters computed at the workpiece surface and applied to the corresponding element in the mesh. Nodal forces in the element due to applied residual stresses are computed and stored to be used later in the assembly of the global RHS vector. Nodal forces from residual stresses are computed and stored for all elements on the surface.

Bulk stresses from the primary process are incorporated in an analogous manner. Limited published data for these profiles is available in the literature; a typical example is shown in Fig. 6 [13]. These stresses are applied to the mesh in a manner analogous to that used for the machining induced stresses.

Once the stresses are applied, assembly of the global stiffness matrix, global right hand side (RHS) vector and application of boundary conditions are done using standard Finite Element techniques.

4 Preliminary Application to Aerospace Components

Analyses were carried out for two aerospace structural parts provided by EADS, the fillet rib and pressure bulkhead shown in Figs. 7 and 8. Both the parts are made of Al7050 and have several pockets, thin walls of different thicknesses, and 5-axis walls.

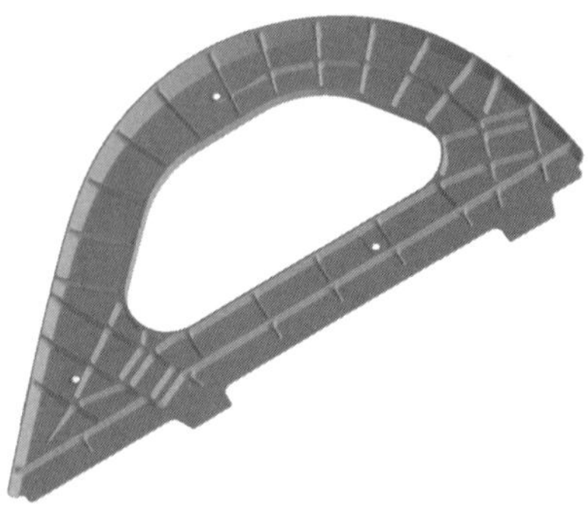

Fig. 7. Fillet rib (1.51 m x 785mm x 38mm)

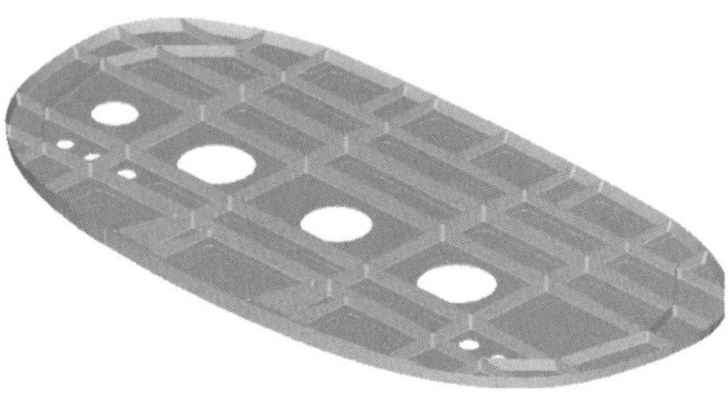

Fig. 8. Pressure Bulkhead (1.63m x 3.14m x 76mm)

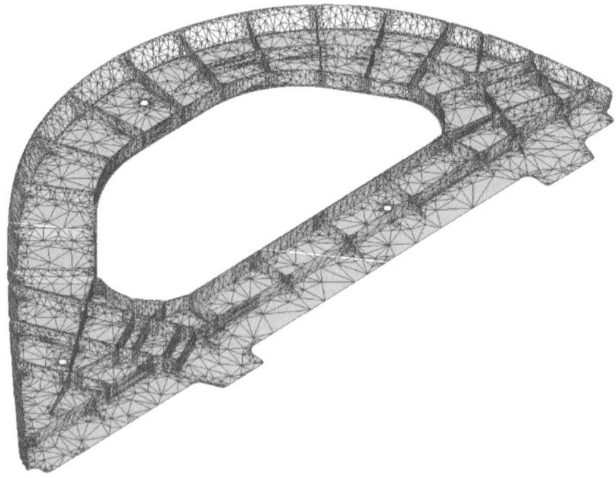

Fig. 9. Mesh for fillet rib.

The mesh for the fillet rib, which contains 22,736 elements and was automatically generated, is shown in Fig. 9. This part is machined from a rectangular block of dimensions 1.62 m x 900mm x 60mm. Distortions computed are shown in Fig. 10. CMM measurements of distortions from a machined component, taken at the points illustrated in Fig. 11, are shown in Fig. 12. Fig. 13 shows the comparison between the measured and predicted distorted shapes. As can be seen, the measured and predicted distortions agree well both qualitatively and quantitatively in this case.

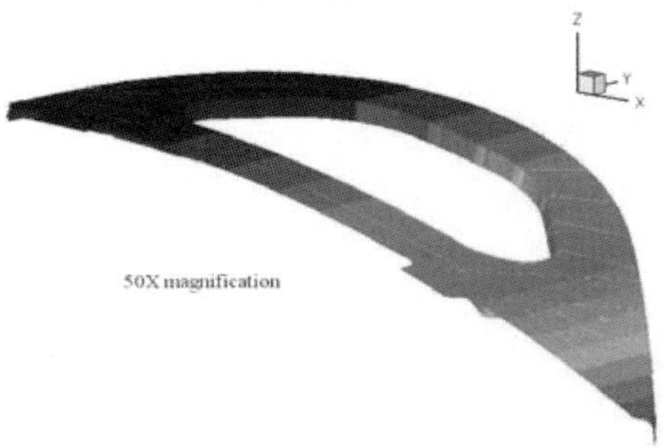

Fig. 10. Predicted distorted shape of fillet rib

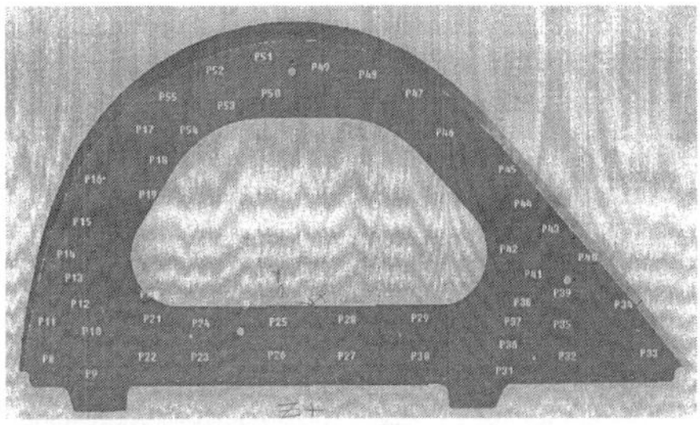

Fig. 11. Locations at which distortion was measured by CMM

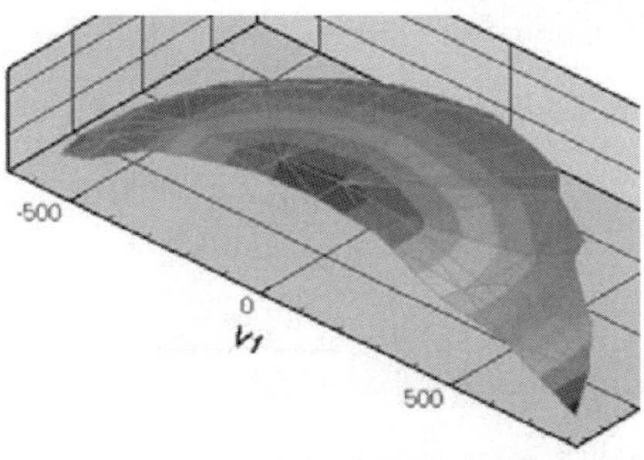

Fig. 12. Surface plot of measured distortion

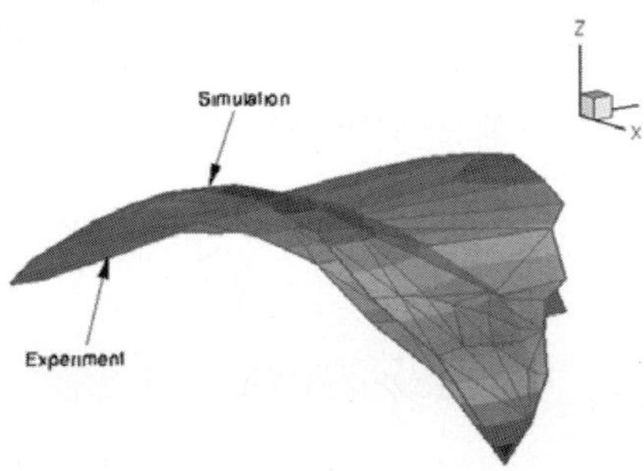

Fig. 13. Comparison of computed and measured distortions for the fillet rib

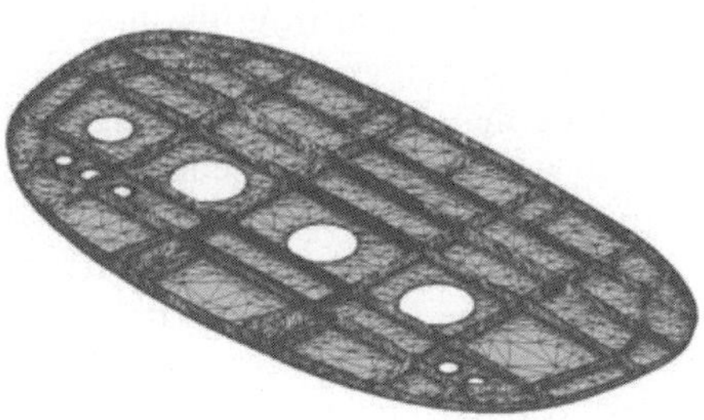

Fig. 14. Pressure bulkhead mesh of 147,769 elements

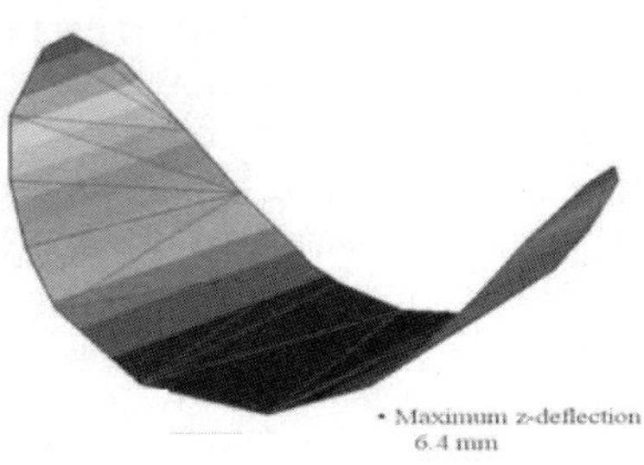

Fig. 15. Predicted distorted shape of pressure bulkhead

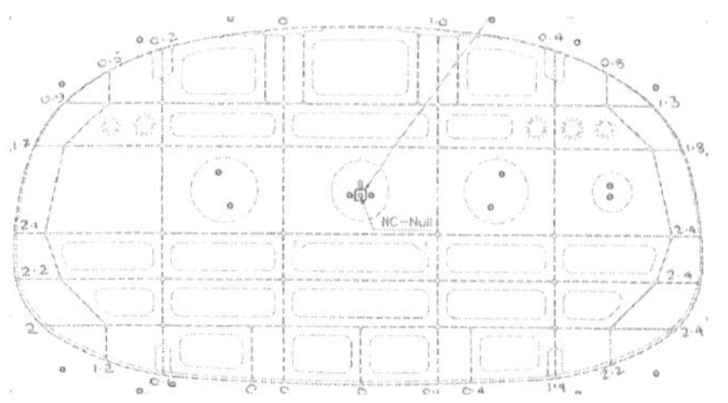

Fig. 16. Locations at which distortion was measured by feeler gauges

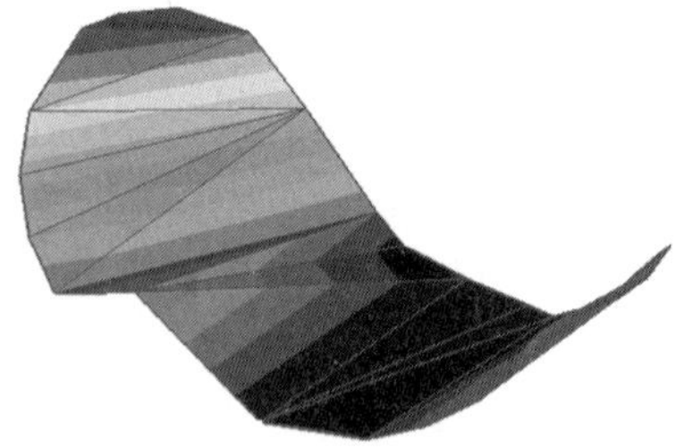

Fig. 17. Measured distorted shape of pressure bulkhead

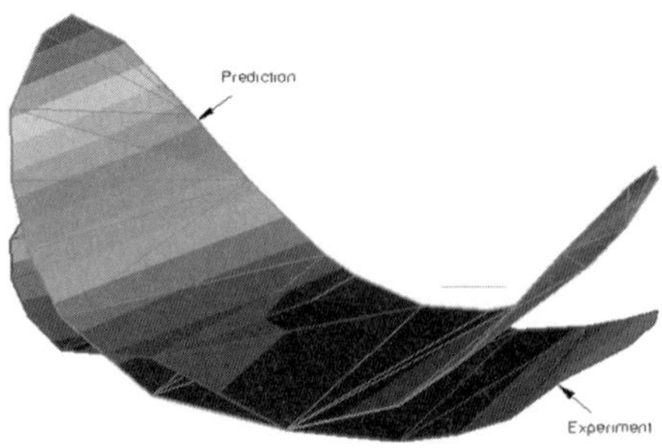

Fig. 18. Comparison of prediction versus measurement for pressure bulkhead

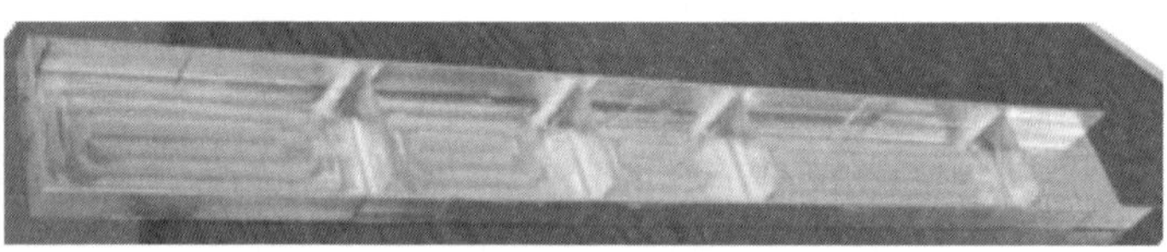

Fig. 19. Machined 800mm x 100mm x 25mm machined part

The mesh for the pressure bulkhead, which contains 147,769 elements, is shown in Fig. 14. The pressure bulkhead was machined from a rectangular block of dimensions 3.33 m x 1.82 m x 100mm. The final part is located 10.0 mm from the bottom of rectangular block. Distortion of the component after machining was measured at several points (see Fig. 16) on the bottom flange along the circumference using feeler gauges. The measured distortion profile is shown in Fig. 17, and a comparison of predicted and measured distortions is shown in Fig. 18. In this case, the measured and computed distortions agree well qualitatively, but the calculated values significantly overestimate the measured values at the outer edges of the part. This is partly due to the geometry of the part; given its large dimensions, a slight errors in distortion near the center would be magnified at the edges due to a parallax effect.

An aerospace componenent 800mm x 100mm x 25mm high was machined from 75mm thick Al7050-T7451 plate material, Fig. 19. The corresponding distorted measurement was performed, Fig 20, and compared with the predicted distorted

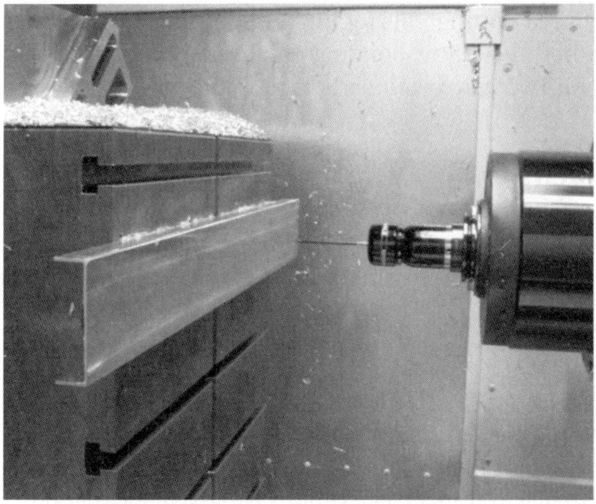

Fig. 20. Distortion measurement of machined part

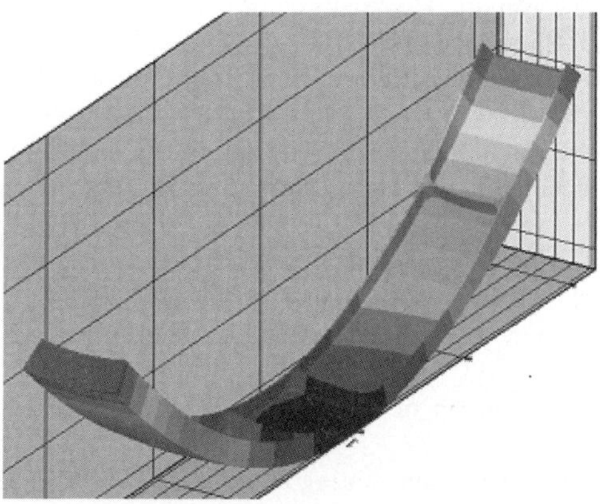

Fig. 21. Predicted distortion of machined part

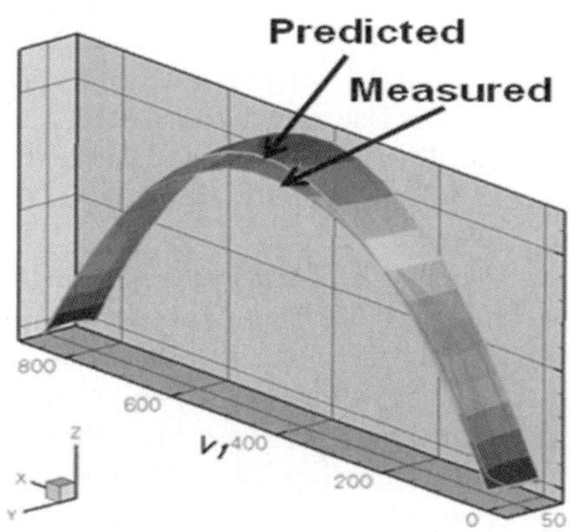

Fig. 22. Comparison of predicted and measured distortion for 800mm long part

configuration, Fig 21 and Fig 22. Excellent agreement between both shape and distortion magnitude are seen.

5 Summary and Conclusions

This paper summarizes a methodology for calculating distortions in thin-walled components due to both bulk and machining induced residual stresses. A tool path analysis program is used to determine the final part geometry, mesh the final part for distortion analysis, and apply stress components. Machining induced stresses are applied based on a database of values computed through finite element analysis for a range of representative cutting and tooling conditions. Measured bulk stresses in the parent billet are stored in a corresponding database. Preliminary validation of the bulk stress component for two aerospace parts is presented.

Acknowledgements

We are grateful to Martin Hand of EADS for valuable comments on this work, and for providing the fillet rib and pressure bulkhead data files and measurement data.

References

1. Stephenson, D.A., Agapiou, J.S.: Metal Cutting Theory and Practice, 2nd edn., pp. 568–569. CRC, Boca Raton (2006)
2. Wiesner, C.: Residual Stresses After Orthogonal Machining of AISI 304: Numerical Calcuation of the thermal Component and Comparison with Experiments. Metall. Trans. A 23, 989–996 (1992)
3. Shirakashi, T., Obikawa, T., Sasahara, H., Wada, T.: Analytical Prediction of the Characteristics Within Machined Surface Layer (1st Report, The Analysis of the Residual Stress Distribution). J. Jpn. Soc. Precis. Eng. 59, 1695–1700 (1993)
4. Shih, A.J., Yang, H.T.Y.: Experimental and Finite Element Predictions of Residual Stresses Due to Orthogonal Metal Cutting. Int. J. Num. Meth. Eng. 36, 1487–1507 (1993)
5. Liu, R., Guo, Y.B.: Finite Element Analysis of the Effect of Sequential Cuts and Tool-Chip Friction on Resdiual Stresses in a Machined Layer. Int. J. Mech. Sci. 42, 1069–1086 (2000)
6. Lundblad, M.: Influence of Cutting Tool Geometry on Residual Stress in the Workpiece. In: Proc. 2002 Third Wave AdvantEdge User's Conference, Atlanta, GA, vol. 7 (2002)
7. Shet, C., Deng, X.: Residual Stresses and Strains in Orthogonal Metal Cutting. Int. J. Machine Tools Manuf. 43, 573–587 (2003)
8. Marusich, T.D., Ortiz, M.: Modeling and Simulation of High-Speed Machining. Int. J. Num. Meth. Eng. 38, 3675–3694 (1995)
9. Marusich, T.D.: Effects of Friction and Cutting Speed on Cutting Force. In: Proc. IMECE (ASME), New York, Paper No. MED-23313, November 11–16 (2001)
10. Sandstrom, D.R., Hodowany, J.N.: Modeling the Physics of Metal Cutting in High-Speed Machining. Machining Science and Technology 2, 343–353 (1998)
11. Childs, T.H.C.: Material Property Needs in Modelling Metal Machining. Machining Science and Technology 2, 303–316 (1998)
12. `http://www.thirdwavesys.com/products`
13. Prime, M.B., Hill, M.R.: Residual stress, stress relief, and inhomogeneity in aluminum plate. Scripta Materialia 46, 77–78 (2002)

Kinematics Analysis for a New-Style Machine Tool Based on 3-PRS Parallel Robot

Zhigang Niu and Ming Lv

College of Mechanical Engineering, Taiyuan University of Technology
79 West Yingze Street, 030024 Taiyuan, China
zgniu@163.com

Abstract. A five-degree-of-freedom hybrid parallel machine tool, composed of a 3-PRS parallel robot and an X-Y series table, is designed on geometry and analyzed on kinematics. The 3-PRS parallel robot consists of three serial chains and a fixed base and a moving platform which can be moved in a pose space corresponding to the three degrees of freedom. This kind of mechanism can be applied to measuring and machining through carrying test set or cutting tool on the moving platform. Both the forward and inverse kinematics models are established based on the kinematics analysis. By means of numerical analysis, a calculation example is performed to verify the correctness of the kinematics models.

Keywords: kinematics analysis, machine tool, 3-PRS, parallel robot.

1 Introduction

As the research on parallel mechanism goes further, a kind of robot including parallel mechanisms has been excogitated in order to overcome the shortage of stiffness of common series robots. The application of parallel mechanism on machine tools is a great innovation and more and more research productions have achieved on the parallel machine tool based on parallel robot [1]. Kinematics analysis is one of the key problems during the researches. In this paper, the kinematics analysis for a new-style machine tool based on 3-PRS parallel robot is given as follows.

The five-degree-of-freedom hybrid parallel machine tool is shown as Fig. 1, which is composed of a 3-PRS parallel robot and a common X-Y series table. The 3-PRS parallel robot belongs to parallel mechanism and consists of a fixed base and moving platform which is connected by three serial chains, each chain containing one active prismatic joint and one passive revolute joint and spherical joint. The geometry of the parallel mechanism is designed with three stands arranged at 120° to each other, and the linkages keep the fixed length. The parallel kinematics mechanism has three degrees of freedom and is equipped with linear direct drive. The moving platform of the parallel mechanism can be moved in a pose space corresponding to the three degrees of freedom. Thus this kind of mechanism can be applied to measuring and machining through carrying test set or cutting tool on the moving platform.

C. Xiong et al. (Eds.): ICIRA 2008, Part II, LNAI 5315, pp. 339–347, 2008.

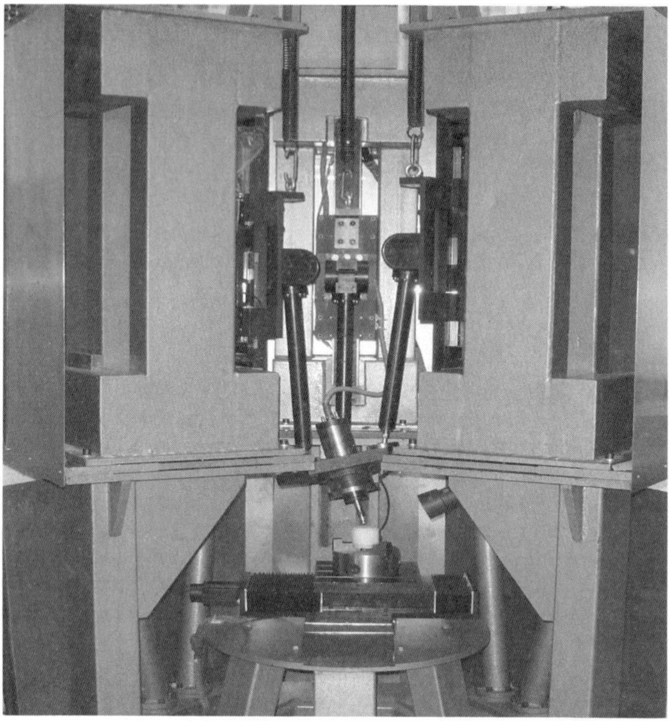

Fig. 1. Prototype of the new-style machine tool based on 3-PRS parallel robot

2 Configuration Model

The coordinate system of the new-style machine tool based on 3-PRS parallel robot is illustrated in Fig. 2. It consists of a conventional X-Y table with two degrees of freedom and a 3-PRS parallel robot with three degrees of freedom. The X-Y table can carry the work piece and provide motions in two horizontal directions. The 3-PRS parallel robot includes two angular orientations in pitch (about the y axis) and yaw (about x-axis) and one linear motion in the vertical direction. The 3-PRS parallel robot is made up of three vertical slider-tracks, three linkages and a moveable platform.

Ball joints C_1, C_2, C_3 is even distributed on the platform where regards the "r" as the radius. The linkages and sliders are jointed together by rotational joints. u_1, u_2, u_3 are orientation vectors of the rotational joints B_1, B_2 and B_3. The plane on which the X-Y table lays, intersects the extending line B_iA_i (i=1, 2, 3) at point A_1, A_2, A_3.They are also even distributed on a circle which regards the "R" as the radius.

The static Cartesian coordinate frame O-XYZ is posited at the geometry centre of equilateral triangle $A_1A_2A_3$ with Z-axis pointing along the vertical direction, X-axis points towards to A_1 and Y-axis points parallel along the line that parallels to A_2A_3.The movable Cartesian coordinate fame, O_1-$X_1Y_1Z_1$, is fixed at the of the geometry centre of equilateral triangle $C_1C_2C_3$ with the same axes directions as the O-XYZ coordinate frame. The length of the linkage is "L". The distances between the

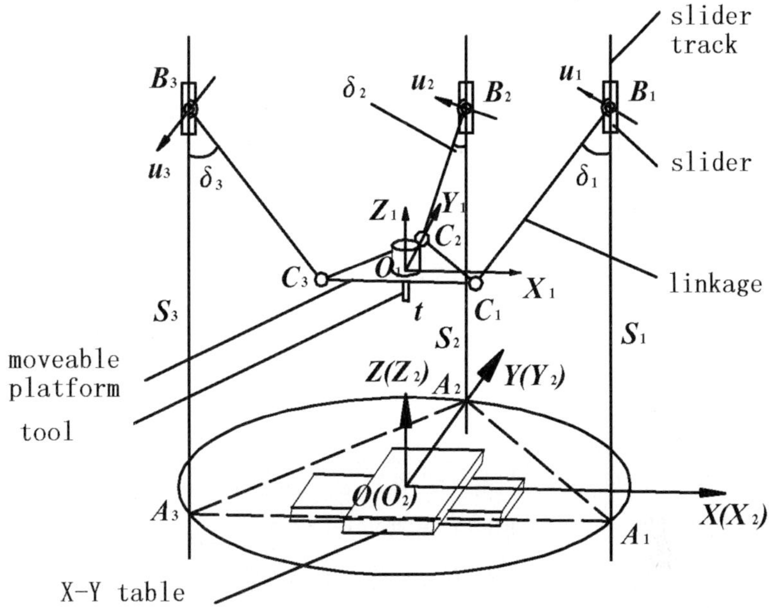

Fig. 2. Coordinate frames of the new-style machine tool based on 3-PRS parallel robot

rotational joints B_1, B_2, B_3 and plane $A_1A_2A_3$ are S_1, S_2, S_3 respectively. The length of the tool (O_{1t}) is lt.

3 Inverse Kinematics Analysis

3.1 Analysis for 3-PRS Parallel Mechanism

Parallel mechanism contains of three degrees of freedom: two angular orientations in pitch (about the y axis) and yaw (about x-axis) and one linear motion in the vertical direction. The inverse kinematics analysis is mainly about the mathematical relationship between the positions and poses factors of the moveable platform and S_1, S_2, S_3.

The transformation matrix T represents spatial location of the movable Cartesian coordinate fame: O_1-$X_1Y_1Z_1$. The orientation unit vectors: $[l_x\ l_y\ l_z]^T$, $[m_x\ m_y\ m_z]^T$ and $[n_x\ n_y\ n_z]^T$ are directional cosines of the x, y, z-axes with respect to the coordinate frame O-XYZ.

$$\mathbf{T}=\begin{bmatrix} l_x & m_x & n_x & x_c \\ l_y & m_y & n_y & y_c \\ l_z & m_z & n_z & z_c \\ 0 & 0 & 0 & 1 \end{bmatrix}=\begin{bmatrix} \mathbf{l} & \mathbf{m} & \mathbf{n} & \mathbf{O_1} \\ 0 & 0 & 0 & 1 \end{bmatrix}=\begin{bmatrix} \mathbf{R_0} & \mathbf{O_1} \\ \mathbf{0} & 1 \end{bmatrix} \tag{1}$$

For the x, y, z-axes are perpendicular to each other, six constraint equations are given below:

$$\begin{cases} \mathbf{l}\cdot\mathbf{l}=\mathbf{m}\cdot\mathbf{m}=\mathbf{n}\cdot\mathbf{n}=1 \\ \mathbf{l}\cdot\mathbf{m}=\mathbf{m}\cdot\mathbf{n}=\mathbf{n}\cdot\mathbf{l}=0 \end{cases} \tag{2}$$

x_c, y_c and z_c are absolute coordinates of O_1, meanwhile the absolute coordinates of C_1,C_2,C_3 are given below:

$$\begin{bmatrix} \mathbf{C_i} \\ 1 \end{bmatrix}_{XYZ} = \mathbf{T}\cdot\begin{bmatrix} \mathbf{C_i^e} \\ 1 \end{bmatrix}_{XYZ}, \quad i=1,2,3 \tag{3}$$

$\mathbf{C_i^e}$ are coordinates of C_1,C_2,C_3 in moveable coordinate system O_1-$X_1Y_1Z_1$.

Plane constraint equation

The movement of linkage $\overline{B_1C_1}$, $\overline{B_2C_2}$, $\overline{B_3C_3}$ are restricted within the plane that is both passed by B_1, B_2, B_3 and perpendicular to u_1, u_2, u_3.

$$\mathbf{u_i}\overrightarrow{C_iB_i}=0, \quad i=1,2,3 \tag{4}$$

Length constraint equation

Let the length of the linkage be "L".

$$\left|\overrightarrow{C_iB_i}\right| = L, \quad i=1,2,3 \tag{5}$$

From (1) (2) (3) (4) (5) , S_1, S_2, S_3 can be derived as follows:

$$\begin{cases} S_1=\sqrt{L^2-(\frac{\sqrt{3}}{2}R-\frac{\sqrt{3}}{2}rl_x+\frac{3}{2}rm_x)^2-(\frac{1}{2}R-\frac{\sqrt{3}}{2}rl_y+\frac{1}{2}rl_x)^2} \\ +\frac{\sqrt{3}}{2}rl_z-\frac{1}{2}rm_z+z_c \\ S_2=\sqrt{L^2-(R+\frac{1}{2}rl_x-\frac{3}{2}rm_y)^2}+rm_z+z_c \\ S_3=\sqrt{L^2-(\frac{\sqrt{3}}{2}R+\frac{\sqrt{3}}{2}rl_x+\frac{3}{2}rm_x)^2-(\frac{1}{2}R+\frac{\sqrt{3}}{2}rl_y+\frac{1}{2}rl_x)^2} \\ -\frac{\sqrt{3}}{2}rl_z-\frac{1}{2}rm_z+z_c \end{cases} \tag{6}$$

For the moveable platform are rigid body, its location can be represented with the coordinates (x_c,y_c,z_c) of O_1 ,the centre of the moveable platform in fixed coordinate system .The pose can be represented by Euler angle α, β, γ. It means that the moveable coordinate frame will round the z-axes, x-axes, y-axes of fixed coordinate frame revolves α, β and γ respectively.

T rotational matrix of the moveable platform pose can be described as follows:

$$\mathbf{R}_1 = \begin{bmatrix} c\alpha c\gamma - s\alpha c\beta s\gamma & -c\alpha s\gamma - s\alpha c\beta c\gamma & s\alpha s\beta \\ s\alpha c\gamma + c\alpha c\beta s\gamma & -s\alpha s\gamma + c\alpha c\beta c\gamma & -c\alpha s\beta \\ s\beta s\gamma & s\beta c\gamma & c\beta \end{bmatrix} \quad (7)$$

In the equation, there are "c=cos" and "s=sin".

For the first three column are directional cosines of the X_1-axes,Y_1-axes,and Z_1-axes with respect to the coordinate frame of O-XYZ, $\mathbf{R}_0$ must be equal to $\mathbf{R}_1$.

$$\mathbf{R}_0 = \mathbf{R}_1 \quad (8)$$

Each element of the left matrix should be equal to right, so equation (6) and (7) can be simultaneous equations. Once α, β, γ and z_c are evaluated, S_1, S_2, S_3 will also be known.

Generally the known variables during the path planning are location of the tool tip and the orientation vector of the tool shaft, "tool-orientation vector". The centre of the moveable platform and the tool tip are located at the opposite ends of the tool shaft, so O1 should be equal to "$O_t+l_tN_t$".

$$\mathbf{O_1} = \mathbf{O_t} + l_t\mathbf{N_t} \quad (9)$$

And then z_c should be equal to "$z_c=z_t+l_t n_{tx}$".

The tool axes is heavy matching with Z_1-axes of the moveable coordinate frame ,what just make the last column of the rotational matrix $\mathbf{R}_1$ be the unit vector of the Z_1-axes, then three equations can be concluded as follows:

$$\begin{cases} \sin\alpha \sin\beta = n_{tx} \\ -\cos\alpha \sin\beta = n_{ty} \\ \cos\beta = n_{tz} \end{cases} \quad (10)$$

From the above three equations, α, β can be known. At last, $\gamma = -\alpha$ [4][5], since the moveable platform can not rotate.

Then, S_1, S_2, S_3 become computable by the simultaneous equations of (6) and (7) .

3.2 Analysis for X-Y Table

First, coordinate frame O_2-$X_2Y_2Z_2$ is fixed at right the centre of the X-Y table with same original location as the fixed coordinate frame O-XYZ. Let (x_t^e, y_t^e, z_t^e) be the orientation vector of the tool tip and $(n_{tx}^e, n_{ty}^e, n_{tz}^e)^T$ be of the tool shaft at sometime . Since the movement of the X-Y table is planar, the included angle of the tool shaft between each axes of the O-XYZ and O_2-$X_2Y_2Z_2$ are completely identical, that is to say $n_{tx}^e= n_{tx}$,$n_{ty}^e= n_{ty}$, $n_{tz}^e= n_{tz}$ .Meanwhile, $z_t^e=z_t$, S_1,S_2,S_3 is already unknown, and constraint equations [6] for the x_c, y_c are listed as below:

$$\begin{cases} x_c = -rm_x \\ y_c = \frac{1}{2}rm_y - \frac{1}{2}rl_x \end{cases} \tag{11}$$

From the equation $\mathbf{O_1}=\mathbf{O_t}+l_t\mathbf{N_t}$, the orientation vector of the tool tip can be concluded.

$$\begin{bmatrix} x_t \\ y_t \end{bmatrix} = \begin{bmatrix} x_c \\ y_c \end{bmatrix} - l_t \begin{bmatrix} n_{tx} \\ n_{ty} \end{bmatrix} \tag{12}$$

Finally, the coordinates of O_2 in the coordinate frame O-XYZ come down to bellow:

$$\begin{cases} x_{o_2} = x_t - x_t^e \\ y_{o_2} = y_t - y_t^e \end{cases} \tag{13}$$

4 Forward Kinematics Analysis

4.1 Analysis for 3-PRS Parallel Mechanism

To synthesize the kinematics of the machine tool ,three coordinates frames are shown in Fig. 1.The absolute coordinates of C_1,C_2,C_3 can be expressed in the following vector forms, when S_1,S_2,S_3 are known. δ_i (i=1,2,3) are angles between linkages and axes.

$$\begin{cases} \mathbf{C}_1 = \left[\frac{\sqrt{3}}{2}(R - Ls\delta_1), -\frac{1}{2}(R - Ls\delta_1), S_1 - Lc\delta_1\right]^T \\ \mathbf{C}_2 = [0, R - Ls\delta_2, S_2 - Lc\delta_2]^T \\ \mathbf{C}_1 = \left[-\frac{\sqrt{3}}{2}(R - Ls\delta_3), -\frac{1}{2}(R - Ls\delta_3), S_3 - Lc\delta_3\right]^T \end{cases} \tag{14}$$

In the equation, there are "*c*=cos" and "*s*=sin".

C_1, C_2, C_3 meet the following constraint conditions, for they are just as long as the sides of the equilateral triangle.

$$\left|\overline{C_1C_2}\right|^2 = \left|\overline{C_2C_3}\right|^2 = \left|\overline{C_1C_3}\right|^2 = 3r^2 \tag{15}$$

Namely,

$$\begin{cases} \left[\frac{\sqrt{3}}{2}(R-Ls\delta_1)-0\right]^2+\left[\frac{1}{2}(R-Ls\delta_1)-(R-Ls\delta_2)\right]^2 \\ +(S_1-Lc\delta_1-S_2+Lc\delta_2)^2=3r^2 \\ \left[0+\frac{\sqrt{3}}{2}(R-Ls\delta_3)\right]^2+\left[(R-Ls\delta_2)+\frac{1}{2}(R-Ls\delta_3)\right]^2 \\ +(S_2-Lc\delta_2-S_3+Lc\delta_3)^2=3r^2 \\ \left[\frac{\sqrt{3}}{2}(R-Ls\delta_1)+\frac{\sqrt{3}}{2}(R-Ls\delta_3)\right]^2+\left[-\frac{1}{2}(R-Ls\delta_1)+\frac{1}{2}(R-Ls\delta_3)\right]^2 \\ +(S_1-Lc\delta_1-S_3+Lc\delta_3)^2=3r^2 \end{cases} \tag{16}$$

In the equation, there are "c=cos" and "s=sin".

Substituting these vectors forms into (14) yields, δ_i (i=1,2,3) are derived, as well as the position and the posture of the parallel part.

4.2 Analysis for X-Y Table

Once the position and posture of the moveable platform is determined by direct kinematics, the absolute coordinates can be derived from equation $\mathbf{O}_1=(\mathbf{C}_1+\mathbf{C}_2+\mathbf{C}_3)/3$, homogeneously, $[x_t\ y_t\ z_t\ ]^T$ can be also computed from equation $\mathbf{O}_1=\mathbf{O}_t+l_t\mathbf{N}_t$:

$$\begin{bmatrix} x_t \\ y_t \\ z_t \end{bmatrix} = \begin{bmatrix} x_c \\ y_c \\ z_c \end{bmatrix} - l_t \begin{bmatrix} n_{tx} \\ n_{ty} \\ n_{tz} \end{bmatrix} \tag{17}$$

Let (x_{o2},y_{o2}) be the x-axes and y-axes coordinates of O_2 in the coordinate frame O-XYZ. Then the coordinates of the tool tip can be expressed as follows:

$$\begin{cases} x_t^e = x_t - x_{o_2} \\ y_t^e = y_t - y_{o_2} \\ z_t^e = z_t \end{cases} \tag{18}$$

5 Numerical Analysis

There may be more than one answer to the kinematics equations, so the proper selection is needed. According to our research group's need, explicit result to the direct kinematics equations is not crucial. Therefore, verification method is applied to verify the correctness of the direct kinematics equation .The verification approach can be done following two steps bellow: first , the value of S_1,S_2,S_3 and δi should be obtained form the inverse kinematics equations, when both the parameters of the mechanism and the posture-location of the tool shaft (so the value of δ_i can be calculated by orientation vector) are given, then S_1,S_2,S_3 and δ_i are considered as inputs and substituted into direct kinematics equations. Whether the direct equation is true or false just depends on whether the equations are equal or not. Similarly, the coordinates of the tool tip in coordinate frame O_2-$X_2Y_2Z_2$ can also be derived form direct kinematics equations, and the same verification can be done in the same way. We define L=550mm, r=110mm, R=165mm, l_t=100mm. Let the orientation vector, $(n_{tx}^e, n_{ty}^e, n_{tz}^e)^T$, be expressed by directional cosines($n_{tx}^e=\cos\theta_x^e$, $n_{ty}^e=\cos\theta_y^e$, $n_{tz}^e=\cos\theta_z^e$) . There are four groups of inputs for $(\theta_x^e,\theta_y^e,x_t^e, y_t^e,z_t^e)$, four groups of absolute coordinate value of S_1,S_2,S_3,$\mathbf{C}_1$,$\mathbf{C}_2$,$\mathbf{C}_3$, which can be computed by inverse kinematics equations, as well as the value of δ_i (i=1,2,3).

$(\boldsymbol{\theta}_x^e,\boldsymbol{\theta}_y^e,\mathbf{x}_t^e, \mathbf{y}_t^e,\mathbf{z}_t^{e)}$ = **(90°,90°,0,0,0)**

$\mathbf{C}_1$ = (110, 0, 100)
$\mathbf{C}_2$ = (-55, 95.262794, 100)
$\mathbf{C}_3$ = (-55, 95.262794, 100)
$S_1 = 647.243103$
$S_2 = 647.243103$
$S_3 = 647.243103$
$\delta_1 = 5.7391°$
$\delta_2 = 5.7391°$
$\delta_3 = 5.7391°$

$(\boldsymbol{\theta}_x^e,\boldsymbol{\theta}_y^e,\mathbf{x}_t^e, \mathbf{y}_t^e,\mathbf{z}_t^e)$= **(80°,85°,20,18,5)**

$\mathbf{C}_1$ = (107.699287, 0, 83.993050)
$\mathbf{C}_2$ = (-55.516907, 96.158104, 104.342300)
$\mathbf{C}_3$ = (-54.061287, -93.636894, 120.947708)
S_1= 631.0
$S_2 = 651.688293$
$S_3 = 667.998840$
δ_1= 5.980127°
$\delta_2 = 5.630956°$
$\delta_3 = 5.935785°$

$(\boldsymbol{\theta}_x^e,\boldsymbol{\theta}_y^e,\mathbf{x}_t^e, \mathbf{y}_t^e,\mathbf{z}_t^e)$ = **(68°,78°,35,25,13)**

$\mathbf{C}_1$ = (99.085274, 0, 62.150478)
$\mathbf{C}_2$ = (-57.648731, 99.850533, 104.154320)
$\mathbf{C}_3$ = (-49.853329, -86.348503, 143.766830)
$S_1 = 608.186401$
$S_2 = 651.903931$
$S_3 = 689.877441$
$\delta_1 = 6.883171°$
$\delta_2 = 5.184815°$
$\delta_3 = 6.817941°$

$(\boldsymbol{\theta}_x^{\,e},\boldsymbol{\theta}_y^{\,e},\mathbf{x}_t^{\,e},\mathbf{y}_t^{\,e},\mathbf{z}_t^{\,e}) = (\mathbf{79°,60°,-42,-7,18})$

$\mathbf{C}_1 = (114.197151, 0, 81.485374)$

$\mathbf{C}_2 = (-52.473091, 90.886063, 65.337471)$

$\mathbf{C}_3 = (-42.619690, -73.819466, 160.600266)$

$S_1 = 629.134033$

$S_2 = 612.049072$

$S_3 = 704.786133$

$\delta_1 = 5.299916°$

$\delta_2 = 6.268522°$

$\delta_3 = 8.338388°$

Ignore impacts of the rounding errors ,we can come down to the conclusion that all groups of the derived answers meet the equations fairly well ,and the inverse-obtained x_t^e, y_t^e, z_t^e are precisely math their original value. From above all, the results of the direct and inverse kinematics equation are consequently well consistent.

6 Summary

This paper presents research works dedicated to kinematics analysis of a five-degree-of-freedom hybrid parallel machine tool. The 3-PRS parallel robot is key part of the new-style machine tool which it can produce two rotations circling x-axes and y-axes, and one translation along z-axes. Direct kinematics model and inverse kinematics model have been made. The kinematics models were proved to be correct by numerical analysis validation.

References

1. Weck, M., Staimer, D.: Parallel Kinematics Machine Tools-Current State Future Potentials. Annals of the CIRP as production systems 15, 671–681 (2002)
2. Company, O., Pierrot, F.: Modeling and Design Issues of A 3-axis Parallel Machine Tool. Mechanism and Machine Theory 37, 1325–1345 (2002)
3. Huang, Z., Kong, L., Fang, Y.: Parallel Robots Mechanism Theory and Control. Mechanical Express, Beijing (1997)
4. Juan, H.: Research on Basic Manufacture Theory of BKX-I NC System and the Development and Application of the NC System. Beijing Institute of Technology, Beijing (2002)
5. Liang, J.: Foundational Research on Precise Kinematics Manufactures Technology. Beijing Institute of Technology, Beijing (1999)
6. Liu, X., Wang, Y.: Kinematics Analysis on Special 3-PRS Parallel Robot. Mechanical Science and Technology 22, 785–787 (2003)
7. Tsai, M.-S., Shiau, T.-N., Tsai, Y.-J., Chang, T.-H.: Direct Kinematics Analysis of A3-PRS Parallel Mechanism. Mechanism and Machine Theory 38, 71–83 (2003)

Safe and Short Tool Length Generation for 3+2 Axis NC Machining of a Ball-End Cutter Using Graphics Hardware

Qingzhen Bi, Han Ding, and Yuhan Wang

State Key Lab. of Mechanical System and Vibration, School of Mechanical Engineering, Shanghai Jiaotong University,
1954 Hua Shan Road, Shanghai 200030, P.R. China
{biqz,hding,yhwang}@sjtu.edu.cn

Abstract. In 3+2 axis NC machining, only three linear axes are executed while 5-axis machine's two rotational axes are locked. Compared with conventional 3-axis machining, the main advantage of 3+2 machining is that it allows use of a shorter cutter. The magnitude of tool deflection and the stability of cutting process strongly depend on the slenderness of the tool. However, the tool overhang length can't be easily shortened because of collision avoidance. In this paper the accessibility cone of a milling cutter is newly defined to generate collision-free cutting orientations. The accessibility cone and safe tool length can be efficiently computed by a novel method using graphics hardware. The proper cutting orientation of 3+2 machining is then obtained by optimizing the safe and shortest tool length. The computational example and cutting experiment of sculptured surface machining confirm the validity of the approach.

Keywords: 3+2 machining; pTool length; Cutting orientation; Access-based machining.

1 Introduction

3+2 axis NC machining is a technique whereby only three linear axes are executed with the cutting tool locked in a titled position using the 5-axis machine's two rotational axes, hence the name, 3+2 axis machining. The fixed cutting tool orientation distinguishes 3+2 axis machining from continuous or simultaneous 5-axis machining. Generally locking the rotary axes generates fewer fluctuations in the feed rate than simultaneous 5-axis machining and results in a more consistent surface finish with lower variations in the cutting force and torque. The other main advantage of 3+2 axis machining is that it allows use of a shorter, more rigid cutter that would not be permissible with conventional 3-axis machining. Since the magnitude of tool deflection and the stability of cutting process strongly depend on the slenderness of the tool, short cutters can improve the rigid of the whole cutting process and significantly reducing deflection and vibration [1, 2]. As a result, higher cutting speed can be achieved without putting excessive load on the cutter and, so increasing tool life and reducing breakages.

C. Xiong et al. (Eds.): ICIRA 2008, Part II, LNAI 5315, pp. 348–355, 2008.

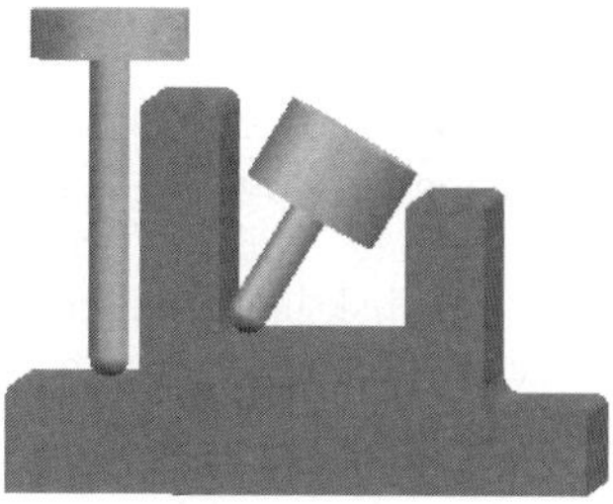

Fig. 1. The different safe tool lengths with different tool orientations

However the tool overhang length can't be easily shortened because the tool holder will collide with the workpiece. Collision avoidance becomes the most important consideration to use a short cutting tool. Though some methods [3-5] are helpful to get collision-free tool path, the shorter tool length has not been considered. The collision-free short cutters of multi-axis NC machining are usually considered in machining simulation process. The minimal cutter extension can be calculated by the simulation software such as Vericut [6]. Kim [7] proposed a method to calculate short and safe cutter length by safe space in NC machining. The problem of these methods is that the safe tool length can only be determined based on a predefined tool path. However the safe and shortest tool length (SSTL) of a tool path is usually determined by the tool orientations as shown in Fig. 1. Therefore the tool orientation is the most important to use a short cutter for 3+2 axis machining.

Recently commodity graphics hard has been enormous improvements in terms of programmability and computational speed [8]. Morimoto [9] proposed a GPU based algorithm to optimize cutting direction and the algorithm conservatively considers collision avoidance. Expired by the existing works, a new GPU-based approach is proposed to efficiently generate safe and short cutter length when tool paths are planned. The SSTL for each accessible orientation is first computed at each CC points. The collision-free tool orientations are then optimized by considering cutter length.

The remainder of the paper is organized as follows. In Section 2, a GPU-based algorithm is proposed to compute accessible cones for CL points of a cutting tool. Section 3 describes a method to compute the SSTL at each CL point for each accessible orientation. Section 4 presents the whole process to obtain optimal tool orientation and SSTL. A computational example is given in Section 5 and Section 6 verifies the example by a cutting experiment. Section 7 draws some conclusions.

2 GPU-Based Accessibility Cone Computation

Since collision avoidance can be viewed approximately as access assurance of the milling cutter at each CL point, collision avoidance at discrete CL points is first considered.

2.1 Basic Concept of Accessibility Cone

Usually a milling tool and tool holder can be regarded as a cylinder with fixed radii respectively to detect global collision as shown in Fig. 2. The CL point of a ball-end cutter is the center of the end half sphere. The tool orientation is represented as $\mathbf{v}_c$ and the cutter length is expressed as l_c. A disk in spatial coordinates can be represented as $D(\mathbf{p},\mathbf{v},r)$, where the three parameters are the center, the direction perpendicular to the disk plane and the radius respectively.

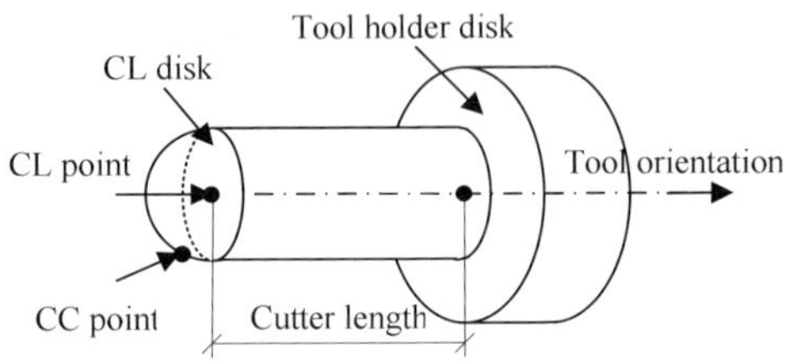

Fig. 2. Model of a ball-end cutter

Definition 1. (The CL Disk of the Milling Cutter Along an Orientation). As shown in Fig. 2, let $\mathbf{p}_c \in \mathbf{R}^3$ be the CL point of a milling tool. The CL disk $CLD(\mathbf{p}_c,\mathbf{v}_c)$ of the milling tool is defined as

$$CLD(\mathbf{p}_c, \mathbf{v}_c) = D(\mathbf{p}_c, \mathbf{v}_c, r_c) \tag{1}$$

where r_c is the radius of the milling tool.

Definition 2. (The Tool Holder Disk of the Milling Cutter Along an Orientation). As shown in Fig. 2. The tool holder disk $THD(\mathbf{p}_c,\mathbf{v}_c)$ is defined as

$$THD(\mathbf{p}_c,\mathbf{v}_c) = D(\mathbf{p}_t, \mathbf{v}_c, r_t) \tag{2}$$

where $\mathbf{p}_t = \mathbf{p}_c + \mathbf{v}_c \bullet l_c$ and r_t is the radius of the tool holder.

Definition 3. (The Complete Visibility Cone of a CL Disk). The view direction $\mathbf{v}_v$ is set as the opposite direction of the tool orientation. A CL disk $CLD(\mathbf{p}_c, \mathbf{v}_c)$ in a set of obstacles S is completely visible in a viewing orientation $\mathbf{v}_v$ if all points of the CL disk are visible when the observer locates outside the bounding sphere of S and $CLD(\mathbf{p}_c, \mathbf{v}_c)$. Complete visibility cone of $CLD(\mathbf{p}_c, \mathbf{v}_c)$, $CVC(CLD(\mathbf{p}_c, \mathbf{v}_c), S)$ is defined as all tool orientations from which $CLD(\mathbf{p}_c, \mathbf{v}_c)$ is completely visible.

The complete visibility cone of a tool holder disk is analogously defined as $CVC(THD(\mathbf{p}_c, \mathbf{v}_c), S)$. Based on the concepts of the CL disk and tool holder disk, the accessibility detection of the milling cutter is conducted to justify the complete visibility of $CLD(\mathbf{p}_c, \mathbf{v}_c)$ and $THD(\mathbf{p}_c, \mathbf{v}_c)$.

Definition 4. (Accessibility Cone at a CL Point). At a CL point, a milling tool is accessible along an orientation $\mathbf{v}_c$ if both the CL disk and the tool holder disk are completely visible. The accessibility cone of the CL point for the milling tool is defined as

$$AC(\mathbf{p}_c, S) = \{\mathbf{d} | \mathbf{d} \in CVC(CLD(\mathbf{p}_c, \mathbf{v}_c), S) \cap CVC(THD(\mathbf{p}_c, \mathbf{v}_c), S)\} \tag{3}$$

2.2 Accessibility Detection

Definition 4 reduces the accessibility detection to problems of check the complete visibility of disks. Taking advantage of robust and efficient performance of a graphics card to implement occlusion query, the complete visibility of the CLD and the THD in each candidate orientation is detected based on the depth representation of obstacles.

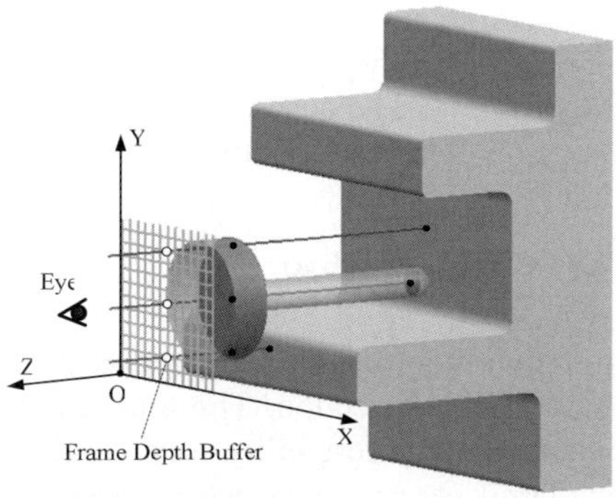

Fig. 3. Complete visibility detection of a CL disk

2.2.1 GPU-Based Visibility Detection

GPU-based algorithm means that the visibility detection of the disks is implemented by the graphics card. The detailed explain about the graphics card can be referred to Ref. [10]. Fig. 3 shows an eye position and screen coordinate system to detect the complete visibility of the CL disk. The orthographic projection mode of OpenGL is used to create the rectangle viewing volume which encloses the disks. Graphical calculations first convert obstacle objects to a set of pixels into the frame buffer where the surface appears. The depth values associated with pixels describe the minimal relative distances between the screen and the objects. Therefore the complete visibility of the CL disk can be detected by depth representation of the CL disk.

2.2.2 Accessibility Detection

Definition 4 shows the accessibility of a cutter is determined by the complete visibility of both CLD and THD of the cutter. With the help of collision query function of the GPU, the accessibility of the cutter in an orientation can be detected by follows.

Algorithm 1. GPU-based accessibility detection for a cutting tool

Step 1. Enable back face culling and standard depth test

Step 2. Set view matrix parameters as described in Section 2.2.1

Step 3. Render obstacle geometry

Step 4. Set the depth function to *GL_GEQUAL* and disable depth writes.

Step 5. Render the CLD. Call an occlusion query to test the number n_{CLD} of rendered pixels. The CL point is not accessible if n_{CLD} is not equal to zero.

Step 6. Render the THD. Call an occlusion query to test the number n_{THD} of rendered pixels. The CL point is not accessible if n_{THD} is not equal to zero. Otherwise, the cutter is accessible to the CL point in the orientation.

2.2.3 Accessibility Cone Computation

The accessibility cone at a CC point represents the set of directions along which the cutting tool is collision free. Theoretically there are infinite directions in the accessibility cone. In practice only some sampled directions in the Gauss Sphere are used to decrease the compute cost. These sampled discrete orientations are regarded as candidate orientations of the accessibility cone.

The algorithm like Ref. [5] is employed to tessellate the Gauss Sphere. The vertexes of the resulted triangle mesh represent a fairly homogenous sampling of the Gauss Sphere and the orientations represented by the vertexes can be regarded as the candidate orientations. The accessibility of a CC point along each candidate orientation is determined by Algorithm 1. The accessibility cone of a CC point will then be obtained by collecting all accessible orientations of the CC point.

3 GPU-Based SSTL Computation

The idea is to find the minimum tool length without collision between tool holder and the part surface in each accessible direction. The tool length is initially set as larger value l_{int} by experience to compute accessibility cones for all CC points. The SSTL of each CC point is computed only for each accessible orientation.

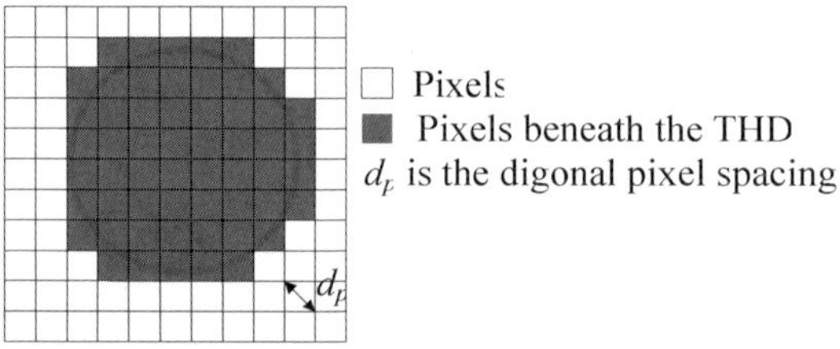

Fig. 4. Pixels beneath the THD

When the obstacles are rendered into a frame buffer, each pixel is associated with a depth value. A depth test guarantees that pixels with larger depth-buffer values are overwritten by pixels with smaller values. Therefore the SSTL can be determined by the pixels of obstacle object beneath the THD. For machining security of tool path, the THD are redefined as

$$THD(\mathbf{p}_c, \mathbf{v}_c) = D(\mathbf{p}_t, \mathbf{v}_c, r_t+d_p/2) \tag{4}$$

where d_p is the diagonal pixel spacing for a resolution to render the scene as shown in Fig. 4 and r_t is the tool holder radius. The depth values of pixels representing the THD are all equal because the THD is perpendicular to the view direction as shown in Fig. 3. The SSTL in the accessible direction is calculated by

$$l_{shortest} = l_{init}\text{-}(d_t\text{-}min(d_i,\ i=1\ldots n_{pixel})) \tag{5}$$

where $l_{shortest}$ is the safe and shortest tool length,

d_t is the depth value of the THD in screen coordinate system,

d_i are the depth values of obstacle pixels beneath the THD,

n_{pixel} is the number of pixels beneath the THD.

4 Tool Orientation and SSTL Optimization

The whole process to optimize the tool orientation and SSTL is described based on Section 2 and Section 3. A series of CL points calculated based on cutter center point representing the cutting trajectory. The computation of SSTL and tool orientation must be applied to each CC point. The GPU-based algorithm to generate SSTL and tool orientation for all CL points is described as follows.

Algorithm 2. GPU-based SSTL and tool orientation generation

```
Input: CO_i: Candidate orientations and i=1,…,n_co,
       CL_j: Successive CL points and j=1,…,n_cl,
       S: Obstacles.
Output: l_sstl: SSTL•TO_sstl: Optimized tool orientation.
l_sstl=l_init. /*Initial tool length*/
FOR (Each CO_i with i=1,…,n_co)
{ Render S
  FOR (Each CL_j with j=1,…,n_cl)
  { Detect accessibility of CL_j for CO_i by Algorithm 1
    IF (CL_j is not accessibility)  CO_i is invalid.
  }/*End of FOR_CL_j */
  IF (CO_i is valid)
  { FOR (Each CL_j with j=1,…,n_cl)
     { Calculate SSTL l_sstl_ij. /* the algorithm in Section
3*/
     }/*End of FOR_CL_j */
     l_sstl_i = max(l_sstl_ij, j=1…n_cl);
  }/*End IF*/
}/*End of FOR_CO_i */
Find the index k with minimal value in l_sstl_i (i=1,…,n_co);
l_sstl= l_sstl_k; TO_sstl = CO_k;
END.
```

5 Computational Examples

The proposed algorithms have been implemented in a prototype system using Visual C++ programming language and OpenGL library. The input to the system is polygonal mesh obstacle model, a group of CL points of a ball end cutter and the cutter model. The system output the tool orientation and SSTL for the CL points. As shown in Fig. 5. The part model consists of 291,506 triangles and represents the shape of a propeller. The maximum radius of the propeller is about 100mm. The example is performed using the graphics card, NVIDIA Quadro NVS 140M. The pixel resolution of the frame buffer is set 1000×1000.

A R3 ball-end cutter is employed for finishing milling. The tool length is initialized to 55mm and the diameter of tool holder is 36mm. The approximation tolerance of the driven surface is set 0.01 mm and the maximal step over distance is set 0.15 mm. 22,122 CL points are obtained as shown in Fig. 5. After 1,026 candidate orientations are achieved, it takes 337.687 seconds to compute the accessibility cone and optimize tool orientation. Six accessible orientations are generated and the accessibility cone is

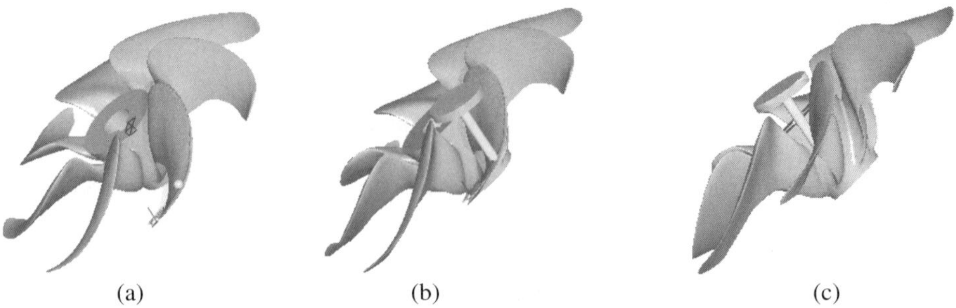

Fig. 5. (a) Accessibility cone, (b) Optimized tool orientation, (c) Optimized SSTL

shown in Fig. 5 (a). The SSTL of the tool path is 37.27 mm and the optimized cutting tool is shown in Fig. 5 (b) and Fig 5 (c).

6 Cutting Experiment

With the collision-free tool orientation and the SSTL generated by the proposed algorithm, the cutting experiment is performed in a five-axis machine tool with a dual-rotary table structure. The tool length in the actual machining process is 40mm because some remained materials still exist in the neighboring leafs. Fig.6. shows the cutting process and the shape after being cut. No collision takes place in the machining process.

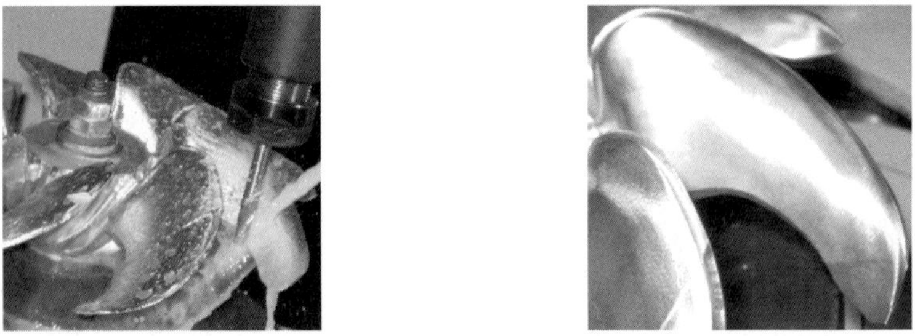

Fig. 6. Cutting process and the shape after being cut

7 Conclusions and Future Work

The SSTL of tool path for 3+2 axis machining of sculpture parts is considered in tool path generation. Based on the newly defined accessibility of a ball-end cutter, a fast and robust algorithm is generated to compute accessible orientations and to optimize SSTL using graphics hardware. The computational example and cutting experiment of sculptured surface machining confirm the validity of the proposed algorithm.The SSTL generation algorithm for a simultaneous 5-axis machining of sculpture parts will be further studied. The tool orientation of the 5-axis machining can be changed more flexibly, which allows use of a shorter cutter compared with 3+2 axis machining.

Acknowledgements

This work is supported by the National Basic Research Program of China under Grant 2005CB724103.

References

1. Salgado, M.A., De Lacalle, L.N.L., Lamikiz, A., Munoa, J., Sanchez, J.A.: Evaluation of the stiffness chain on the deflection of end-mills under cutting forces. International Journal of Machine Tools and Manufacturing 45, 727–739 (2005)
2. De Lacalle, L.N.L., Lamikiz, A., Sanchez, J.A., Salgado, M.A.: Effects of tool deflection in the high-speed milling of inclined surfaces. International Journal of Advanced Manufacturing Technology 24, 621–631 (2004)
3. Ilushin, O., Elber, G., Halperin, D., Wein, R., Kim, M.S.: Precise global collision detection in multi-axis NC-machining. Computer-Aided Design 37, 909–920 (2005)
4. Yin, Z.P., Ding, H., Xiong, Y.L.: Visibility theory and algorithms with application to manufacturing processes. International Journal of Production Research 38, 2891–2909 (2000)
5. Balasubramaniam, M., Laxmiprasad, P., Sarma, S., Shaikh, Z.: Generating 5-axis NC roughing paths directly from a tessellated representation. Computer-Aided Design 32, 261–277 (2000)
6. CGTech Company, http://www.cgtech.com
7. Kim, S.J.: Short and safe tool setting by safe space in NC machining. International Journal of Advanced Manufacturing Technology 33, 1017–1023 (2007)
8. Owens, J.D., Luebke, D., Govindaraju, N., Harris, M., Krüger, J., Lefohn, A.E., Purcell, T.J.: A Survey of General-Purpose Computation on Graphics Hardware. Computer Graphics Forum 26, 80–113 (2007)
9. Morimoto, K., Inui, M.: A GPU based algorithm for determining the optimal cutting direction in deep mold machining. In: Proceeding of the 2007 IEEE international symposium on assembly and manufacturing, pp. 203–208. IEEE press, Michigan (2007)
10. Shreiner, D., Woo, M., Neider, J., Davis, T.: OpenGL Programming Guide: The Official Guide to Learning OpenGL. Addison-Wesley Professional, Reading (2005)

Analysis of Clamping within a Fixing System

Matthias Klärner[1], Jürgen Leopold[2], and Lothar Kroll[1]

[1] Chemnitz University of Technology, Institute of Mechanical and Polymer Engineering, Chemnitz, Germany

[2] Fraunhofer Institute for Machine Tools and Forming Technology (IWU), Chemnitz, Germany

Abstract. The complex workpiece-fixing behaviour during machining is essential for the fixture development process, especially when using innovative intelligent Piezo-electric clamping systems being very susceptible to transverse forces. Therefore, the loads acting on fixture components have been analysed and a model for predicting the reaction forces due to clamping and process loads is presented. First, a complex finite element model is used to obtain detailed information about the behaviour during the process. Second, a faster model with fewer elements is developed, validated and used for the variation of process parameters. Finally, both results are combined to an analytical model. This empiric equation allows to predict the reaction forces depending on several process parameters. The usability of this method has been exposed by modelling shape grinding of a nozzle guide vane.

Keywords: Clamping Force, Grinding, Finite Element Method, Fixture.

1 Introduction

The ability to establish and secure desired positions is significantly affecting the effectiveness of a fixture system [19]. Further on, product differentiation increases the need of highly efficient, flexible, accurate and automatic fixing systems in industry. Especially in the aerospace and automotive sector the number of low volume, high value and difficult-to-handle products is increasing[6,13,14].

Specialised fixtures only are economic within a mass production and cannot be reconfigured easily. Otherwise, the complex design and construction of modular fixtures are very time-consuming and expensive, with problems in repeatability and positioning accuracy[21,28]. Quality and precision cannot be controlled and influenced actively during the manufacturing process.

Moreover, an iterative improvement of fixture prototype designs is still common and causes high development costs[19]. At the same time the workpiece-fixture contact condition, workpiece distortion caused by cutting and clamping forces and deformation of the work holding tools still enjoy research effort[6].

As a basis of all development processes, the forces acting upon the fixing components during the manufacturing process have to be analysed. Consequently, an

C. Xiong et al. (Eds.): ICIRA 2008, Part II, LNAI 5315, pp. 356–367, 2008.

effective modelling and simulation method for the prediction of the workpiece-fixture behaviour during machining is required. It enables the possibility of fixture optimisation, too[24,23,22].

2 Finite Element Models

The finite element (FE) mesh has been developed dividing the nozzle-guide vane (NGV) into components: the blades, the outer and the inner frame (figure 1).

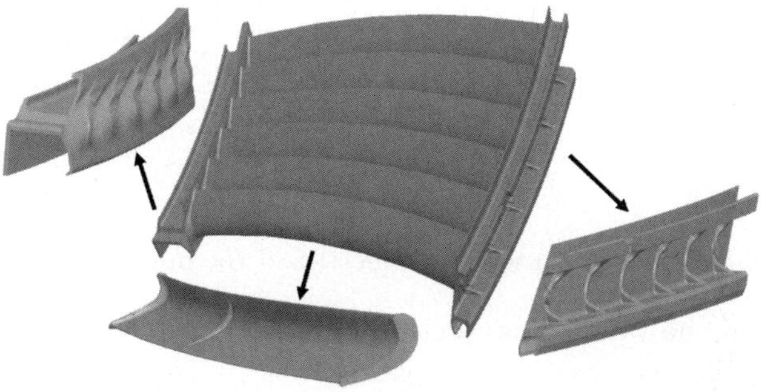

Fig. 1. Division of the NGV into three components

Simplified parametric cross section geometries and parameter optimisation lead to a simple FE-model. This inductive method of modelling has been completed by summarizing the results within an analytical model.

2.1 Complex FE-Model vs. Parametric FE-Model

Importing the geometry from CAD data, the model has been meshed using tetrahedron and hexahedron elements. As already mentioned, the part has been cut into pieces, meshed separately with the same amount and position of nodes on the contacting surfaces. This lead to a model with about 550000 elements, a mixture of eight-noded isoparametric 3D brick elements with trilinear interpolation and four-noded tetrahedral elements.

Less elements cause decreasing computation times and enlarge the capabilities of the variation of process parameters. After analysing the characteristic cross section parameters (e.g. area, second moment of inertia) of the three parts of the workpiece, suitable simplified cross section forms have been chosen (figure 2). Several curvatures have been neglected and wall thicknesses have been assumed to be constant. Moreover the blades were reasonably substituted using a simple parallelogram cross section geometry. All together 30 parameters were necessary to describe the simplified geometry of the whole workpiece.

As an important next step, the equations of the area, the centre of area and the second moment of inertia have been developed depending on the dimensions for all three cross section geometries by subdividing each cross section into simple triangles, rectangles and parallelograms (table 1).

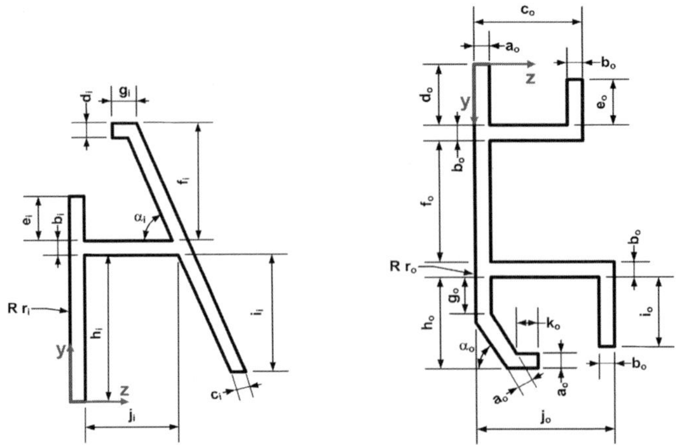

Fig. 2. Simplified cross section geometries of the inner and outer frame

The values for the whole cross section geometry have been evaluated by summation of all subareas.

$$A = \sum_k \operatorname{sgn}_k A_k \qquad I_{yy/zz/yz} = \sum_k \operatorname{sgn}_k I_{yy/zz/yz_k} \tag{1}$$

Based on the reference values from the CAD model, all geometric parameters have been optimised comparing the real part and the parametric model:

Table 1. Second moment of inertia of simple subareas

	rectangle	triangle	parallelogram
	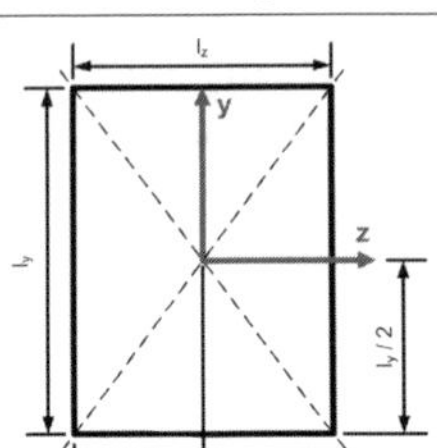	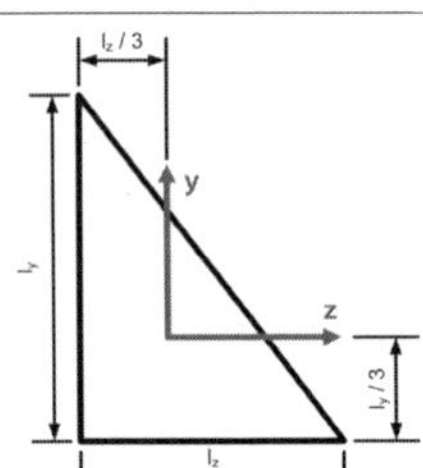	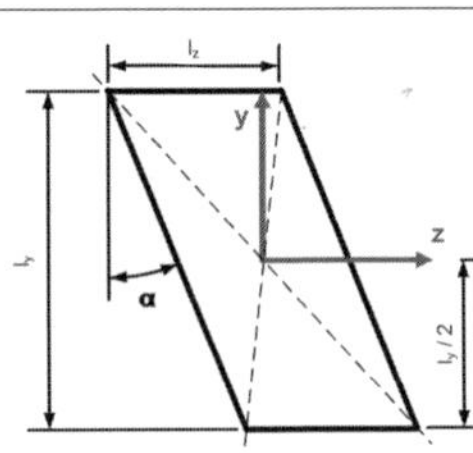
$\mathbf{A_k}$	$l_{y_k} l_{z_k}$	$\frac{l_{y_k} l_{z_k}}{2}$	$l_{y_k} l_{z_k}$
$\mathbf{I_{yy_k}}$	$\frac{l_{y_k} l_{z_k}^3}{12} + A_k \left(z_{s_k} - z_S\right)^2$	$\frac{l_{y_k} l_{z_k}^3}{36} + A_k \left(z_{s_k} - z_S\right)^2$	$\frac{l_{y_k} l_{z_k}}{12}\left[l_{y_k}^2 \tan^2\alpha + l_{z_k}^2\right] \ldots + A_k(z_{s_k} - z_S)^2$
$\mathbf{I_{zz_k}}$	$\frac{l_{y_k}^3 l_{z_k}}{12} + A_k \left(y_{s_k} - y_S\right)^2$	$\frac{l_{y_k}^3 l_{z_k}}{36} + A_k \left(y_{s_k} - y_S\right)^2$	$\frac{l_{y_k}^3 l_{z_k}}{12} + A_k \left(y_{s_k} - y_S\right)^2$
$\mathbf{I_{yz_k}}$	$-A_k \left(y_{s_k} - y_S\right)(z_{s_k} - z_S)$	$\frac{l_{y_k}^2 l_{z_k}^2}{72} - A_k(y_{s_k} - y_S)(z_{s_k} - z_S)$	$\frac{-l_{y_k}^3 l_{z_k} \tan\alpha}{12} \ldots - A_k \left(y_{s_k} - y_S\right)(z_{s_k} - z_S)$

- the second moments of inertia related to the centre of area I_{yy}, I_{zz} and I_{yz}
- the principal moments of inertia I_1 and I_2 and their orientation φ
- the area of the cross section A

The starting values have been chosen approximating the geometry of the real part. Further on, an optimisation procedure using least square fitting has been used. A boundary condition for the inclination angle of the blades has been set.

Again, the parameters have been determined for each of the three parts separately. Considering the criteria described above, the relative error in comparison to the real part was 5% for the bounding geometries. Due to the boundary condition of the inclination angle, the relative error of the blades' principal moments of inertia was about 10%. The deviation of the blades has been considered negligible due to their small influence on the reaction forces.

Based on the estimated parameter values, the simplified FE-model has been developed in MSC.Marc.®Mentat®. Enabling fast modifications, a script for automatic mesh generation has been generated.

Finally, the parametric FE-model consists of about 17000 eight-noded 3D brick elements, which is about 3% of the amount of elements of the complex model. The similar model geometries are shown in figure 3.

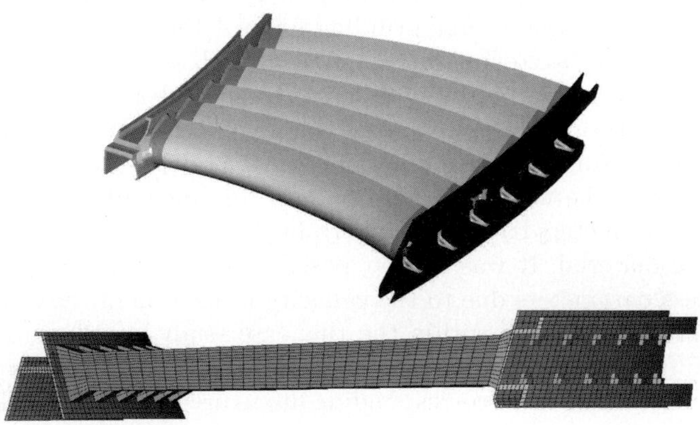

Fig. 3. Complex model vs. parametric model - geometry

2.2 Evaluation of Boundary Conditions

2.2.1 Grinding Forces

"Kinematic actions in grinding are constrained series of statistically irregular single engagements that are dependent upon the structure of the cutting area, the motion values and the geometric properties. ... The basic models are mainly based on tests with conventional abrasives .... Therefore the applicability is limited to machining conditions that are usually employed in conventional grinding processes." [5] "As grinding is a very complex manufacturing process with a large number of characteristic quantities which influence each other, the reproducibility is critical." [26]

Table 2. Theoretical Models of Grinding Forces

KLOCKE [12]	$F'_n = \int_0^{l_g} k_p \cdot A_{cu}(l) \cdot N_{kin}(l)\ \mathrm{d}l$
HUANG and CHENG [11]	$F'_n = N_t\ L_s\ p\ \overline{h}_g^2 \sin\Theta\ \tan\Theta$ $F'_t = \frac{\pi}{4}\ N_t\ L_s\ p\ \overline{h}_g^2 \sin\Theta$
BÖGE [3]	$F_t = k_c \cdot A = k_c \cdot a_e\ f_l\ \frac{v_{ft}}{v_c}$
BRINKSMEIER *et al.* [5], TÖNSHOFF [26] SALJE[20],WERNER [27]	$F'_n = c_{wp} \cdot c_{gw} \cdot \left(\frac{1}{q}\right)^{e_1} \cdot a_e^{e_2} \cdot d_{eq}^{e_3}$
DECNEUT [7], ONO [18], WERNER[27]	$F'_n = K_f \cdot \left(\frac{v_{ft}}{v_c}\right)^{2\varepsilon-1} \cdot a_e^{\varepsilon} \cdot d_{eq}^{1-\varepsilon}$

For small feed rates the grinding forces can be "resolved into three component forces, namely, normal grinding force F_n, tangential grinding force F_t and a component force acting along the direction of longitudinal feed, which is usually neglected because of its insignificance ". ...The tangential grinding force is ...much lower than the normal grinding force. "[15] Furthermore the normal grinding force caused by cooling lubricants is as high as the usual normal grinding force or even higher.[1,9] A lot of different basic models of grinding forces can be found in literature (table 2).None of the given theoretical models could be used for the evaluation of the grinding forces. All models include specific parameters depending on the workpiece material and/or machining conditions. These characteristic parameters have to be determined experimentally for each process and workpiece material. It was neither possible to measure the grinding forces nor the process parameters due to the capacity utilisation of the manufacturer.

Furthermore, the process within the this case study is unique due to shape grinding of different complex and variable grinding areas and a super-alloy workpiece. As a result, there is no corresponding literature for assuming these process

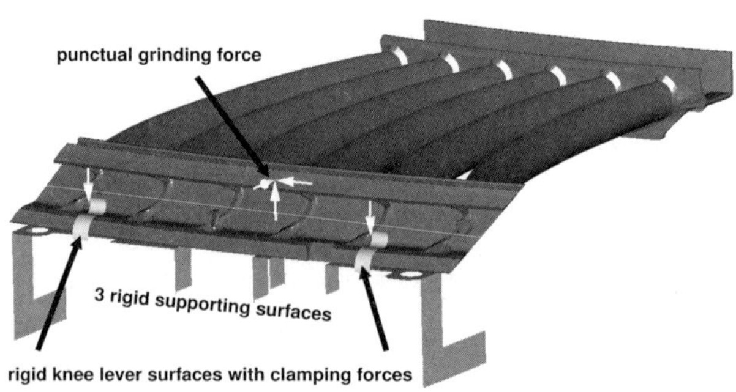

Fig. 4. Complex model with two punctual clamping forces on rigid contact surfaces and one single point load representing the grinding force

parameters. All publications either deal with simple grinding processes (e.g. face grinding) or use conventional workpiece materials.

Due to the lack of experimental data or comparable parameters for the theoretical grinding force models, an overview of corresponding projects has been carried out. Considering the major conclusions drawn by NIEWELT[17] and MEIER[16] while investigating surface grinding of Nickel based alloys similar to the material within this case study and comparing other relevant literature ([5],[8],[10],[15] and [25]), related grinding forces have been reasonably assumed for the current setup.

Two possibilities of load application have been tested. First, the forces have been applied on a solid contact body representing the grinding wheel geometry and touching the deformable workpiece, which is moving along the grinded area. Due to the discretization of the workpiece geometry and the small displacement compared to the grinding wheel diameter, the contact area is restricted to two nodes. Based on these results, the grinding forces have been modeled as equidistant static point loads on the grinded areas (figure 4). This reduces the computation time by avoiding the iteration processes of the contact algorithms.

It should be pointed out that all point loads are singularities in the FE-model causing higher deformations and stresses than the real process. These peaks are limited to a small area surrounding the point load, thought the main focal points - reaction forces on the clamping mechanism - are not affected.

2.2.2 Fixture-Workpiece-Contact

Currently, knee levers are used for clamping of the workpiece. Based on the given tightening torque of the screws, the estimation of the clamping forces, using BÖGE's approach of the screw preload force [4] and the law of the lever, lead to clamping forces. To avoid plastic deformation due to the clamping forces, the contact stress is limited to the yield tensile strength. Thus the maximum clamping force has been ascertained with the help of the HERTZian contact equations [2].

Within the FE-models, the surrounding surfaces of the fixture are represented by rigid contact bodies surfaces (figure 4). The clamping normal forces F_{cnf} have been applied to one single node per knee lever. This node has been coupled to the surface representing the rigid contact body. Furthermore, the node displacement in both horizontal directions has been fixed to withstand the transverse contact forces. Finally, the supporting areas are simply fixed by displacement boundary conditions.

2.2.3 Heat Effects

Grinding is a process with a significant thermal load upon the workpiece. Furthermore, different fixing principles (e.g. piezoelectric actuators) have a very high thermal sensitivity. Nevertheless, the heat conductivity of the workpiece was not taken into account due to the small heat affected zone and the cooling lubricants flooding the workpiece during the grinding process. Though, the influence on the fixing points has been neglected as well as the thermal expansion of the workpiece.

3 Simulation Results

3.1 Verification of the Parametric Model

The parametric model has been verified by comparing two types of simulation results. First, single point loads have been applied on the workpiece fixed by displacement boundary conditions, neglecting contact problems, friction and fixture stiffness. The maximum total displacements close to the loaded nodes have been compared (figure 5). The results are corresponding for all applied loads except the first and the last increment. This inaccuracy is caused by the replacement of the blade geometry with a simple parallelogram and its influence upon the stiffness on the connected frames. Except the outer load locations, the relative error is less than 2.5%.

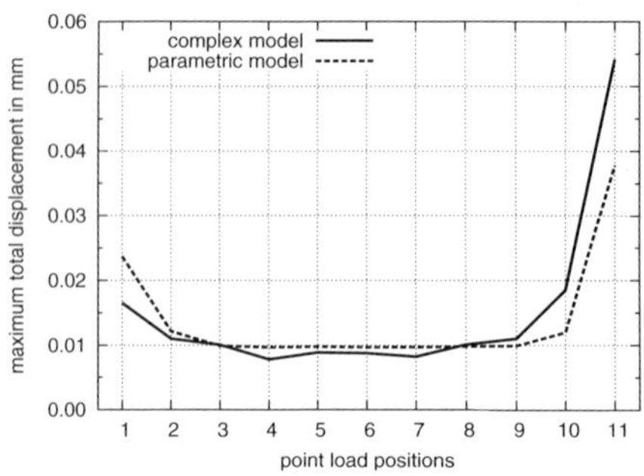

Fig. 5. Maximum total displacement at point load position

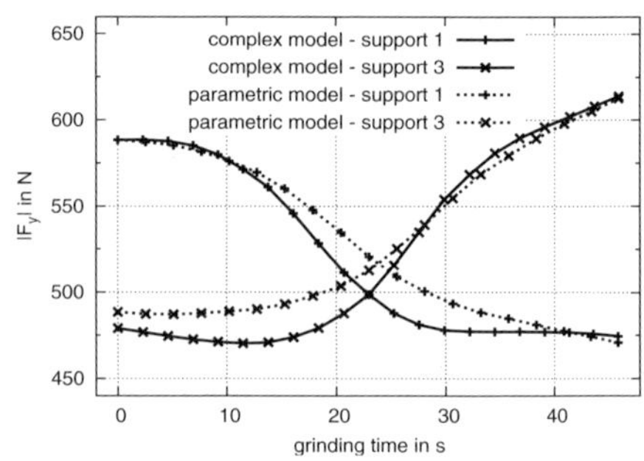

Fig. 6. Normal reaction forces on supporting surface

Secondly, fixture-workpiece-contact has been considered, too, evaluating the reaction forces acting on the knee levers due to the grinding loads. In general, the forces show the same curve paths with similar absolute values. The normal forces acting on the knee levers remain constant throughout the whole process in both models. In contrast, the transverse forces on the knee levers as well as all force components acting on the supporting surfaces show a time dependency.

As an example, the reaction forces on the supporting areas one and three during load case five have been compared (figure 6). The curve progression for the results of both models are similar in most cases but not equal. For all loadcases and fixture components the approximation of the contact normal forces is almost accurate. It is possible to show tendencies of the transverse forces with the help of the parametric model but not exact values.

3.2 Parameter Variation

The main influencing parameters on the reaction forces are the coefficient of static friction, the grinding forces and the clamping forces. These parameters have been varied using the parametric model.

The friction coefficient has been reasonably assumed to be $\mu = 0.2$. Considering other surface finishes ($\mu = 0.4$) and coated supporting surfaces ($\mu = 0.05$), the friction coefficient has been varied. The normal forces acting on both knee levers remain constant throughout the whole process, due to the direction of the acting grinding forces. The transverse preload forces on both knee levers due to the clamping loads show a linear dependency on the static coefficient of friction. Equally, the time dependent force components caused by the grinding process are rising. Figure 7 shows the force paths for the transverse forces. It is reasonably assumed that the amplitude of the reaction forces caused by the clamping loads is linear dependent on the friction coefficient.

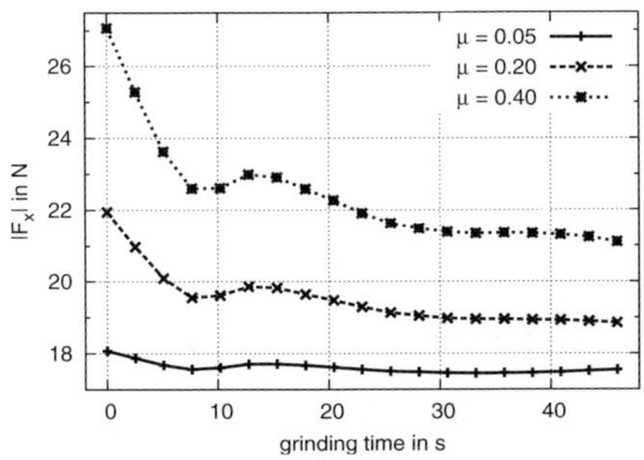

Fig. 7. Variation of friction coefficient

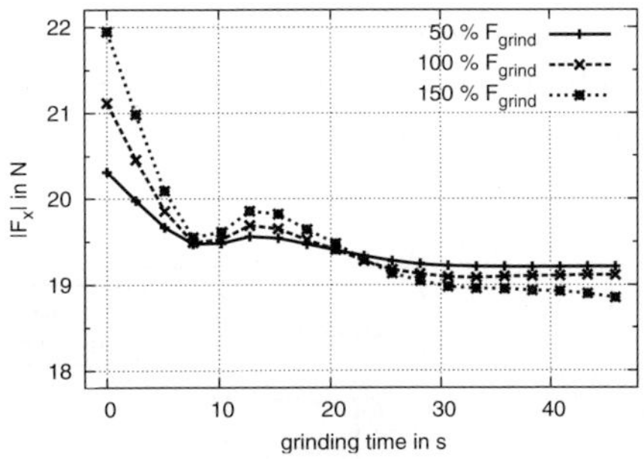

Fig. 8. Variation of grinding forces

In addition, simulations have been done with 50% and 150% of the assumed grinding forces. Again, the normal forces remain stable whereas the transverse forces acting on both knee levers (figure 8) are varying. The amplitude of the dynamic force component is linear dependent on the grinding forces. Lastly, the clamping force has been decreased 25% three times (figure 9).

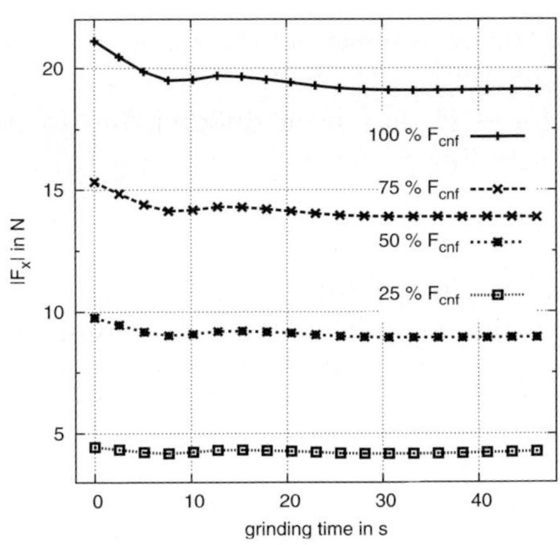

Fig. 9. Variation of clamping forces: transverse force on knee lever

Predictably, the static share of the reaction forces is linear dependent on the clamping forces. Decreasing clamping forces cause decreasing reaction forces in all directions naturally. The amplitude of the dynamic transverse reaction forces caused by the grinding process is also changing, dependent on the clamping forces. This dependency is reasonably assumed to be linear. The combination of both effects leads to a non-linear dependency of the transverse reaction forces on the clamping preloads.

4 Analytical Model

An analytical model has been developed exemplary for the transverse force in x-direction being applied on one knee lever. To ensure the accuracy of the model, it is based on one curve path taken from the complex model. Furthermore, the results of the parameter variation with the parametric model have been used to consider the dependencies on grinding load, clamping forces and the coefficient of static friction (figure 10).

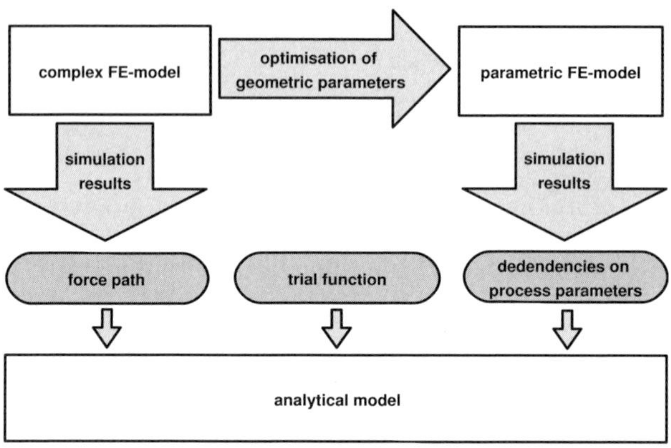

Fig. 10. Development of the analytical model

The total reaction force F_x has been divided due to its causes - clamping preloads $F_{x_{preload}}$ and grinding forces $F_{x_{grind}}$ (figure 11).

$$F_x(t) = F_{x_{preload}} + F_{x_{grind}}(t) \tag{2}$$

The reaction forces due to the grinding loads are evaluated by eliminating the constant preload force component. Moreover, this curve has been approximated by a sine function, leading to the basic form of the empirical model (figure 12):

$$F_x(t) \approx F_{x_{preload}} + a \cdot \sin(b \cdot t + c) + d \tag{3}$$

All four parameters within the approximation function are determined with a curve fitting procedure. The preload force has been taken from simulation results.

The parameters b and c are influencing period and phase shift of the function but are not dependent on the clamping loads, the grinding forces or the friction coefficient. Once determined for one force path, they remain stable.

Scaling is done by the parameters a and d. Referring to the results of section 3.2, the amplitude a of the sine approximation is linear dependent on the grinding

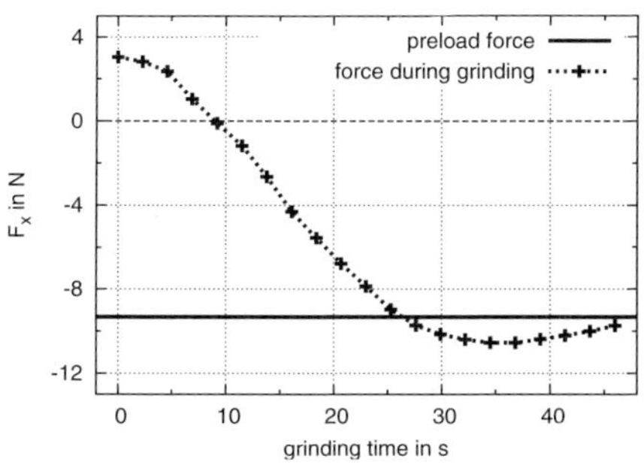

Fig. 11. Reaction forces on a knee lever caused by preload and grinding forces

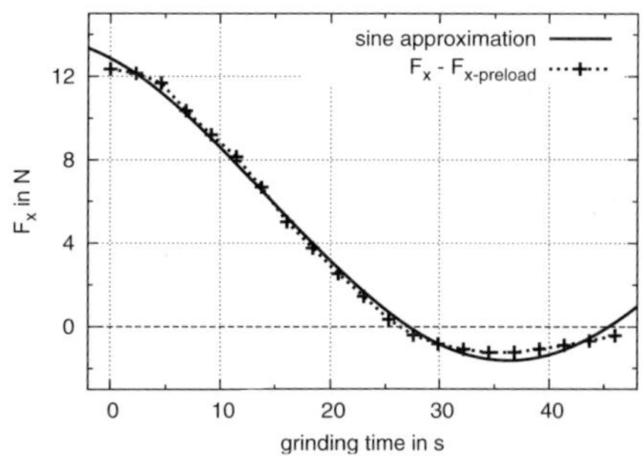

Fig. 12. Time dependent reaction force due to grinding loads and its sine approximation

forces as well as on the clamping forces and on the friction coefficient. Moreover the same dependencies have been assumed for the vertical shift d. Lastly, a, d and the preload forces are again linear dependent on the static coefficient of friction.

To predict the reaction forces due to changing process parameters, one exact reference force path (measured or taken from the simulation results with the complex model) has been scaled. Scaling factors referring to clamping forces, grinding loads and friction coefficient of the reference curve (indexed with *ref*) are introduced.

$$k_{clamp}\left(F_{cnf}\right) = \frac{F_{cnf}}{F_{cnf_{ref}}} \quad k_{grind}\left(F_{grind}\right) = \frac{F_{grind}}{F_{grind_{ref}}} \quad k_{frict}\left(\mu\right) = \frac{\mu}{\mu_{ref}} \tag{4}$$

A combination of the basic model (3) and the scaling factors (4) leads to the final analytical model:

$$\begin{aligned} F_x\left(F_{cnf}, F_{grind}, \mu, t\right) =& k_{clamp}\left(F_{cnf}\right) \cdot k_{frict}\left(\mu\right) \cdot \ldots \\ & \left\{F_{x_{preload}} + k_{grind}\left(F_{grind}\right) \cdot \left[a \cdot \sin\left(b \cdot t + c\right) + d\right]\right\} \end{aligned} \tag{5}$$

5 Summary and Outlook

Using different FE-models, a method is presented which allows to predict the reaction forces depending on different grinding parameters. A complex FE-model with a huge number of elements has been created followed by a parametric model with similar mechanical properties but less elements. Therefore, the cross sections have been simplified with optimised geometric parameters based on the second moments of inertia.

The results of the complex model provided detailed information of the workpiece-fixture behaviour during the process. An analysis of the influencing process parameters has been carried out with the fast but less accurate parametric model resulting in scaling factors. Combining the accurate force path, the scaling factors and a sine trial function, an analytical model has been developed. It provides the opportunity to forecast the reaction forces within a certain range of grinding parameters.

The usability of the method has been exposed by forecasting the transverse reaction forces acting on knee levers fixing a NGV during shape grinding.

Nevertheless, further investigations need to be carried out on this field. The most important pending issue is the validation of the complex FE-model with experimentally measured values. In addition, the complex model can be improved using time dependent grinding force profiles from ongoing research activities to get information about the dynamic behaviour of the workpiece-fixture system. Spring-damper elements can be used to consider the deformable behaviour of the fixture components. Moreover, the fast parametric model can be combined with optimisation algorithms to improve the locations of the fixture components and to minimise clamping forces. Lastly, the analytical model in combination with control software/hardware facilitates real time process simulation for possibly active clamping components.

Acknowledgement

This research work has been tutored by Prof. Dr.-Ing. habil. Reiner Kreißig, Institute of Applied Mechanics and Thermodynamics, Chemnitz University of Technology and Dr.-Ing. habil. Jürgen Leopold, Fraunhofer Insitute for Machine Tools and Forming Technology, Chemnitz which is gratefully acknowledged. Moreover, this work has been supported by the European Union within the integrated project AFFIX.

References

1. Beck, T.: Kühlschmierstoffeinsatz beim Schleifen mit CBN. PhD thesis, RWTH Aachen, Aachen (2001)
2. Beitz, W., Grote, K.-H. (eds.): Dubbel - Taschenbuch für den Maschinenbau, 20th edn. Springer, Heidelberg (2001)
3. Böge, A.: Das Techniker Handbuch. Vieweg Verlag, Braunschweig (1999)
4. Böge, A.: Vieweg Handbuch Maschinenbau. Vieweg Verlag, Braunschweig (2004)
5. Brinksmeier, E., Tönshoff, H.K., Czenkusch, C., Heinzel, C.: Modelling and optimization of grinding processes. Journal of Intelligent Manufacturing 9 (4), 303–314 (1998)
6. AFFIX consortium. Affix - aligning, holding and fixing flexible and difficult to handle components (2006), http://www.affix-ip.eu
7. Decneut, A.: Verantwoorde Keuze van de Slijpvoorwaarden. PhD thesis, Katholieke Universiteit te Leuven (1974)
8. Gromann, K., Mühl, A.: Simulation and Realization of Adaptive Control Constraint in Path Grinding. Production Engineering 9 (1), 29–32 (2002)
9. Heinzel, C.: Methoden zur Untersuchung und Optimierung der Kühlschmierung beim Schleifen. PhD thesis, Universität Bremen (1999)
10. Hoffmeister, H.W.: Simulation of grinding processes with fea. In: CIRP International Workshop on Modeling of Machining Operations (2005)
11. Huang, Z.Y., Chen, G.: Derivation of grinding force of online roll grinder. Journal of Iron and Steel Research International 12 (5), 18–20 (2005)

12. Klocke, F.: Fertigungsverfahren 2, 4th edn. VDI-Buch. Springer, Berlin (2005)
13. Leopold, J., Poppitz, A., Klärner, M., Schmidt, A.-K., Berger, J.: Interaction between machining and new fixturing principles for aerospace structures. International Journal of Material Forming (2008)
14. Leopold, J., Poppitz, A., Klärner, M., Clauß, D., Bandoli, M., Merlo, A., Gimenez, M., Larranaga, J.: Investigations to New Fixturing Prnciples For Aerospace Structures. In: Vollertsen, F. (ed.) APT 2007, International Conference on Applied Production Technology, Bremen, Germany, pp. 173–189. Bremer Institut für Angewandte Strahltechnik (2007)
15. Li, Z.C., Lin, B., Xu, Y.S., Hu, J.: Experimental studies on grinding forces and force ratio of the unsteady-state grinding technique. Journal of Materials Processing Technology 129 (1-3), 76–80 (2002)
16. Meier, A.: Bearbeitung von metallischen gasturbinenwerkstoffen durch tiefschleifen und drahterodieren. research report, Fraunhofer-Institut für Produktionsanlagen und Konstruktionstechnik, Berlin, Berichte aus dem Produktionstechnischen Zentrum Berlin (1997)
17. Niewelt, W.: Planschleifen von Nickelbasis-Legierungen. PhD thesis, TU Berlin, Institut für Werkzeugmaschinen und Fertigungstechnik (1995)
18. Ono, K.: Analysis of the Grinding Force. Bulletin of the Japan Society of Grinding Engineers 1 (1961)
19. Ratchev, S., Huang, W., Phuah, K., Liu, S., Becker, A.A.: Fea-based simulation for dynamic fixture-workpiece behaviour during grinding processes. CIRP Journal of Manufacturing Systems 34(4), 309–317 (2005)
20. Salje, E.: Kennzahlen und Gesetzmäßigkeiten beim Schleifen. Research report, Technische Hochschule Aachen (1952)
21. Shen, Y., Shirinzadeh, B.: Qualitative analysis and quantitative evaluation of fixturing. Robotics and Computer Integrated manufacturing 18, 335–342 (2001)
22. Tan, E.Y.T., Senthil-Kumar, A., Fuh, J.Y.H., Nee, A.Y.C.: Modeling, Analysis and Verification of Optimal Fixturing Design. IEEE Transactions on Automatic Science and Engineering 1(2), 121–132 (2004)
23. Tao, Z.J., Senthil-Kumar, A., Nee, A.Y.C.: A Computational Approach to Optimum Clamping Synthesis of Machning Fixtures. International Journal of Production Research 37(15), 3495–3517 (1999)
24. Tao, Z.J., Senthil-Kumar, A., Nee, A.Y.C., Mannan, M.A.: Modelling and experimental investigation of a sensor-integrated workpiece-fixture system. International Journal of Computer Applications in Technology 10(3/4), 236–250 (1997)
25. Teicher, U., Künanz, K., Chattopadhyay, A.B.: Grinding of titanium alloy by single layered cbn and diamond grinding wheels. In: CIRP International Workshop on Modeling of Machining Operations (2005)
26. Tönshoff, H.K., Peters, J., Inasaki, I., Paul, T.: Modelling and simulation of grinding processes. CIRP Annals 41(2), 677–688 (1992)
27. Werner, G.: Kinematik und Mechanik des Schleifprozesses. PhD thesis, RWTH Aachen (1971)
28. Xionga, C.-H., Lib, Y.-F., Rongc, K., Xiong, Y.-L.: Qualitative analysis and quantitative evaluation of fixturing. Robotics and Computer Integrated Manufacturing 18, 335–342 (2002)

A Novel Dual-Cam Linkage Drive Automatic Tool Changer for Horizontal Machining Center

Ming Cong[1], Jing Liu[1], and Quanpu Li[2]

[1] Dalian University of Technology, Dalian, Liaoning, China
[2] Dalian Machine Tool Group Corp., Dalian, Liaoning, China
congm@dlut.edu.cn, jingjun040930@yahoo.cn

Abstract. In this paper, a novel automatic tool changer for horizontal machining center is presented. The mechanism and working principle of the automatic tool changer are introduced. Push-pull rod and tool changer run synchronously driven by dual-cam linkage. The key structure, dual-cam linkage, is analyzed and designed in details. Cam curves of two sets of cams, one of which drives push-pull rod and another drives tool changer, are selected by way of comprehensive evaluation. The transmission unit is designed. An application example of this novel automatic tool changer in MDH65 Horizontal Machining Center is presented and motion simulation is carried out. The result shows that the novel dual-cam linkage automatic tool changer works more efficiently and reliably than general with rational matching design of two sets of cams.

Keywords: ATC. Dual-cam linkage. Cam curve. Comprehensive evaluation. Motion simulation.

1 Introduction

Automatic Tool Changer (ATC) is a system that automatically performs tool exchange between the spindle and the tool magazine of a machining centre. It plays an important role in reducing the machine idle time, which can improve work efficiency and reliability significantly.

Various types of ATC with quite different working principles have been applied in machining centers. Yan and Chen studied the configuration synthesis of machining centers with tool change mechanisms and the classification of automatic tool changers in [1] and [2]. Reference [3] investigated types and design characteristics of automatic tool change mechanism. According to the difference of drive mechanism for tool changer, it mainly includes two types of ATC, one of which is hydraulic drive ATC, another is mechanical cam drive ATC. Reference [4] compared those two type of ATC and indicated that the latter has more advantage because of higher efficiency and reliability. A tool changer driven by double-follower cam gear, which can be used in both vertical and horizontal machining center, was researched on in [5]

Based on the investigation of existing types of ATC and research on ATC working process[6], a novel type of ATC driven by dual-cam linkage is considered for horizontal machining center.

C. Xiong et al. (Eds.): ICIRA 2008, Part II, LNAI 5315, pp. 368–377, 2008.

2 The Dual-Cam Linkage Drive ATC

Generally, there are two parts participating in tool exchange in a machining center with ATC. A push-pull rod in spindle is used to push or pull the tool holder, so that the tool in the front-end of spindle would be clamped or unclamped, and a tool changer is used to exchange tools between the spindle and tool magazine. Tool changer and push-pull rod should work sequentially, otherwise serious problems, for example, damage to tools, spindle and magazine, may occur.

2.1 Mechanism of Dual-Cam Linkage Drive ATC

A typical cam drive ATC used popularly is shown in Fig. 1. The two parts participating in tool exchange are driven separately. In tool push-pull part, the push-pull rod is driven by hydraulic pressure, and the tool in the front-end of spindle will be clamped or unclamped according to the movement of push-pull rod. In the tool exchange part, the power is from a motor, and the tool changer is controlled by cams. In order to ensure the two parts work sequentially, several limit and proximity switches are used to coordinate the positions of push-pull rod and tool changer. In this way, the process of tool exchange is complex, so it costs much time and the reliability is difficult to ensure.

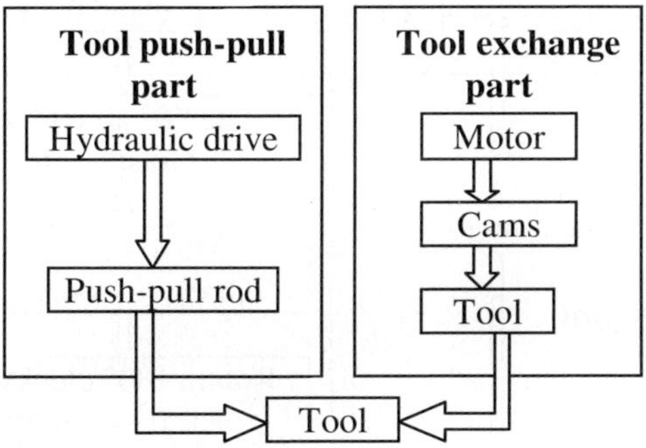

Fig. 1. The typical cam drive ATC

The novel type of dual-cam linkage drive ATC could resolve above problems. The schematic diagram of dual-cam linkage ATC mechanism is shown in Fig. 2.

As shown in Fig. 2, Tool push-pull part and toll exchange part are driven by one motor. One power line is motor, cam I, push-pull rod, disk spring and tool, and the other power line is motor, coupling, transmission unit, cam II, tool changer and tool. These two parts would work synchronously driven by one motor. This structure can simplify tool exchange process and save time remarkably, and rational design of dual-cam linkage can ensure that the working timing of two parts match with each other perfectly, so tool exchange would be more accurately and reliability.

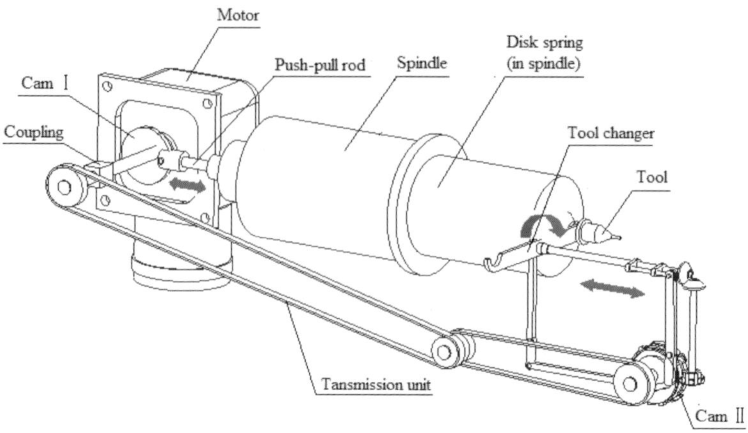

Fig. 2. The schematic diagram of dual-cam linkage drive ATC

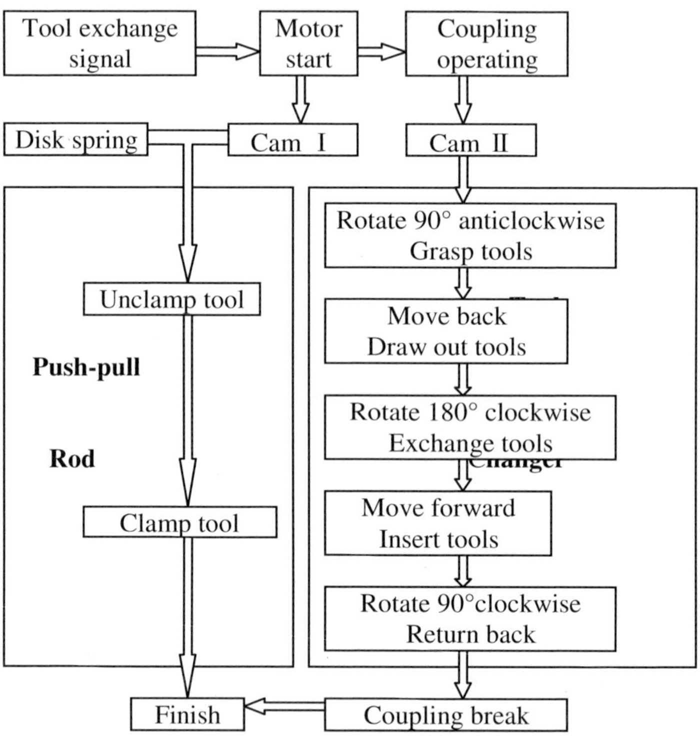

Fig. 3. The working principle of dual-cam linkage drive ATC

2.2 The Working Principle of Dual-Cam Linkage Drive ATC

The main innovation of dual-cam linkage drive ATC is the application of a new mechanism, in which tool push-pull part and tool exchange part are driven by one motor synchronously. The working principle is shown in Fig. 3.

Push-pull rod in the spindle is controlled by cam I and disk spring, to clamp or unclamp the tool which is fixed in the front-end of spindle. Cam II is composed of two cams, a slot cam inlaid on one side of a globoid cam. The slot cam controls the translation movement of tool changer, which can draw tool out from or insert tool into spindle. The globoid cam controls the rotation movement of tool changer, which can exchange tools between tool magazine and spindle. When machining center gives tool exchange signal, motor starts, then push-pull rod and tool exchange manipulator will work in timing separately controlled by cam I and cam II, which are driven by the same motor. Therefore, the process and control are simple, which make it possible to realize reliable operation and save tool exchange time.

3 Design of Dual-Cam Linkage

In design, dual-cam linkage is the most challenging part. The movement of cam I and cam II must match with each other perfectly to insure high reliability, and the power transmission unit between motor and cam II should be designed reasonably based on the structure of machining center.

3.1 The Matching Design for Cam Timing Chart

According to the functional requirements of cams in dual-cam linkage drive ATC, the types of cams are selected, shown in Table 1.

Table 1. Cams in Dual-Cam Linkage

Number	Cam type	Follower type	Function
I	Plate cam	Translating	Translation motion of push-pull rod
II	Slot cam	Oscillating	Translation motion of tool changer
	Globoid cam	Indexing	Rotation motion of tool changer

Supposed the transmission ratio of two sets of cams is 1:1. In other words, two sets of cams can be regarded as located on a same axis. In order to realize coordinated motion of push-pull rod and tool changer, the cam timing chart are designed as Fig. 4 based on the working principle of dual-cam linkage drive ATC.

ϕ_c is angular displacement of the cams. ϕ_f is linear or angular displacement of the cam followers. It is mm for translating follower of plate cam, and it is deg for oscillating follower of slot cam and indexing follower of globoid cam.

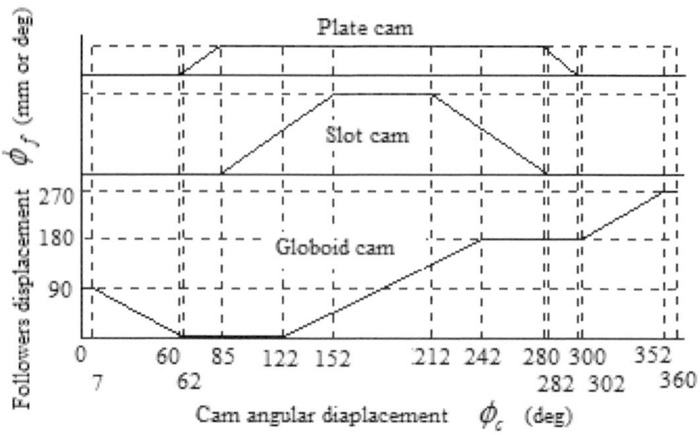

Fig. 4. Cam timing chart

In a tool exchange cycle, the process is as follows:

1. Indexing follower rotates 90°anticlockwise and drives tool changer to grasp tools while globoid cam rotates from ϕ_c =7°to ϕ_c =62°.

2. Plate cam pushes push-pull rod to unclamp the tool in the front-end of spindle while it rotates from ϕ_c =60°to ϕ_c =85°

3. Oscillating follower drives the tool changer to draw out tools from spindle and tool magazine while slot cam rotates from ϕ_c =85°to ϕ_c =152°.

4. Indexing follower rotates 180°clockwise and drives tool changer to exchange tools between spindle and tool magazine while globoid cam rotates from ϕ_c =122°to ϕ_c =242°.

5. Oscillating follower drives the tool changer to insert tools into spindle and tool magazine while slot cam rotates from ϕ_c =212°to ϕ_c =282°. Then, the slot cam involutes

6. Disk spring pushes push-pull rod back to clamp the tool assembled into spindle, and plate cam rotates from ϕ_c =280°to ϕ_c =300°, then involutes.

7. Indexing follower rotates 90°clockwise and drives tool changer to return to former condition while globoid cam rotates from ϕ_c =302°to ϕ_c =352. Then, the globoid cam involutes.

3.2 The Analysis and Optimum Design of Cam Curve

Cam curve is closely related to the kinematics characters, dynamic performance, efficiency and service life of cam mechanism. It's important to select optimum cam curve for different working periods. The main features of cam curve are as follows:

Dimensionless maximum velocity V_m: It is related to maximum momentum, according to $P=mv$, where P is momentum, m is mass, and v is velocity. V_m has influence on pressure angle and size of cam. If m is large, it's necessary to choose the cam curve, of which V_m is small.

Dimensionless maximum acceleration A_m: It is related to maximum inertial force, according to $f=ma$, where f is inertial force, m is mass, and a is acceleration. The extrusion force between cam and follower increases with increase of A_m, and the amplitude of vibration force increases too. If velocity curve is discontinuous, A_m would be infinite, and impact vibration will occur. It is reliable to choose a cam curve, of which A_m is small, in high-speed cam.

Dimensionless maximum jerk J_m: It is the differential of acceleration with respect to time. J_m is mainly related to the vibration of follower. If acceleration jumps on one point, J_m is large in this point and strenuous vibration appears. To reduce vibration, it is better to choose a cam curve, of which J_m is small.

In cam curve design of dual-cam linkage, the mainly requirements are:

1. All cams should run sequentially and smoothly.

2. The plate cam and slot cam have no-impact and less vibration in operation to avoid destructing tools.

3. The indexing precision and accurate positioning of globoid cam should be improved to ensure tool exchange accuracy

4. Considered the service life of globoid cam, thin ridge must be avoided.

To avoid rigid impact caused by velocity jump and flexible impact caused by acceleration jump is the basic principle in selecting cam curve. It is required that the features V_m, A_m and J_m are as small as possible, but there is no cam curve, of which the features can be all small. So an optimum design method of cam curve, comprehensive evaluation of cam curve, is presented.

Comprehensive evaluation is based on fuzzy theory and maximum degree of membership principle[7]. All factors related to the project would be concerned, and the solution comes from comprehensive evaluation of them. The process of cam curves optimum design in dual-cam linkage is as follows:

1. According to cam curve design standard and practical design experience, candidate set of cam curve is founded, which includes polynomial curve, modified trapezoid curve (MT), modified sine curve (MS), and modified constant velocity curve (MCV)[8].

2. Consider the features of cam curve V_m, A_m and J_m as evaluation factors. They are specified in Table 2.

3. Through comparing the mainly requirements of cam in dual-cam linkage and the effect aspect of every cam feature, and analyzing the evaluation factors, fuzzy subsets are established. Practical design experience is also invited.

4. Present membership satisfied grade of each cam curve in candidate set.

5. Based on set theory, select optimum cam curve for each cam in dual-cam linkage. The result is shown in Fig. 5.

Table 2. Features of Cam Curve

Cam curve	V_m	A_m	J_m	Application
Polynomial	1.88	5.77	60.00	High speed and heavy load
MT	2.00	4.89	61.43	High speed and light load
MS	1.76	5.53	69.47	High speed and moderate load
MCV	1.28	8.01	201.4	Low speed and heavy load

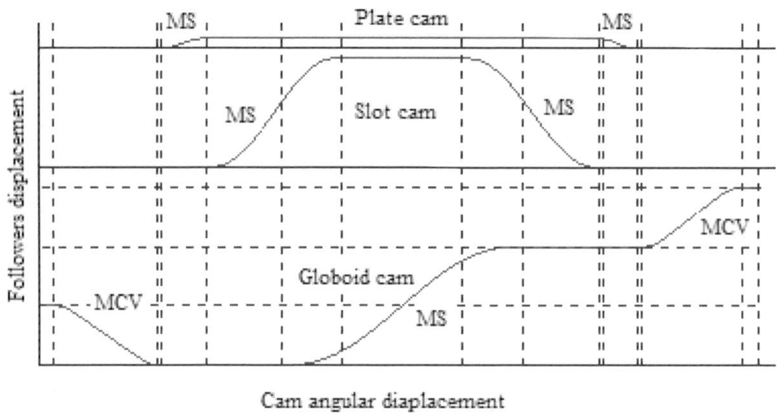

Fig. 5. The result of optimum design for cam curve

Compared with Fig. 4 and Fig. 5, it shows that modified sine curve (MS) is selected for plate cam and slot cam, and modified constant velocity curve (MCV) and modified sine curve (MS) are selected for globoid cam in their different working periods.

3.3 The Design of Transmission Unit

In dual-cam linkage drive ATC, two sets of cams are driven by one motor, so the transmission unit between them must be designed on the basis of the concrete structure of machining center. In a general way, as shown in Fig. 2, the motor is fixed near the rear end of spindle, and the power from motor pass through speed reducer to drive cam I axis directly. Then, the transmission unit should transfer power from cam I axis to cam II axis.

Because of the indexing operation of globoid cam, the torque of cam II axis appears positive-negative changes in one cycle, which tends to induce fluctuation. It is necessary to ensure the cam II axis runs smoothly, so that it is possible to give full scope to the indexing precision of globoid cam, and the slot cam gets stable operation to avoid breakage when drawing tool out from or assembling tool into spindle. So neither the chain transmission with pulsation nor gear transmission with interval is suitable. The solution is to choose synchronous belt, which is with constant velocity and non-slip, as the transmission unit.

The arrangement of synchronous belt transmission is dependent on the concrete structure of machining center. If the size of machining center is large, it is permissible to design multiple level synchronous belt transmission as shown in Fig. 2.

4 The Application Example

Dual-cam linkage drive ATC has been applied in MDH65 Horizontal Machining Center. The ATC structure is similar to the one shown in Fig. 2. The cams are designed according to the above analysis, and the design result is shown in Fig. 6. Transmission unit is constituted by two level synchronous belt. The motor is fixed near the rear end of spindle. Based on the limitation of the structure of MDH65, a set of cam-linkage mechanism including a couple of bevel gears is proposed to drive tool changer.

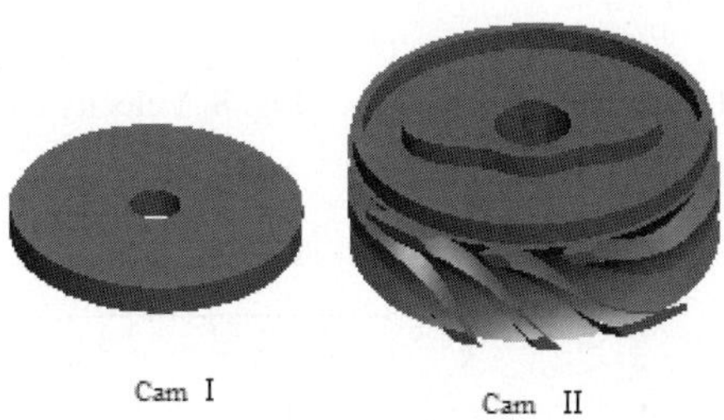

Fig. 6. The cams

Based on the virtual prototype technology, a motion simulation of the ATC is carried out. Supposed a tool exchange cycle time is 2 seconds, we get motion curves of two sets of cams from motion simulation. The displacement curve diagram of cams is shown in Fig. 7. The displacement curves are continuous and smooth, without jump, and match with Fig. 5.

As shown in Fig. 8, the velocity curves of cams are all continuous. Slot cam and globoid cam velocity curves are smooth. There are two cusps in plate cam velocity curve, but one happens in middle time of plate cam pushing push-pull rod and the other happens in middle time of disk spring pushing push-pull rod back, so they wouldn't cause impact when tool holder unclamps or clamps the tool. From velocity curves, no rigid impact would occur to cause damage.

As shown in Fig. 9, it is acceleration curve diagram of cams. We can see there are several cusps in plate cam and globoid cam acceleration curves. They would cause flexible impact and can't be avoided easily, but that is acceptable in a certain range.

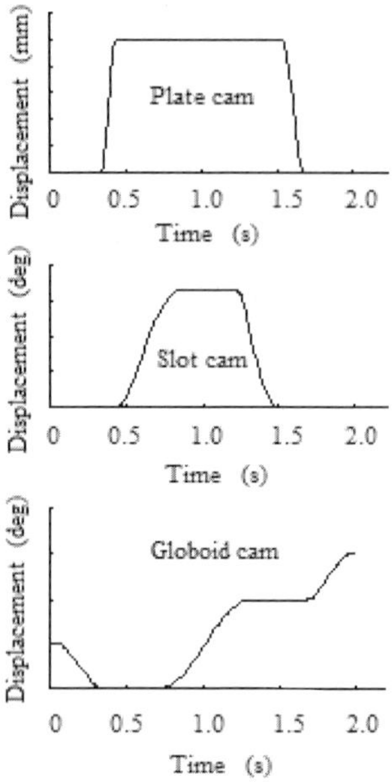

Fig. 7. Displacement curve

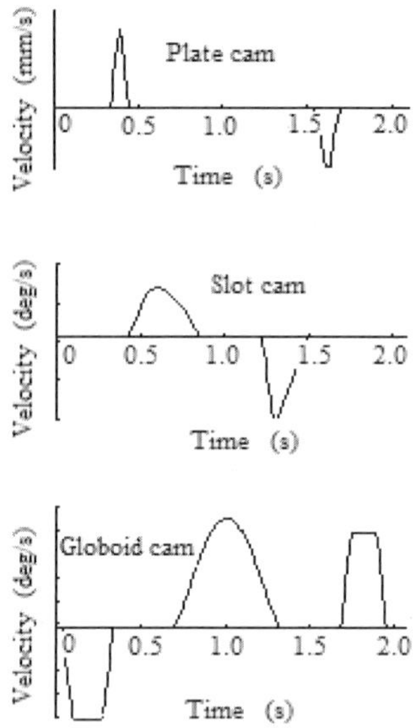

Fig. 8. Velocity curve

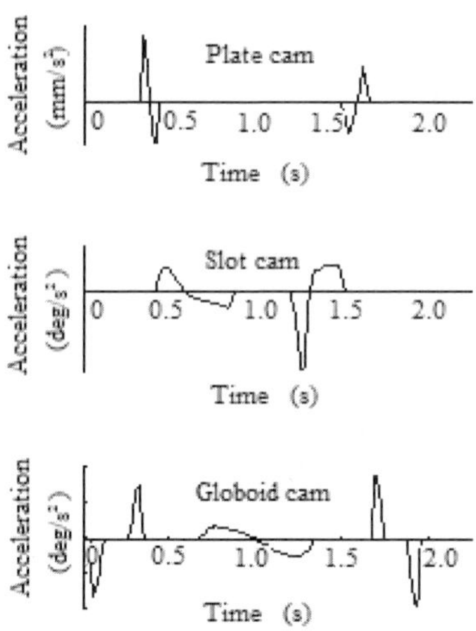

Fig. 9. Acceleration curve

The result of motion simulation shows that every part of the ATC has noninterference; two sets of cams work in coordination; tool exchange process is accurate and reliable. In practical test, the number of normal tool exchange operation times has reached 20000 and the minimal tool to tool change time (T-T) is 2 seconds.

5 Conclusion

In this paper, a novel dual-cam linkage drive ATC is derived based on the typical cam drive ATC. The mechanism and working principle are described. Analysis and design of key structure, dual-cam linkage, are introduced in details. The method comprehensive evaluation is invited in cam curve design. An application example is presented for demonstrating this new type of ATC, and motion simulation is carried out. The result shows that dual-cam linkage drive ATC works normally applied in horizontal machining center. It simplifies tool exchange process remarkably through dual-cam linkage. Tool exchange efficiency and reliability are improved. Along with the development of machine tool industry, this new type of ATC has a wide application prospect.

Acknowledgments

This work is supported by National Natural Science Foundation of China by Grant No.50675027, and Dalian Municipal Science and Technology Commission by Grant No.2006A12GX003. The authors are grateful to the industrial partner, Dalian Machine Tool Group Corp., who produced MDH65 Horizontal Machining Center, and made dual-cam linkage drive ATC used in this study. And thank all people made contribution in this study.

References

1. Chen, F.C., Yan, H.S.: Configuration syntheses of machining centers with tool change mechanisms. International Journal of Machine Tool & Manufacture 39, 273–295 (1999)
2. Yan, H.S., Yiou, C.W., Chen, F.C., Chang, P.: On the classification of automatic tool changers for machining centers. In: Proceedings of ASME 1995 Design Engineering Technical Conferences, Boston, USA, vol. 1, DE(82), pp. 931–936 (1995)
3. Liu, J.H., Zou, H.J.: Types summary and design characteristics of automatic tool change mechanism of machine center. Machine design and research 17(3), 49–52 (2001)
4. Wang, K.S., Zhang, H.C., Yang, Q.-D.: The comparison of cam type and hydraulic drive type about ATC of machining centers. Modular Machine Tool & Automatic Manufacturing Technique 9, 38–41 (1995)
5. He, W., Xia, F.L., Tang, X.F.: Researches on cam gear vertical & horizontal tool changing manipulator. Modular Machine Tool & Automatic Manufacturing Technique 12, 17–19 (2003)
6. Liu, J.H.: Research on the scheme design methodlogy for machining centers based on topological structure and tool changing motion characteristics. Doctoral dissertation of Shanghai Jiao tong University (2006)
7. Peng, Z.Z., Sun, Y.Y.: Fuzzy Mathematics And Applications. Wu Han University Press (2007)
8. Rothbart, H.: Cam Design Handbook. McGraw-Hill Professional, New York (2003)

Scheduling Mixed-Model Assembly Lines with Cost Objectives by a Hybrid Algorithm

Binggang Wang, Yunqing Rao, Xinyu Shao, and Mengchang Wang

The State Key Laboratory of Digital Manufacturing Equipment and Technology, Huazhong University of Science and Technology, Wuhan, Hubei, China
ryq@hust.edu.cn

Abstract. This paper is concerned about how to optimize the input sequence for a mixed-model assembly line (MMAL) with limited intermediate buffers. Three optimization objectives are considered simultaneously: minimizing the total production rate variation, the total setup, and the total assembly cost. The mathematical model is presented by incorporating the three objectives. Since the problem is NP-hard, a hybrid algorithm based on genetic algorithm (GA) and simulated annealing (SA), is proposed for solving the model. The performance of the proposed algorithm is compared with a genetic algorithm for different-sized sequencing problems in MMALs that consist of different number of machines and different production plans. The computational results show that the proposed hybrid algorithm finds solutions with better quality and often needs a smaller number of generations to converge to a final stable state, especially in the case of large-sized problems.

Keywords: Mixed-model assembly line, Scheduling, Hybrid algorithm, Genetic algorithm.

1 Introduction

Mixed-model assembly line is a type of production line where various and different models of the same products are inter-mixed to be assembled on the same line. The MMAL considered in this paper can be described as follows: it is a conveyor system, in each stage of the line, there is only one machine. Between every two successive machines j and j-1 , there exists a buffer with the size B_j, and jobs obey the FIFO (first in first out) rule in each buffer. Each job is to be sequentially processed on through the first machine to the last one. If there is no buffer space available for a completed job on one machine, then this job must remain on that machine until either a buffer space or the machine in the next stage becomes available. At any time, no job can be processed on more than one machine, while no machine can process more than one job simultaneously. In order to maximize the utilization of a MMAL, many researchers have investigated the sequencing problem.

To make the sequencing results more reasonable and practicable, much research work has done on multi-criteria sequencing problem in MMAL. Bard et al. [1] developed a mathematical model that involved two objectives: minimizing the overall line length and keeping a constant rate of parts usage, and a tabu search method was

C. Xiong et al. (Eds.): ICIRA 2008, Part II, LNAI 5315, pp. 378–387, 2008.

proposed for solving the model. Hyun et al. [2] considered three practically important objectives: minimizing total utility work, keeping a constant rate of parts usage and minimizing total setup cost, which was solved using genetic algorithm by proposing a new genetic evaluation and selection mechanism, called Pareto stratum-niche cubicle. A SA method was proposed by McMullen and Fraizer [3] for solving the model used by McMullen [4] and the SA was compared with the tabu search method in [4]. The same problem was also solved by McMullen [5-7] by using another three methods: genetic algorithms, Kohonen self-organizing map, and ant colony optimization, respectively, and also the three method were compared with the SA and the tabu search methods.To minimize the weighted sum of tardiness and earliness penalties and to balance the production flow of the flexible assembly line, Guo et al. [8] developed a bi-level genetic algorithm to solve the scheduling problem. Tavakkoli-Moghaddam et al. [9] applied a memetic algorithm to solve a multi-criteria sequencing problem model for a MMAL, which is a weighted sum of the three objectives: total utility work, total production rate variation, and total setup cost according to their relative importance weights. Yu et al. [10] proposed a multi-objective genetic algorithm to schedule a flexible assembly line with the objectives of leveling the parts usage rate and minimizing the makespan.

It can be seen from above, though many research work has done on sequencing problem in MMALs, to our best knowledge, few work was on the sequencing problem in the MMAL described above with the three important optimization goals simultaneously: total production rate variation, total setup, and total assembly cost. In this paper, we consider the three objectives simultaneously.

The remainder of this paper is organized as follows: Section 2 presents the mathematical models. The proposed hybrid algorithm is described in Section 3. Case studies and discussions are reported in Section 4. The last section is the conclusions.

2 Mathematical Models

In this paper, the concept of minimum part set (MPS) is applied. MPS is a vector representing a product mix, such that $(d_1, d_2,\ldots, d_M)=(D_1/h, D_2/h,\ldots, D_M/h)$, where d_m is the number of product type m to be assembled in one period, D_m is the number of products type m needs to be assembled during the entire planning horizon, h is the greatest common divisor factor of $D_1, D_2,\ldots, D_M$ This strategy operates in a cyclical manner.

2.1 Minimizing the Total Production Rate Variation Cost

This problem can be formalized as below, which is improved according to the model proposed by Miltenberg[11].

Minimizing:

$$\sum_{i=1}^{I}\sum_{m=1}^{M}\left(v_{im}\left|\sum_{l=1}^{i}\frac{x_{lm}}{i}-\frac{d_m}{I}\right|\right) \tag{1}$$

Subject to:

$$\sum_{m=1}^{M} x_{im} = 1, \quad \forall i, \tag{2}$$

$$\sum_{i=1}^{I} x_{im} = d_m, \quad \forall m, \tag{3}$$

$$x_{im} = 0, \ or, \ 1, \ \forall i, m \tag{4}$$

where v_{im} is the sequence-dependent production rate variation cost for the product model m in the ith position of the sequence. The first term in the objective function is the production ratio of model m until the ith product is produced. The second term is the demand ratio of model m. x_{im} is 1 if model m is assigned at the ith position in a sequence; Otherwise, x_{im} is 0. Equation (2) is a set of position constraints indicating that every position in a sequence is occupied by exactly one product. Equation (3) imposes the restriction that all the demands must be satisfied in terms of MPS.

2.2 Minimizing the Total Setup Cost

The mathematical model used by Tavakkoli-Moghaddam and Rahimi-Vahed [9] is adopted in this paper.

Minimize:

$$\sum_{j=1}^{J} \sum_{i=1}^{I} \sum_{m=1}^{M} \sum_{r=1}^{M} X_{imr} C_{jmr} \tag{5}$$

Subject to:

$$\sum_{m=1}^{M} \sum_{r=1}^{M} X_{imr} = 1, \quad \forall i, \tag{6}$$

$$\sum_{i=1}^{I} \sum_{r=1}^{M} X_{imr} = d_m, \quad \forall m, \tag{7}$$

$$X_{imr} = 0, or, 1, \quad \forall i, m, r \tag{8}$$

$$\sum_{m=1}^{M} X_{imr} = \sum_{p=1}^{M} X_{(i+1)rp}, \quad i = 1, ..., I-1, \quad \forall r, \tag{9}$$

$$\sum_{m=1}^{M} X_{Imr} = \sum_{p=1}^{M} X_{1rp}, \quad \forall r, \tag{10}$$

where C_{jmr} is the setup cost required when model type is changed from m to r at machine j and X_{imr} is 1 if model type m and r are assigned, respectively, at the ith and $(i+1)$th position in a sequence; Otherwise, X_{imr} is 0. Equation (6) is a set of position constraints indicating that every position in a sequence is occupied by exactly one product. Equation (7) imposes the restriction that all the demands must be satisfied in terms of MPS. Equation (9) and (10) ensure that the sequence of products must be maintained while repeating the cyclic production.

2.3 Minimizing the Total Assembly Cost

Extending from the models in literature [12], the mathematical model for this objective is formulated as follows:

Minimize:

$$c_l\left(S_{P(I)J} + A_{P(I)J}\right) \tag{11}$$

Subject to:

$$S_{P(1)1} = 0 \tag{12}$$

$$S_{P(1)j} = S_{P(1)j-1} + A_{P(1)j-1}, \; j = 2,3,...J \tag{13}$$

$$S_{P(i)j} = \max\left\{S_{P(i)j-1} + A_{P(i)j-1}, S_{P(i-1)j} + A_{P(i-1)j}\right\}, \; i = 2,3,...B_{j+1} + 1 \tag{14}$$

$$S_{P(i)j} = \max\left\{S_{P(i)j-1} + A_{P(i)j-1}, S_{P(i-1)j} + A_{P(i-1)j}, S_{P(i-B_{j+1}-1)j+1}\right\}, \; i > B_{j+1} + 1 \tag{15}$$

where c_l is the sequence-independent assembly cost per unit time. $S_{P(I)J}$ is the starting time of the last product $P(I)$ processed on the last machine J. $A_{P(I)J}$ is the processing time of the last product on the last machine.

3 Algorithms for Solving the Model

3.1 Notations

POPSIZE	the maximum number of individuals in one population
P_c	probability of crossover operation
P_m	probability of mutation operation
l	length of Markov chain
l_{max}	maximum length of Markov chain
P_a	probability of inferior solution being accepted
q	times of the current best solution remains unchanged
q_{max}	maximum times of the current best solution remains unchanged
α	cooling rate.

3.2 Hybrid Algorithm Procedures

The procedures of the proposed algorithm are described as follows.

Step1: Generate an initial population, *Pop*(0).

Step2: Calculate each individual's fitness value in *Pop*(0), let the best solution and its objective function value be the global best S^* and C^*, respectively, determine the initial temperature t_0, and let generation g=0.

Step3: If the terminating condition is satisfied, then output S^* and C^*, otherwise, continue the following steps.

Step4: Selection operations.
Step5: Crossover operations.
Step6: Mutation operations.
Step7: Metropolis sampling process, using each individual in the temporary population after Step6 as the initial solution. Then a new temporary population, $p^t(g)$, is formed.
Step8: Calculate each individual's fitness value in $p^t(g)$, and update S^* and C^* if necessary.
Step9: Keep the best individual.
Step10: Let $g=g+1$, $t_g=\alpha\times t_{g-1}$. go to Step3.

3.3 Implementation of the Hybrid Algorithm

The details of implementation of the proposed algorithm are described as follows.

(1) Encoding scheme: Job permutation based encoding scheme is widely used in many literatures for sequencing problem in MMALs, so it is also adopted in this paper.

(2) Initial population: To maintain large population diversity, individuals are generated randomly to form the initial population. When generating the individuals, the number of each type of products in each individual can not break the constraints on the demands in MPS.

(3) Fitness calculation: In order to let the individual with smaller objective function value has more chance to survive, the fitness value is calculated as follows:

$$f(i,m,j)=1/F(i,m,j)\,. \tag{16}$$

where, $f(i,m,j)$ and $F(i,m,j)$ is the fitness and objective function value, respectively, of a feasible solution.

(4) Initial temperarure: Let Boltzman constant be 1, initial temperature can be calculated from the following [13]:

$$to=\Delta F/ln(P_a^{-1})\,. \tag{17}$$

$$\Delta F=F_{max}-F_{min}\,. \tag{18}$$

where, F_{max} and F_{min} is the maximum and the minimum objective function value respectively in $Pop(0)$.

(5) Termination criterion: For comparison's convenience, a maximum generation number, G, is set as the stopping criterion.

(6) Selection operation: Proportional selection based on fitness values is used in this paper. This process is repeated until *POPSIZE* solutions are selected.

(7) Crossover operation: The Modified order crossover (*modOX*) operator is adopted in this paper. The parents for performing crossover operation are selected by probability, P_c. After crossover operation, the best two among the four solutions, two parents and two offsprings, are selected to replace the original two parents.

(8) Mutation operation: To improve the solutions' diversity, mutation operations are made on the selected individuals, controlled by probability, P_m. Here, the *INV* mutation operator is adopted.

(9) Metropolis sampling process: Using each individual, S, in the temporary population, $p^t(g)$, as the initial solution, a local search process is performed. The scheme has the following working steps:

① Let l=0, current best solution $S^{*'}=S^*$, q=0, current state $S^{'}(0)=S$.
② Generate a new solution, $S^{'}$, from S using *INV* mutation operator described in Section 3.3.7, calculate $\Delta C^{'}=C(S^{'})-C(S)$.
③ If $\Delta C^{'}<0$, accept $S^{'}$, let $S^{*'}= S^{'}$, q=0, moreover, if $C(S^*)> C(S^{'})$, let $S^* = S^{'}$□If$\Delta C^{'}>0$, accept $S^{'}$ by the probability of P_a, if $S^{'}$ is accepted, let $S^{'}(l+1)=S^{'}$, $q=q+1$, else let $S^{'}(l+1)=S^{'}(l)$.
④ Let $l=l+1$. If termination condition ($q>q_{max}$ or $l>l_{max}$) satisfied, continue the following steps, else go to ②.
⑤ Replace S with $S^{*'}$.

(10) Keep the best: In order to avoid losting the best solution, after Step7, if $C(S^*)>C(S^{*'})$, let $S^*= S^{*'}$, else, replace the worst solution (with the biggest objective value) in the population obtained after Step7 with S^*.

3.4 GA Algorithm

For testing the performance of the proposed hybrid algorithm, a genetic algorithm is designed. The procedures of the GA can be inherited from Section 3.2 by deleting Step7, "determine the initial temperature t_0" in Step2 and "$t_g=\alpha\times t_{g-1}$" in Step10, and it can be implemented by deleting the corresponding parts in Section 3.3.

4 Case Studies and Discussions

The proposed hybrid algorithm and the GA are coded in C++ and implemented on an IBM ThinkPad (Intel (R) Celeron (R) M, CPU 1.70 GHz, 768M). Various experiments have been conducted to measure the performance of the proposed hybrid algorithm and the GA. And, the performance has been compared with each other. Each experiment is repeated 30 times. The experimental data is listed in the following Table 1 to Table 4.We make all the experiments under the following assumptions:

①All the sequence-dependent production rate variation costs, v_{im}, are the same and equal to 1.
②The sequence-independent assembly cost per unit time, c_l, is set to 1 for the sake of computational convenience.
③All the buffer sizes are equal to 1.

Table 1. MPS

Products	P1	P2	P3	P4	P5
MPS1	2	1	3	2	2
MPS2	3	4	4	2	2
MPS3	3	5	2	6	4

Table 2. Setup cost

Products	P1	P2	P3	P4	P5
P1	0	2	3	1	2
P2	1	0	1	3	2
P3	2	1	0	2	1
P4	3	2	2	0	3
P5	2	1	1	2	0

Table 3. The assembly time for different products on different machines

Product	Machine code																			
	1	2	3	4	5	6	7	8	9	10	11	12	13	14	15	16	17	18	19	20
P1	4	6	8	9	5	6	8	9	8	7	5	5	6	7	8	8	3	4	5	6
P2	2	5	6	8	4	5	7	9	6	8	9	5	4	4	5	6	7	8	9	9
P3	3	4	6	7	9	6	8	7	6	9	9	6	6	5	6	7	7	6	7	8
P4	2	3	4	4	4	5	7	8	8	9	6	7	7	5	6	6	7	8	8	9
P5	3	5	7	8	9	7	6	8	8	8	9	9	6	4	5	5	5	6	8	8

Table 4. The algorithm parameters

Parameters	GASA	GA
POPSIZE	50	50
G	150	150
P_c	0.85	0.85
P_m	0.20	0.20
l_{max}	20	none
q_{max}	3	none
P_a	0.15	none

Firstly, the small-sized problem is considered, in which the total number of machines in the MMAL and that of the five types of products need to be assembled in one period are small. Assuming that the MMAL has 4 machines and the total demand is 10, as listed in MPS1. Computational results by the hybrid algorithm and the GA are shown in Table 5 , respectively. Fig. 1 shows their convergence curves. It can be seen, for small-sized problems, the best solution obtained by the hybrid algorithm has 1.5 percent improvement over that obtained by the GA. From Fig. 1, it can be also find that both the two algorithms can converge to the optimal within 8 generations.

Secondly, when the number of machines in the MMAL and the total demand of all the products in MPS2 increase to 10 and 15, respectively, the computational results of the two algorithms are also listed in Table 5, and the convergence curves are demonstrated in Fig. 2. The solution quality of the hybrid algorithm is better than that of the GA by 1.63 percent. The number of generations needed to converge to the optimal is 22 for the hybrid algorithm and 87 for the GA.

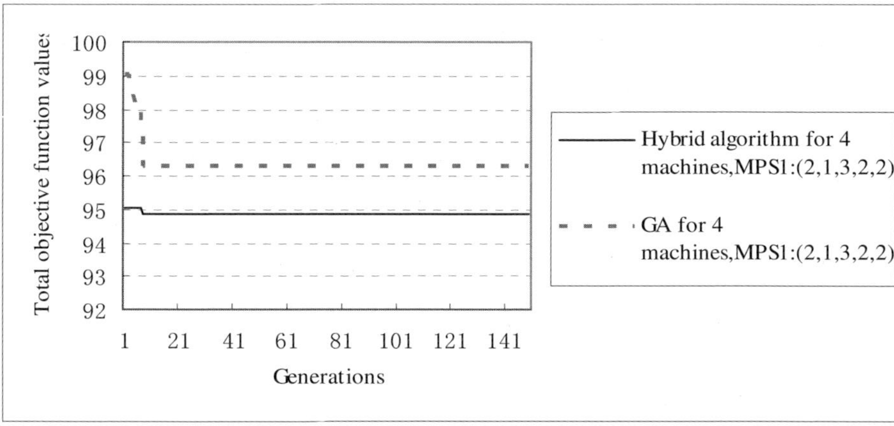

Fig. 1. Convergence curves for 4 machines and MPS1

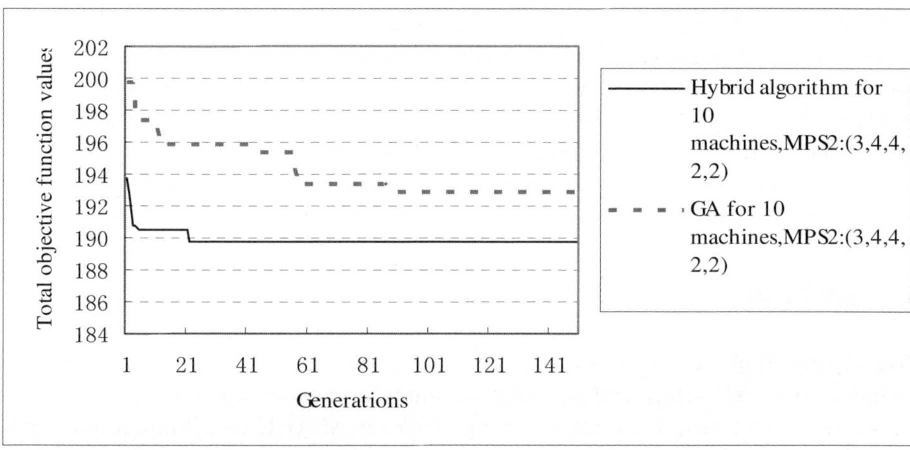

Fig. 2. Convergence curves for 10 machines and MPS2

Table 5. Computational results

machines	MPS	Total objective function values		Best solutions	
		Hybrid algorithm	GA	Hybrid algorithm	GA
4	(2,1,3,2,2)	94.8587	96.3008	4333552114	4433211553
10	(3,4,4,2,2)	189.783	192.924	443223552332111	443232155233112
20	(3,5,2,6,4)	304.7	312.752	44222344442215555311	44422231142553214455

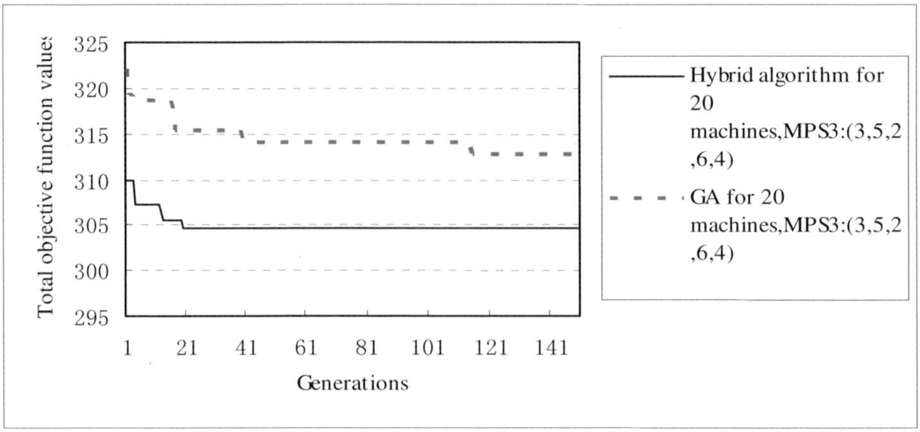

Fig. 3. Convergence curves for 20 machines and MPS3

Finally, for the large-sized case, there are 20 machines in the MMAL and the total demand in MPS3 is 20. The last line in Table 5 shows the computational results of the two algorithms. Fig.3 shows their convergence processes. The ratio of improvement increases to 2.57 percent in terms of solution quality and the number of generations needed for the hybrid algorithm to converge to the final stable state is much smaller than that for the GA, which is 20 for the former and 115 for the latter. To summarize, we can conclude that the hybrid algorithm also performs better than the GA.

5 Conclusions

Considering three cost-related objectives, minimizing the total production rate variation, the total setup, and the total assembly cost, simultaneously, we describe the mathematical model for sequencing problem in MMAL with limited intermediate buffers. A hybrid algorithm is proposed to solve the model and the algorithm performance is compared with a GA. Three computational efforts are made by the two algorithms for different sequencing problems in MMALs, each has different MPS and different number of machines. The computational results show that the hybrid algorithm can always converge to the final stable state within a smaller number of generations than the GA, especially in the case of large-sized problems and the proposed hybrid algoritm performs better than the GA in terms of the solution quality for all the test problems, and we can have more improvement as the problem size increases.

Acknowledgments. This research work is supported by 863 High Technology Plan Foundation of China under Grant No. 2007AA04Z186 and National Natural Science Foundation of China under Grant No. 50775089.

References

1. Bard, J.F., Shtub, A., Joshi, S.B.: Sequencing Mixed-Model Assembly Lines to Level Parts Usage and Minimizing Line Length. International Journal of Production Research 32(10), 2431–2454 (1994)
2. Hyun, C.J., Kim, Y., Kim, Y.K.: A Genetic Algorithm for Multiple Objective Sequencing Problems in Mixed Model Assembly Lines. Computers and Operations Research 25(7/8), 675–690 (1998)
3. McMullen, P.R., Frazier, G.V.: A Simulated Annealing Approach to Mixed-Model Sequencing with Multiple Objectives on a JIT Time. IIE Transactions 3(8), 679–686 (2000)
4. McMullen, P.R.: JIT Sequencing for Mixed-Model Assembly Lines with Setups Using Tabu Search. Production Planning and Control 9(5), 504–510 (1998)
5. McMullen, P.R.: An Efficient Frontier Approach to Addressing JIT Sequencing Problems with Setups Via Search Heuristics. Computers and Industrial Engineering 41, 335–353 (2001)
6. McMullen, P.R.: A Kohonen Self-Organizing Map Approach to Addressing a Multiple Objective, Mixed-Model JIT Sequencing Problem. International Journal of Production Economics 72, 59–71 (2001)
7. McMullen, P.R.: An Ant Colony Optimization Approach to Addressing a JIT Sequencing Problem with Multiple Objectives. Artificial Intelligence in Engineering 15, 309–317 (2001)
8. Guo, Z.X., Wong, W.K., Leung, S.Y.S., Fan, J.T.: A Genetic-Algorithm-Based Optimization Model for Scheduling Flexible Assembly Lines. International Journal of Advanced Manufacturing Technology (2007), doi:10.1007/s00170-006-0818-6
9. Tavakkoli-Moghaddam, R., Rahimi-Vahed, A.R.: Multi-Criteria Sequencing Problem for a Mixed-Model Assembly Line in a JIT Production System. Applied Mathematics and Computation 181, 1471–1481 (2006)
10. Yu, J.f., Yin, Y.H., Chen, Z.N.: Scheduling of an Assembly Line with a Multi-Objective Genetic Algorithm. International Journal of Advanced Manufacturing Technology 28, 551–555 (2006)
11. Miltenburg, J.: Level Schedules for Mixed-Model Assembly Lines in Just-In-Time Production Systems. Management Science 35(2), 192–207 (1989)
12. Wang, L., Zhang, L., Zheng, D.Z.: An Effective Hybrid Genetic Algorithm for Flow Shop Scheduling with Limited Buffers. Computers & Operations Research 33, 2960–2971 (2006)
13. Metropolis, N., Rosenbluth, A., Rosenbluth, N., Teller, A., Teller, E.: Equation of State Calculations by Fast Computing Machines. Journal of Chemical Physics 21, 1087–1092 (1953)

Design and Implement of Synchronizing Dual-Drive Gantry Based on Multi-axes Motion Control Card

JianZhou Quan[1,2], Yuhui Wang[1], and ZhouPing Yin[1]

[1] State Key Laboratory of Digital Manufacturing Equipment and Technology, Huazhong University of Science and Technology, Wuhan, 430074, P.R. China
[2] Air Force Radar Academy,Wuhan,430019,Hubei Province China
quanjianzhou@sohu.com, wyh@mail.hust.edu.cn, yinzhp@mail.hust.edu.cn

Abstract. The present paper deals with the development and implementation of synchronizing controller for dual-drive servo system that is often used for high speed and precision gantry system, in which two primary axes aligned in parallel are synchronously driven by independent servo motors. To achieve satisfactory positioning accuracy and reduce the synchronization error between the two parallel axes, a new control scheme for accurate synchronous in motion control, is proposed by combining feedforward control, feedback control and cross-coupled control. The scheme is implemented using multi-axes motion control board. Experimental results illustrate that the scheme improves effectively the performance.

Keywords: Dual-drive; synchronous compensation control; multi-axes motion control card.

1 Introduction

Among the various configurations of long travel and high precision Cartesian robotic systems, one of the most popular is the H-type which is more commonly known as the moving gantry stage. In this configuration, driving mode of the dual axes is a recommendable one in manufacturing machine, industrial robot, IC wire bonder, surface chip mounter, etc., where two motors are mounted on two parallel slides and move the gantry simultaneously in tandem. This mode has many advantages comparing with that driven by a single motor. It can significantly increase the system rigidity and overall thrust for driving the stage. This layout can also improve the system dynamics, speed and accuracy for large gantry-type stage.

The application domain of the moving gantry stage is rapidly expanding because of the increasingly stringent requirements arising from developments in precision engineering and nanotechnology. To-date, there is not one precision machine manufacturer who does not provide for a moving gantry stage in one form or another.

Although this layout has potential advantages, it does not come without additional concerns. The level of synchronization may become crucial for the pair of parallel axes due to the coupling restriction. This implies that precise control is required, which aims not only to achieve satisfactory positioning accuracy but also to eliminate

C. Xiong et al. (Eds.): ICIRA 2008, Part II, LNAI 5315, pp. 388–397, 2008.

the synchronization error between the two parallel axes. In addition to the required performance, safety is another major concern, as damage may occur when significant synchronization error or control failure takes place. Therefore, appropriate synchronous control techniques and safety protection schemes are demanded to achieve satisfying accuracy and avoid potential hazards.

In conventional control systems, the ways of synchronous moving control are usually the series connection (i.e. Master-Slaved Motion Control) and parallel connection (i.e. Main-Main Control)[1]. The first scheme assigns one motor as the master and the other as the slave. The command signal is only transmitted to the master, and the slave simply tracks the motion of the master. Although the structure of dual position servo system is the same and designed independently, the servo lag brings synchronous error. The second scheme addresses explicitly the possibly different dynamics of the two motors. Two motors are assigned to the same axis in the same coordinate system. The motors use an identical desired trajectory commanded for the motion. Each servo loop of the two motors then has the responsibility of keeping the actual trajectory as closely as possible to the commanded trajectory. However, similar to the master–slave scheme, due to lacking communication, any error caused by disturbances in one loop is corrected only by this loop, while the other loop may carry on its own correction. In practice, the mechanical coupling strengthens the effect of this disturbance, so resulting in asynchronous moving for dual axes.

Cross-coupling control (CCC), firstly introduced and structured to reduce the contour error by Koren in 1980[2], is a potential solution for the aforementioned problem by sharing the feedback information of both control loops. The principle of CCC is that looking upon the synchronous control for dual-axial/multi-axial driven independently as a whole, viz. multiple inputs multiple outputs system. Recently, other types of CCC have also been reported to achieve desired contouring performance [3-5]. However, the design of the compensators in the classical CCC, intending to modify the command of velocity or torque, is very difficult because it will influence the stability of individual axial positioning control loops. Moreover, it is not able to cope with systems using the position mode feed drive, which is the most commonly used control configuration in industry.

Since the 1990s, with the rapid development of DSP chips and the improving reliability of industrial computer (IPC), the combined IPC and DSP configuration motion controller has been widely used in engineering practice. This scheme is powerful enough to provide good control for the many standard systems. However, the classical master-slave control or/and parallel connection control can only provide for the multi-axes synchronous motion, it is hardly meet the requirements of high speed and high-precision synchronization motion for gantry movement stage.

In this paper, A new control scheme combining feedforward control□feedback control and cross-coupled control, for accurate synchronous in motion control, is proposed. The scheme is implemented using multi-axes motion control card and compared to other control schemes currently available.

The rest of the paper is organized as follows. Section II presents a mathematical model of servo systems which will be used in many of the control components.

Section III gives the principles and details of the development of the proposed crossed-coupling composite controller. Implemented method based on multi-axes motion control card is covered in Section IV. Experimental results under the various scenarios are presented in Section V.

2 System Description

Although different kinds of motors may be used in the construction of a gantry motion system, depending on the precision and cost requirements, they are intrinsically similar. Synchronous control technique aims at zero synchronization errors for the two parallel servomotors.

2.1 Brief Description of a Typical Gantry Stage

A typical synchronous drive system is shown in Fig.1. The gantry (Y axis) slides along the two side linear guides and are driven with two ball screws/motors which are arranged in parallel to provide a joint thrust in the X direction. It consists of two servo motors, two ball screws, linear guides and slide tables. The feed drive system of each axis includes the single-phase AC servomotor, 20mm/pitch ball screw, and linear guide. The feed drive servo for each axis uses 400W YASKAWA AC servo motor. Position sensing is provided by 2048 pulse/rev optical encoders in which its signal is multiplied by 4 times after quadrature decoding and then sent to multi axes motion control board.

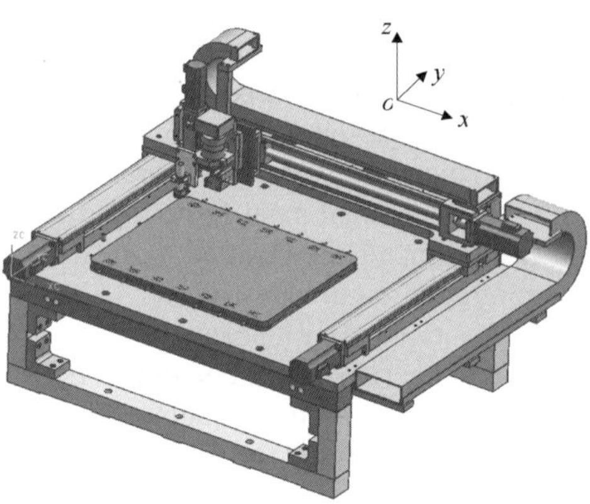

Fig. 1. Configuration of the dual servomotor driven system

2.2 Modeling of Coupled System

The kinematics of the parallel servomotor system with Y-axis is analyzed. One motor yields a linear displacement x_1, while the other yields a linear displacement x_2. Ideally $x_1 = x_2$, but they may differ owing to different dynamics exhibited by each of the motor, and also the dynamic loading present due to the translation of the slider along the gantry as illustrated in Fig. 2. The characteristics of the Y-axis components are assumed to be time-invariant and homogeneous, and the kinematics analysis is limited to X-direction [6]. Some denotations are defined as follows:

M_1 inertia of the slide of the servo motor and screw
M_2 inertia of the slide of the servo motor and screw
M_b mass of the X-axis components
B_1 viscosity coefficient of the slide of the servo motor 1
B_2 viscosity coefficient of the slide of the servo motor 2
x_1 displacement of the slide of the servo motor1
x_2 displacement of the slide of the servo motor2
x_b displacement of X-axis components
$u_1(t)$ torque voltage input of the servo motor 1
$u_2(t)$ torque voltage input of the servo motor 2
f_c friction force
f_k deformed force of the X-axis components in Y- direction

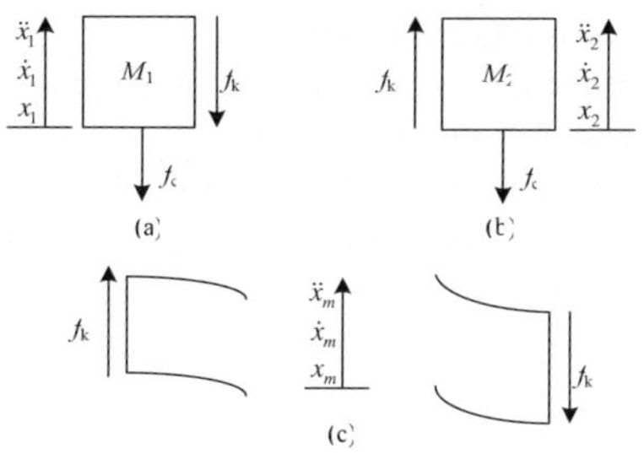

(a) the slide of the motor 1 (b) the slide of the motor 2
(c) the Y-axis components

Fig. 2. Free body diagrams

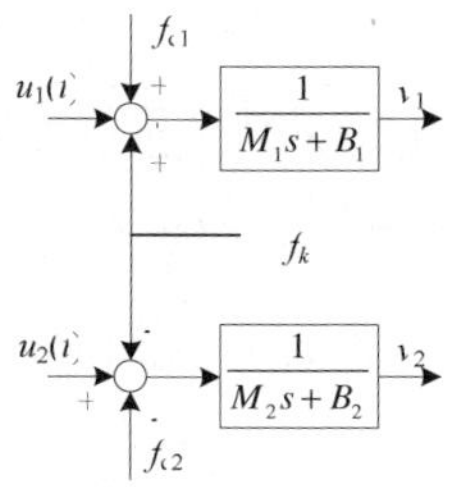

Fig. 3. The controlled plant of the parallel dual servomotor system

As shown in Fig. 2, for equilibrium of the force, the dynamic equations of the two slides are given respectively by

$$M_1 \frac{d^2 x_1}{dt^2} + B_1 \frac{dx_1}{dt} = u_1(t) - f_c - f_k \quad (1)$$

$$M_2 \frac{d^2 x_2}{dt^2} + B_2 \frac{dx_2}{dt} = u_2(t) - f_c - f_k \quad (2)$$

From equations (1) and (2), the controlled plant can therefore be given as in Fig. 3.

3 Design of the Synchronous Control System

3.1 Conventional Synchronal Control Scheme

The block diagram of conventional synchronous control scheme is shown in Fig. 4, where the gray box represents the controlled plant presented in Fig. 3. Two motors are assigned to the same axis in the same coordinate system. A supervisory motion program drives the gantry along the axis through the two motors simultaneously. The motors use an identical desired trajectory commanded for the motion. Each servo loop of the two motors then has the responsibility of keeping the actual trajectory as closely as possible to the commanded trajectory, since each of them has its own individual servo loop. Presuming all motors have tight servo loops, this method provides a tight and smooth link between the motors for the gantry. The main problem with this form of control is due to the transient synchronization error between the motors which is inevitable due to their inequality in characteristics and the environmental uncertainties. The situation can be even more severe when the two motors are coupled with a mechanism, by causing the motors to oppose each other in a non-synchronization state.

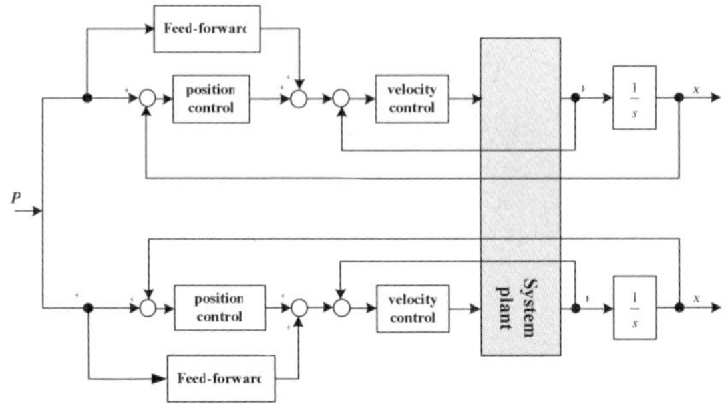

Fig. 4. Conventional dual axes synchronous control scheme

3.2 Description of the Proposed Control Structure

By using the synchronous error compensation controller to couple the two axes, we propose a novel control structure as shown in Fig.5. P^* is the desired position command of both axes. For each axis of the system, the control block diagram contains a position loop in which P^*_1 and P^*_2 are the modified position commands of each axis and P_1 and P_2 are the actual position or position feedback of the motors respectively.

The synchronous compensation controller forms two extra position loops, which are used to modify the position command of each axis. The inputs of this controller are the position synchronous error ε_P between dual axes position output and the velocity synchronous error ε_v between dual axes velocity output. The output variable is added into position reference for single axis, acts as a compensation control. Based on the concept of multi-loops cascade control, to modify the position reference command does not influence the stability of individual axial positioning control loops.

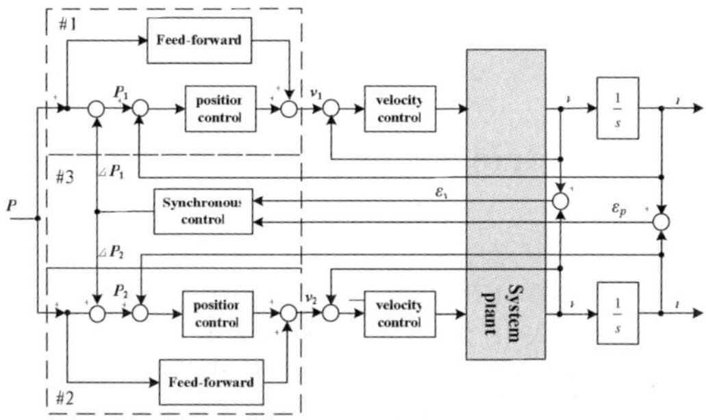

Fig. 5. Block diagram of the position synchronous drive system

From the above description, it is known that the parameters of the speed controllers, feed-forward controller and position feedback controller, are determined in prior to guarantee the stability and the tracking performance. The position loop is designed based on the PID control algorithm for improving the control performance. By considering the essential causation that produces position tracking error, a velocity and acceleration feed-forward compensating controller is used to this system. And then the position servo lag is reduced in advance. By tuning the gains of feed-forward, we can increase the tracking performance and guarantee that the control effort is within the system driving limitation.

3.3 Design of the Compensation Controller

As is indicated before that the transient synchronization error between two motors is inevitable due to their inequality in characteristics and the environmental uncertainties. However, this can be improved by adding the synchronous controller (Fig. 5) to coordinate the movement of the motors. Also, the strong mechanical coupling limits the relative movement of the two motors so that the synchronization error is expected to be small.

The position synchronous error ε_P and the velocity synchronous error ε_v, can be expressed as:

$$\begin{bmatrix} \varepsilon_p \\ \varepsilon_v \end{bmatrix} = \begin{bmatrix} P_1 - P_2 \\ v_1 - v_2 \end{bmatrix} \tag{3}$$

The output variable is added into position reference for single axis.

$$\begin{bmatrix} \Delta P_1 \\ \Delta P_2 \end{bmatrix} = \begin{bmatrix} \varepsilon_p & \varepsilon_v \\ -\varepsilon_p & -\varepsilon_v \end{bmatrix} \begin{bmatrix} K_x \\ K_v \end{bmatrix} \tag{4}$$

where K_x, K_v are controller gains for synchronous error compensation.

The modified reference position commands for the servo control loops are then represented as

$$\begin{bmatrix} P^*_1 \\ P^*_2 \end{bmatrix} = \begin{bmatrix} P^* - \Delta P_1 \\ P^* + \Delta P_2 \end{bmatrix} = P^* - \begin{bmatrix} \varepsilon_p & \varepsilon_v \\ -\varepsilon_p & -\varepsilon_v \end{bmatrix} \begin{bmatrix} K_x \\ K_v \end{bmatrix} \tag{5}$$

4 Real-Time Axes Control System Implementation

The experimental setup for the present study is shown in Fig.1 while Fig.6 presents the system architecture of experimented setup. Turbo PMAC-PCI board provided by the delta tau data systems Inc. is used to implement the control system, which is an industrial motion control card with an on-board DSP. This card is different from most motion control cards in that it is possible not only to download user written programs to the card directly but also to modify the control structure [7].

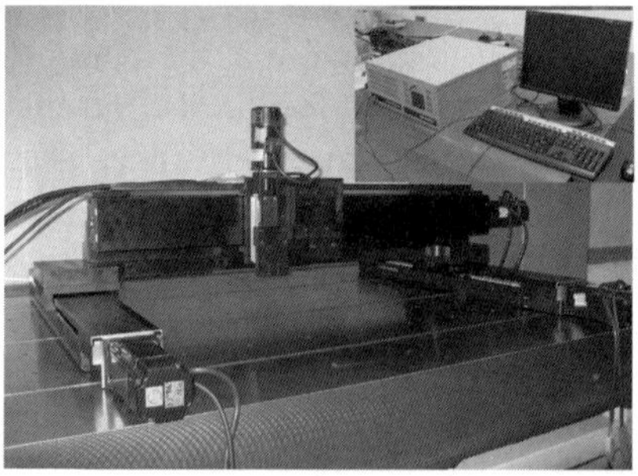

Fig. 6. The system architecture of experimented setup

To achieve our control structure, three axis channels are taken up, which is #1, #2 and #3 respectively, as shown in Fig.5. Two axes channel #1 and #2 is used to realize position control for each axis and the third channel #3 is used to realize synchronous error compensation control respectively. It is important to establish compensation controller model. This controller should adopt mast-slave control model, and the input command is the first axis's actual displacement viz. the feedback of the first motor axis #1, feedback is the second axis's actual displacement, viz. the feedback of the second motor axis #2. At the same time, its output does not positive governing actual motor, but is to modify two servo motor's position reference command to realize the two axle synchronization.

In our practical application, two kinds of movement control schemes be used, viz. mast-slave mode used during jogging and homing moves, the new control structure used during the high speed automatic movement by completing the two axes synchronization control. For equipment's security concern, the monitor routine to the third channel's following error, namely the synchronization error has carried on the real-time monitoring. As the synchronous error bigger than that some given value, system would force to shutdown: servo loop opened, zero output commanded.

5 Experimental Results

In this section, experiments are carried out to verify the effectiveness of the proposed control method. Two experiments are considered, i.e., the conventional independent axis control without synchronous compensator for the parallel servomotor system, and the motion control for the same servo system with synchronous compensator. In these experiments, two desired trajectories with S-curve speed profile planning are considered as shown in Fig.7 and Fig.8 respectively. For the first case, the parameters for the command are the position r = 240 *mm*, the maximum velocity $v_{\max}$ = 500 *mm/s,* the maximum acceleration $a_{\max}$ = 8 m/s^2 and the average acceleration a_{ave} is 5 m/s^2. For the second condition, the maximum acceleration $a_{\max}$ is 14 m/s^2, the average acceleration a_{ave} is 10 m/s^2, and other parameters remain unchanged.

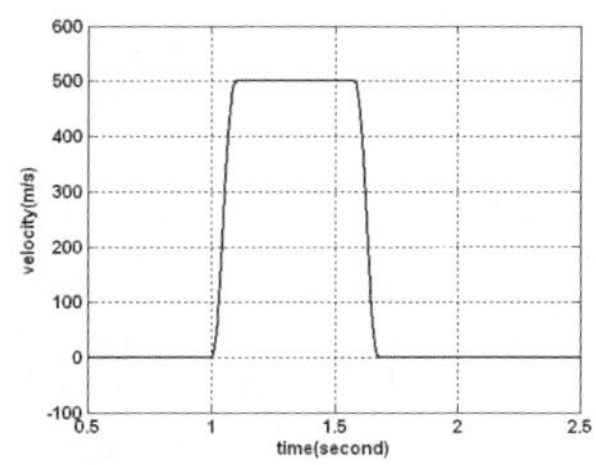

Fig. 7. The desired speed trajectories with S-curve planning at a_{ave}= 5 m/s^2

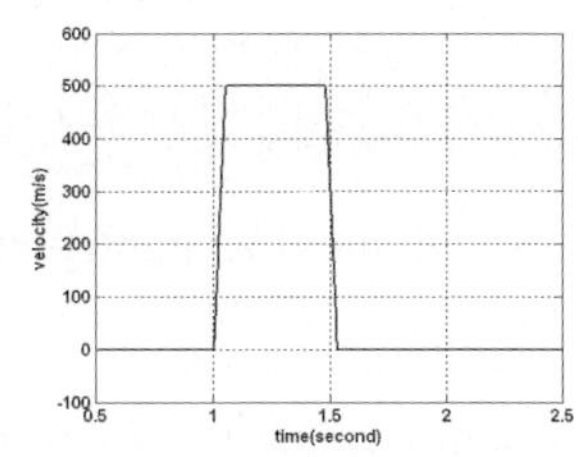

Fig. 8. The desired speed trajectories at a_{ave}= 10 m/s^2

The synchronization error response of the parallel servomotor system is shown in Fig.9 and Fig.10 respectively. As can be seen, the transient synchronization error also enhance gradually with the acceleration increasing, but the register maximal synchronous error with compensator to be smaller than that without compensator. This is especially true during acceleration and deceleration.

It is clear that the proposed synchronized control scheme provides slightly better performance in terms of synchronization error and its variance than the conventional independent axis control.

Moreover, for both cases the steady-state synchronization errors can reach 1μm.

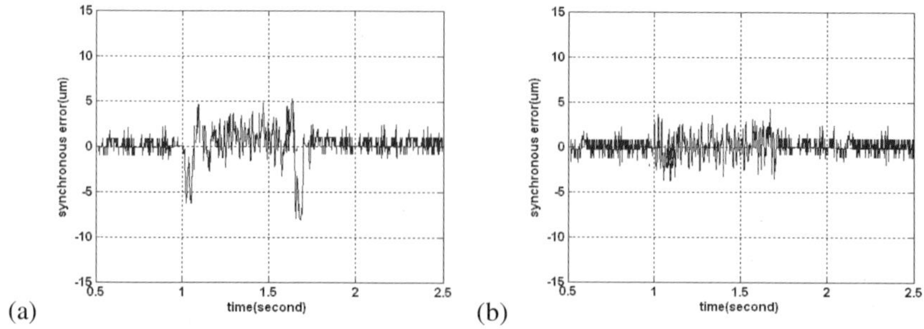

Fig. 9. Synchronous error at a_{ave}= 5 m/s^2: without compensation control. with compensation-control

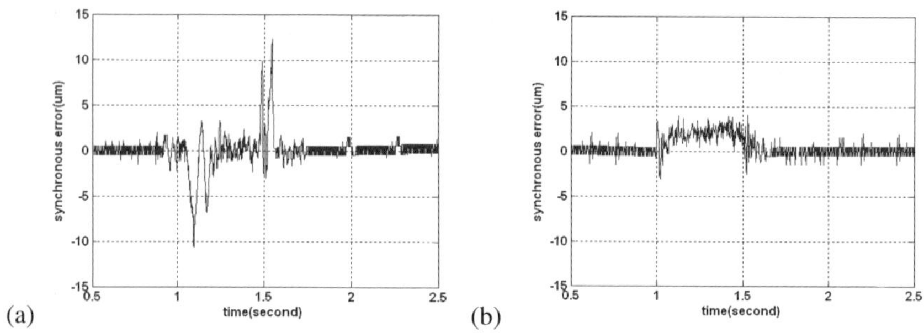

Fig. 10. Synchronous error at a_{ave}= 10 m/s^2: (a) without compensation control; (b) with compensation control

6 Conclusions

The synchronous motion control of moving gantry stages for precision applications has been addressed in this paper. A novel control scheme combining feed-forward, feedback and synchronous error compensation control is presented. The scheme has been implemented and compared to control schemes currently available for this purpose. Experimental results illustrate the enhanced performance of the fully coordinated control scheme with respect to tight trajectory tracking purposes.

Acknowledgements

The work is supported by the Natural Science Fund of China (NSFC) (Project No 50625516), the National Fundamental Research Program (973) (Project No. 2003CB716207) and the 863 program of China under Grant No. 2006AA04A110.

References

1. Lorenz, R.D., Schmidt, P.B.: Synchronized Motion Control for Process Automation. In: Proceedings of the 1989 IEEE Industry Applications Annual Meeting, pp. 1693–1698 (1989)
2. Koren, Y.: Cross-coupled Biaxial Computer Control for Manufacturing Systems. ASME Tans. Journal of Dynamic Systems, Measurement and Control 102, 265–272 (1980)
3. Chen, S.L., Liu, H.L.: Contouring Control of Biaxial Systems Based on Polar Coordinates. IEEE/ASME Trans. Mechatron 7, 329–343 (2002)
4. Shih, Y.-T., Chen, C.-S., Lee, A.-C.: A Novel Cross-Coupling Control Design for Bi-Axis Motion. International Journal of Machine Tools and Manufacture 42, 1539–1548 (2002)
5. Tsai, M.C., Hsieh, M.F., Yao, W.S.: Synchronous Control of Linear Servo Systems for CNC Machine tools. In: Proceedings of the 2003 European Control Conference, Cambridge (2003)
6. Tan, K.K., Lim, S.Y., Huang, S., Dou, H., Giam, T.S.: Coordinated Motion Control of Moving Gantry Stages for Precision Applications Based on An Observer-Augmented Composite Controller. IEEE Trans. Control Syst. Technol. 12(6), 984–991 (2002)
7. TURBO PMAC User's Manual, Delta Tau Data Systems Inc. (2004)

Tools for Simulation Based Fixture Design to Reduce Deformation in Advanced Fusion Welding

F. Sikström, M. Ericsson, A.-K. Christiansson, and K. Niklasson

University West, Dep of Engineering Science, SE 46186 Trollhattan, Sweden

Abstract. The traditional fusion welding and fixture simulations are performed using advanced finite element simulation tools, commonly used are e.g. MSC.Marc, ANSYS, ABACUS and COMSOL Multiphysics. These simulations are made one at a time and separately due to heavy calculation load for each case. Such an approach does not give a full description of the integrated work piece and fixture behaviour. We propose a strategy to decrease the computational time and solve the problem accurately enough for industrial needs. Focus of the simulation result is on residual deformation. The work piece is a simplified component composed by metal sheets, and rigid and loose clamping was investigated. Simulation results give the size of forces and deformations in the clamped edge. Deformation measurements are performed using 3D-scanning of the work piece after cooling and released from fixture, same situation as in the FE-simulations. The proposed strategy has shown to be useful and is industrially competitive due to reduced engineering manpower, computation time, and need for practical experiments. The strategy is to use full off-line programming where computer aided robotics for weld sequencies is integrated with finite element modelling in order to obtain weld parameters and fixture design.

1 Introduction

Increased use of robotised fusion welding is crucial for obtaining high efficiency in automated joining of metallic parts. A number of supporting technologies can further improve the performance of such welding, and this paper considers Off-Line Programming (OLP) of robot paths, Finite Element (FE)-simulations of interactions between welded work piece and fixture, and simulated feedback control for generation of optimised weld parameters. These engineering technologies are performed in advance to assure the quality of the weld and to reduce the need for costly and time consuming trials. The novelty of this paper lies in the combined use of these tools. Simulations of weld and fixture are normally performed one at a time since they are numerically heavy. They are also working in different time domains, from micro to macro scale. Another problem is that different software often is used without any integration and sharing of results. These facts call for more efficient methods and this paper presents how reliable simplifications can be made. The approach described is generic, however when

C. Xiong et al. (Eds.): ICIRA 2008, Part II, LNAI 5315, pp. 398–407, 2008.

it comes to applications, this paper considers laser welding of titanium sheets to form a simplified three-dimensional component.

Computer Aided Robotics (CAR) simulations have been used during some decades to simulate robot motions and to generate robot code off-line, see e.g. [1,2]. The research focus has been to generate optimal trajectories. Another focus has been to use CAR simulations as a visulation tool. CAR is a graphical tool for manufacturing simulations that can be used in several applications, such as the OLP of robots, tele-operation of robots and the simulation of general kinematic systems. The OLP of robots using a graphical simulation tool was first demonstrated in the beginning of the 1980s. Developments in computer technology have significantly improved the precision of OLP. The simulation of the production of a component makes it possible to test, verify and optimise robot motions and to design fixtures and automation equipment before the real production process begins, see e.g. [3,4]. Accessibility, collisions and timing can be verified before expensive machine tools and robots are purchased. Further, production accuracy can be improved by using OLP of robots, thus avoiding the complexity inherent in manually programming a robot in three dimensions with a high degree of accuracy. The most commonly used method to program a robot is still that an operator jogs the robot arm to each coordinate pose in space, a procedure that is both error-prone and heavily dependent on the experience and skill of the operator. The application of three-dimensional computer graphic tools for production planning makes it possible to achieve high degrees of accuracy for complex parts, see e.g. works presented in [5,6]. Several CAR software exist on the market, e.g. IGRIP, RobCAD and GRASP. All CAR software work with similar approach involving, [1]:

1. Geometrical, kinematic and dynamical modelling of the robot cell
2. Programming of the robot
3. Simulation of the robot program
4. Downloading to the physical robot
5. Final test of robot program in physical robot

The softwares considered in this work are MSC.Marc for FE-simulations of weld and fixture for thermal and mechanical properties; Comsol Multiphysics for FE-simulations for OLP of weld parameters; IGRIP for robot paths; MATLAB for model calibration; LabVIEW for data acquisition and control signals; and finally a MySQL database for data logging in experimental verification.

This paper is organised as follows: Section 2 presents combined use of OLP of robot paths, feedback control of weld power and fixture simulations; Section 3 describes the experimental setup, measurements and results, and Section 4 concludes and discusses.

2 Off-Line Programming of Robot Paths and Weld Parameters

This section presents the two different fields for simulation, CAR and Finite Element Analysis (FEA), and concludes how these can be combined.

2.1 Off-Line Programming of Robot Paths

In the first step the robot cell is modelled using both external Computer Aided Design (CAD) software and the CAR software directly. Complex parts, such as the workpiece to be welded, are normally first modelled in the CAD software and then exported to the CAR software. The geometric and kinematic models of the robot cell are usually made directly in the CAR software.

In step two, robot trajectories are generated by defining torch locations and orientations. The weld parameters (e.g. laser power and welding speed for laser welding) are connected to each welding location. These parameters are normally determined in a Weld Procedure Specification (WPS). In the work presented in this paper these parameters are imported from the FEA, see Section 2.2.

In the third step the robot program is simulated to detect and eliminate possible collisions between the weld torch and the workpiece as well as robot singularities. Then a calibration of the simulation cell is performed. This can include several sub steps such as calibration of the tool centre point, workpiece calibration, and signature calibration of the robot. When everything fulfills specifications the robot program is exported to the specific robot manufacture language and downloaded to the physical robot and finally a test run is performed. Left part of Fig. 1 shows a snapshot from simulation software IGRIP, where a verification component is welded. Right part of the figure shows the corresponding physical cell setup.

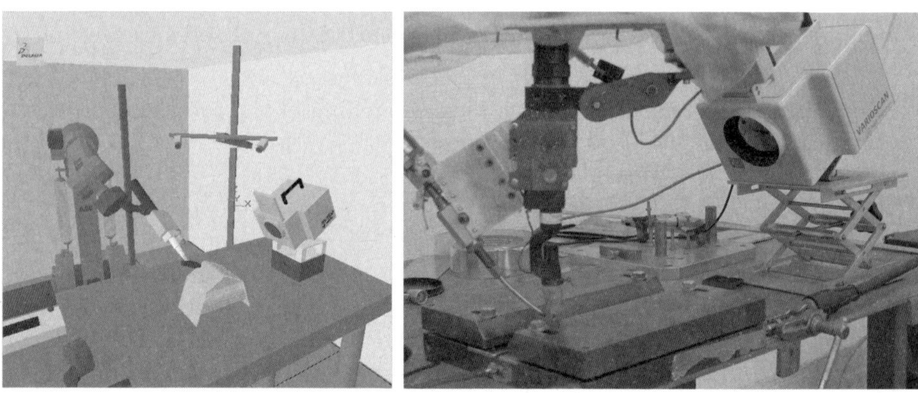

Fig. 1. Left: Simulation model from IGRIP and Right: Experimental cell setup (N.B. different work pieces in the figures)

The fixture is a critical part for the collision check during the test of the robot program. Normally the fixture is a passive component without any active elements. However if active elements are used these can be simulated using both kinematic models and signal communication between robot and fixture control system. These signals can be used as boundary conditions in the FE-simulations of the weld process in order to design an optimal fixture in this respect, e.g. to turn on and off loads.

One common problem during programming of robots is to find the best operation sequence for the robot, e.g. finding the fastest operation sequence or the sequence that results in minimal distorsion in a certain point. This distorsion is most often the main issue in welding applications, and it requires a lot of combined skill and knowledge of the programmer. The development of integrated CAR- and FE-simulation offers an efficient aid in increased understanding of the complex situation.

2.2 Off-Line Programming of Weld Parameters

Conventionally the designer sets a desired WPS to constrain the set of weld parameters into a limited domain in order to assure weld properties. Parameters within this domain are then used for the specific workpiece considered. This approach usually guarantees a certain degree of weld quality for the nominal weld situation but it does not really take into account perturbations in the process. In physical welding of complex geometry workpieces these perturbations have to be considered as the normal situation, since they always are present whatever precautions are made. Possible perturbations are variations in the shape and nature of the welded structure, e.g. the influence of heat sinks like fixtures, temporary buckling restraints, chill blocks or abrupt changes in symmetry of the geometry causing changes in the thermal and mechanical boundary conditions. One way to mitigate the adverse effect of a priori known perturbations is to include them in the simulation from start. The proposed method is to use simulation models to find varying weld parameters that are optimised to mitigate the effect of perturbations from the nominal weld situation, the situation for which the WPS is specified, [7]. It is however important to be within the process window defined by the WPS. Next subsection gives an example of how this can be done.

Weld Power Control. Robot coordinates and the nominal welding parameters are exported from the CAR-model to the FE-model where a heat and residual stress prediction is made.

Some of the most important considerations to take in welding are, as mentioned before, residual geometrical deformations and stress together with defective weld joint quality. These phenomena often result in costly and unwanted rectification actions afterwards in order to guarantee a proper design and quality that fulfils the manufacturing specification. Both residual deformation and stress occur from a mismatch of transient thermal strains during the passage of the weld heat source. The magnitude of these effects depend primarily on the specific thermal energy input of the weld process, i.e. the energy per unit length of weld [8]. One focus is thus to maintain the depth of penetration but still keep the energy input at a limited value. This can be done by varying the parameters that control the power input within the limits of the WPS. The basic idea for weld penetration control is that the geometry of the fusion zone, which is the zone that has been melted during the process, can be influenced by variations in the weld power and that change in the temperature on the topside of the work piece indicates changes in the fusion zone. The effect of increased weld power

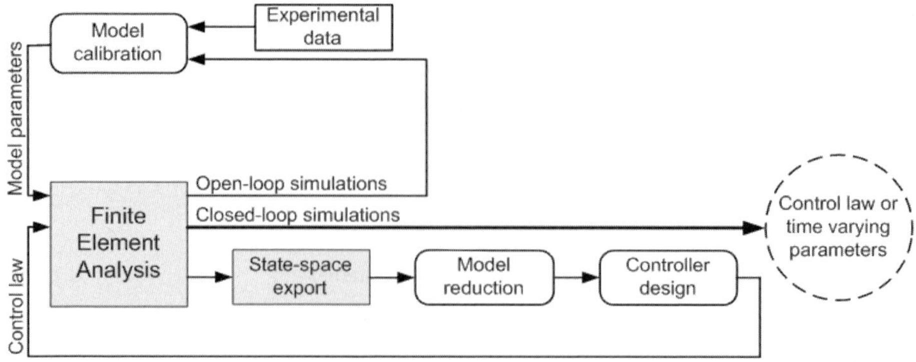

Fig. 2. Illustration of the coordinated use of the softwares MATLAB (white round corner boxes) and Comsol (grey sharp corner boxes)

is mainly higher heat input and consequently a deeper weld penetration [8]. By configuring one or more sensors that move together with the weld torch fixed relative the centre of the weld pool it is possible to detect changes in the temperature caused by perturbations experienced by the process. The task is to establish the dynamic relation between the actuating weld power signal and the temperature sensor readings. By knowing this relation it is possible to design a model based controller that will mitigate the effect of the perturbation and maintain a full penetration weld with a specific thermal energy input that is just enough to perform a high quality weld. This basic idea can be applied off-line in a FE-simulation. By applying a calibrated heat source model and a sensor model to a heat transfer simulation in the fashion described above one can find a control law to regulate the specific thermal energy input. This method has been applied and evaluated and also proven to be successful. FE-simulations of welding have been performed in COMSOL Multiphysics from COMSOL AB according to Fig. 2. For model based controller design a linearized state-space representation of the FE-model was exported to MATLAB from MathWorks Inc. Model order reduction was computed in MATLAB to find a low order representation of the dynamic relation between actuator and sensor. This low order model was then used to synthesise a model based controller. This controller in turn was implemented in COMSOL Multiphysics so that the closed-loop behaviour could be simulated and analysed. MATLAB was also used to calibrate and validate the FE-model by way of comparing available experimental data and simulation results. The result from this computing is a control law that can be used for implementation in the physical weld system or used as OLP of optimised weld parameters.

One specific problem during FE-simulations of welding is the need of a fine mesh density around the weld pool to be able to catch the high temperature gradient. User defined functions were developed in MSC.Marc to generate the moving mesh. This mesh follows the weld pool and ficilitates for faster simulations, however not shown here.

2.3 Fixture Simulations

Another important issue is to find methods to simplify the FE-modelling of fixtures and investigate how accurate they are. Two different models have been designed in this analysis. First a full 2D-reference model was created, which simulates the sliding of the work piece at the clamping due to the welding procedure. The model also comprises the transient thermal warm-up of the fixture. The mesh density needed to keep the discretization errors low was determined.

Second a 2D simplified model was created and validated by comparing the results with those of the reference model. The simplification is made by modelling the fixture using superelements (SE). The main problem was that SEs could only be used in mechanical analyses, not in coupled thermal-mechanical analyses. It has been found that a SE-matrix created in a mechanical analysis can be imported to a coupled analysis. In that way it was possible to do a coupled analysis with SEs but the thermal analysis did not comprise the SEs. The SE-method was straightforward and it was rather easy to establish a general instruction compared to the reference model. The results were also in good agreement with the results from the reference model.

A 3D-reference model was also created, see left part in Fig 3. As for the 2D-reference model it simulates the sliding of the work piece at the clamping due to the welding procedure. The model also comprises the transient thermal warm-up of the fixture. The mesh density needed to keep the discretization errors low was investigated and determined.

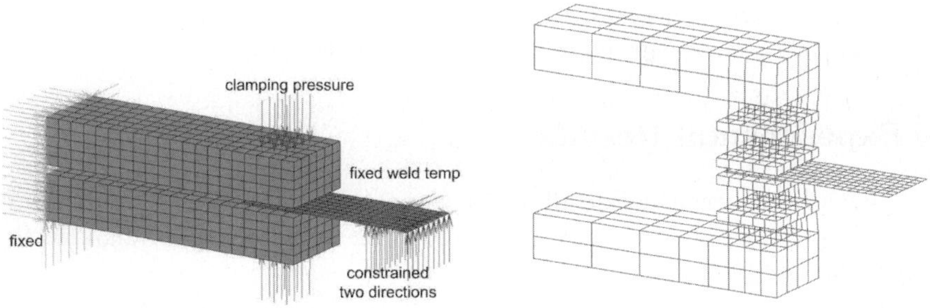

Fig. 3. Left: Reference model in 3D and Right: Superelement model in 3D (superelements not shown)

A 3D SE-model was created, see right part of Fig. 3. A new problem turned up. The thermal solution of the SE-connection nodes did not always converge. If it converged the node temperatures became as expected zero. This problem was solved by applying a boundary condition with fix temperature to the connection nodes. The heat flow to the fixture was again simulated with a separate thermal model of the fixture (thermal fixture) connected to the work piece with thermal links. It was again found that the thermal mesh density can be rather coarse and still simulate the thermal flow with good accuracy.

Comparisons of the stress results to the reference model showed not identical but very similar results. The reason for the differences between the models is mainly that the SE-model has a much coarser mesh of the thermal fixtures, which results in a little more uneven and slower warm-up. Another difference is that the SE-model does not simulate the temperature expansion of the fixture, which increases the contact pressure forces a little. What remains to do in the integrated simulation of the fixture and workpiece interaction is to test the SE-method on an industrial 3D-model.

2.4 Combined Off-Line Programming

An interface protocol between the CAR-software and the FE-software was developed allowing exchange of information. Fig. 2.4 shows a block chart of the principle. The same workpiece geometry was used in both softwares. The principle is that the workpiece to be manufactured is created in a CAD software and is then, using either a direct translator or a neutral interface, such as IGES or Step, imported to the CAR-software. Here the engineer plans the production, following the steps described in Section 2.1. A robot trajectory is generated. The weld trajectories are then exported to the FE software, where the thermal history, residual stresses and distortion are predicted. An optimisation can also be performed to reach a full penetration weld with minimised distortion further described in Section 2.2. A result of such optimisation is a time varying weld power parameter. This power signal is then transferred to the robot, together with the program for the robot motion. The robot program is finally downloaded to the robot control system and a test weld can be performed.

The simplifications described in the former sections can be used to facilitate for efficient integrated workpiece and fixture simulations.

3 Experimental Results

Trials have been performed in different respects to validate the strategies presented. Experimental setups are perfomed with data logging of signals. Some experiments are presented here.

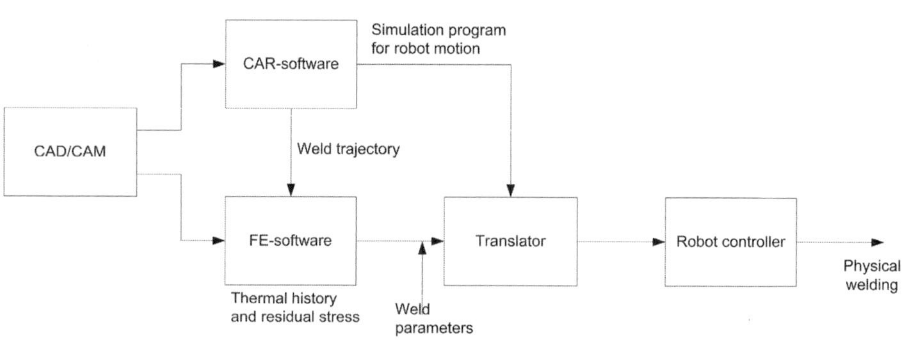

Fig. 4. Illustration of the integration between the CAR- and FE-softwares

3.1 3D-Scanning

3D-scannings have been used to capture geometrical displacements corresponding to residual deformations. The measurement was used to validate thermo-mechanical simulation results presented in [11]. The 3D-scanner is the commercial system ATOS 2/400 (Advanced TOpometric Sensor) developed by the German company GOM (Optical Measuring Techniques), see left part in Fig. 5 (also modelled in left part in Fig. 1). Optical 3D-scanning could under right conditions serve as a tool for quality control in welding manufacturing. It can detect imperfections in the joint and unpredicted distortion. Left part of Fig. 6 is a colour-scaled presentation of displacement from measured data and the right part is a similar presentation of predicted displacement calculated from FE-simulations. There is in general a good agreement in the distribution and the overall trend of displacement between these data sets. Optical 3D-scanning systems generally have limitations due to reflection problem when they are used to scan shiny metal surfaces, but the most important finding is that it is possible to collect 3D-data with sufficient quality to capture the weld process. This was done to validate the FE-model used in the OLP strategy.

3.2 Thermal Imaging

Temperature measurements during welding are described in e.g. [10]. This approach of performing thermal imaging was used to capture the temperature development during welding in order to have data for calibration and validation of the heat transfer and the heat source model [9]. One assumption is that this heat source model calibration on a simplified nominal weld situation is approximately valid also for more complex geometries. In the measurement experiment a bead on plate weld was made on a plain plate corresponding to a nominal weld situation specified in a WPS. Right part of Fig. 1 shows the experimental

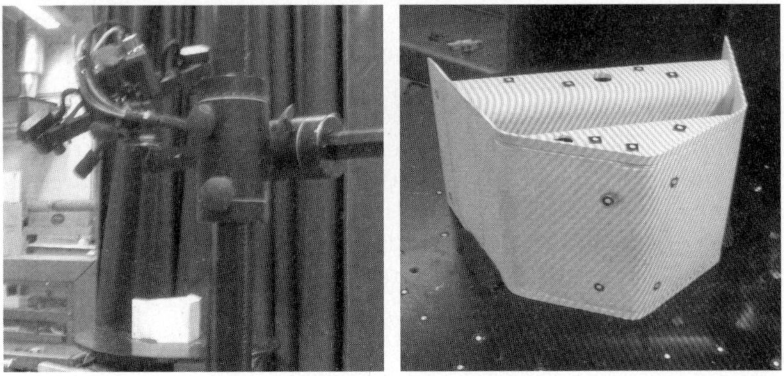

Fig. 5. Left: The Atos system setup with component at bottom, projector and cameras mounted on the tripod. Right: The component lit with fringe pattern from the Atos projector

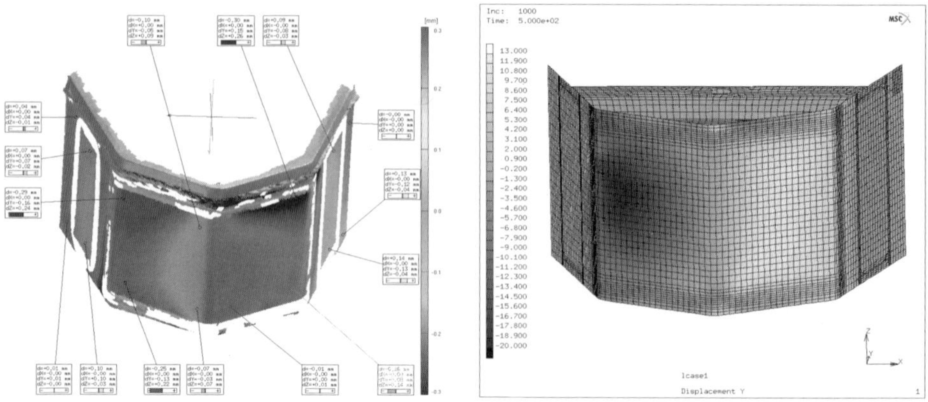

Fig. 6. Presentation of the displacement. Left: the displacements from measurements by the Atos system and right: from the simulations.

setup with a robot, plate in fixture and infrared camera. From this experiment temperature data along a line crossing the peak temperature in the centre of the heat source perpendicular to the weld direction was extracted. This data is easily comparable with corresponding simulation data. An infrared camera from JENOPTIK Group GMbH, called VARIOSCAN model 3021-ST was used. Further analysis of the temperature data was made in MATLAB. An optimisation routine was then successfully used to find model parameters by minimising the residual between measured and simulated values [9].

4 Conclusions

The conclusions are that the methods presented work well in real situations and that further work for more robust industrialisation will be beneficial for the welding community. In short, it is shown successful off-line programming of weld scheduling and robot motion, of weld parameters, and of fixture simulation and work piece interaction. Further work is planned for more integration of different softwares and for design of physical demonstrators to visualise the concept. The results are encouraging to do further extensions in the field of active fixturing and sensoric control of fusion welding, since the integrated simulations indicate what fixturing and what sensors would be beneficial. The development of integrated computer aided robotics (CAR) with finite element (FE) simulation has also shown to be an efficient tool for understanding advanced weld situations.

Acknowledgement

This research work is supported in part by grants from the European Union within the Integrated Project AFFIX (IP NMP2-CT-2006-026670-AFFIX), which is gratefully acknowledged.

References

1. Bolmsjö, G., Olsson, M., Brink, K.: Off-line programming of GMAW robotic systems - a case study. International Journal for the Joining of Materials 9(3), 86–92 (1997)
2. Walter, S.: Simulation and Calibration for off-line-programming of industrial robots. Paper 54 in Proc. of Computer Technology in Welding, Paris (1997)
3. Nof, S.Y.: Off-line programming of robots. In: Handbook of industrial robotics. Wiley, New York (1985)
4. Ting, Y., Lei, W.I., Jar, H.C.: A path planning algorithm for industrial robots. Computers and Industrial Engineering 42(2-4), 299–308 (2002)
5. Ericsson, M., Nylen, P.: A look at the optimisation of robot welding speed based on process modeling. Welding Journal (Miami, Fla) 86(8), 238–244 (2007)
6. Ericsson, M., Nylen, P., Berglund, D., Lin-Peng, R.: Three dimensional simulation of robot path, heat transfer and residual stresses of a welded part with complex geometry. International Journal for the Joining of Materials 17(2), 42–51 (2005)
7. Sikstrom, F., Christiansson, A.K.: Modelling for feedback control of weld penetration - applied to gas tungsten arc welding. In: Proc. Reglermöte 2008, Luleaå, Sweden (2008)
8. Connor, L.P.: Welding handbook. Welding Technology, vol. 1. American Welding Society, Miami (1987)
9. Sikström, F., Christiansson, A.K., Lennartson, B.: Simulation for design of automated welding. In: IEEE Eurocon 2007, Warsaw, Poland, pp. 2263–2270 (2007)
10. Henrikson, P., Ericsson, M.: Non-contact temperature measurements using an infrared camera in aerospace welding applications. In: ASM Proceedings of the International Conference: Trends in Welding Research, Phoenix, AZ, United States, ASM International, pp. 930–935 (2002)
11. Sikström, F., Ericsson, M., Nylen, P., Christiansson, A.K.: 3D-scanning for weld distortion measuring. In: Conference Record - IEEE Instrumentation and Measurement Technology Conference, Sorrento, Italy, pp. 2132–2137 (2006)

Modeling of Machining Error Propagation Network for Multistage Machining Processes

Daoyu Liu and Pingyu Jiang

State Key Laboratory for Manufacturing Systems Engineering, Xi'an Jiaotong University, Xi'an 710049, China
dyliu@mail.xjtu.edu.cn, pjiang@mail.xjtu.edu.cn

Abstract. Due to the complicated interactions among different stages in multistage machining processes (MMPs), it is important and necessary to explore the inherent mechanism of machining error propagation for improving product quality. As for this issue, a machining error propagation network (MEPN) of MMPs is proposed in this paper, in which machining form feature (MFF) of workpeice, machine tool, fixture and cutting tool (That is machining element, ME) are defined as different network nodes. The associated relationship among different nodes is mapped by graph theory, according to the results of CAPP of workpiece. Based on this, complex networks theory is introduced to analyze the characteristics of the established MEPN, and several measuring indices of error propagation at different nodes are proposed to quantify the interactions among different nodes. At last, a box part of missile launcher is used to illustrate the proposed method.

Keywords: Multistage machining processes (MMPs); machining error propagation network (MEPN); complex networks; machining form feature; synthesized propagation index (SPI).

1 Introduction

As for the multistage machining processes (MMPs), the quality attributes of workpiece at a stage node are often affected by the output quality of their preceding stages. Therefore, quantifying the quality linkage across stages is a key issue to improve machining quality in MMPs. In order to explore the error propagation behavior of MMPs, the machining error flow was described by Luo et al. [1] with iterated mapping and catastrophe theory, but they didn't provide physical model of error propagation. Hu [2] proposed the stream of variation theory for automotive body assembly. Mantripragada et al. [3] established a state transition model of variation propagation for achieving robust design of assembly processes. Jin and Shi [4] provided a physical model of the sheet metal assembly for dimension control with state space theory. Ding et al. [5] extended Jin's model to be a general case and studied the diagnosisability of multistage manufacturing processes. Huang et al. [6] established a machining variation propagation model to describe the variation stack-up in MMPs. Zhou et al. [7] provided an explicit variation propagation model with differential motion vectors. Djurdjanovic and Ni [8] also offered an explicit dimensional error

C. Xiong et al. (Eds.): ICIRA 2008, Part II, LNAI 5315, pp. 408–418, 2008.

propagation model, but they didn't consider machine tool error. Loose et al. [9] established a mapping relationship model between typical process faults and product quality attributes through a kinematics analysis for MMPs with general fixture layouts.

According to the above description, we can see that there are various kinds of complicated interactions among different stages and their quality attributes. At the same time, quality attributes are also determined by many machining process elements, such as machine tool, cutting tool and fixture etc. Therefore, it is almost impossible to establish a physical or statistical model to describe all these interactions. Complex network theory [10,11], as an effective method to analyze system complexity, has been widely applied to many different fields, such as social networks, information networks, technological networks and biological networks [12,13]. It is noted that the machining process flow of workpiece can be regarded as a complex system due to the complex interactions among different stages. Therefore, the complex networks are introduced to describe these interactions and open out the error propagation rule in MMPs. Here, quality attributes of workpiece and their machining process elements (That is machine tool, cutting tool and fixture) are regarded as different network nodes, based on this, a machining error propagation network (MEPN) is established with graphic theory, and then its some characteristics are discussed in detail.

2 Machining Error Propagation Network of MMPs

2.1 Related Definition

Regarding the MEPN, some rules and concepts are first defined as follows.

Rule1: Machining form features (MFFs) of workpeice and their machining elements (MEs) are regarded as the nodes of network, the associated relationship among different nodes are defined as the edges of network. Here, the associated relationship among different MFFs contains locating and evolving relationship.

Rule 2: The edges of network have direction, if node *i* affects node *j*, the direction is $i \rightarrow j$, else $j \rightarrow i$. For example, the status of node *j* (quality attribute) is influenced by node *i* (quality attribute) and *k* (machine tool), the direction of edges among them are connected by $i \rightarrow j$ and $k \rightarrow j$, respectively.

Rule 3: In order to quantify the interactions among different nodes, the weight of edge is also introduced into the MEPN.

According to the above rules, the MEPN can be represented in the following.

$$G = (V, E, W) \tag{1}$$

Where $V = \{v_1, v_2, \cdots, v_N\}$ denotes node set consisting of MFFs and MEs; $E = \{e_1, e_2, \cdots, e_p\}$ denotes edge set, and e_i $(i = 1, 2, \cdots, p)$ denotes the mapping relationship among different nodes; $W = (w_1, w_2, \cdots, w_p)$ denotes weight set of different edges, and w_i $(i = 1, 2, \cdots, p)$ quantifies the coupled interactions between v_i $(i = 1, 2, \cdots, N)$ and v_j $(j = 1, 2, \cdots, N)$. It should be noted that the initial

MEPN derived from the results of CAPP is modeled in this study. Therefore, it is reasonable to assume that if there is associated relationship between two different nodes i and j, w_{ij} is 1, else w_{ij} is 0.

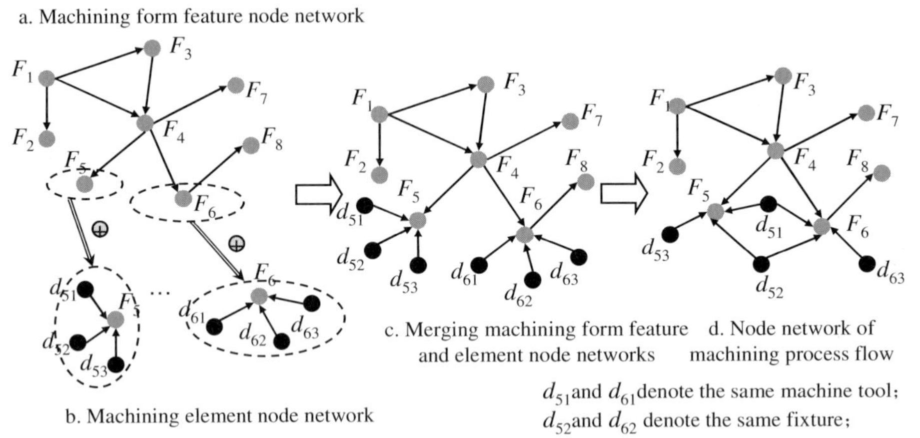

Fig. 1. The modeling procedure of MEPN

2.2 Modeling Procedure of MEPN

Based on the above description, the modeling procedure of the MEPN is provided, as shown in Figure 1.

Step 1: Extracting MFFs of workpiece to establish machining form feature (MFF) network. Assume that $F=\{F_1,\cdots,F_n\}$ (n is the number of MFFs) denotes the MFF set of workpiece, here, MFF is defined as a network node. Based on this, the associated relationship between two different nodes is defined as a directed edge. The MFF network is defined as follows.

$$G_F =< F, E_F > \tag{2}$$

Where E_F denotes the directed edges and $E_F=\{e_{F1},\cdots,e_{Fm}\}$ (m is the number of directed edges).

Step 2: Constructing MFF oriented ME network. Assume that there is F_i and its ME set is denoted with $D_i=\{d_{i1},\cdots,d_{is}\}$ (s is the number of MEs), the associated relationship between the F_i and its MEs is defined as a directed edge. The ME network is defined in the following.

$$G_{Di} =< \{F_i, d_{ij}\}, E_i > \; i=1,\cdots,n \; ; \; j=1,2,\cdots,s \tag{3}$$

Where E_i denotes the directed edges of F_i and its MEs, and $E_i=\{e_{i1},\cdots,e_{is}\}$.

Step 3: Combining the MFF network with the ME network as follows.

$$G'=<V',E'>=G_F \cup G_{D1} \cup \cdots \cup G_{Dn}$$
$$=<F,E_F> \cup <\{F_1,D_{1j}\},E_1> \cup \cdots \cup <\{F_n,D_{nj}\},E_n> \quad (4)$$

Where $V'=\{F_1 \cup \cdots \cup F_n \cup D_{1j} \cdots \cup D_{nj}\}(j=1,\cdots,s)$ and $E'=\{e_1,\cdots,e_r\}(r=1,\cdots,m+ns)$.

Step 4: Merging the repeated ME nodes to generate the MEPN. The repeated ME nodes are the nodes who are used to machine several different MFFs. The size of the achieved MEPN G shown in eq. (1) is achieved as follows.

$$N=4n+m-\frac{1}{2}\sum_{i,j\in N_i,i\neq j,k\in N_k}(r_{ki}*r_{kj}) \quad (5)$$

Where n denotes the number of MFFs; m denotes the number of locating datum features of initial blank of workpeice; N_i and N_j denote MFF set and ME set respectively; $r_{ki}*r_{kj}$ denotes whether MFF i and j are machined by the same ME k or not. If the MFF i is machined by the ME k, r_{ki} is 1, else 0. In the same way, r_{kj} is also set. For example, there are 44 MFFs and 4 initial locating datum features for a box part of missile launcher, according to eq. (5), the size of the MEPN is achieved as follows, $N=44\times4+4-\frac{1}{2}\times198=81$.

3 Some Characteristics of MEPN

3.1 Basic Parameters of MEPN

In order to explore the structural property of the above MEPN, some basic parameters are defined as follows.

Definition 1: The in-degree of node i of the MEPN is written as k_i^{in}, which describes the influence of other nodes on node i.

$$k_i^{in}=\sum_j a_{ji} \quad (6)$$

Where a_{ji} denotes the directed edged from node j to i, and its value is determined by influence weight of node j on i.

Definition 2: The out-degree of node i of the MEPN is written as k_i^{out}, which describes the influence of node i on other nodes.

$$k_i^{out} = \sum_j a_{ij} \tag{7}$$

Where a_{ij} denotes directed edged from node i to j, and its value is determined by influence weight of node i on j.

Definition 3: The degree of node i of the MEPN is written as k_i, which describes the importance of node i to some extent.

$$k_i = k_i^{in} + k_i^{out} \tag{8}$$

Definition 4: The clustering coefficient of node i of the MEPN is written as c_i, which describes the connectivity degree of sub-network oriented for i. The bigger c_i is, the larger opportunity of machining error propagation among these different nodes is.

$$c_i = \frac{\sum_{r=1}^{k'} \sum_{s=1}^{k'} d(n_r, n_s)}{k'(k'-1)} \tag{9}$$

Where k' denotes the neighbor nodes of the node i, and $d(n_r, n_s)$ denotes the coefficient of the associated relationship between node r and s. If there no relationship between node r and s, $d(n_r, n_s)$ is 0.

Definition 5: The average coefficient of the MEPN is written as C, which describes the connectivity degree of the MEPN. Bigger C is, larger opportunities of machining error propagation among different nodes are.

$$C = \frac{1}{N} \sum_{i=1}^{N} c_i \tag{10}$$

Definition 6: The average shortest path length of the MEPN is written as L, which describes the average length of machining error propagation path. Shorter average length is, frequenter the interactions among different nodes are.

$$L = \frac{1}{M} \sum_{i,j \in N, i \neq j}^{N} d_{ij} \tag{11}$$

Where d_{ij} is the shortest path connecting node i and j; and M is the number of shortest paths of the MEPN. If there is directed edge connecting nodes i and j, d_{ij} is summed, else d_{ij} is not summed.

3.2 Measuring Indices of MEPN

On the basis of the above definitions, the measuring indices of the MEPN are provided as follows.

Definition 7: Loading degree (LD) of node i is written as l_i, which describes the possibility of error propagation from other neighbor nodes to node i.

$$l_i = \sum_{j \in N_i} k_j^{in} = \sum_{j=1}^{M} a_{ji}(k_j^{in} + 1) \tag{12}$$

Definition 8: Extending degree (ED) of node i is written as e_i, which describes the possibility of error propagation from node i to its neighbor nodes.

$$e_i = \sum_{j \in N_i} k_j^{out} = \sum_{j=1}^{M} a_{ij}(k_j^{out} + 1) \tag{13}$$

Definition 9: Activating degree (AD) of node i is written as f_i, which describes the occurring possibility of error propagation at node i in the MEPN.

$$f_i = \frac{1}{(N-1)(N-2)}\left[100 \times \left(\sum_{i,j \in N, j \neq k} \frac{n_{jk}(i)}{n_{jk}}\right) + \frac{(N-1)(N-2)}{N}\right] \tag{14}$$

Where n_{jk} is the number of shortest paths connecting node j and k, while $n_{jk}(i)$ is the number of shortest paths connecting node j and k through i.

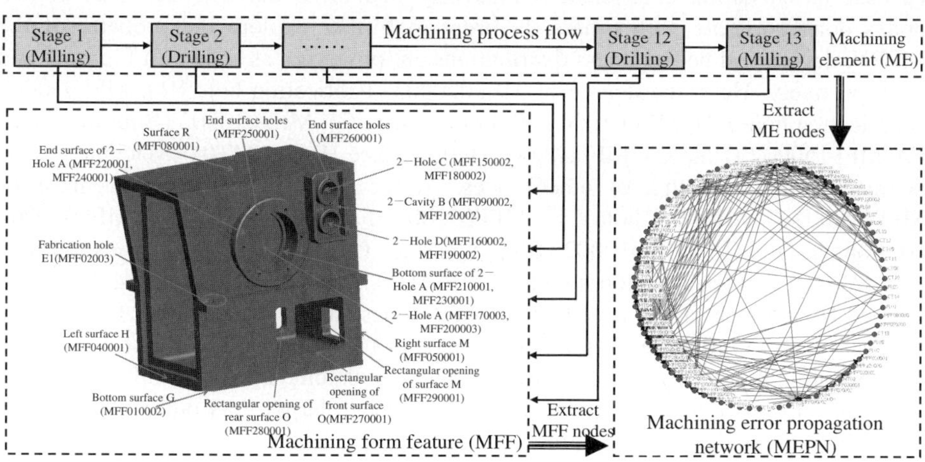

Fig. 2. Machining form features and machining process flow of box part

Definition 10: Synthesized propagation index (SPI) of node i is written as I_i, which is used to identify and quantify the key nodes of the MEPN.

$$I_i = (l_i + e_i) f_i \tag{15}$$

4 An Example

4.1 Topology of MEPN for Box Part

4.1.1 MFFs of Box Part and Their MEs

A box part of missile launcher is used to verify the proposed method, its MFFs and machining process flow are shown in Figure 2. There are 13 different machining stages. The number of the extracted MFFs of the box part is 44, and there are 4 initial locating datum surfaces. The MFFs and their MEs are first coded by coding rules. According to the modeling procedure of MEPN in section 2.2, a topology of MEPN of box part is established, as shown in Figure 3, and the size of the MEPN is 81 according to eq. (5). The number of MFFs, machine tool, cutting tool and fixture nodes are 48 (44 MFFs and 4 initial locating datum features), 9, 14 and 10, respectively.

4.1.2 Topology Property of MEPN

Regarding the topology of the MEPN, some basic parameters of it are provided, which are listed in Table 1.

From the Table 1, the shortest path length of the MEPN is 2.12, which is less than 2.28. And the clustering coefficient of MEPN is 0.056, which is less than 0.085. It can be seen that the MEPN has small-world property, but it is not small world network, because its clustering coefficient is relatively smaller. It may be that most of ME nodes don't correlate with others. In order to further explore the property of the MEPN, degree and betweenness distributions are observed, as shown in Figure 4 and 5, respectively. Here, the degree of MFF020003 (Fabrication hole E1), MFF030003 (Fabrication hole E2), MFF010001 (Bottom surface G), MFF010002 (Bottom surface G), MFF150002 (Hole C), MFF040001 (Left surface H) and MT04 (Machine tool 4) is much larger than that of other nodes. At the same time, the betweenness of MFF020003 (Fabrication hole E1), MFF030003 (Fabrication hole E2), MFF010001 (Bottom surface G), MFF010002 (Bottom surface G), MFF020002 (Fabrication hole E1), MFF030002 (Fabrication hole E2), MFF150002 (Hole C) and MFF040001 (Left surface H) is much larger than that of other nodes. It can be seen that these nodes have substantive influence on the performance of the MEPN. In fact, bottom surface G, fabrication holes E1 and E2 are used as locating datum surfaces at different stages for many times, so the degree of these nodes is much larger than others, which consists with the principle of machining process concentration.

Based on the above observation, some measuring indices defined at section 3.2 are used to further explore the propagation characteristics of the MEPN. The results are listed in Table 2.

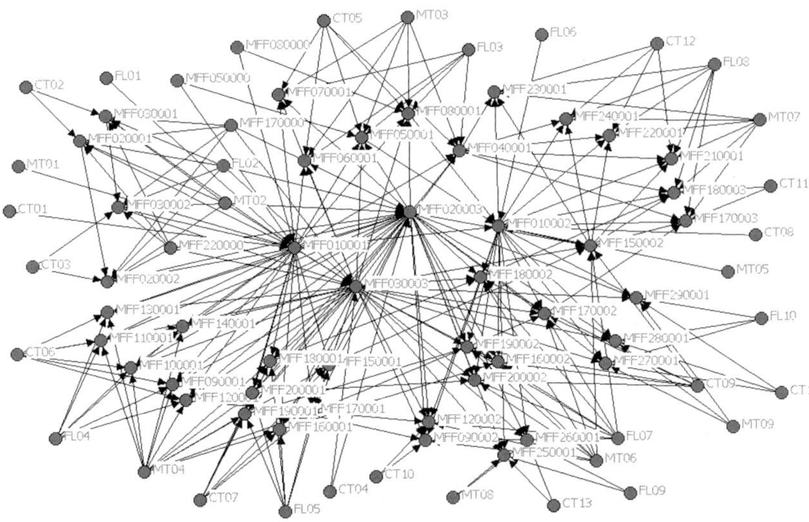

Note that: MFFxxxxxx denotes machining form feature node, MTxx denotes machine tool node, CTxx denotes cutting tool node, and FLxx denotes fixture node.

Fig. 3. The topology of machining error propagation of box part

Table 1. Basic parameters of MEPN

Type	Size	Shortest path length	Clustering coefficient	Degree
MEPN	81	2.12	0.056	3.44/3.44
Random network	81	2.28	0.085	6.88

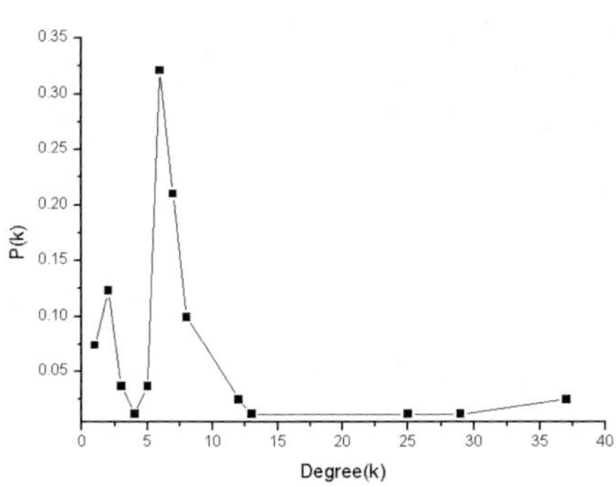

Fig. 4. Degree distributions of MEPN

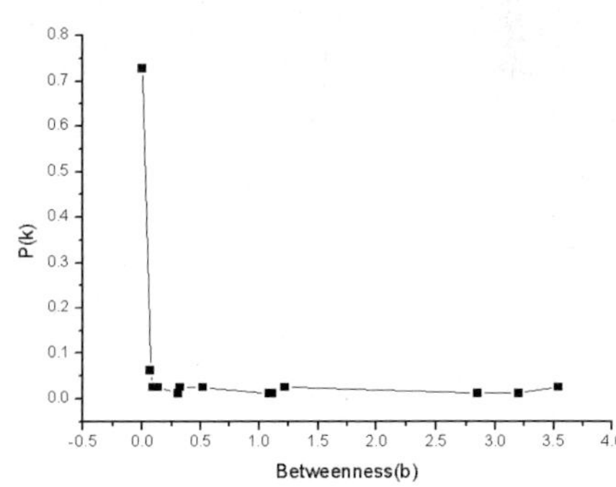

Fig. 5. Betweenness distributions of MEPN

4.2 Results

From the Table 2, we can see that the SPI of MFF010001 (Bottom surface G), MFF020003 (Fabrication hole E1), MFF030003 (Fabrication hole E2) and

Table 2. Measuring indices of MEPN (Top 25)

No.	Node name	LD	ED	AD	SPI
1	MFF010001	5	122	3.213	408.051
2	MFF020003	19	52	3.554	252.334
2	MFF030003	19	52	3.554	252.334
4	MFF010002	25	27	2.861	148.772
5	MFF020002	18	31	1.230	60.270
5	MFF030002	18	31	1.230	60.270
7	MFF040001	25	6	1.098	34.038
8	MFF150002	21	6	1.130	30.510
9	MFF080001	26	20	0.532	24.472
9	MFF050001	26	20	0.532	24.472
11	MFF150001	25	7	0.319	10.208
12	MFF170002	33	1	0.144	4.896
12	MFF180002	33	1	0.144	4.896
14	MFF030001	11	2	0.336	4.368
14	MFF020001	11	2	0.336	4.368
16	MFF180001	25	2	0.105	2.835
16	MFF170001	25	2	0.105	2.835
18	MFF200001	25	1	0.082	2.132
18	MFF160001	25	1	0.082	2.132
18	MFF120001	25	1	0.082	2.132
18	MFF190001	25	1	0.082	2.132
18	MFF090001	18	1	0.082	1.558
23	MT02	0	70	0.012	0.84
23	FL02	0	70	0.012	0.84
25	CT04	0	62	0.012	0.744

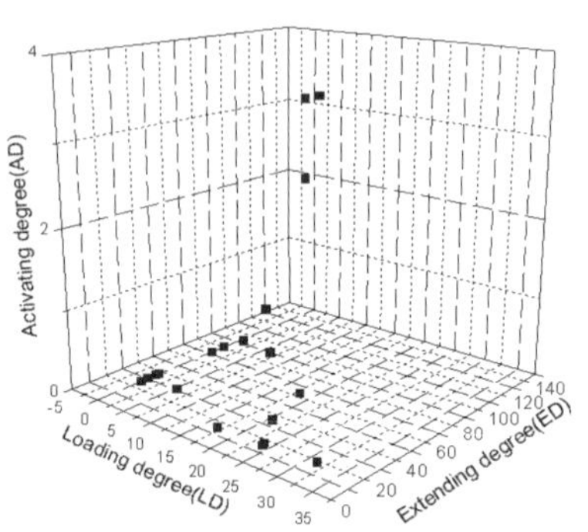

Fig. 6. Error propagation space of MEPN

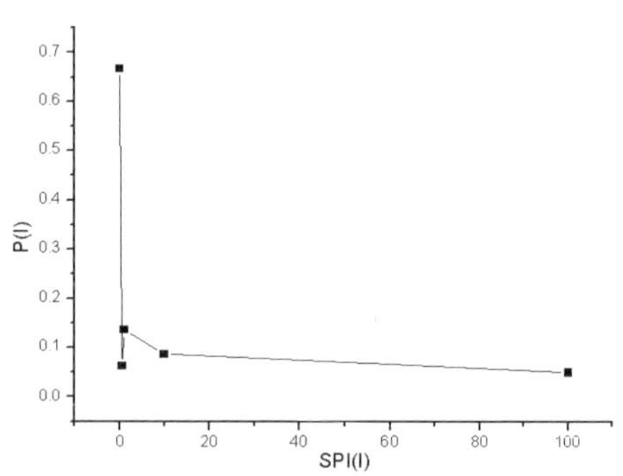

Fig. 7. SPI distribution of nodes for MEPN

MFF010002 (Bottom surface G) is much larger than others. Once quality defects of these nodes occur, the quality defects will be widely propagated to the machining process flow. In order to further observe the SPI distribution of MEPN, the plots of error propagation space and SPI distribution are shown in Figure 6 and 7, respectively.

We can see that there are only a few nodes having higher SPI. In Figure 7, the five points denotes five intervals including [100,∞], [10,100], [1,10], [0.5,1] and [0,0.5] respectively. In addition, it should be noted that the SPIs of the MT02, FL02 and CT04 are relatively small, but they have great influence to the MEPN. It is because that the values of their EDs are very larger in the MEPN. Therefore, these nodes also have to be monitored strictly in order to prevent their error from propagating to the MEPN.

5 Conclusions

In this paper, a MEPN of MMPs is firstly proposed to describe the behavior of machining error propagation in MMPs. Its modeling procedure is then discussed in detail. The MFFs of workpiece and their MEs are defined as different network nodes, the associated relationship among MFFs and MEs are defined as different network edges. Shortest path length, clustering coefficient and degree distributions of the MEPN are observed. The results show that the MEPN has the small world property, but is not small world network. Based on this, the measuring indices of the MEPN are established, and the SPI is used to quantify the propagation effect of different nodes, which provide a basis for identifying key nodes of the MEPN. At last, a box part of missile launcher is used to illustrate the proposed method.

Acknowledgment

The research reported in this paper is supported by both the National Basic Research Program of China with Grant No.2005CB724106 and the support of national 863 High-Tech R&D Program with Grant No.2007AA00Z108. We hereby thank them for the financial aids.

References

1. Luo, Z., Wang, J., Jia, K., Quan, Y., Zheng, L.: Machining error flow model in manufacturing processes. Chin. J. Mech. Eng. 30(1), 112–118 (1994) (in Chinese)
2. Hu, S.J.: Stream of variation theory for automotive body assembly. CIRP Ann-Manuf. Technol. 46(1), 1–6 (1997)
3. Mantripragada, R., Whitney, D.E.: Modeling and controlling variation propagation in mechanical assemblies using state transition models. IEEE Trans. Robot. Autom. 15(1), 124–140 (1999)
4. Jin, J., Shi, J.: State space modeling of sheet metal assembly for dimensional control. J. Manuf. Sci. Eng.-Trans. ASME. 121(11), 756–762 (1999)
5. Ding, Y., Ceglarek, D., Shi, J.: Fault diagnosis of multistage manufacturing processes by using state space approach. J. Manuf. Sci. Eng.-Trans. ASME 124(2), 313–322 (2002)
6. Huang, Q., Shi, J., Yuan, J.: Part dimensional error ant its propagation modeling in multi-operational machining processes. J. Manuf. Sci. Eng.-Trans. ASME 125(2), 55–262 (2003)

7. Zhou, S., Huang, Q., Shi, J.: State space modeling for dimensional monitoring of multistage machining process using differential motion vector. IEEE Trans. Robot. Autom. 19(2), 296–309 (2003)
8. Djurdjanovic, D., Ni, J.: Dimensional errors of fixtures, locating and measurement datum features in the stream of variation modeling in machining. J. Manuf. Sci. Eng.-Trans. ASME 125(4), 716–730 (2003)
9. Loose, J.-P., Zhou, S., Ceglarek, D.: Kinematic analysis of dimensional variation propagation for multistage machining processes with general fixture layouts. IEEE Trans. Autom. Sci. Eng. 4(2), 141–152 (2007)
10. Watts, D.J., Strogatz, S.H.: Collective dynamics of 'small-world' networks. Nature 393, 440–442 (1998)
11. Barabasi, A.-L., Albert, R.: Emergence of scaling in random networks. Science 286, 509–512 (1999)
12. Newman, M.E.J.: The structure and function of complex networks. SIAM Rev. 45(2), 167–256 (2003)
13. Boccaletti, S., Latora, V., Moreno, Y., Chavez, M., Hwang, D.-U.: Complex networks: structure and dynamics. Phys. Rep. 424, 175–308 (2006)

Research on Design Method and Application of FPGA-Based Motion Control

Dong Liu, Xuesong Mei, Tao Tao, and Youqing Zhou

School of Mechanical Engineering
Xi'an Jiaotong Unviersity
710049 Xi'an Shaanxi P.R. China
xsmei@mail.xjtu.edu.cn

Abstract. A novel approach for development of FPGA-based motion control system in MATLAB/Simulink environments was proposed. The specialized software tools System Generator in Matlab/Simulink environments, related design procedure and system architecture are presented. According to the approach, an integrated development platform which consists of MATLAB/Simulink, FPGA experimental board and *X-Y* servo table has been established. The interpolator, acceleration/deceleration controller unit and PID controller of motion control system are implemented to validate the approach and platform. The experiments show that the approach and development platform have characteristics of integrated architecture and rapid development.

Keywords: FPGA; motion control; MATLAB/Simulink; System Generator.

1 Introduction

The increasing demand on better position accuracy and quicker motion velocity of servo-mechanism requires higher sampling rates (servo update period), quicker computation capacity and more system resource. The controller based on digital signal processor (DSP) are one of most popular commercial motion control platform, such as PMAC [1], but their implementation of higher servo period and algorithm adjustment is strictly restricted due to the fixed system hardware structure and sequential computation architecture. Field Programmable Gate Array (FPGA) has the high-speed parallel computation ability and flexible programming through large quantity of configurable resources and internal integrated high-speed coprocessor. A novel FPGA-based motion controller can overcome DSP's drawbacks to implement rapid and flexible design for motion control system. In these years, some work has been done on the research and application of FPGA-based motion control, First in servo control strategy and equipments: Zhao et al. [2] implemented control equipment FPGA-based for small-scale robot using FPGA, where they utilized the high-integration of FPGA to complete small-size hardware, and authors evaluated the design in terms of area, power, and speed. Li and Hu [3] proposed a parallel PID algorithm with Fuzzy gain conditioner on FPGA and investigated the simulation-based approach. For the velocity planning of CNC machine tools, Wook and Kim [4] analyzed the digital convolution method in FPGA hardware. Chen and Lee [5] realized FIR filter to implement

C. Xiong et al. (Eds.): ICIRA 2008, Part II, LNAI 5315, pp. 419–430, 2008.

acceleration/deceleration control. Osorni-Rios [6] showed a low cost, computationally efficient, on-line operation and hardware implementation through the multiplier-free recursive algorithm for computing the polynomial-based profile. On the interpolation research, Yau et al. [7] presented an FPGA-based motion control to improve the overall computation performance for NURBS interpolation and servo control. Oldknow and Yellowed [8] implemented three-dimensional dynamic interpolation in FPGA.

In above cited works, the design flow and methodology about FPGA have the similar design process and application methodology, that is: control algorithm is develop firstly, and then control strategy in FPGA is represented with Hardware Describe Language (HDL) or schematic circuit diagram, finally verified by simulation and experiment. With the increase of design complexity, the difficult of simulation and implement increase continually. Aiming at modeling and simulation of FPGA in Matlab/Simulink plant which has powerful functions, Xilinx Company developed a new software tool System Generator (SG), a toolbox in the Matlab/Simulink environment. It provides a library of blockset representing functions which can be implemented in an FPGA. Also it can convert the created model into HDL code automatically. Make FPGA designs efficient and rapid.

This paper presents a novel approach for the design, simulation and implementation of control algorithms for motion control systems using SG in Matlab/Simulink. This approach makes full use of FPGA and the SG to provide the platform with the characters of integrative architecture and rapid development. In this text, the development environment and design procedure about SG is introduced firstly. Then the model of *X-Y* servomotor table is discussed in Section III. The circular and linear interpolator, acceleration/deceleration unit, general PID controller are completed by using SG in Matlab/Simulink in Section IV. The result of simulation and experiment are also presented in this section. A conclusion follows in Section V.

2 FPGA-Based Motion Control System

2.1 System Generator

System Generator is a system-level modeling and design tool from Xilinx that enables the use of the MATLAB/Simulink design environment for FPGA design. It is composite of FPGA functional blockset (as shown in Fig. 1) and other complementary utility tools. The blocks provide abstractions of mathematical, logic, memory, and DSP functions that can be used to build sophisticated signal processing, control and other systems et al. The SG library related to control system includes 5 sections [9]:

1. Basic Elements: Includes standard building blocks for digital logic (*delay, mux, counter, register,* etc).
2. Control Logic: Includes blocks used for control circuitry and state machines.
3. Math: Includes blocks that implement mathematical functions (*adder, multiplier, relational, negate*).
4. Memory: Includes memories (*RAM, ROM, FIFO*, etc).
5. Tools: Includes utility blocks (automatic code generation, resource estimation, Hardware co-simulation, etc).

Like other Simulink blocksets, SG blocksets are he blocks can be connected in the Simulink block editor to create functional models of a dynamical system. And SG allows designs to be composed of a variety of ingredients: Data flow models, traditional hardware design languages (VHDL, Verilog, and EDIF), and functions derived from the MATLAB programming language. And the design can be used side-by-side, simulated together, and synthesized into working hardware. It should be noted that the fundamental scalar signal type in Simulink is double precision floating point, but all the mathematical operations in FPGA are done by fix-point format. For each function operation, the precision must be given in the *M-N* format where *M* is the integer number bits and *N* is the faction bits. Therefore, the connection between Xilinx blocks and non-Xilinx blocks is provided by *gateway* blocks. The *gatewayin* converts a double precision signal into a Xilinx signal, and the *gatewayout* converts a Xilinx signal into double precision automatically.

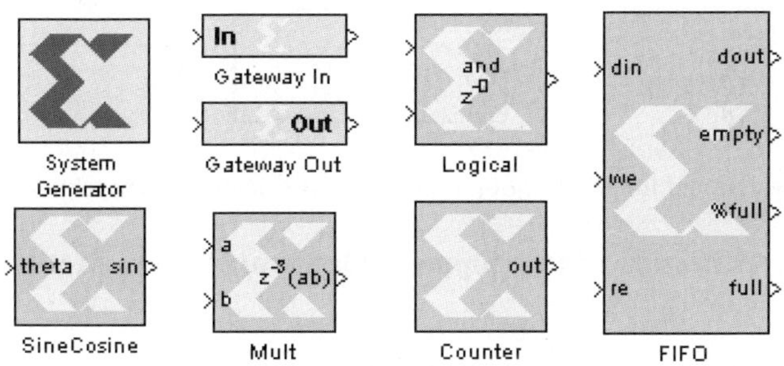

Fig. 1. System Generator blocksets

2.2 FPGA-Based Motion Control System Development Procedure Using SG

The characteristic of SG is modeling and simulation of FPGA in Matlab/Simulink, and generating HDL automatically. The main design procedure can be divided into two stages. Firstly, the system is designed and tested in MATLAB/Simulink. Secondly, the HDL code is generated automatically and implemented into the FPGA with the programming files. The flow diagram (as shown in Fig. 3) explained the design procedure in detailed.

Firstly, the targeted control object is modeled by using Simulink blockset or s-function. Then the control algorithm is developed using SG blocks only, and the SG-based controller is connected to the Simulink model blockset by "*GatewayIn*" and "*GatewayOut*" blocks. The third step is the simulation of the complete system in Simulink. Once the simulation performance in Simulink is acceptable, the design enters the next stage. Following step is to generate HDL code automatically with the "*System Generator*" block. After this step, a configuration file is obtained can g program FPGA device. In some cases, some modifications of the system maybe required, finally can implement optimal performance through readjusting partial parameters.

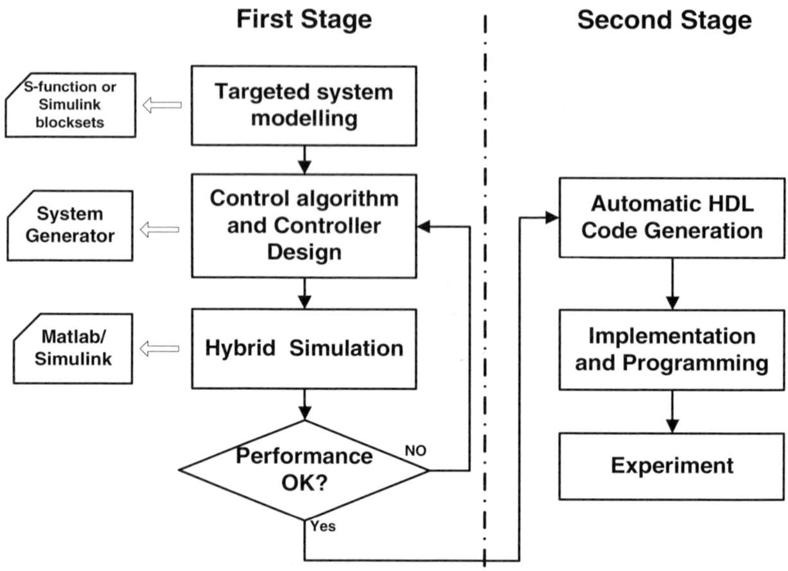

Fig. 2. Design and implementation process of motion control system development

2.3 System Architecture of Development Platform of Servo Motion Control System

The developing platform for the servo motion control system is shown in Fig. 2. It is composed of four parts: PC, FPGA experimental board, servo amplifier and *X-Y* table. PC provides the integrated development environment in which can model, design and simulate. The controller is realized on FPGA experiment board. The amplifier converts pulse control signal to current signal applied to motor armature. *X-Y* table is controlled object. Because FPGA can integrate processing units and related peripheral logic in hardware, it can provide a high integrated system-on-chip solution. In this design, interpolator, acceleration/deceleration unit, PID controller and peripheral

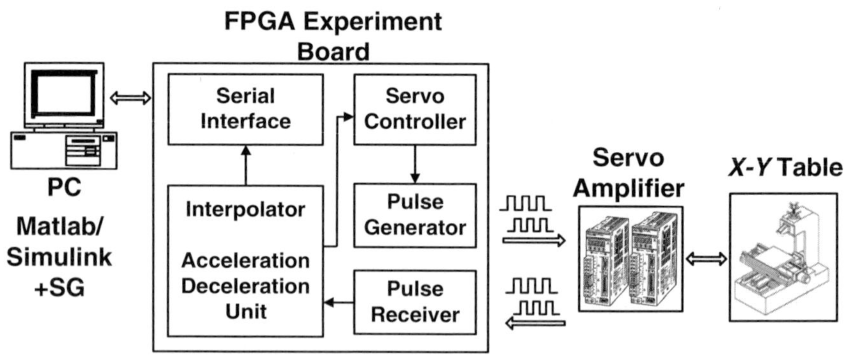

Fig. 3. Architecture of servo table control system platform

interface logic are implemented in one chip. Small hardware size and low power consumption are realized. Furthermore, the difficulty of board-level hardware design is lowed and the system reliability is increased.

3 Modeling of Pulse *X-Y* Servo Table

The work area of *X-Y* servo table studied in this paper is 300 *mm*×300 *mm*. The worktable is driven by *X*-axis which is above the *Y*-axis. Each axis is driven by a ball screw coupled to a permanent-magnet synchronous motor (PMSM) and a servo amplifier. The pitch of ball screw is 10*mm*. Moving elements are supported by roller-type guideway. An incremental encoder mount on the motor shaft to supply velocity feedback signal whose highest resolution is 131072 pulses per round. And 1 μm resolution linear scale along with each axis generate position feedback signal.

Simplifying the close loop control system consisting of an amplifier, a servomotor and the *X″Y* table, and the AC motor can transfer to DC motor in control model when using vector control. So the servo system model can be expressed as three equilibrium equations [10]. (e.g. current equilibrium equation, servomotor dynamics equilibrium equation and servo-table dynamics equilibrium equation). And can obtain the block diagram of the close loop control system of the *X≷Y* table as shown in Fig. 4. where L_a is the inductance of the motor, R_a is the resistance of the motor, K_t is the toque constant of the motor, K_e is the counter electromotive force of the motor, K_e is current loop feedback gain, K_b is velocity loop feedback gain, K_N is position loop feedback gain, $J(J_x,J_y)$ is the moment of inertia of the drive train, H is transmission ratio, K_g is the pitch of the ball screw, $K_{st}(K_x,K_y)$ is the stiffness of the transmission elements, $B(B_x,B_y)$ is the construction dampness of the transmission elements, and $M(M_x,M_y)$ is the mass of the table. The parameter value gave in Table 1. G_p , G_v and G_c are respectively position, velocity and current controller to regulate the position, velocity and current loops.

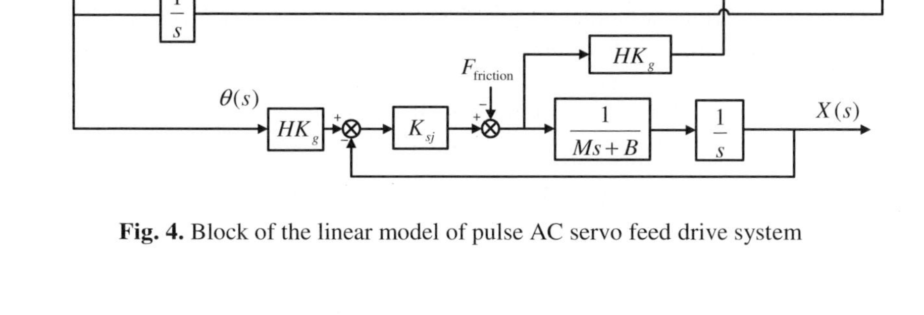

Fig. 4. Block of the linear model of pulse AC servo feed drive system

Table 1. Servomotor system parameter

Parameter	Value	Unit	Parameter	Value	Unit
J_x	2.93×10^{-2}	Kg . m2	K_e	0.18	V/rad
J_y	1.55×10-2	Kg . m2	K_g	10×10-3	m/rad
B_x	1.5×104	Kn . m/s	K_{st_x}	0.41×106	N/m
B_y	8.2×104	kN . m/s	K_{st_y}	2.2×107	N/m
R_s	1.05	Ω	K_b	1	V/A
L_a	0.037	H	K_a	1	V/rad
K_t	0.797	N . m/A	H	1	—

4 Design of Motion Controller Based FPGA

To obtain more accurately and more quickly, the interpolator, acceleration/deceleration unit and servo-controller must be appropriate and efficient. The general control architecture is depicted in Fig. 5. The interpolator is applied to generate coordinated movement of separately driven axes of motion. The acceleration/deceleration controller smoothes motion velocity in start-down stage and at a corner when paths change direction. The servo-controller is to reduce the axial position errors to follow the desired trajectory. In popular commercial motion system, the typical interpolators are linear and circular interpolator. Velocity profile is based on polynomial functions, such as, linear and S-curve. The common servo-controller is PID controller. These designs will be given respectively as follow.

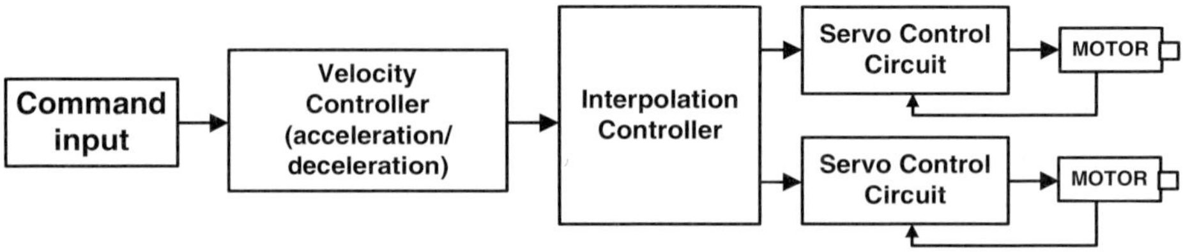

Fig. 5. Architecture of motion control system

4.1 Linear and Circular Interpolator

Despite the tremendous development in CNC system, linear and circular interpolations continue to be the standard motions of modern CNC machines. The interpolation mainly adopts sample-data method, when servo control system is close-loop or semi close-loop. The calculation procedures are as follows:

The computation formula of the coordinate X_{i+1}, Y_{i+1} in linear interpolation:

$$\begin{cases} X_{i+1} = X_i + KX_e \\ Y_{i+1} = Y_i + KY_e \end{cases}, \text{ where } K = FT/L \tag{1}$$

The computation formula of the coordinate X_{i+1}, Y_{i+1} in circular interpolation at clockwise direction:

$$\begin{cases} X_{i+1} = \cos\alpha X_i - \sin\alpha Y_i \\ Y_{i+1} = \cos\alpha Y_i + \sin\alpha X_i \end{cases}, \text{ where } \alpha = FT/R \tag{2}$$

where X_{i+1}, Y_{i+1} represent the successive point, X_i, Y_i denote the current point, F is max feedrate, T is sampling period. R is circular radius.

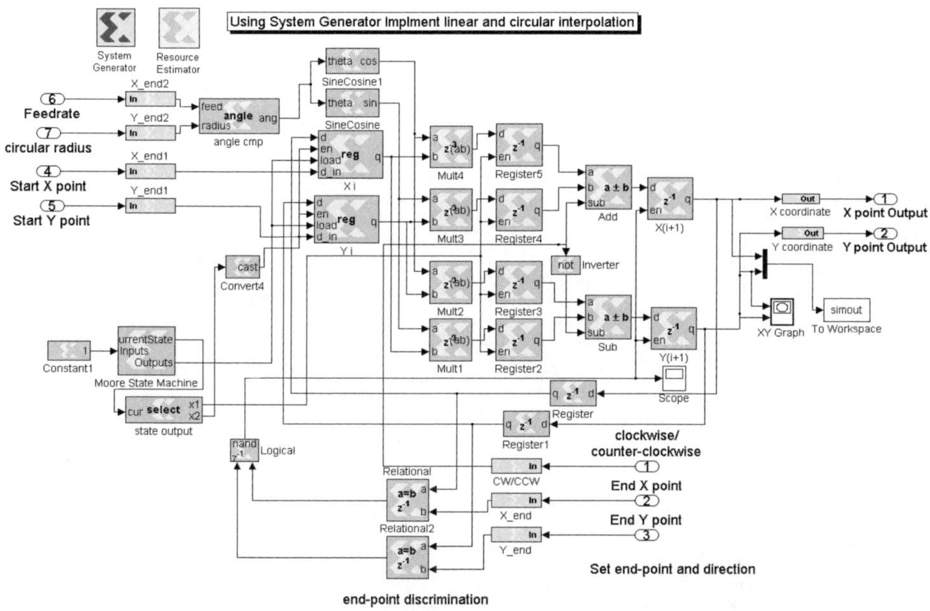

Fig. 6. Linear and circular interpolator

Equation (1) and (2) is composed of multiply, add, divide and trigonometric function, and the blocks needed exist in the SG library, the complex sinusoidal and cosinoidal function can replace by RAM-based lookup table. Linear and circular interpolator represent in SG model shown as Fig. 6, the model includes two parts: 1) interpolation computation: the linear and circular interpolation increment computation; 2) end-point discrimination: decide to cease the interpolation process when motion reaches the end-point.

In comparison with the conventional methods, the SG design approach provides many advantages in particular. Firstly, the SG blocks can exactly represent the hardware model running the algorithm, and that is that the modeling of the algorithm is also the implementation of algorithm. Therefore a lot of design time is saved, and the conversion error between modeling and implementation is not existed. Second, the parameters and architectures of controller and controlled object can conveniently adjust. The simulating and experimental result can easily be obtained in MATLAB/Simulink. The total design is rapid, efficient and flexible.

4.2 Acceleration/Deceleration Unit

The majority acceleration/desecration algorithms are referred to the polynomial types nowadays. They mainly rely on software methods and cost large CPU computational time. Digital convolution method can efficiently achieve similar performance as polynomial method [11], and can be implemented by FPGA easily. The schematic diagram of digital convolution illustrated in Fig. 7(a). The sequence *H1* and *H2* carry out convolution manipulation. The time length of *H1*is nT_s, and magnitude is V_{max}, *H1* denotes the velocity command. The time length of *H2* is n_aT_s and magnitude is $1/n_aT_s$, it represents the acceleration/deceleration control command. After convolution manipulation, the result shows as sequence *H3*, time duration from *0* to n_aT_s is trapezoidal acceleration time, $n_aT_s - nT_s$ is constant speed time, $nT_s + n_aT_s$ is the deceleration time equal to the acceleration time. The parabolic sequence is obtained by Two-level convolution manipulation (shown as Fig. 7(b)), so the acceleration/deceleration is a second-order parabolic velocity profile.

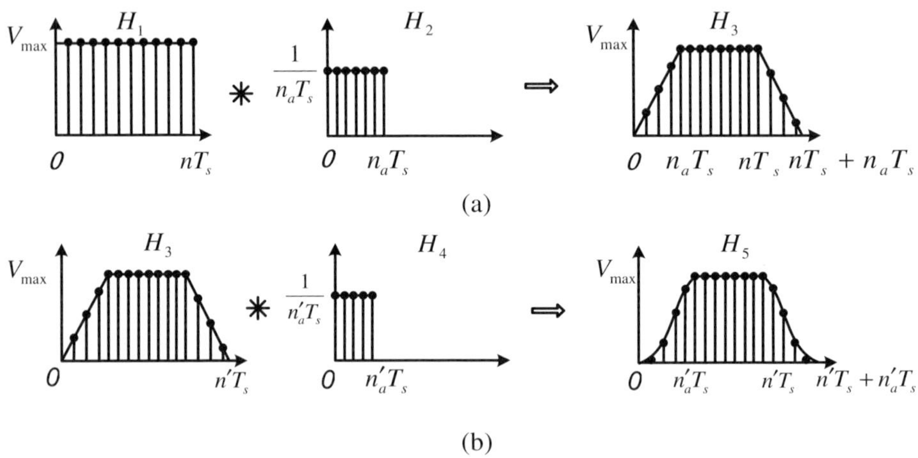

Fig. 7. Result of a constant federate by performing digital convolution

SG model of one-level digital convolution shows as Fig. 8. The model mainly is composed of two parts: (1) one-level digital convolution, (2) deceleration-point computation. The primary functional blocks of digital convolution include: two *AddSub*, two *Register*, one *Slice*, and one *m*-bit *Addressable Shift Buffer*. In the one-level convolution, the output of current velocity = (*input register* + *accumulative register* – *m*-bit *shift register*) / *m*, when *m* is an integer power of 2, the divider can replace by *Slice*. At acceleration stage (acceleration duration should be *m* times of the servo update periods), the output of *shift register* is 0, so output of velocity gradually increase (*1/m×velocity command*) in every cycle. When the acceleration is completed, the output of *shift register* change into the value of *velocity command*, so the output of velocity is the value of *velocity command*. According to the acceleration, when motion close to the deceleration-point (function of deceleration-point computation part),

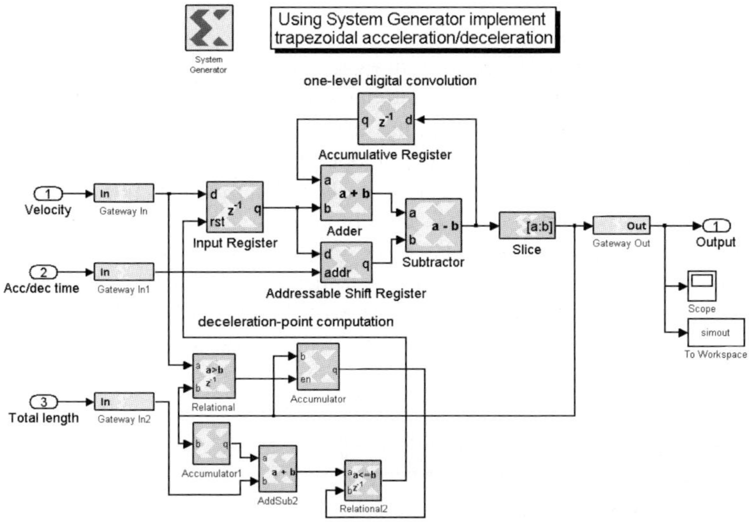

Fig. 8. Using SG implement linear acceleration/deceleration

the velocity command is set to 0, but *shift register* hold output. so the velocity output gradually decrease (*1/m×velocity command*) in every cycle. Finally reach to the end-point when velocity decreases to 0.

4.3 PID Controller

The PID algorithm is commonly applied for servo control loop (current loop, velocity loop and position loop). The controller is described as a differential equation:

$$u(t) = K_p\left[e(t) + \frac{1}{T_i}\int_0^t e(t)dt + T_d \frac{de(t)}{dt} \right] \tag{3}$$

where K_p is proportional gain, T_i is the integral time constant and T_d is the derivative time constant. For a small sample interval T, this equation can be turned into a difference equation by discretization. The difference equation is given as:

$$u(n) = K_p e(n) + K_i \sum_{j=0}^{n} e(n) + K_d (e(n) - e(n-1)) \tag{4}$$

where $K_i = K_p T/T$ is the integral coefficient, and $K_d = K_p T_d / T$ is the derivative coefficient. Equation (4) is called the "position algorithm". But "incremental algorithm" is more applied in engineering practice. Show as Equation 5.

$$u(n) = u(n-1) + \Delta u(n) = u(n-1) + K_0 e(n) + K_1 e(n-1) + K_2 e(n-2)$$

$$\text{where} \begin{cases} K_0 = K_p + K_i + K_d \\ K_1 = -K_p - 2K_d \\ K_2 = K_d \end{cases} \tag{5}$$

The incremental algorithm can avoid the accumulation of all past errors *e(n)* and can realize smooth switching from manual to automatic operation [12]. The equation (5) can be decomposed into its basic arithmetic operations, then implement by FPGA easily. The architecture of controller includes serial and parallel architecture [13]. For a parallel design, each basic operation has its own arithmetic unit, all operation carry out simultaneously. For serial design, all operations share only one adder and one multiplier and perform sequentially. Fig. 9 shows parallel design of the PID incremental algorithm. The architecture is mainly composed of combinational logic. The design requires 3 adders, 3 multipliers and 4 registers. Error signal *e(n)* of the last cycle is latched at register *REG1*, thus becomes *e(n−1)* in this cycle. In the same manner, *e(n−2)* and *u(n−1)* are recorded at *REG3* and *REG4* by latching *e(n−1)* and *u(n)* respectively. And then obtain the control output variable *u(n)* through hardware operation.

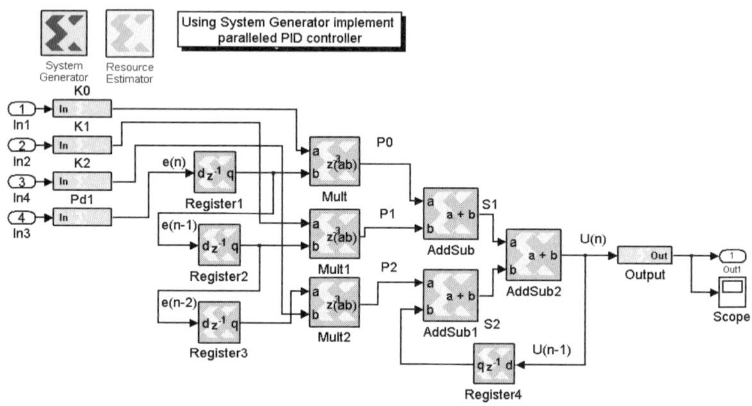

Fig. 9. Parallel design of incremental PID algorithm

4.4 Simulation and Experiment

Each module is simulated to ensure function and accuracy firstly, and then the integrated simulation model is built to examine connection among modules after the full design is accomplish. Once the performance of simulation is acceptable, the modeling of interpolator, acceleration/deceleration control and servo-controller can be implemented to HDL through automatic code generation of SG. In practical experiment, some controller parameters need be readjusted by repeated experiments to improve the control algorithm performance. The total prototype is implemented on the Spartan-3E [14] board. The syntheses results show an average 28% FPGA usage, equivalent to 140,000 system gates. The experiments show that the maximum motion errors do not exceed 15μm under the condition that the maximum velocity is 12 *m/min*. The minimum servo update cycle can reach 600 μs. The experimental results of signal axial trapezoidal acceleration/deceleration with velocity 200 *mm/s*, sampling time T=0.40 *ms* is shown in Fig. 10. The results of circular motion with tangent velocity 200 *mm/s*, radius of 150 *mm* and sampling time is T=0.40 *ms* is gave in Fig 11.

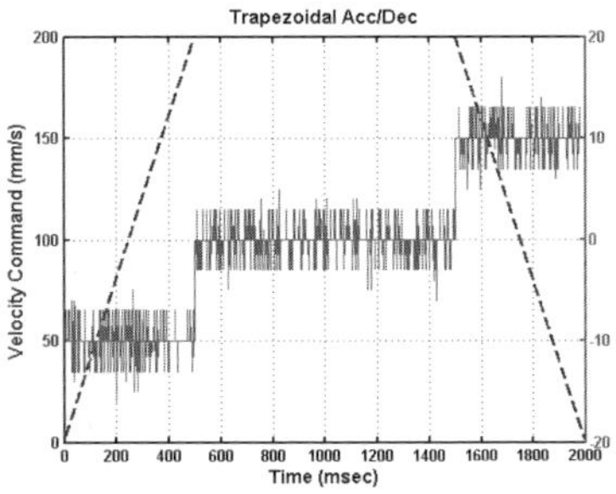

Fig. 10. Velocity profile experiment

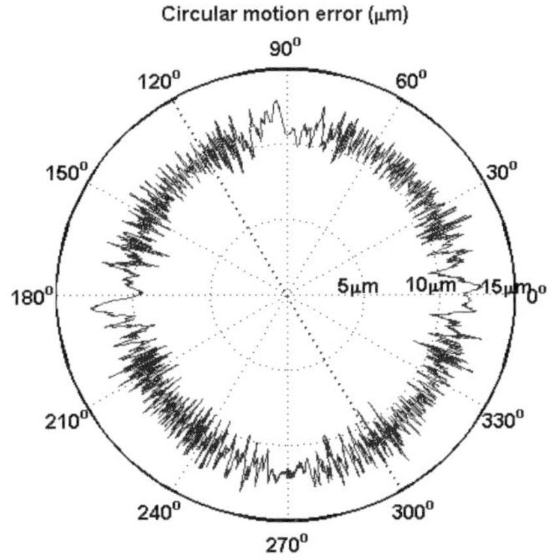

Fig. 11. Circular interpolation experiment

5 Conclusions

This paper designs and implements a new pulse motion control platform based on FPGA. A novel approach to design, simulate and implement FPGA motion control system has been proposed by using specialized tools System Generator in Matlab/Simulink. Simulation and experiment prove that interpolation algorithm, acceleration/deceleration control and servo-controller can be completed through this approach. This approach can reduce develop time largely and ensure the simulation model represent exactly the hardware model to run the algorithm. This approach can help rapid design control system algorithms and motion system prototype develop.

References

1. Tau, D.: Turbo PMAC-Lite PCI Data Sheet, http://www.deltatau.com
2. Zhao, W., Kim, B.H., et al.: FPGA Implementation of Closed-Loop Control System for Small-Scale Robot. In: Advanced Robotics 2005 ICAR 2005 Proceedings 12th International Conference, pp. 70–77 (2005)
3. Li, J., Hu, B.S.: The Architecture of Fuzzy PID Gain Conditioner and Its FPGA Prototype Implementation. In: Proceedings of 2nd IEEE International Conference on ASIC, pp. 61–65 (1996)
4. Wook, J.J., Kim, Y.K.: FPGA based acceleration and deceleration circuit for industrial robots and CNC machine tools. Journal of Mechatronics 12(4), 635–642 (2002)
5. Chen, C.-S., Lee, A.-C.: Design of acceleration/deceleration profiles in motion control based on digital FIR filters. International Journal of Machine Tools and Manufacture 38, 799–825 (1998)
6. Alfredo, R.: Osornio-Rios, et al.: FPGA implementation of higher degree polynomial acceleration profiles for peak jerk reduction in servomotors. Robotics and Computer-Integrated Manufacturing (April 2, 2008)

7. Yau, H.T., Lin, M.T., Tsai, M.S.: Design and implementation of Realtime NURBS interpolator using a FPGA-based motion controller. In: Proceedings of the IEEE International Conference on Mechatronics, pp. 56–61 (2005)
8. Oldknow, K.D., Yellowley, I.: PGA-based servo control and three-dimensional dynamic interpolation. IEEE/ASME Transactions on Mechatronics, 10(1), 98–110 (2005)
9. Xilinx Inc.: System Generator User Guide, `http://www.xilinx.com`
10. Mei, X.S., Tsutsumi, M., et al.: Study of the friction error for a high-speed high precision table. International Journal of Machine Tools & Manufacture 41, 1405–1415 (2001)
11. Jeon, J.W., Ha, Y.Y.: A Generalized Approach for the Acceleration and Deceleration of Industrial Robots and CNC Machine Tools. Transcation on Industrial Electronics 47(1), 133–139 (2000)
12. Isermann, R.: Digital Control Systems. Springer, New York (1989)
13. Samet, L., Masmoudi, N., et al.: A Digital PID Controller for Real Time and Multi Loop Control: a comparative study. In: Proceedings of 1998 IEEE International Conference on Electronics, Circuits and Systems, pp. 291–296 (1998)
14. Xilinx Inc.: Spartan-3E FPGA Family: Complete Data Sheet, `http://www.xilinx.com`

A Method of Change Management in Error Analysis for Multistage Machining Processes

Feng Jia, Pingyu Jiang, and Daoyu Liu

State Key Laboratory for Manufacturing Systems Engineering, Xi'an Jiaotong University, Xi'an, Shaanxi 710049, China
jiafeng.1983@stu.xjtu.edu.cn, pjiang@mail.xjtu.edu.cn, dyliu@mail.xjtu.edu.cn

Abstract. In this paper, a reference framework is proposed for managing the error variation in multistage machining processes (MMPs). In MMPs, quality attributes of workpiece may be subject to many different process elements, such as fixture error, machine tool error, etc. It is a key issue to manage the machining error variation cased by these elements for improving the final quality of product. An information management method is firstly provided, which is used to manage the basic information of MMPs. Based on this, a control and management method of error variation is established. Here, grey-model theory and least square method are used to analyze the rule of error variation at single process and in MMPs respectively. The grey-model theory is used to predict the changes of quality attributes, and then the least square method is used to explore the associated relationship between the change of the quality attributes and the working condition of machining equipment.

Keywords: Change management; grey model; least square method; principal component analysis (PCA).

1 Introduction

In multistage machining processes (MMPs), it is known that the error variation is very complex due to the interactions between the different quality attributes and their machining elements. There are many kinds of process information reflecting quality status of workpiece at different stages. How to manage the information is a key issue for improving the final quality of workpiece.

Thierry et al.[1]presented that organizational change management is concerned with realizing strategies using models, methods and prescriptions that seek to guide the three key elements of strategic management process: strategic analysis, strategic choice and strategic implementation. Change management has been widely applied in engineering fields in the world. Cao and McHugh [2] argued that any change program characterized by diversity and interaction of activity change should be managed as a whole by using multiple methods in one intervention. The application in change management for process quality control is different from commerce application. It is considered that the problem about error variation is objective. The man factor is neglected factitiously. So error variation is introduced due to fault of machining elements (such as machine, material, method, environment, etc.), which directly affects the machining quality of workpiece.

C. Xiong et al. (Eds.): ICIRA 2008, Part II, LNAI 5315, pp. 431–439, 2008.

In order to monitor and manage the fluctuation of quality attributes at different stages, partial least square model has been applied widely in the manufacturing process (Song et al.[3], Fu et al.[4]). Du and Tang [5] adopted principal component analysis to control and diagnose for multivariate quality. It can be seen that these methods focus on monitoring the machining quality of product.

In this study, a grey model is used to predict the status of current stage according to the machining information of previous stages. But this method can not identify the error sources if abnormal changes are detected. Here, least square method is adopted to solve this problem, which can get the associated relationship between machining errors and their error sources.

2 The Model of Information Management

2.1 The Classification and Structure of Features

In the multistage machining processes, we should integrate the design field and manufacture field to ensure the feasibility of the manufacture. So the features of workpiece not only contain the form features, but also contain the precision information related to the manufacturing. The classification and structure of the features are composed of the information of design, technology and manufacture. In the MMPs, the quality attributes of the features that will be controlled and managed are the geometric, dimension and roughness etc. The dimension of the features is a comparatively important quality factor. The form feature includes the step, plane, ring, hole, trough and chamfer. The features of workpiece could be described according to the form classification, which can be described in eq. (1).

$$F_k = \{ f_k \quad P_k \} (k = 1, 2, \cdots, n) \tag{1}$$

Where F_k denotes the feature k of the workpiece; denotes the form feature; denotes the precision feature.

2.2 The Variation of Characteristics in MMPs

At design phase, the form feature and precision feature are the final standard of the product. At manufacturing phase, the various features are machined with the different process activities. To the different process activities, there are different precision features and dimension feature respectively. We propose a concept, named as the intermediate feature $F_k = \{ f_k \quad P_k \}$, which consists of different precision features and dimension features. A full feature chain is composed of these intermediate characteristics. When this chain is executed exactly, we can achieve the target what we design. So for analysing the propagation rule of the feature quality, the description of the feature chain is necessary. The chain is simplified to be a kind of linear transmission. Besides the direct relationship there are several location relationships. For example, as shown in figure 1, the relationship among sub-activity 11 to 13 is the propagation relationship, and between sub-activity 11 and 31 is the location relationship. So we can conclude that the variation relationships of the features quality in MMPs include two kinds of relationships, that is, the direct propagation and the indirect propagation.

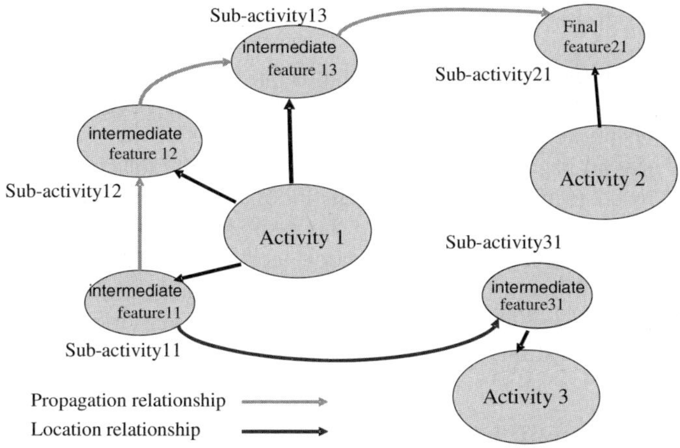

Fig. 1. Variation propagation relationship among different characteristics

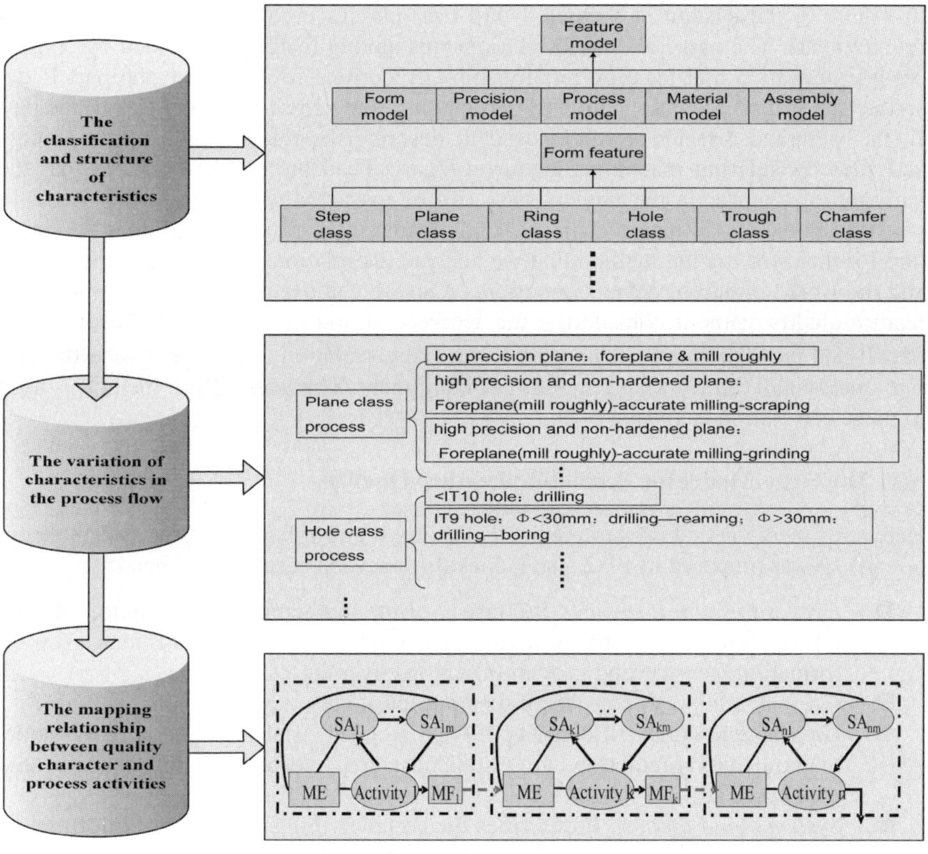

Fig. 2. The model of information management

2.3 The Mapping Relationship between Features and Process Activities

To manage the machining information, it should be noted that the process activities are associated with corresponding features. Weighted directed graph is used to describe the relationship among process activities. In the same way, to the variation of features, there are propagation relationship and location relationship. Here, e-QC controller [6] is used to manage and control the quality status of different features, working condition status of equipment and the associated relationship among different stages. The information management model consists of all e-QC controllers, as shown Figure 2. Based on the classification and variation of features, a database is founded to support the mapping relationship. The process activities can be separated into many activities consisting of different sub-activities (SA).

3 The Model of Quality Characteristics Management

3.1 The Method of Characteristics Quality Management

In Figure 3, the system is separated into four parts according to different function requirements. The part I about the relationships among features is defined by considering propagation and location relationships. According to the part I, the part II describes the mapping relationship between features and activities. According to the part II, the weighted directed graph is used to describe the relationship among process activities considering machining feature of part. Then the part III denotes that the variation of features in the process flow can be extracted according to the part I. In part III, the complete feature chain of single feature of part, which provides the structure for the error tracing method that we analyze the relationships between the feature and the work condition, is very important. Also we can use grey-model to predict the feature quality without considering the work condition of equipment. According to part II and part III, part IV is proposed to make correlation analysis between the feature quality and the working condition of equipment. The least square method is used to make correlation analysis.

3.2 The Grey-Model for Predicting Feature Quality

Here, grey theory is first used to predict the quality status of features. Grey system theory (Deng [7]) was proposed in 1982, and it consists of several basal parts (Chen [8]).

➊ *Grey information theory.* It consists of the mathematical description of grey information that information cognitive model, information element, grey information measure and grey information cover etc.

➋ *Grey set theory.* It consists of the concept of grey fuzzy set .

➌ *Grey methodology.* It consists of Grey Related Analysis method, grey-model method, grey prediction, grey statistics, grey clustering, grey decision and grey control.

➍ *System cloud theory.* It describes the complex things about poor information, multi-factor, uncertainty, that consists of grey screening, trend relational analysis, grey dynamic modelling etc.

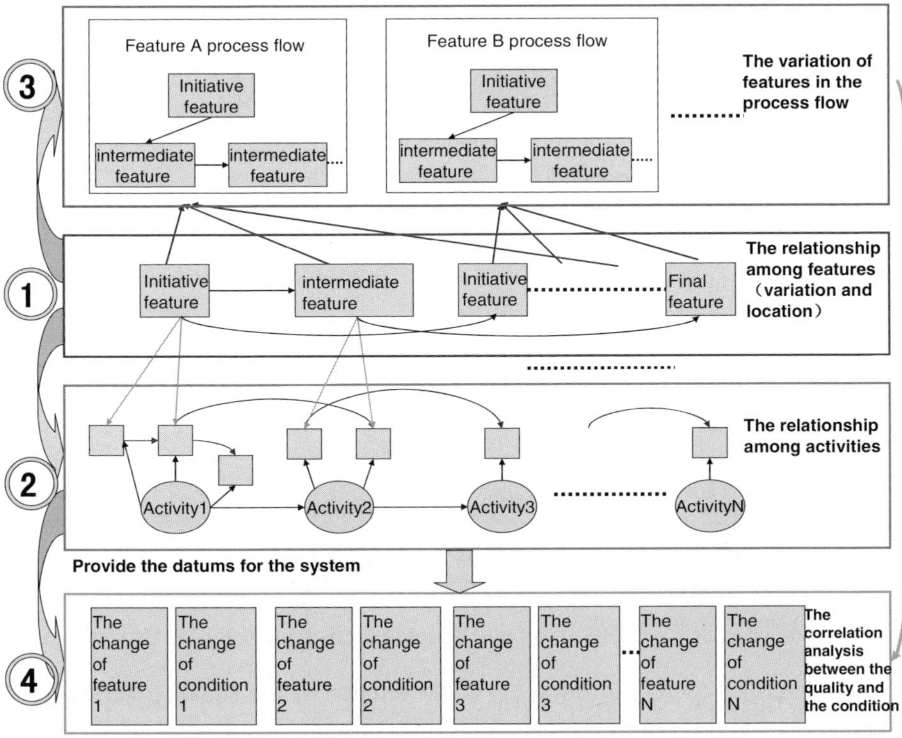

Fig. 3. A reference framework of change management in MMPs

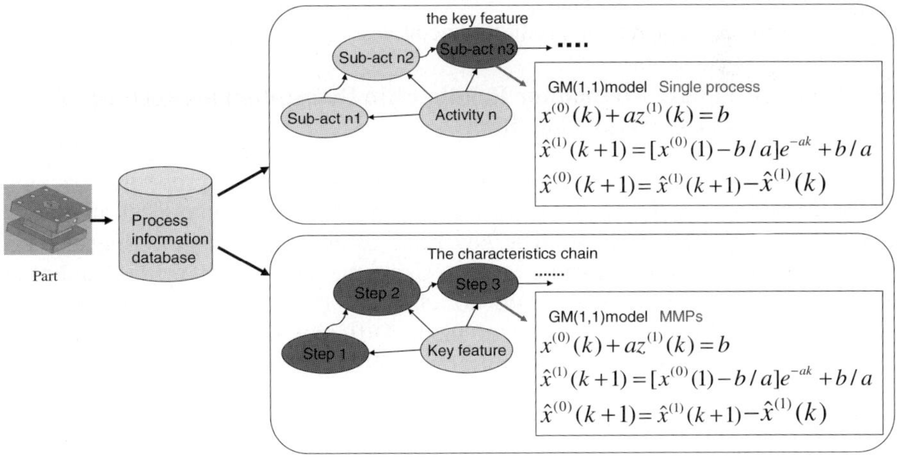

Fig. 4. Predicting quality status of feature with grey model

As shown in Figure 4, we make prediction for single machining process and multistage machining processes respectively. The GM(1,1) is a typical first order grey differential equation model.

Step1 $$x^{(1)}(k)=\sum_{r=1}^{k}x^{(0)}(r)\ (k=1,2,\cdots,n) \tag{1}$$

Step2 $$x^{(0)}(k)+az^{(1)}(k)=b\ \ (k=1,2,\cdots,n) \tag{2}$$

Step3 $$z^{(1)}(k)=0.5\left[x^{(1)}(k)+x^{(1)}(k-1)\right]\ (k=1,2,\cdots,n) \tag{3}$$

$$y_N=\left[x^{(0)}(2)\quad x^{(0)}(3)\quad x^{(0)}(4)\quad \cdots \quad x^{(0)}(n)\right] \tag{4}$$

$$B=\begin{bmatrix}-z^{(1)}(2) & 1\\ -z^{(1)}(3) & 1\\ \vdots & \vdots\\ -z^{(1)}(n) & 1\end{bmatrix} \tag{5}$$

$$\hat{a}=(B^TB)^{-1}B^Ty_N \text{ or } \hat{a}=\left[a,b\right]^T \tag{6}$$

Step4 $$\hat{x}^{(1)}(k+1)=\left[x^{(0)}(1)-b/a\right]e^{-ak}+b/a \tag{7}$$

$x^{(0)}=\left[x^{(0)}(1),x^{(0)}(2),\cdots,x^{(0)}(n)\right]$ denotes a raw time series as process quality data. $x^{(1)}$ denotes 1-AGO. Equation (7) is the solution of the equation (2), and then equation (8) can reduce $\hat{x}^{(1)}$ to $\hat{x}^{(0)}$. In multistage machining processes prediction, the application of the GM(1,1) is successful due to the trend of $x^{(0)}$. But in the single process prediction, the effect is not good enough. So it is necessary that preprocessing $x^{(0)}$ to be trend to improve the prediction accuracy.

3.3 The Least Square Method for Relationship Description between Error Variation and Working Condition

When the error occurs, we must identify its error sources to improve the machining quality. In this study, the least square method and principal component analysis are proposed to solve this problem. The key issue of error tracing is finding the main factors affecting the current feature quality. Using the least square method and principal component analysis to analyse the correlation, we can get the coefficient matrix and then get the distribution model of them. Different input (work condition) has different output (feature quality) and different coefficient matrix. Through experiment with different inputs, the coefficient matrix for corresponding input can be collected to compose the coefficient set.

In Figure 5, the frame consists of three parts. $S_i=[\Delta V_i,\Delta Ap_i,\Delta f_i,\Delta Vc_i,\Delta J_i,\Delta O_i]$ denotes the input set of this model, and S_i consists of machining tool speed variable quantity ΔV_i, cutting parameter variable

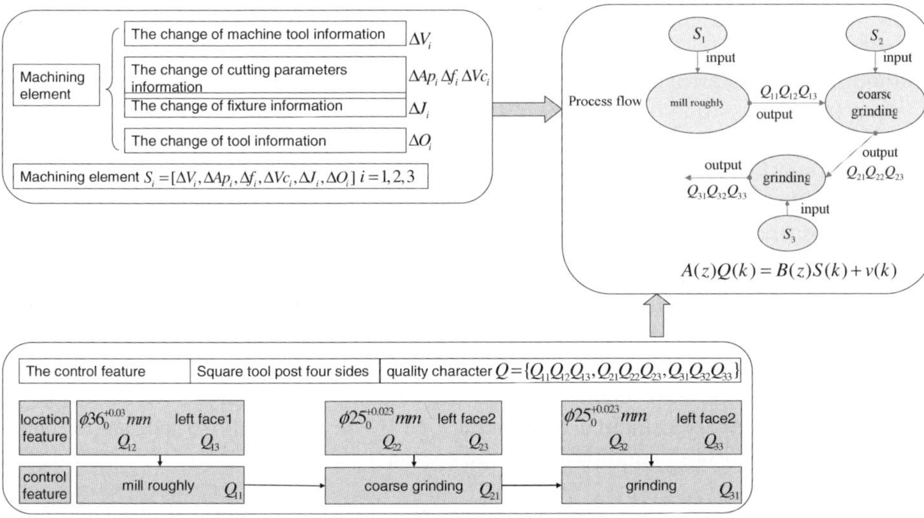

Fig. 5. The frame of least square method for MMPs

quantity $\Delta Ap_i\ \Delta f_i\ \Delta Vc_i$, fixture parameter ΔJ_i and tool parameter ΔO_i. We suppose that the influence of tool and fixture can be neglected. Thus, S_i can be simplified as $S_i = [\Delta V_i, \Delta Ap_i, \Delta f_i, \Delta Vc_i]$. $\Delta Q = [\vec{Q}_1, \vec{Q}_2, \cdots, \vec{Q}_n]$ denotes the output set of this model, here, n denotes the number of processes. $\vec{Q}_i = [Q_{i1}, Q_{i2} \cdots Q_{ik}]$ consists of current feature quality and several locating feature quality. For example, as shown in figure 5, Q_{11} is current feature , and the hole Q_{12} and left face1 Q_{13} are the locating features.

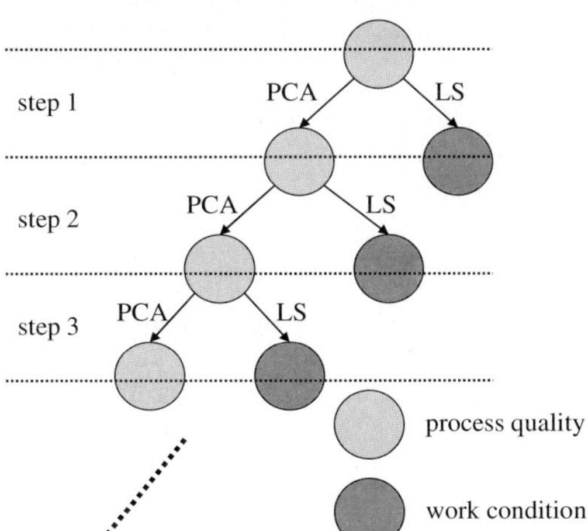

Fig. 6. Error source decomposition

In the practical application, we divide the data processing into two processes as shown in Figure 6. In the step 1, we analyze the working conditions with least square method to find the error source firstly. If current working conditions are normal, we analyze the process quality with the principal component analysis (PCA) to find the most likely influencing factors in former process activities. Then repeat the step1. The working condition is the end node of error source decomposition. In the end the error sources can be decomposed until we find what results in the error happened.

The steps of data processing are shown in Figure 7.

A. Standardizing processing of quality data;
B. Built the function of least square between current quality information and current working condition information;
C. If we can not find the error source at step B, we decompose the error source to the related process features with principal component analysis;
D. Examine every principal component one by one with step B and step C until find the working condition what we expect.

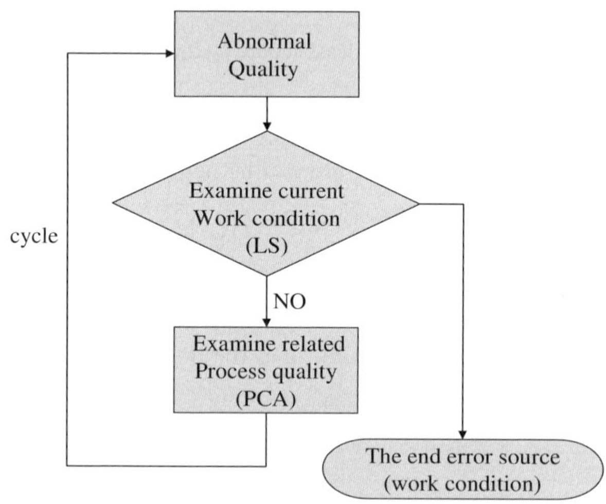

Fig. 7. The procedure of analyzing error source

4 Conclusions

In this paper, an error change management model is proposed. It consists of process information management, process quality prediction and error tracing modules, etc. For process information management module, it is a key issue that the associated relationship among the different stages is mapped according to machining form features of workpiece. In order to analyze the change trend of quality attributes among different stages, grey method is used to model the associated relationship among different stages and predict the next process. A decomposition method is proposed to error tracing analysis, in which least square method and principal component analysis (PCA) are used to find the error source. The PCA is adopted to analyze the current factors, and the least square model is used to analyze the former factors. Based on this, error sources can be identified accurately.

Acknowledgements

The research presented in this paper is under the support of national 863 High-Tech R&D Program (Grant No.: 2006AA04Z149), the National Basic Research Program of China (No. 2005CB724106) and the Program for New Century Excellent Talents in University by China Ministry of Education (No. NCET-04-0928).

References

1. Joel, T., Mccarthy, L., Tranfield, D.: A Structural and Evolutionary Approach to Change Management. Comput. Math. Org. Theor. 8, 337–364 (2002)
2. Cao, G., McHugh, M.: A systemic view of change management and its conceptual underpinnings. Systematic Practice and Action Research 18(5), 475–490 (2005)
3. Song, K., Jang, P., Cho, H., Jun, C.: Partial least square-based model predictive control for large-scale manufacturing processes. IIE Trans. 34, 881–890 (2002)
4. Fu, D., Su, L.i., Wang, Y.: The application of least square in precision cylindrical grinding. In: Federation for Information Processing (IFIP). Knowledge Enterprise: Intelligent Strategies In Product Design, Manufacturing, and Management, vol. 207
5. Wang, K.G., Wozny, M., Fang, M.: pp. 749–754. Springer, Boston (2006)
6. Du, F., Tang, X.: Multivariate quality control and diagnose based on the Principal Component Analysis. Manuf. Autom. 08, 10–13 (2006) (in Chinese)
7. Jiang, P.Y., Liu, D.Y., Feng, J.: A Change Management Framework: Managing the Error Variation in Multi-stage Machining Processes. In: The 7th World Congress on Intelligent Control and Automation, Chongqin, China, June 25-27 (accepted, 2008)
8. Deng, J.: Control problems of grey systems. Systems & Control Letters 1(5), 288–294 (1982)
9. Chen, M.Y.: Grey dynamic modeling and prediction control of macroeconomic systems. In: Proceedings of the IFAC Workshop on Modeling Decision and Game with Application to Social Phenomena, pp. 77–86. Chinese Association of Automation for IFAC, Beijing (1986)

Research on the Thermal Error of the 3D-Coordinate Measuring Machine Based on the Finite Element Method

Shuanghui Hao, Jizhu Liu, Baoyu Song, Minghui Hao,Weifeng Zheng, and Zili Tang

School of Mechatronic Engineering ,Harbin Institute of Technology, Harbin, 150001, China
liu_jizhu@yeah.net

Abstract. 3D-coordinate Measuring Machine (CMM) is affected by various heat sources in high-speed measuring, which results in deformation of the machine and measurement errors. This paper makes a theoretical analysis on the thermal error produced during the CMM's work process. And the thermal deformation of CMM is analyzed with Finite Element Method (FEM). A thermal error compensation model is also established by multi-body theory. Meanwhile integral mean value theorem is used to establish a mathematical model of the thermal expansion of the drive screw, and the CMM measurement accuracy is improved.

Keywords: CMM, Thermal Error, Finite Element Analysis.

1 Introduction

The development of modern manufacturing technology has made higher requirement for speed and precision to CMM. With the accelerating pace of production, CMM is usually required to achieve high precision under various circumstances. In order to increase the precision of CMM, people put more and more emphasis on the study of its thermal error[1-2]. There are two basic approaches to decrease thermal error and increase measuring precision: Error prevention method and Error compensation method. The former has a great limitation and it usually costs too much. And the latter is an effective and economical method[3]. The sources of the thermal error of CMM mainly consist of the following two aspects: the internal heat sources of CMM (warming of the electromotors for axes X, Y and Z; friction of the ball screws installed in the directions X, Y and Z; friction of the bearings and so on); the external heat sources of CMM (warming of the electrical sources, change of the environment temperature). These two factors affect the measurement precision of CMM synthetically[4]. In this article, change of the temperature distributing of CMM caused by internal thermal sources is mainly studied as well as the thermal error. The forms and traits of the deformation of CMM are analyzed and error compensation model is established. In addition, the thermal expansion is systematically analyzed and particularly calculated with the integral mean value theorem and a good result has been attained.

C. Xiong et al. (Eds.): ICIRA 2008, Part II, LNAI 5315, pp. 440–448, 2008.

2 Finite Element Analysis

The CMM(400mm×400mm×400mm)studied in this paper has a gantry structure, linear rails and ball-screws. Figure 1 shows the Structure of the CMM.

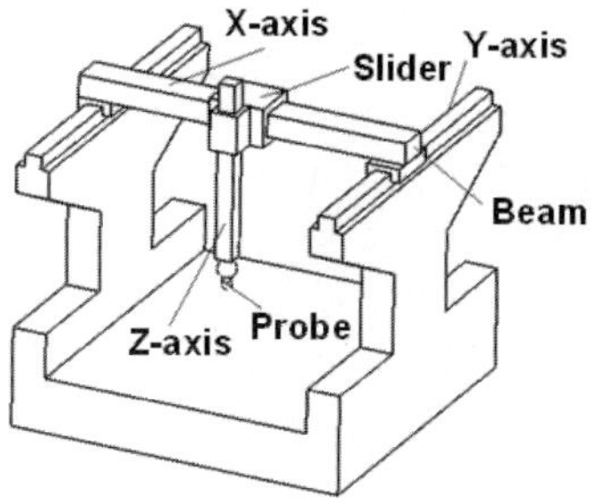

Fig. 1. Structure of the CMM

Thermal analysis includes two main parts: Steady-state heat transfer analysis and Instantaneous-state heat transfer analysis. The former is used to analyse the effect of steady thermal load to the system or components. And the latter refers to the heating or cooling process of a system. In this process, the system's temperature, heat flux□boundary conditions and internal energy changed obviously with time. The form and traits of the thermal errors of the CMM are observed by virtue of steady-state analysis. And then the instantaneous-state analysis is carried through to analyse the deformation during the machine's work process. The thermal characteristics of the components of the CMM are chosen as showed in Table 1.

Table 1. Thermal Parameters of the CMM

Components	Working Platform	Beam	Z-Axis	Screw	Rail
Material	Granite			Chrome Steel	Chrome-Nickel Steel
Density (kg/m^3)	2700			7710	7820
E (GPa)	120			206	207
Poisson Rate	0.21			0.28	0.27
Heat Conduction Coefficient (W/m·K)	1.73～3.98			22	15.2
Heat Capacity(J/kg·K)	800			460	463
Heat Expassion Coefficient (10^{-6}/K)	5~9			11.2	14.5

With regard to the selection of the thermal loads, is mainly considered the radiation of the electromotors in the article. Through the experiments it's known that the temperature of the output shaft reaches 39.3°C when the environmental temperature is 21°C and the temperature change of the output shaft tends to stabilization in the meantime. So the temperature is imposed as loads upon the joint part between the CMM

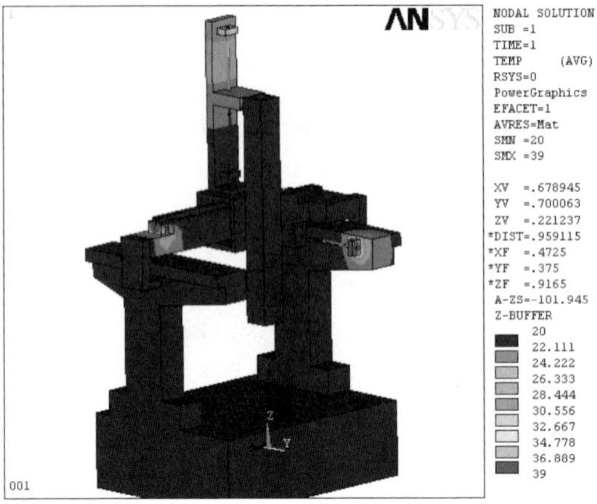

Fig. 2. Steady-state temperature distributing contour of the CMM

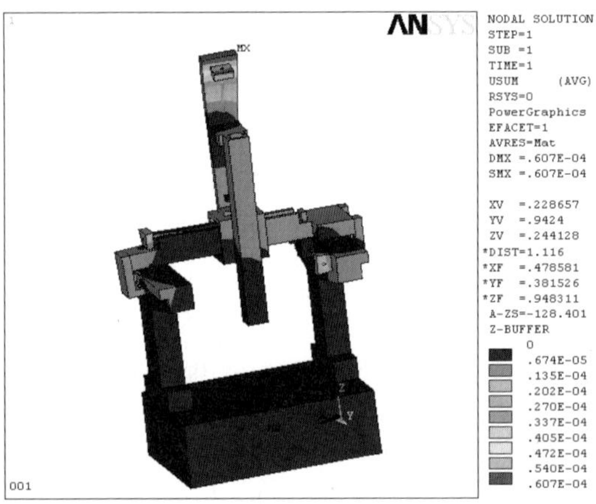

Fig. 3. Contour of the steady-state thermal deformation of the CMM

and the output shaft, then the steady-state temperature distributing contour of the CMM is obtained, which showed in Figure 2.

Loading the temperature data of the steady-state thermal analysis (as body loads, in Figure 2) on the model of the CMM, then changed element type and analysis type, restricting all the freedoms of the bottom of the working platform, and then solved the steady-state structure's thermal deformation, which is showed in Figure 3.

Observing the Figure 3, we can see that the two main deformation forms of the CMM are: thermal expansion and thermal bend. And regarding the influence on the precision of the CMM, the thermal expansion plays a more important role. The deformation has close relations with the internal heat sources.

3 Modeling for the Error with Multi-body Theory

There are many modeling ways for the thermal errors of the CMM, for instance, error compounding, pre-design of the technics frame, FEM, multiple linear regression, artificial neural network, etc. Multi-body theory is adopted in this paper to establish the thermal error model of the CMM through the method of error compounding.

According to the topological structure multi-body system includes open-loop system and close-loop system, and the basic concept is the element analysis and synthesized with the integer.

First of all, the CMM system was divided into two embranchments: measuring embranchment and part embranchment.

Measuring embranchment includes: 0-inertia reference frame; 1-working platform and column; 2-electromotor screw driving system in direction Y; 3- electromotor screw driving system in direction X; 4-beam; 5- electrical motor screw driving system in direction Z; 6-sliding sheath and holder in direction Z; 7-probe.

Part embranchment includes: 0- inertia reference frame; 1- working platform and column; 8-parts

All the body systems are established as showed in Figure 4.

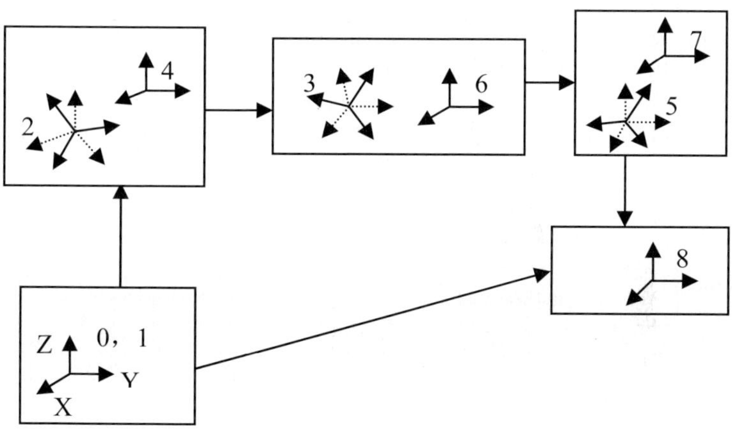

Fig. 4. Body Systems of the CMM

The dashed in Figure 4 denotes ideal coordinates systems and the real line denotes the practical coordinates systems. The working platform and the column belong to the part embranchment are steadily fixed on the ground. Therefore the body coordinates system of body 1 coincides with the inertia reference frame. The ideal moving reference coordinate system of body 8 coincides with the body coordinates system of body 1. Because temperature change of body 8 is not in consideration, the relative position error also not, i.e., there's only one position vector between body 8 and body 1 $\{P_{8x}, P_{8y}, P_{8z}\}^T$.

As for the measuring embranchment the coordinates system of body of body 1 likely coincides with the inertia reference frame. Body 2 is the ball-screws' driving system in direction Y. The position vector between its ideal moving reference frame and the body coordinates system is $\{P_{2x}, P_{2y}, P_{2z}\}^T$. The actual moving reference frame rotates toward the ideal moving reference frame with the perpendicularity errors ε_{2px} and ε_{2pz}. The ideal moving reference frame of body 4 (the beam) coincides with the body coordinates system of body 2. And there's an error δ_{4py} between the beam's realistic moving reference frame and its ideal one. Body 3 is the ball-screws' driving system in direction X. And the position vector between its ideal moving reference frame and body 4 is $\{P_{3x}, P_{3y}, P_{3z}\}^T$. The actual moving reference frame rotates toward the ideal moving reference frame with the perpendicularity errors ε_{3py} and ε_{3pz}.

Body 6 is the slider and the holder in axis Z. Its ideal moving reference frame coincides with the body coordinates system of the adjacent body 3. And there's an error δ_{6px} between the actual one and the ideal one. The position vector between the ideal moving reference frame of the ball-screws' driving system of body 5 and the body coordinates system of body 6 is $\{P_{5x}, P_{5y}, P_{5z}\}^T$. There are perpendicularity errors ε_{5px} and ε_{5py} between actual one and the ideal one. Body 7 is the probe. Its ideal moving reference frame coincides with body 5. And there's an error δ_{7pz} between the actual one and the ideal one.

The thermal errors includes position error and move error. According to Finite Element Analysis, the deformation of the CMM is mainly reflected on the form of thermal expansion and heat bending. The position errors between the bodies can be obtained by analyzing the errors between every two bodies. Of these, δ_{6px}、δ_{4py} and δ_{7pz} concentratively reflect the thermal expansion of the whole CMM, including heat stretch of the beam, ball-screws' thermal expansion, expansion of the probe, etc. ε2px、ε5px、ε3py、ε5py、ε2pz and ε3pz concentratively reflect the heat bending and leaning in the three directions. The CMM move error parameters are shown in Table 2.

Table 2. Move error parameters of the CMM

Art of the error	linear displacement error			angle displacement error		
direction	X	Y	Z	A	B	C
body 4	δ_{4sx}	δ_{4sy}	δ_{4sz}	ε_{4sx}	ε_{4sy}	ε_{4sz}
body 6	δ_{6sx}	δ_{6sy}	δ_{6sz}	ε_{6sx}	ε_{6sy}	ε_{6sz}
body 7	δ_{7sx}	δ_{7sy}	δ_{7sz}	ε_{7sx}	ε_{7sy}	ε_{7sz}

According to the relation of the coordinates systems as shown in Figure 4, the vector deviation matrix of the radius vector of the probe's actual position $\{t_7\}=\{m,n,h\}^T$ and the theoretical measuring points $\{w_8\}=\{X_w, Y_w, Z_w\}^T$ can be established as below (indicated as $\{e_{tw}\}$):

$$\begin{bmatrix}\{e_{tw}\}\\0\end{bmatrix}=\left(\prod_{6}^{0}\left([AJK]_p[AJK]_{pe}[AJK]_s[AJK]_{se}\right)\right)\begin{bmatrix}\{t_7\}\\1\end{bmatrix}-\left(\prod_{1}^{0}\left([AJK]_p[AJK]_{pe}[AJK]_s[AJK]_{se}\right)\right)\begin{bmatrix}\{w_8\}\\1\end{bmatrix}$$

Thereinto:

$[AJK]_p$ indicates the transformation matrix of the position vector of ideal moving reference frame and the body coordinates systems of bodies.

$[AJK]_s$ indicates the transformation matrix of the displacement vectors of the adjacent bodies.

$[AJK]_{pe}$ and $[AJK]_{se}$ indicate the counterchange matrix of the position and move errors of the adjacent bodies. Each of them includes 3 linear displacement errors and 3 angle displacement errors. $[AJK]_{pe}$和$[AJK]_{se}$ can be obtained through the coordinates transformation of the homogeneous matrix, shown as below:

$$[AJK]_{pe} = \begin{bmatrix} 1 & -\varepsilon_{kpz} & \varepsilon_{kpy} & \delta_{kpx} \\ \varepsilon_{kpz} & 1 & -\varepsilon_{kpx} & \delta_{kpy} \\ -\varepsilon_{kpy} & \varepsilon_{kpx} & 1 & \delta_{kpz} \\ 0 & 0 & 0 & 1 \end{bmatrix}$$

$$[AJK]_{se} = \begin{bmatrix} 1 & -\varepsilon_{ksz} & \varepsilon_{ksy} & \delta_{ksx} \\ \varepsilon_{ksz} & 1 & -\varepsilon_{ksx} & \delta_{ksy} \\ -\varepsilon_{ksy} & \varepsilon_{ksx} & 1 & \delta_{ksz} \\ 0 & 0 & 0 & 1 \end{bmatrix}$$

Substituted the error parameters into the coordinates transformation matrix, then carried out the coordinates transformation, and finally obtained the measuring errors of the CMM.

4 The Thermal Expansion Modeling of the Ball-Screws

We have established the model of the thermal error of the CMM with the multi-body theorem. When all the error parameters are being determined, the confirmation of the error parameters value of each part is very important. This paper takes the ball-screws in the direction X of the CMM as an example, and does research on the thermal expansion of the ball-screws.

We impose heat quantity Q on an end of the ball-screws. Meanwhile there is convection and radiation recuperation between the ball-screws and the surrounding environment. But because these forms of heat exchange exert little impact on the ball-screws, only the heat of the end of the ball-screws is taken into consideration. Thus, due to the impact of the heat quantity Q, the thermal stretch of the ball-screws caused by the rise of the temperature is:

$$\Delta L = a_t \int_0^L [\theta(x) - \theta_0] dx \tag{1}$$

herein, a_t——coefficient of linear thermal expansion, we consider it as a constant to the screws.

L——length of the ball-screws;
x——position on the ball-screws;
$\theta(x)$ ——temperature distribution along the length of the screws;
θ_0——prime temperature
Utilize the integral mean value theorem referring to expression (1), we have:

$$\theta(\xi) - \theta_0 = \frac{\int_0^L [\theta(x) - \theta_0] dx}{L} \tag{2}$$

Here we call $\theta(\xi)$ temperature's mean value. Then the relative thermal expansion of the ball-screws is:

$$\Delta L = a_t [\theta(\xi) - \theta_0] L \tag{3}$$

Herein, ξ——some point in the range of [0, L], indicated in Figure 4.

We can see from expression (3): There's at least one point ξ' s temperature $\theta(\xi)$ on the ball-screws that can express the thermal expansion ΔL of the ball-screws.

Whether the point ξ has uniqueness and invariability, we'll try to draw a conclusion through finite element calculation and comparison.

First of all, use the finite element calculation. Impose temperature stepping load 30ºC on an end of the ball-screws. The prime temperature of the screws is defined as 20ºC. The size, material and every physical parameter of the ball-screws are the same as the definition of the CMM. Time is defined as 1200 seconds. It is solved by 100 substeps. And then change the analysis type, i.e. change the thermal analysis to the structural analysis, obtaining the deformation condition of the ball-screws at each certain time.

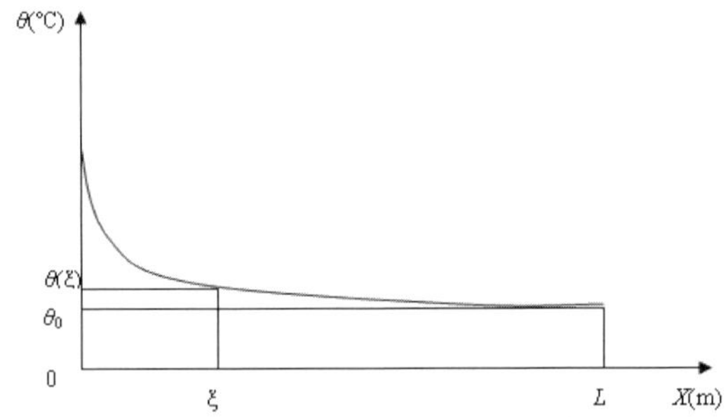

Fig. 5. Curve of temperature-position distribution of the ball-screws

Extracting the data of the ball-screws' deformation, time and temperature in the length direction and drawing the curve of temperature-position, we can obtain the integral mean value at each certain time. And according to the data we can make the relation curve of mean value temperature and the end's temperature (see Figure 6) and the relation curve of heat transfer length and the end's temperature (see Figure 7).

Fitting the curve in Figure 6 and applying Lagrange interpolation to the curve in Figure 7, we can obtain the expression for calculating the expansion quantity.

Comparing the expansion quantity with the quantity obtained through finite element method, we can gain the curve of comparison error, as shown in Figure 8.

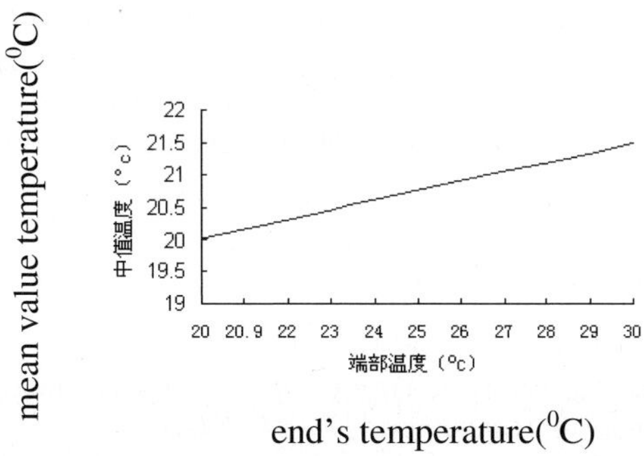

Fig. 6. Mean value temperature and the end's temperature

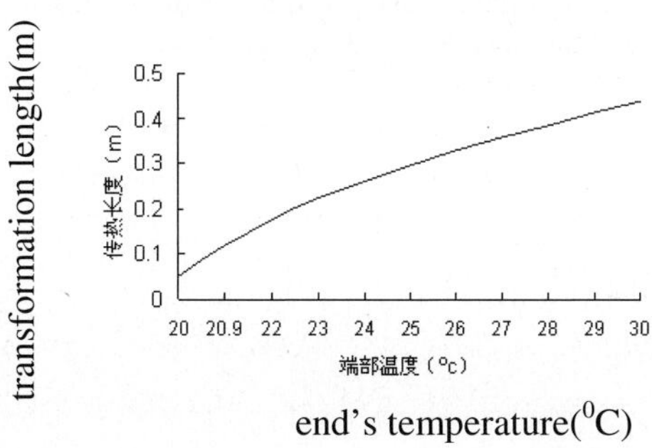

Fig. 7. Relation curve of the transformation length and the end's temperature

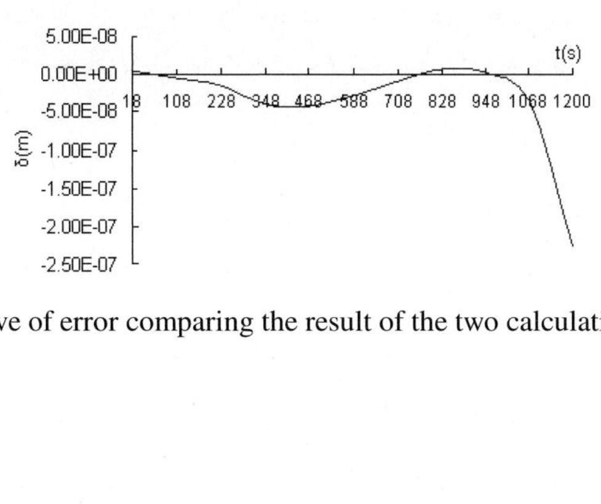

Fig. 8. Curve of error comparing the result of the two calculating method

5 Conclusion

In this paper we use FEM to analyse the thermal error of the CMM and obtain the form and traits of its thermal deformation. And according to the characteristics of the deformation we establish the simulation of the thermal error with multi-body theorem. Meanwhile we analyse the expansion of the ball-screws of the CMM and describe the thermal expansion of the CMM with integral mean value theorem, which can be a theoretical base for the calculation of the thermal errors of the CMM. This is good for the compensation of the thermal error and increase the measurement precision of the CMM.

References

1. Zhan, Y., Le, Q., Jia, M.: Error and error compensation technology of machine tools. Journal of Fujian University of Technology 4, 75–84 (2004)
2. De Nijs, J.F.C.: Modeling of a coordinate measuring machine for analysis of its dynamic behavior. Annals of the CIRP 37, 507–510 (1988)
3. Huang, P.S.: On-line Error Compensation of Coordinate Measuring Machines. International Journal of Machine Tools and Manufacture 35(5), 725–738 (1995)
4. Kim, S.K., Cho, D.W.: Real-time estimation of temperature distribution in a ball-screw system. Int. J. Mach. Tools Manufact. 37(4), 325–327 (1997)

Dynamic Stability Analysis of a Novel Forging Manipulator

Changya Yan and Feng Gao

State Key Laboratory of Mechanical System and Vibration, Shanghai Jiao Tong University, Shanghai, 200240, China
{yanchangya,fengg}@sjtu.edu.cn

Abstract. The dynamic stability problem of heavy-duty mobile forging manipulators is of great importance for both designing purpose and working task planning. In this paper, a new stability measure named as Force-Moment Ratio Stability is presented. This measure regards the complex multi-rigid body system of the mobile manipulator as a whole and incorporates all static and dynamic factors into consideration. The process of formulation together with the dynamic model of a novel forging manipulator shows this measure is physically meaningful and applicable to dynamic mobile systems subject to inertial, external forces and moments under any kind of motion trajectories. The performance and effectiveness of the measure is demonstrated through a practical implement in the designing of a heavy-duty mobile manipulator used in integrated heavy forging center.

Keywords: Stability measure, Dynamic stability, PKM, Dynamic modelling, Forging manipulator.

1 Introduction

Heavy-duty mobile manipulator with Parallel Kinematic Mechanism(PKM)[1] is an important part of integrated manufacturing system such as an open-die forging center. The so-called forging manipulator [2,3] in forging workshop can handle heavy ingot as weight as 200+ tons and can move by tracks or tires and be in coordination control with hydraulic press so as to realize programmable forging process (see Fig. 1). This huge machine's tip-over accidents about any sides under any circumstances are unacceptable and may cause disasters. Many previous literatures have tried to propose a suitable stability criterion for tip-over stability evaluation of such mobile manipulators. In [4], the shortest distance between the projection of the center of mass on horizontal plane and the projected support boundary was used as a measure of the system's static stability. In [5,6] the author proposed an energy-based approach which used the minimum work required to tip-over a vehicle to measure the stability. However [4-6] only considered static stability while ignoring dynamic effects. [7] proposed a method to complete tasks quickly and decrease dynamic forces and torques which may destroy the stability of the system on the basis of motion trajectory optimization, but they didn't propose a clear evaluation criterion. The Zero Moment Point(ZMP) [8-10] was presented and used for planning of the motion of a redundant

C. Xiong et al. (Eds.): ICIRA 2008, Part II, LNAI 5315, pp. 449–458, 2008.

mobile manipulator, but did not provide any specific indication about the system's instability and not sensitive to top-heaviness. [11,12] reported another measure named Force-Angle margin, which is applicable to systems subject to inertial and external forces and with the assumption of low velocities. In [13] the author introduced a kinematic reconfiguration method to enhance system's tip-over stability, the method was built upon the force-angle measure and was intended for quasi-static systems. Literature [14,15] proposed another stability criterion based on the required energy for placing center of mass into a so-called equilibrium plane such that the whole moment exerted on the system was minimized. This method takes the dynamic effects such as inertial forces into account with the assumption that the directions of the external forces, inertial forces and torques relative to mobile base during imaginary rotation of the system are fixed. However Energy-Equilibrium Plane method may possibly fail in predicting the occurrence of critical stability due to the fixed direction assumption during imaginary rotation [16]. [16,17] proposed a new stability measure named as Moment-Height Stability(MHS) measure used for wheeled mobile manipulator, which is sensitive to the height of center of mass and can be implemented with limited computation effects. In engineering, a simplified stability evaluation measure called Stability Factor Method developed in heavy loader machines such as crane or log loader is used due to its simplicity and directness. Stability Factor method gives the compare of two different moments' action to the support boundary, but loses its useability in many circumstances, for example, when the destabilizing moment is zero or very small. Force-Angle measure [11-13] and MHS measure [16,17] are calculated on the basis of the resultant forces and moments of the system, then the details of the stabilizing moments and destabilizing moments caused by different dynamic factors of rigid bodies are missing during the summing process.

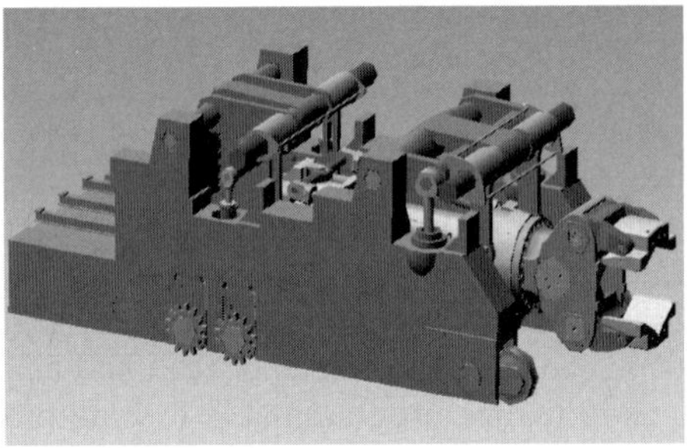

Fig. 1. A new type mobile forging manipulator SJTU-200

In this paper, to solve the dynamic stability problem of a new-type forging manipulator SJTU-200, we proposed a new Force-Moment Ratio Stability measure. Section 0 reveals the mechanical configuration of SJTU-200 and presents its kinematic and dynamic model. In section 0 the tip-over problem of this kind of forging manipulator is modelled, afterwards the FMRS measure is thoroughly disclosed based on the analyzing of all kinds of static and dynamic factors which can impact the mobile system's stability. The process of formulation shows the stability measure is physically meaningful and can better reflect the system's dynamic behaviour than other measures with low computational costs. Then this measure's normalization is discussed.

Section 0 presents a practical implement case on forging manipulator SJTU-200, the proposed FMRS measure is proved to be effective both in theory and in practice. Finally section 0 gives the summary.

2 Modeling of the Forging Manipulator

Fig. 2 shows that the serial-parallel mechanism is obtained by parallel concatenation of 3 complex limbs E_1, E_2, E_3. The simple open kinematic chain associated with E_1-limb is denoted by $E_1[1_A \equiv 0-2_A-3_A-4_{A1}(4_{A2})-5_A-6_A \equiv 6]$, where $4_{A1}, 4_{A2}$ are connected in parallel with link $3_A, 5_A$ respectively, so as to form a parallelogram loop chain; 0 denotes the reference frame (fixed platform) and $1_A \equiv 0$ means link 1_A is integrally fixed on the reference frame; 6 denotes the mobile platform and $6_A \equiv 6$ means link 6_A is integrally fixed on the mobile platform. The other two limbs are denoted respectively by $E_2[1_B \equiv 0-2_B-3_B-4_{B1}(4_{B2})-5_B-6_B \equiv 6]$ and $E_3[1_C \equiv 0-2_C-3_C-(4_{C1}-5_{C1}-6_{C1})[(4_{C2}-5_{C2}-6_{C2})]-7_C \equiv 6]$. The complex limbs E_2 ,E_3 share 5 links as $1_B \equiv 1_C, 2_B \equiv 2_C, 3_B \equiv 3_C, 4_{B1} \equiv 4_{C1}, 4_{B2} \equiv 4_{C2}$. In limb E_3 there is a loop chain in which serial chain $(4_{C1}-5_{C1}-6_{C1})$ and $(4_{C2}-5_{C2}-6_{C2})$ are connected in parallel with link $3_C, 7_C$ respectively.

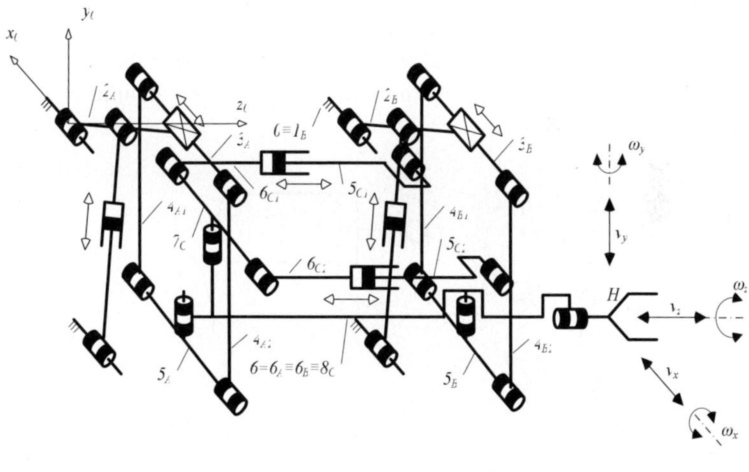

Fig. 2. The hybrid serial-parallel mechanism of the forging manipulator

Simply by inspection and analysis, it can be observed that the mobile platform has 6 D.O.F.s . For each limb *i*, we define its joint vector space as $U_i = \{q_{i1}, q_{i2}, ..., q_{ij}\}$, here *j* denotes the number of joints in limb *i*. When $i = 1,2$, $j = 1,2,3,4,5$, when $i = 3$, $j = 1,2,...,7$. The geometric constraints imposed by the limbs on the motion of the moving mobile platform give, for the ith limb, the following set of k general relations as

$$f_{ik}(q_{ij}) = w_k \qquad i = 1,2,3;\ k = 1,2,...,6\ , \tag{1}$$

where q_{ij} ($j \times 1$ matrix) represents the linear or angular displacements in the joint space of the ith limb and $w_1, w_2, \cdots, w_6$ represent the parameters used to describe the spatial position and orientation of the moving platform.

By differentiating Eq.(1) with respect to time, and let J_i represent Jacobian Matrix, it leads to

$$\omega_k = \dot{w}_k = J_i \dot{q}_{ij}\ , \tag{2}$$

where $\dot{q}_{ij} = \left[\dot{q}_{i1}, \dot{q}_{i2}, \cdots, \dot{q}_{ij}\right]^T$ is the velocity vector of joints in i[th] limb, $\omega_k = \left[\omega_1, \omega_2, \cdots, \omega_6\right]^T = \left[\dot{w}_1, \dot{w}_2, \cdots, \dot{w}_6\right]^T$ is the velocity vector of the moving platform.

Giving a feasible motion trajectory of the moving platform, in the whole joint space we have $\det(J_i) \neq 0$, so the velocity vector of joints $\dot{q}_{ij}$ is computed as

$$\dot{q}_{ij} = J_i^{-1} \omega_k\ . \tag{3}$$

As we have already got the knowledge of velocity vector $\dot{q}_{ij}$ of each link, then we can use forward iteration method to compute the linear acceleration of center of mass and angular acceleration from the first link to the last link. The flow of forward iteration which is the first procedure of Newton-Euler formulation is a regular algorithm which is often listed in text books and literatures, so we ignore the details here. Then the linear acceleration $\dot{v}_g$ of center of mass of jth link and its angular acceleration $\dot{\omega}_j$ are obtained.

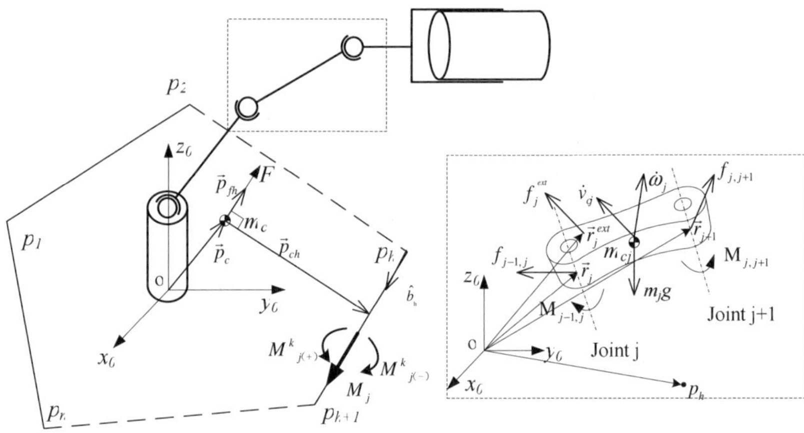

Fig. 3. Mobile manipulator and its support polygon

3 Force-Moment Ratio Dynamic Stability Measure

Fig. 3 shows a general 3-D mobile manipulator system, the support polygon is shaped by ground contact points $p_1, p_2, \ldots p_n$ .Let $\vec{p}_h$ denote the location of the hth ground contact point in base frame (o-$x_0y_0z_0$), the unit vector on hth tip-over axis $\overline{p_h p_{h+1}}$ is denoted by $\hat{b}_h$, whose direction is such defined that all unit vectors make a closed clockwise loop. So the hth unit vector can be computed as

$$\hat{b}_h = \frac{\vec{p}_{h+1} - \vec{p}_h}{\left\| \vec{p}_{h+1} - \vec{p}_h \right\|} \quad (h = 1, 2, \ldots, n-1) \qquad \hat{b}_n = \frac{\vec{p}_1 - \vec{p}_n}{\left\| \vec{p}_1 - \vec{p}_n \right\|} \ . \tag{4}$$

Then we compute the moment M_j^{ph} acted on point p_h by ith limb (for simplicity, in the following notation we omit mark i when the computation is obviously about ith limb), and we have

$$M_i^{ph} = \sum\nolimits_j M_j^{ph} = \sum\nolimits_j \left((\vec{p}_h - \vec{r}_{mcj}) \times m_j (\vec{v}_{cj} + \vec{g}) + I_j \dot{\omega}_j + \omega_j \times I_j \omega_j \right) \ , \tag{5}$$

where $\vec{r}_{mcj}$ is the position vector of center of mass of jth link and I_j is the internal tensor matrix with respect to base frame (o-$x_0y_0z_0$), and I_j is computed as $I_j = R_j \overline{I}_j R_j^T$, wherein R_j represents the rotation matrix of the body frame of jth link with respect to base frame, and $\overline{I}_j$ represents the inertial tensor matrix of jth link in its body frame. $\vec{g}$ is the vector of gravity acceleration. Then the moment acted on the hth tip-over axis $\overline{p_h p_{h+1}}$ by the ith limb is the projection of M_i^{ph} on the unit vector $\hat{b}_h$, as

$$M_i^h = M_i^{ph} \cdot \hat{b}_h \ . \tag{6}$$

As we can see from Eq.(5) and (6), when the mobile platform is moving, each link is under the action of inertia force, inertia moment and gravity, these actions exert on the fixed platform through the concatenation of links and generate three moment components to the hth tip-over axis denoted by $\mathrm{M}^1{}_j$, $\mathrm{M}^2{}_j$,and $\mathrm{M}^3{}_j$ respectively, as

$$\begin{aligned} M^1{}_j &= (m_j (\vec{p}_h - \vec{r}_{mcj}) \times \dot{v}_{cj}) \cdot \hat{b}_h \\ M^2{}_j &= (I_j \dot{\omega}_j + \omega_j \times I_j \omega_j) \cdot \hat{b}_h \ \cdot \\ M^3{}_j &= (m_j (\vec{p}_h - \vec{r}_{mcj}) \times \vec{g}) \cdot \hat{b}_h \end{aligned} \tag{7}$$

If the kth (k=1,2,3) moment component $M^k{}_j > 0$, then $M^k{}_j$ belongs to stabilizing moment to hth tip-over axis and is marked by $M^k{}_{j(+)}$, otherwise if $M^k{}_j < 0$, $M^k{}_j$ marked by $M^k{}_{j(-)}$ belongs to destabilizing moment. The ith limb's resultant stabilizing moment to hth tip-over axis $\overline{p_h p_{h+1}}$ is computed as

$$M^h_{i(+)} = \sum_{j=1}^k \sum_{m=1}^n M^m_{j(+)} \quad (n \le 3) \ , \tag{8}$$

the resultant destabilizing moment to hth tip-over axis by ith limb is computed as

$$M^h_{i(-)} = \sum_{j=1}^k \sum_{m=1}^n M^m_{j(-)} \quad (n \le 3) \ , \tag{9}$$

the resultant moment to hth tip-over axis generated by all limbs is computed as

$$M^h = \sum_i M^h_i = \sum_i (M^h_{i(+)} + M^h_{i(-)}) \ . \tag{10}$$

The location of the system's center of mass m_c in base frame is denoted by $\vec{p}_c = (x_c, y_c, z_c)^T = f(q)$,wherein q represents the joint variables of the manipulator's actuated joint space, so $\vec{p}_c$ is the function of the system configuration. A normal vector $\vec{p}_{ch}$ of the hth tip-over axis through m_c shown in Fig.3. is computed as

$$\vec{p}_{ch} = (I - \hat{b}_h \hat{b}_h^T)(\vec{p}_{h+1} - \vec{p}_c) \ , \tag{11}$$

where I is 3×3 unit matrix. Let $\hat{p}_{fh}$ be a unit vector which is perpendicular to both of $\vec{p}_{ch}$ and $\hat{b}_h$, then $\hat{p}_{fh}$ can be computed as

$$\hat{p}_{fh} = \left(\hat{b}_h \times \vec{p}_{ch}\right) / \|\vec{p}_{ch}\| \ . \tag{12}$$

Suppose that $\vec{F}$ is an imaginary force exerted on the center of mass, the direction of $\vec{F}$ is parallel to $\hat{p}_{fh}$ and it satisfies the following equation

$$M^h_{i(+)} + M^h_{i(-)} + \vec{p}_{ch} \times \vec{F} = 0 \ , \tag{13}$$

then the magnitude of $\vec{F}$ can be computed as

$$\|\vec{F}\| = \|M^h\| / \|\vec{p}_{ch}\| \ . \tag{14}$$

$\vec{F}$ is physically meaningful, as can be seen from Eq.(13), it is not only determined by the system's resultant moment, but also related to the location of center of mass, the position and orientation of tip-over axis. If $M^h > 0$, the system is stable, suppose to make the system go to critical stability situation, then the minimum force of all the possible imaginary forces exerted on the center of mass is $\vec{F}$. If $M^h < 0$,the system goes to unstable, in this case $\vec{F}$ represents the minimum forces of all the possible imaginary forces to make the system reverse back to the critical stability situation. Here the first auxiliary stability index about one tip-over axis is proposed, name it as Force Stability margin K_f , K_f about the hth tip-over axis is defined as

$$K_{fh} = \mathrm{sgn}(M^h)\|\vec{F}\| \quad (h = 1, 2, ..., n) \ , \tag{15}$$

where $\mathrm{sgn}(M^h) = \begin{cases} 1 & if\ M^h > 0 \\ -1 & if\ M^h < 0 \end{cases}$.

Force Stability margin K_f describes the system's stability margin from the view of resultant moment and mass distribution. However the information about the dynamic behaviors of the system's components and their respective influences on the stability about tip-over axis is missing due the summing process of all forces and moments. Then another stability adjustment index named Moment Ratio K_d is proposed, as

$$K_{dh} = \frac{\left\|M^h(+)\right\|}{\left\|M^h(+)\right\| + \left\|M^h(-)\right\|}, \tag{16}$$

where $M^h(+)$ and $M^h(-)$ can not be zero simultaneously.

It should be noted that K_{dh} shows the weight of the stabilizing "strength" in the sum of the absolute values of these two kinds of "strength" which have contrary functions to the system's stability. Combined Eq.(15) with (16), a new dynamic stability measure named Force-Moment Ratio Stability measure(FMRS) is proposed. The FMRS measure to a certain hth tip-over axis is defined as

$$K_{sh} = K_{fh} K_{dh} \ . \tag{17}$$

And the FMRS measure of the whole system is defined as:

$$K_s = \min_h (K_{fh} K_{dh}) \quad (h = 1, 2, ..., n) \tag{18}$$

To compute the Force-Moment Ratio Stability measure, one must thus have the knowledge of the supporting boundaries, the knowledge of the location of center of mass, the knowledge of the external forces and moments exerted on every rigid body of the system, and knowledge of the rigid body's linear and angular accelerations. All of these can be figured out from the system's dynamic model, and are all measurable quantities on a real system equipped with appropriate sensors. All mobile manipulator should have a nominal state (i.e. initial state), in which the manipulator is in home position and keeping statically stable and energy saving. The Force-Moment Ratio Stability measure is normalized as

$$K_{FMRS} = \frac{K_{fh} K_{dh}}{K_{fh_{nom}} K_{dh_{nom}}} \tag{19}$$

where $K_{fh_{nom}}$ and $K_{dh_{nom}}$ are the nominal values for K_{fh} and K_{dh} when the system is in initial state.

4 Case Study

Fig. 1 shows a perspective view of a forging manipulator with hydraulic driving system, which has a mobile truck moveable back and forth on tracks and a gripper support suspended by articulated linkages of the mobile truck. Fig. 4 shows the configuration of the gripper support and its suspending mechanism. To manipulate heavy forged pieces, the gripper which holds the forged piece is adapted for spatial 6 -D.O.F mobility. The design has a maximum 200 (Tons) loading capacity with 400 (T.m) maximum moment capacity. The maximum static stability factor which is the ratio of the maximum static resetting moment (stabilizing moment) to maximum moment capacity in the turning point of the front wheel is designed to be around 5.6 . According to this criterion, the Force-Moment Ratio Stability measure is implemented to evaluate the system's overall dynamic stability under extreme working tasks. For simplicity, the details of configuration parameters of the hybrid linkage mechanism are omitted.

In this case the truck moves on a straight line with the maximum load and moment capacity at velocities and accelerations shown in Fig. 5. Three positions of the gripper are considered: the home position, the rear side of home position to which the relative distance in front and rear direction is -0.6 m, and the front side of home position with a corresponding relatively distance for +0.6 m. The configuration with gripper at

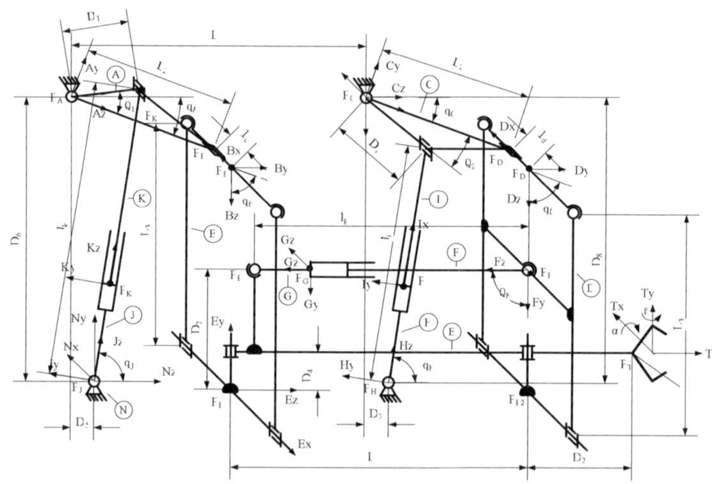

Fig. 4. Mechanism configuration of the forging manipulator

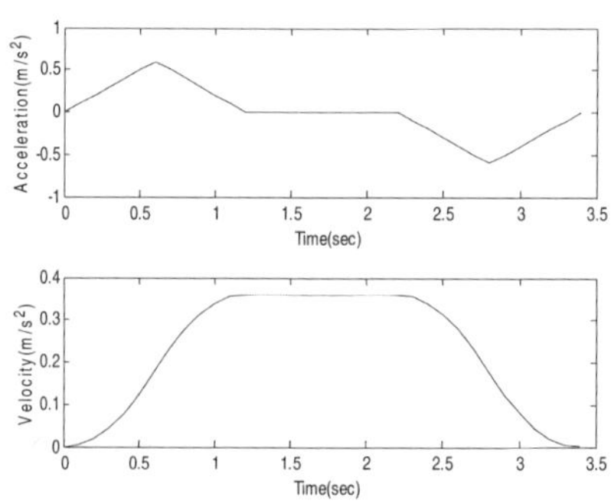

Fig. 5. Acceleration and velocity of truck moving on straight line

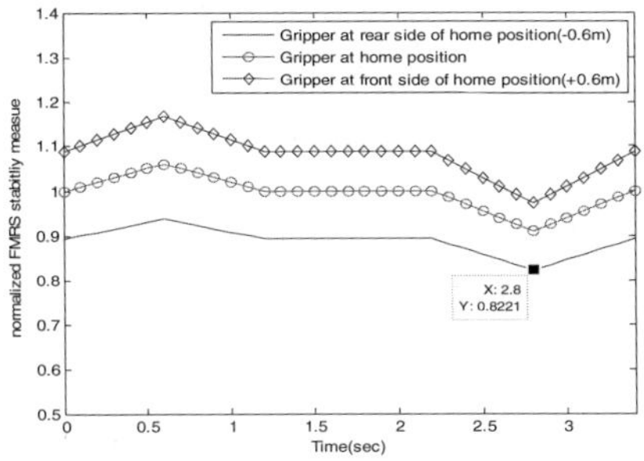

Fig. 6. Dynamic stability curves about the tip-over axis of front wheel

home position is regarded as nominal state in which the static safe stability factor about the front tip-over axis is around 5.6. The FMRS measure curves during the movement of the truck are shown in Fig. 6. It can be observed when the gripper is at the most front side the stability is relatively lower, and the lowest stability occurs at t=2.8 s, when the truck has the highest deceleration which makes every components of the system subject to the biggest inertia force heading forwardly, that causes the decreasing of stability about the front wheel. In this case, the lowest stability is about 82.21% of the nominal state's stability, which means the whole system still has enough stability margin in such a extreme maneuver, so the design is safe.

5 Summary

In this paper, a new Force-Moment Ratio stability measure is proposed. It is applicable to analyze and evaluate the dynamic stability problem of heavy-duty mobile manipulators with complex mechanisms. This measure is not only sensitive to static factors such as top-heaviness, mass distributions and support polygon etc, but also can describe the dynamic influence factors such as the dynamic comparison between stabilizing and destabilizing moment in complex mobile systems, especially in high-velocity and high-acceleration motion modes. Furthermore, this measure needs limited computational cost. The simulation study for evaluating the dynamic stability of a heavy-duty forging manipulator under extreme working conditions shows its effectiveness in designing and evaluating such kind of mobile manipulators.

Acknowledgements

The support of this work by The National Basic Research Program (2006CB705400) and the Natural Science Foundation of China (60534020) is gratefully acknowledged.

References

1. Merlet, J.P.: Parallel Robots, pp. 12–13. Springer, Heidelberg (2006)
2. Schubert, P.K.: Forging manipulator: United States, SMS Hasenclever Maschinenfabrik GmbH & Co. KG, Dusseldorf DE (1989)

3. Westermeyer, W.N.: Process and apparatus for operating a press unit. United States, Pahnke Engineering GmbH & Co.KG, Dusseldorf DE (1995)
4. McGhee, R.B., Iswandhi, G.I.: Adaptive locomotion of a mulitilegged robot over rough terrain. IEEE Trans. Syst. Man Cybernetics 9(4), 176–182 (1979)
5. Messuri, D., Klein, C.: Automatic Body Regulation for Maintaining Stability of a Legged Vehicle During Rough-Terrain Locomotion. IEEE Journal of Robotics and Automation 1(3), 132–141 (1985)
6. Nagy, P.V., Desa, S., Whittaker, W.L.: Energy-Based Stability Measure for Reliable Locomotion of Statically Stable Walkers: Theory and Application. International Journal of Robotics Research 13(9), 272–287 (1994)
7. Dubowsky, S., Vance, E.E.: Planning Mobile Manipulator Motions Considering Vehicle Dynamic Stability Constraints. In: Proceedings of the IEEE International Conference on Robotics and Automation, pp. 1271–1276 (1989)
8. Sugano, S., Huang, Q., Kato, I.: Stability criteria in controlling mobile robotic systems. In: Proc. IEEE/RSJ Int. Conf. on Intelligent Robots and Systems, pp. 832–838 (1993)
9. Huang, Q., Sugano, S., Tanie, K.: Motion planning for a Mobile Manipulator Considering Stability and Task Constraints. In: Proceedings of the IEEE International conference on Robotics and Automation, pp. 2192–2198 (1998)
10. Kim, J., Chung, W.K., Youm, Y., et al.: Real-time ZMP compensation method using null motion for moblile manipulators. In: Proc.of the IEEE Int. Conf. On Robotics and Automation, pp. 1967–1972 (2002)
11. Papadopoulos, E.G., Ray, D.A.: A new measure of tip over stability margin for mobile manipulators. In: Proceedings of the IEEE international conference on robotics and automation, pp. 3111–3116 (1996)
12. Papadopoulos, E.G., Rey, D.A.: The Force-Angle Measure of Tip over Stability Margin for Mobile Manipulators. Journal of Vehicle Systems Dynamics 33, 29–48 (2000)
13. Iagnemma, K., Rzepniewski, A., Dubowsky, S., et al.: Mobile Robot Kinematic Reconfigurability for Rough-Terrain. In: Proceedings SPIE's International Symposium on Intelligent Systems and Advanced Manufacturing, vol. 4196-47 (2000)
14. Ghasempoor, A., Sepehri, N.: A measure of stability for mobile based manipulators. In: Proceedings of the IEEE international conference on robotics and automation, pp. 2249–2254 (1995)
15. Ghasempoor, A., Sepehri, N.: A Measure of Stability for Mobile Manipulators With Application to Heavy Duty Hydraulic Machines. ASME Journal of Dynamic Systems, Measurement and Control 120, 360–370 (1998)
16. Ali, S., Moosavian, A., Alipour, K.: Stability Evaluation of Mobile Robotic Systems Using Moment-Height Measure. In: Proc. of the IEEE Int.Conf. on Robotics, Automation and Mechatronics, pp. 97–102 (2006)
17. Ali, S., Moosavian, A., Alipour, K.: Moment-Height Tip-Over Measure for Stability Analysis of Mobile Robotic Systems. In: Proceedings of the 2006 IEEE/RSJ International Conference on Intelligent Robots and Systems, pp. 1356–1361 (2006)

Intelligent Clamping Fixture in General

Peter Košťál, Karol Velíšek, and Radovan Zvolenský

Institute of Production Systems and Applied Mechanics,
Faculty of Materials Science and Technology,
Slovak University of Technology,
Rázusova 2, 91724 Trnava,
Slovak Republic
peter.kostal@stuba.sk, karol.velisek@stuba.sk,
radovan.zvolensky@stuba.sk

Abstract. The majority of actual production are small or middle batch character. Thence, using of flexible production systems has lot of advantages. Their new generation fixture devices different from classical fixtures not only by design but also by its properties. One from the ways of supplementary time reducing is an suitable fixture using and supplementary operations automation. Using of proper fixture will increase the production quality, the productivity and reduce the production costs. The fixture provide clamping of workpiece on machine desk, so as the workpiece have the right position toward tool. This position must be retain in machining time too. The fixture design are dependent on the batches of production. In small batches we use the fixtures designed from modular system and in large batches we can use the dedicated fixtures. Their new generation fixture devices different from classical fixtures not only by design but also by its properties. In standard production are mechanical peripheries (for example fixtures) controlled and monitored by operators. In automated production must these mechanical peripheries working in automated mode too. In time of work cycle these devices works automatically, without operator intervention and cooperate with other devices of production system.

Keywords: flexible manufacturing, clamping fixture, intelligent manufacturing, intelligent clamping fixture, fixture design.

1 Introduction

In these days is manufacturing customer oriented. Product ranges are widened and innovative cycles are shortening. The products are changing the shape, material and there are fill up with new functions. Short innovative cycle needs changing of actual manufacturing structure to the flexible cell aided manufacture structure. By those manufacturing strategy traditional material are loosing on their importance. Manufacturing time and its shortening is coming to be important. Manufacturing strategy which is time oriented needs also change of manufacturing structure to the manufacture in manufacturing cells, or lines. Flexible manufacturing cell manufacture is the most important philosophy in last time. This manufacturing philosophy is based on:

C. Xiong et al. (Eds.): ICIRA 2008, Part II, LNAI 5315, pp. 459–465, 2008.

- manufactured products likeness,
- manufacturing progress likeness.

Product likeness recognition allows its grouping according to the used manufacturing machines. By manufacture of such products group is possible to reach economical effect which is coming to the high series or mass production. Flexible manufacturing cell is opened manufacturing unit with transparent producing process. Such manufacturing cells are representing these days trend in manufacturing development and productivity increasing.

One possibility how to decrease additional manufacturing times is selection of proper clamping device such as automation of similar helping activities. Work piece have to be clamped, to disable its possible movements, which can be created by external forces (cutting forces for example). Work piece position regarding to the tool have to be defined during realization of whole technological process. In many cases necessary to lead the tool during some part of technological process. Such function is usually insured by fixture device.

Using of proper fixture device type will lead to the quality increasing, manufacturing time decreasing and whole manufacturing process effectiveness increasing. In many cases is using of proper clamping device necessary because of realization of some technological operation.

Specific design of clamping device depends on asking manufacturing series. In case of low number series can be used universal fixture devices, or also simple modular fixtures can be used. In case of production in large series or in case of mass production are often used special one purpose fixtures, which are designed and optimized for one concrete work piece type. Or they are designed for small range of work pieces. Clamping systems than has these basic functions:

- work piece positioning and clamping in coordinate system of manufacturing device,
- prevention of work piece deformation, which can be created by actions of external forces,
- in come cases in necessary to realize tool leading by fixture design.

These clamping fixture functions are realized by using of positioning, clamping and bearing elements. These elements can be placed separately on some part of technological device, or they are placed such a complex set in form of clamping device, which is placed as single part on technological device.

2 "Intelligent" Manufacturing Systems

Automation process is basic condition for manufacture intensification and flexible reaction to the customer requirements. Main trends of todays manufacturing process research includes integration, flexibility and intelligence. According to the unceasing research in machinery production, the using of computing technique is not enough for other development of manufacturing systems. It is also not effective to use classical automated devices and flexible manufacturing systems. For other effectiveness increasing is necessary to research of new generation manufacturing systems. These new generation manufacturing systems will include new intelligent functions, which will ensure its self control of some manufacturing process parameters. Such self control function will also ensure constant optimization based on actual data coming from system surrounding. Very important task will be realized by self organization system, which will organize whole manufacturing process following to the defined target functions. All subsystems of intelligent manufacturing system have to include elements proper for realization of intelligence. Running of such systems in praxis, can eliminate the most unreliable element of manufacturing systems – the operator. Main requirements needed for integration of such intelligent systems will be shortening of manufacturing time, higher manufacturing productivity, high effectiveness and minimal need of worker intervention in to the manufacturing process. Present automated manufacturing devices are equipped by various manufacturing and helping devices which are automated on various design level. Using of intelligent manufacturing systems is based on effectiveness of all its subsystems, which were used for system building. From this reason, new intelligent manufacturing system is designed together with whole its subsystems. This is made because such designed subsystems will not prevent to the effective using of whole intelligent manufacturing system.

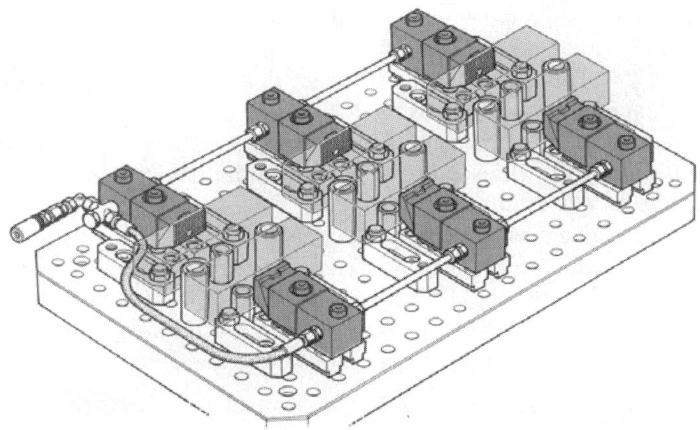

Fig. 1. Pneumatically operated clamping fixture

Category of flexible manufacturing systems includes one or more technological work places with its automated control. Basic classification of such systems is possible according to the number of technological work places. Or these systems can be classified according to the system flexibility. Intelligent manufacturing systems are able to adapt to the unexpected events, which can be done in the system, or in its surrounding. Base of complex manufacturing automation is not only automation of technological process, but there is also important automation in field of transport, manipulation, feeding, control, tool changing, fixture changing, storage system and many other activities.

3 New Generation of "Intelligent" Clamping Fixtures

Main target of every manufacturing process is creating of some product in asked quality. There are some differences between manufacture in automated production systems and manufacture in conventional production systems. These differences are standing in problematic of operation elimination from the production system. Automated manufacturing systems have to be able to provide long term needed quality level. This quality level has to be reached without labour intervention. That means, that all automated manufacturing systems subsystems are dealing on outcome quality realization. For quality realization in automated manufacturing systems it is necessary to create proper single functions composition, which are created between single subsystems. The exact time coordination of such function is very important. In such process it is very important to respect the dynamic of the system. Development of new manufacturing machines generation needs that such machines and systems have to be equipped by proper clamping systems. Such clamping systems and devices are usually developed and designed in the same time as production machines. This is done because bad clamping device can decrease using properties of whole machine. Clamping device effectiveness is affecting to the effectiveness of whole production machine or manufacturing system.

Fixture device is clamping work piece on technological devices. Such clamping operation has to be realized that way, that exact position between the tool and work piece have to hold. This position has to exact during whole technological process realization. Clamping devices are using for reason of quality and effectiveness increasing. Such quality and effectiveness increasing is also leading to the decreasing of production costs. In many cases using of proper fixture device is needed also for reason of better manufacturability. There is a wide number of technological operation which can not be realized without proper clamping device. Design of used clamping device is also based to the production series. In case of low series production are usually used universal clamping devices, which can be little adapted for each production machine. In low series production can be also used fixtures with modular design. Such modular clamping devices are usually not very expensive.

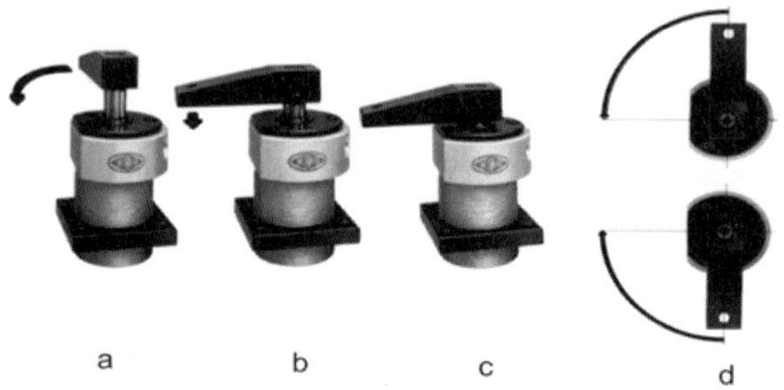

Fig. 2. Clamp with linear and rotational feed

That why, also the price of final product is also not very high. In case of high series production and mass production are usually used one purpose clamping devices or specialized fixture systems, which are characterized by high effectiveness. Such fixture system can ensure also some advanced function such as cooperation with control system of manufacturing devices. In case of its using in high series production or mass production, the price of such devices is not a problem, because such high price is compensated by effectiveness increasing. According to the rising use of low series production, there is an effort to reach same mass production economical effect also in low series production. That means, that producers are making great researches about decreasing of production costs.

In this production segment are with effort used flexible manufacturing systems of various levels. Its using has wide range of advantages. Such manufacturing systems have to be equipped by proper fixture devices, what will lead to the maximal using of the machine. Such new generation clamping systems are different not by its design but also by advanced functions.

In standard production are all mechanical peripherals controlled by machine operation. In case of automated production it is needed, that all peripheries will work and cooperate in one fully automated mode. That means, that all peripheries have to equipped by its own acting units (pneumatic actuators, electric actuators, hydraulic actuators), but they have to be also equipped by sensors. Sensors will monitor single technological operation, and they will also monitor internal stay of whole clamping system and its single elements. In the same time, clamping systems have to be able to communicate with superior control system (usually control system of production machine). Control system will coordinate fixture activity and in case of some failure, the control system will correctly react to this situation. Many of modern clamping systems are providing such control function, but in these days there is not such clamping system on the market, which will include all needed functions. Needed functions such are clamping cycle monitoring, internal stay of the clamping device monitoring. Such complex clamping systems are in these days in stay of researches, and they are known as intelligent clamping fixtures.

Main areas of intelligent fixtures application are following:

- clamping during cutting system,
- clamping during assembly operations,
- clamping during measuring and control operations,
- clamping during functional exams.

Intelligent clamping systems are able to offer many advanced (intelligent) functions such as:

- forces and torque measuring,
- clamping cycle monitoring,
- single functional parts monitoring,
- other job oriented functions.

The purpose of forces and torque monitoring, which are acting to the clamped work piece is to monitor certain clamping during manufacturing operation. This monitoring also guard work piece before deep deformation or before surface damage. Clamping force regulation can be realized very simple by using of pneumatic or hydraulic actuator. In this case is clamping force bound with the pressure, which is acting to the piston. Such clamping force can be measured and regulated by regulation of the pressure. When exact measurement of clamping force is needed, we can use special sensors, which will be placed on the clamps body. Clamping cycle monitoring defends before not correct clamping of the work piece. So, clamping cycle monitoring process protects the machine, tool, clamping device and also the work piece.

In case of single functional parts monitoring of clamping device, the system has information about function of single system elements. Automated production and assembly are areas in which can be used clamping systems of new generation. Area of automated assembly is one of most complex operation in the manufacturing process and every possibility how to increase the effectiveness is a great addition. Very important area of flexibility increasing is an using of intelligent clamping systems and also to this area belongs automated tool changing system and system of end effectors identification.

4 Conclusion

These days production is characterized by increasing of manufacturing quality. This quality increasing have to be realized together with manufacturing costs reduction. For such process, proper clamping device is needed. Modern manufacturing device needs using of clamping device which is on some suitable level. In other case, all machine manufacturing abilities are not used.

In automated manufacture is needed, that also other helping actions have to be realized automatically. To these actions also belongs clamping. Condition to the using of automated clamping systems is using of intelligent clamping systems.

These clamping systems are taking the clamping process to the higher level and they also ensures better manufacturing conditions stability control. They also ensures higher and more equal manufacturing quality. Nevertheless to the price of such intelligent clamping device, these devices are leading to the manufacturing costs cut down. Manufacturing costs cut down will be showed mostly in shorten manufacturing time, stoppage cut down and also in work productivity increasing.

Acknowledgment

This paper was created thanks to the national grants:

VEGA 1/3193/06 - **Multifunctional** ***manufacturing and assembly cell.***

VEGA 1/3164/06 - ***Using of intelligent fixtures in manufacturing and assembly processes.***

References

1. Danišová, N., Fidler, B., Charbulová, M.: Návrh kontrolného zariadenia na sledovanie kvality výrobkov typu uzavretých nádob. Design of checking device for quality monitoring of products type of closed cases. Vedecké práce MtF STU v Bratislave so sídlom v Trnave 23, 21–27 (2007); ISSN 1336-1589. - Č. 23
2. Danišová, N., Velíšek, K.: Intelligent manufacturing and assembly system. In: Machine Design: On the Occasion of the 47th Anniversary of the Faculty of Technical Sciences. 1960-2007, pp. 413–416. Faculty of Technical Sciences, Novi Sad (2007)
3. Danišová, N.: Intelligence in roboted assembly. In: RaDMI 2007: Proceedings on CD-ROM of 7th International Conference Research and Development in Mechanical Industry - RaDMI 2007, Belgrade, Serbia, 16-20 September 2007, pp. 569–574. High Technical Mechanical School of Trstenik, Trstenik (2007); ISBN 86-83803-22-4

4. Drstvenšek, I., Ficko, M., BaliČ, J.: Relational database as a cogitative part of an intelligent manufacturing system. J. mater. process. technol. 157/158, 114–122 (2004) [Print ed.] [COBISS.SI-ID 9191446], http://dx.doi.org/10.1016/j.jmatprotec.2004.09.021
5. Drstvenšek, I., Ficko, M., Pahole, I., Balič, J.: A model of simulation environment for prediction and optimisation of production processes. J. mater. process. technol. [Print ed.], 155/156, 1641–1646 (2004) (November 2004), http://dx.doi.org/10.1016/j.jmatprotec.2004.04.315 [COBISS.SI-ID 8811030]
6. Hrušková, E.: Selection efficiency of parametrical designed elements. In: Annals of MTeM for 2007 & Proceedings of the 8th International Conference Modern Technologies in Manufacturing, 4th-5th October 2007, pp. 191–194. Technical University of Cluj-Napoca, Cluj-Napoca (2007)
7. Charbulová, M., Pecháček, F.: Modular clamping systems. In: RaDMI 2007: Proceedings on CD-ROM of 7th International Conference Research and Development in Mechanical Industry - RaDMI 2007, Belgrade, Serbia, September 16-20, 2007, pp. 149–153. High Technical Mechanical School of Trstenik, Trstenik (2007)
8. Javorová, A., Matúšová, M.: Chápadlo priemyselného robota ako upínač obrobkov (Robot gripper as a workpieces fixture.) In: Materials Science and Technology [online] (2005); ISSN 1335-9053. - Roč. 5, č. 1 [cit. 2005-03-29]
9. Košt'ál, P., Matúšová, M., Velíšek, K.: Modeling of clamping fixtures. In: MicroCAD 2007: Section L: Production Engineering and Manufacturing Systems / nadát. International Scientific Conference, March 22-23, 2007, pp. 109–115. University of Miskolc, Miskolc (2007)
10. Košt'ál, P., Mudriková, A.: Hmotné a informačné toky v pružnej výrobnej bunke (Material and data flow in flexible manufacturing cell.) In: Materials Science and Technology [online] (2007). ISSN 1335-9053 - Roč. 7, č. 3
11. Matúšová, M., Hrušková, E.: Modular fixture design for flexible manufacturing. In: Annals of MTeM for 2007 & Proceedings of the 8th International Conference Modern Technologies in Manufacturing, 4th-5th October 2007, pp. 267–270. Technical University of Cluj-Napoca, Cluj-Napoca (2007); ISBN 973-9087-83-3
12. Mudriková, A., Košt'ál, P., Velíšek, K.: Material and information flow in flexible manufacturing cell In: Annals of DAAAM and Proceedings of DAAAM Symposium. - ISSN 1726-9679. - vol. 18(1). Annals of DAAAM for 2007 & Proceedings of the 18th International DAAAM Symposium Intelligent Manufacturing & Automation: Focus on Creativity, Responsibility, and Ethics of Engineers: Croatia, Zadar 24-27th, - Vieden̆: DAAAM International Vienna, 2007, pp. 485–486 (October 2007)

Kinematics Analysis for a 4-RPR Parallel Mechanism of the Milling of the Big Radius Spherical Fiducial Surface

Xiaoliang Wang, Hang Li, Jishun Li, Yujun Xue, and Sangang Yao

Henan Key Laboratory of Modern Mechanical Design and Transmission System,
Henan University of Science and technology, Luoyang, China
Wangxl327@163.com

Abstract. Kinematics characteristics of a 4-RPR (The 4-RPR paralle machine based on the theory on parallel robot was brought forward to realize a mechanism swinging around virtual axes. Its dimension and moment of inertia are so small that the continuous processing of rollers could be gotten) parallel machine of the milling of the big radius spherical fiducial surface of the cylindrical roller-bearing of high-speed railway are analyzed in this paper. According to the characteristics of micro-motion, direct and inverse kinematics equations are formulated using differential transformation, and Jacobian matrix of the input /output displacement is derived, which can be considered as a constrant matrix over the entire range of minute motion. Direct and inverse velocity equation and acceleration equation are also obtained explicitly which carry out that the kinetic plane swings aroung virtual axes. This research work provides theoretical foundations for the continuous milling of the big radius spherical fiducial surface.

Keywords: Paralle machine, Parallel robot, Virtual axes, Cylindrical roller-bearing, Jacobian matrix.

1 Background Knowledge

It is popular to use the method of mold grinding at home and abroad when a cylindrical roller-bearing of high-speed railway is proceeded, however it couldn't realize a continuous processing. It's needed to make axis of the roller to swing around a fixed axis and the roller rotate around self- axes at the same time in order to realize a continuous processing, which needs a mechanism swinging around a fixed axis. Because a diameter of spherical fiducial surface of cylindrical roller-bearing exceeds five meters, the dimension of a swinging mechanism must be very huge, which makes moment of inertia become great and limit the swinging speed. This mechanism isn't practical. In view of this situation, a 4-RPR paralle mechanism based on the theory on parallel robot was brought forward to realize a mechanism swinging around virtual axes. Its dimension and moment of inertia are so small that the continuous processing of rollers could be gotten [1-3].

C. Xiong et al. (Eds.): ICIRA 2008, Part II, LNAI 5315, pp. 466–474, 2008.

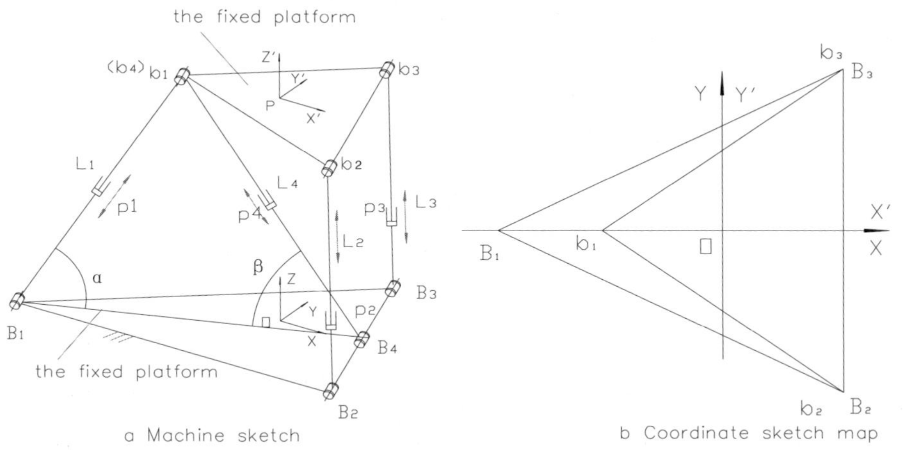

Fig. 1. 4-RPR Machine sketch

2 4-RPR Structure Design

Such as figure 1 show,the fixed and kinetic platform of the 4-RPR Structure both adopt triangle layout. And the fixed platform is the Equilateral triangle and its side is t_1 long. The kinetic platform is the Isosceles triangle and its two equilateral sides are t_2 long($2t_2>t_1$) .The revolute connect the pole piece(L_1,L_2,L_3) with the top points of the kinetic platform. And there is a prismatic on the every pole using p_1,p_2,p_3,to express separately. There is another pole L_4 between the points b_1 and B_4 witch Increases the stability of the structure. In the initial state, the pole L_2 and L3 and the fixed platform are virtical. The angle between the pole L_1 and the line B_1B_4 is α and it is β between the pole L_4 and the line B_1B_4.And the pole L_2 and L_3 are both l long and the pole L_1 and L_4 are respective l_1 and l_4 long [2][6].

Degrees of Freedom Analysis for a 4-RPR Parallel Mechanism

In the parallel institutions, the pole l1 and l2 have the same movements.so one of them is virtual bound. There is a complex hinge on the point b1.

The formula of the freedom degrees of the Parallel institutions as follows:

$$F = 6(n-1-g) + \sum_{i=1}^{g} f_i$$

In this formula, n is the total number of components; g is the number of the kinematic pair; and f_i is the number of degrees of freedom of the kinematic pair i.

Get rid of the virtual bound and increase the complex hinge, and we can account the freedom degrees of the Parallel institutions:

$$F = 6\times(8-1-8)+9 = 3$$

3 Kinematics Analysis for a 4-RPR Parallel Mechanism

3.1 4-RPR Parallel Mechanism Homogeneous Transformation Matrix

In the initial state, set the fixed reference frame OXYZ and the kinetic reference frame PXY′Z′ such as figure 1 showing. The transformation matrix for transforming the moving reference frame PX′Y′Z′to the fixed reference frame OXYZ is :

$$T = Rot(y,\theta)Trans(a,0,b)$$

$$Trans(a,0,b) = \begin{bmatrix} 1 & 0 & 0 & a \\ 0 & 1 & 0 & 0 \\ 0 & 0 & 1 & b \\ 0 & 0 & 0 & 1 \end{bmatrix} \tag{1}$$

$$Rot(y,\theta) = \begin{bmatrix} \cos\theta & 0 & \sin\theta & 0 \\ 0 & 1 & 0 & 0 \\ -\sin\theta & 0 & \cos\theta & 0 \\ 0 & 0 & 0 & 1 \end{bmatrix} \tag{2}$$

So

$$T = \begin{bmatrix} \cos\theta & 0 & \sin\theta & a\cos\theta + b\sin\theta \\ 0 & 1 & 0 & 0 \\ -\sin\theta & 0 & \cos\theta & b\cos\theta - a\sin\theta \\ 0 & 0 & 0 & 1 \end{bmatrix} \tag{3}$$

In coordinate system PX′Y′Z′, the homogeneous coordinates of the point b_1, b_2, b_3 are, respectively,

$$\left.\begin{aligned} b_1^{'} &= [\frac{-\sqrt{3}}{3}t_1, 0, 0, 1]^T \\ b_2^{'} &= [\frac{\sqrt{3}}{6}t_1, \frac{-t_1}{2}, 0, 1]^T \\ b_3^{'} &= [\frac{\sqrt{3}}{6}t_1, \frac{t_1}{2}, 0, 1]^T \end{aligned}\right\} \tag{4}$$

So, in coordinate system OXYZ, the homogeneous coordinates of the point b_1, b_2, b_3 are:

$$b_i = Tb_i^{'} \qquad (i = 1,2,3) \tag{5}$$

When the Pose of the kinetic platform establishes,the iverse equation of the 4-RPR parallel mechanism is:

$$l_i^2 = \|b_i - B_i\|^2 \qquad i = 1,2,3,4 \tag{6}$$

The ponderance form is :

$$l_i^2 = (b_{ix} - B_{ix})^2 + (b_{iy} - B_{iy})^2 + (b_{iz} - B_{iz})^2 \tag{7}$$

3.2 4-RPR Parallel Mechanism Differential Homogeneous Transformation Matrix and the Characteristic Matrix

In the initial state, the kinetic reference frame PX′Y′Z′ Moves around the virtual axis angle $\Delta\theta$ which equivalents that it moves respectively along X-axis and Z-axis Δa and Δb long and spin around Y-axis $\Delta\theta$ [4][5].

$$\mathrm{T} + \mathrm{dT} = \mathrm{Trans}(\Delta a, 0, \Delta b)\mathrm{Rot}(y, \Delta\theta)\ \mathrm{T}$$

$$\text{So}\quad \mathrm{dT} = [\mathrm{Rot}(y, \Delta\theta)\mathrm{Trans}(\Delta a, 0, \Delta b) - \mathrm{I}] \tag{8}$$

$$\because \lim_{\Delta\theta \to 0} \sin\Delta\theta \to \Delta\theta \qquad \lim_{\theta \to 0} \cos\Delta\theta \to 1 \ (\Delta\theta \text{ is very small})$$

$$\therefore Trans(\Delta a, 0, \Delta b) = \begin{bmatrix} 1 & 0 & 0 & \Delta a \\ 0 & 1 & 0 & 0 \\ 0 & 0 & 1 & \Delta b \\ 0 & 0 & 0 & 1 \end{bmatrix} \tag{9}$$

$$Rot(y, \Delta\theta) = \begin{bmatrix} 1 & 0 & \Delta\theta & 0 \\ 0 & 0 & 0 & 0 \\ -\Delta\theta & 0 & 1 & 0 \\ 0 & 0 & 0 & 0 \end{bmatrix} \tag{10}$$

According to formula(3)(8)(9)(10),we can figure out:

$$dT = \begin{bmatrix} -\Delta\theta\sin\theta & 0 & \Delta\theta\cos\theta & \Delta a + (\Delta b + b\cos\theta - a\sin\theta)\Delta\theta \\ 0 & -1 & 0 & 0 \\ -\Delta\theta\cos\theta & 0 & -\Delta\theta\sin\theta & \Delta b - (\Delta a + a\cos\theta + b\sin\theta)\Delta\theta \\ 0 & 0 & 0 & -1 \end{bmatrix}$$

$$\therefore (\Delta b_{ix}, \Delta b_{iy}, \Delta b_{iz}, 0)^T = dT(b_{ix}', b_{iy}', b_{iz}', 1)^T \tag{11}$$

In the initial state, the directions of the fixed reference frame OXYZ and the kinetic reference frame PX'Y'Z' are same, so $\sin\theta=0$, $\cos\theta=1$. Ignore high-end infinitesimal and we can figure out:

$$
\left.
\begin{aligned}
dT &= \begin{bmatrix} 0 & 0 & \Delta\theta & \Delta a + b\Delta\theta \\ 0 & -1 & 0 & 0 \\ -\Delta\theta & 0 & 0 & \Delta b - a\Delta\theta \\ 0 & 0 & 0 & -1 \end{bmatrix} \\
\Delta b_1 &= \begin{bmatrix} \Delta a + b\Delta\theta \\ 0 \\ \frac{\sqrt{3}}{3} t_1 \Delta\theta + \Delta b - a\Delta\theta \\ -1 \end{bmatrix} \\
\Delta b_2 &= \begin{bmatrix} \Delta a + b\Delta\theta \\ \frac{t_1}{2} \\ -\frac{\sqrt{3}}{6} t_1 \Delta\theta + \Delta b - a\Delta\theta \\ -1 \end{bmatrix} \\
\Delta b_3 &= \begin{bmatrix} \Delta a + b\Delta\theta \\ -\frac{t_1}{2} \\ -\frac{\sqrt{3}}{6} t_1 \Delta\theta + \Delta b - a\Delta\theta \\ -1 \end{bmatrix} \\
\Delta b_4 &= \begin{bmatrix} \Delta a + b\Delta\theta \\ 0 \\ \frac{\sqrt{3}}{3} t_1 \Delta\theta + \Delta b - a\Delta\theta \\ -1 \end{bmatrix}
\end{aligned}
\right\} \tag{12}
$$

According to formula(7), we can figure out:

$$l_i \Delta l_i = (b_{ix} - B_{ix})(\Delta b_{ix} - \Delta B_{ix}) + (b_{iy} - B_{iy})(\Delta b_{iy} - \Delta B_{iy}) + (b_{iz} - B_{iz})(\Delta b_{iz} - \Delta B_{iz}) \tag{13}$$

For the pole L_1,L_2,L_3, L_4, Δli=0(i=1,2,3,4).According to the geometric relations such as the figure 1 showing,we can introduce:

$$\left.\begin{array}{ll} \Delta B_{1y} = \Delta B_{2y} = \Delta B_{3y} = \Delta B_{4y} = 0 & \\ \Delta B_{1x} = \Delta P_1 \cos\alpha & \Delta B_{1z} = \Delta p_1 \sin\alpha \\ \Delta B_{2x} = \Delta B_{3x} = 0 & \Delta B_{4z} = \Delta P_4 \sin\beta \\ \Delta B_{2z} = \Delta B_{3z} = \Delta P_2 & \Delta B_{4x} = -\Delta P_4 \cos\beta \end{array}\right\} \tag{14}$$

Suppose:

$$\left.\begin{array}{ll}
K_{11} = \dfrac{b_{1x} - B_{1x}}{(b_{1x} - B_{1x})\cos\alpha + (b_{1z} - B_{1z})\sin\alpha} & \\
K_{12} = \dfrac{b_{1z} - B_{1z}}{(b_{1x} - B_{1x})\cos\alpha + (b_{1z} - B_{1z})\sin\alpha} & \\
K_{13} = \dfrac{(b_{1x} - B_{1x})b + (b_{1z} - B_{1z})\left(\dfrac{\sqrt{3}t_1}{2} - a\right)}{(b_{1x} - B_{1x})\cos\alpha + (b_{1z} - B_{1z})\sin\alpha} & \\
K_{23} = \dfrac{(b_{2x} - B_{2x}) - (b_{2z} - B_{2z})\left(\dfrac{\sqrt{3}t_1}{6} + a\right)}{b_{2z} - B_{2z}} & K_{21} = \dfrac{b_{2x} - B_{2x}}{b_{2z} - B_{2z}} \\
K_{41} = \dfrac{b_{1x} - B_{1x}}{(b_{1z} - B_{1z})\sin\beta - (b_{1x} - B_{1x})\cos\beta} & K_{24} = \dfrac{b_{2y} - B_{2y}}{b_{2z} - B_{2z}}\dfrac{t_1}{2} \\
K_{42} = \dfrac{b_{1z} - B_{1z}}{(b_{1z} - B_{1z})\sin\beta - (b_{1x} - B_{1x})\cos\beta} & \\
K_{43} = \dfrac{(b_{1x} - B_{1x})b + (b_{1z} - B_{1z})\left(\dfrac{\sqrt{3}t_1}{2} - a\right)}{(b_{1z} - B_{1z})\sin\beta - (b_{1x} - B_{1x})\cos\beta} &
\end{array}\right\} \tag{15}$$

According to formula(12)(13)(14)(15), we can figure out:

$$\begin{cases} \Delta P_1 = K_{11}\Delta a + K_{12}\Delta b + K_{13}\Delta\theta \\ \Delta P_2 = K_{21}\Delta a + K_{22}\Delta b + K_{23}\Delta\theta + K_{24} \\ \Delta P_3 = K_{21}\Delta a + K_{22}\Delta b + K_{23}\Delta\theta - K_{24} \\ \Delta P_1 = K_{41}\Delta a + K_{42}\Delta b + K_{43}\Delta\theta \end{cases}$$

$$\therefore \text{Jacoby matrix}: J^{-1} = \begin{bmatrix} K_{11} & K_{12} & K_{13} & 0 \\ K_{21} & 1 & K_{23} & K_{24} \\ K_{21} & 1 & K_{23} & -K_{24} \\ K_{41} & K_{42} & K_{43} & 0 \end{bmatrix} \text{which is Constant matrix}$$

3.3 The Inverse and Positive Solution of Pose of the 4-RPR Parallel Mechanism and the Analysis of the Speed and Acceleration

$$\text{According to Jacoby matrix matrix}: J^{-1} = \begin{bmatrix} K_{11} & K_{12} & K_{13} & 0 \\ K_{21} & 1 & K_{23} & K_{24} \\ K_{21} & 1 & K_{23} & -K_{24} \\ K_{41} & K_{42} & K_{43} & 0 \end{bmatrix}, \text{ we}$$

can figure out the Inverse solution of the 4-RPR Parallel Mechanism.

$$P(\Delta P_1, \Delta P_2, \Delta P_3, \Delta P_4)^T = J^{-1}Q(\Delta a, \Delta b, \Delta\theta)^T \tag{16}$$

Suppose:

$$K = -K_{11}K_{43} + K_{11}K_{23}K_{42} + K_{21}K_{12}K_{43} - K_{21}K_{13}K_{42} - K_{41}K_{13}$$

$$\therefore J = \frac{1}{K}\begin{bmatrix} K_{43}+K_{23}K_{42} & \frac{1}{2}(K_{12}K_{43}-K_{13}K_{42}) & \frac{1}{2}(K_{12}K_{43}-K_{13}K_{42}) & -(K_{12}K_{23}-K_{13}) \\ -(K_{21}K_{43}+K_{41}K_{23}) & \frac{1}{2}(K_{12}K_{43}-K_{13}K_{42}) & \frac{1}{2}(K_{12}K_{43}-K_{13}K_{42}) & K_{11}K_{23}-K_{21}K_{13}) \\ -(K_{21}K_{43}+K_{41}K_{23}) & \frac{1}{2}(K_{11}K_{42}-K_{41}K_{12}) & \frac{1}{2}(K_{11}K_{42}-K_{41}K_{12}) & -(K_{11}K_{43}-K_{12}K_{21}) \\ 0 & \frac{K}{2K_{24}} & \frac{K}{2K_{24}} & 0 \end{bmatrix}$$

So the positive solution of the 4-RPR Parallel Mechanism:

$$Q(\Delta a, \Delta b, \Delta\theta)^T = JP(\Delta P_1, \Delta P_2, \Delta P_3, \Delta P_4)^T \tag{17}$$

According to formula (15)(16),the inverse and positive solution of The speed of the 4-RPR Parallel Mechanism are respective :

$$\left.\begin{aligned}
&\frac{dP}{dt}=J^{-1}\frac{dQ}{dt}\\
&\frac{dQ}{dt}=J\frac{dP}{dt}\\
&\frac{dP}{dt}=\begin{bmatrix}\frac{d\Delta P_1}{dt} & \frac{d\Delta P_2}{dt} & \frac{d\Delta P_3}{dt} & \frac{d\Delta P_4}{dt}\end{bmatrix}^T\\
&\frac{dQ}{dt}=\begin{bmatrix}\frac{d\Delta a}{dt} & \frac{d\Delta b}{dt} & \frac{d\Delta \theta}{dt} & 0\end{bmatrix}^T
\end{aligned}\right\}$$

According to formula(15)(16), the inverse and positive solution of the acceleration of the 4-RPR Parallel Mechanism are respective :

$$\left.\begin{aligned}
&\frac{d^2P}{dt^2}=J^{-1}\frac{d^2Q}{dt^2}\\
&\frac{d^2Q}{dt^2}=J\frac{d^2P}{dt^2}\\
&\frac{d^2P}{dt^2}=\begin{bmatrix}\frac{d^2\Delta P_1}{dt^2} & \frac{d^2\Delta P_2}{dt^2} & \frac{d^2\Delta P_3}{dt^2} & \frac{d^2\Delta P_4}{d^2t}\end{bmatrix}^T\\
&\frac{d^2Q}{dt^2}=\begin{bmatrix}\frac{d^2\Delta a}{dt^2} & \frac{d^2\Delta b}{dt^2} & \frac{d^2\Delta \theta}{dt^2} & 0\end{bmatrix}^T
\end{aligned}\right\}$$

4 Conclusion

Kinematics characteristics of a 4-RPR parallel mechanism of the milling of the big radius spherical fiducial surface are analyzed in this paper. Direct and inverse kinematics equations are formulated using differential transformation, and Jacobian matrix of the input /output displacement is derived, which can be considered as a constrant matrix over the entire range of minute motion. Direct and inverse velocity equation and acceleration equation are also obtained explicitly which carry out that the kinetic plane swings aroung virtual axes. This research work provides theoretical foundations for the continuous milling of the big radius spherical fiducial surface.

References

1. Hua, Y.H.: A number of technical research on cylindrical roller-bearing of high-speed railway. Master paper of Henan University of Science and technology, 32–34 (2004)
2. Wang, M.F., Li, H.: Study on large radius of spherical fiducial surface of bearing of high-speed railway forming base on virtual axis. In: Proceeding of International Technology&Innovation Conference 2006. Herts SG1 2AY, The Institution of Engineering and Technology (2006)

3. Chen, C., Fan, S.W.: Kinematics Analysis for a 4-DOF parallel Microcompulator. Journal of University of Electronic Science and Technology of China 36(1) (2007)
4. Zhang, T., Xie, C.X.: Robotics. South China University of Technology Press, GuangZhou (2004)
5. Yang, Y., Tamio, A.: Manipulation kinematics on dexterous hands considering pure rolling contacts us passive joints. Chinese Journal of Mechanical Engineering 18(3), 361–365 (2005)
6. Song, L.B., Zhang, J.L., Lu, T.S.: Direct and Inverse Kinematic Analysis of a Leg-wheeled Passive Wheel Mobile Robot—Ice-skater Robot. Journal of Donghua University 20(3), 27–31 (2003)

Development of a 3D High-Precise Positioning System Based on a Planar Target and Two CCD Cameras

Jinjun Li[1,2], Hong Zhao[1], Tao Jiang[1], and Xiang Zhou[1]

[1] State Key Laboratory for Manufacturing Systems Engineering, Xi'an Jiaotong University, Xi'an 710049
[2] Xi'an Research Inst. of Hi-tech, Hongqing Town, Xi'an 710025
lixy6228@sohu.com

Abstract. Three-dimension positioning and coordinates measuring is the key technique in modern manufacturing, reverse engineering, automation, precision measurement and computer aided surgery. This paper presents a positioning system based on a planar target and two CCD cameras. The binocular stereo vision measuring principle is proposed. Planar scene geometry and the Direct Reference Plane (DRP) method for the calibrated cameras are discussed. The 3D plane can be reconstructed according to the DRP method and 3D coordinates of the contact head on Planar Target can be directly computed according to rigid geometric transformation. We also develop a new three-step calibration method for matrices and distortion factors of the two cameras using coplanar feature points. Further results of calibrating and measuring are verified experimentally.

Keywords: Binocular Stereo Vision, 3D High-precise Positioning System, VCMM, Planar Target, Direct Reference Plane.

1 Introduction

Three-dimension positioning and coordinates measuring is the key technique in modern manufacturing, reverse engineering, automation, precision measurement and computer aided surgery. In past several decades, most research focused on space target location and tracking. Generally there are many methods to measure the position and orientation of the pose, such as the Global Positioning system (GPS) [1], the mechanical arm localization system, the ultrasonic localization system and the optical positioning system, among those the optical positioning technique have the higher degree of accuracy [2,3]. Macellari, V. firstly developed the COSTEL system which can monitor human motion in the 3D space using linear CCD camera [4]. Abdel-Aziz and Karara firstly measured the 3D points using the DLT method and the CCD Image sensor [5]. Subsequently there are much more research findings [6-8].

In recent years, the 3D coordinates vision measurement becomes a newly technique in the measurement domain and has been developed rapidly. Some vision coordinates measurement machines (VCMM) were developed by several companies. i.e.Leica in Switzerland and METRONOR Company in Norway [9-11]. Those VCMMs, generally belonging to non-Cartesian coordinate system and being unrestricted by the guide

C. Xiong et al. (Eds.): ICIRA 2008, Part II, LNAI 5315, pp. 475–484, 2008.

way, are mostly used in measuring as a batch due to installing and calibrating complexly. Other companies in America, Switzerland, Norway and Belgium, have developed portable vision coordinate measurement machines (PVMM) [12-13]. Some researches have also been done by Tianjing University, Shanghai University and Haerbin Industrial University in China [2,14,15]. Because the PVMM mostly capture the images of the hand-held probe and the man-made mark points using single camera, Perspective-n-Point camera pose determination, popularly called the PnP problem, must be solved [16]. Therefore some control points must be designed accurately, i.e. three control points must be collinear in the reference. Also the probe images may be susceptible to the mal-condition and external noise, i.e. point brilliance and ambient light illumination [12-15].

In order to overcome these problems, a new portable 3D high-precise positioning system bases on a planar target and two CCD cameras, is developed. A briefly description for this system is in Section 2. In Section 3, Planar Scene Geometry and the Direct Reference Plane (DRP) method are discussed, and a new three-step method for calibrating the matrices and distortion factors of the binocular stereo vision system is developed. The 3D plane can be reconstructed according to the DRP method and 3D coordinates of the contact head on Planar Target can be directly computed according to rigid geometric transformation. In Section 4, further results of calibrating and measuring are verified experimentally.

2 System Configuration and Key Component Designing

The proposed system consists of a special planar target, two high-resolution CCD cameras, a special module for calibration, a notebook PC host and a software package in Fig. 1. We adopt the cross optical axes structure [17]. Because there is a angle between the double optical axes, z_l and z_r, we can flexibly adjust the distance and lean between two cameras. We also use two high-performance CCD cameras with wide frame, large filed views and short-focus lenses. The angle between each optical axis and baseline is from 30°to 60°, and the angular filed of view is controlled within 20°.

The planar target, the most important part, consists of a target panel, some light spots, a probe and a set of lengthening bar. There are 10 fixed index points on the target panel. Because only three non-collinear points are used, those 10 index points are redundant, which may ensure that measuring results are stable and reliable when some part of planar target is not in the field of views and some points have defect. Each index point consists of 9 super-high intensity infrared or homochromous light-emitting diodes (LEDs). The intensity of those LEDs is stable and uniform and apparently higher than that of ambient light. The sub-pixel mean centre of 9 light spots is made as the centre of each index point in order to improve measurement accuracy [18,19]. Then the traditional problems, i.e. the spot distortion and low-accuracy recognition of the spot centre induced by oversize light-emitting area, can be solved preferably [20,21]. The extension bar with different length may be connected at the bottom of the planar target and a trigger probe is connected at the front of the extension bar. Therefore it can be applied to measuring 3D invisible points, discontinuous surface and large-scale object. Special Module, cooperating with the planar target, is suitable to the on-line and high-accuracy calibration.

The 3D high-precise positioning will undergo four stages of processing:

1. The high-accuracy calibration for binocular stereo vision system;
2. Synchronously capturing target images using two CCD cameras and preprocessing the captured images;
3. Recognizing LED spots and the sub-pixel center of the index points;
4. Matching and reconstructing.

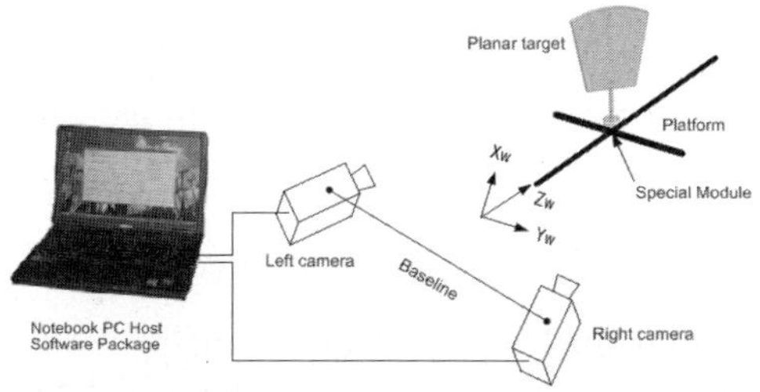

Fig. 1. The compact configuration of 3D high-precise positioning system

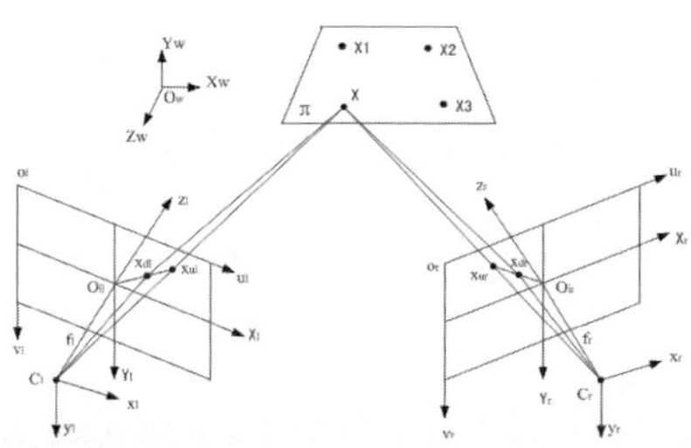

Fig. 2. A binocular stereo vision system of cross optical axes. An object point X in the world coordinate frame $O_w X_w Y_w Z_w$ is imaged the ideal projected point X_{ul}, X_{ur} and the actual projected point X_{dl}, X_{dr} in two camera coordinate frame $C_l x_l y_l z_l$ and $C_r x_r y_r z_r$. C_l and C_r represent the coordinates of the left and right camera centre in the world coordinate frame respectively. f_l and f_r represent the left and right focal length respectively.

3 System Model and 3D Positioning Method

In this section, we will present measuring principles of binocular stereo vision, Planar Scene Geometry and linear reconstruction method. Also a new three-step calibration method will be presented.

3.1 Binocular Stereo Vision Measuring Principles

In Fig.2, a stereo vision system of cross optical axes is presented with the non-linearity of lens distortion under the pinhole camera model. Under the ideal (non-distorted) pinhole projection, we can describe the central projection mapping from world coordinates to camera coordinates as [22]

$$\begin{pmatrix} \lambda_c X_{uc} \\ \lambda_c \end{pmatrix} = P_c \begin{pmatrix} X \\ 1 \end{pmatrix} = K_c [R_c \mid T_c] \begin{pmatrix} X \\ 1 \end{pmatrix} \tag{1}$$

where, $c = l, r$ subscripts which represent the left and right camera respectively, P_c is 3×3 projected matrix, R_c , T_c are the rotation matrix and translation matrix, n_{cx}, n_{cy} are the number of pixels of the unit length in the camera coordinate frame, s_c is the skew, $(u_{c0}, v_{c0})^T$ is the coordinate of the image centre, K_c is the intrinsic matrix, $K_c = ((n_{cx}^{-1} f, s_c, u_{c0}), (0, n_{cy}^{-1} f_c, v_{c0}), (0,0,1))^T$.

The linear triangulation method is the direct analogue of the DLT method described in [22]. The homogeneous scale factor is eliminated by across product to give three equations for each image point, of which two are linearly independent. Then an equation of the form $AX = 0$ can be composed, as

$$AX = \begin{bmatrix} x_{ul} p_{3l}^T - p_{1l}^T \\ y_{ul} p_{3l}^T - p_{2l}^T \\ x_{ur} p_{3r}^T - p_{1r}^T \\ y_{ur} p_{3r}^T - p_{2r}^T \end{bmatrix} \begin{bmatrix} X_w \\ Y_w \\ Z_w \end{bmatrix} = 0 \tag{2}$$

where two equations have been included from each image, giving a total of four equations in four homogeneous unknowns. This is a redundant set of equations. If we have P_l, P_r, X_{ul} and X_{ur}, a world point X can compute by solving the set of equations of the form $AX = 0$. Several ways were discussed in [22].

For real (non-pinhole) lenses equations (1) and equations (2) will not hold due to the design and assemble deviation. Generally the important deviations are the radial distortion and tangential distortion. The correspondence relation between the ideal projected point X_{u} and the actual projected point X_{d} is written as

$$\begin{bmatrix} x_d(x_d^2 + y_d^2) & x_d(x_d^2 + y_d^2)^2 & 3x_d^2 + y_d^2 & 2x_d y_d \\ y_d(x_d^2 + y_d^2) & y_d(x_d^2 + y_d^2) & 2x_d y_d & x_d^2 + 3y_d^2 \end{bmatrix} \begin{bmatrix} k_1 \\ k_2 \\ d_1 \\ d_2 \end{bmatrix} = \begin{bmatrix} x_d - x_u \\ y_d - y_u \end{bmatrix} \tag{3}$$

where, $(x_u, y_u)^T$ is the ideal image position (which obeys linear projection), $(x_d, y_d)^T$ is the actual image position after distortion, k_1 , k_2 are the first and second coefficient of the radial distortion, d_1, d_2 are the coefficient of the tangential distortion, r_d is the radial distance $\sqrt{x_d^2 + y_d^2}$ from the centre to the actual image position.

According to equations (3), we can compute the distorted coefficients k_1, k_2, d_1, d_2 and the ideal image position $(x_u, y_u)^T$. The two cameras are then effectively again linear devices.

3.2 Planar Scene Geometry and Linear Reconstruction

Suppose the camera matrices are those of the calibrated stereo vision system with the world origin at the left camera

$$P_{El} = K_l[I \mid 0], \quad P_{Er} = K_r[R \mid t] \tag{4}$$

and the world plane π_E has coordinates $\pi_E = (n, d)^T$ so that for points on plane $n\widetilde{X} + d = 0$ [23]. Consider three (non-collinear) 3D points $X_{i=1,2,3}$ which lies on the plane π_E and is visible in two views $x_{l,i=1,2,3}$, $x_{r,i=1,2,3}$. The image points are related by the homography H as $x_{l,i} = Hx_{r,i}$. Given the homography, we may reconstruct the planar scene. For the calibrated stereo vision system, the following relationship holds

$$H = \lambda(I + (nC_l + d)^{-1}(C_r - C_l)n) \tag{5}$$

The unknown scale λ may be determined directly from the homography H. Equation (5) may be rewritten as

$$\widetilde{H} = \lambda^{-1}H - I = (nC_l + d)^{-1}(C_r - C_l)n \tag{6}$$

Since the matrix $\widetilde{H}$ has rank 1, H has the double eigenvalue λ.

As with 3D lines, the orientation of the plane, i.e. its normal n, can be derived given the plane π_E. The vanishing points $(0, v_1)^T$, $(0, v_2)^T$ of the lines $L_1 = (X_1, X_2), L_2 = (X_1, X_3)$ are given as (see fig. 3)

$$v_1 = (x_{l,1} \times x_{l,2}) \times (x_{r,1} \times x_{r,2}), \quad v_2 = (x_{l,1} \times x_{l,3}) \times (x_{r,1} \times x_{r,3}) \tag{7}$$

Consequently, the plane's normal is $n = v_1 \times v_2$.

Given n and λ, the remaining parameter is d. From equation (6), we can hold

$$d = ((C_r - C_l)n^T - n^T C_r \widetilde{H})\widetilde{H}^{-1} \tag{8}$$

This is a linear method for reconstructing the plane π_E from the three (non-collinear) 3D points and the same points in the two views.

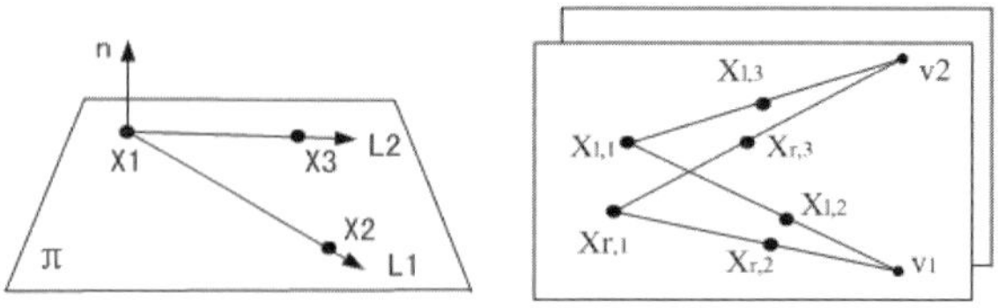

Fig. 3. The three non-collinear 3D points $X_{i=1,2,3}$ define uniquely the plane. Two stabilized images $x_{l,i=1,2,3}$, $x_{r,i=1,2,3}$ are shown on the right.

3.3 Calibration of Binocular Stereo Vision

Camera calibration is a crucial problem for vision measurement system. The precision of the vision measurement system mainly rests with the accuracy of the camera calibration parameters [24]. The goal of camera calibration is to develop a mathematical model of the transformation between world points and observed image points resulting from the image formation process. The parameters which affect this mapping can be divided into four categories: a) intrinsic matrices K_l, K_r; b) rotation matrices R_l, R_r and translation matrices T_l, T_r; c) distortion parameters, k_1, k_2, d_1, d_2, in two cameras; and d) the rotation matrix R and the translation matrix T between two camera frames. Many techniques and some studies concerning calibration have been presented in the last few years [25-28]. These different approaches can be classified as: linear techniques, nonlinear optimization techniques and two-step techniques. Each of those has advantages and disadvantages. We present a new calibration method for binocular stereo vision using a movable calibration plane target as following:

The first step is linear parameter estimation of intrinsic matrix of single camera, based on the ideal (non-distorted) pinhole projection. We use a set of coplanar feature points and the center of the world frame is on the planar target. Then these feature points have coordinates of the special form $X = (X_w, Y_w, 0)^T$. Eqn.(1) may be simplified to (for example, left camera)

$$\lambda_l [x_{ul}, y_{ul}, 1]^T = K_l [r_{l1}, r_{l2}, T_l][X_w, Y_w, 1]^T = H[X_w, Y_w, 1]^T \tag{9}$$

Where r_1, r_2 are the first two columns of the rotation matrix R. The matrix $H = K[r_1, r_2, T]$ is a linear transformation of the homogeneous coordinates $[X_w, Y_w, 1]^T$ to the homogeneous coordinates $[x, y, 1]^T$. Multiplying both sides by the skew-symmetric matrix $\hat{x}$, we may eliminate λ (for $\hat{x}x = 0$) and yields [29]

$$\hat{x} H [X_w, Y_w, 1]^T = 0 \tag{10}$$

We can be solved (up to a scalar factor) linearly from such equations if at least four points on the plane are given. Since r_1, r_2 are orthonormal vectors, we obtain two equations that the calibration matrix K has

$$h_1^T K^{-T} K^{-1} h_2 = 0, \quad h_1^T K^{-T} K^{-1} h_1 = h_2^T K^{-T} K^{-1} h_2 \tag{11}$$

These equations are quadratic in the entries of K . Now we can recover $S = K^{-T} K^{-1}$ linearly from the equations above, as usual, using the SVD. Once S is known, K can be retrieved, in principle, using the Cholesky factorization. If we have at least three images of the plane, we can obtain five unknowns of the matrix K.

The second step is nonlinear estimation of the intrinsic matrix and distortion factors based on maximum likelihood criterion. For a world plane, the maximum likelihood estimation of camera parameters can be obtained by minimizing the following functional $\sum_{i=1}^{n} dis_i(K, r_1, r_2, T, X_i)$, where $dis_i(K, r_1, r_2, T, X_i)$ is the distance of the coplanar points X_i, from the corresponding optical ray generated by its projection points and the center of camera. Given an initial estimation of K and n coplanar feature points, $[r_1, r_2, T]$ can be obtained. Then we can get the equation of the initial guess of distortion parameters. Given n point correspondences, by stacking eqn. (3), we can obtain $AD = Q$, where $D = [k_1, k_2, d_1, d_2]$ and A is $2n \times 4$ matrix and Q is $2n \times 1$ matrix. With the initial guess of all the camera parameters, we can estimate the complete set of parameters by minimizing the following functional $\sum_{i=1}^{n} dis_i(K, k_1, k_2, d_1, d_2, r_1, r_2, T, X_i)$.

The third step is to compute the rotation matrix and the translation matrix between two cameras. Now we suppose the world origin is the center of the left camera. In the second step, we obtained the extrinsic matrices $[R_{l,i}, T_{l,i}]$, $[R_{r,i}, T_{r,i}]$ ($i = 1, 2, \cdots, m$ present m positions of the calibration plane). The rotation matrix R and the translation matrix T in equa.(4) can be presented

$$R = R_{r,i} R_{l,i}^{-1}, \qquad T = T_{r,i} - R_{r,i} R_{l,i}^{-1} T_{l,i}^{-1}, \quad i = 1, 2, \cdots, m \tag{12}$$

From eqns.(16), we obtain the initial guess of R and T. Then the maximum likelihood estimation can be obtained by minimizing the following functional [30]

$$\sum\sum \left\| X_{ul,ij} - \widehat{H}_l(R_{l,i}, T_{l,i}, X_{ij}) \right\| + \left\| X_{ur,ij} - \widehat{H}_r(R, R_{l,i}, T, T_{l,i}, X_{ij}) \right\| \tag{13}$$

where $X_{ul,ij}$, $X_{ur,ij}$ are the image coordinates of the feature point (j) at the position (i), $\widehat{H}_l$, $\widehat{H}_r$ are transformation relations from the world frame to the left and right camera respectively. Also minimizing is solved with the Levenberg-Marquardt Algorithm.

4 Experiments and Results

The performance of our proposed system has been tested through both simulation and experiments with real data.

Spatial configuration of the simulation experiments is showed in Fig.1. Two CCD cameras with lenses of 17 mm focal length were calibrated. The Special Module was fixed at a numerical control platform and may be moved in the direction of X, Y and Z axis by a step length. The planar target was placed at the Special Module in different orientations. We tested 100 world points and 20 different orientations of each point. In Table 1 and 2, all of the estimated camera parameters are displayed. The planar scene geometry and linear reconstruction algorithm was applied to the input images. We recognized the LED image spots using Canny Algorithm and Least-squares ellipse fitting method. We carried out 3D reconstruction from three correspondence points captured by the calibrated two cameras. The experimental result in Fig.4 shows that our system has achieved a measuring stability precision of 0.047mm, 0.039mm and 0.061mm in the direction of X, Y and Z axis respectively in 300mm×300mm×500mm measuring range. The developed system, with portable type, easier assembles and operation, high speed, high precise, wide range and flexibly, can be applied to measuring 3D invisible points and discontinuous surface, the car underpan and body, the plane wing and airframe, the workshop platform at field, and testing the dynamic trace of the mechanical arm, inverse engineering in NC machining.

This work was supported by National Basic Research Program of China (2005CB724106), and the National Natural Science Foundation of China (50575169).

Table 1. Calibration results of the cameras

Parameter	Left	Right	Parameter	Left	Right
f /mm	17.28±0.25	17.16±0.21	s	-0.0015±0.0003	-0.0015±0.0003
u_0 /pixel	641.25±0.72	640.8±0.87	v_0 /pixel	511.84±0.54	512.42±0.64
n_x	0.0052	0.0052	n_y	0.0052	0.0052
k_1	-4.37e-008	-3.78e-008	k_2	5.79e-013	4.54e-013
d_1	-8.30e-005	-6.31e-005	d_2	8.75e-006	6.77e-006

Table 2. Calibration results of the sensor

	0.9416	-0.0032	0.3369		21.4916
R	0.0038	0.9998	-0.0025	T	208.4779
	-0.3366	0.0026	0.9416		-44.2711

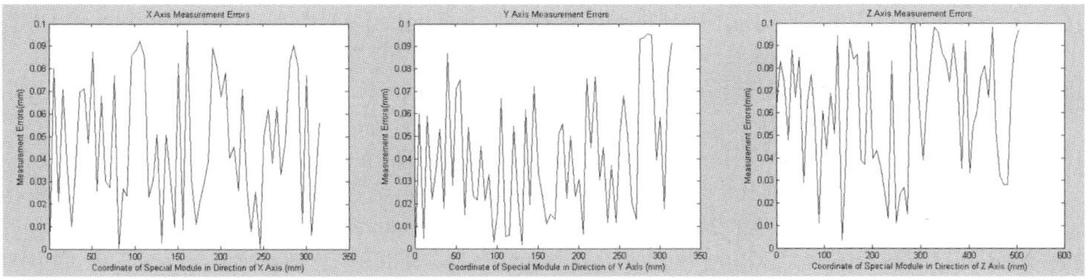

Fig. 4. Measurement errors in the direction of X, Y and Z axis respectively

References

1. Cannon, M.E.: Kinematic Positioning Using GPS Pseudorange and Carrier Phase Observations, UCSE Reports No.20019, Department of Geomatics Engineering. The University of Calgary (1987)
2. Jian, W.: Three-Dimensional High Precise Optical Positioning Technique and its Clinical Application, Doctor Dissertation, pp. 3–18. Tsinghua University (2004)
3. Lyndon, N.S., Melvyn, L.S.: Stereo Vision Technology for Object Measurement. In: Hunt, M.A., Price, J.R. (eds.) Machine Vision Applications in Industrial Inspection XI, Proceedings of SPIE-IS&T Electronic Imaging, vol. 5011, SPIE (2003)
4. Macellari, V.: COSTEL: a computer peripheral remote sensing device for 3-dimensiona monitoring of human motion. Med. Biol. Eng. Comp. 21, 311–318 (1983)
5. Wong, K.W.: Mathematical formulation and digital analysis in close-range photogrammetry. Photogrammetric Eng. Remote Sensing 41, 1355–1373 (1975)
6. Toyohiko, H., Rika, K., Michio, M.: Calibration of Linear CCD Cameras Used in the Detection of the Position of the Light Spot. IEICE Trans. INF. & SYST. 76(8), 912–918 (1993)
7. Gazzani, F.: Performance of a 7-parameter DLT method for the calibration ofstereo-photogrammetric systems using 1-D transducers. Biomed. Eng. 14, 476–482 (1992)
8. Qingchao, W., GuoQing, Z., Qing, Z.: On DLT Method for CCD Camera Calibration. In: Proceedings of ICSP 1996 (1996)
9. Yandong, C., Xueyou, Y.: Machine Vision Testing system for the white body of car. In: Light Automobile Technique, vol. 12 (2001)
10. Prenninger, J.P., Vincze, M., Gander, H.: Contactless position and orientation measurement of robot end effectors. In: Proceedings of IEEE on Robotics and Automation, vol. 180 (1993)
11. Vincze, M., Prenninger, J.P., Gander, H.: A laser tracking system to measure position andorientation of robot end effectors under motion. Int. J. Robotics Res. 13(4), 305 (1994)
12. Heeren, T.A.G., Veldpaus, F.E.: An optical system to measure the end effector position for on-line control purpose. Int. J. Robotics Res. 11(1), 53 (1992)
13. Brown, J., Dold, J.: V-STARS—A System for Digital Industrial Photogrammetry. In: Optical 3D Measurement Techniques Congress, Vienna (1995)
14. Fengshan, H., Hui-fen, Q.: Single camera 3D coordinate vision measuring system using a light pen. Opto-Electronic Engineering 34(4), 69–72 (2007)
15. Changying, L., Dong: Optical Probe Pose Estimation in the Vision Measurement. Journal of Harbin Institute of Technology 38(10) (October 2006)

16. Hongwu, Y., Yihu, Z.: PnP Problem Revisited. Journal of Mathematical Imaging and Vision 24, 131–141 (2006)
17. Ke, Z., Mianhao, Z.: Construction of the nonlinear model for binoculars stereo vision system. Transducer and Micro-system Technologies 25(10), 21–37 (2006)
18. Jianfei, M., Rong, X., Weilong, D.: A Compound and Robust Algorithm for Ellipse Detection. In: Proceedings of the 16th International Conference on Artificial Reality and Telexistence–Workshops (ICAT 2006). IEEE Computer Society Press, Los Alamitos (2006)
19. Kenichi, K.: Ellipse Fitting with Hyper-accuracy. IEICE Trans. Inf. Syst. E89-D(10), 2653–2660 (2006)
20. Chao, B.: Problems About Measurement of Super-high Intensity LED. Chinese Journal of Liquid Crystals and Display 18(4), 24–250 (2003)
21. Zhibi, Z.: Analysis on the Luminous Characteristics of InGaAlP LEDs. Chinese Journal of Liquid Crystals and Display 18(6), 450–453 (2003)
22. Richhard, H., Andrew, Z.: Multiple View Geometry in computer vision. Cambridge University Press, Cambridge (2003)
23. Carsten, Rother: Linear Multi-View Reconstruction of Points, Lines, Planes and Cameras using a Reference Plane. In: Proceedings of the Ninth IEEE International Conference on Computer Vision (ICCV 2003). Computer Society, IEEE (2006)
24. Qiaoyu, X., Dong, Y., Rensheng, C., Yan, H.: Accurate Camera Calibration with New Minimizing Function. In: Proceedings of the 2006 IEEE International Conference on Robotics and Biomimetics, Kunming, China, December 17-20 (2006)
25. Wei, G.Q., De Ma, S.: Implicit and explicit camera calibration: Theory and experiments. IEEE Trans, Pattern Anal. Mach. Intell 16, 469–480 (1994)
26. Ito, M.: Robot vision modelling camera modelling and camera calibration. Adv. Robotics 5, 321–335 (1991)
27. Tsai, R.Y.: A versatile camera calibration technique for high-accuracy 3D machine vision metrology using oH-the shelf TV cameras and lenses. IEEE Int. J. Robot. Automat. RA-3, 323–344 (1987)
28. Weng, J., Cohen, P., Herniou, M.: Camera calibration with distortion models and accuracy evaluation. IEEE Trans. Pattern Anal. Mach. Intell 14, 965–980 (1992)
29. Yi, M., Stefano, S., Jana, K.: An Invitation to 3-D Vision From Images to Geometric Models. Springer, Now York (2004)
30. Zhidong, D., Jianjun, L., Jingdan, Z.: Three-dimensional Modeling Approach Based on Stereo Vision. Journal of System Simulation 19(14) (2007)

Research on TOC Accounting Based Decision Making of Products Pricing

Qiong Liu, Gang Zhou, and Chaoyong Zhang

State Key Laboratory of Digital Manufacturing Equipment and Technology,
Huazhong University of Science and Technology, Wuhan, Hubei Province, China
qiongliuq@sina.com.cn

Abstract. In order to help enterprises to make a competitive strategy of price, a TOC accounting based decision making model of products pricing is proposed. A function between sales and prices is taken into account in a product decision-making model for the first time. The function between sales and prices could be yielded by statistical analyzing or forecasting. If an enterprise has much historical date on sales and price, BP neural network is adopted to get the function. Otherwise, polynomial fitting method is adopted. Genetic algorithm is adopted to solve the decision making model of products pricing and an optimized price is yielded. The validity of proposed model and algorithm are verified by corresponding with case studies.

Keywords: TOC accounting; decision making of products pricing; Genetic algorithm; Back-Propagation Neural Network, polynomial fitting method.

1 Introduction

The product pricing is a very sensitive element. It might affect the sales and profits. The pricing should facilitate both the promotion of sales and making profits. At the same time it should consider the customers' acceptance. The product pricing is heavily based on the accounting system. Currently there are two major different accounting systems. One is the widely used system, Traditional Accounting method. The other is TOC (Theory of Constrains) Accounting. Some Literatures[1-2] pointed out that in the current business condition Traditional Accounting method might cause corporate making mistakes on decision-making. However TOC accounting is simple and easy to calculate. It is more suitable for enterprise decision-making. Some scholars [1-2] have used TOC accounting in the product-mixing decision. However there were many hypotheses such as unchanged price of the product and less than market demands' sales in these studies. These hypotheses might not be consistent with the current oversupplying market and frequent price fluctuations etc. Therefore, it is very important to study TOC accounting based pricing when the sales changes with the price.

The rest of the paper is constructed as follows. Section 2 is devoted to introduce the TOC accounting system. Section 3 proposes a TOC accounting based productions pricing model and it's solution. Section 4 presents a computational test to indicate the process of pricing and validate the proposed model and algorithm. Finally a conclusion and future research fields are outlined.

C. Xiong et al. (Eds.): ICIRA 2008, Part II, LNAI 5315, pp. 485–494, 2008.

2 The TOC Accounting and Its Application

In order to measure the performance of enterprises, the TOC accounting [2] breaks the traditional cost accounting concept and proposes three major measurable indicators, namely: effective output, inventory and operating costs, shown in Figure 1. The profit of enterprises= effective output -operating expenses. The ratio of profits and the inventory is the Return on Investment (ROI) in the TOC. TOC figures that the enterprise as a whole to evaluate the effect of improvement, not just local. Stocks and operating costs could be reduced, but can not be reduced below zero. Only the effective output could continue to grow. TOC accounting [2-3] only distributes the cost of the direct materials costs on a variety of products. According to TOC accounting, how the fixed costs distribute on various products is meaningless.

TOC accounting is not the same as the traditional accounting. Some methods of calculating the cost in the TOC accounting are not allowed by in the traditional financial accounting system. Therefore, TOC accounting currently is only used in the in – house decision making.

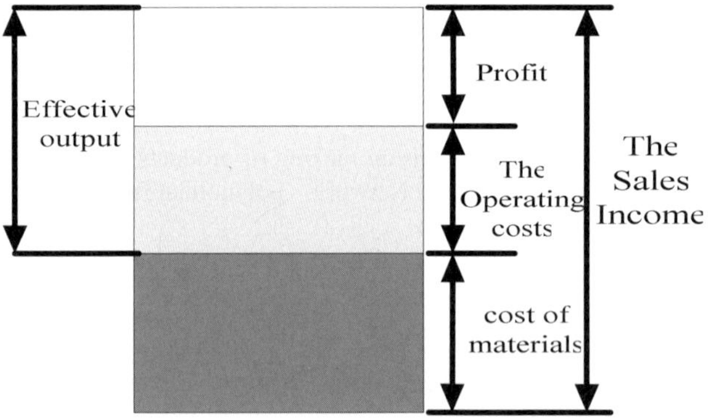

Fig. 1. The effective output in the TOC accounting

At present, TOC accounting is used in the decision making of product-mix for enterprises [3-4]. The literature [4] compared the ABC (ABC) accounting and the TOC accounting in the product-mix decision and concluded that the ABC accounting is better for long-term product-mix decision, and the TOC accounting was better for short-term product-mix decision. Currently all the studies of TOC accounting based decision making of products [4-5] assume that the prices are constant and the sales volume is less than the market demand. The relationship between corporate profits and production of different products is studied under this premise. However, the price of products has a direct impact on sales, thus affects the profits of corporate. Therefore pricing of product will ultimately affect the product mix programmed. Therefore, for the in-house decision-making, the pricing of products is more important than the product-mix. So, it is very important to study the decision-making of pricing in the condition of the sales of products changing with price. This study will help enterprises to make a competitive price strategy.

3 TOC Accounting Based Decision Making of Products Pricing

In order to model the TOC accounting based pricing, the modal of the product-mix decision in the reference [4] is modified. Firstly, the hypothesis of unchanged price in reference [4] is cancelled. So the price of product is variable. Secondly, the function of sales of products with its price is established. Then modal of decision making of products pricing is proposed as following.

$$\text{MAX} \quad Y = \sum_{i=1}^{Np}(p_i - c_{i0})X_{i1} - \sum_{j=1}^{N_A}\sum_{k=1}^{3} c_{jk}Q_{jk} \tag{1}$$

$$\text{ST} \quad \sum_{i=1}^{N_p} X_{ik}q_{ijk} \le Q_{jk} \qquad \forall j,k \tag{2}$$

$$X_{i1} \le D_i X_{i3} \qquad \forall i \tag{3}$$

$$X_{i1} \ge 0 \qquad \forall i \tag{4}$$

$$X_{i1} = X_{i2} \times B_i \qquad \forall i \tag{5}$$

$$X_{i3} = 0 \text{ Or } 1 \qquad \forall i \tag{6}$$

$$D_i = f(p_i) \tag{7}$$

Where Y is the objective function, the corporate profit; i: Item No. of the products, i=1,2...... N_p ; N_p: The number of product categories; j :Operating No., j=1, 2...... N_A ; N_A :The number of types of operations; k :The operating level,(k =1 says Products unit level, k =2 says batch level, k =3 says Product level); q_{ij1} :the number of operation j consumed by producing unit of product i; q_{ij2} :the number of operation j consumed by producing a batch of product i; q_{ij3} :the number of operation j consumed by producing product i; B_i :Bulk of the products i; Q_{jk} :available capacity of an operation j on the operating level k; c_{i0} :material costs consumed by producing unit of product i; c_{jk} :the unit cost of operations j on the implementation of the operating level k ; D_i :market demand of product i ; p_i :The selling price of product i ; X_{i1} :the Production volume of product i in a given time period; X_{i2} :the Production batches of product i in a given time period; X_{i3} is the strategy variable. If the company decides to produce product $i$in a given time period, then X_{i3} =1; otherwise X_{i3} =0.

In this model, from the objective function value Y it can be found that all kinds of enterprises operating costs are direct fixed costs but are not distributed to each product, which is in line with the standards of TOC accounting. In order to get greater profit, the enterprise needs to develop suitable price decision-making.

In order to make a competitive decision on pricing, the enterprises should follow the following steps shown in Fig 2.

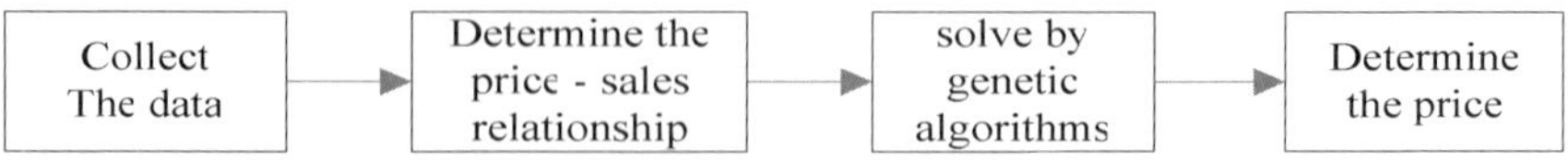

Fig. 2. Steps of decision-making of pricing

Firstly, the enterprise needs to be aware of various factors that impact the enterprises' sales, like Brand awareness x_1 , consumption level x_2 , market saturation x_3 , the size of the market x_4 , the price and others might have a great impact on the product sales. Then collect relevant data. After the enterprise could do some correlation analyze to identify the most important factor and at the same time cancel some irrelevant factors or remove some unreasonable data.

Because different enterprises in different periods have or can collect different amount of data, if an enterprise has many historical market data, regression method can be used to get the relationship between the demand and the relevant variables. As the relationship is nonlinear, the BP neural network [6] is adopted to do multiple nonlinear regression analysis to get the function of the price and the demand. Otherwise, polynomial fitting method could be adopted to forecast the relationship between the price and the demand.

It has been proved that a threshold, at least one hidden layer with a linear output of the network, can approach any non-linear continuous mapping, in Figure 3.

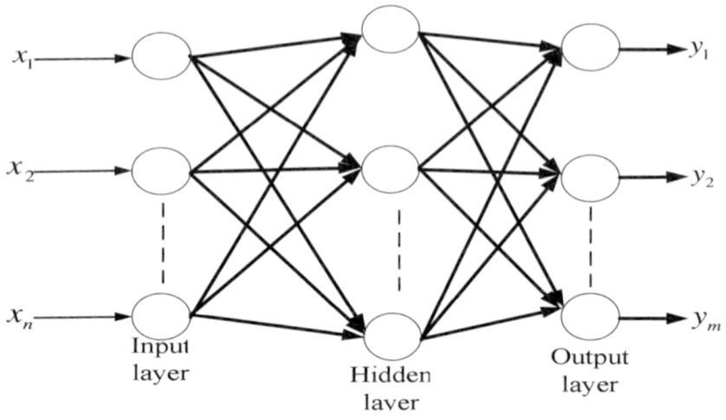

Fig. 3. BP Neural network structure

If BP neural network is adopted, the floors layer of the network general is firstly considered to only have a hidden layer. Only if a hidden layer whit many hidden nodes still could not improve network performance, the number of hidden layer could be increased. The input and output nodes are determined by the variable dimension. The BP neural network in this paper has only one hidden layer. The transmission functions of the nerve cell were selected TANSIG function and PURELIN function, Anti-function of the BP network is set TRAINLM.

However when enterprises have relatively few data on the market demand, or there are some errors in the data, the BP neural network is invalid. In this case, only the factor of price is considered to affect the market demand. It is relatively easy to get the market demands in several price points by qualitative analysis. Therefore, Polynomial fitting could be adopted to get the function between the market demand and the price in the whole range of prices. If a group of the product prices and the corresponding sales is given $\{(x_i, y_i), i=1, 2, ..., N\}$, polynomial model [7] is adopted to describe the data set. The fitting goal is to minimize the χ^2 in (9) .such as the type (8): strike parameters $a_1, a_2, \ldots, a_n, a_{n+1}$.

$$y(x) = f(a,x) = a_1 x^n + a_2 x^{n-1} + ... + a_n x + a_{n+1} \tag{8}$$

$$\chi^2(a) = \sum_{i=1}^{N} \left(\frac{y_i - (a_1 x_i^n + a_2 x_i^{n-1} + ... + a_n x_i + a_{n+1})}{\Delta y_i}\right)^2 \tag{9}$$

If the order of Polynomial is too low, the fitting effect might be bad. If the order of polynomial is too high, it might cause over fitting, the errors are also included in the calculation.

Due to lacking of original accurate data of price and sales, a higher order of Polynomial could not make a better fitting effect. Therefore, second or third order polynomials are adopted in practice.

After determining the relationship between the sales and the price $D_i = f(p_i)$, genetic algorithms [8] is used to solve the model (1). The problem is a limited constraint of non-linear programming problem; the non-binding for the situation should be excluded or use the method of increasing the penalty function to make it an unlimited bound and non-linear problem.

4 An Example

Some product-related data of an enterprise are shown in table 1.In order to help managers quickly make decision on pricing; it is not needed necessary to distribute the operating costs according to TOC accounting. Therefore, Effective price which is sale price minus material costs could be used to instead of the actual sale price of product according to TOC accounting. The effectively price can directly indicate the profits of enterprises. For simplifying, all prices in the rest of the paper are the effective prices.

The enterprise produces two types of products A and B. The price, which is actual sale price minus the cost of materials, of products A and B are P_A and P_B respectively. The sales of product A, y_A could not affect the sales of product B, y_B. Brand awareness x_1, consumption levels x_2, market saturation x_3, the size of the market x_4, and product prices are the main factors affecting demands. The higher the brand awareness x_1 of enterprise, the more demands are. The higher the level of consumption x_2 , the more demands are. The higher the degree of market saturation x_3, the less demands are. The highest scores for x_1 and x_3 are both ten. The bigger the size of the market x_4 , the more demands are. The original dates are show in table 2.

Table 1. Product-related data

	Operating	Cost Driver	Product A	Product B	Capacity (10,000)	Budget Costs (Million)	Unit Cost (Yuan)
Products unit level	Human	Working hours	0.5	1	24	48	2
	Machines	Working hours	1	0.5	24	144	3
Products level	Drawings	The number	100	200	300	3	100

In order to use MATLAB to generate two BP neural networks, all data are pre-treated into [0 1] range. The input data of the first network are x_1 , x_2 , x_3 , x_4 and P_A , the output data of the first networks is y_A . The input data of the second networks are x_1 , x_2 , x_3 , x_4 and P_B , the output data of the second networks is y_B . The data in the table 2 are used to train the network. The number of iterative and the hidden layer of hidden nodes are adjusted to meet the requirements. The number of iterative is 100 and the hidden layer of hidden nodes is 9 in the first network. And the number of iterative is 100 and the hidden layer of hidden nodes is 11 in the second network. After training the network, the current market situation: $x_1 = 10$, $x_2 = 1140$, $x_3 = 9.5$, $x_4 = 1000$ etc are put into the trained neural networks. Then the function of sales with the current price, $D_i = f(p_i)$, is yielded. Inputting some price points in the range to the neural networks, can get some sale points corresponding to price, and then draw the graphics of the function showed in fig 4.

In order to solve modal of decision making of products pricing in formula (1), The genetic algorithm is adopted, gets the optimal pricing and the corresponding sales of two types of products A and B. Initial population is 100,the number of iterative is 100, cross-rate is 0.9, the mutation rate is 0.1. Therefore the enterprise could get the largest profits of 2.416 million Yuan if both products A and B are produced and the effective price for both products are P_A =13.8(Yuan), P_B =15.6(Yuan) respectively. In this case the sales of both products are y_A =15.80 (million) and y_B =14.01(million).

On the other hand, if a company has no relative data, it is still possible for the company to make decision on pricing. It is relatively easy for a company to forecast the sales of products at certain prices shown in tables 3 and 4. The enterprise forecasts the minimum sales volume, most likely sales and the largest sales volume according

Table 2. The original data

o	x_1	x_2 (Yuan)	x_3	x_4 (million)	P_A (Yuan)	y_A (million)	P_B (Yuan)	y
	9.8	950	9	970	11	21	13	7
	10	1140	9.5	1000	9	24	11	0
	9.5	600	8.8	600	14	16	16	2
	7	940	8.5	680	10	22	12	8
	8	1080	9.2	1400	14	17	16	3
	6.8	770	7	1200	12	19	14	5
	9	890	7.5	642	10	20	12	6
	10	730	9.7	483	11	19	13	5
	7	850	7.4	700	12	18	14	4
0	8	970	6.8	750	13	17	15	3
1	9	680	6.5	800	14	16	16	2
2	8	780	7.3	720	12	18	14	4

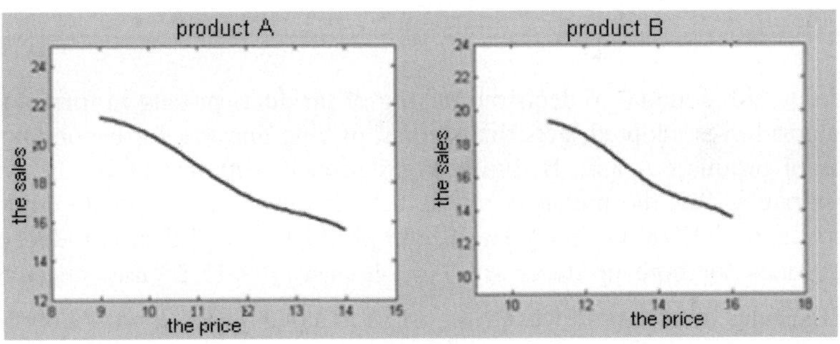

Fig. 4. The relationship between the current price and sales

to the certain product prices (that is sale price minus the cost of materials). The formula (10) is adopted to accurately forecast the sales of the products A and B in a given category of the sales price, as seen table 3, 4.

$$\text{Sales} = (\text{the minimum sales+the largest sales}+4\times\text{the most likely sales})/6 \qquad (20)$$

Based on the data of the tables 3 and 4, MATLAB programming is used to do the polynomial fitting. The quadratic polynomial fitting is adopted and the fitting results are shown in Figure 5.

Table 3. The relationship of Prices-sales (A)

Price(P_A) (Yuan)	the minimum sales (million)	the most likely sales (million)	the largest sales (million)	the sales (y_A) (million)
9	20	24	27	23.83
11	15	20	23	19.67
12	14	18	22	18
14	12	16	19	15.83

Table 4. The relationship of Prices-sales (B)

Price (P_B) (元)	the minimum sales (million)	the most likely sales (million)	the largest sales (million)	the sales (y_A) (million)
11	14	18	23	18.17
13	10	14	19	14.17
14	8	13	18	13
16	7	11	15	11

In order to solve modal of decision making of products pricing in formula (1), The genetic algorithm is adopted, gets the optimal pricing and the corresponding sales of two types of products A and, B. Initial population is 100,the number of iterative is 100, cross-rate is 0.9, the mutation rate is 0.1.Therefore the corporate could get the largest profits of 2.1778 million Yuan if both products A and B are produced and the effective prices for both products are P_A =14(Yuan), P_B =12.2(Yuan) respectively. In this case the sales of both products are y_A =15.82 (million) and y_B =15.68(million).

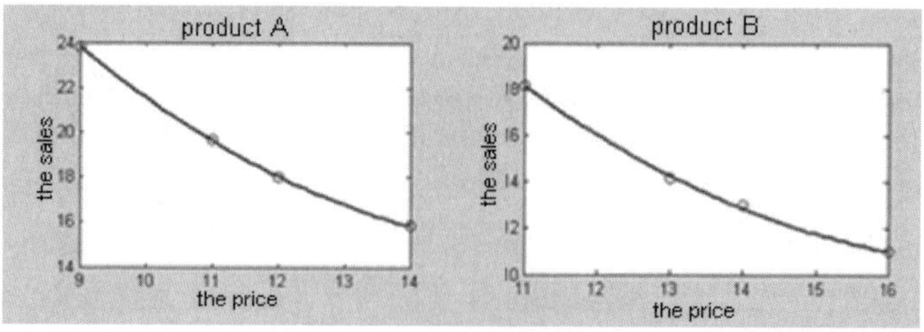

Fig. 5. The relationship of Prices-sales

5 Conclusion

TOC accounting is different from the traditional accounting. As it is not needed necessary for TOC to distribute the fixed costs and calculate the unit costs, the managers could quickly make decision on product pricing and help company make profits. According to the computational results in this paper, if an enterprise has more relevant data, then the function of the sales with the price could be generated by the BP neural network. Based on the assessment of the current market conditions: Enterprise brand awareness is very high, the local consumption level x_2 = 1,140 Yuan; products in a saturated market x_3 = 9.5; the market size x_4 = 10000000, the company could make the conclusion that the enterprise could get the most profit 2.416 million Yuan if the company produces product A of 158,000 pieces and sale it at unit effective price of 13.8 Yuan and produces product B of 140,100 pieces and sale it at unit effective price of 15.6 Yuan. For other enterprises that have few data, it is possible to get the function of the sales with the price by the polynomial fitting. The company could make the conclusion that the enterprise could get the most profit 2.1778 million Yuan if the company produces product A of 158,200 pieces and sale it at unit effective price of 14 Yuan and produces product B of 156,800 pieces and sale it at unit effective price of 15.82 Yuan.

This paper proposes TOC accounting based decision making model of products pricing, firstly taking the function between sales and prices into account in a product decision-making model. It also does research on the application of the model in the enterprise, verify the validity of the model, get the conclusions that this model can help enterprise develop the right price and get the maximum benefit in a the highly competitive market environment.

Acknowledgement

This work is supported by National High-Tech Research and Development Program of China Grant # 2007AA04Z190 and # 2007AA04Z10, National Natural Science Foundation of China Grand # 50705036.

References

1. Ma, G.F., Tu, M.Z., Shi, Z.Z.: The history of costing method based TOC accounting of in strategic decision-making research. Industrial Engineering and Management 3, 115–120 (2005)
2. Zhang, L.H., Jiang, W.B.: TOC accounting. Industrial Engineering 4, 51–56 (2005)
3. Cao, D.B., Wang, J., Sun, Y.: Theory of Constraints-U.S. manufacturing secret weapon. Industrial Engineering and Management 6, 22–26 (2001)
4. Fu, A.: Theory of Constraints and Activity-Based Costing: Can we get the best of both worlds? Business Review 2, 67–74 (2000)
5. Robert, K., Charles, S.: Comparative analysis of utilizing activity-based costing and the theory of constraints for making product-mix decisions. International Journal of Production Economics 63, 1–7 (2000)

6. Wang, C.Y., Tang, Y.C., Liu, T.: Study on forecasting smooth-surface blasting effects based on BP neural network. Journal of Liaoning Technical University 1, 73–75 (2005)
7. Yang, C., Liu, R.Z., Yang, Z.Y.: Master MATLAB. Beijing University of Aeronautics and Astronautics Press, Beijing (1997)
8. Qiao, W., Wang, B., Sun, J.: Uncertain Job Shop scheduling problems solved by genetic algorithm. Computer Integrated Manufacturing Systems 12, 2452–2455 (2007)

A Genetic Algorithm for Integration of Process Planning and Scheduling Problem

Xinyu Li, Liang Gao, Guohui Zhang, Chaoyong Zhang, and Xinyu Shao

The State Key Laboratory of Digital Manufacturing Equipment and Technology
Huazhong University of Science and Technology, Wuhan, Hubei, China
gaoliang@mail.hust.edu.cn

Abstract. Traditionally, process planning and scheduling for parts are carried out in a sequential way, where scheduling is done after process plans have been generated. Considering the two functions are usually complementary, there is a great potential to integrate them more tightly so that greater performance and higher productivity of a manufacturing system can be achieved. In this paper, a genetic algorithm-based approach has been developed to facilitate the integration and optimization of these two functions. To improve the optimized performance of the genetic algorithm-based approach, efficient genetic representations and operator schemes have been developed. Experiment studies have been conducted. The experimental results show that the proposed approach is a promising and very effective method for the integration of process planning and scheduling.

Keywords: Integration of process planning and scheduling, Process planning, Scheduling, Genetic algorithm.

1 Introduction

Process planning and scheduling are two of the most important sub-systems in manufacturing system. A process plan specifies raw materials or components what are needed to produce a product, processes and operations which are necessary to transform those raw materials into the final product. It is the bridge of the product design and manufacturing. The outcome of process planning is the information of manufacturing processes and the identification of the machines tools and fixtures. And, most jobs may have a large number of alternative process plans. Scheduling plans receive process plans as their input and their task is to schedule the operations on the machines while respecting the precedence relations given in the process plans. It is the link of the two production steps which are the preparing processes and putting them into action [1]. There is a strong relationship between process planning and scheduling.

In the beginning research of computer integrated manufacturing system (CIMS), some researchers have found that the integration of process planning and scheduling (IPPS) is very important to the development of CIMS. Chryssolouris and Chan [2] were the first to propose the preliminary idea of the integration of process planning and scheduling. Beckendorff [3] used alternative process plans to improve the flexibility of manufacturing system. Khoshnevis and Chen [4] introduced the concept of

C. Xiong et al. (Eds.): ICIRA 2008, Part II, LNAI 5315, pp. 495–502, 2008.

dynamic feedback into the integration of process planning and scheduling. The integration model which was proposed by Zhang [5] and Larsen [6] extended the concepts of alternative process plans and dynamic feedback. And it also gave expression to the methodology of hierarchical approach. Some earlier works of the integration strategy have been summarized in [7].

More recently, Lee and Kim [8] presented the nonlinear process planning model which was based on the genetic algorithm. Kim and Park [9] used a symbiotic evolutionary algorithm for the integration of process planning and job shop scheduling. Tan and Khoshnevis [10] presented a mixed integer programming model to solve process planning and scheduling problems. Li and McMahon [11] used a simulated annealing-based approach for flexible process plans.

In this paper, a genetic algorithm based approach has been developed to facilitate the integration and optimization of this problem. Through experimental studies, the merits of the approach can be shown clearly.

2 Problem Formulation

The IPPS problem can be defined as follows [12]:

Given a set of n parts which are to be processed on machines with operations including alternative manufacturing resources, select suitable manufacturing resources and sequence the operations so as to determine a schedule in which the precedence constraints among operations can be satisfied and the corresponding objectives can be achieved.

The most popular criteria for scheduling include makespan, job tardiness and the balanced level of machine utilization, while manufacturing cost is the major criterion for process planning [13]. In this paper, scheduling is often assumed as job shop scheduling, and makespan is used as the criteria.

Job shop scheduling problem (JSP) has been proved to be a NP-hard problem. The problem in this paper is more complicated than JSP. It is also known as a NP-hard problem. When for large problems, it can not be found the exact solution in the reasonable time. So, in this paper, a genetic algorithm based approach has been used to solve it.

3 Genetic Algorithm for IPPS

3.1 Representation

Each chromosome in scheduling population consists of two parts with different length as shown in Fig.1. The first part of chromosome is the alternative process plan string (B-string). The positions from 1 to n in this string represent the job from 1 to n. The number in the ith position represents the alternative process plan of the ith job which has been chosen.

The second part of chromosome is the scheduling plan string (A-string). In this paper, the scheduling encoding is the operation-based representation, which is made up of the Genes (The fist number is the jobs' number and the second number is the alternative machine).

For the first number in the Genes, it is represented by a permutation of the operations. Different appearances of this number in the chromosome represent different operations of the job, and the sequence of the appearances of this number is the same with the sequence of the operations of the job. The important feature of representation is that all offspring formed by crossover are feasible solutions. It is assumed that there are n jobs, and qi is the number of operations of the process plan which has the most operation numbers among all the alternative process plans of the ith job. Then the length of the A-string is equal to $\sum q_i$. The number of appearances of i in the A-string is equal to the number of operations of the alternative process plan which has been chosen. Based on this principle, the composition elements of A-string are determined. If the number of the elements is less than $\sum q_i$, all the other elements are filled with 0. One A-string is generated by arraying all the elements randomly. And the B-string is generated by choosing the alternative process plan randomly for every job.

For the second number of gene is the alternative machine for each operation. It denotes the selected machine set of the corresponding operations of all jobs. Assuming the *h*th operation in the selected alternative process plan of job *i* can be processed by a machine set $S_{ih} = \{m_{ih1}, m_{ih2}, \ldots, m_{ihc_{ih}}\}$. The *i*th part of this string can be denoted as $g_{i1} g_{i2} \cdots g_{ih} \cdots g_{iq_i}$, and g_{ih} is an integer between 1 and c_{ih} and it means that the *h*th operation in the selected alternative process plan of job *i* is assigned to the g_{ih}th machine $m_{ihg_{ih}}$ in S_{ih}. If the number of the operations of the selected alternative process plan of job *i* is *p* and *p* is less than q_i, $g_{ip} \cdots g_{iq_i}$ are equal to 0.

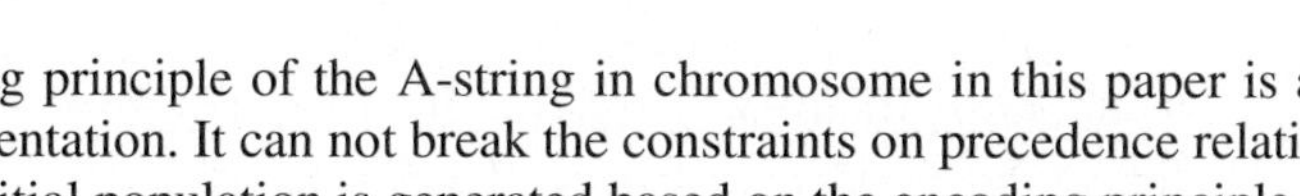

Fig. 1. The chromosome of the integration

3.2 Initialization

The encoding principle of the A-string in chromosome in this paper is an operation-based representation. It can not break the constraints on precedence relations of operations. The initial population is generated based on the encoding principle.

3.3 Crossover and Mutation

(1) Crossover

The procedure of the crossover for scheduling is described as follows:

Step 1: Select a pair of chromosomes P1 and P2 by the selection scheme and initialize two empty offspring: O1 and O2;

Step 2: crossover the B-strings of P1 and P2 and get the B-strings of O1 and O2;

Step 2.1: Compare the B-string of P1 with the B-string of P2, if the element of P1 is the same as P2, record the value and position of this element. This process is repeated until all the elements of B-string have been compared;

Step 2.2: The recorded elements in B-string of P1 in *Step* 2.1 are appended to the same positions in O1; the recorded elements in B-string of P2 in *Step* 2.1 are appended to the same positions in O2. The other elements (they are the different elements between P1 and P2) in B-string of P2 are appended to the same positions in O1; the other elements in B-string of P1 are appended to the same positions in O2.

Step 3: in order to match the B-strings of O1 and O2 and avoid getting unlawful O1 and O2, the A-strings of P1 and P2 are crossovered as follows:

Step 3.1: If the values of the first numbers of Genes in A-string of P1 are the same as the recorded positions in B-string, these Genes (include (0, 0)) are appended to the same positions in O1 and they are deleted in P1; if the values of the first numbers of Genes in A-string of P2 are the same as the recorded positions in B-string, these Genes (include (0, 0)) are appended to the same positions in O2 and they are deleted in P2.

Step 3.2: Get the numbers of the remaining Genes in A-strings of P1 and P2, n_1 and n_2. If $n_1 \geq n_2$, for O1, it implies that the number of empty positions in O1 is bigger than the number of remaining elements in P2. So, $n_1 - n_2$ empty positions in O1 are selected randomly and be filled with (0, 0). Then, the remaining elements in A-string of P2 are appended to the remaining empty positions in O1 seriatim. For O2, $n_1 \geq n_2$ implies that the number of empty positions in O2 is smaller than the number of remaining elements in P1. So, $n_1 - n_2$ (0,0) are selected randomly in O2 and are set to empty. And then, the remaining elements in A-string of P1 are appended to the empty positions in O2 seriatim; if $n_1 < n_2$, the procedure is reversed.

Step 4: Then, two valid offspring O1 and O2 are achieved.

One example is showed in Fig. 2.

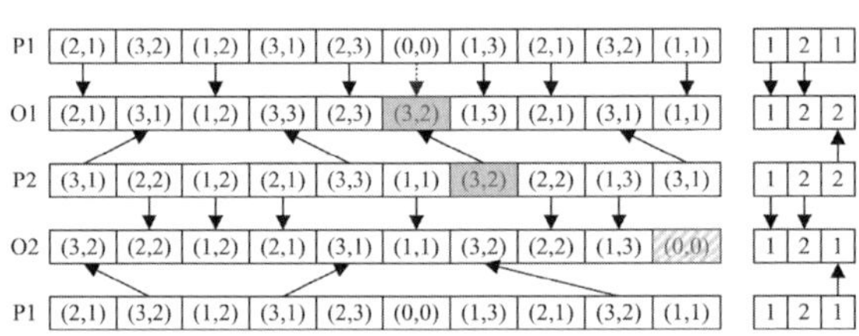

Fig. 2. The crossover operation

(2) Mutation

In this paper, three mutation operators have been used. The first one is two-point swapping mutation, the second one is changing one job's alternative process plan, and the third one is the mutation of alternative machines. In the evolution procedure, one operator has been chosen randomly in every generation.

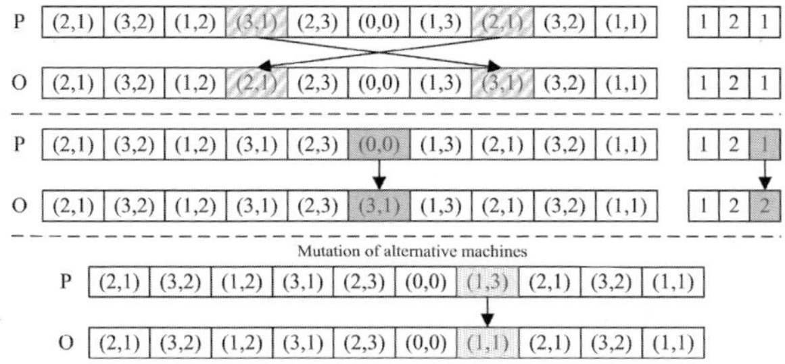

Fig. 3. Mutation operation

The procedure of the second mutation (changing one job's alternative process plan) for scheduling is described as follows:

Step 1: Select one chromosome P by the selection scheme;
Step 2: Select one point in the B-string of P randomly;
Step 3: Change the value of this selected element to another one in the selection area (the number of alternative process plans);
Step 4: Judge the number of the operations of the selected job's alternative process plan which has been changed. If it has been enlarged, a new chromosome O is generated by changing the margin (0, 0) which are selected randomly to the job's number in the A-string of P seriatim; if it has been lessened, a new chromosome O is generated by changing the margin job's number which are selected randomly in the A-string of P to (0, 0) seriatim.

The mutation of alternative machines is applied in order to change the alternative machine represented. One element in the A-string is randomly chosen from the selected individual. Then, this element is mutated by altering the machine number (the second number of Gene) to another one of the alternative machines at random. One example of mutation is showed in Fig. 3.

4 Experimental Studies

Two experiments are presented to illustrate the proposed method for integrated process planning and scheduling. And in this paper, the makespan is used as the objective. The integration model has been compare with no integration model. No integration means that there is only one process plan for each job (In this paper, each job chooses the first alternative process plan as its process plan in the no integration model.).

4.1 Experimental Studies

4.1.1 Problem 1

Experiment 1 is adopted from Sundaram and Fu [14]. In this experiment, one problem is constructed with 5 jobs and 5 machines, and the makespan is used as the objective. Each part undergoes four different operations in a specified order.

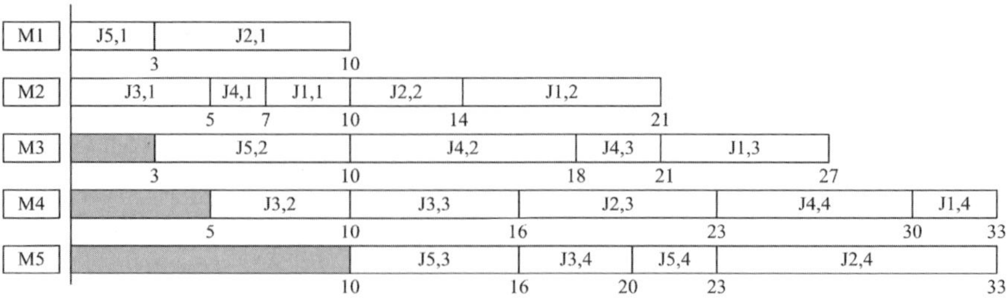

Fig. 4. Gantt chart of experiment 1 (Makespan = 33)

Using the proposed approach, the best value obtained is 33 compared with the value of 38 obtained using the heuristic reported by Sundaram and Fu [14]. Palmer [15] used simulated annealing (SA) for this problem and obtained the same result of 33. The advantage of the proposed approach compared with the SA approach is the availability of multiple solutions that injects some flexibility into the decision-making process. If the best solution produced can not be implemented due to machine breakdown or tardiness in delivery of raw material, the decision-maker can resort to other solutions that can provide the same optimal or near-optimal solutions without run the whole process again. In the SA approach, only one solution is produced for every run. Fig.4 illustrates Gantt chart of this problem for scheduling.

4.1.2 Problem 2

Experiment 2 is adopted from [16] which has considered the outsourcing machine. In this experiment, four problems are constructed with 8 jobs and 6 machines, and the makespan is used as the objective. And in this paper, the outsourcing machine was not considered. Table 1 shows the experimental results, and Fig.5 illustrates Gantt chart of the first problem in this experiment. In this experiment, each job chooses the first alternative process plan as its process plan in the no integration model.

Table 1. The experimental results of experiment 2

Problem	Parts	Operation	Machine	Makespan	
				Integration	No Integration
1	8	20	6	23	31
2	16	40	6	43	57
3	32	80	6	84	111
4	64	160	6	168	219

Based on the experimental results of experiment 2, the makespan of scheduling of no integration is worse than the integration model. And the integration model can get better scheduling plans.

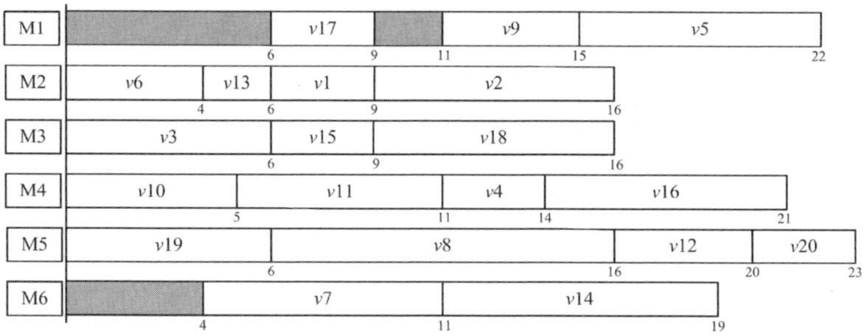

Fig. 5. Gantt chart of the first problem in experiment 2 (makespan=23)

5 Conclusion

In traditional approach, process planning and scheduling are regarded as two separate tasks and performed sequentially. However, the functions of the two systems are usually complementary. Therefore, the research on the integration of process planning and scheduling is necessary. This paper has developed a genetic algorithm-based approach to facilitate the integration and optimization of these two systems. To improve the optimization performance of the proposed approach, the efficient genetic representations and operator schemes have been developed. Experimental studies have been used to test the approach, and the comparison has been made. The experimental results show that the proposed approach is a promising and very effective method in the research of integration of process planning and scheduling.

With the approach developed in this work, it would be possible to increase the efficiency of manufacturing systems. One future work is to apply the proposed approach to practical manufacturing systems. The increased use of this approach will probably enhance the performances of future manufacturing systems.

Acknowledgements. This research work is supported by the National High-Tech Research and Development Program of China (863 Program) under grant No.2007AA04Z107 and 2006AA04Z131.

References

1. Sugimura, N., Hino, R., Moriwaki, T.: Integrated Process Planning and Scheduling in Holonic Manufacturing Systems. In: IEEE International Symposium on Assembly and Task Planning Soft Research Park, vol. 4, pp. 250–254. IEEE Press, New York (2001)
2. Chryssolouris, G., Chan, S., Cobb, W.: Decision Making on The Factory Floor: An Integrated Approach to Process Planning and Scheduling. Robot. Comput.-Integr. Manuf. 1(3-4), 315–319 (1984)
3. Beckendorff, U., Kreutzfeldt, J., Ullmann, W.: Reactive Workshop Scheduling Based on Alternative Routings. In: Proceedings of Conference on Factory Automation and Information Management, pp. 875–885. CRC Press, Inc., Florida (1991)

4. Khoshnevis, B., Chen, Q.M.: Integration of Process Planning and Scheduling Function. In: Proceedings of IIE Integrated Systems Conference & Society for Integrated Manufacturing, pp. 415–420. Industrial Engineering & Management Press, Atlanta (1989)
5. Zhang, H.C.: IPPM-A Prototype to Integrated Process Planning and Job Shop Scheduling Functions. Annals of the CIRP 42(1), 513–517 (1993)
6. Larsen, N.E.: Methods for Integration of Process Planning and Production Planning. Int. J. Comput. Integr. Manuf. 6(1-2), 152–162 (1993)
7. Tan, W., Khoshnevis, B.: Integration of Process Planning and Scheduling – A Review. J. Intell. Manuf. 11, 51–63 (2000)
8. Lee, H., Kim, S.S.: Integration of Process Planning and Scheduling Using Simulation Based Genetic Algorithms. Int. J. Adv. Manuf. Technol. 18, 586–590 (2001)
9. Kim, Y.K., Park, K., Ko, J.: A Symbiotic Evolutionary Algorithm for The Integration of Process Planning and Job Shop Scheduling. Comput. Oper. Res. 30, 1151–1171 (2003)
10. Tan, W., Khoshnevis, B.: A Linearized Polynomial Mixed Integer Programming Model for The Integration of Process Planning and Scheduling. J. Intell. Manuf. 15, 593–605 (2004)
11. Li, W.D., McMahon, C.A.: A Simulated Annealing – Based Optimization Approach for Integrated Process Planning and Scheduling. Int. J. Comput. Integr. Manuf. 20(1), 80–95 (2007)
12. Guo, Y.W., Li, W.D., Mileham, A.R., Owen, G.W.: Applications of Particle Swarm and Optimization in Integrated Process Planning and Scheduling. Robot. Comput.-Integr. Manuf. (2008), doi:10.1016/j.rcim.2007.12.002
13. Li, W.D., Gao, L., Li, X.Y., Guo, Y.: Game Theory-Based Cooperation of Process Planning and Scheduling. In: Proceeding of CSCWD, pp. 841–845. IEEE Press, New York (2008)
14. Sundaram, R.M., Fu, S.S.: Process Planning and Scheduling. Comput. Ind. Eng. 15(1-4), 296–307 (1988)
15. Palmer, G.J.: A Simulated Annealing Approach to Integrated Production Scheduling. J. Intell. Manuf. 7(3), 163–176 (1996)
16. Lee, Y.H., Jeong, C.S., Moon, C.: Advanced Planning and Scheduling with Outsourcing in Manufacturing Supply Chain. Comput. Ind. Eng. 43, 351–374 (2002)

Variable Neighborhood Genetic Algorithm for the Flexible Job Shop Scheduling Problems

Guohui Zhang, Liang Gao*, Xinyu Li, and Peigen Li

The State Key Laboratory of Digital Manufacturing Equipment and Technology
Huazhong University of Science & Technology, Wuhan, 430074, China
gaoliang@mail.hust.edu.cn

Abstract. Flexible job shop scheduling problem (FJSP) is an important extension of the classical job shop scheduling problem, where the same operation could be processed on more than one machine. A Variable Neighborhood Genetic Algorithm (VNGA) is proposed for the problem with makespan criterion, consisting of a combination of the variable neighborhood search (VNS) and genetic algorithm (GA). Variable neighborhood search is adopted to improve the quality of individuals of GA before injecting them into the population and strengthen the local search ability. Two different neighborhood structures are used in the VNS. Representative flexible job shop scheduling benchmark problems are solved using the VNGA. Computational results show that the proposed algorithm is efficient and effective.

Keywords: Genetic Algorithm, Variable Neighborhood Search, Flexible job shop scheduling.

1 Introduction

The classical Job-shop Scheduling Problem (JSP) is one of the most difficult problems in this area [1]. The JSP has been proven to be NP-hard [2]. In the real manufacturing systems, an operation could be allocated to a suitable machine from an alternative machines set. It is known as the Flexible Job-shop Scheduling Problem (FJSP). The FJSP is a generalization of the classical JSP. And the FJSP is also NP-hard. Each machine may be capable of performing more than one type of operations. The problem of scheduling jobs in FJSP could be decomposed into two sub-problems: the routing sub-problem, which is assigning each operation to a machine selected out of a set of capable machines and the scheduling sub-problem, which consists of sequencing the assigned operations on all machines in order to obtain a feasible schedule minimizing the predefined objective function.

Bruker and Schile [3] were the first to address this problem in 1990, they develop a polynomial graphical algorithm for a two jobs problem. However exact algorithms are not effective for solving FJSP and for large instances. In recent years several heuristic procedures and meta-heuristics have been developed for

* Corresponding author.

C. Xiong et al. (Eds.): ICIRA 2008, Part II, LNAI 5315, pp. 503–512, 2008.

FJSP. Kacem et al. [4] used tasks sequencing list coding scheme and developed an approach by localization (AL) to find promising initial assignment. Then, dispatching rules were applied to sequence the operations. Dauzére-Pérès et al. [5] proposed different tabu search heuristic approach and neighborhood structure based on disjunctive graph to solve the FJSP. Mastrolilli and Gambardella [6] proposed some neighborhood functions for the FJSP. Ho et al. [7] proposed an architecture for learning and evolving of FJSP to improve the computational time and quality of solutions. Gao et al. [8] combined the GA and a variable neighborhood descent (VND) for solving the FJSP, the VND was adopted to strengthen the local search ability. In this paper, a hybrid genetic algorithm (GA) and variable neighborhood search (VNS) is used to solve the FJSP. An improved chromosome representation method is used to express the machine selection and operation sequencing information for different type FJSP. And under the framework of the GA, the VNS is applied to each newly generated offspring to improve its quality before injecting it into the population. There were two neighborhood structures for VNS, moving one operation and moving two operations respectively.

2 Problem Description

The flexible job shop scheduling problem could be formulated as follows.

- There is a set of n jobs $J = \{J_1, \ldots, J_n\}$ to be processed. Each job J_i consists of a predetermined sequence of operations. Each job J_i may have different operation number. However, there has the same operation number for the classical JSP.
- There is a set of m machines $M = \{M_1, \ldots, M_m\}$. For each operation O_{ij} , there is a set of alternative machines set M_{ij} of performing it. Then each job could be processed more than once on the same machine. The processing time of each operation on each machine is predefined.
- All jobs are released at time 0. All machines are available at time 0. The machine of executing each operation is non preemption. And each machine could perform at most one operation at any time. There are no precedence constraints among operations of different jobs. The objective in this paper is to find a schedule with shortest makespan, where the makespan of a schedule is the time required for all jobs to be processed in the job shop according to the schedule.

According to Kacem *et al.* [4], If $M_{ij} \subset M$, it is partial FJSP (P-FJSP). Each operation could be processed on one machine of subset of M. If $M_{ij} = M$, it is total FJSP (T-FJSP). Each operation could be processed on any machine of M. With the same number of machines and jobs, the P-FJSP is more difficult to solve than the T-FJSP [4].

In order to describe the algorithm more easily, we give an illustrative instance of FJSP. In Table 1, there are 2 jobs and 5 machines. In the table, the "-" means that the machine can't execute the corresponding operation, i.e., it does not belong to the subset of compatible machines for that operation. This instance presents a P-FJSP.

Table 1. An instance of FJSP

Job	*Operation*	M_1	M_2	M_3	M_4	M_5
J_1	O_{11}	2	6	5	3	4
	O_{12}	-	8	-	4	-
J_2	O_{21}	3	-	6	-	5
	O_{22}	4	6	5	-	-
	O_{23}	-	7	11	5	8

3 A GA for FJSP

3.1 Representation of Individuals

Chromosome representation is important to find solutions in a heuristic or meta-heuristic algorithm. Better chromosome representation is well designed, no infeasible solutions will be produced after genetic recombination and the algorithm could expect to be more efficient by avoiding the use of a repair mechanism. Chen et al. [1] divided the chromosome into two parts: A-string and B-string. A-string denotes the routing policy of the problem, and B-string denotes the sequence of the operations on each machine, but this method need to consider the order of operations and require a repair mechanism. Kacem et al. [4] represented the chromosome by an assignment table representation. A data structure of the assignment table must necessarily describe the set of all machines. This increases the overall time complexity due to the presence of redundant assignments. Ho et al. [7] also divided the chromosome into two strings, the first string represents the operation order and the second string represents the machine by an array of binary values. This structure can represent the problem clearly and conveniently, but the binary-coded increases the memory space and the operation is not convenient, so when the scale of problem is oversized, the memory space and computational time will increase tremendously [9]. In this paper, an improved chromosome representation is used. The chromosome representation has two components (called MSOS): Machine Selection (MS) and Operation Sequence (OS), in Fig. 1.

Machine selection part: We use an array of integer values to present machine selection. The length L is the sum of all operations of all jobs. Each integer value equals to the index of alternative machines set of each operation. For instance, in Fig.1, M_2 is selected to process operation O_{12} because the index

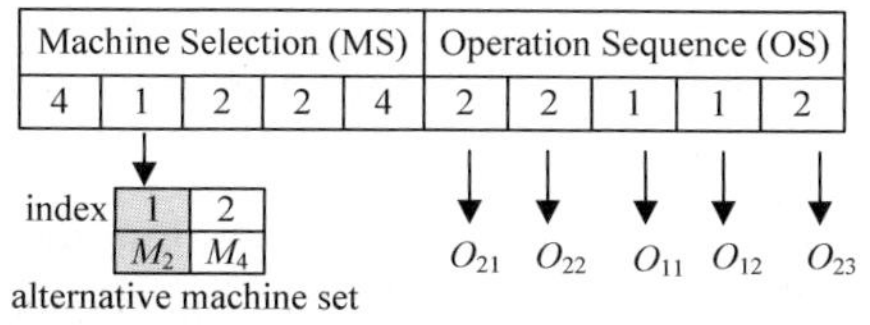

Fig. 1. The structure of MSOS representation

in the alternative machines set of processing operation O_{12} is 1. If only one machine could be selected to some operations, the value is 1 in the machine selection array.

Operation sequence part: We use the operation-based representation, which defines all operations for a job with the same symbol and then interpret them according to the order of occurrence in the sequence of a given chromosome. The length is L too. It can avoid creating an infeasible schedule through replacing each operation by the corresponding job index. In Table 1. J_1 has two operations O_{11}, O_{12}; J_2 has three operations O_{21}, O_{22}, O_{23}. In Fig.1, reading the data from left to right and increasing operation index of each job, the operation sequence 2-2-1-1-2 depicted could be translated into a list of ordered operations: O_{21}-O_{22}-O_{11}-O_{12}-O_{23}.

3.2 Selection

The task of selection is that better individuals are chose and moved into a mating pool for reproduction. The chosen individuals could be reproduced once or more times in different literature. The roulette wheel selection is a fitness-based approach. The objective fitness value that is achieved by decoding chromosome must be repaired for solving FJSP. In order to overcome the scaling problem of the direct fitness-based approach, tournament approach is adopted in our paper. And the number of tournament approach is three. Three individuals are randomly chosen from parent population, and three objective values are directly compared to select the best individual to move into the mating pool.

3.3 Crossover

The goal of the crossover is to obtain better chromosomes to improve the result by exchanging information contained in the current good ones. According to the chromosome having two components, two kinds of crossover operators are used for both MS and OS respectively.

Machine Selection Part: For the alternative machines of each operation could be different, the machine must be included in the alternative machine set of the corresponding operation through the process of crossover. The crossover operator of MS performs on two machine selection parts and results in two new machine selection parts each of which corresponds to a new allocation of operations to machines. Uniform crossover was adopted in our paper. An integer num was generated randomly between $[0, L-1]$. Then num integers were generated randomly between $[0, L-1]$. Swap the allele in the two MS chromosomes according the num integers orderly. We only changes some elements' value, their preceding constraints are not be changed. Therefore, the individuals after crossover are also all feasible.

Operation Sequence Part: The coding of OS is based on operation-representation. The each value in the OS is equal to the index of each job. So in this study, we adopt a improved Precedence Preserving Order-based crossover (POX) for the operation sequence [10]. The POX works as follows.

Step 1: Generate two sub-job set J_{s1}/J_{s2} from all jobs and select two parent individuals as OS_1 and OS_2 randomly;

Step 2: Copy any element in OS_1/OS_2 that belong to J_{s1}/J_{s2} into two child individuals $OS_1^{'}/OS_2^{'}$, and retain in the same position in $OS_1^{'}/OS_2^{'}$;

Step 3: Delete the elements that are already in the sub-job J_{s1}/J_{s2} from OS_2/OS_1;

Step 4: Orderly fill the empty position in $OS_1^{'}/OS_2^{'}$ with the remnant elements of OS_2/OS_1;

3.4 Mutation

The goal of the mutation is to enhance the diversity of population by introduced some extra variability into the population. Mutation usually works on a single chromosome and creates another chromosome through alteration of the value of a string position or exchange of the values of two string positions etc.

Machine Selection Part: MS mutation operator only changes the assignment property of the chromosomes. We select the shortest processing time from alternative machine set to balance the workload of the machines. MS mutation is described as follows.

Step 1: Select one individual from population;

Step 2: Read the chromosomes of the individual from left to right and generate a probability value randomly; if all the chromosomes have been read, then end the procedure;

Step 3: If probability value less than or equal the mutation probability then go to Step 4; otherwise, go to Step 2;

Step 4: Select the shortest processing time from the alternative machines set to assign it to the mutation position;

Operation Sequence Part: The OS mutation probability is the same as the MS mutation probability. If one position in the OS chromosome is to be mutated, then another position is randomly generated in $[0, L-1]$ to exchange with it. According to our chromosome representation, the new individual is a feasible solution all the same.

4 Variable Neighborhood Search

The convergence speed of simple GA is relatively slow. One promising approach for improving the convergence speed to improved solutions is the use of local search in GA [8]. A good local search method is adopted to improve the quality of individuals of GA before injecting them into the population and strengthen the local search ability.

Variable neighborhood search (VNS) is a relatively recent meta-heuristic which relies on iteratively exploring neighborhoods of growing size to identify better local optima with shaking strategies [11]. VNS is based on a simple principle: systematic change of neighborhood within a possibly local search. Contrary to other meta-heuristics based on local search methods, VNS does not follow a trajectory but explores increasingly distant neighborhoods of the current incumbent solution, and jumps from this solution to a new one if and only if an improvement has been made [11]. So favorable characteristics of the incumbent solution will be kept and used to obtain promising neighboring solutions.

4.1 Basic VNS

The procedure of basic VNS is presented in Fig. 2. Let us denote a finite set of pre-selected neighborhood structures with N_k, $(k = 1, ..., k_{max})$, and with $N_k(s)$ the set of solutions in the kth neighborhood of s. Most local search heuristics use one neighborhood structure, i.e., $k_{max} = 1$. The main step could possibly be iterated until some other stopping condition is met such as maximum number of iterations or maximum number of successive iterations without improvement of best solution. Often successive neighborhood will be nested. Observe that point s' is generated at random in step (2)(a) in order to avoid cycling, which might occur if any deterministic rule was used [11].

---

procedure: Basic VNS
input: parameters
output: a best solution s
begin
  Initialization.
  Select the set of neighborhood structures N_k, k=1,...,k_{max}, that will be used in the search; find an initial solution s; choose a stopping condition;
  Repeat the following until the stopping condition is met:
    (1) Set k=1;
    (2) Until k=k_{max}, repeat the following steps:
      (a) Shaking. Generate a point s` at random from the $k^{th}$ neighborhood of $s$ ($s$` $\in N_k(s)$);
      (b) Local search. Apply some local search method with s` as initial solution; denote with s`` the so obtained local optimum;
      (c) Move or not. If this local optimum is better than the incumbent one, move there (s=s``), and continue the search with N_1 (k=1); otherwise, set k=k+1;
end

Fig. 2. The procedure of Basic VNS

4.2 Neighborhood Structure

Changing of neighborhood within a possibly local search is the basic principle. So how to define the effective neighborhood around an initial solution is crucial in VNS. In this paper, two neighborhoods were adopted, i.e., $k_{max} = 2$. The two neighborhoods are based on the concept of critical path. The detailed description of defining the critical path and neighborhood might see ref. [6]. The makespan of a solution is defined by the length of its critical paths, in other words, the makespan could not be reduced while maintaining the current critical paths. In order to get a new solution with smaller makepan, the existent critical paths one by one must be identified and broken. Moving different number critical operation on the critical path could get different neighborhoods. In this paper, two neighborhoods are used by moving one operation and two operations respectively.

Neighborhood of type I. Neighbor solutions could be generated by moving one critical operation on the critical path. This kind of neighborhood is named as type I.

In this paper, the proposed neighborhood of Zhang [13] is used, which was proposed for JSP problems. And the efficient and effectiveness of the neighborhood is proved in ref. [13]. It is also used for the FJSP problem by moving one operation in Fig. 3. The procedure of generating neighbor solutions is described as following.

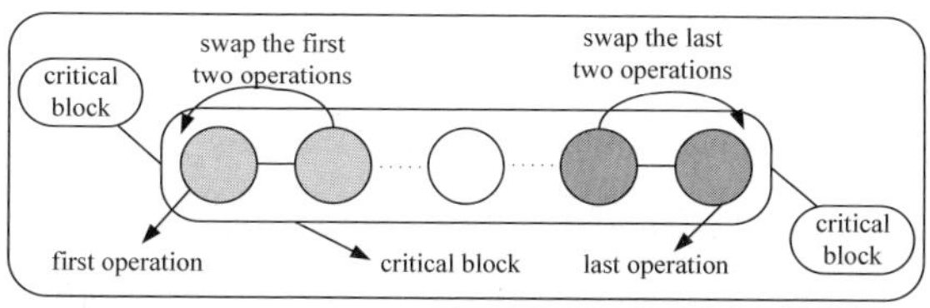

Fig. 3. Neighborhood of type I

(1) In each block, the first (last) operation is inserted into the internal operation within the block.

(2) In each block, the internal operation is moved to the beginning or the end of the block.

(3) If a block contains only one operation, then no swap is made.

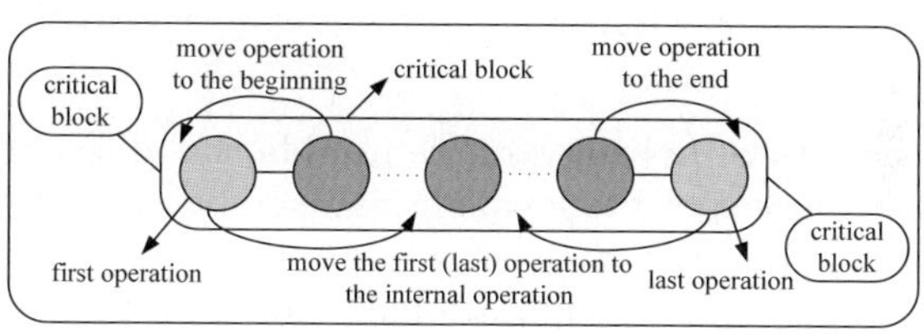

Fig. 4. Neighborhood of type II

Neighborhood of type II. Neighbor solutions could be generated by moving two critical operations on the critical path. This kind of neighborhood is named as type II. In this paper, we use the neighborhood approach of Nowicki and Smutnicki [14]. It is defined swapping between two operations on the critical path in Fig. 4.

The rules of swapping two operations on the critical path are as follows.

(1) If the first (last) block contains more than two operations, we only swap the last (first) two operations in the block. Otherwise, if the first (last) block contains only two operations, these operations are swapped.

(2) In each block, we only swap the last two and first two operations.

(3) If a block contains only one operation, then no swap is made.

A larger neighborhood would bring a greater computational load because more neighbor solutions have to be created, evaluated and compared [8]. So we only used two type neighborhoods to improve the efficiency of local search. Firstly, the type I repeatedly works until the local optimum is met. Then once an improved solution is found in the type II, the type I is used again for local search.

4.3 Framework of the Hybrid VNGA

The framework of the proposed hybrid variable neighborhood search genetic algorithm is illustrated in Fig. 5.

```
procedure: Variable Neighborhood Search Genetic Algorithm (VNGA)
input: FJSP data set, GA parameters
output: a best solution s
begin
  Initialization;
    Generate initial population using MSOS chromosome represent method;
    Set GA parameters;
  Decoding each individual to get the objective value and Evaluate ;
  Repeat the following until the stopping condition is met:
    MS crossover by uniform crossover and OS crossover by POX;
    MS mutation by the shortest processing time and OS mutation;
    Improve the solution s by VNS;
    Select individuals to generate a new population by tournament selection;
    Decoding each individual to get the objective value and Evaluate ;
  end
  output solutaion
end
```

Fig. 5. The framework of the proposed VNGA

Under the framework of hybrid variable neighborhood search and genetic algorithm, the convergence speed to local optima is improvement with the variable neighborhood search. However, the computation time may be increased, moving two operations is much more computationally complex than moving only one. In this paper, the two neighborhoods is adopted from other literature, they have proved that the two neighborhoods is effective and efficiency. Hence, the entire computational time would be increased a little, but the near optimal solution could be improved significantly.

5 Computational Results

To illustrate the effectiveness and performance of the proposed hybrid algorithm, representative benchmark instances from Brandimarte which includes 10 problems have been selected and tested. The proposed algorithm was implemented in C++ on a Pentium IV running at 1.8 GHz. The population size is 100, crossover probability is 0.7, and mutation probability is 0.01. In order to evaluate the efficacy of the computational results, the test problems were run 5 times consecutively.

Table 2. The Computational results

Problem	$n \times m$	(LB,UB)	Ho&Tay		VNGA		
			C_M^*	AV(C_M)	C_M^*	AV(C_M)	CPU
MK01	10×6	(36,42)	40	41.5	40	40	2.6
MK02	10×6	(24,32)	29	29.1	26	26	3.8
MK03	15×8	(204,211)	N/A	N/A	204	204	1.1
MK04	15×8	(48,81)	67	67.34	60	60	8.2
MK05	15×4	(168,186)	176	178.1	173	174.8	8.3
MK06	10×15	(33,86)	67	68.82	58	60.5	18.6
MK07	20×5	(133,157)	147	152.9	144	145.8	17.9
MK08	20×10	(523)	523	523.34	523	523	1.2
MK09	20×10	(299,369)	320	327.74	311	311	38.6
MK10	20×15	(165,296)	229	235.72	201	203.9	40.3

In Table 2, $n \times m$ denotes the problem scale. (LB, UB) denotes the optimal makespan if known, otherwise, the best lower and upper bound found to date. AV(C_M) stands for the average makespan. C_M^* denotes the best makespan. Ho&Tay is the approach proposed by Ho and Tay [7]. VNGA is our proposed hybrid algorithm. Column CPU times fives the sum of the average computer independent CPU time out of five runs to compute all the solutions of each data set. From Table 2, the results indicate that our proposed algorithm outperforms Ho's approach in all problems. Totally, we found 7 new better solutions than Ho's. And 2 instances of Mk01 and Mk08, their makespan found by the VNGA are equal to the Ho's algorithm. And from the CPU time, the computational speed is quick.

6 Conclusions

In this paper, the hybrid variable neighborhood genetic algorithm (VNGA) is proposed to solve the FJSP. Variable neighborhood search is adopted as local search method to improve the quality of individuals of GA before injecting them into the population and strengthen the local search ability. At the same time, two different neighborhoods by moving one operation and two operations respectively are used. Computational results show that the proposed algorithm is efficient and effective. In the future, design more effective local search strategy is remarkable.

Acknowledgement

This project is supported by 863 High Technology Plan Foundation of China under Grant No.2006AA04Z131, 2007AA04Z107. 973 National Basic Research Program of China under Grant No.2004CB719405.

References

1. Chen, H., Ihlow, J., Lehmann, C.: A genetic algorithm for flexible job-shop scheduling. In: IEEE International conference on Robotics and Automation, Detroit, vol. 2, pp. 1120–1125 (1999)
2. Graey, M.R., Jonmson, D.S., Sethi, R.: The complexity of flow shop and job shop scheduling. Mathematics of Operational Research 1, 117–129 (1976)
3. Brucker, P., Schile, R.: Job-shop scheduling with multi-purpose machines, Computing. Computing 45(4), 369–375 (1990)
4. Kacem, I., Hammadi, S., Borne, P.: Approach by localization and multiobjective evolutionary optimization for flexible job-shop scheduling problems. IEEE Transactions on Systems, Man and Cybernetics 32(1), 1–13 (2002)
5. Pérès, D., Paulli, E.: An integrated approach for modeling and solving the general multi-processor job-shop scheduling problem using tabu search. Annals of Operations Research 70, 281–306 (1997)
6. Mastrolilli, M., Gambardella, L.M.: Effective neighborhood functions for the flexible job shop problem. Journal of Scheduling 3(1), 3–20 (2000)
7. Ho, N.B., Tay, J.C., Edmund, M.K.L.: An effective architecture for learning and evolving flexible job shop schedules. European Journal of Operational Research 179, 316–333 (2007)
8. Gao, J., Sun, L.Y., Gen, M.: A hybrid genetic and variable neighorhood descent algorithm for flexible job shop scheduling problems. Computers & Operations Research 35(9), 2892–2907 (2008)
9. Liu, H.B., Abraham, A., Grosan., C.: A Novel Variable Neighborhood Particle Swarm Optimization for Multi-objective Flexible Job-shop Scheduling Problems. In: 2nd International Conference on Digital Information Management, pp. 138–145 (2007)
10. Lee, K., Yamakawa, T., Lee, K.M.: A genetic algorithm for general machine scheduling problems. International Journal of Knowledge-Based Electronic 2, 60–66 (1998)
11. Hansen, P., Mladenović, N.: Variable neighborhood search: Principles and applications. In: Glover, F.W., Kochenberger, G.A. (eds.) Handbook of Metaheuristics. Kluwer Academic Publishers, Dordrecht (2003)
12. Zhang, C.Y., Li, P.G., Guan, Z.L., Rao, Y.: A tabu search algorithm with a new neighborhood structure for the job shop scheduling problem. Computers & Operations Research 34, 3229–3242 (2007)
13. Nowicki, E., Smutnicki, C.: A fast taboo search algorithm for the job shop problem. Management Science 42(6), 797–813 (1996)

Intelligent Robot Manipulator's Application in the Racking of Drill Pipe

Kui Zhou, Ding Feng, Chaobin Huang, Peng Wang, Jin Liu, and Shouyong Li

School of Mechanical Engineering, Yangtze University, Jingzhou, Hubei 434023, China
{Ding Feng,fengd}@yangtzeu.edu.cn, fengd0861@yahoo.com

Abstract. The racking of drill pipe, loading and unloading are all completed through the automated manipulator; the degree of manipulator automation also reflects the wellhead mechanization and automation. Take intelligent robot technology into manipulator on the wellhead device, It is of great significance to improve the degree of automation, improve labor productivity, reduce production costs and improve working conditions, reduce operating risk in process of the well drilling. Drill pipe emissions-system based on emission frame in the form of pipe finger can be divided into the kinds of radial, parallelism and X-Y. The composition of drill-pipe operating system which used to the wellhead will be compared with the composition of the human body structure.

Keywords: Intelligent robot, Manipulator, Drill pipe, Mechanization.

1 Introduction

Modern oil drilling operations are mostly in the oceans, deserts and hills, where the environment field are extremely difficult. In order to lessen the labor intensity of the drilling workers, improve the working environment and the safety factors to production, the drilling equipment automation requirements are increasingly to be higher, particularly mechanization on the wellhead device and automation requirements, it has become one of the key factors focus on considering of a design to drilling machine. In the process of drilling, it needs to make the drill pipe move from the well head to emissions or from emissions to the well head, which is the operation of the drill pipe emissions. They are high-risk, high repeatability and high labor intensity, time-consuming, intensive labor power consumption. The key of mechanization and automation on wellhead operations to oil-drilling rig is whether does the degree of automation to the drill pipe operating system high or low, and the main equipment of well head drill pipe operating system is manipulator, the drill pipe emissions, handling and so on all through the automated machinery manipulator to complete, Hence, the degrees of manipulator automation also indirectly reflects the extents on mechanization and automation to the wellhead.

The Wellhead manipulator is one of the industrial machinery manipulators, because of the rapid development of the technology on industrial machinery manipulator, there still not have be a unified and clear definition on manipulator so far in the world. International Organization for Standardization(ISO) define to the manipulator is: A reprogrammable and multifunctional manipulator, devised for the transports of

C. Xiong et al. (Eds.): ICIRA 2008, Part II, LNAI 5315, pp. 513–521, 2008.

masteries, parts, tools or specialized Systems, with varied and programmed movements, with the aim of carrying out varied tasks [1]. China's national standards-GB/T12643-90 will also defined industrial machinery manipulator as an operation machine which can automatic positioning control, re-programming, multifunctional, multi-freedom [1]. It can carry materials, parts or maintaining the tools used to complete the various operations tasks. Manipulator can replace some or all of the manual labor, at present the world's advanced manipulator, can simulate human's arm motion to complete more complicated operations. Modern manipulator as a new technology of the field of automatic control, is the edge discipline in multi-disciplinary integration field, it is one of the fastest growing technology in today's high-tech field, and has become an important part in modern production.

As the successful development of the third generation intelligent robots, thence, the robot not only has the capability of perception, but also with the ability of memory, independent judgment and reasoning and decision-making, to complete more complex movements. Its "intelligent" lies on possessing the work function in line with the coordination of the outside world -objects, environment and people [2]. From the mode of control, the intelligent robot differs from the industrial robots on the "teaching, reproduction" , differ from the remote-control robot on the "main - subordinate operation" , but to operate self-regulatory in the way of "cognitive - adaptation".

Take intelligent robot technology into manipulator on the wellhead device, it is of great significance to improve the degree of automation, improve labor productivity, reduce production costs and improve working conditions, reduce operating risk in process of the well drilling.

2 The Ways to Racking of Drill-Pipe

The 1940s, people began to explore an effective way to make the drill pipe operate mechanization, thereby resulting emissions system to the drill pipe, also realized emissions-automatic discharge operation of the drill pipe from wellhead to emission frame in the drilling process, and to avoid the direct contact on people and the drill pipe, to accelerate the pace of trip drilling, particularly to play an important role on reducing operating costs in offshore drilling. In the 1980s, a variety of different designs of vertical drill pipe emissions system began to appear. That mainly due to the impact of relevant national standards, particularly the standards of Norway Petroleum Institute: the drilling rig operating in the territorial waters of Norway must be equipped with drill pipe emissions in fully automated system, power slips and the breaking device to automation.

Drill pipe emissions-system based on emission frame in the form of pipe finger can be divided into the kinds of radial, parallelism and X-Y. [3]

1. The kinds of radial (Fig. 1)

It uses for the drill pipe emissions system early, most used for many small drilling rig. The principle is that hydraulic-driven emission frame rotate to drive the drill pipe.

2. The kinds of parallelism (Fig. 2)

It uses in the form of a more extensive large-scale drill, mainly due to be deposited larger number of drill pipe, drill collar and casing, and it can achieve a perfect coordinate

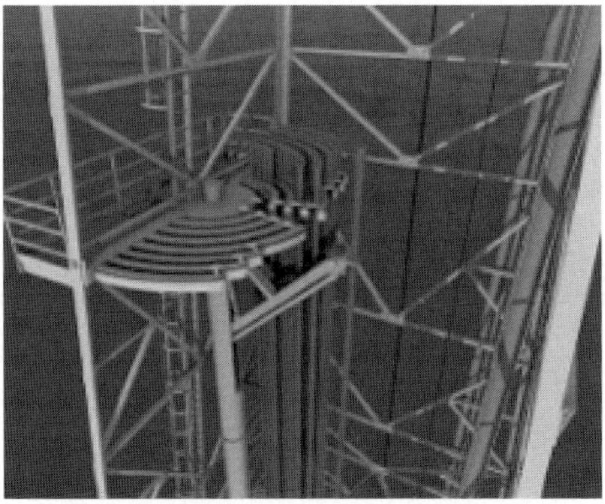

Fig. 1. Radial type drill pipe emissions graph

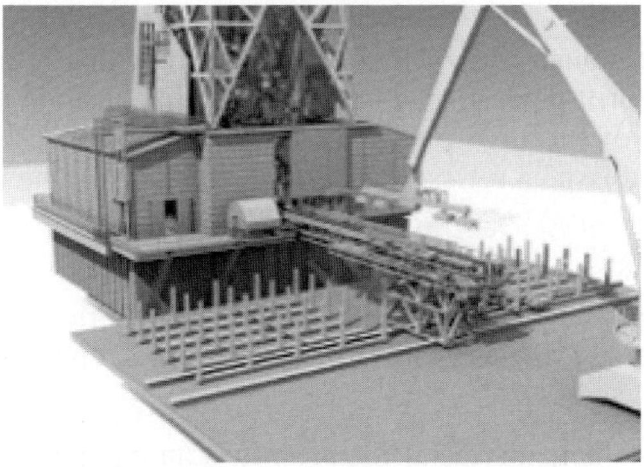

Fig. 2. X-Y-type drill pipe emissions graph

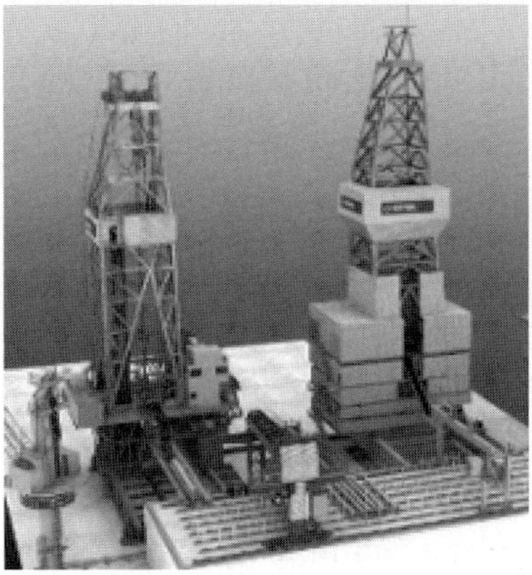

Fig. 3. Parallel - type drill pipe emissions graph

with the horizontal drilling pipe operating system. With this structure, two sets of emission system can be installed in orbit at the same time, and two sets of system can work independently, and don't affect each other, so it's more applicable to coupled-head frame drilling rig. The coupled-head frame drilling rig more use in the ocean and become an application development trend.

3. The kinds of X-Y (Fig. 3)
At present, Most of the emissions system to the drill pipe uses such structures.

3 The Manipulator Operating System on Intelligent Robot

The composition of drill pipe operating system on the wellhead to emission drill pipe can be compared with the human body structure (Fig. 4). It can be divided into four parts [4]:

1. The control part
It's equivalent to the human brain and nervous system, which is the central part of the operating system to drill pipe, it used to processing information and judgment to the control information of the drill pipe operating system and feedback's information from the sensors, and issue a series of motion instructions to the implementation part (mechanical arm).

2. The operative part
It's equivalent to the human's hand-foot, transfer the electrical signals from the control part into the mechanical energy to drive the mechanical part operating.

3. The examination part
It's equivalent to the human's facial features, it is an equipment of sensing devices and be used to detect manipulator movements and action, to achieve the measurement, monitoring and feedback for the results to the coil out of the manipulator of the campaign.

4. The mechanical part
It is equivalent to the human's bones, an organization can realize the emission to drill pipe.

The existing the name of "drill pipe emission to wellhead automation" and "manipulator drill pipe system", which are talking about here some of manpower, with some control (such as SCM, PLC, etc.)are all replaced by the implementation and mechanical parts to instead of the human brain and the sensors connected with the control part to replace the cognitive of man(visual, tactile, etc.) to achieve the total process of the drill pipe emissions from wellhead (Fig. 5).

3.1 The Error Analysis to Positional Manipulator

Drill pipe emissions manipulator run in its specific path, the precision of the implementation at the end arrived at pinpoint designated eventually which is an important criterion to measure whether the quality of the work manipulator superior or inferior. Compared to the general precision mechanical, the absolute precision of the

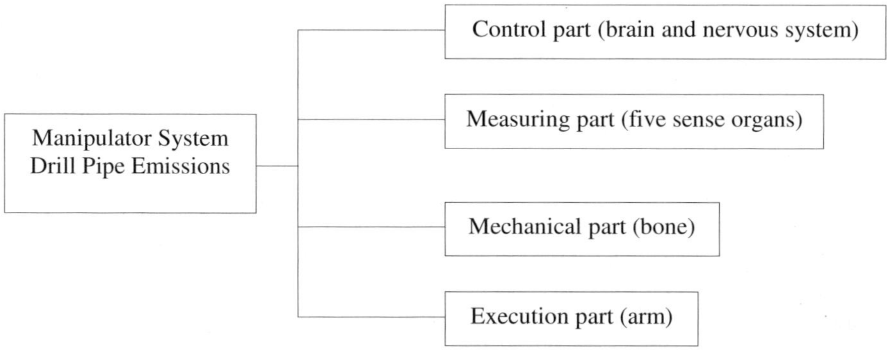

Fig. 4. Intelligent manipulator and human body structure comparison chart

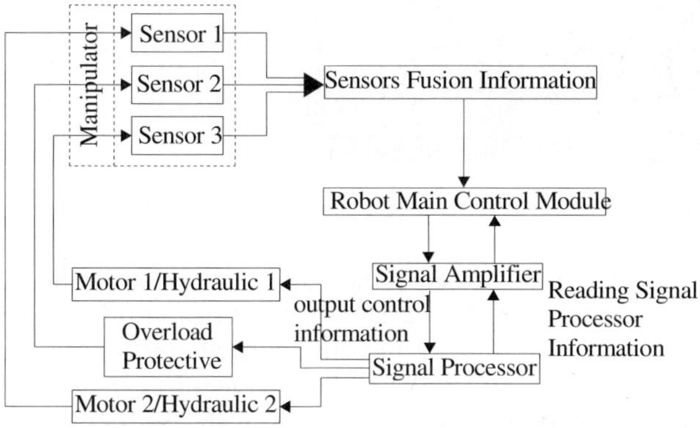

Fig. 5. Intelligent robot control principle

manipulator is very low. Two main reasons: the one that known as the error on geometry, the manufacturing error when processing mechanical components, the error on assembly or installation, the error on level parameters for cause of the deviation to the encoder, which shows as the error on D-H parameters at last; The another that called as the error on non-geometry, the flexible of joint, the deflection of arm, changes on temperature, the worn out of various parts, The error due to gravity or the power generated form the movement, the error in the transformation calculation and so on. The main factors which cause positional error are servo system error, the error on the deformation to level, the error in mechanical drive, the error from the temperature and so on. By compensation of these errors can improve the absolute precision.

4 The Manipulator to Intelligent Robot in the Application of Drill-Pipe Emissions

At present, the drill pipe emissions systems have many types, including a simple manipulator on the drilling platform, as well as the complex emissions system of 2 or 3 manipulator arms (Fig. 6). These systems can lift the drill pipe to stay, and some are even able to lift a casing with the diameter of ø508mm (20 inches) .These systems can be considered as the two-or-three-arm robot between the wellhead and emission frame .The operators in the closed control room to operate the system through computer or other electronic devices .

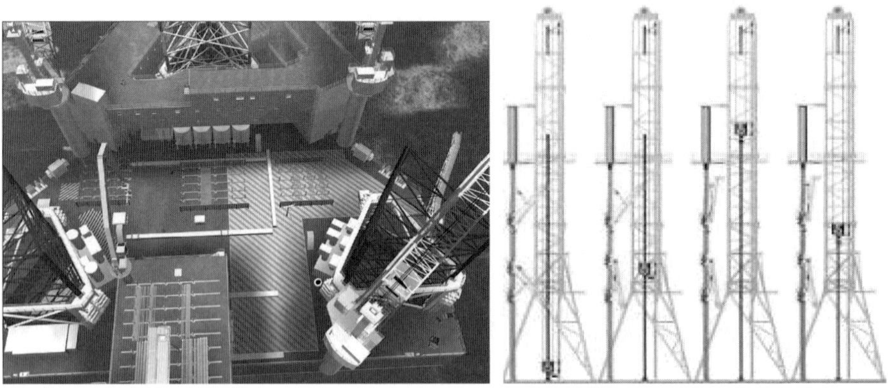

Fig. 6. Ordinary drill pipe emissions manipulator and 2-arm drill pipe emissions manipulator

The two-or-three-arm robot manipulator [6] is developed as the main mechanical power tools in the 1960s, intended to use for the floating drilling rig that the manpower shortage to take the drill pipe from the wellhead to the location of the drill pipe emissions. These drill pipe emissions will be operated by on-site team personnel, in fact, to be usually an increase in members in the team, so they aren't industrial manipulator.

The basic problem of the drill pipe emissions is that if the running and pulling process of the drill pipe can't realize automation, then it is impossible to replace the people's many operations, So almost the all trying to take the manipulator to running and pulling of the drill pipe are the combined operation on mergence between drill pipe emissions and iron driller, or use a computer to control two separate devices. Two of the cases are the drill pipe operation and the overall iron driller.

In order to effect the automation on the process of the all drilling operation when the drill pipe running and pulling, basically use a twist - rotating device to automatically complete the drill pipe operation. The drill pipe operation machine has a function to twist - rotation, which formed a relatively entire drill pipe robot, People even can imagine, it is a very tall "person", its arm can seize the drill pipe and reverse it, And through turning left or right to move the drill pipe from the wellhead onto the catheter bent frame. Both methods have the same effects under the drilling function, and abolish the normal personnel staff in teams and groups on drilling platform and the derrick hand.

4.1 Applications

One company developed a drill pipe emissions manipulator (Fig. 7). It can achieve movements of the drill pipe and casing through remote control on the drilling platform and in line with the drilling operations. The manipulator equipped with the hydraulic drive is made from hydraulic and pneumatic industrial manufacturing companies in Arlington, Texas. It includes a 40 horsepower power machine (electric motor or diesel engine) driven two-stage hydraulic pump, a 120 gallons (454kg) of the reservoir tank, a return pipeline filters and several inhalation pipeline filters (Table. 1) .

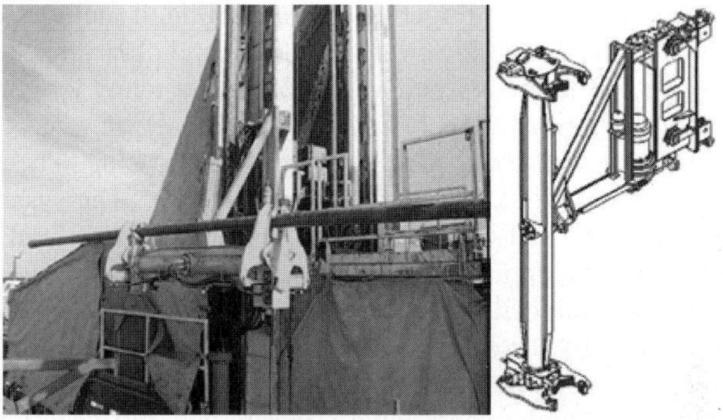

Fig. 7. Drill pipe emissions manipulator

This manipulator is equipped at the traveling pedestal with the chain of driving. The function of the traveling pedestal is: To move the tubes in line with the drilling operations, rat holes to tie with single joint and coordinate with the drill pipe under loading party and casing operations and so on. The end of retractable arm is an adjustable nose. The components of nose are following: the positioning conductor pipe, the distant controlled latch with the drill pipe lock into conductor pipe. In order to adapt to the different dimensions of the pipes, the size of conductor pipe can be changed, and the conductor pipe can be controlled by the distant controlled situation. After the nose clamp pipe, the manipulator can be pushed forward and backward lateral movement, so that the pipe can be moved to any position of the drill platform.

RA-D automated drilling rig, the key part is lighter-weight manipulator drill pipe operating system, it can operate and transport all kinds of drill pipe, and control drill pipe emissions through intelligent control system on computer, making the drill pipe emissions in right drilling orders. Keeping pipe frame is placed at the drilling platform. The carrying devices are able to transport the keeping pipe frame equipped with drill pipe to the manipulator at horizontal position, the manipulator will transfer the drill pipe within head frame.

Table 1. Drill pipe emissions manipulator performance parameters

Series	400	1500	4000	4000HD
Lifting Capacity	400lbs	1500 lbs	4000 lbs	4000 lbs
Jaw Range	$4^1/_2$"	$3^1/_2$"~$10^3/_4$"	$3^1/_2$"~$10^3/_4$"	$3^1/_2$"~$10^3/_4$"
Pipe Length Capacity	20m	20 m	20 m	30 m
Breakout Torque Capacity	—	12000ft-lbs	12000ft-lbs	12000ft-lbs
Estimated Weight	1000lbs	3500lbs	3800lbs	3800lbs
A special set of jaws are required for larger diameter tubular up to $10^3/_4$"				

According to Petroleum Engineer report, U.S. Varco company developed a kind of SRS-2 radial pipe emissions system, both with the function of iron drilling, in addition to tripping operations, the drill pipe also can be racked and moved drill collar from the pipe setback to wellhead or from the wellhead to pipe setback, And do not need to drill under derrick hand and platform driller. The system includes an assembly rotating positive and negative 180 column, two-piece removing arm (each one upper and lower) and one kind of radial fingerboard. In addition, it includes expanded range of vertical column, the upper and lower arm, carriage and claw, check ring, upper and lower rotation device and trajectory and so on. There are many long troughs fixed up with radial layout in fingerboard, accessing to pipe setback in tank. Long- removing arm can take up the pipe setback in 31m, drill collar and casing. The lower removing arm can be lift to 10m in height, lifting capacity to 97.5kN. The system has been applied to offshore platforms, self-elevating, semi-submersible and land drilling rig, Up to August in 1996. We have applied four sets in using.

The configured automatic drilling system (CADS) is a representative new technology developed by Maritime Hydraulics Company. The offshore drilling platform in Norway uses the programmable drill pipe handling system developed by Maritime Hydraulics company to achieve operational programmed, not need to operate winch, the top drive, drill pipe treatment plants and slips, just only for one person on drilling platform. In addition, there is a set of E-Tally automatic measuring and recording system to record the drill specifications, as well as models from unloading number and the size of the uncoupling torque, can also record the drilling location in the entire underground drill pipe and place in proper order in pipe setback after pipe. At the same time a manually operated backup system is fixed up. Because don't need manual control operation, it reduces the drilling time and trips 55 post vertical column each hour.

5 Conclusions

Summing up the situation of domestic and international, intelligent manipulator has completely changed the traditional way of bit feeding and completely replaces the function of the derrick hand and platform driller. Intelligent manipulator has been application abroad for many years and the production efficiency and safety are both improved at a significant extent. In terms of the domestic situation, the continued rise in international oil prices has brought unprecedented opportunities for development to the oil drilling machinery in China, research and develop the high-performance manipulator will meet the needs of domestic oil production soon. It increases production efficiency and safety in a wide margin and to promote the developments of unmanned automation drilling rig, to promote the modernization of oil production process.

References

1. Peng, N.: Research on the Charge/Discharge Manipulator of Friction Welding Geological Drill Stem. D. China Coal Research Institute (2006)
2. Graf, B., Pfeiffer, K., Staab, H., Ipa, F.: Mobile Robots for Offshore Inspection and Manipulation. In: J. International Petroleum Technology Conference, pp. 4–6 (December 2007)

3. Liu, W., Cui, X., Zhang, F.: Development and Typical Structure of Pipe Racking System. J. Oil Field Equipment 36, 74–77 (2007)
4. Cheng, X., Zhang, Z.: Application of Manipulator in Well Head Mechanical Unit. J. Science & Technology Information 5, 24–25 (2007)
5. Zhou, D.: The Research of Intelligent Robot and Motion Control System Based on the Embedded System. D. Chengdu University (2007)
6. Mark, D.: Hansen/Weatherford International, Egill Abrahamsen/Weatherford. Improving Safety Performance Through Rig Mechanization. J. Society of Petroleum Engineers 27 February–1 March (2001)

A Novel Six-Axis Heavy Force Sensor

Sheng Lin, Wei Liu, Yongqing Wang, Zhenyuan Jia, and Fuji Wang

Key Lab. for Precis. and Non-tradit. Mach. Technol. of Minist. of Edu.,
Dalian Univ. of Techno., 116024 Dalian, China
linsheng138@yahoo.com.cn

Abstract. The measurement of six-axis force is the base of coordinate control, but there are still no six-axis heavy force sensors in most of big load operation equipments for the contradiction of six-axis and heavy force. So with combining the parallel load sharing principle and the principle of six-axis force measurement of Stewart structure, a novel method of six-axis heavy force measurement is presented. Based on the new method, a finite element model of six-axis heavy force piezoelectric sensor is established, and then the static and dynamic simulations are made. Results indicate that there are good load sharing effectiveness and dynamic characteristic with six-axis heavy force sensor. In the end, the structure parameters are optimized with respect to the ability of load sharing, and the result indicates that the ability of load sharing is improved obviously after optimization.

Keywords: six-axis; heavy force; sensor; simulation; optimization.

1 Introduction

Heavy force sensor is defined as the sensor with carrying capacity in the range of 10 - 2000kN, which is usually used in heavy machinery. Furthermore, the heavy force sensors with the carrying capacity of more than 100MN are needed in many heavy load manipulators. However, these are usually one-axis and with the supporting type, and the heavy force sensor of supporting type is so difficult to produce that it can only be made in a few countries. The thought of load sharing in parallel originated from 1960s. After that, adhesion type heavy force is developed in America, Canada and Germany etc. Professor Shen Jiuheng researched the heavy force sensor of adhesion type [1] in the industrial university of Beijing in 1980, which has been used widely in many steel rolling machine. However, these sensors above can only measure force in one axis. Six-axis force sensor is one of the hot issues in measurement and control field in recent 20 years, and there are some typical structure such as cross-shape structure [2], twin-head type structure [3], Stewart structure [4], etc. But these six-axis sensors can not measure heavy force, and there are no the report about the six-axis heavy force at present.

Based on the principle of parallel load sharing, a new type of six-axis heavy force sensor is presented in this paper. By load sharing, a little of the six-axis heavy force shares on the sensor, and then the six-axis heavy force acted on the arm of the manipulator can be deduced by the little six-axis force. Simulation of static and dynamic characteristics is conducted to verify the effectiveness of the proposed approach.

C. Xiong et al. (Eds.): ICIRA 2008, Part II, LNAI 5315, pp. 522–529, 2008.

2 Measurement Principle of Six-Axis Heavy Force

There are two methods to measure heavy force at present: one method is improving the load-bearing ability, the other one is load sharing. However, it is difficult to improve the ability of load-bearing of six-axis force sensor due to the complicated structure, so the load sharing thought can be used to design the six-axis heavy force sensor based on the structure of Stewart.

A six-axis heavy force sensor based on the Stewart structure is shown in Fig.1. Stewart structure is composed of an upper platform and a lower platform connected with six legs, where the connections are composed of spherical joints [5]. The coordinate frame {b} and {B} in Fig.1 are attached to the centers of the upper and the lower platform [6]. The centers of the Spherical joints are, respectively, denoted by b_i and $B_i(i=1$ to $6)$. Then the platform geometry is described by vectors $\vec{b}_i$ and $\vec{B}_i$ $(i=1,...,6)$.

In the novel six-axis heavy force sensor, the upper platform and lower platform are fixed to the manipulator in parallel mode, which is shown in Fig.2, where the dotted line represents the arm of manipulator. When the manipulator catches a work piece, six-axis reaction force denoted $\vec{F}$ is acted on the arm. However, only a little of the force denoted $\vec{F}'$ is delivered to the six-axis heavy force sensor because most of $\vec{F}$ is applied on the arm. According to the screw theory [7], the force equilibrium equation of Stewart structure can be expressed as

$$\vec{F}'=f_1\$_1+f_2\$_2+f_3\$_3+f_4\$_4+f_5\$_5+f_6\$_6 \tag{1}$$

where f_i denotes the axial force acted on the ith leg ; $\$_i$ denotes the unit linear vector of the ith leg in the coordinate system {B}, $\$_i=S_i+\in S_{0i}$, $S_i\bullet S_i=1$, $S_i\bullet S_{0i}=0$, $S_{0i}=\vec{b}_i\times S_i$; $\vec{F}'$ denotes the six-axis force acted on the upper platform, and $\vec{F}'=[F_x,F_y,F_z,M_x,M_y,M_z]^T$, equation(1) can be written to matrix form

$$\vec{F}'=[G_f^F]\vec{f} \tag{2}$$

where $\vec{f}=[f_1,f_2,f_3,f_4,f_5,f_6]^T$; $[G_f^F]$ presents the influence coefficient matrix, which can be described by

$$[G_f^F]=\begin{bmatrix} S_1 & S_2 & S_3 & S_4 & S_5 & S_6 \\ S_{01} & S_{02} & S_{03} & S_{04} & S_{05} & S_{06} \end{bmatrix} \tag{3}$$

where $S_i=\dfrac{\vec{b}_i-\vec{B}_i}{|\vec{b}_i-\vec{B}_i|}$, $S_{0i}=\vec{B}_i\times S_i=\dfrac{\vec{B}_i\times\vec{b}_i}{|\vec{b}_i-\vec{B}_i|}$.

It is well known that the matrix $[G_f^F]$ can be determined unique according to the structure parameter. Therefore, it is very easy to determine $\vec{F}'$ from the equation (2). After $\vec{f}$ is measured. Deformation value of six legs is denoted as the vector $\overline{\Delta l} = (\Delta l_1, \Delta l_2, \Delta l_3, \Delta l_4, \Delta l_5, \Delta l_6)$, and then $\overline{\Delta l}$ can be obtained by the measured vector $\vec{f}$. Thus the increment of the upper platform position denoted $\phi = (\Delta_x, \Delta_y, \Delta_z, \theta_z, \theta_y, \theta_x)$ can be obtained by forward kinematics of the Stewart structure. In the end, force analysis of the manipulator arm is made with taking the displacement of upper platform as boundary condition, then we get the six-axis force $\vec{F}''$, which is the resultant force of six-axis heavy force $\vec{F}$ acted on the arm and the force $\vec{F}'$.Then, the six-axis heavy force $\vec{F}$ is obtained.

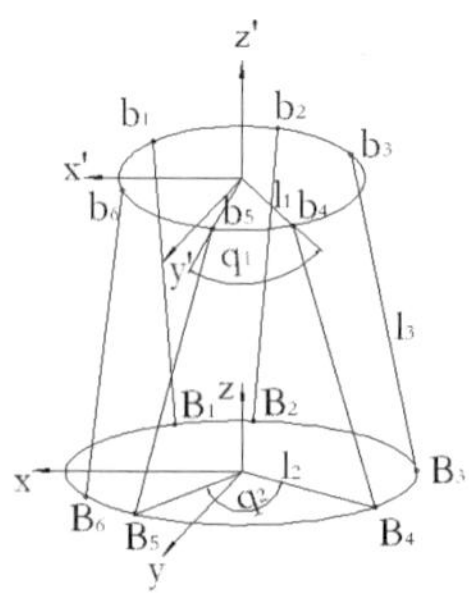

Fig. 1. The Stewart platform

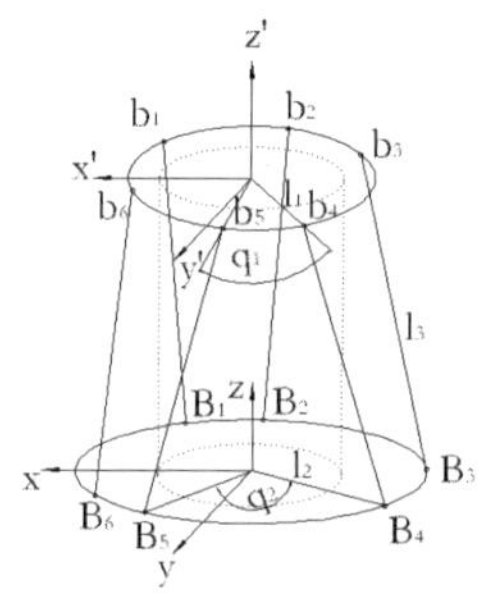

Fig. 2. The Stewart platform with load sharing

3 Simulation

3.1 Static Analysis of Six-Axis Heavy Force

Piezoelectric quartz is selected as the sensitive element of the six-axis heavy force sensor. In order to test whether the pressure of the piezoelectric quartz is in permissible stress range, a finite element model shown in Fig.3 is established. The geometric parameters of the sensor are given by

$$l_1=0.11\text{m},\ l_2=0.14\text{m},\ l_3=0.2\text{m},\ q_1=40°,\ q_2=80°.$$

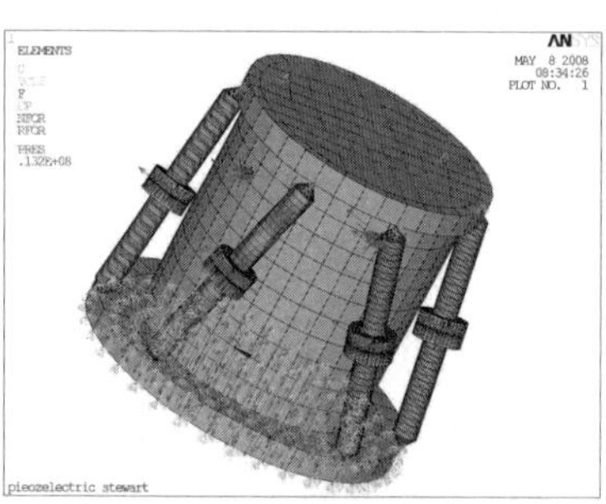

Fig. 3. The finite element model

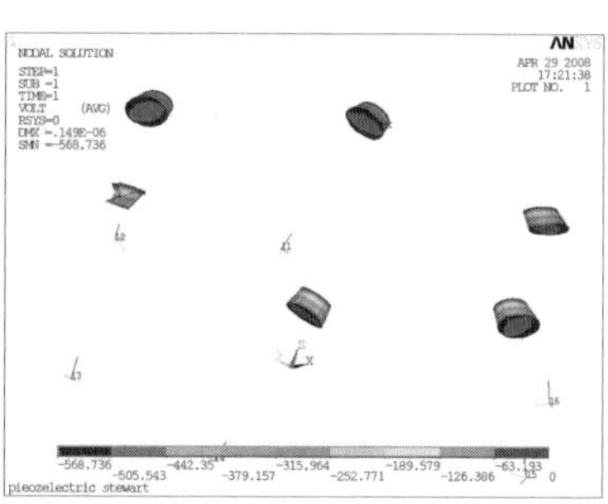

Fig. 4. The cloud picture of voltage

where l_1 denotes the upper platform radius, l_2 denotes the lower platform radius, l_3 denotes the length of each leg, q_1 denotes the angle between b_1 and b_2, q_2 denotes the angle between B_1 and B_2. When 500kN the force is acted on the arm along z axis, the cloud picture of piezoelectric quartz voltage is shown in Fig.4. The result of the simulation shows that the maximum of the voltage is 569mV, and the maximum of pressure on the piezoelectric quartz is 10.2N/mm^2, which is within the range of permissible pressure.

3.2 The Relationship between the Load Sharing Ability and Size

It is difficult to develop a six-axis heavy force sensor with large dimension, so we can reduce the size of sensor as a scale and find the relationship between the load sharing ability and the ratio of size increasing. Then the load sharing ability can be calculated by testing sensor with little size. In order to getting the internal force of six legs directly, the finite element model is simplified as Fig.5. The size of the simplified model and the force acted on the arm are amplified in the same scale, and the magnification is denoted as r. Then the internal force of the first leg is analyzed. The change law of f_1 with r is shown in Fig.6, which shows that f_1 increases with r linearly. Thus we can conclude that the ability of load sharing is a constant with the amplification of the size in the same ratio.

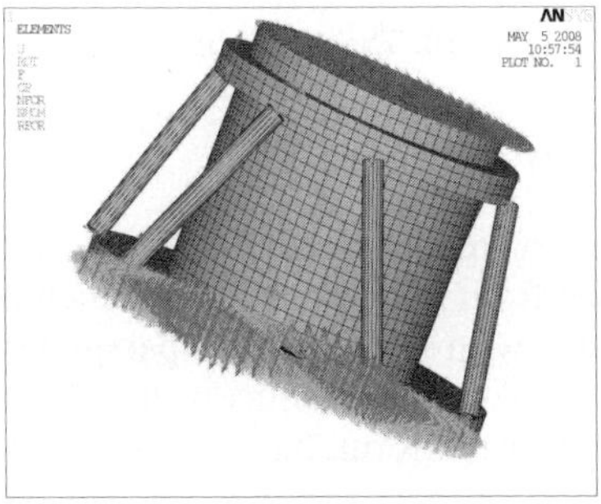

Fig. 5. The simplified finite element model

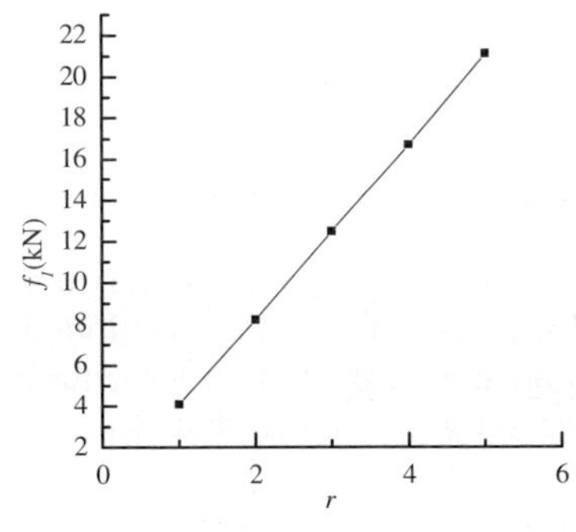

Fig. 6. The Change law of f_1 with r

3.3 Modal Simulation Analysis of the Six-Axis Heavy Force Sensor

Impact load may occur during the manipulator working, so the dynamic characteristic of sensor is very important. In order to minimize the computational time, modal analysis is done to the simplified model shown in Fig.5. With all the degrees of freedom of the lower platform constrained, the four orders natural frequency of the six-axis heavy force sensor can be obtained by simulation, which are 2551.1Hz, 2552.0Hz, 3648.8Hz, 6339.9Hz, respectively. Results show that the first order natural frequency is greater than 1000Hz, which meets the design requirements. The main vibration mode is shown from Fig.7 to Fig.10, and they are vibration along x axis, vibration along y axis, torsion vibration around z axis and vibration along z axis, respectively.

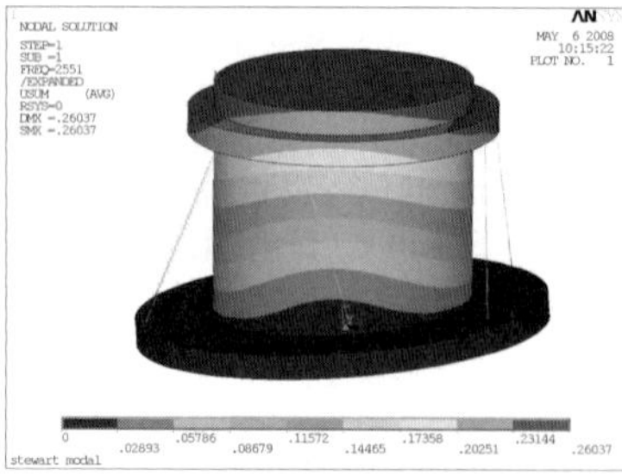

Fig. 7. The first order mode

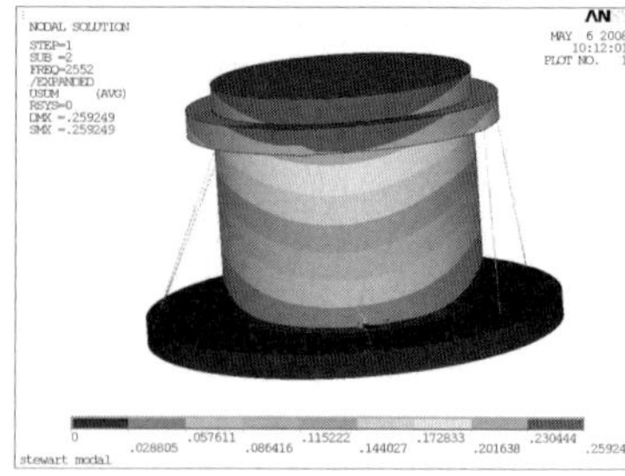

Fig. 8. The second order mode

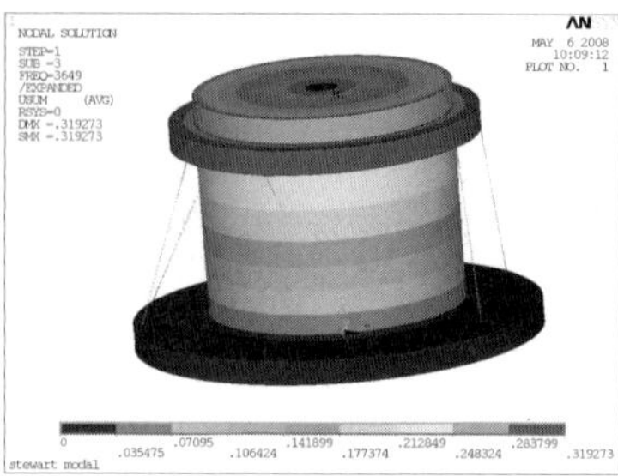

Fig. 9. The third order mode

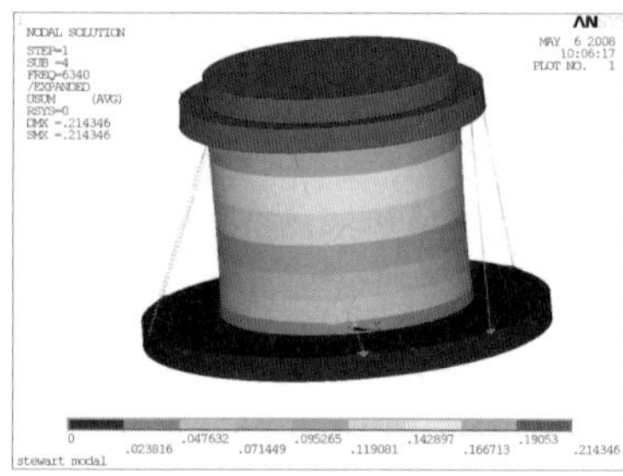

Fig. 10. The fourth order mode

3.4 Influence of Structure Parameter on Natural Frequency

Based on the simulation data, the curve of the structure parameter and the first order natural frequency denoted f_{1st} is plotted as shown from Fig.11 to Fig.15, which reflects the change law of the first order natural frequency with each structure parameter.

These figures reveal that two structure parameters, the radius of upper platform and the distance between upper platform and lower platform, have great influence on the first order natural frequency.

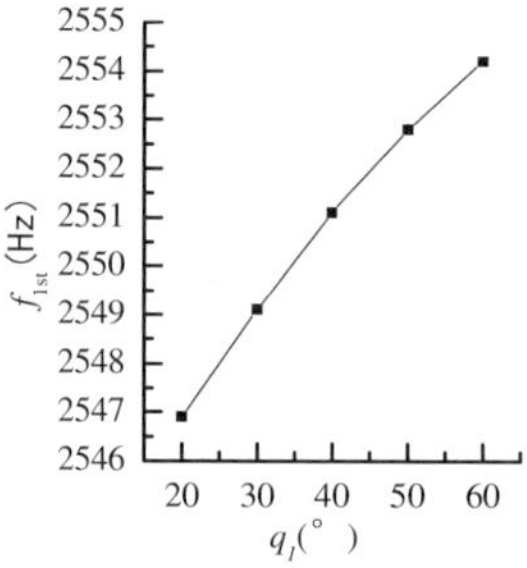

Fig. 11. The influence of q

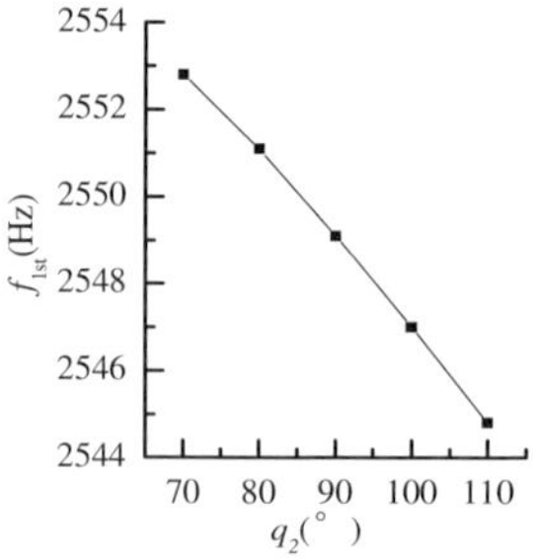

Fig. 12. The influence of q

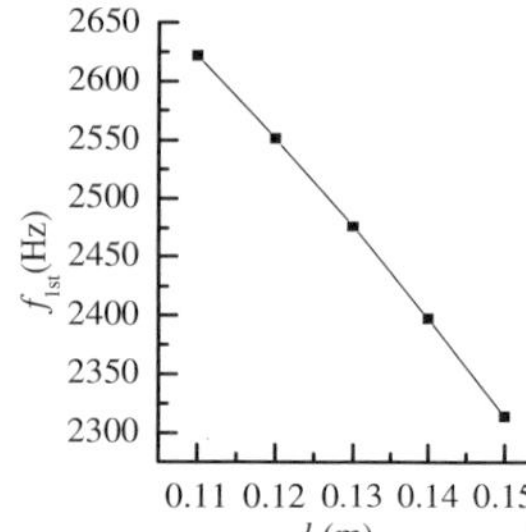

Fig. 13. The influence of l_1

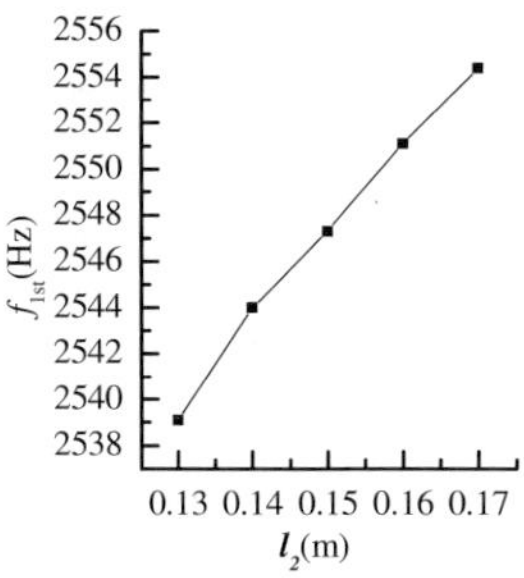

Fig. 14. The influence of l_2

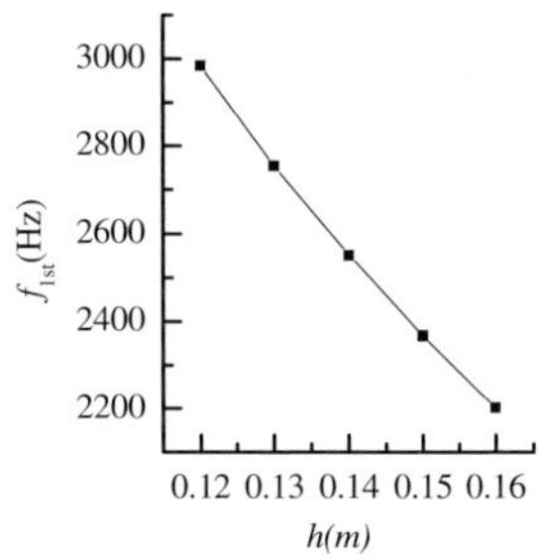

Fig. 15. The influence of h

4 The Optimization of Structure Parameter

The load sharing ability is the most important performance of six-axis heavy force sensor, and the maximum internal force of the six legs reflects the ability of load sharing directly, so it is selected as the objective function, which is denoted as $f(\vec{x})$. The first order natural frequency is taken as the constraint, which is denoted as $g(\vec{x})$. The five parameter of Stewart structure denoted as $\vec{x} = [l_1, l_2, l_3, q_1, q_2]$ are defined as the design variables, then the problem of optimization is given by

$$\begin{cases} \min f(\vec{x}) \\ s.t. 1000 - g(\vec{x}) \le 0 \end{cases} \tag{4}$$

After the structure parameters of the six-axis heavy force sensor is optimized with the zero-order method, the optimization results are listed in Tab.1 with the convergence histories depicted in Fig.16. According to the structure parameter after optimization, a new finite element modal is shown in Fig.17. It is noticed that when 500kN force along z axis is acted on the new modal, the maximum internal force of the six legs is only 391N, which is 24% of the value before optimization.

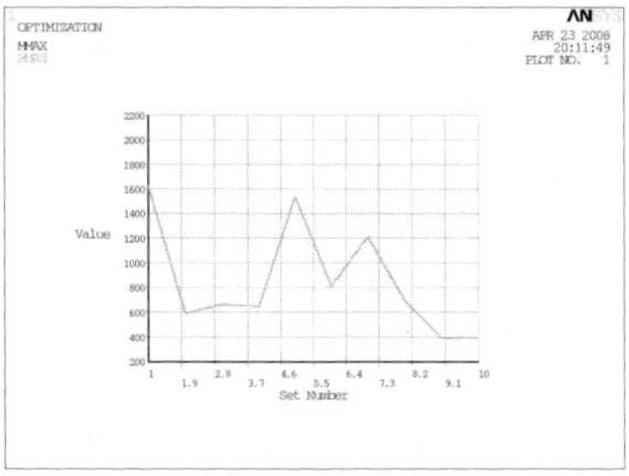

Fig. 16. Convergence histories

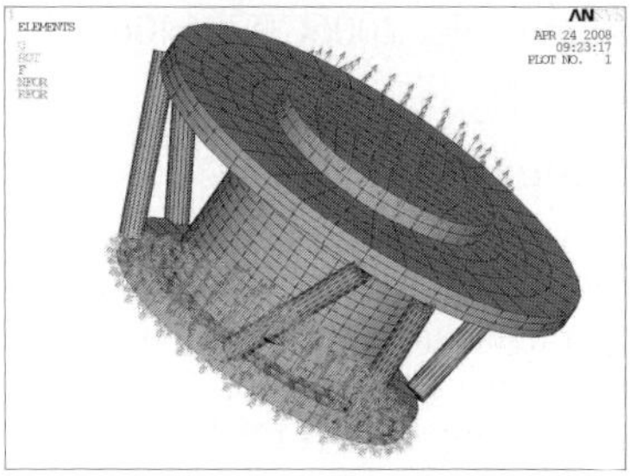

Fig. 17. The model after optimization

Table 1. Chart of optimization results

l_1	l_2	l_3	q_1	q_2	$g(\bar{x})$	$f(\bar{x})$
0.20m	0.14m	0.15m	17°	51°	1462Hz	391.04N

5 Conclusions

A measurement method of six-axis heavy force is presented with combining the parallel load sharing principle and the principle of six-axis force measurement, which provides important reference for the study of six-axis heavy force sensor. The conclusions are drawn as follows:

- The acquired process of the six-axis heavy force is given: Firstly, the reaction force of the upper platform to the arm of the manipulator is calculated; secondly, the displacement of the upper platform is deduced by forward kinematics; finally, the six-axis heavy force is obtained by analyzing the part of the manipulator between the upper platform and the lower one.
- Force analysis is made to the finite element model with piezoelectric quartz. 500kN force along z axis is acted on the model, and the pressure acted on the surface of piezoelectric quartz is 10.2N/mm^2, which is in the permissible preasure range. Furthermore, if the sizes of the Stewart structure and the arm of the manipulator are amplified in the same scale, the ability of load sharing is a constant.
- By the modal analysis with the finite element modal, four order natural frequencies of the sensor are obtained; The first order natural frequency is 2551Hz, which meets the design requirements of more than 1000Hz. The influence of the structure parameter on the natural frequency is analyzed.

After the optimization of the structure parameter, the ability of load sharing is improved, the maximum internal force of the six legs is only 24% of the value before the optimization.

Acknowledgments

This paper is supported by the National Basic Research Program of China 973 Project under Grant No. 2006CB705406.

References

1. Shen, J.H.: The New Development of Heavy Force Measurement Technique –Adhesion and Super miniature Type of Heavy Force Sensors. J. Engineering Science 3, 22–27 (2001)
2. Yoshikawa, T., Miyazaki, T.: A six-axis force sensor with three-dimensional cross-shape structure. In: 1989 IEEE International Conference on Robotics and Automation, pp. 249–255. IEEE Press, Scottsdale (1989)
3. Kaneko, M., Nishihara, T.: Twin-head Type Six-axis Force Sensors. In: 1993 IEEE/RSJ International Conference on Intelligent Robots and Systems, pp. 991–996. IEEE Press, Yokohama (1993)

4. Kerr, D.R.: Analysis, Properties and Design of a Stewart-platform Transducer. J. Mech. Transm.Autom. Des. 111, 25–28 (1989)
5. Khalil, W., Besnard, S.: Self Calibration of Stewart-Gough Parallel Robots without Extra Sensors. J. In: 1999 IEEE Transactions on Robotics and Automation, pp. 1116–1121. IEEE Press, Minneapolis (1999)
6. Chul-Goo, K.: Closed-form force sensing of a 6-axis force transducer based on the Stewart platform. J. Sensors and Actuators 90, 31–37 (2001)
7. Huang, Z., Zhao, Y.S., Zhao, T.S.: The Grid: Advanced Spatial Mechanism. Higher Education, Beijing (2006) (in Chinese)

Research on Benefits Distribution of Fourth Party Logistics Based on Nonprofit Organization

Qiong Liu and Tingting Li

State Key Laboratory of Digital Manufacturing Equipment and Technology
Huazhong University of Science and Technology, Wuhan 430074, P.R. China
qiongliuq@sina.com

Abstract. In order to implementing fourth party logistics and avoiding interest conflict between third party logistics and fourth party logistics, fourth party logistics must be a nonprofit organization. Therefore, the benefits distribution of fourth party logistics among its third party logistics is one of the critical issues. A Nash equilibrium model of fourth party logistics based on nonprofit organization is proposed and the game theory is adopted to analyses the distribution relationship among third party logistics. A utility function is constructed to evaluate the effectiveness of third-party logistics providers, and distribution factor is gotten using Analytic Hierarchy Process (AHP). Finally an example of Wuhan logistics market is taken to prove the validity of the proposed model. This distribution scheme takes into account the distribution of individual rational and collective rational principle, and it is valid in benefits distribution of fourth party logistics based on nonprofit organization.

Keywords: Fourth party logistics; Benefits distribution; Nash model; Utility function; Third party logistics.

1 Introduction

The concept of fourth party logistics was proposed by Anderson Consulting in 1998[1-2]. At the present time the study on fourth party logistics is still in its initial stage at home and abroad, mainly focusing on its concept、features、operation mode、transport planning and so on. Professor Robert Lieb of Northeastern University [3] mentioned the important role and application prospects of fourth party logistics in large-scale manufacturing enterprises; indicated that the fourth party logistics providers should be consultant firm or IT company. Reference [4] expounded the different viewpoints of the consultant firm and third party logistics provider on fourth party logistics and pointed out the relationship between fourth party logistics and third party logistics service providers. Tsinghua University Professor Chen [5] established the directed graph model with multi-dimension weight, researched the transport planning of fourth party logistics, sought the shortest distance of transportation tasks so as to achieve lower costs. Reference [6] adopted clustering algorithm to group tasks of reverse logistics to achieve economies of scale and proposed an algorithm of optimization to match reverse logistics tasks with logistics resource.

C. Xiong et al. (Eds.): ICIRA 2008, Part II, LNAI 5315, pp. 530–538, 2008.

Fourth party logistics assigns logistics tasks to appropriate third party logistics service provider by controlling information and integrating logistics tasks and resources. It integrates demands of logistics on the number of cross-industry customers, optimize the entire supply chain. Thus the operation costs are reduced and profits are increased. Fourth party logistics and third party logistics are all want to get more profits while the total profits is certain. Therefore, there is a question about benefits distribution between fourth party logistics and third party logistics. Benefits distribution is the key about fourth party logistics. How to distribute the benefits concerns the stability of fourth party logistics, and is also the guarantee of its active cooperation.

Nash model has been widely used in the benefits distribution and many other fields. Reference [7] used Nash model in equilibrium analysis of pricing and outsourcing capability in order to minimize costs and maximize profits. Referring to the principle that the income is in direct proportion to the investment, and using Nash Negotiation Model, Professor Sun [8] put forward a feasible solution to the non-technical problem of the benefit allocation in Manufacturing Grid. This solution not only realized reasonable benefit allocation, but also proposed a technical means to control and manage the non-technical factors. Therefore Nash model is adopted to analyze the benefits distribution of fourth party logistics alliance in this paper.

2 The Operation Mode of Fourth Party Logistics Based on Nonprofit Organization

Fourth party logistics based on nonprofit organization is the powerful combination and complementary forms of cooperation responding to market opportunities quickly. Putting the interest of fourth party logistics outside the logistics interest group can avoid the competition between third party logistics and fourth party logistics and might promote application of fourth party logistics. In order to reach economies of scale and reduce investments on reverse logistics, the concept of fourth party reverse logistics based on nonprofit organization was brought [9].

Fig.1 is one of the common forms of fourth party logistics based on nonprofit organization. In order to reduce the logistics cost, fourth party logistics must have an advanced logistics information-network platform, which could integrate logistics resource and tasks [10]. It is not needed for a fourth party logistics to invest logistics facilities such as transportation vehicles and other equipment, but to collect the information on scattered logistics needs and logistics resources, and then integrates them into large-scale logistics tasks through cluster analysis and rearranges the logistics task so to reduce costs and increase profits. Therefore, the increased margin made by integrated operation could be distributed among all participators of third party logistics providers.

Fourth party logistics based on nonprofit organization is a network configuration consisting of third party logistics service providers and logistics-demand enterprises which are took as the main participants in game theory. Every participant wants to realize their own profits maximum, so the respectively different ideas are took as the strategy space in game theory. Every participant receives different earnings, which constitutes their own utility function. All of these are in line with the basic requirements of game theory.

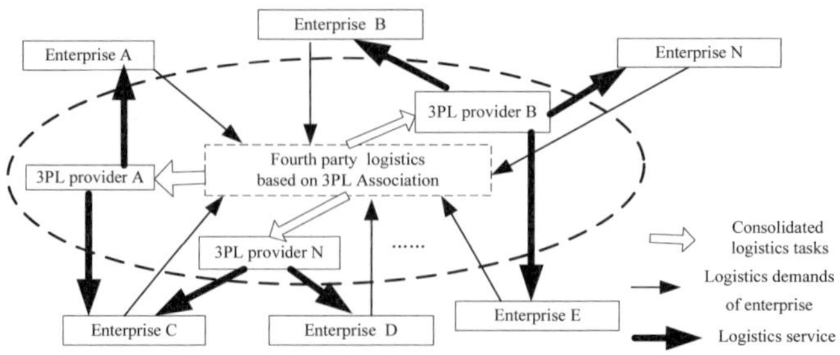

Fig. 1. Fourth party logistics based on 3PL association

3 Nash Model of Fourth Party Logistics Based on Nonprofit Organization

The primarily focus of benefits distribution is the profits generated by the fourth party logistics. A good distribution scheme should meet the following criterions:

(1) All profits made by 4PL must be distributed among its participators;

(2)The distribution scheme must be fair for all participators and encourage all members to take part in the alliance.

Suppose there are two 3PL providers A and B who can make profit m_0 and n_0 respectively called conflict point. In order to reduce costs and increase profits, they hope to form a fourth party logistics. By integration of resources and operations, the total profit of the fourth party logistics is increased, as the curve I in fig.2. All profits should be distributed between A and B because the fourth party logistics is nonprofit organization. If 3PL provider B gets profits q, the provider A can only get profits m_0. If provider B gets profits n_0, the provider A can increase its profits to p.The flowing equation is exist: $m_0 + q = n_0 + p$.

Both provider A and B expect that the profits they gets from fourth party logistics are larger than the profits they can make before joining the party. In another word, the benefits distribution scheme must guarantee the distributed profit to A be above point T(including T) in curve I and the profit to B be below point S(including S)in curve I. Therefore the segment of ST in curve I is the reasonable distribution scheme for both A and B, called Pareto Improvement interval.

According to the Nash model of two parties, there must be a negotiated solution between the two parties A and B (a point in ST segment) at which the distributed profits are accepted by both parties. However, both parties always hope to get distributed profits as many as possible. It is impossible to improve the distributed profits of A and B at the same time. In other words, if the distributed profits for party A are increased, the distributed profits for B will be reduced. The starting point for cooperation between the two parties is the minimum profits when unallianced, that is the point of conflict (point (m_0, n_0)) .If the distributed profit is below this point, the negotiation will break down and the cooperation will end. That constitutes the feasible set of negotiation. In this case, the feasible set is the distributed profits for party A and B.

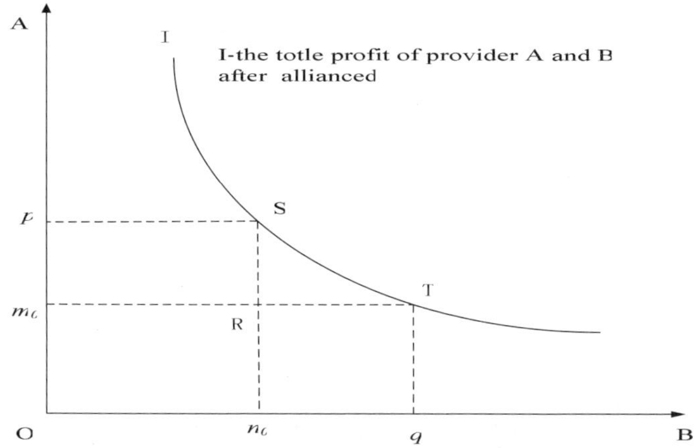

Fig. 2. Pareto improvement about two third party logistics alliance

In the negotiations involved two parties, the feasible set P can be expressed as:

$$P=\{\ (m,n)\mid m\geq m_0, n\geq n_0,\ \ (m_0,n_0):\text{the point of conflict}\}$$

Nash believed that the negotiation solution should satisfy the individual rationality, the joint rational symmetry, the linear invariability and the irrelevant selectivity. Under these five axioms limit, Nash proved the following theorem:

The only rational negotiation solution (m_1,n_1) should satisfy the following condition:

$(m_1,n_1)\in P$, P: the feasible set $m_1\geq m_0, n_1\geq n_0$ (not inferior to the point of conflict), and maximize the value of $(m_1-m_0)(n_1-n_0)$.

Nash model of negotiation has been extended to be used in multi-parties cooperation. So it can be adopted in fourth party logistics based on nonprofits organization.

4 Benefits Distribution Model of Fourth Party Logistics Based on Nonprofit Organization

Suppose the total number of 3PL who joins the 4PL is n and the 4PL could make total profits $v(N)$. All profits should be shared among all participators of 3PL. The utility function of the third party logistics provider i is u_i .which is the function of distribution value. All utility functions of third party logistics providers are mutually independent. Before joining the 4PL, the profit of third party logistics provider i is d_i, which is the lower bound of strategy for each third party logistics provider. The benefits distributed for 3PL i is x_i .The benefits distribution vector is $X=\{x_1,x_2,...x_n\}$.

Based on the above supposition, Nash model for the cooperation between two parties is extended to n parties. That is:

$$Max\prod_{i=1}^{n}[u_i(x_i)-u_i(d_i)]. \quad (1)$$

Since fourth party logistics based on nonprofit organization has a certain similarity with virtual enterprise and dynamic alliance, the principle of benefits distribution is also similar. The basic principles are as following [11]:

1) All profits of fourth party logistics based on nonprofit organization must be shared by all participators of third party logistics providers, that is:

$$\sum_{i=1}^{n} x_i = v(N) \; . \quad (2)$$

2) Based on the game theory, in order to guarantee the stability of the alliance, fourth party logistics must ensure all participators get more profits than they did before. Otherwise the third party logistics providers would not join the alliance.

$$d_1 + d_2 + ... + d_n \le v(N) \; . \quad (3)$$

3) After joining the alliance, each participator of 3PL expects more profit than he did before.

$$x_i \ge d_i \; . \quad (4)$$

4) It is unfair that some participants could get large amount of profits while the others get nothing.

The key issues for the benefits distribution model of fourth party logistics based on nonprofits organization is the construction of utility function.

Based on the analysis about utility function in Nash equilibrium [12], the utility function should meet the following conditions:

(1)It is the function of profits obtained;
(2)It must satisfy the diminishing effectiveness of the border;
(3)The benefits distributed increases as the distribution factor increase;
(4)The utility value is zero in point of conflict.

Based on the above conditions, the utility function could be as: $u_i = (x_i)^{\alpha_i/(\alpha_1+...+\alpha_n)}$. The function satisfies the conditions listed. dx_i has little impact on u_i when x_i is small, otherwise the impact is large.

Based on the above conditions, the utility function takes this kind of form: $u_i = (x_i)^{\alpha_i/(\alpha_1+...+\alpha_n)}$. The function satisfies the conditions listed, and dx_i has a smaller impact on u_i when x_i is smaller; otherwise it is bigger. It is in line with the requirements of the utility function.

In order to create the utility function $u_i = (x_i)^{\alpha_i/(\alpha_1+...+\alpha_n)}$, the distribution factor α_i must be known. Analytic Hierarchy Process (AHP) is adopted to determine the distribution factor. Considering the operation features of fourth party logistics based on nonprofit organization, the evaluation factors for AHP are the strength and the scale of 3PL providers, the contribution to the benefits of 4PL and the risk undertaken. Let factor set $U = \{$ the strength and scale, the contribution to benefits, the risk undertaken $\} = \{p_1, p_2, p_3\}$. According to the different impact of each factor, the factors are given a corresponding weights. $A = \{w_1^0, w_2^0, w_3^0\}$ .The evaluation set is $V = \{$ low, lower, medium, higher, high $\}$, which can be quantified as $V = \{1,3,5,7,9\}$. Here, number "1" stands for low. Therefore the distribution factors of third party logistics providers are obtained and the utility function is yield. Finally the Nash model is as follows:

$$Max\sum_{i=1}^{n}(x_i)^{\alpha_i/(\alpha_1+...+\alpha_n)} . \tag{5}$$

s.t.

$$x_1 + x_2 + ... + x_n = v(N) . \tag{6}$$

$$d_1 \le x_1 \le v(N) . \tag{7}$$

$$......$$

$$d_n \le x_n \le v(N) . \tag{8}$$

5 Case Study

The logistics market in Wuhan is taken as an example [13] .There are about 30 third party logistics service providers, and the average asset is about 6.0632 million yuan, their average annual income is 19.5591 million yuan. The income of each provider is shown in Table 1. In order to reduce operation costs, these third party logistics service providers hope to set up a fourth party logistics based on nonprofit 3PL alliance. Due to information sharing and resources consolidating, the operation cost could be reduced. According to reference [14], the current logistics costs could be reduced by about 10% from present costs, and the profit of the company could be increased about 7% by applying information technology and other management tools. Therefore, it is reasonable to estimate that 9% of increasing in profits could be created by implementing the 4PL alliance. The increased benefits, which is 21.3172 million Yuan, increase a little in this foundation, let it be 9%, be distributed amount its 3PL providers.

Suppose the benefits distributed to each third party logistics be $x_1, x_2, ...x_{30}$ respectively. The Nash model is created. The distribution factors are shown in Table 2.

Table 1. Comparison of third party logistics provider Benefits

3PL i	d_i/thousand yuan	x_i/thousand yuan	growth rate %
1	650.7	703.1	8.89
2	623.8	670.1	8.29
3	828.5	911.8	10.63
4	697.7	769.0	11.01
5	604.7	652.6	7.90
6	465.4	501.0	7.63
7	598.4	635.0	7.92
8	326.9	340.6	5.93
9	381.2	399.9	6.58
10	521.7	549.3	7.35
11	828.3	907.4	10.89
12	841.7	920.6	10.61
13	509.6	533.8	7.75
14	758.3	819.6	9.51
15	942.1	1045.9	12.21
16	759.8	823.9	9.89
17	400.3	415.3	6.41
18	478.2	514.1	7.51
19	429.8	450.4	7.29
20	905.9	1006.3	11.95
21	430.4	467.6	7.71
22	573.5	619.6	8.04
23	631.1	687.7	8.97
24	514.9	542.7	5.39
25	860.6	958.0	11.30
26	699.5	773.4	105.6
27	512.0	547.1	7.88
28	748.7	817.4	9.12
29	1038.0	1206.3	16.15
30	975.0	1127.2	15.6

After obtaining the distribution factors, the genetic algorithm adopted to solve the Nash model. In this case GATOOL in Matlab is adopted to solve the model. The computational results are shown in Table 1.

According to the computational results, each 3PL provider after jointing the 4PL could get more profits than it was. The growth rates correspond with the scales of 3PL providers and its contribution to the benefits. Larger scale the 3PL provider is and greater contribution to the alliance the 3PL make, larger benefits growth rate the 3PL has, vice versa. The distribution results could encourage individuals to participate in the alliance and maintain the stability of fourth party logistics alliance. Therefore, the proposed Nash equilibrium model of fourth party logistics based on nonprofit organization could get a reasonable benefits distribution.

Table 2. Distribution factors of third party logistics provider

3PL i	distribution factor	3PL i	distribution factor
1	4.28	16	5.03
2	4.08	17	2.54
3	5.56	18	3.13
4	4.69	19	2.74
5	3.97	20	6.13
6	3.05	21	2.82
7	3.87	22	3.76
8	2.07	23	4.19
9	2.44	24	3.31
10	3.35	25	5.84
11	5.52	26	4.73
12	5.61	27	3.34
13	3.29	28	4.98
14	4.99	29	7.36
15	6.37	30	6.87

6 Conclusion

Although fourth party logistics has been proposed for a long time, it is only a concept. The operation mode and benefits distribution have not been solved. It has not been used widely in practice. Aiming at benefits distribution, the key issue of fourth party logistics, this paper makes some original study on the benefits distribution by using Nash model. The validity of the proposed algorithm of benefits distribution is verified by the logistics market in Wuhan. At present, only the strength and the scale, the contribution to the benefits and the risk undertaken are considered as the distribution factor. Further research would take account other factors so as how to ensure the fair of benefits distribution. In addition, other utility functions will be considered in the future study.

Acknowledgment

This work is supported by National High-Tech Research and Development Program of China Grant # 2007AA04Z190, National Natural Science Foundation of China Grand # 50705036 and National High-Tech Research and Development Program of China Grant # 2007AA04Z107.

References

1. Fleischmann, M., Bloemhof-Ruwaard, J.M., Dekker, R., et al.: Quantitative models for reverse logistics: a review [J]. European Journal of Operational Research 103, 1–17 (1997)
2. Rogers, D.S., Tibben-Lembke, R.S.: Going backwards: reverse logistics trends and practices. The University of Nevada, Reno, Center for Logistics Management, Reverse Logistics Council (1998), http://www.rlec.org

3. Lieb, R.C.: The Use of Third-Party Logistics Service by Large American Manufacturers. Journal of Business Logistics 13(2), 29–42 (1992)
4. Hoffman, K.C.: Just What Is a 4PL Anyway? Global Logistics & Supply Chain Strategy 8 (2000), http://www.glscs.com/archives/8.00.4PL.htm?adcode75
5. Jianqing, C., Wenhuang, L., Xiu, L.: The Directed Graph Model with Multi-Dimensions in the Fourth Party Logistics and Its Algorithm. Industrial Engineering and Management 3, 45–48 (2003)
6. Jingjing, Y.: Research on forth party reverse logistics and its key techniques [D]. Thesis for Master Degree, Huazhong University of Science and Technology((2007)
7. Dube, P., Liu, Z., Wynter, L., et al.: Competitive equilibrium in e-commerce: Pricing and outsourcing. Computers & Operations Research 34, 3541–3559 (2007)
8. Haiyang, S., Tao, Y., Lilan, L.: The Research of Benefit Allocation for Manufacturing Grid. Modular Machine Tool & Automatic Manufacturing Technique 9, 110–112 (2004)
9. Qiong, L., Jingjing, Y.: Research on fourth party reverse logistics based on nonprofit organization [C/OL]. In: IEEE International Conference on Automation and Logistics, Jinan, China, pp. 2846–2850 (2007), http://ieeexplore.ieee.org/xpl/freeabs_all.jsp?isnumber=4338503&arnumber=4339066&count=614&index=562&fromcon
10. Qiong, L., Shouling, C., Jingjing, Y.: Research on forth- party logistics service platform based on SOA [J]. Machinery Design & Manufacture 9, 210–212 (2007)
11. Weidong, F., Jian, C.: Study on the Proport ion Making for Profit/Risk Allocation within Virtual Enterperises. Theory and Practice of Systems Engineering 4, 46–49 (2002)
12. Baoming, L.: Utility Function and Nash Equilibrium. Mathematics in Economics 17(4), 21–28 (2002)
13. Jitao, Y., Eping, S., Weixsheng, X.: Analysis about the Present Situation of Wuhan Modern Logistics Industry. Journal of Whhan University of Science and Engineering 18(2), 64–66 (2005)
14. Decheng, W.: How manufacturing Company to Develop the Third Profit Resource. Logistics Technology 4, 6–8 (2002)

Design of Acceleration Feedforward and Study of Calibration Algorithm

Wei Teng, Yunfei Zhou, Xiaoqing Li, and Liangliang Yang

School of Mechanical Science & Engineering, Huazhong University of Science & Technology, Wuhan, 430074, Hubei Province, China
tengwei1981@tom.com

Abstract. This paper introduces a new acceleration feedforward control strategy. The proposed feedforward control consists of a feedforward coefficient and a delay element. A calibration algorithm is provided which calculates the feedforward coefficient and delay time accurately based on experiments. And a detailed calibration process is described. The feedforward control can make model-based feedforward design simple and can gain high tracking performance. Experimental results demonstrate the feasibility and effectiveness of the proposed feedforward control strategy and calibration algorithm.

Keywords: Acceleration feedforward; Feedforward coefficient; Delay time; Calibration algorithm.

1 Introduction

In high-performance position servo system, high orientation precision, non-overshooting orientation process and as quick a dynamic response as possible are required. Generally, feedback-feedforward control strategy is utilized to achieve the above goals [1-2]. As shown in Fig.1, a feedback-feedforward loop consists of:

- third-order profile planning [3-5]: the representation of the nominal acceleration, nominal velocity and nominal position based on motion restrictions such as maximal velocity, motion distance etc.,
- feedforward loop [6-9]: the calculation of nominal acceleration with feedforward coefficient to drive the plant in advance,
- controller: the regulation of position error,
- plant: the actuation device (e.g. a linear motor with air bearing),
- feedback loop [10]: the introduction of the actual position into controller to compensate for unknown disturbances.

In many motion controllers, model-based feedforward is proposed. This feedforward action can improve tracking performance greatly as long as the feedforward model approximates the plant inverse sufficiently well. In practice, some disadvantages make the model-based feedforward difficult as follows: ①Inherent delay time in digital system can not be well identified because the power amplifier and position

C. Xiong et al. (Eds.): ICIRA 2008, Part II, LNAI 5315, pp. 539–547, 2008.

measurement are not ideal [11]. ②For high order control system, the inverse model of the plant will be complicated, which will bring much noise [6]. ③Motion damping of the plant is not accurate enough because the viscous degree of suspension and the friction can not be calculated exactly [12].

Based on model-based feedforward design, this paper will propose a new acceleration feedforward control strategy consisting of a feedforward coefficient and a delay element to overcome the disadvantages above. In Section 2 how the new feedforward strategy works is illuminated. And a calibration algorithm calculating the feedforward coefficient and delay time is provided in Section 3, followed by the calibration process in Section 4. Then, experimental platform, motion parameters and intermediate data will be listed and experimental results will be analyzed in Section 5, which demonstrate the feasibility of the feedforward strategy and calibration algorithm. Finally, conclusions are drawn in Section 6.

2 Design of Acceleration Feedforward

In the motion control system described as Fig.1, the plant is driven by the feedforward force *ffd_out* calculated from Eq. (1). The feedback loop consists of a controller, a power amplifier, a plant and position measurement. The controller includes a PID, a 2nd low-pass filter and a notch filter. The plant is a linear motor suspended by air bearing with transfer function $1/ms^2$. The acceleration feedforward loop consisting of the feedforward coefficient M and delay element is described as

$$ffd\_out = acceleration \times M \times e^{-s(2T-t)} . \tag{1}$$

M is not the actual mass of actor of the linear motor and it will be calculated accurately according to the calibration algorithm in Section 3.

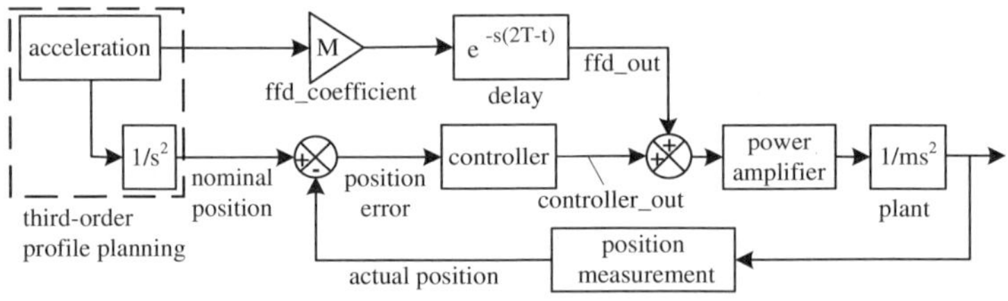

Fig. 1. Motion control diagram with acceleration feedforward for electromechanical system

As an inertial electromechanical system, the plant has an inherent lag time in responding to the feedforward force. If the plant is expected to reach a certain nominal position at τ time, the nominal acceleration instruction should be sent out at τ-t time, with t as the inherent lag time of the plant. In digital system, t is not the very integral number of sampling period so that the nominal acceleration should be sent out two sampling periods ahead of the corresponding nominal position. There is a redundant time resulting from the difference between the advance time and the lag time. So a delay element with transfer function in S-domain $e^{-s(2T-t)}$ is designed to counteract this redundant time. To accomplish the delay element in digital system conveniently, the transfer function is substituted by first-order lag element defined as

$$H_{delay}(s) = \frac{1-(2T-t)s/2}{1+(2T-t)s/2}, \tag{2}$$

with t as the inherent lag time of the plant, T the sampling period and $2T$-t the delay time of the delay element.

Tustin transformation is adopted to achieve the discretization in digital system. And the transfer function of the delay element in Z-domain is described as

$$H_{delay}(z) = \frac{B_0 + B_1 z^{-1}}{1 + A_1 z^{-1}}, \tag{3}$$

with

$$A_1 = \frac{-T+t}{3T-t}, \quad B_0 = \frac{-T+t}{3T-t}, \quad B_1 = 1. \tag{4}$$

3 Calibration Principle and Calibration Algorithm

Due to the existence of the disadvantages in Section 1, a calibration algorithm should be introduced to calibrate the feedforward coefficient and delay time in this section. The coupling relationship between the feedforward loop and feedback loop can be minimized even eliminated by the calibration, which will obtain an optimal feedforward coefficient and delay time. Then all the disadvantages will be overcome.

3.1 Calibration of Feedforward Coefficient

Suppose the feedforward coefficient is not accurate enough, the feedforward force will be too short or redundant to make the plant reach the nominal acceleration accurately. So the controller will export a force due to the existence of the feedback loop to compensate the feedforward force accordingly. If the controller output can be transferred to the feedforward force as many as possible, the plant will be driven quite appropriately to move. Also the controller output will be minimized during accelerating or decelerating process. A converted mass $\triangle$*ffd_mass* is calculated by the controller output with the corresponding nominal acceleration in a calibration process according to the equation

$$\Delta ffd\_mass = \frac{\sum_{i=1}^{n}(acceleration_i \times controller\_out_i)}{\sum_{i=1}^{n}(acceleration_i \times acceleration_i)} . \tag{5}$$

with i denoting the sampling point, n the total number of sampling points in a calibration process. Then, the new feedforward coefficient will be obtained based on the old one with the $\triangle ffd\_mass$ described as

$$M = M + \Delta ffd\_mass . \tag{6}$$

3.2 Calibration of Delay Time

As mentioned in Section 2, the advance time of two sampling periods is longer than the inherent lag time of the plant, which will lead to fluctuations on controller output during accelerating or decelerating process. Jerk, the derivative of the nominal acceleration, can influence the time of the feedforward force acting on the plant. The coupling relationship between the jerk and controller output is calculated as the following equation

$$\Delta ffd\_cross = \frac{\sum_{i=1}^{n}(jerk_i \times controller\_out_i)}{\sum_{i=1}^{n}(jerk_i \times jerk_i)} . \tag{7}$$

And then the delay time in the delay element can be updated as

$$t_{delay} = t_{delay} + \Delta ffd\_cross / M , \tag{8}$$

where the t_{delay} behind the equal sign is the previous delay time. The redundant advance time resulting from the difference between the advance time of two sampling periods and the lag time of the plant can be counteracted by the t_{delay}, which makes the controller output as small as possible during jerk.

4 Calibration Process

A calibration routine is adopted to eliminate the motion chanciness of samples, consisting of four motion steps: from 0 to 0.02m, return to 0, from 0 to -0.02m and return to 0. All the nominal acceleration and controller output signals are sampled during the calibration process to determine the feedforward coefficient and delay time as described in Eq. (5) to (8). The calculation process is executed circularly until the $\triangle ffd\_mass$ is less than 0.1kg. The detailed calibration process is shown in Fig.2.

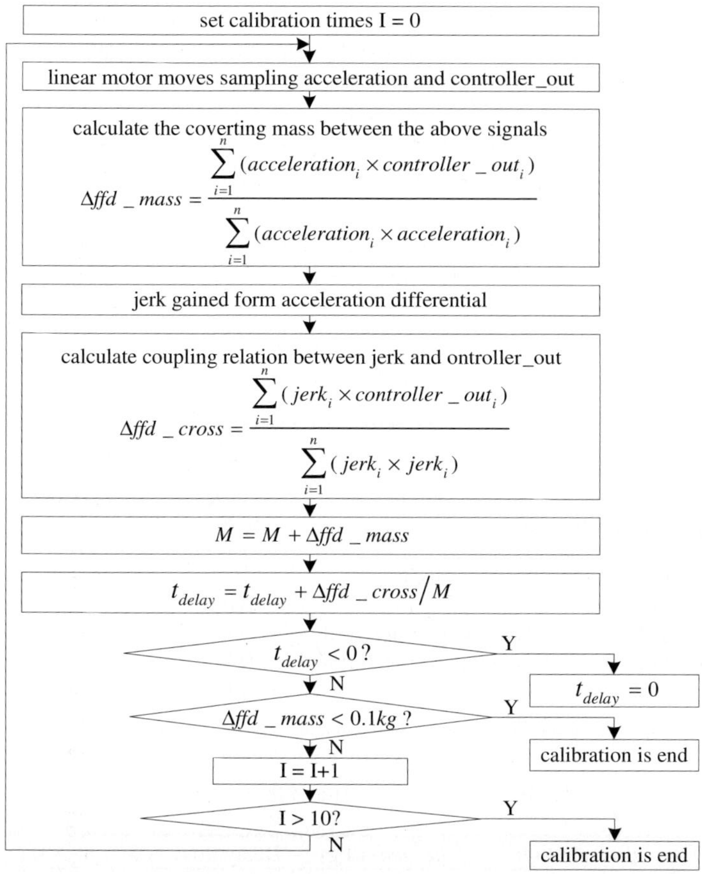

Fig. 2. Process of experimental calibration

5 Experimental Results

The experimental platform consists of a linear motor equipped with an encoder whose resolution is 1 micron to measure the actual position. The motion parameters are list in Table 1. First, Fig.3 shows the comparison between the position errors with feedforward control and without that. Obviously the latter has more impulsion and longer settling time. Second, the calibration process in Section 4 is executed and finished after three times, considering the initial values of the feedforward coefficient and delay time as zero in experiments. Fig.4 shows the controller output without any feedforward control. From Fig.4 to 7, the controller output becomes smaller and smaller during three calibration processes and Fig.7 shows the final result when the $\triangle ffd\_mass$ is less than 0.1kg. The variation of controller output illuminates that the dynamic characteristic becomes better and better as the feedforward coefficient and delay time become more and more optimal. The intermediate data of three calibration processes are shown in Table 2. After the feedforward coefficient is calibrated accurately, a test is done to show the importance of the delay element only. The fluctuation of actual acceleration with delay element shown in Fig.9 is smaller than that without delay element shown in Fig.8. That is because the difference between the advance time of two sampling periods and the inherent lag time of the plant has been well counteracted by the delay element. Finally, the plant moves from 0 to 0.06m with the actual mass in feedforward control, and then with the calibrated feedforward coefficient and delay time according to the principle above. Comparing the two craves in Fig.10, it is obvious that the latter position error has better effect on dynamic response, which suggests that feedforward control with the actual mass only can not get the optimal control effect.

Table 1. Parameters of controller and filters

Parameters	Value	Unit
Sampling period	400e-6	s
Gain	110e3	N/m
Integral frequency	0.5	Hz
Differential frequency	7	Hz
Frequency of 2nd low-pass filter	68	Hz
Damping of 2nd low-pass filter	0.68	/
Pole and zero frequency of notch filter	69 69	Hz
Pole and zero damping of notch filter	0.06 0.01	/
Max jerk	200	m/s^3
Max acceleration	2	m/s^2

Table 2. Intermediate data of three calibrations

Time of calibration	$\triangle$*ffd_mass*(kg)	Delay time $\triangle$*ffd_cross/M* (s)
1	16.3702	213e-6
2	3.896	-49e-6
3	0.082	12e-6

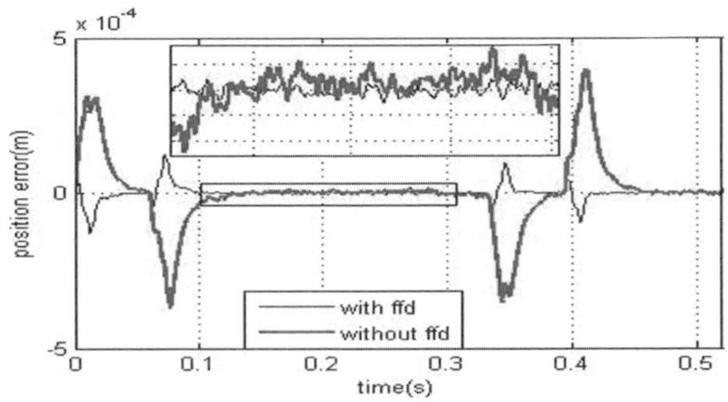

Fig. 3. Position error with and without acceleration feedforward

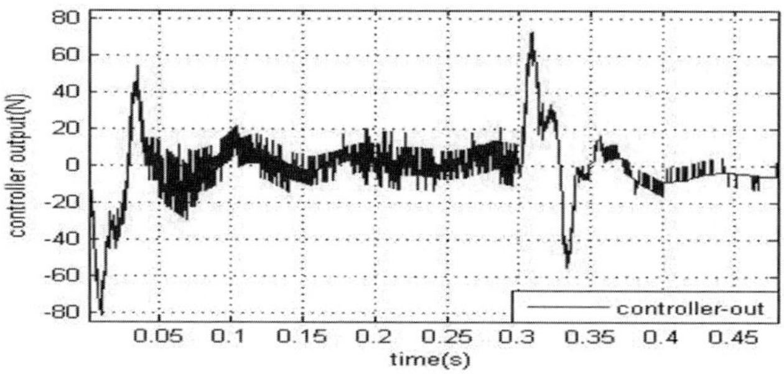

Fig. 4. Controller output without feedforward control

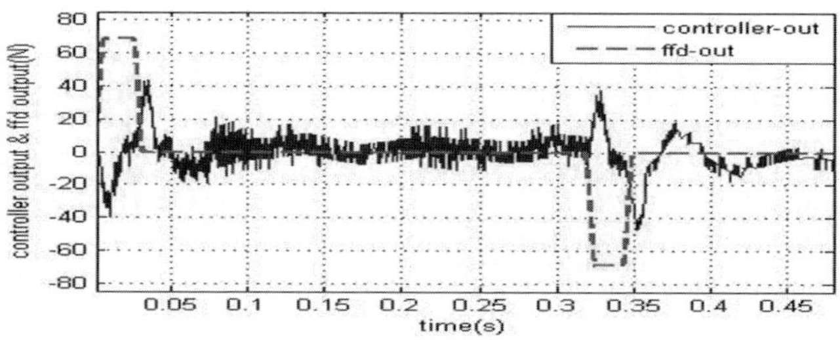

Fig. 5. Feedforward force and controller output after the first calibration

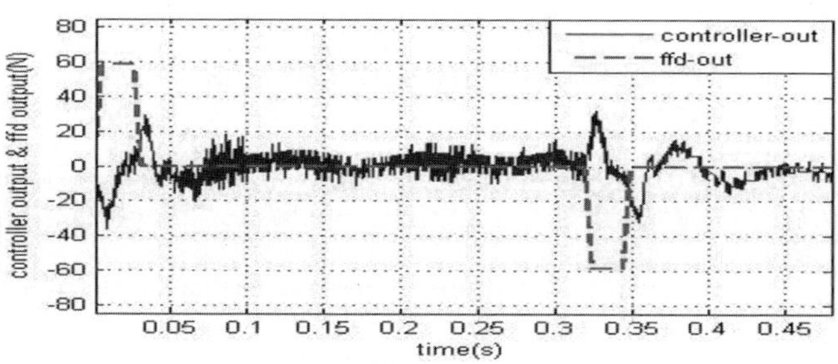

Fig. 6. Feedforward force and controller output after the second calibration

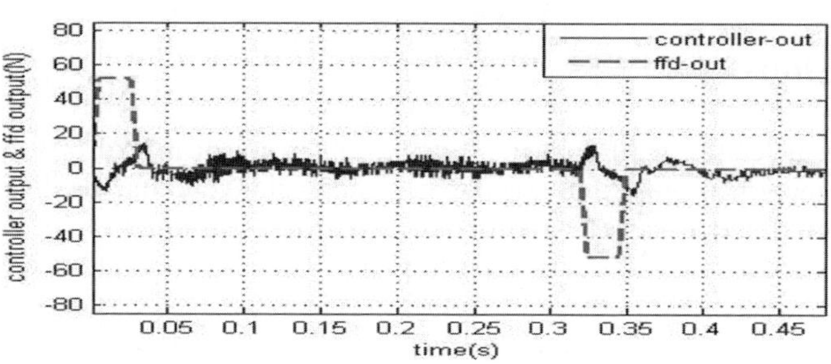

Fig. 7. Feedforward force and controller output after the third calibration

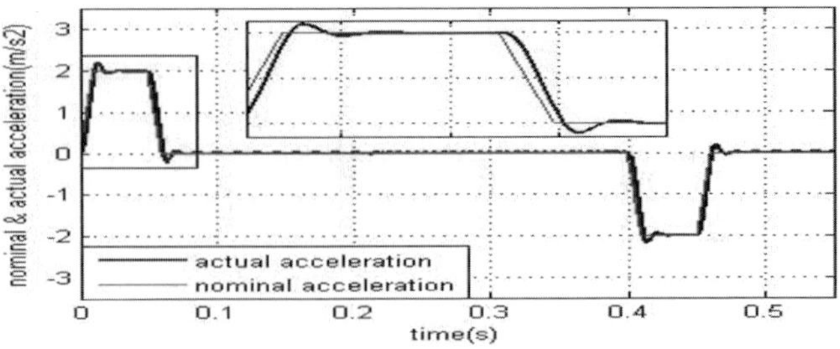

Fig. 8. Nominal acceleration and actual acceleration without delay element

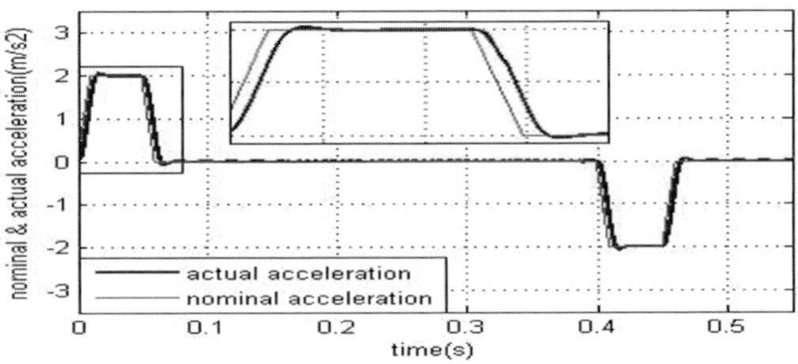

Fig. 9. Nominal acceleration and actual acceleration with delay element

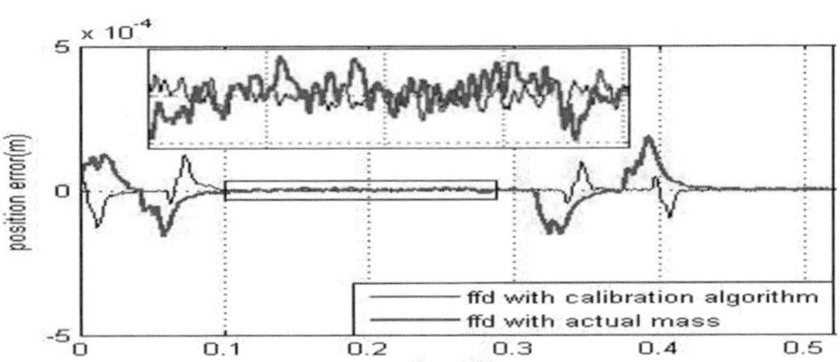

Fig. 10. Position error with actual mass and with calibration algorithm

6 Conclusions

An acceleration feedforward control strategy consisting of a feedforward coefficient and delay element is proposed in this paper, which can overcome the disadvantages of the conventional model-based feedforward control. A calibration principle on the feedforward coefficient and delay time is given, and the calibration process is executed based on experiments to validate the effectiveness of the acceleration feedforward control strategy. Through the calibration algorithm, with the optimal feedforward coefficient and delay time, the non-overshooting orientation process is realized; the motion impulsion during acceleration or deceleration process is minimized; and the settling time is shortened effectively. The calibration algorithm can be applied in practice widely to gain high control performance.

Acknowledgments

The authors are very grateful for the financial support from the National Natural Science Foundation of China (No. 507775088).

References

1. Lin, C.Y., Tsao, T.C.: Nano-Precision Dynamic Motion Control. In: Proceeding of the SPIE, p. 66480H (2007)
2. Yang, P.H., Alamo, B., Andeen, G.B.: Control Design for a 6 DOF E-beam Lithography Stage. In: Proceeding of the American Control Conference, VA, Arlington, June 25-27, pp. 2255–2260 (2001)
3. Dijkstra, B.G., Rambaratsingh, N.J., Scherer, C.: Input design for optimal discrete-time point-to-point motion of an industrial XY positioning table. In: Proceedings of the 39th IEEE conference on decision and control, Sydney, Australia, pp. 901–906 (2000)
4. Mu, H.H., Zhou, Y.F.: Profile Generation Algorithm and Implementation for High Accuracy Motion. In: Proceeding of the 2006 IEEE International Conference on Robotics and Biominetics, Kunming, China, pp. 549–554 (2006)
5. Roover, D., Sperling, F.: Point-to-point Control of a High Accuracy Positioning Mechanism. In: Proceedings of the American Control Conference 1997, Albuquerque, NM, USA, pp. 1350–1354 (1997)
6. Boerlage, M., Steinbuch, M., Lambrechts, P.F.: Model based feedforward for motion systems. In: Proceedings of the IEEE international conference on control applications (CCA), Istanbul, Turkey, pp. 1158–1163 (2003)
7. Kang, M.S., Yoon, W.H.: Acceleration feedforward control in active magnetic bearing system subject to base motion by filter-XLMS algorithm. J. Control System Technology. 14(1), 134–140 (2006)
8. Suzuki, Y.: Acceleration feedforward control for active magnetic bearing systems excited by ground motion. J. Control Theory and Applications. 145(2), 113–118 (1998)
9. Lambrechts, P.F., Boerlage, M., Steinbuch, M.: Trajectory planning and feedforward design for electromechanical motion systems. J. Control Engineering Practice 13, 145–157 (2005)
10. Tam, M.S.W., Cheung, N.C.: A high speed high precision linear drive system for manufacturing automation. In: Applied Power Electronics Conference and Exposition, Sixteenth Annual, vol. 1(4-8), pp. 440–444. IEEE, Los Alamitos (2001)
11. Venkatesan, G.: Modelling feedback control adjustment to control output product quality. In: Proceeding of American Control Conference, vol. 6, pp. 5049–5053 (2002)
12. Milasinovic, D.D.: Rheological-dynamical analogy: Prediction of damping parameters of hysteresis damper. J. Solids and Structures 44, 7143–7166 (2007)

Research on Acceleration and Deceleration Control Algorithm of NC Instruction Interpretations with High-Order Smooth

Fang Song, Shuanghui Hao, Minghui Hao, and Zhimin Yang

School of Mechatronics Eng., Harbin Institute of Technology, Harbin, 150001, China
songfang2005@163.com

Abstract. In order to solve the vibration problem of flexible system which the control order of CNC servo system is four orders or over four orders, one of the mainly effective methods is the characteristic of high-order smooth of the acc/dec (acceleration and deceleration) control instructions. According to the control theory of linear acc/dec, a novel acc/dec control algorithm based on moving-average is presented in this paper. The continuity of the acceleration curve can be obtained by using the proposed algorithm. Further, the curve of Jerk will also be continuous by extending the proposed algorithm. In practice, this algorithm is simple and needn't solve the high-order equation. By extending this algorithm, the high-order smooth acceleration instruction can be achieved that is the important meaning to improve the machining accuracy of CNC system.

Keywords: NC instruction; acc/dec control; high-order smooth; moving-average algorithm.

1 Introduction

At present, the research and development of CNC system are mainly from the mechanical or mathematical point of view. Servo system, as an independent branch, is developing paralleled with CNC system. Due to profession division there is some unreasonable effect to the whole machine tool. When requiring the high-speed and high-precision, CNC system will make shock and vibrate which will lead to low positioning accuracy with the acceleration increasing more and more. The researchers found that the main reasons [1-2] of leading to the above disadvantages are the discontinuity and high-order non-differentiability of the acceleration instruction, so the cubic S-curve acc/dec control algorithm based on linear acc/dec control algorithm was developed to solve these problems of the shock and vibration[3]. Although the cubic S-curve acc/dec control algorithm is strict logic, continuity and differentiability, to some extent, can be used to solve the problem of the acceleration continuity. Because the interpolation cycle is constant to meet the boundary condition of the velocity, acceleration and position at the same time at the end, the cubic equation must be calculated, which will generate vast codes. However the computation is not easy to MCU in practical engineering application and the real time is bad. Currently, the general

C. Xiong et al. (Eds.): ICIRA 2008, Part II, LNAI 5315, pp. 548–557, 2008.

solution to this problem is either acceleration jump or lengthening positioning time to meet the boundary condition of the terminal point, which would impact CNC system performance at the high speed[4]. Furthermore, For the fourth-order or exceeding fourth-order flexible system, in order to solve these phenomena of the shock and vibration, only to increase the order of the S-curve acc/dec control algorithm to match that of the system. Because the S-curve acc/dec control algorithm lacks of expandability [5], which will make algorithm calculation more complex.

In order to improve CNC system performance, the key issues such as instruction high-order differentiability, expandability and performability under the boundary condition should be well solved. In the paper, a novel moving average acc/dec control algorithm is proposed to solve these key issues. This control algorithm has advantage of expandability and simple calculation. For the high-order control system, the algorithm is repeatedly extended to achieve the high-order differentiability of CNC instruction interpretation.

2 Linear acc/dec Control Algorithm

Moving average acc/dec control algorithm is based on linear acc/dec control algorithm, so it must ensure that position, speed and acceleration meet the boundary condition at first when the linear acc/dec control algorithm running to the end of program segment. The principle of the linear acc/dec control algorithm is shown in figure 1.

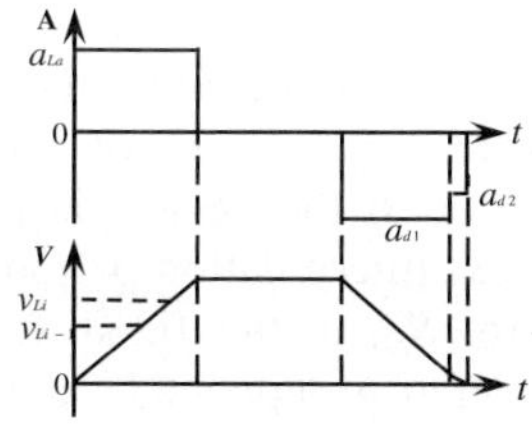

Fig. 1. Linear acc/dec control

When the starting point of speed and position is known, at the Nth interpolation cycle the formula of the acceleration, velocity and location are expressed as follows:

$$\begin{cases} a_{LN} = a_L \\ v_{LN} = v_{LS} + a_{LN} NT \\ S_{LN} = S_{LS} + v_{LS} NT + \dfrac{a_{LN} N^2 T^2}{2} \end{cases} \tag{1}$$

where a_{LN}, v_{LN} and S_{LN} are acceleration, velocity and location at the Nth interpolation cycle, respectively. v_{LS} and S_{LS} are velocity and position of the starting point, respectively. N is the iterative step number.

a_L is the maximum acceleration of the system in the equation (1). Due to the interpolation cycle T is constant, the velocity, acceleration and position should be ensured to satisfy their respective constraint condition. Under this condition, the iterative step number N may be decimal fraction, so the iterative step number must be adjusted to being round number before calculating the maximum actual acceleration again during the acc/dec state.

2.1 The Calculation of the Acceleration during the Acceleration State

According to the starting velocity v_{LS} and the instruction feed velocity v_{Lf}, the acceleration step number n_a can be achieved from equation (2).

$$n_a = \frac{|v_{Lf} - v_{LS}|}{a_L T} \tag{2}$$

It is important that the actual system acceleration could not exceed the theory system acceleration and the acceleration step number N_a should be up to round number, namely, $N_a \geq n_a$. Based on equation (2), the actual acceleration a_{La} in the acceleration state can be obtained:

$$a_{La} = \frac{v_{Lf} - v_{LS}}{N_a T} \qquad (a_{La} \leq a_L) \tag{3}$$

2.2 The Calculation of the Acceleration during the Deceleration State

Firstly, the deceleration point is predicted according to the rule of acc/dec, the distance of the deceleration course S_d is computed firstly. Then judge if the rest distance of current interpolation point is less than S_d or not and confirm if the system comes into the deceleration course or not. If the answer is positive, the system will begin decelerating at the start of the next interpolation period. Here, the start position is S_{Ld} at the deceleration course (here, S_{Ld} is the fixed value). During the deceleration course, the theoretical acceleration a_L is depicted by the formula(4):

$$a_L = \frac{v_{Le}^2 - v_{Ld}^2}{2(S_{Le} - S_{Ld})} \tag{4}$$

Where, S_{Le}, S_{Ld}, v_{Le} and v_{Ld} are the final position, the initial position, the finial velocity and the initial velocity at the deceleration state respectively. Meanwhile, v_{Ld} is just the instruction feedrate v_{Lf}. The deceleration step number n_d (n_d may be decimal fraction which is the same as n_a) at the deceleration state may be expressed as:

$$n_d = \frac{2(S_{Le} - S_{Ld})}{(v_{Le} - v_{Ld})T} \tag{5}$$

Different from the acceleration state, in the deceleration state, besides the deceleration step must be round number and the actual acceleration should not exceed the system maximum acceleration, the position and the velocity of the end point should reach the given value at the same time.

In the deceleration state, only to adjust acceleration can not meet the requirement of the instruction control. The reasons are explained as follows.

The actual acceleration a_{Ld} in the deceleration state can be expressed as :

$$a_{Ld} = \frac{v_{Le} - v_{Ld}}{N_d T} \qquad (a_{Ld} \le a_L) \tag{6}$$

a_{Ld} is inducted into formula(4). In formula (4), v_{Ld}□ v_{Le} and S_{Ld} are fix value. If the equation comes into existence, S_{Le} must be changed. But if S_{Le} is changed, the final position will be changed. This is ambivalent.

For solving this problem resulted from the contradiction, two different accelerations a_{d1} and a_{d2} are used to decelerate in the deceleration state, respectively. Besides, the two accelerations should be being within the system maximum acceleration. Calculated as follows:

(1) The position S_{Le1} and the velocity v_{Le1} in the (N_d-1)th step are calculated by using the acceleration a_{d1} and then they are taken as the starting point of the position and velocity in the N_d th step in the deceleration state.

$$S_{Le1} = S_{Ld} + v_{Ld} T(N_d - 1) + \frac{a_{d1} T^2 (N_d - 1)^2}{2} \tag{7}$$

$$v_{Le1} = v_{Ld} + a_{d1} T(N_d - 1) \tag{8}$$

(2) With the acceleration a_{d2} decelerating to the N_d th step, the end point of the position and the velocity are expressed as:

$$S_{Le} = S_{Le1} + v_{Le1} T + \frac{a_{d2} T^2}{2} \tag{9}$$

$$v_{Le} = v_{Le1} + a_{d2} T \tag{10}$$

(3) According to the equation (7)~(10), the acceleration a_{d1} and a_{d2} can be respectively expressed as:

$$a_{d1} = \frac{-v_{Le} T - v_{Ld}(2N_d - 1)T + 2(S_{Le} - S_{Ld})}{(N_d - 1) N_d T^2} \tag{11}$$

$$a_{d2} = \frac{v_{Le}(N_d + 1)T + v_{Ld}(N_d - 1)T - 2(S_{Le} - S_{Ld})}{N_d T^2} \tag{12}$$

3 Moving Average acc/dec Control Algorithm

The specific solving process of the moving average acc/dec control algorithm is shown in figure 2. In the figure 2, n is the moving average step, v_L is the velocity with the linear acc/dec control, v_J is the actual velocity after moving average processing and a_J is the actual acceleration by differentiating moving average velocity with respect to the time.

The main mind of acc/dec control algorithm based on moving average method is: This algorithm is based on linear acc/dec mode to dispose the velocities of all the discrete points obtained by linear acc/dec mode. Then, compute the new acceleration by the processed velocity. At last, the displacement will be expressed by the former obtained velocity and acceleration. The acceleration obtained by this method changes continuous, so the change of the velocity is steady during the acc/dec interval. figure.2 shows the process to obtain the new velocity by the use of the control algorithm based on moving average. Meanwhile, n, v_L, v_J, and a_J are the step number of moving average, the velocity of linear acc/dec mode, the practical velocity that the velocity of linear acc/dec mode is processed by moving average and the practical acceleration obtained by the practical velocity respectively.

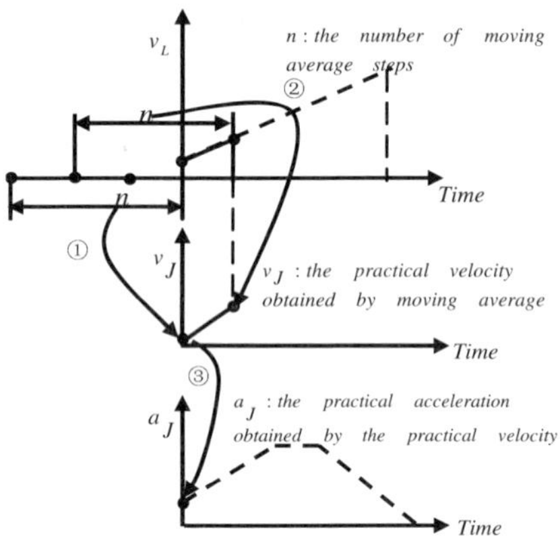

Fig. 2. Acc/dec control algorithm based on moving average

3.1 Moving Average Velocity Before n -1 Interpolation Cycles

As shown in figure 2, the initial velocity of the moving average algorithm is equal to that of the linear acc/dec control algorithm, Namely, $v_{J0} = v_{L0}$. In the next n -1 interpolation cycles, the moving average velocity of the i th interpolation cycle can be expressed as:

$$v_{Ji} = \frac{(n-i)v_{J0} + \sum_{j=1}^{i} v_{Lj}}{n} \quad (i = 1,2,\cdots,n-1) \tag{13}$$

where v_{Li} that is the transient velocity of the i th interpolation cycle is computed iteratively by the linear acc/dec control algorithm.

3.2 Moving Average Velocity from n to N Interpolation Cycle

If N is the total interpolation cycle step number used to finish this procedure of processing with the linear acc/dec algorithm, then the moving average velocity of the ith interpolation cycle can be expressed as:

$$v_{Ji} = \frac{\sum_{j=i-n+1}^{i} v_{Lj}}{n} \quad (i = n, n+1,\cdots,N) \tag{14}$$

3.3 Moving Average Velocity Delay *n*-1 Interpolation Cycle

After the linear acc/dec operation completion, the running velocity is equal to the end point velocity v_{Le}. Compared with the linear acc/dec/ algorithm, the moving average algorithm has some delay time and the delay cycle is n-1 cycles. In the n-1 delay interpolation cycles, the moving average velocity of the ith interpolation cycle can be expressed as:

$$v_{Ji} = \frac{\sum_{j=i-n+1}^{N} v_{Lj} + (i-N)v_{Le}}{n} (i = N+1,..., N+n-1) \tag{15}$$

After every interpolation cycle the moving average velocity v_{Ji} has been obtained, differentiating v_{Ji} with respect to the time t then gives the transient acceleration of moving average acc/dec algorithm, and the transient position S_{Ji} also can be obtained.

$$a_{Ji-1} = \frac{v_{Ji} - v_{Ji-1}}{T} \tag{16}$$

$$S_{Ji} = S_{Ji-1} + v_{Ji-1}T + \frac{a_{Ji-1}T^2}{2} \tag{17}$$

4 Extended Moving Average acc/dec Control Algorithm

The first-order moving average processing based on the linear acc/dec control algorithm can only ensure the curve of the acceleration being continuous, which is the same as the S curve acc/dec control algorithm but the calculation of the first-order moving average is more simple than the S curve control algorithm. Transient acceleration rate of change J reflects the relationship between the machine tool response speed and the running stationary. So in order to ensure the acceleration rate of change being continuous, the first- order moving average control algorithm should be extended. Namely, the second-order moving average processing should be done, whose solution procedure is shown in figure 3.

As shown in figure 3, n' is the number of the second-order moving average steps, v_J is the first moving average velocity, v_{JJ} is the actual velocity after the second moving average and a_{JJ} is the actual acceleration by differentiating v_{JJ} with respect to running time. Based on the assumption that the first moving average velocity v_{Ji} is known during the ith interpolation cycle, moving average velocity in different interpolation cycle would be analyzed detailed as follows.

4.1 Moving Average Velocity Before *n'*-1 Interpolation Cycles

As shown in figure 3, the initial velocity of the second-order moving average algorithms is equal to that of the first-order moving average algorithms, namely, $v_{JJ0}=v_{J0}$. In the next n' -1 interpolation cycle, the moving average velocity of the i th interpolation cycle can be expressed as:

$$v_{JJi} = \frac{(n'-i)v_{JJ0} + \sum_{j=1}^{i} v_{Jj}}{n'} \quad (i = 1,2,..., n'-1) \tag{18}$$

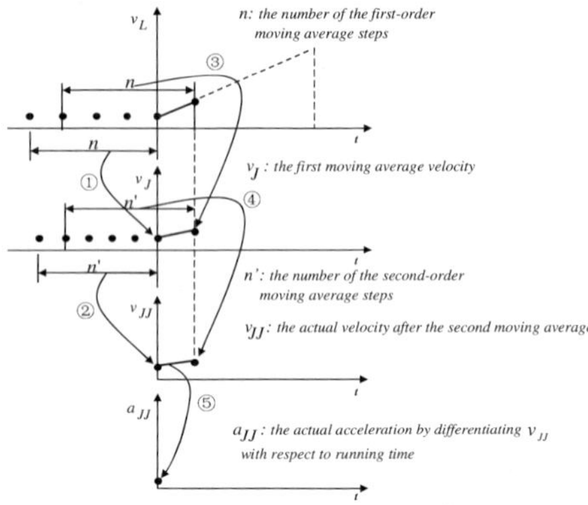

Fig. 3. Quadratic moving average acc/dec control algorithm

4.2 Moving Average Velocity from *n'* to *N*+*n*+1 Interpolation Cycle

If *N* is the total interpolation cycle used to finish this procedures of processing with the linear acc/dec control algorithm and *n* is the moving average step number, then the moving average velocity of the *i* th interpolation cycle can be expressed as:

$$v_{JJi} = \frac{\sum_{j=i-n'+1}^{i} v_{Jj}}{n'} (i = n', n' + 1, ..., N + n - 1) \tag{19}$$

4.3 Moving Average Velocity with Delay n' -1 Interpolation Cycle

After the first-order moving average finishing, the second-order moving average does not start immediately. There exists some delay between them, and the delay cycle is *n'*-1 cycles. Then moving average velocity of the *i*th interpolation cycle can be expressed as:

$$v_{JJi} = \frac{\sum_{j=i-n'}^{N+n-1} v_{Jj} + (i - N - n) v_{Je}}{n'} \quad (i = N + n + 1, ..., N + n + n' - 1) \tag{20}$$

where v_{Je} is the terminal velocity of the first-order moving average processing.

After the second-order moving average velocity, v_{JJi} has been obtained, differentiating v_{JJi} with respect to the time *t* then gives the transient acceleration of the second-order average acc/dec control algorithm. So the transient position S_{JJi} also can be obtained.

$$a_{JJi-1} = \frac{v_{JJi} - v_{JJi-1}}{T} \tag{21}$$

$$S_{JJi} = S_{JJi-1} + v_{JJi-1} T + \frac{a_{JJi-1} T^2}{2} \tag{22}$$

Acceleration curve is continuous and velocity curve is smooth under the moving average acc/dec control algorithm. This ensures that velocity, acceleration and position are all within the constraints every moment to ensure the processing accuracy.

5 Simulation Analysis of the Moving Average acc/dec Control Algorithm

In order to verify the validity of the moving average acc/dec control algorithm, the algorithm has been simulated and analyzed using the MATLAB simulation software. During the simulation, the motion displacement S is set to be 10mm, the feed velocity F is set to be 100mm/s, the maximum acceleration a_{max} is set to be 3000mm/s^2, the interpolation cycle T is set to be 0.001s, the initial velocity v_s and the terminal velocity v_e are set to be zero, respectively, and the moving average step number of the first-order n and second- order n' are set to be $n=n'=8$. The linear acc/dec control algorithm, the first-order moving average and the second-order moving average acc/dec control algorithm have been used to simulation analysis. Figure 4 shows the simulation curve of the displacement, velocity, acceleration and acceleration rate of change.

As shown in figure 4, with the linear acc/dec control algorithm, the acceleration and acceleration rate of change jump with a rush in the velocity transition point. After dealing with a moving average, the curve of the acceleration is smooth, but the acceleration rate of change still has some jump compared with that of the acceleration rate of change with the linear acc/dec control algorithm is slight. After the second moving average processing, the acceleration is smooth and the acceleration rate of change is continuous except for existing n-1 interpolation cycles delay which is shorter than that caused by general control algorithm.

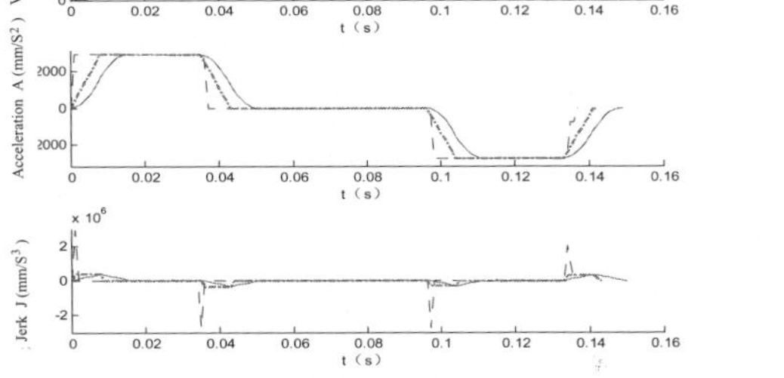

Fig. 4. Compare of linear, simple and quadratic moving average acc/dec algorithm

6 Experiments of the Moving Average acc/dec Control Algorithm

For evaluating the capability of the moving average acc/dec control algorithm, an AC servo experimental system based on MCU is built up, which uses NEC's uPD70F3184 MCU as its core controller and the method of embedded system design is used to design the NC instruction modular. The experimental system architecture as shown in figure 5(a) and the figure 5(b) is the photo of the structure of the experimental system.

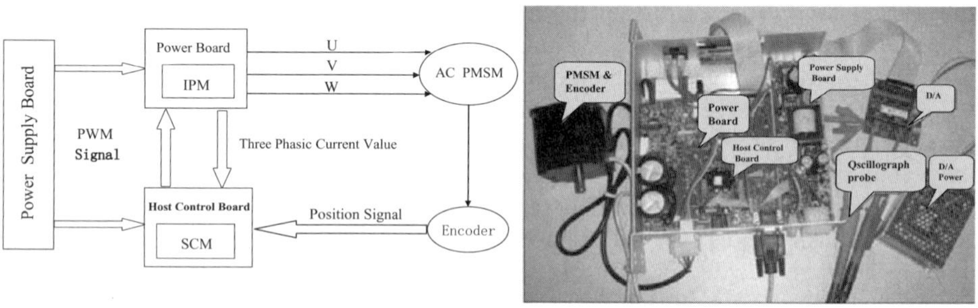

(a)system work principle chart (b) practical experiment equipment chart

Fig. 5. Chart of experiment equipment configuration

Table 1. Machining parameters

Displacement	4 mm	4000000 LSB
Maximum velocity	10 mm/s	10000 LSB/Ts
Maximum acceleration	50 mm/s^2	50 LSB/Ts^2
Initial velocity	0.676 mm/s	676 LSB/Ts
Terminal velocity	0.676 mm/s	676 LSB/Ts
Interpolation cycle	0.001 s	1 Ts

During the course of testing, the timer interrupt is set to be one interpolation cycle. Namely, the control cycle is equal to the interpolation cycle. And to meet the MCU control and computing needs of the whole integer, the selected parameter units should be converted into the relationship between the resolution (LSB) and control cycle (T_s) to ensure the adequate accuracy of the control calculation. Besides, the values of the selected parameters are up to three orders of magnitude. The selected parameters are shown in table 1.

The first-order and second-order moving average acc/dec control algorithms are used to be experimental study, during the experiment, the moving average step number is 16 and 32 respectively. Figure 6 is the curves of the velocity and acceleration.

As shown in figure 6, the curves of the velocity and acceleration are continuous and smooth, after which have been processed by moving average acc/dec control algorithm. The experimental results agree well the control algorithm simulation results, which also verify that the algorithm simulation is valid indirectly.

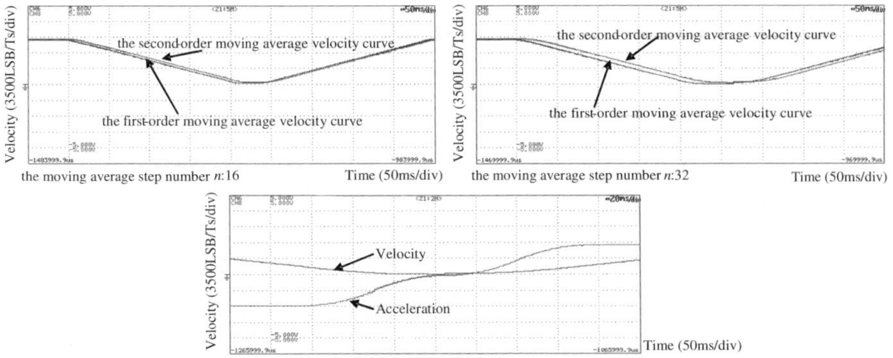

Fig. 6. Velocity/acceleration curves after moving average:(a) velocity curve of moving average steps 16 (b) velocity curve of moving average steps 32 (c) velocity and acceleration curve of Fig.6-b processed by quadratic moving average

7 Conclusions

Theoretical analysis of the moving average acc/dec control algorithm and algorithm simulation using MATLAB as simulation tool are presented in this paper. The experimental results verify the algorithm can be a good solution to the machine vibration problem of the high-order NC system during the high-speed and high-precision processing. The vibration is generated from the limitations of the NC instruction interpretation due to the general control algorithms lack of expandability in order. The moving average acc/dec control algorithm, based on the linear acc/dec control algorithm, is used to process the velocity by the method of moving average, which are simple and expandability. Besides, the curve of acceleration rate of change is smooth by moving average processing to the velocity. For the high-order control system, the algorithm is repeatedly extended to achieve the NC instruction interpretation high-differentiable.

References

1. Bin, W., Zhe, L.: Preshaped input commands applied to minimizing the vibration of a multiple-modes system. J. Journal of Beijing Polytechnic University 20(3), 97–102 (1994)
2. Xingui, G., Decai, W., Congxin, L., et al.: A rapid and accurate positioning method with linear deceleration in servo system. J. International Journal of Machine Tools & Manufacture 42, 851–861 (2002)
3. Shuang, C., Zexiang, L.: Applied motion control technology, pp. 279–297. Electric Industry Press, M. Beijing (2006)
4. Jeon, J.W., Ha, Y.Y.: A generalized approach for the acceleration and deceleration of industrial robots and CNC machine tools.C. IEEE Transactions on industrial electronics 47(1), 133–139 (2000)
5. Erkorkmaz, K., Altintas, Y.: High speed CNC system design. Part I: jerk limited trajectory generation and quintic spline interpolation. J. International Journal of Machine Tools & Manufacture 41, 1323–1345 (2001)

A Novel Auto-focusing Method Applied to Micro Manipulation System

Chaohui Wang, Guang Guo, Xin Zhang, and Peng Ye

School of Mechanical Engineering, Xi'an Jiaotong University, Xi'an, 710049, China
jlab@mail.xjtu.edu.cn

Abstract. The MEMS (Microelectromechanical Systems) technology is a new interesting research direction which aims to manufacture and assembly of micro-systems. The research of micro assembly robot has significances of academy and commerce. In the paper the theory and related key technologies of micro-assembly robot based on computer microscope vision feedback were investigated. To enlarge the manipulation area, a novel method of microscope focusing automatically was studied. The focusing process was carried out in cursory step and accurate one. The coarse focusing was based on the image gray histogram while the accurate one compared the width of image edges. Theory analysis and experiments showed that this algorithm enlarged the microscope focusing depth, with the advantages of simplicity and good real time performance.

Keywords: Microscope vision; image preprocessing; auto focusing.

1 Introduction

Micro manipulation is identified to operate micro objects in microcosmic field. Micro robots with micromanipulators, control systems, microscope systems to explore microcosm are urgently demanded. Micro robots are widely used in fields such as precision assembly, fiber alignment, IC bonding and detecting, biologic engineering, biological cells manipulating, microsurgery and so on.

Micro assembly is one of the most important tasks for current micro-robot. An optical microscope is typically used to observe micro assembly with a micro hand. Considering micro assembly with microscope, the scene structure is relatively constant and the operation object is known which, makes it easy to realize rapid image recognition. In its high scale magnification, the focusing range is limited and the finger tips may often go out of the sight. In this paper a novel auto focusing method of microscope to enlarge the manipulation area is studied. The focusing process is carried out in coarse step and accurate one, respectively. The coarse focusing is based on the image gray histogram, while the accurate one is based on comparison with the width of image edges.

2 Image Preprocessing on Focusing

In the process of collecting images using a microscope, noise is usually introduced by several factors, such as uneven lighting, light intensity changing, diffraction effecting,

C. Xiong et al. (Eds.): ICIRA 2008, Part II, LNAI 5315, pp. 558–565, 2008.

nonlinear photovoltaic conversion, micro-device surface quality, and so on. For this reason, the best image is not obtained according to focusing evaluation function. Especially when micro-scenes move closer to the range of microscope depth of field, evaluation parameters are often disturbed in a particular range by the random image noise. To enable the calculation results of focusing evaluation function be accurately and rapidly reflected by system defocusing information, as far as possible to eliminate random noise, it is necessary to preprocess the serial images acquired in the process of focusing or the images near the focal plane.

To reduce the noise influence on the quality of image and improve device performance, a suitable denoising technology is proposed. According to features of microscopic image of micro manipulation system, on the effect of eliminating noise effectively and maintaining the edge, median filtering algorithm for microscopic image processing is adopted, which meets the system requirements.

Fig. 1 shows the original image (a) and the filtering image of micromanipulator (b). By experiments, the square window of 3*3 plays a satisfying denoising effect.

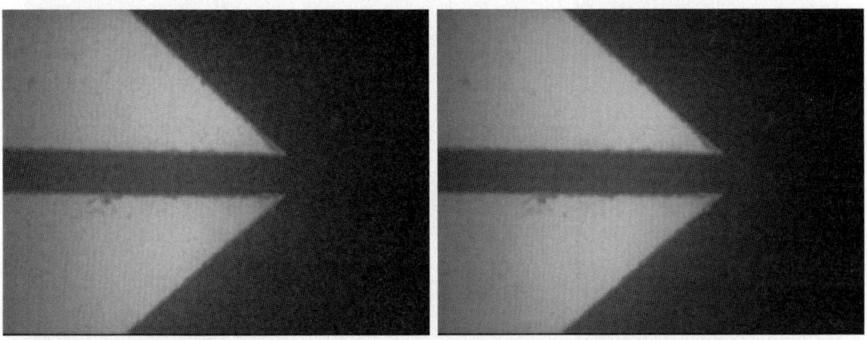

(a) Original image (b) Median filtering image

Fig. 1. Comparison Original image with Median filtering image of micromanipulator

3 Two-Grade Focusing Algorithm

Auto focusing based on digital image processing is that, the same operation scene at different locations under microscope objective lens will ultimately determine the clearest image, by real-time image acquisition and image sequence analysis as well as comparison. The scene position corresponding to this image can be considered in the range of microscope depth of field. Whether the operation scene is located in the depth of field or not is entirely determined by image quality. Therefore, it is critical to choose a suitable focusing evaluation function.

To describe conveniently, in this paper the operation zone in the range of the microscope depth of field is defined as "clear image zone"; the zone outside the scope of depth of field where we may distinguish background scene and regional operation targets is defined as "fuzzy image zone"; If it continues to move out of the depth of field, the zone where the image would not be totally identified is called as "no image zone". Fig. 2 shows serial images of micromanipulator at different locations under a microscope.

Generally speaking, research on microscope auto focusing algorithm is about how to adjust the operation scene from "fuzzy image zone"(b) to "clear image zone"(c). However, for micro manipulation, the relatively large operating zone in the direction perpendicular to microscope optical axis is required, thus it is necessary to research microscope auto focusing issues from "no image zone"(a) to "clear image zone"(c).

After repeated comparison study, we present a novel type of two-grade focusing algorithm: cursory focusing and accurate one. The evaluation function of cursory focusing is based on image gray histogram which makes it quickly guide the operation scene to "fuzzy image zone". And the evaluation function of accurate one is based on detection of image edge width, by which the operating scene according to prior information to enter a local area or not, in accordance with changes of image edge in this area, finally to let the operation scene enter "clear image zone".

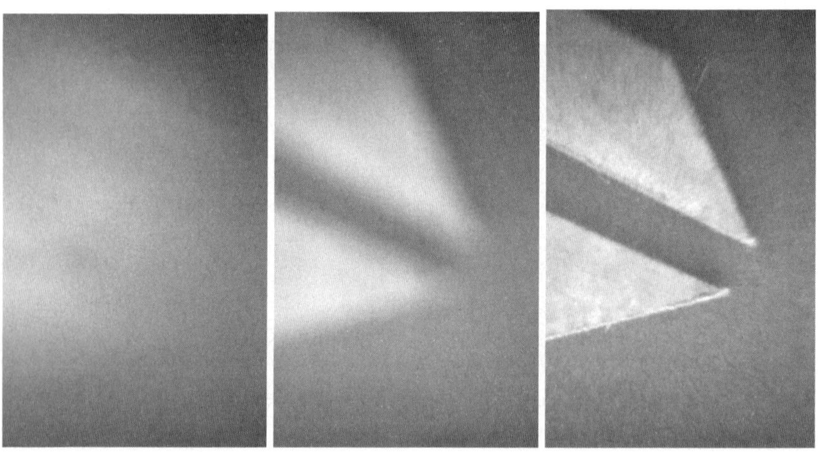

(a) no image zone (b) fuzzy image zone (c) clear image zone

Fig. 2. Images of micromanipulator at different locations under a microscope

The evaluation function of microscope cursory focusing is determined as the statistical characteristic value (variance σ^2) of whole image gray histogram. That is to say, the two digital images I_1 and I_2 are generated by the same scene at different microscope defocus plane, while the variance of image gray histogram is σ_1^2 and σ_2^2, respectively. If $\sigma_2^2 > \sigma_1^2$, image I_2 is considered closer to focal plane than image I_1, that is, image I_2 is more clear than image I_1.

Table 1 is the statistic of image gray histogram for Fig. 2. In the table, $\bar{s}$ is the mean value of image gray distribution; σ^2 is the variance. These data are obtained by calculating figures of whole image gray distribution.

Table 1. Comparision of image gray histogram statistical figures

microscope image	no image zone (a)		fuzzy image zone (b)		clear image zone (c)	
gray histogram statistical figures	$\bar{s}_1$	σ_1^2	$\bar{s}_2$	σ_2^2	$\bar{s}_3$	σ_3^2
	134.8498	1474.592	138.6928	2110.064	136.394	2383.551
change rate	---	---	2.85%	43.12%	-1.66%	12.96%

In Table 1 it can be noticed that the mean value of image gray histogram changes a little when operation scene moves from a(no image zone) to b(fuzzy image zone), then to c(clear image zone). However, the variance has an obvious change. Especially when moving from a(no image zone) to b(fuzzy image zone), σ^2 has increased by 43.12%, a significant change. Obviously, the variance σ^2 is appropriate as the evaluation function of the microscope cursory focusing.

Table 1 also indicates that the variance value of gray histogram compared c (clear image zone) to b (fuzzy image zone) has only increased by 12.96%. If image is more complex or the noise distributing image is bigger, the change between them is not significant. So the evaluation function is not suitable for the entire focusing process.

After the target object entering the fuzzy image zone, although the scene is still quite fuzzy, micro-manipulation information obtained from image has accumulated enough. To take full use of the information, high accurate focusing algorithm should be researched. Micro-manipulation of digital image researched has been summarized in this paper, as follows two characteristics: 1) the image is generally composed of two kinds of gray elements: background scene and target object; 2) target object (including micro-gripping hand and spare parts to be assembled) has the regular geometric figures. Using these two characteristics, a simple and efficient accurate focusing algorithm--comparing the width of image edge is proposed.

According to the principle of the edge detection, the focusing steps for microscope accurate focusing algorithm are designed as follows. Fig.3 shows images in the process of auto focusing. Fig.3 (a) is the image of operation scene entered "fuzzy image zone".

Step 1, smoothing the first microscopic digital image Fig.3 (a) by the local average method.

Step 2, obtaining the gradient matrix of image in x direction (or y direction) by computing the first order differential operator in x direction (or y direction).

Step 3, computing the gradient matrix in x direction (or y direction) with the neighborhood average method.

Step 4, selecting the threshold Ω to transform gradient matrix. The element in gradient matrix, whose value is greater than Ω, is taken as 1, otherwise as 0. Ω can be obtained by statistical computing the mean value of low frequency component in gradient matrix, or by prior information.

Step 5, acquiring the longest line segment l_0 whose value is 1 continuously in the x direction (or y direction). The image region where l_0 is located is the research region of focusing process. Fig. 3(b) shows the location of l_0.

Subsequently, moving a small distance again to the microscope focusing direction, then the second image is collected. At this time the line segment l_1 whose value is 1 continuously can be directly acquired at the region of l_0 located. l_1 is shown in Fig. 3(c). If $l_1 < l_0$, the micro lens would be moved continuously in the same direction, then l_2 is acquired...... until $l_i \approx l_{i-1}$, that is, the process of microscope accurate focusing is achieved.

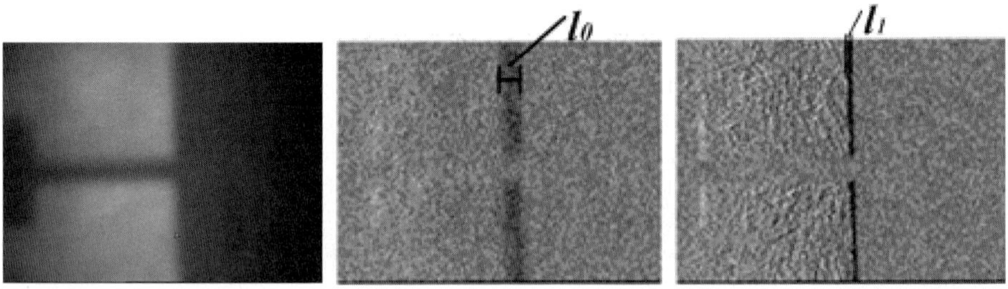

(a) (b) (c)

Fig. 3. Images in the process of auto focusing

The entire algorithm only carries out global calculation for the first image, and then partial image is disposed in the process of focusing and contrast. If prior information is sufficient, the first image can be merely disposed with partial image, which greatly reduces the computation of image processing and solves the bad real-time problem in the focusing process.

4 Experiment and Discuss

The microscope auto focusing software for micro-robot is developed successfully in this paper. The bottom module of software realizes the control of each step motor controller and power supply, and the top module realizes the basic functions which the micro manipulation requires. By step motor driving micro lens to translate in the optical axis direction, microscope digital image of operation scene is collected in real-time. At the start of experiment, an operation scene under the microscope lens is in the state of microscope out-of-focus. Using cursory focusing algorithm, the microscope lens is moved up and down to guide micro ripping hand moving from "no image zone" to "fuzzy image zone". Then to the process of accurate focusing, the operation scene entered "clear image zone" where the target object and background scene can be distinguished clearly.

In the experiment, based on microscope magnification (3 times lens), the step of cursory focusing and accurate one is determined. The step of cursory focusing is 2mm, while the step of accurate one is 0.5mm. Table 2 and Fig. 4 show changes of focusing evaluation function in the process of focusing. As the microscope lens dropped to 26 mm, the value of σ^2 is not significantly increased, and then the process of focusing is entering accurate focusing.

Table 2. Experimental results in the process of focusing

P: microscope lens position (mm) $\bar{s}$: mean value of image gray distribution

σ^2 : variance of image gray distribution

P	0	2	4	6	8	10	12
$\bar{s}$	68.59	68.59	68.25	68.32	68.59	68.67	68.66
σ^2	1967.39	2006.67	2020.33	2038.49	2065.88	2111.95	2122.55
P	14	16	18	20	22	24	26
$\bar{s}$	68.81	68.52	68.01	68.15	67.94	67.99	67.18
σ^2	2146.97	2151.04	2155.28	2176.17	2198.43	2215.05	2201.8
P	28	30	32	34	36	38	40
$\bar{s}$	66.77	66.54	66.51	65.67	64.98	66.26	65.08
σ^2	2200.41	2214.15	2228.76	2215.85	2207.39	2234.02	2253.34

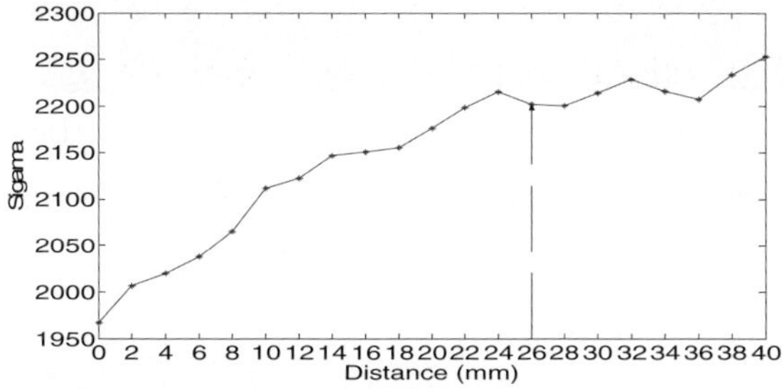

Fig. 4. Changes of σ^2 in the process of focusing

In the process of accurate focusing, by calculating first order differential of the original image in the x direction, gradient array is revealed. Using the sequence composed of selecting gradient array's 300th row to the 450th row of 100th line, the width of image marginal zone is obtained. Table 3 shows the changes of marginal width in the process of accurate focusing.

Table 3. Changes of marginal width value in process of accurate focusing

P: microscope lens position (mm) W: marginal width

P	26	26.5	27	27.5	28	28.5	29	29.5	30	30.5
W	71	68	63	58	55	50	47	44	42	41
P	31	31.5	32	32.5	33	33.5	34	34.5	35	35.5
W	40	38	37	36	32	31	29	26	24	23
P	36	36.5	37	37.5	38	38.5	39	39.5	40	40.5
W	21	19	17	15	14	11	9	7	7	8

It's about 40mm that microscope lens moves from initial position to final position at the end of focusing. Therefore, the actual focusing range is up to about 80 mm, which realizes large-scale focusing.

Fig. 5 shows several typical experimental images in the process of auto-focusing.

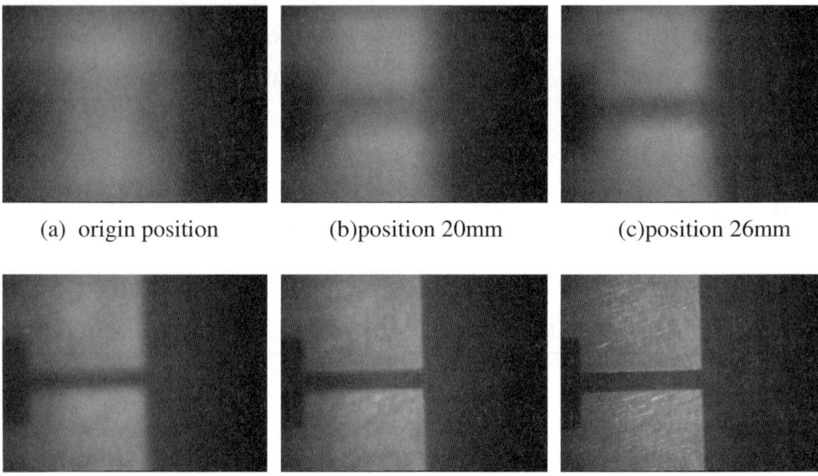

(a) origin position (b)position 20mm (c)position 26mm

(d)position 34mm (e) position 40 mm (f)position 42 mm

Fig. 5. Typical images in the process of auto-focusing

5 Conclusion

A large-scale auto focusing method applied to micro manipulation system has been presented and analyzed. Two-grade focusing algorithm, cursory focusing and accurate one, is proposed. The algorithm is not only greatly increasing the microscope focusing scale, but also simple and real-time. Theoretical analysis and experimental results have proved that this method of auto focusing for micro assemble robot is successful, and meets the demands of micro manipulation.

Acknowledgements

This research was supported by the National Natural Science Foundation Project "A Research of Blood Micro-processing System Based on MEMS Technology" (No.50775177).

References

1. Pfeifer, T., Freudenberg, R., Dussler, G.: Quality control and process observation for the micro assembly process[J]. Measurement 30(1), 1–18 (2001)
2. Wang, C., Jiang, Z., Chen, W.: Micro Assembly Operation System on Microscope. Information and Control 31(7), 724–727 (2002)

3. Fatikow, S., Benz, M.: A microrobot-based automated micromanipulation station for assembly of microsystems. Computer in Industry 36, 155–162 (1998)
4. Woern, H., Seyfried, J., Fahlbusch, S.: Flexible Microrobots for Micro Assembly Tasks. In: International Symposium on Micromechatronics and Human Science, pp. 135–143 (2000)
5. Xu, W.L., Yang, T.W., Tso, S.K.: Dynamic control of a flexible macro-micro manipulator based on rigid dynamics with flexible state sensing. Mechanism and Machine Theory 35(1), 41–43 (2000)

Simulation and Development Environment for Digital Controlled PMSM Servo System

Shuanghui Hao, Weifeng Zheng, Minghui Hao, Jie Liu, and Hong Li

School of Mechatronics Eng., Harbin Institute of Technology, Harbin, 150001, China
hitren1982@163.com

Abstract. The robotic manipulator with digital controlled PMSM servo system has many advantages: low weight, fast response, high load rate, low power consumption, low probability of damage (less bumping). To get high-powered and low-cost PMSM servo system for robotic, a simulation and development environment based on personal computer is present in this paper. The environment is integrated with the platform of control code identifying and executing, IPM model and motor model. Realization of this method which can be used to simulate the servo control code with closed-loop and stakeout the wave of key parameters will greatly reduce the time and cost in developing system and improve the performance of system. In this paper, the arithmetic of RPN and Runge-Kutta are introduced in detail. And then, the validity and the feasibility of environment are verified by simulation and experimental results. Also, the control parameters gotten through the environment are successfully used in the high speed/high positioning PMSM servo system.

Keywords: PMSM servo system; closed-loop simulation; Reverse Polish Notation; Runge-Kutta.

1 Introduction

Robotic manipulator is a focus issue in the field of robotics. The Fig.1 is the single link manipulator designed by David Wange in Canada Waterloo University. The digital controlled PMSM (permanent magnetism synchronization motor) servo system which has the advantages of high-speed, high-efficiency, high-precision, fast-response, and low-power-waste is often applied to be robotic controller. PMSM servo system plays an important role in the robotic control.

For digital controlled PMSM servo system, the control code in MCU completes the computation in each circle to support its digital closed-loop control. So the performance and effect of the system are directly determined by the quality of code, control parameters and control methods. Consequently, the control code plays an important role in system. The quality and precision will get worse if the control code is not reliable and rational [1]. Moreover, with the development of technology and economy, the research achievements are required to become industrialization as soon as possible. So the research on the simulation and development environment for digital controlled PMSM servo system will be of high application value and social economy effect.

C. Xiong et al. (Eds.): ICIRA 2008, Part II, LNAI 5315, pp. 566–575, 2008.

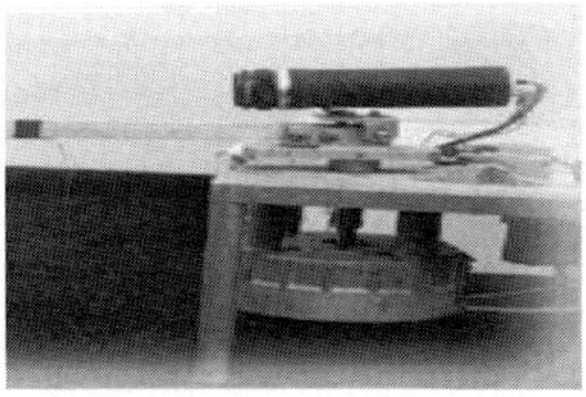

Fig. 1. The single link manipulator designed by David Wange

The structure of digital controlled PMSM servo system is shown in Fig.2. For the system, the movement of PMSM is actuated by the intelligent power model (IPM) on the mother board, which is integrated with insulated gate bipolar transistor (IGBT), drive circuits and protect circuits. The IPM provides the three-phase voltage for the PMSM. They give birth to the three-phase currents together with magnetic field which is rounding. Then it drives the rotor of PMSM to run. The three-phase current of PMSM is measured by the hall-effect sensors. And the angle of rotor is gained by the encoder. And then, the signal of current and angle is transmitted to the MCU on the main board. The MCU which is used to control the PMSM is the core of PMSM servo system. It carries out the signal collecting and computation to realize the control method. Subsequently, it produces the control voltage signal of PWM (Pulse Width Modulation).

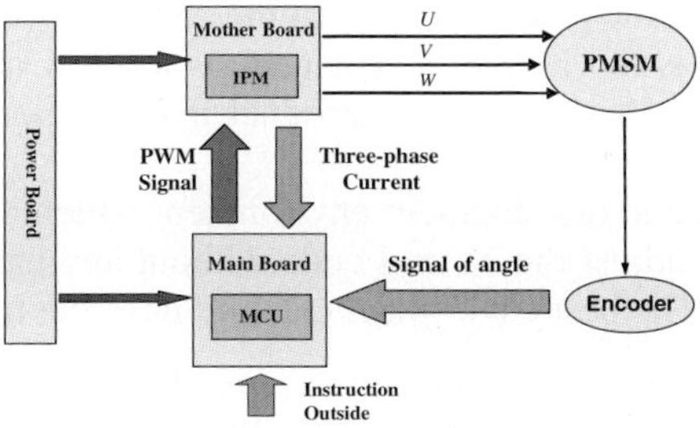

Fig. 2. Structure diagram of PMSM servo system

The control code of digital controlled PMSM servo system in the MCU includes the parts of position computation, velocity computation, current computation and vector transformation, which are shown in the Fig.3. The MCU executes a large amount of code to carry out the close-loop control by interrupt in fixed circle. It finishes the computation in every circle to produce the signal of PWM.

For the PMSM servo system, the hardware is same each other, and its function and control effect are achieved by the software of system mainly. Consequently, the engineers should attach importance to the points below when programming, choosing the control methods and selecting the control parameters [2].

(1)Reliability: the control code has to achieve a large amount of computation. The rate and precision of computation are required to be high. The engineers should make sure that the result is correct and precise. Meanwhile, the control code is required to finish all the control and computation in the fixed time.

(b)Rationality: the control code should incarnate the control models of PMSM servo system, and the parameters should meet the demand of the control to make the control methods and parameters get the best effect.

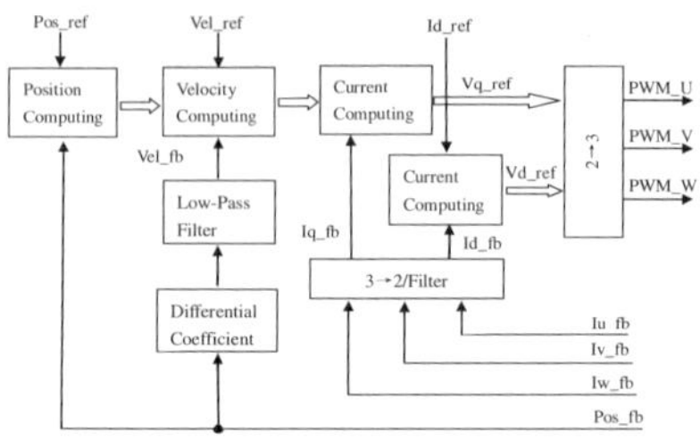

Fig. 3. Structure diagram of servo control code

2 Simulation and Development Environment

In the real application, engineers should evaluate, optimize and adjust the software, and then implement digital system by virtue of their experience and professional judgment to improve the system and make it more reliable and rational. At the present time, the control code needs to be tested on the hardware from time to time, and then engineers find and judge the problem to adjust the control code. It brings the problems that the develop circle is too long, the efficiency is too low and the cost is too high. Subsequently, it induces that most servo product into a vicious circle of low quality and slow market.

Hence, a simulation and development environment which can be used to simulate, evaluate, optimize and adjust the control code without any hardware becomes necessary for the engineers. The best environment should have the functions below:

1) It can identify the control code and execute the code with simulation.
2) It possesses of the motor model and IPM model, so that it can simulate to execute the code with closed-loop.
3) It has the platform to implement the basic function. And then, it can evaluate, optimize and adjust the control code of system.

At the present time, the simulation tools used to develop the PMSM servo system have no the function above. The integrated development environment of MCU has the function of simulation. It can be used to execute the program with single step, fulltime and breakpoints to observe the variables of registers. But it is limited to track the computation with localization and single circle. It can't simulate the control code in multi-circle without the feedback of controlled object. So it can not be used to evaluate the reliability and rationality of system. Usually, the simulation software, such as MATLAB is used to simulate the control models and design results of the servo system [3]. The MATLAB has the simulation model library, physic model library, advanced math method and powerful computation function, but it can't be used to simulate the control code directly. And it can't evaluate the precision of computation and optimize the control models and parameters.

In order to improve the develop status of control code. For this paper, it's an exploration for the improvement of the program test. This method's realization will make the time and cost of PMSM servo system's development reduce greatly.

1) It can simulate the control code without any hardware instead of executing the code in the MCU.
2) To some extent, it can be used to evaluate the rate and precision of computation, the control models and parameters instead of engineer.
3) It can optimize the parameter automatically. To some extent, it can be used to modify and debug the control code instead of engineer.

The method proposed in this paper will achieve the functions above. The concrete realization of control code identifying, PMSM model building and IPM mode building will be introduced in present paper.

3 Implement of Simulation and Development Environment

3.1 Identifying and Executing of Environment

The simulation platform is different from the traditional platform when it simulates to execute the control code of system. Instead of building the C language or assemble language to binary code, the control code is read into the platform first, and then the key information is distilled which includes the variable, program structure, program control, function transferred. After finishing the disposition of the control code, the platform simulates to compute according to the information together with code. The processes of distilling and simulating are regarded as identifying and executing of control code. The processes of it are shown in Fig.4.

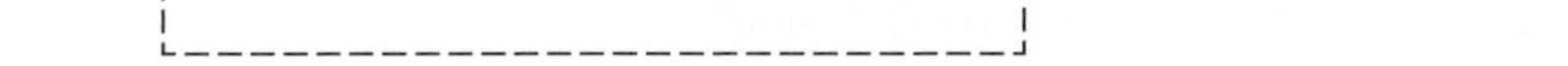

Fig. 4. Processes of the control code simulation

Identifying and executing the control code is the important part of the environment. The processes of the function are as follows:

a) Code disposing
b) Key information distilling
c) Whole variable information distilling
d) RPN (Reverse Polish Notation)algorithm
e) Computation simulating
f) Simulation results displaying

The algorithm of RPN is used to solve the problem of arithmetic. It transforms the arithmetic expresses to the RPN expresses and makes it easy to simulate the computation of the control code.

3.2 Differential Equations Building and Solving

To get the feedback signal and execute the control code in close-loop, the motor model should be built and its differential equation should solve. Building the d-q axis equivalent model of PMSM is to analyze the static performance. And it also can be used to analyze the dynamic performance.

Considered the reciprocity of mechanical and electrical system, the differential equation of mechanical movement and electromagnetic filed should be solved. So we can get the differential equations as follows:

$$\begin{cases} \frac{d}{dt}i_d = \frac{1}{L_d}u_d - \frac{R}{L_d}i_d + \frac{L_q}{L_d}p\omega_r i_q \\ \frac{d}{dt}i_q = \frac{1}{L_q}u_q - \frac{R}{L_q}i_q - \frac{L_d}{L_q}p\omega_r i_d - \frac{\lambda p\omega_r}{L_q} \\ T_e = p[\lambda i_q + (L_d - L_q)i_d i_q] \\ \frac{d}{dt}\omega_r = \frac{1}{j}(T_e - F\omega_r - T_m) \\ \frac{d}{dt}\theta = \omega_r \end{cases} \tag{1}$$

$$\begin{cases} u_d = \sqrt{\frac{2}{3}}[u_A \cos p\theta + u_B \cos(p\theta - \frac{2}{3}\pi) + u_C \cos(p\theta + \frac{2}{3}\pi)] \\ u_d = \sqrt{\frac{2}{3}}[-u_A \sin p\theta - u_B \sin(p\theta - \frac{2}{3}\pi) - u_C \cos(p\theta + \frac{2}{3}\pi)] \end{cases} \tag{2}$$

where R is the equivalent resistance of d and q axis, λ is the flux of magnetic pole.

To achieve the processes of the motor, the differential equation should be solved. In this paper, the algorithm of RungeKutta is adopted to achieve the results of motor's differential equation .It is to obtain the key parameters of motor in each circle, such as the current of d-q axis, velocity and angle of rotor. And then the current of three-phase would be gotten by through 2/3 transform. The current of three-phase and angle can be returned to system as the feedback value.

3.3 IPM Modeling

In real application, the IPM model is the bridge of the control code and motor model. The MCU gets the time value by computation, which is corresponding to the voltage value of PWM. And then, the PWM signal is produced by the special model embedded in MCU for the motor control. According to the special model for the motor control and the IPM model, the three-phase voltage pulse can be got by the time value of PWM. Subsequently, the voltage pulse would be sent to the motor model.

The servo system executes the control code in circles to achieve the close-loop control. The time of circle is fixed. According to the characteristics above, the environment simulates to execute the control code in circles with the feedback value and

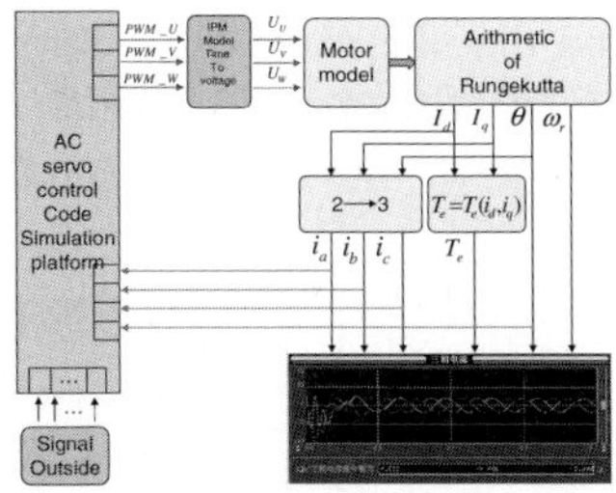

Fig. 5. Structure of the environment

reference outside. Meanwhile, the key parameters can be recorded and shown by the virtual oscillograph to observe the control effect. The structure of environment is shown in Fig.5.

4 Validation of Motor Model

4.1 Validation of Motor Model

The parameters of motor validated in this paper are as follows: R=1.8Ω, p=4, Ld=7e-3H, Lq=7e-3H, F=0Nm, λ=6.65e-2 Wb, J=3.1625e-5 kg·m2 . The interface of the simulation and development environment is shown in Fig.6.

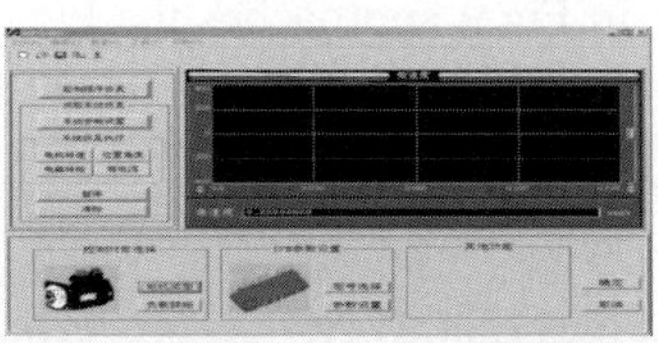

Fig. 6. Interface of environment.

4.2 Validation of Motor Model

Take the input of motor as three-phase voltage of sine wave in MATLAB and the environment of this paper respectively. Its peak value is 80V, frequency is 100Hz and load torque is 2Nm. The Structure diagram for motor model simulation in MATLAB is shown in Fig.7.

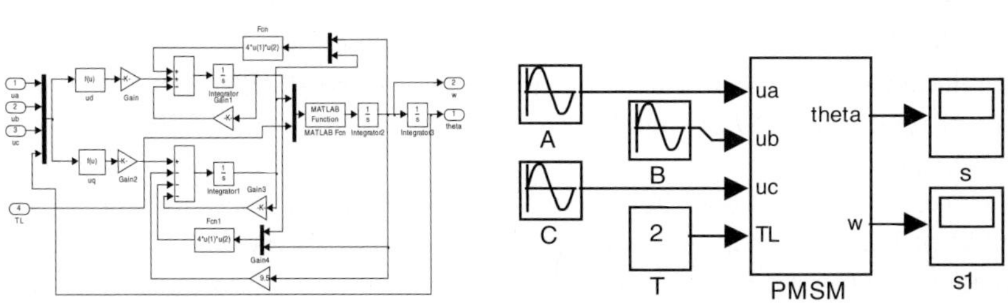

Fig. 7. Structure diagram for motor model simulation in MATLAB

From the Fig.8, we can find that the wave of velocity of environment approaches the result of MATLAB, and both of them are 157rad/s. It is accord with the relative theory. So it figures out that the motor model of environment is rational.

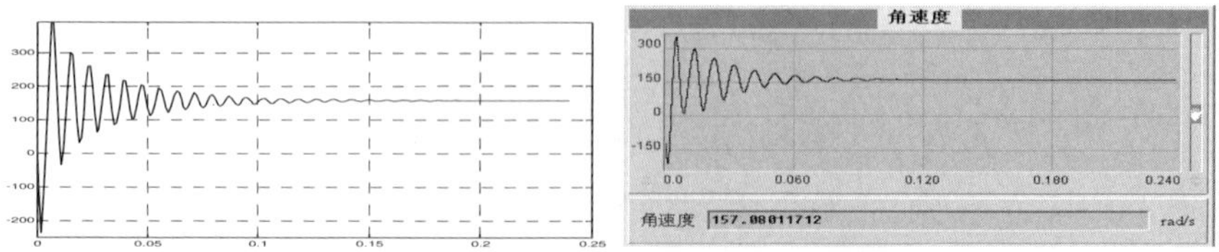

Fig. 8. The result of simulation by MATLAB and environment

4.3 Feasibility of Motor Model for the Three-Phase Voltage Pulse

According to the modulate principle, we get the three-phase voltage pulse which is equivalent to three-phase voltage of sine wave. Take them as the input of motor model in this environment, and the other parameters are the same. The result of simulation is as follows:

4.4 Validation of Closed-Loop Simulation

The velocity wave of motor in Fig.9 approaches the Fig.8. All of them are 157rad/s. We can get the conclusion that the input of motor model can be the three-phase voltage pulse. It indicates that the output of IPM model can be the motor model in this environment.

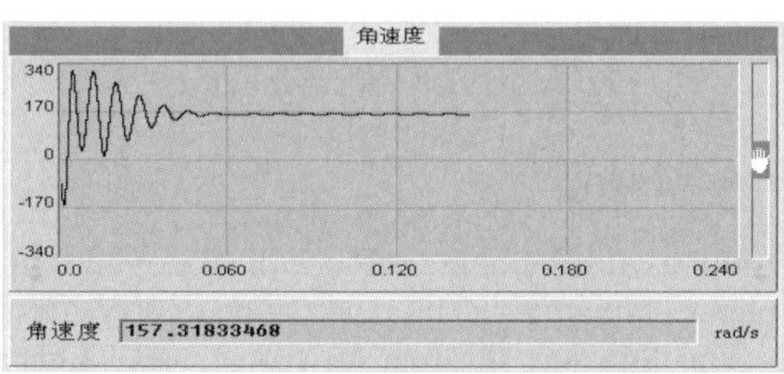

Fig. 9. The result of simulation by environment with three-phase voltage pulse

The equipment of experiment is the digital controlled PMSM servo system. Take the current reference of D axis and Q axis as 1A and 0A respectively, and then take the electric angle as 0.

In Fig.10, we can find that the current output of U phase in equipment approaches the output of that in the environment, and the last value of them are 1A. The experimental equipment is shown in Fig.11.

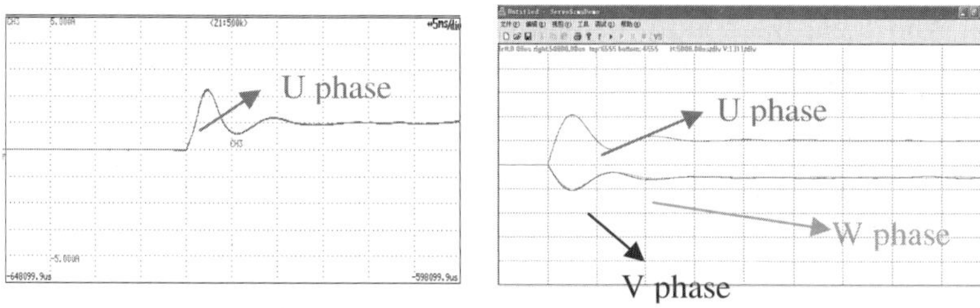

Fig. 10. The result of experiment and environment

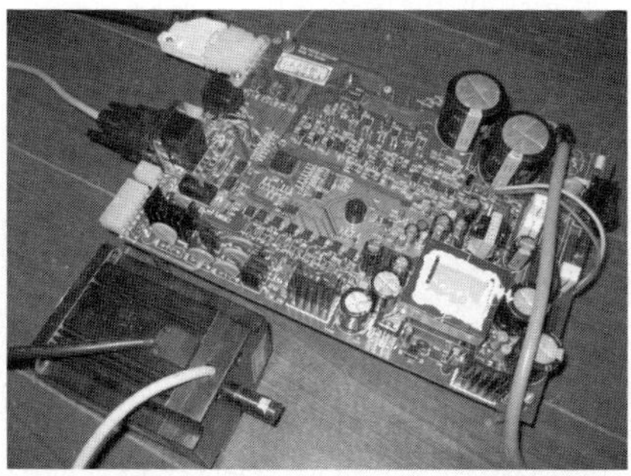

Fig. 11. The experimental equipment of PMSM servo system

When the velocity of PMSM servo system is set to 4000rpm, the outputs of three phases in the equipment and environment are shown as follows:

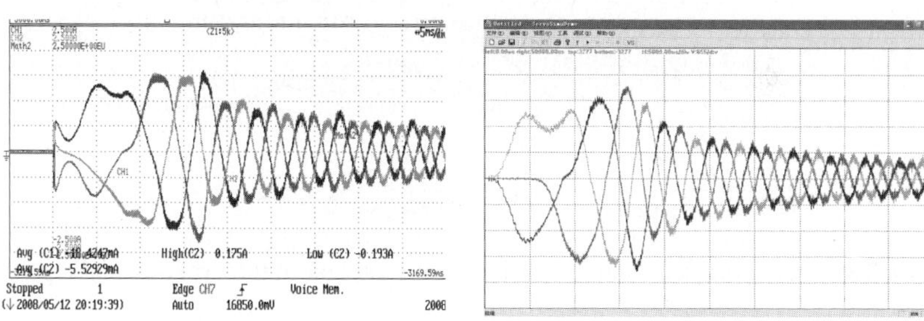

Fig. 12. The output of three phase in equipment and environment

5 Experiments of High Speed/High Precision Positioning System

High speed/high precision positioning system is widely used in the robotic. It requires the PMSM servo system to be excellent in response and positioning. So the control parameters of system are of great importance. Through the simulation and development environment, we can get the best control parameters without any hardware in

advance. And then, the control parameters would be used in the real experimental equipment (high speed/high precision positioning PMSM servo system).
In the High speed/high precision positioning system, the velocity reference is dealt with as the Fig.13.

With the control parameters gotten by the simulation and development environment, the current of q axis and the position error integral of the experimental equipment are shown as Fig.14.

Comparing the Fig.13 and Fig.14, we can find that the real system needs 5ms to achieve the positioning, and the time of velocity reference is 4ms in all. Hence, it can achieve the high speed/high positioning with the 12000 times per minute. The acceleration is higher; the range of movement is larger. The high speed/high precision positioning system meets demand of the scatter-gun robotic.

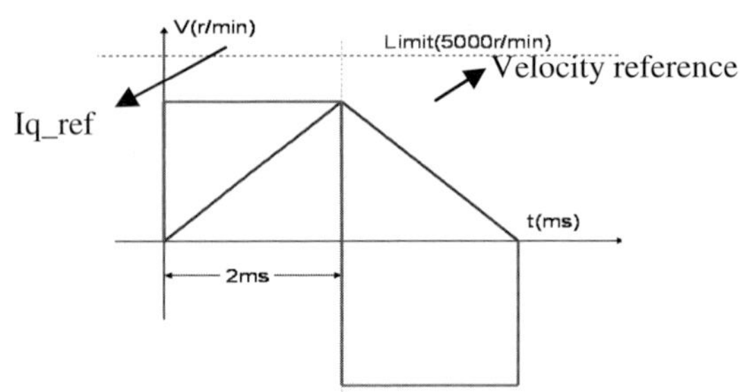

Fig. 13. The velocity reference of experimental equipment

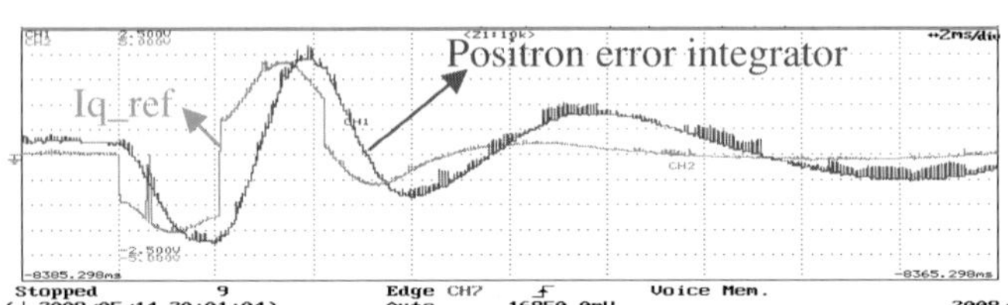

Fig. 14. The current of q axis and the position error integral of the experimental equipment

6 Conclusion

In this paper, a simulation and development environment is proposed for the digital controlled PMSM servo system, which can simulate and debug the control code without any hardware. It will bring many benefits for the development of PMSM servo system. Also, the research dealt with in this paper has brought robotic manipulators one step nearer to its engineerisation and practicality.

The validity and feasibility of environment are verified by comparing the simulation results of this environment with MATLAB, and validated by the experimental results.

References

1. Jabbar, M.A., Phyu, H.N., Zhejie, L., Chao, B.: Modeling and numerical simulation of a brushless permanent magnet DC motor in dynamic conditions by time-stepping technique. IEEE Transactions on Industry Application 40(3), 763–770 (2004)
2. Petrovic, V., Ortega, R.: Design and implementation of an adaptive controller for torque ripple minimization in PM synchronous motors. IEEE Trans. On PE. 15(5), 871–876 (2000)
3. Kim, Y.S., Choi, Y.K., Lee, J.H.: Speed-sensorless vector control for permanent-magnet synchronous motors based on instantaneous reactive power in the wide-speed region. IEE Proc.-Electr. Power Appl. 152(5), 1343–1349 (2005)
4. Lee, S.-B.: Closed-Loop Estimation of Permanent Magnet Synchronous Motor Parameters by PI Controller GainTuning. IEEE Transitions On Energy Conversion 21(4), 863–870 (2006)
5. Su, Y.X., Zheng, C.H., Duan, B.Y.: Automatic Disturbances Rejection Controller for Precise Motion Control of Permanent-Magnet Synchronous Motors. IEEE Transactions on Industrial Electronics 52(3), 814–823 (2005)
6. Konghirun, M., Xu, L.: A Fast Transient-Current Control Strategy in Sensorless Vector Controlled Permanent Magnet Synchronous Motor. Power Electronics, IEEE Transactions 21(5), 1508–1512 (2006)

Development of SOA Based Equipments Maintenance Decision Support System

Xiangang Cao[1,2] and Pingyu Jiang[1,2]

[1] State Key Laboratory for Manufacturing Systems Engineering, School of Mechanical Engineering, Xi'an Jiaotong, University, Xi'an, Shaanxi 710049, China
[2] School of mechanical engineering, Xi'an University of Science and Technology, Xi'an Shanxi 710054, China
caoxg@xust.edu.cn, pjiang@mail.xjtu.edu.cn

Abstract. Nowadays equipment maintenance represents a significant and important task to ensure that plant facilities continue to function properly, so an Integrated Intelligent Equipment Maintenance Decision(IIEMD) platform based on Service Oriented Architecture(SOA) environment is studied and developed to support collaborative maintenance decision, remote equipment diagnosis, and so on. Firstly, an ontology-supported hybrid conceptual architecture of IIEMD is provided. Secondly, SOA based layered IIEMD framework architecture is given. Thirdly, an ontology based knowledge base construction method, mixed inference process combining RBR and CBR studied. Last, based on the previous theory studies, an equipments maintenance decision support system prototype was developed.

Keywords: Equipment maintenance; decision support system; rule-based reasoning; case-based reasoning; ontology.

1 Introduction

Nowadays maintenance systems operate on very complex industrial equipments. Factories are capital-intensive requiring highly sophisticated and automated production equipments. Further more, the industry is realizing that the efficient use of industrial assets is a key issue in supporting company competition. In this context, efficiency means producing good quality products without interrupting the production for unnecessary breakdowns. Research has shown that a company can easily increase 20% of its operating cost if it does not maintain its production equipment properly1. Hence, A demand for improvements on system productivity, availability and safety is increasing, as well as product quality and customer satisfaction. Taking into account the trend for decrease in profit margins, the importance of implementing efficient maintenance strategies becomes unquestionable. In this picture the maintenance function plays a critical role in a company's ability to compete on the basis of cost, quality and delivery performance and maintenance is taken into account in production requirements2.

It is important to develop equipment maintenance systems to prevent equipment failures and unexpected breakdowns. Now, an equipment maintenance system should

C. Xiong et al. (Eds.): ICIRA 2008, Part II, LNAI 5315, pp. 576–582, 2008.

be Internet/web-enabled, intelligent, agile and adaptable. It consists of adaptable machine monitoring components, network based diagnostics, prognostic system to keep manufacturing operation machines in good operating condition. Besides effective monitoring of the machine statuses and the good diagnosis and maintenance analysis to ensure that equipment continues to function properly, further more, the company maintenance, economics and business systems must be harmonized to communicate with each other and to produce the essential key figures needed for both strategic and day-to-day business decisions3. Due to a lack of efficient inter-operation among the plant software systems, research on "highly-integrated" e-maintenance systems, which meet overall demands, is a promising research area4. There is also a lack of cooperative systems formal models. This is why the efficiency of cooperation within a complex computerized remote system (with several different tools, with a particular cooperation algorithm...) is still a preoccupation for industrialists who are users of these systems5. The challenge to manage to predict failures and disturbances, and to estimate the remaining lifetime of components, mechanical systems and integrated systems is an extremely tough one for researchers and engineers. An effective and efficient predictive-based machine condition prognosis is necessary for modern plants, many methods are studied on this678. Further more, an intelligent maintenance system must collect, extract, and manage adequate domain knowledge constantly. Therefore, there are many research focusing on it, especially using rule-based reasoning, cased-based reasoning methods to improve expert systems91011. but does not yet exist system for above due to the inconsistent set of heterogeneous models used by the different designers of partial maintenance processes, also different companies12. In order to perform the above-mentioned various tasks, this study of our research was to develop distributed cooperative intelligent maintenance platform that proposes a set of decision help tools for different maintenance activities in a distributed environment.

Although many systems and tools have been developed in the maintenance, effectively and dynamically designing, implementing and updating these systems, especially in distributed cooperative intelligent maintenance applications, is still a challenging task. In this research, an Integrated Intelligent Equipment Maintenance Decision(IIEMD) platform based on Service Oriented Architecture(SOA) environment is studied and developed.

This paper is divided into five sections. In Section 2, an conceptual IIEMD architecture , which integrates rule-based-reasoning (RBR) and case-based reasoning (CBR) method, are described. In Section 3, we describe the architecture of IIEMD system based on SOA. Section 4 reveals some key technologies. Finally, the conclusions are drawn in Section 5.

2 The Conceptual Architecture of IIEMD

In this paper, IIEMD is an ontology-supported hybrid system where it has dual reasoning logics, RBR, CBR technique for equipments maintenance decision service to improve the overall maintenance performance. Figure 1 illustrates its architecture and shows how it interacts with User Interface and Backend Process.

Inference engine process the user's request through Rule module, Case module, Data interface module, Ontology based knowledge base give model or case information, simulation analysis base, product measure data are also included. The IIEMD employ two or more representations of expertise to emulate reasoning in some domain. First, RBR are very good at making decisions where the domain knowledge is very well structured and defined. Because of this, RBR can be used to reason from first principles to arrive at a general conclusion. RBR tend not to perform well when the domain knowledge is ill-conditioned, poorly-structured, or sparse. In these instances, a CBR module emulates the very human-like practice of re-using past experiences and problem solutions to synthesize new solutions to new problems. Collections of past problems and their associated solutions are stored as cases. When given some search criteria, it tries to find the case or cases that most closely match the criteria according to some evaluation algorithm. The most popular algorithm is called Nearest Neighbor. The strength of CBR is that if the adapted solution works, it is rolled back into the case base as new knowledge -- therefore the more a CBR module is used, the more it learns.

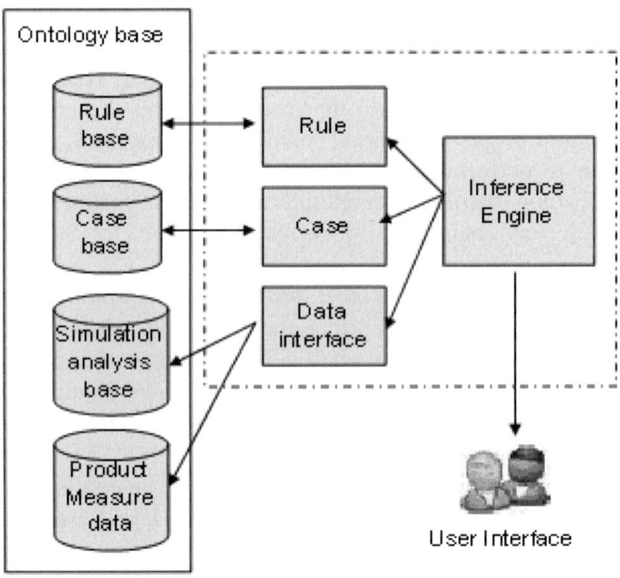

Fig. 1. The conceptual architecture of IIEMD

CBR can be thought of as a type of RBR, though in CBR the emphases is on the contents of the knowledge issues as opposed to the emphases on the mechanism of reasoning in RBR. Thus in CBR one is typically interested in the kind of content should cases have, what type of adaptation strategies etc. In IIEMD system, the aim is to attempt to model components that was not matched to model in the RBR stage by comparing the features of this component with all components (cases) previously modeled by the system and stored in a case base with the aim of adapting the solution method (model) used in solving the most similar component to the current unsolved component.

3 SOA Based IIEMD Architecture

Service-oriented architecture (SOA) is a Web-based, standards-driven, modular architecture that promises to deliver pervasive integration for real-time business agility. The optimum implementation architecture for SOA is a component-based architecture. Many will be familiar with the concepts of process and entity component, and will understand the inherent stability and flexibility of this component architecture, which provide a one to one mapping between business entities and component implementations.

Our SOA based IIEMD framework architecture, which can realizing comprehensive data presentation and synthesis, continuous assessment of equipment health, maintenance and repair decision; can integrating other system or integrating each other, shows in fig 2.

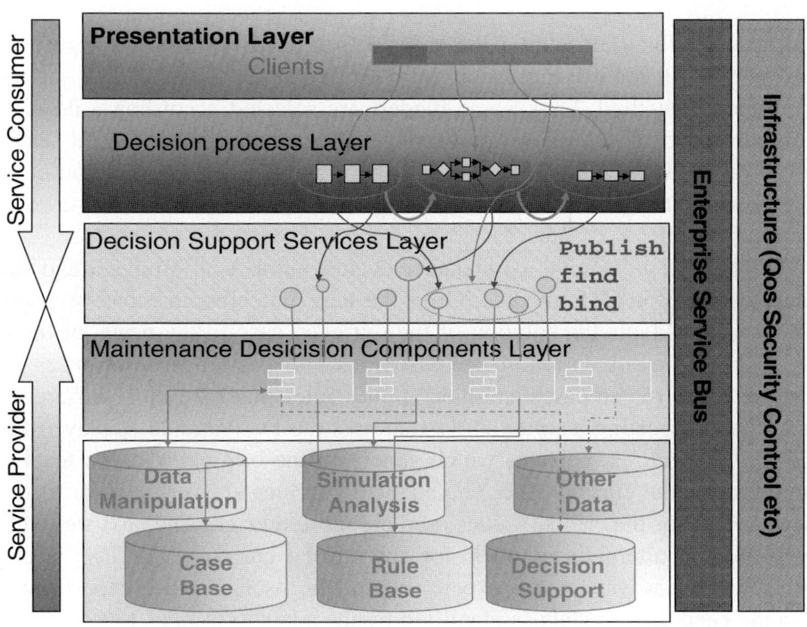

Fig. 2. The Architecture of SOA based IIEMD

The architecture defined should not be exclusive to any specific hardware implementations, operating systems, or software technology. In this maintenance system, Main functions show below:

The maintenance presentation and decision process layers. This is the decision facing solution which consumes services from one or more service providers and integrates them into the maintenance or other business processes.

The decision support services layer. This provides a bridge between the implementations and the consuming maintenance decision support applications, creating a ogical view of sets of decision services which are available for use, invoked by a common interface and management architecture.

The maintenance decision component layer. This describes the various components supporting the implemented applications, influence engine, etc.

Through this architecture, maintenance decision tools (all are defined as WEB Services) may register, get information about other tools, distribute information to other tools and so on through UDDI, WSDL. So it provides a transparent, seamless and automated decision process in a unified way, independently of its origin, equipment manufacturer, integrator, end-users.

4 Key Technologies

4.1 Inference Process

How to integrate the RBR and CBR is a key factor in IIEMD system. Figure 3 shows how it operates in identifying an appropriate model for a given data set with the mixed inference method. First, some models are selected according a dataset, if no model is identified for a certain dataset, the CBR is evoked. The method selected for case retrieval in IIEMD is the Nearest Neighbor algorithm. The selection of the features in the similarity function and their weights is fundamental for the success of the application for CBR.

The numbers of preventive maintenance events, number of failures, trend value are the main features for CBR module, Once the best matching case has been retrieved the CBR system adapts the solution of the retrieved case to the needs of the current dataset. Thus at the adaptation phase, CBR looks for prominent differences between the current and retrieved cases and then applies rules that take those differences into account when suggesting a solution. System uses the Derivational Replay Adaptation technique which reuses the rules which generated the original solution to produce a new solution for the current case. The adaptations rules are very similar to the RBR rule base except for the critical values used are more relaxed. The next step in CBR is the evaluation of alternative models for solving the current case. This step can be performed in two ways: for the expert and for the user. For the expert the system displays the candidate models as identified by the adaptation rules together with their features for the current case. The system also displays the identified cases from retrieval. The expert can then make judgment about the model to select. For the user the system provides recommended model(s) based on the evaluation process. This is carried out by comparing the results of adaptation with the results of retrieval. If there is no matching model then no model is recommended. If there are more than one matching model, the system recommends the first ranked model by the retrieval nearest neighbor mechanism.

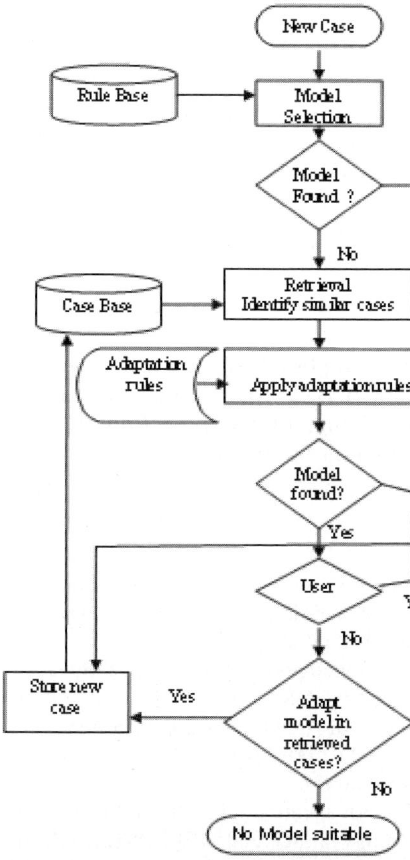

Fig. 3. The mixed inference method of IIEMD

4.2 Ontology Based Knowledge Base

In our system, one main challenge is to match the semantic web concept to the maintenance and maintenance decision function for system. In this way, information used over internet must be specified in ontology. The ontology represents the knowledge in internet, defining in a formal way the concepts of the different domains and relationships, with ability to perform reasoning over this knowledge. On this research, we use the standard CRIS (Common Relational Information Schema) defined by MIMOSA to define ontologies. CRIS represents a static view of the data, a part of OSA-CBM standard was developed around MIMOSA13. CRIS that provides coverage of the information (data) that will be managed within a condition based maintenance system. It defines a relational database schema with about 200 of tables approximately for machinery maintenance information. In short, CRIS is the core of MIMOSA which aim is the development and publication of open conventions for information exchange between plant and machinery maintenance information system. Above it, we give the rule base description base OWL. So we investigate the way to improve these ontology defined in XML language to other richer semantic ontology languages as RDF or OWL.

5 Conclusions

This work proposes a IIEMD system in SOA infrastructure that intends to provide distributed maintenance decision support. Further more, this effort is performed within a flexible architecture concept to provide flexible data and information management and maintenance decision where core concepts such as The Architecture of SOA based IIEMD are followed. Next step, other decision methods, like the neural network, support vector machine, etc, will be integrated.

Acknowledgement

The research reported in this paper is supported by both the National Basic Research Program of China with Grant No. 2005CB724106 and the Program for New Century Excellent Talents in University by China Ministry of Education with Grant No. NCET-04-0928. We hereby thank them for the financial aids.

Reference

1. Bengtsson, M.: Standardization issues in condition based maintenance. In: Proceedings of the 16th International Congress on Condition Monitoring and Diagnostic Engineering Management, Vaxjo University, Sweden, pp. 27–29 (2003)
2. Crespo Marquez, A., Gupta, J.N.D.: Contemporary Maintenance Management: Framework and Supporting Pillars. Omega 34(3), 325–338 (2006)
3. Zhang, W., Halang, W., Diedrich, C.: An Agent-based Platform for Service Integration in E-Maintenance. In: Proceedings of ICIT 2003, IEEE International Conference on Industrial Technology, vol. 1, pp. 426–433 (2003)
4. Li, Y., Chun, L., Nee, A., Ching, Y.: An agent-based platform for Web-enabled equipment predictive maintenance. In: Proceedings of IAT 2005 IEEE/WIC/ACM International Conference on Intelligent Agent Technology, Compiègne, France, pp. 132–135 (2005)
5. Saint-Voirin, D., Lang, C., Zerhouni, N., Guyennet, H.: Cooperative systems modelling, example of a cooperative e-maintenance system. In: Proceedings of CIRA 2005, Computational Intelligence in Robotics and Automation, Espoo, Finland, pp. 439–444 (2005)
6. Dong, Y.L., Gu, Y.J., Yang, K., Zhang, W.K.: A combining condition prediction model and its application in power plant. In: Proceedings of 2004 International Conference on Machine Learning and Cybernetics, Shanghai, China, vol. 6, pp. 3474–3478 (2004)
7. Wang, W.Q., Golnaraghi, M.F., Ismail, F.: Prognosis of machine health condition using neuro-fuzzy systems. J. MECH SYST S. 18, 813–831 (2004)
8. Yam, R., Tse, P., Li, L., Tu, P.: Intelligent predictive decision support system for condition-based maintenance. J. Int. J. Adv. Manuf. Technol. 17, 383–391 (2001)
9. Maf, S., Magv, F.: Designing reusable rule-based architectures with design patterns. J. Exper. Sy. Ap. 23(4), 395–403 (2002)
10. Chou, J.-S., Tsao, Y.-J.: Web-based CBR system applied to early cost budgeting for pavement maintenance project. J. Exper. Sy. Ap. 2, 1–14 (2008)
11. Xia, Q., Rao, M.: Dynamic case-based reasoning for process operation support systems. J. Eng. App. Art. 12(3), 343–361 (1999)
12. Léger, J.B., Morel, G.: Integration of maintenance in the enterprise: Towards an enterprise modeling based framework compliant with proactive maintenance strategy. J. Prod. Plan. C. 12(2), 176–187 (2001)
13. OSA-CBM v3.1 Standard, `http://www.mimosa.org/`

Fuzzy Synthetic Evaluation Approach of Reliability for Condition Monitoring System

Youmin Hu, Bo Wu*, and Pongxin Yi

School of Mechanical Science & Engineering, Huazhong University of Science and Technology, Wuhan, PRC., 430074
youmhwh@163.com

Abstract. Condition monitoring system (CMS) is now widely used in engineering fields. It plays an important role if it's reliable. But many factors affect reliability of CMS. The traditional reliability theory and approach or fuzzy reliability theory and approach can only assess how one of these factors affects CMS's reliability. More comprehensive reliability evaluation theory and approach need be developed to assess the reliability of CMS, as well as to analyze impact factors of reliability of CMS. Fuzzy synthetic evaluation theory is becoming a new method of assessing or decision making step-by-step and used broadly in many fields. Based on fuzzy synthetic evaluation and reliability theory, this paper studies the fuzzy synthetic evaluation approach of reliability of CMS and proposes a new method to evaluate reliability of CMS. It first reviews recent development in the study of reliability of CMS, then a fuzzy synthetic evaluation model of reliability for CMS is built, and a practical paradigm is given to show the application of proposed fuzzy synthetic evaluation for reliability of CMS and some conclusions are presented.

Keywords: Fuzzy reliability, fuzzy synthetic evaluation, modeling of fuzzy reliability, impact factors of fuzzy reliability, condition monitoring system.

1 Introduction

Condition monitoring technology ensures reliable operation of monitored objects and is widely used. Researchers have made a lot of research on theory and application approach in theoretical basis and realization measures of condition monitoring technology, etc. for many years. Many important achievements have been made [1-2].

Research on reliability of CMS has not been stressed enough during technical development of condition monitoring technology. Many users and researchers have a wrong conception that failures and accidents can be predicted and anticipated as long as CMS exists. That is to say, they think that CMS is very reliable and can predict latent failures and prevent accidents. From 2000 to 2002, the author participated in a project and experienced several cases related to monitoring system. The facts prove that there are questions of reliability of CMS as well as a critical problem of design and maintenance of CMS [1].

* Corresponding author.

C. Xiong et al. (Eds.): ICIRA 2008, Part II, LNAI 5315, pp. 583–592, 2008.

It is a pity that there is little research on reliability of CMS in many relevant documents. Not to say monographs which systematically introduce reliability of CMS.

Keywords of "reliability & condition monitoring" are respectively searched in materials of the recent ten years in database of IEEE, Elsevier (Science Direct Onsite), Kluwer Online and SpringerLink, etc. Only 4 documents [3-6] related to reliability of CMS are found. In which document[3] mainly discusses how to use condition monitoring technology to improve reliability of industrial equipment; document[4] mainly discusses reliability and risk of characteristic used in CMS; document[5] mainly analyzes reliability for maintenance system based on condition monitoring technology; document [6] mainly discusses remote condition monitoring technology focused on reliability. It indicates that there is still rare research specifically on reliability of CMS in occident.

Topics of "reliability & condition monitoring" are searched in database from January 1990 to April 2003 in www.cnki.net and www.cqvip.com. 45 documents related to reliability for condition monitoring (supervision and control) system are found (ref. to [1]). In which 27 documents discuss service reliability and on-site service experience introduction of condition monitoring (supervision and control) system, and 18 documents discuss inherent reliability and theoretical research (system reliability modeling, calculation and evaluation approach of reliability, as well as reliability design method, etc.)

The analysis of the found documents and materials indicates: Though Europe and the US lead the research on reliability technology in the world; little material shows that a lot of specific research has been made on reliability for condition monitoring (supervision and control) system. In nearly 13 years from 1990 to 2003, only 45 domestic documents discuss reliability for condition monitoring (supervision and control) system, only about 5 documents per year. Most of these 45 found documents are involved in experience introduction (covering 60% of total documents), only 40% are documents of theoretical research, and documents really published in high-level transactions or core periodicals cover merely 20% of all found documents.

The research content of the found 45 domestic documents is mainly about service reliability and inherent reliability for condition monitoring (supervision and control) system. Research on service reliability mainly analyzes methods to improve system reliability in use, maintenance and environmental impact, etc. of system. Research on inherent reliability mainly discusses methods to enhance system reliability in system structure design, component selection and software development, etc. The research is mainly based on classical reliability engineering theory. The system reliability models built in theoretical research are all based on probability model of two-state logical assumption (i.e. it is assumed that the system has only two working states: normal and failure). Mathematical knowledge in documents besides [7,8] is all probability theory; besides probability theory, documents [7,8] apply graph theory in reliability modeling of CMS for the first time.

Analysis documents found, CMS as the technology guarantee for safe and reliable operation of modern industrial system is widely used now. However, insufficient importance is attached to reliability research on CMS, and there is so little reliability research on CMS that it can hardly meet the requirements of CMS. The paper plans to systematically research the reliability synthetic evaluation of CMS, offer a fuzzy synthetic evaluation approach for reliability of CMS, and prove reasonableness and validity of the approach by examples.

The first part introduces the research background and reviews domestic and foreign research. The second part introduces the mathematical basis of fuzzy synthetic evaluation approach. The third part integrates examples and proposes the fuzzy synthetic evaluation approach for CMS. The fourth part is the summary.

2 Mathematical Basis—Fuzzy Synthetic Evaluation

Fuzzy synthetic evaluation can make a synthetic evaluation on objects affected by many factors[9-10]. For the evaluated objects as a whole, assign an evaluation index—non-negative real number to each object according to the given conditions, then carry out ordering and optimization on the basis of this index. The general process of fuzzy synthetic evaluation goes as follows.

2.1 Building Factor Set, Alternative Set (Evaluation Set) and Weight Set

$$U = \{u_1, u_2, \cdots, u_m\} \tag{1}$$

Where, U refers to factor set, u_i $(i = 1, 2, \cdots, m)$ represents each impact factor.

$$V = \{v_1, v_2, \cdots, v_n\} \tag{2}$$

Where, V refers to evaluation set, v_i $(i = 1, 2, \cdots, n)$ represents various possible evaluation results.

In order to show the importance of the impact of each factor to evaluated objects, assign a non-negative real number smaller than 1, a_i $(i = 1, 2, \cdots, m)$ ($\sum_{i=1}^{m} a_i = 1$) , to each factor as the corresponding weight value. Call set

$$\underset{\sim}{A} = \{a_1, a_2, \cdots, a_m\} \tag{3}$$

as weight set. Each weight value is generally determined according to the need of actual engineering problems subjectively.

2.2 Single Factor Fuzzy Evaluation

Investigating and evaluating the degree of membership of evaluated objects to each factor in alternative sets from the aspect of one factor is called single factor fuzzy evaluation. If evaluation is based on u_i, its degree of membership to v_j is recorded as r_{ij}, then the evaluation result of NO. i factor u_i is shown as:

$$\underset{\sim}{R}_i = \frac{r_{i1}}{v_1} + \frac{r_{i2}}{v_2} + \cdots + \frac{r_{in}}{v_n} \tag{4}$$

Obviously it is a fuzzy subset of alternative set V recorded as

$$\underset{\sim}{R}_i = \{r_{i1}, r_{i2}, \cdots, r_{in}\} \tag{5}$$

Then the evaluation set of all the factors in factor sets can constitute a fuzzy matrix as below:

$$\underset{\sim}{R} = \begin{bmatrix} r_{11}, r_{12}, \cdots, r_{1n} \\ r_{21}, r_{22}, \cdots, r_{2n} \\ \vdots \\ r_{m1}, r_{m2}, \cdots, r_{mn} \end{bmatrix} \tag{6}$$

Call formula（6）as single factor fuzzy evaluation matrix.

2.3 Fuzzy Synthetic Evaluation

It can be inferred from single factor evaluation matrix $\underset{\sim}{R}$ that row i of $\underset{\sim}{R}$ reflects the degree of impact of factor i on evaluated objects in selecting each alternative factor, and column j of $\underset{\sim}{R}$ reflects the degree of impact of all the factors on evaluated objects in selecting alternative factor j. If the impact degree of each factor on evaluation object is taken into comprehensive consideration, then the synthetic impact of all factors on alternative factor j can be reflected by the weight sum of factors of all lines in column j, i.e.

$$b_j = \sum_{i=1}^{m} a_i r_{ij} \quad (j = 1, 2, \cdots, n) \tag{7}$$

from which fuzzy matrix $\underset{\sim}{B} = (b_1, b_2, \cdots, b_n)$ can be obtained. $\underset{\sim}{B}$ is called fuzzy synthetic evaluation set, b_j $(j = 1, 2, \cdots, n)$ is called fuzzy synthetic evaluation index, when it refers to the comprehensive consideration of all impact factors, the degree of membership of evaluated objects to factor j in the alternative set is evaluated. Considering fuzzy matrix $\underset{\sim}{B}$ as the composition of $\underset{\sim}{A}$ and $\underset{\sim}{R}$, i.e.

$$\underset{\sim}{B} = \underset{\sim}{A} \bullet \underset{\sim}{R} \tag{8}$$

In this formula, "$\circ$" represents fuzzy relation calculation, here it can be taken as fuzzy matrix multiplied by "$\bullet$". Therefore we have

$$\underset{\sim}{B} = \underset{\sim}{A} \bullet \underset{\sim}{R} = (a_1, a_2, \cdots, a_m) \bullet \begin{bmatrix} r_{11}, r_{12}, \cdots, r_{1n} \\ r_{21}, r_{22}, \cdots, r_{2n} \\ \vdots \\ r_{m1}, r_{m2}, \cdots, r_{mn} \end{bmatrix} = (b_1, b_2, \cdots, b_n) \tag{9}$$

where $b_j = \overset{m}{\underset{i=1}{\vee}} (a_i \wedge r_{ij})$ $(j = 1, 2, \cdots, n)$.

2.4 Evaluation Index Processing

$\underset{\sim}{B}' = (b_1', b_2', \cdots, b_n')$ is obtained after normalization processing of synthetic evaluation set matrix $\underset{\sim}{B}$, take the evaluation index b_j' after normalization processing as weight number, calculate weighted mean evaluation index according to the formula below

$$V = \frac{\sum_{j=1}^{n} (b_j')^k v_j}{\sum_{j=1}^{n} (b_j')^k} \tag{10}$$

In this formula k refers to weighted index, normally it is taken as 2.

If the alternative factor is a fuzzy language variable, then language fuzzy quantities can be represented by relevant appropriate digital quantities respectively, e.g. {good, above average, average, under average, bad} = {5, 4, 3, 2, 1}, and processed by weighted mean method.

3 CMS Reliability Fuzzy Synthetic Evaluation

In engineering practice, there are many factors which may impact CMS, including not only technological factors, but also many non-technological factors such as environmental factors, economic factors and even human factors, etc. A single or more reliability indices is not capable to contain all factors possible to impact system reliability. The definition of traditional reliability index has not taken into consideration the impact of various factors on system reliability, not to mention the inspection of impact degree of some factors on a certain index.

In this section, taking CMS as an example, the theory of fuzzy synthetic evaluation will be used to study the issue of synthetic evaluation on fuzzy reliability of CMS and establishing a synthetic evaluation approach on reliability of CMS.

3.1 Impact Factor Set

The reliability of CMS are usually affected by many factors, such as the degree of the advanced technologies, complication degree of the system, maintenance level, working environment status, personnel technology quality and economic factors and etc. Thus, factor sets of CMS can be set up to carry out fuzzy synthetic evaluation are:

$$U = \{u_1, u_2, u_3, u_4, u_5, u_6\} \tag{11}$$

where U —Factor set affects the reliability of CMS;

u_1 to u_6 refer respectively the advanced technology, complication degree, the maintenance status, the working environment status, operation of CMS and the technical quality of the maintenance personnel, investment of the establishment and maintenance of CMS.

3.2 Alternative Set—Reliability Index Set

Various factors in the alternative set represent various possible evaluations for the generalized reliability level of CMS. The generalized reliability of CMS covers the performance of CMS, such as classic reliability, fuzzy reliability, maintenance, usability, anti-disturb, creditability, safety and etc.. The evaluation on generalized reliability of CMS can be expressed with indices of very high, higher, high, low, lower and very low. Since the indices are fuzzy language variation, for the purpose of convenience for the calculation, give them a digital quantity separately, such as to adopt ten point system evaluation: very high=10; higher=8; high=6; low=4; lower=2 and very low=1. Thus, the alternative set of the fuzzy synthetic evaluation is

$$V = \{v_1, v_2, v_3, v_4, v_5, v_6\} = \{10, 8, 6, 4, 2, 1\} \tag{12}$$

where V —reability evaluation alternative set of CMS;

v_1 to v_6 refer respectively generalized reliability evaluation indices 1 to 6 of CMS, $v_1 = 10$ (very high), $v_2 = 8$ (higher), $v_3 = 6$ (high), $v_4 = 4$ (low), $v_5 = 2$ (lower), $v_6 = 1$ (very low).

3.3 Weight Sets

The importance degree of influence of each factor in the factor set for CMS fuzzy synthetic evaluation is different to the system reliability. In order to reflect the importance degree of influence of factors to the reliability, the following sets up weight set that reflect factor's degree of importance. The factor's degree of influence on reliability can be classified into six ranks, i.e. very great, greater, great, small, smaller and very small. The six ranks reflecting importance degree of influence on generalized reliability is also the fuzzy language variable, which should be processed the same as the elements in index set, give a corresponding digital quantity to each rank that should also be evaluated with ten point system: very great=10; greater=8; great=6; small=4; smaller=2 and very small=1. Therefore, the weight set should be:

$$A = \{very\ great,\ greater,\ great,\ small, smaller,\ very\ small\} = \{10,\ 8,\ 6,\ 4,\ 2,1\} \tag{13}$$

As for the CMS of mixer, the value for the importance degree of influence of the six factors in the factor set that affect system reliability should be one of elements in the weight set , detailed value should be determined by expert grade. The expert grade see table 3.1.

We invited 10 experts (designers, supervisors, users and maintainers) to respectively fill the expert grade table for degree of importance. For shortly , we just collect the results as table 3.1. In the table 3.1, adopt arithmetic mean for every each row of data, thus can obtain weight set corresponding with the factor set as follows:

Table 3.1. Expert grade summary for degree of importance June 20, 2003

Impact factors	Expert									
	1	2	3	4	5	6	7	8	9	10
Technological advance	8	6	6	6	6	6	6	6	8	8
Complexity degree	10	10	10	10	10	10	10	10	10	10
Maintenance	10	6	6	6	6	6	8	6	8	6
Environment	1	8	4	4	6	4	4	6	4	4
Personnel ability	2	10	6	6	6	6	6	6	4	6
Fund invested	10	8	6	6	6	6	6	8	6	6

$$\underset{\sim}{A}_u = \{a_1, a_2, a_3, a_4, a_5, a_6\} = \{6.6, 10, 6.8, 4.5, 5.8, 6.8\} \quad (14)$$

where $\underset{\sim}{A}_u$ —weight set corresponding with factor set;

a_i —degree of influence of factor $u_i (i = 1,2,3,4,5,6)$ on reliability for the CMS of mixer.

Then normalize $\underset{\sim}{A}_u$, and the $\underset{\sim}{A}_u$ after normalization is the weight set corresponding with factor set.

$$\underset{\sim}{A}_u = \{a_1, a_2, a_3, a_4, a_5, a_6\} = \{0.1692, 0.2469, 0.1679, 0.1111, 0.1432, 0.1679\} \quad (15)$$

3.4 Single-Factor Fuzzy Evaluation

After setting up the factor set and alternative set, the single-factor fuzzy evaluation then can be carried out. The so-called single-factor fuzzy evaluation refers to determine the fuzzy relationship between factors in the factor set and all the elements in alternative set, and build grade of membership of factors in factor set to the evaluation index in alternative set, i.e. the grade of membership of factors affecting CMS reliability to the reliability evaluation index. This fuzzy relationship is generally expressed by the grade of membership r_{ij} (r_{ij} indicates the grade of membership of No. i factor in factor set to the j evaluation index in alternative set). Therefore, the core of single-factor fuzzy evaluation is to determine the grade of membership r_{ij} . In engineering, determination for grade of membership can also adopt expert grade, the detailed steps are as follows.

Firstly design an experts grade table 3.2 for the grade of membership, and invite relevant experts (designers, supervisors, users and maintainers) to fill the table, then deal with the data, such as $r_{11}(1)$ (the grade of membership of the first factor filled by the first expert to the evaluation index) filled by experts as follows: take arithmetic mean of all the data as the final result, i.e.:

Table 3.2. Expert grade summary of grade of membership

Date: June 2003

Impactfactors	Reliability evaluation rank					
	Very high	High	High	Low	Low	Very low
Technological advance	0.21	0.30	0.24	0.13	0.08	0.04
Complexity degree	0.13	0.14	0.18	0.25	0.18	0.11
Maintenance	0.24	0.30	0.17	0.11	0.09	0.09
Environment	0.19	0.14	0.21	0.22	0.16	0.08
Personnel ability	0.27	0.21	0.22	0.15	0.08	0.07
Fund invested	0.17	0.34	0.20	0.13	0.09	0.06

$$r_{ij} = \frac{\sum_{n=1}^{p} r_{ij}(n)}{p} \tag{16}$$

Where i —factors number in the factor set, $i = 1,2,3,4,5,6$;

j—evaluation index number in the alternative set, $j = 1,2,\cdots,6$;

p —number of experts filling the table.

Fill the data being processed according to formula (16) into table 3.2 as the required table for grade of membership. The single-factor evaluation matrix is built according to table 3.2 as follows:

$$\underset{\sim}{R} = \begin{bmatrix} r_{11}, r_{12}, \cdots, r_{1n} \\ r_{21}, r_{22}, \cdots, r_{2n} \\ \vdots \\ r_{m1}, r_{m2}, \cdots, r_{mn} \end{bmatrix} = \begin{bmatrix} 0.21\ 0.13\ 0.24\ 0.19\ 0.27\ 0.17 \\ 0.30\ 0.14\ 0.30\ 0.14\ 0.21\ 0.34 \\ 0.24\ 0.18\ 0.17\ 0.21\ 0.22\ 0.20 \\ 0.13\ 0.25\ 0.11\ 0.22\ 0.15\ 0.13 \\ 0.08\ 0.18\ 0.09\ 0.16\ 0.08\ 0.09 \\ 0.04\ 0.11\ 0.09\ 0.08\ 0.07\ 0.07 \end{bmatrix} \tag{17}$$

3.5 Fuzzy Synthetic Evaluation Matrix

The above single-factor evaluation only involves the fuzzy relationship between single factor in factor set and evaluation index in alternative set, the importance degree of influence of each factor on reliability hasn't been considered. Comprehensively considering the importance degree of each factor on reliability, we can set up the fuzzy synthetic evaluation set as follows:

$$\underset{\sim}{B} = (b_1, b_2, \cdots, b_n) = \underset{\sim}{A} \bullet \underset{\sim}{R} = \begin{bmatrix} 0.1629 \\ 0.2469 \\ 0.1679 \\ 0.1111 \\ 0.1432 \\ 0.1679 \end{bmatrix}^T \bullet \begin{bmatrix} 0.21\ 0.13\ 0.24\ 0.19\ 0.27\ 0.17 \\ 0.30\ 0.14\ 0.30\ 0.14\ 0.21\ 0.34 \\ 0.24\ 0.18\ 0.17\ 0.21\ 0.22\ 0.20 \\ 0.13\ 0.25\ 0.11\ 0.22\ 0.15\ 0.13 \\ 0.08\ 0.18\ 0.09\ 0.16\ 0.08\ 0.09 \\ 0.04\ 0.11\ 0.09\ 0.08\ 0.07\ 0.07 \end{bmatrix} \tag{18}$$

$$= (0.2469\ \ 0.1679\ \ 0.2469\ \ 0.1679\ \ 0.2200\ \ 0.2000)$$

Implement normalization for the above formula and get:

$$\underset{\sim}{B}' = (b_1', b_2', \cdots, b_6') = (0.1954\ \ 0.1329\ \ 0.1954\ \ 0.1329\ \ 0.1812\ \ 0.1622) \tag{19}$$

3.6 Evaluation Results

As for the above normalized fuzzy synthetic evaluation set $\underset{\sim}{B}'$, the evaluation index can be processed with the method of second weighted mean ($k = 2$) according to formula (10), thus the fuzzy synthetic evaluation results can be obtained for the CMS reliability of mixer.

$$V = \frac{\sum_{j=1}^{n} (b_j')^2 v_j}{\sum_{j=1}^{n} (b_j')^2} = 5.36 \tag{20}$$

Observing the above calculation, after comprehensive consideration of advanced technology, complex system structure, system maintenance level, system working environment, technical quality of operating and maintenance personnel, as well as investment adopted by the CMS of mixer, the general reliability of the entire system (performances as classical reliability, fuzzy reliability, maintainability, usability, anti-disturbing, creditability and stability, etc.) is between high and low, and is more closer to high level.

4 Conclusion

There are many factors that affect CMS reliability. It is impossible to evaluate influence of all factors on CMS reliability by traditional reliability research methods. Only with fuzzy synthetic evaluation, influence of impact factors on CMS reliability and combined influence of all factors can be comprehensively evaluated so as to help design, use, and maintenance of CMS as well as system reliability improvement.

Acknowledgements

This research was supported in part by National Natural Science Foundation of China(Grant NO. 50575087) and the National Key Basic Research Special Found of China (Grant NO. 2005CB724101).

References

1. Hu, Y.: Reliability of condition monitoring system. [Doctoral dissertation] Wuhan. Huazhong University of Science & Technology (2003)
2. Muller, A., et al.: On the concept of e-maintenance: Review and current research. Reliab. Eng. Syst. Safty 93(8), 1165–1187 (2008)
3. Siyambalapitiya, D.J.T., Mclaren, P.G.: Reliability improvement and economic benefits of on-line monitoring systems for large induction machines. IEEE transactions on industry applications 26(6), 1018–1025 (1990)
4. Cempel, C., Natke, H.G., Yao, J.T.P.: Symptom reliability and hazard for systems condition monitoring. Mechanical Systems and Signal Processing 14(3), 495–505 (2000)
5. Saranga, H., Knezevic, J.: Reliability prediction for condition-based maintained systems. Reliability Engineering and System Safety 71, 219–224 (2001)
6. Márquez, F.P.G., Schmid, F., Collado, J.C.: A reliability centered approach to remote condition monitoring: A railway points case study. Reliability engineering and system safety 80, 33–40 (2003)
7. Youmin, H., Runsheng, D., Shuzi, Y.: Reliability analysis of concentrated monitoring and control system. Joural of Vibration, Measurment & Diagnosis 23(3), 6–9 (2003)
8. Youmin, H., Runsheng, D., Shuzi, Y.: Reliability analysis for monitoring and measuring system with hierarchy and redunancy structure. Chinese Journal of Mechanical Engineering 39(8), 110–115 (2003)
9. Utkin, L.V., Gurov, S.V.: A general formal approach for fuzzy reliability analysis in the possibility context. Fuzzy sets and systems 83, 203–213 (1996)
10. Cai, K.-Y.: System failure engineering and fuzzy methodology: an introductory overview. Fuzzy sets and systems 83, 113–133 (1996)
11. Wu, N.E.: Reliability of reconfigurable control system: a fuzzy set theoretic perspective. In: Proceedings of the 36th conference on decision and control 1997, pp. 3352–3356 (1997)
12. Wu, H.-C.: Fuzzy reliability analysis based on closed fuzzy numbers. Information sciences 103, 135–159 (1997)
13. Bing, L., Meilin, Z., Kai, X.: A practical engineering method for fuzzy reliability analysis of mechanical structures. Reliability engineering and system safety 67, 311–315 (2000)
14. Nachtmann, H., Chimka, J.R.: Fuzzy reliability in conceptual design. In: 2003 proceedings annual reliability and maintainability symposium, pp. 360–364. IEEE, Los Alamitos (2003)

The Condition Monitoring and Performance Evaluating of Digital Manufacturing Process

Xuefeng Chen, Bing Li, Hongrui Cao, and Zhengjia He

State Key Lab. for Manufacturing Systems Engineering, Xi'an Jiaotong University, Xi'an 710049, PRC
chenxf@mail.xjtu.edu.cn

Abstract. Spindle assembly is one of the most important components of digital manufacturing equipments. It is key problem to monitor and evaluate its performance to assure the normal process. Aiming at the bearings which damage most easily in spindle system, a new time-frequency analysis method called S transform is studied, time-frequency distribution of vibration signals collected from spindle is obtained, and a singular value decomposition method is employed to condense the time-frequency matrix data so that the fault features can be extracted quantitatively. Simulation and experimental studies have demonstrated that the proposed method may identify the running state of spindle bearing accurately. Thus a new technique for the evaluation of spindle serving performance of digital manufacturing equipments is provided.

Keywords: Digital manufacturing S transform Bearing Spindle.

1 Introduction

As the outcome of manufacturing technologies and information technologies, digital manufacturing has become the kernel of advanced manufacturing technologies and a breakthrough to reach the commanding height in the competition of manufacturing technologies for all the countries. CNC equipments play a crucial role in digital manufacturing with the orientation of high precision and efficiency. Great loss caused by suspended operation of machine tool necessitates reliability, machining quality and working performance of the CNC equipments. It is necessary to have real-time monitoring on working condition of the CNC equipments. Studies at home and abroad lay emphasis on working condition monitoring and quality control in the machining process, and regard them as important technological bases for high-quality digital manufacturing [1, 2].

Spindle assembly is one of the most important components of CNC equipments. It drives rough parts or cutting tool to form the surface of the work piece when the machine tool is in operation. Service performance of the spindle assembly has an important effect on machining quality and efficiency of the machine tool. Conditions of spindle bearing such as precision will affect the performance of the spindle assembly directly. For example, with the increase of rotational speed, DN value of rolling

C. Xiong et al. (Eds.): ICIRA 2008, Part II, LNAI 5315, pp. 593–603, 2008.

bearing in many motorized spindle has reached the millions, which complicate the working conditions of rolling bearings. Therefore, monitoring and diagnosis of spindle bearings in production is an important step for machining precision in digital manufacturing [3, 4].

The spindle bearing of the machine tool is under the cutting forces of different directions, which results in unsteady dynamic signals. In addition, characteristic information is not obvious and easy to be drowned by the noise for initial failure. Therefore, the study adopts a new time-frequency analysis method and a singular value decomposition method for analyzing initial failure of spindle bearings. S transform, a new time-frequency analysis method, is proposed by Stocwkell who studied geophysics in Canada in 1996 and further discussed in 2007 [5,6]. S transform combines the merits of Fourier transform and wavelet transform. It is an extension of continuous wavelet transform with Morlet wavelet as the basic wavelet. Its basic function is the product of harmonic waves and Gaussian function. Harmonic wave just has dilation transform in time domain, while Gaussian Function has dilation and translation, whose time-frequency resolution is related to frequency, that is, high frequency resolution at lower frequency and high time resolution at higher frequency. S transform doesn't have the shortcomings of fixed window of short-time Fourier transform and Cohen cross terms. S transform is directly related to Fourier transform and provides resolution based on frequency instead of scale. In addition, S transform includes phase factor and retains absolute phase feature of every frequency. The study shows that S transform has no phase shift and possess better time-frequency distribution which reflect abrupt changes of signals more directly and clearly. It has been successfully applied to mechanical fault diagnosis, power quality disturbance monitoring and seismic exploration signal analysis, etc [7, 8]. However, time-frequency representation got from S transform does not provide fault features quantitatively. The present study adopts a singular value decomposition method to condense the data and extract the fault features, which can effectively identify the fault of the outer ring of spindle bearings.

2 S Transform Theory

2.1 One-Dimensional Continuous S Transform

Fourier transform $X(f)$ of Signal $x(t)$ is

$$X(f) = \int_{-\infty}^{+\infty} x(t)e^{-j2\pi ft}\mathbf{d}t \tag{1}$$

This transform establishes an access from the time domain to frequency domain for the signal. $X(f)$ indicates total intensity of any sinusoidal frequency f included in $x(t)$ by using sine basis functions. It is the average statistic and cannot reflect the change of signal frequency with the passage of time. And it is not characterized by time frequency localization.

Supposing $w(t)$ is the window function of limited width with τ as the center, short-time Fourier transform of signal $x(t)$ is produced by Fourier transform of windowed signal $x(t)w(t-\tau)$.

$$\mathrm{STFT}_x(f,\tau)=\int_{-\infty}^{+\infty}x(t)w(t-\tau)e^{-j2\pi ft}\mathbf{d}t \tag{2}$$

This transform maps signal $x(t)$ into two-dimensional time-frequency plane (τ, f) and provides information about time domain and frequency domain of the signals. Short-time Fourier transform is a time-frequency localization analysis with fixed time window and form. Once the window function $w(t)$ is chosen, resolution in different time-frequency plane is invariable. However, short-time Fourier transform cannot meet the requirements in analyzing non-stationary signal as reflecting signal's high-frequency component requires narrow time window while low-frequency component requires wide time window.

$$w(t)=\frac{1}{\sigma\sqrt{2\pi}}e^{-\frac{t^2}{2\sigma^2}} \tag{3}$$

If the window function is defined as normalized Gauss window with the time-optimal localization and parameter σ is variable,

$$\sigma(f)=\frac{c}{|f|}, \qquad k>0 \tag{4}$$

Then, $\sigma(f)$ is similar to the scale factor in wavelet transform. The lower the signal's frequency f , the larger $\sigma(f)$. Here $w(t)$ is a wide window with high frequency resolution; on the contrary, $\sigma(f)$ becomes smaller when frequency f becomes larger, that is, the narrow window is in use to meet the demand of time resolution for high-frequency signal. c is a constant and decides width of Gauss window function and thus controls time and frequency resolution.

By substituting (3) and (4) into (2) and one-dimensional continuous S transform formula for signal $x(t)$ can be obtained

$$S(f,\tau)=\int_{-\infty}^{+\infty}x(t)\frac{|f|}{c\sqrt{2\pi}}e^{-\frac{(\tau-t)^2f^2}{2c^2}}e^{-j2\pi ft}\mathrm{d}t \tag{5}$$

The above-mentioned S transform can also be obtained from frequency domain calculation and its corresponding formula is as follows [9]

$$S(f,\tau)=\int_{-\infty}^{+\infty}X(\alpha+f)e^{-\frac{2\pi^2c^2}{f^2}\alpha^2}e^{j2\pi\alpha\tau}\mathbf{d}\alpha \qquad f\neq 0 \tag{6}$$

where $X(\alpha)$ is Fourier transform of $x(t)$. Stockwell also provides inverse transform of S transform, that is

$$x(t)=\int_{-\infty}^{+\infty}\left[\int_{-\infty}^{+\infty}S(f,\tau)\mathbf{d}\tau\right]e^{j2\pi ft}\mathbf{d}f \tag{7}$$

2.2 One-Dimensional Discrete S Transform

As for discrete signal $x[kT]$ with the length of N where T is sampling interval and $k=0,1,\ldots,N-1$, let $f\rightarrow\frac{n}{NT}$, $\tau\rightarrow kT$, $\alpha\rightarrow\frac{m}{NT}$ in Eq. (6), discrete S transform will take the following form

$$S\left[\frac{n}{NT},kT\right]=\sum_{m=0}^{N-1}X\left[\frac{m+n}{NT}\right]e^{-\frac{2\pi^2c^2m^2}{n^2}}e^{\frac{j2\pi mk}{N}} \qquad n=1,\ldots,N-1 \tag{8}$$

In case $n=0$, expressions of discrete form can be obtained as,

$$S[0,kT]=\frac{1}{N}\sum_{m=0}^{N-1}x\left[\frac{m}{NT}\right] \tag{9}$$

A complex time-frequency matrix (S matrix) can be obtained from signal $x[kT]$ with S transform. Its row and column correspond to frequency value and sampling time respectively. The row vector reflects change of amplitude and phase of certain frequency component with the passage of time, while the column vector reflects information such as amplitude and phase of different frequency component at certain time of sampling.

Similarly, discrete form of S inverse transform can be obtained from Eq. (7)

$$x[kT]=\sum_{n=0}^{N-1}\left\{\frac{1}{N}\sum_{k=0}^{N-1}S\left[\frac{n}{NT},kT\right]\right\}e^{\frac{j2\pi nk}{N}} \tag{10}$$

3 Singular Value Decomposition of Time-Frequency Matrix

Two-dimensional time-frequency representation of S transform can reflect time domain and frequency domain of signal simultaneously but cannot provide information about the fault features quantitatively. For this reason, it is not convenient to use in practice. And further information extraction is needed. The singular value decomposition method is employed to condense the time-frequency matrix data so that the fault features can be extracted from non-stationary signals conveniently.

As for discrete signal $x[kT]$ with the length of N where sampling interval $f_s = 1/T$ and $k = 0,1,...,N-1$, matrix $\boldsymbol{S}$ **of** $M \times N$ where analyzing frequency $f_N = f_s/2$ and $M = N/2$ can be obtained with S transform. At this time, by extracting spectral data (column vector) at the time of $T_i = iT$ and its former $T_{i-1}, T_{i-2}, ..., T_{i-K+1}$ from matrix S, matrix $\boldsymbol{A}_i$ can be formed, that is

$$A_i\left[\frac{n}{NT}, kT\right] = \left|S\left[\frac{n}{NT}, (i-(K-k))T\right]\right| \qquad k = 1,2,...,K \tag{11}$$

Make a singular value decomposition of matrix $\boldsymbol{A}_i$, that is

$$\boldsymbol{A}_i = \boldsymbol{U}_i \boldsymbol{D}_i \boldsymbol{V}_i^T \tag{12}$$

where $\boldsymbol{U}_i$ and $\boldsymbol{V}_i$ are matrix of $M \times M$ and $K \times K$ respectively which represent singular matrix. Here $\boldsymbol{U}_i \boldsymbol{U}_i^T = 1$ and $\boldsymbol{V}_i \boldsymbol{V}_i^T = 1$. $\boldsymbol{D}_i$ is diagonal matrix of $M \times K$. Its diagonal elements $d_1^i, d_2^i, ..., d_p^i$ ($d_1^i \geq d_2^i \geq ... \geq d_p^i$, $p = \mathbf{min}(M, K)$) are singular values of matrix $\boldsymbol{A}_i$. As to the time after T_i, i.e. $T_{i+1}, T_{i+2}, ..., T_N$, same method can be used to get corresponding $M \times K$ matrix $\boldsymbol{A}_{i+1}, \boldsymbol{A}_{i+2}, ..., \boldsymbol{A}_N$, and singular value matrix $\boldsymbol{D}_{i+1}, \boldsymbol{D}_{i+2}, ..., \boldsymbol{D}_N$ can be obtained by singular value decomposition. By taking the first order of every singular value matrix, the vector can be formed.

$$\mathbf{P} = [d_1^i, d_1^{i+1}, ..., d_1^N] \tag{13}$$

The first-order singular value vector $\boldsymbol{P}$ is the information after condensing matrix S. It can reflect features of matrix S to some extent. Features of non-stationary signals can be extracted by analyzing the tendency of $\boldsymbol{P}$.

4 Simulation Signal Analysis

This part will make use of simulation signal to test the S transform and singular value decomposition method to extract the fault features. By constructing simulation signal $y(t) = 4\cos(2\pi 10t)$ with 1000Hz as the sampling frequency and 1024 as the data length, and superposing impulse response signal on $y(t)$ every 128 points, the signal shown in Fig.1(a) can be obtained. Combined time-frequency distribution and contour map of the signal can be obtained with S transform as illustrated in Fig. 1(b) and 1(c).

It can be seen that steady low-frequency components of 10Hz in simulation signals and high-frequency impulse signals are separated distinctly. Spectral peak at high frequency corresponds with impulse signal and steady frequency band at low frequency corresponds with frequency component of 10Hz with nearly invariable amplitude value regardless of time.

By using singular value decomposition method to condense the data of matrix S and letting $K = 5$, variation curve of one-order singular value can be obtained as illustrated in Fig. 2(a) where peak position of the singular value represents the time of impulse. By making spectrum analysis as shown in Fig. 2(b), frequency of impulse signals (7.8Hz) can be extracted. Therefore, by making use of the S transform and singular value decomposition method, low-frequency and high-frequency components can be separated distinctly and the frequency of impulse signals can be extracted.

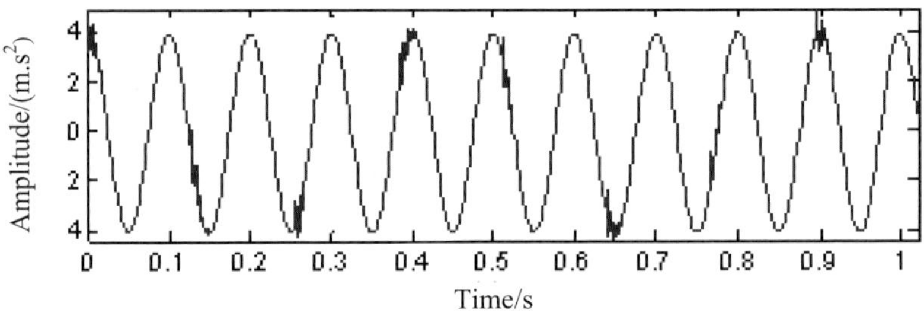

(a) The original signal

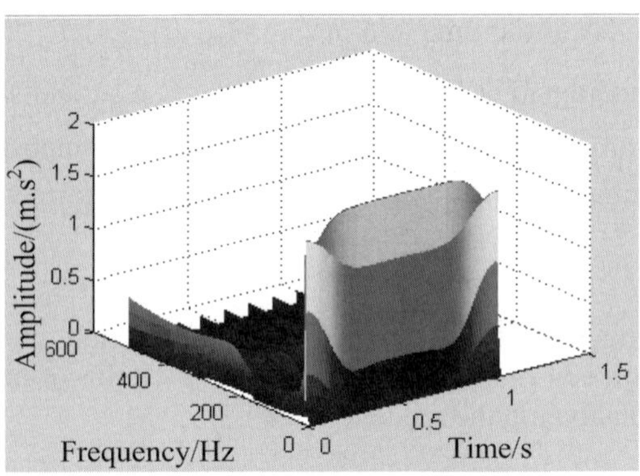

(b) time-frequency distribution

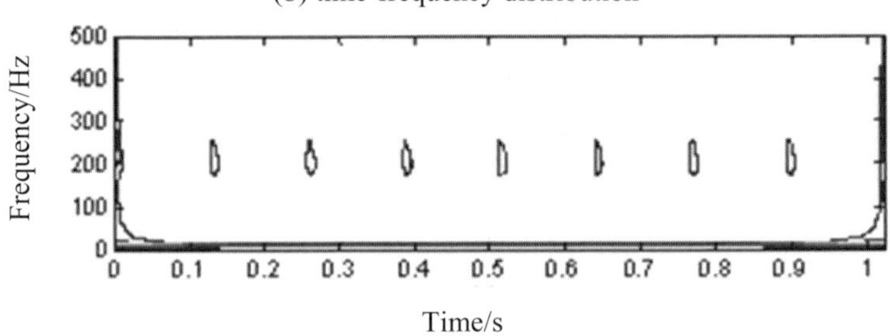

(c) The contour map

Fig. 1. S transform of the simulating signal

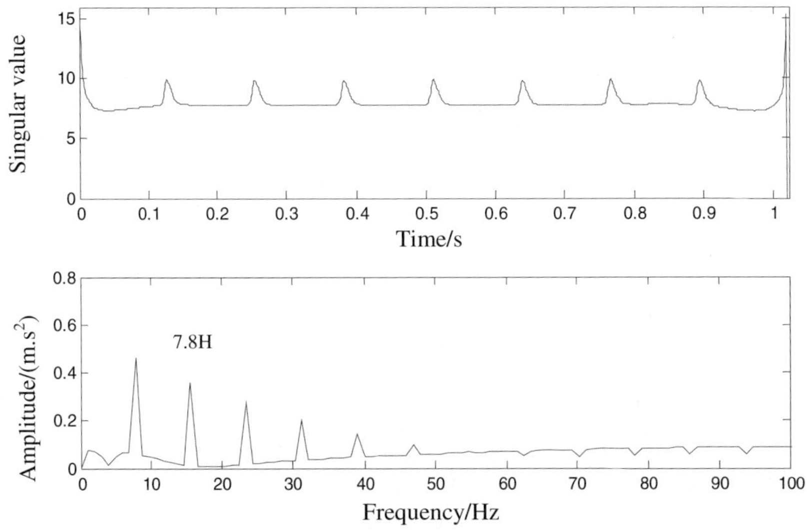

Fig. 2. (a) Variation curve of one-order singular value (b) Spectrum

5 Illustration in Application

A triaxial CNC milling machine has been in service for years. There is so much vibration in machining process that quality of the work piece, especially surface roughness cannot meet the requirement. This milling machine consists of spindle system, feed system, driving system, cooling and lubrication system. As the spindle system bears most of the cutting force, and its dynamic performance is directly reflected by the surface quality of the work piece by the cutting tool, it is crucial to monitor running state of the spindle.

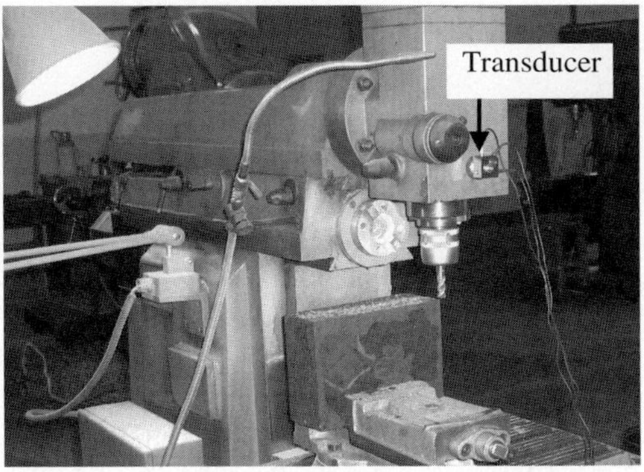

Fig. 3. Vibration test of the spindle

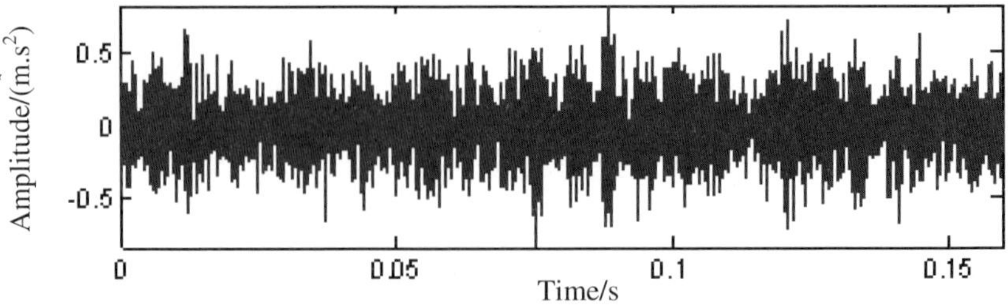

(a) The original signal

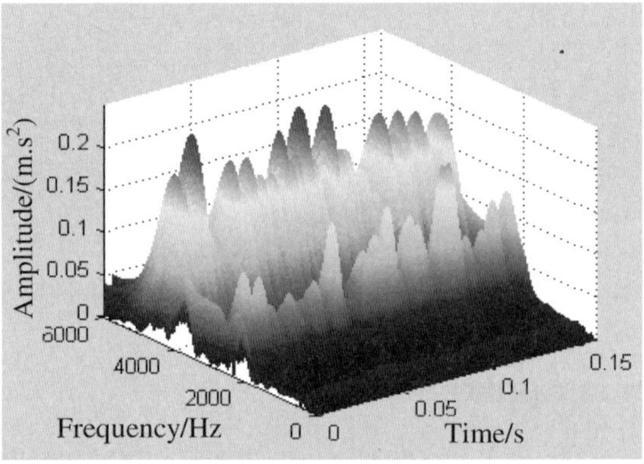

(b) time-frequency distribution

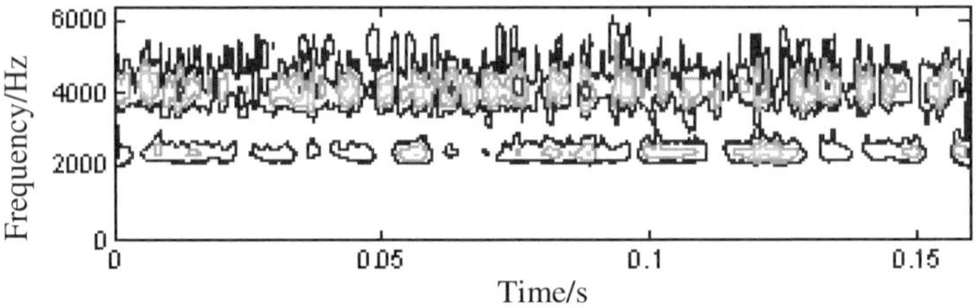

(c) The contour map

Fig. 4. S transform of vibration signal of the spindle box

In the experiment, high-speed steel end mill with straight handle and three edges were used for conventional milling of specimen which was steel 45#. Rotational frequency of the spindle in the machine tool was 19.5Hz. Feed speed was 160mm/min. Both the cutting depth and width were 2mm. A three-way acceleration transducer LC0110 was used to detect vibration signals of the spindle box with 12.8Hz as the sampling frequency. Sony EX was used to collect the data. Installation of the transducer is shown in Fig. 3.

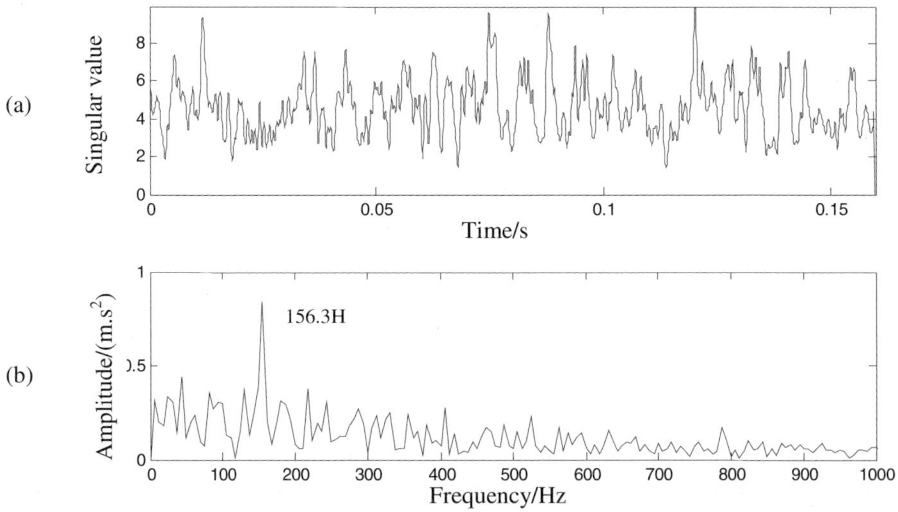

Fig. 5. The spingdle box (a) variation curve of one-order singular value (b) Spectrum

Fig. 4(a) is vibration signals of the spindle box in Y direction. Due to the noise in milling processing, vibration signals are in disorder as useful signals are drowned. By mapping signals in time domain into time-frequency domain with S transform, time-frequency distribution can be obtained as Fig. 4(b) shows. Many evident spectral peaks with certain period can be observed. Contour map in Fig. 4(c) denotes that frequency components of this vibration signal are mainly distributed in the high-frequency range from 4000Hz to 5000Hz.

By using singular value decomposition method to condense the data of matrix S in the spindle box and letting $K = 5$, variation curve of one-order singular value can be obtained. Spectrum analysis is made as illustrated in Fig. 5. An obvious spectral peak exists at the point of 156.3Hz in the spectrogram.

As this frequency is close to damage feature frequency (158.7Hz) of outer ring of the spindle's front bearing, we can decide that the outer ring of the spindle bearing has been damaged. The parameter of this bearing is shown in Table 1.

Table 1. Parameters of spindle's front bearing 32211

Type	Inner diameter	Outer diameter	Roller diameter	Number of roller	Contacting angle
32211	55mm	100mm	12mm	19	22.5°

Spindle bearing is an important part in the spindle assembly. Abrasion of the spindle bearing is an important source of forced excitation which would change the dynamic performance of the spindle assembly and increase the relative vibration between the cutting tool and work piece, consequently influencing machining quality of the work piece. Identification of spindle bearing faults can provide an important basis for tracing the machining errors in digital manufacturing.

6 Conclusion

Digital manufacturing is the kernel of advanced manufacturing technologies as well as the platform for the other advanced manufacturing technologies. It is necessary to have on-line maintenance and support for digital equipments to ensure their secure, reliable and efficient operation and smooth digital manufacturing process. In addition, it can test whether the digital equipments' output accords with their normal functions to ensure the quality of the product. It is of great significance for digital manufacturing.

Quantitative description and analysis are indispensable for digital manufacturing. The key is to improve the digital manufacturing technologies from combination of quantitative analysis and experience to comprehensive digitization which consequently optimizes the parameter and configuration. Spindle bearing is a key component of CNC equipments and its service performance is closely related to machining precision of the CNC equipments. By using the singular value decomposition method in combination with S transform of time-frequency analysis, the present study efficiently realizes quantitative fault diagnosis of spindle bearing of the CNC equipments and provides a theoretical basis and practical way for monitoring and diagnosis of service performance of spindle assembly in the CNC equipments.

Acknowledgments. This work is supported by National Basic Research Program of China (No. 2005CB724106) and National High Technology Research and Development Program (No. 2007AA04Z410).

References

1. Nakkiew, W., Lin, C.W., Tu, J.F.: A new method to quantify radial error of a motorized end-milling cutter/spindle system at very high speed rotations. International Journal of Machine Tools & Manufacture 46, 877–889 (2006)
2. Peng, Z.K., Chu, F.L.: Application of wavelet transform in machine condition monitoring and fault diagnostics: a review with bibliography. Mechanical Systems and Signal Processing 18, 199–221 (2004)
3. Cao, Y.Z., Altinatas, Y.: Modeling of spindle-bearing and machine tool systems for virtual simulation of milling operations. International Journal of Machine Tools & Maufacture 47, 1342–1350 (2007)
4. Gagnola, V., Bouzgarroua, B.C., Raya, P.: Model-based chatter stability prediction for high-speed spindles. International Journal of Machine Tools & Maufacture 47, 1176–1186 (2007)
5. Stockwell, R.G., Mansinhal, L.R., Lowe, P.: Localization of the complex spectrum: the S transfor. IEEE Transactions On Signal Processing 17, 998–1001 (1996)

6. Stockwell, R.G.: A basis for efficient representation of the S-transform. Digital Signal Processing 17, 371–393 (2007)
7. Rehorn, A.G., Sejdic, E., Jiang, J.: Fault diagnosis in machine tools using selective regional correlation. Mechanical Systems and Signal Processing 20, 1221–1223 (2006)
8. Chilukuri, M.V., Dash, P.K.: Multiresolution S-Transform-Based Fuzzy Recognition System for Power Quality Events. IEEE Transactions on power delivery 19, 323–330 (2004)
9. Schimmel, M., Gallart, J.: The inverse S-transform in filters with time-frequency localization. IEEE Transactions On Signal Processing 53, 4417–4422 (2005)

Research on Measurement Entropy-Based of Equipment Management Complexity and Its Application in Production Planning

Jiansheng Liu[1], Haining Tu[1], Hua Zhang[1], Fangchen Xia[1], and Daoyuan Yu[2]

[1] School of Mechanical and Electronic Engineering, Nanchang University, Nanchang, 330031
[2] School of Mechanical Science and Engineering , Huazhong University of Science and Technology, Wuhan 430074

Abstract. With the management development, the complexity has been a basic character of equipment management. It directly affects the impact of the equipment management whether or not the complexity of equipment management can be analyzed and controlled. From the view of information theory point, an information-theoretic approach is applied to study the complexity measurement of equipment management, and an entropy-based measurement model is constructed. Additionally, as an application, the proposed theoretical model is used to investigate the effectiveness of production planning, where the concepts of mean degeneration velocity and the similarity are introduced to quantitatively evaluate the effectiveness of production planning. Examples show that the proposed method is feasible for the feasible analysis and performance evaluation of product planning.

Keywords: Equipment management-complexity measurement-information entropy-product planning.

1 Instruction

Information is contact with manufacturing system closely, and the complexity of information reflects the complexity of manufacturing system at certain extent. In recent years, research & application on manufacturing execution system have been a pop project which is pay attention to by scientists [1][2]. To deal with the complexity of manufacturing execution system, in general one way is to reduce, avoid or eliminate the complexity of manufacturing execution system [3], another is qualitative analysis, which is researched by some scientists, looking forward to predict and control it [4][5].

Equipment management is one of important component of shop floor management. The complexity of manufacturing process leads to directly the complexity of equipment management, and the complex information affects the equipment management and its optimization to a certain extent. Lack of disposal strategy will result in the cases as follows: the equipment may fail to finish the manufacturing assignment, guarantee the product quality, and control production costs. In addition, it can also affect the whole production stability of shop floor. At present, most scientists focus on

C. Xiong et al. (Eds.): ICIRA 2008, Part II, LNAI 5315, pp. 604–611, 2008.

the model and decision analysis on the equipment management based on ideal information environment [6] [7]. As the ideal condition is inexistent under the complex statement of equipment, the model built based on ideal condition becomes meaningless though the model may be optimized perfectly. Thus, it is very necessary to research and analyze the complexity on equipment management. By measurement, it can firstly actively analyze equipment management complexity, evaluate the model validity, improve and optimize equipment management capability. On the other hand, it can provide method for feasible evaluation of business related with equipment management.

2 Analysis of Complexity

Equipment managers always expect to get the equipment information in time and accurately to guarantee the correctness and validity of decision. Essentially, in view of information theory, the equipment manufacturing process can be looked as the process of information generation, information collection, information transfer, information storage and so on. As an actual manufacturing cell, the equipment is not only the actual executive object of manufacturing task, but also the information feedback unit. It is obvious that the equipment information complexity has become one of the basic equipment attributes. The generating reasons of equipment information complexity is multidimensional, and it concludes all the followings: (1) Because information dynamically change with time, its principle of motion is difficult to be mastered and controlled. (2) Artificial factors: as human intervention is inevitable in the equipment manufacturing process, management decision reference information, actual direction of information flow, and the information interrelation, are uncertain. Furthermore, the managers have different technical levels, and hold the different conception and method on equipment management subjectively. (3) The whole production process is accompanied with production complexity, and production process is unstable, such as working procedure delay, limiting in production capability, too many orders to be finished, quality problems and output instability can directly lead to equipment management complexity. (4) Accessory and parts instability, as work program inconsequence, accessory reaching randomly, delivery period changing and order demands changing. (5) The equipment itself is instable: just like equipment fault, aging, improper operation and contingency, and so on. (6) Material defer and quality faults.

Information all above constitutes complex information circumstance, and it also directly leads to equipment management complexity. Thus, it is obvious that equipment management complexity means amount of uncertain information states for equipment management.

3 Complexity Measurement

3.1 Complexity Description Based on Information Entropy

Let x represents equipment state and x_i represents the ith possible state, numeric assemblage(x_1, x_2, x_3 ,…,x_n) is formed, and $p(x_i)$ denotes occurrence probability corresponding to state x_i, and the probability distributing assemblage is $(p(x_1), p(x_2), p(x_3), \ldots, p(x_n))$ then equipment information entropy can be defined as:

$$E(x) = -\sum_{i=1}^{n} P(x_i) \ln P(x_i) \tag{1}$$

with $P(x_i)>0$, $\sum P(x_i)=1$, $(\iota=1,2,\ldots,n)$.

It can be concluded from the definition above that information entropy is equipment state probability function, and it can be used to depict equipment uncertainty extent. The equipment uncertainty extent will be higher as the E（x）is bigger. Information entropy has many important properties: (1) Extremum: the information entropy reaches maximum, when equipment states occurring probability tends to homogenization, while equipment state is most uncertain at the same time; (2)Certainty : When n=1,equipment run in only one state x_1, here minimal information entropy is zero, while equipment state is certain. The value of information entropy reflects equipment management flexibility, bigger entropy value means bigger equipment management flexibility and smaller rigidity. On the contrary, smaller entropy denotes to smaller equipment flexibility and bigger rigidity. Therefore, it is not wise for us to take the view that the smaller information entropy is better.

3.2 Complexity Measurement

The equipment management complexity includes anticipative controllable complexity and dynamic uncontrollable complexity. The former is to depict amount of information of the equipment anticipative controllable state. While the latter is to describe the amount of information the runaway state needs during the equipment process. Under general circumstance, equipment anticipative controllable state mostly relates to equipment management pattern and actual operation directly. Accordingly, equipment anticipative controllable complexity can be also denominated as pattern complexity. Thereby the measurement of equipment anticipative controllable complexity can be transferred to that of information states included by equipment static management and operation items. As a state away from the management object, the equipment uncontrolled state mostly happen in dynamic equipment operation process, such as “equipment faults”, “materials lack”, “operation delay”, and so on, they can be obtained by actual observation in equipment operation process.

The key to calculate equipment complexity is state confirmation and its dividable granularity. In this paper, the state is defined as idiographic discrete event. The state confirmation is based on its generation mechanism, for the discrete manufacturing enterprise, equipment anticipative controllable state is induced by product diversity, processing variation and multivariate management pattern, then it can probably posses states as “product manufacturing”, “equipment startup”, “states detection”, “preventive maintenance”, “lubricant maintenance” and “planning maintenance” and so on.

State granularity division is based on management requirements and calculation convenience as well as practicability. For example, to achieve equipment fine-management, the “product manufacturing” state can be divided into “product A manufacturing”, “product B manufacturing”, “C product manufacturing”, and so on.

The "preventive maintenance" state can be divided into "first-level maintenance" and "second-level maintenance" states based on its complexity. While "states detection" can be divided into "infrared thermograph detection", "precision detection" and "tremble detection" and so on.

3.3 Complexity Measurement Model

Equipment complexity defines the extent of equipment complexity; it is a measurement for equipment complexity. According to the complexity measurement strategy, suppose that the number of anticipative equipment controllable state is $n_{c,}$ and the states are independent. Thus, according to the equation (1), the equipment controllable complexity degree can be given in:

$$E_c = -\sum_{i=1}^{n_c} P_i \ln P_i \tag{2}$$

If the number of uncontrolled equipment states in manufacturing process is n_d, and states are independent, based on equation (1), the equipment uncontrollable complexity degree can be written as:

$$E_d = -\sum_{j=1}^{n_d} P_j \ln P_j \tag{3}$$

Then, due to formula (2) and formula (3), the equipment total complexity can be given by:

$$E = E_c + E_d$$

or

$$E = -\sum_{i=1}^{n_c} P_i \ln P_i - \sum_{j=1}^{n_d} P_j \ln P_j \tag{4}$$

Where p_i is probability of equipment controllable state, and p_j is probability of equipment uncontrolled state, and

$$1 \le i \le n_c, 1 \le j \le n_d;$$

$$\sum P_i + \sum P_j = 1$$

4 Application in Product Management

For a long time, most relative reports put more focus on optimal model and arithmetic. To optimize production planning is emphasized, while the executive validity of production planning is ignored. In fact, the execution of production planning ties up to equipment closely, dynamic changing of equipment states brings obvious time-limit character to production plan. Just like, the production planning in some period time may depart from the planned management goal slowly with time under the effect of equipment state changing, what's more, suppose the production planning period is long, it may probably depart from the planned goal absolutely some time, and the direct result will be an absolute forfeiture of executive capability. Thereby, however optimal the production planning is made, it will do nothing to the executive effect. On this foundation, measurement technology on equipment management complexity is used in production management in this paper, and offered a valid tool and method for the feasible analysis and performance evaluation of product planning.

4.1 Feasible Analysis of Production Planning

The foundation of feasible analysis of production planning is based on the developing trend of equipment management uncontrolled state and its uncontrolled extent. Supposing no uncontrolled state exists, the production planning is feasible, and the whole operation can be executed according to it. While what will do if uncontrolled state exists? What are the corresponding developing trend and its extent? Could the production planning be executed any more? In another word, which degree the plan has departed from the production goal absolutely and when needs to be adjusted again? These are the problems to be solved necessarily. So it can conclude that the evaluation for producing plan feasibility can transfer to measurement for average velocity of equipment uncontrolled state.

In view of time, equipment dynamic uncontrolled complexity generates from the transformation from equipment controllable information to uncontrolled one (in another word, degenerate from normal state to abnormal state), that is, to transfer from anticipative controllable complexity to dynamic uncontrolled complexity. So, the executive capability of production planning can be evaluated, if only the transformation velocity between anticipative controllable complexity and dynamic uncontrolled complexity. It's easy to know that average equipment complexity uncontrolled rate corresponds to average dynamic generation rate of uncontrolled complexity, analyzed from equipment runaway process. The random uncontrolled complexity of equipment can be computed with formula （3） . Supposing dynamic runaway state inspecting period is Δt , then in a stated period T, equipment uncontrollable complexity is :

$$E'_d = -\frac{T}{\Delta t}\sum_{j=1}^{n_d} \mathrm{P}_j \ln \mathrm{P}_j \tag{5}$$

The complexity average uncontrollable velocity caused by equipment abnormity is:

$$V_d = \frac{E'_d}{T} = -\frac{1}{\Delta t}\sum_{j=1}^{n_d} \mathrm{P}_j \ln \mathrm{P}_j \tag{6}$$

Analyzing the result of formula （6） , if V_d is bigger, it shows that equipment average uncontrollable velocity is bigger, and the performance of production planning is inferior. The equipment state may probably change in short time, the result is that production planning departs from the planned object. On the contrary, if V_d is smaller, it means that equipment state will not do much effect on the production plan though it has some slight fluctuation during the executing period.

4.2 Evaluation for Producing Executive Effect

Executive effect of production planning is another index of evaluation for production planning. Generally speaking, it is to judge the similar degree of actual executive result and anticipative result after the production planning is executed in some period. According to equipment management complexity, evaluation for production planning executive effect can be defined in this way: It's a similar degree between the remaining controllable complexity and the anticipative controllable complexity, of which, after a period of time, equipment anticipative controllable complexity partly transferred to dynamic uncontrolled complexity. It depicts the similar degree of actual object and planned object, and it also reflects the executive effect of production planning.

Supposing in some time (T), detecting interval is Δt , then equipment controllable complexity is:

$$E'_c = -\frac{T}{\Delta t}\sum_{i=1}^{n_c} \mathrm{P}_i \ln \mathrm{P}_i \tag{7}$$

Form formula (5) and formula (7) , the complexity similar degree can be calculated by the following formula (8) :

$$P = \frac{E'_c - E'_d}{E'_c} = \frac{\frac{T}{\Delta t}\sum_{i=1}^{n_c} \mathrm{P}_i \ln \mathrm{P}_i - \frac{T}{\Delta t}\sum_{j=1}^{n_d} \mathrm{P}_j \ln \mathrm{P}_j}{\frac{T}{\Delta t}\sum_{i=1}^{n_c} \mathrm{P}_i \ln \mathrm{P}_i} \tag{8}$$

5 Examples and Analysis

Taking an engine plant as the example, this plant divides a whole duty day into morning shift, middle shift and night shift. Take one week (including five duty days) as a statistical period , analyze equipment discrete event, of which relates to this plant includes the following ones: mechanic manufacturing, lubricant maintenance and 5S, equipment startup (warm-up) , preventive maintenance, planning maintenance, materials waiting, plug up line and equipment faults. According to the definition of equipment states, take the equipment discrete events as equipment states and calculate every state generation rate bases on equipment management data of one week, and time interval is $\Delta t = 1$ hour. According to the statistical data and complexity formula, the statistical probability calculative results are shown in Table 1 and Table 2:

Table 1. Equipment uncontrollable complexity

State	Time(m)	Probability	Complexity
Material waiting	170	0.023611	0.08845
pop up line	68	0.009444	0.04403
Short-time stop	25	0.003472	0.01966
time-delay for tools changing	80	0.011111	0.05000
time-delay for plan adjusting	110	0.015278	0.06388
equipment faults	280	0.038889	0.12627

Table 2. Equipment controllable complexity

State	Time(m)	Probability	Complexity
crank processing	1444	0.200556	0.32223
link rod processing	1400	0.194444	0.31842
cylinder-cover processing	1347	0.187083	0.31359
lubricant maintenance and 5S	60	0.008333	0.03990
equipment startup	50	0.006944	0.03451
preventive maintenance	150	0.020833	0.08065
equipment idle state	660	0.091667	0.21905

According to data in table 1 and table 2, with formula (6) and formula (8), P can be counted as P=0.761196, it means that approximately 23.28% information depart from equipment management object everyday under the circumstance disturbance, and V_d=0.39229, of which it executes according to plan 2.5 days a week, thereby, it can execute according to plan in the former three days, while renewing the producing plan is needed by the fourth day. So, taking further analysis of the causes, primary factors are equipment faults, material waiting and plan adjusting time being too long, these factors take great proportion in whole uncontrolled complexity, the respective data are 32.19%, 22.55% and 16.28%. Then corresponding strategy can be made as strengthening equipment maintenance, depressing fault rate, improving equipment utilization ratio, improving the capability of material inventory control and transportation, decreasing material waiting time and strengthening stuff skills training, improving working efficiency, cutting time of equipment adjusting, and so on.

6 Conclusion

With the globalization of market competition, product requirement is whole determined by customers, and personal requirement of the product is more individual. Represented by uncertainty, the complexity is notable in the modern production process. Comparing with the past, the equipment management is more complex. In this paper, the equipment complexity is divided into the controllable complexity and uncontrollable one, and the measurement model of equipment complexity is also constructed using the information entropy. Additionally, two evaluation indexes are presented by applying the proposed approach into the production management of shop floor, which are the mean degeneration velocity and the similarity of production planning. The proper period of the production planning can be calculated by analyzing the complexity average invalidation rate, which the departure from management object can be effectively controlled. Most importantly, by evaluating the similarity, the equipment states and reasons that lead to the declination of the management object are analyzed, and the way will be found to solve the problems. The proposed model can offer an important method for the feasible analysis and performance evaluation of product planning.

Acknowledgements

This research is supported by the Project of China 863 plan, China (Grant No. 2007AA040701). This support is greatly acknowledged.

References

1. Rodriguez-Toro, C.A., Tate, S.J., Jared, G.E.M., Swift., K.G.: Complexity metrics for design (simplicity+simplicity=complexity). Proceedings of the Institution of Mechanical Engineers, Part B, Engineering MANUFACTURE 217(5), 721–725 (2003)
2. Frizelle, G., Richards, H.: Tacking industrial complexity: the ideas that make a difference. In: Proceedings of the 2nd International Conference of Manufacturing complexity Network, Cambridge, UK (2002)
3. Efstathiou, J.: The utility of complexity. Manufacturing Engineer 81(2), 73–76 (2002)
4. Mawby, D., Stupples, D.W.: Deliver complex projects successfully by managing uncertainty. In: Proceedings of the Conference on Complexity and Complex Systems in Industry, Warwick, UK, pp. 155–166 (2000)
5. Yunqing, R., Janet, E.: Entropy-Based Measurement of Manufacturing System Complexity and its Application in Scheduling. Chinese Journal of Mechanical Engineering 42(7), 8–13 (2006)
6. Guo, L., Lianmin, G., Fumin, C.: Research on Equipment Maintenance Optimization Based on Reliability. Chinese Mechanical Engineering 18(4), 419–423 (2007)
7. Moon, J.-F., Yoon, Y.T., Lee, S.-S.: Reliability-centered maintenance model to managing power distribution system equipment. In: 2006 IEEE Power Engineering Society General Meeting (2006)

Error Compensation of Indoor GPS Measurement

Zhongzheng Liu, Zhigang Liu, and Bingheng Lu

Xi'an Jiaotong University
State Key Laboratory for Manufacturing Systems Engineering (710049)

Abstract. Indoor GPS measurement system is a dramatic new type of coordinate measuring system emerging in recent years and has great application prospects. In this paper the mathematic model of Indoor GPS system is derived. Based on the model, an analysis of the errors for the measuring system is presented, and then a simple method to compensate the measurement system errors is proposed with the relevant algorithm designed. Through computer simulation, the compensation model is verified. Simulation results demonstrate the evaluation of compensation method.

Keywords: Indoor GPS Error compensation Coordinate measuring system.

1 Introduction

In recent years, large-scale three-dimensional measurement systems have played increasingly important role in the field of geometric measurement. Indoor GPS measurement system, proposed by Metris, is a dramatic new type of coordinate measuring system. Synthesizing frontage intersection principles of theodolites and the principles of GPS, this system utilizes laser transmitters outputting infrared light instead of satellites. If one receiver could obtain two or more transmitters signals, measured values (azimuth and elevation) can be calculated. Then based on frontage intersection principles the coordinates of the receiver can be obtained. Thus, receiving the infrared light emitted by transmitters, users are able to calculate their position independently. By establishing a factory wide coordinate system, all measurement tasks such as inspection, tracking, and monitoring can be coordinated in ways only imagined up to now. Non-contact measurement, large measurement range, high precision and low environment requirement make this system have a vast application prospect. For example, Metris's Indoor GPS system, called Constellation^{3Di}, has been used in many applications such as aircraft assembly, automatic production line and robot navigation. Boeing has also utilized this system for the assembly of Boeing 777 and drilling robot navigation.

Because of the novel concept of Indoor GPS system, there is few research on it. Like all the large-scale coordinate measuring systems, the measuring accuracy of this system is an important issue need to be considered. Therefore, the purpose of this paper is to analyze and compensate the errors of this measurement system on the basis of the ideal model of Indoor GPS measurement system.

C. Xiong et al. (Eds.): ICIRA 2008, Part II, LNAI 5315, pp. 612–619, 2008.

2 Ideal Model of Indoor GPS Measurement System

Indoor GPS system is composed of laser transmitters, receivers, probes, software, and receiver circuits. Laser transmitters are high-speed revolving platforms with two laser planes as shown in Fig.1.

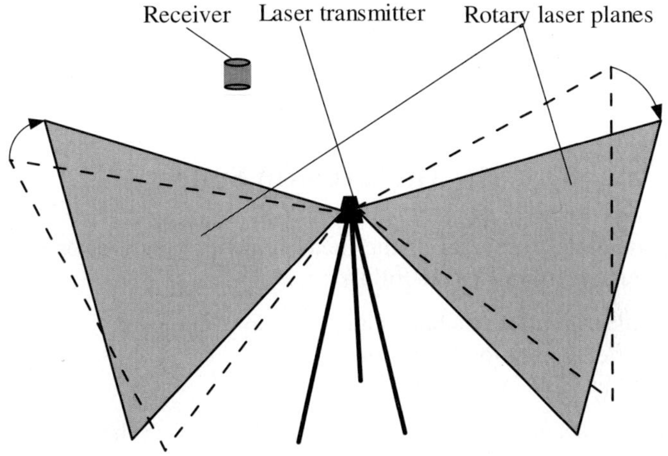

Fig. 1. Laser transmitter

Suppose there is a laser plane L_1 with initial normal vector $\boldsymbol{N} = (A, B, 1)$ and spin center $\boldsymbol{T}(T_x, T_y, T_z)$, whose spin axis is parallel to z axis of the coordinate system. When the laser plane rotates θ degrees around its spin axis, it also rotates θ degrees around z axis. At this point, the normal vector of L_1 can be calculated by equation (1).

$$\mathbf{N}_\theta = \mathbf{R}_\theta \mathbf{N} \quad . \tag{1}$$

where $\mathbf{R}_\theta$ is the rotation matrix, $\mathbf{R}_\theta = \begin{bmatrix} \cos\theta & -\sin\theta & 0 \\ \sin\theta & \cos\theta & 0 \\ 0 & 0 & 1 \end{bmatrix}$.

Suppose one measured point is $\boldsymbol{P}(x, y, z)$. Let the rotation angle of plane L_1 be θ_1 degrees as it passes through point P. Because point P and T are both in plane L_1, $\overline{PT}$ and $\mathbf{N}_{\theta 1}$ have the following relationship.

$$\mathbf{N}_{\theta 1} \bullet \overline{PT} = 0 \quad . \tag{2}$$

where $\overline{PT} = \left(x - T_x, y - T_y, z - T_z\right)^T$.

If P is passed through by the laser planes of n transmitters distributed in space, 2n equations can be derived. That is, measured point P satisfies:

$$(\mathbf{R}_i \mathbf{N}_i) \bullet (\mathbf{P} - \mathbf{T}_i) = 0 \quad . \tag{3}$$

where

i is laser plane index, $i=1,2\cdots 2n$;
P is the coordinates of measured point, $\mathbf{P} = (x, y, z)^T$;
$\mathbf{T}_i$ is the spin center of the ith laser plane, $\mathbf{T}_i = (T_{xi}, T_{yi}, T_{zi})^T$;
$\mathbf{N}_i$ is the initial normal vector of the ith laser plane, $\mathbf{N}_i = (A_i, B_i, 1)^T$;
$\mathbf{R}_i$ is the rotation matrix where the ith laser plane passes through point P.

Solving equations (3) with least square method, the position of P can be obtained. Theoretically, two laser transmitters, meaning four laser planes, are sufficient to determine the spatial position of unknown points. So, in the latter simulation only two transmitters are used.

3 Errors Analysis of the Measurement System

Based on the mathematic model of the measurement system, error sources are analyzed. Measurement errors exist as follows:

1. $\mathbf{R}_i$, angle measurement has biases and random component;
2. $\mathbf{N}_i$, transmitter calibration has biases;
3. $\mathbf{T}_i$, transmitter setup has biases.

The positioning accuracy of measured points depends on these three terms above. To minimize the measurement error, the errors of these terms must be eliminated or minimized. Because of the restriction of present condition and costs, the improvement of these three aspects above is limited. In this case, error compensation technique could be utilized to improve measurement accuracy.

4 Error Compensation Model

From the measurement model, it is observed that measurement is performed through these five parameters $\boldsymbol{N}(A, B, 1)$, $\boldsymbol{T}(T_x, T_y, T_z)$ and measured angle θ. The angle could be measured with high accuracy. And the five system parameters could be determined by calibration. In actual measurement, the unknown calibration error is often influenced by such factors as angle measurement error, calibration target error and solution error, and is synthetical reflection of these errors. Because of this, there is always somewhat systematic error leading to biases of measurement results. Therefore, it is essential to study on the method to compensate the calibration error and correct measurement results effectively.

Represent equation (3) as follows.

$$\left(\begin{bmatrix} \cos\theta_i & -\sin\theta_i & 0 \\ \sin\theta_i & \cos\theta_i & 0 \\ 0 & 0 & 1 \end{bmatrix}\begin{bmatrix} A_i \\ B_i \\ 1 \end{bmatrix}\right) \bullet \left(\begin{bmatrix} x \\ y \\ z \end{bmatrix} - \begin{bmatrix} T_{xj} \\ T_{yj} \\ T_{zj} \end{bmatrix}\right) = 0 \ . \tag{4}$$

The ith laser plane has five calibration parameters, that is, the normal vector A_i, B_i and the spin center T_{xi}, T_{yi}, T_{zi}. Let the calibration values be $\tilde{A}_i$, $\tilde{B}_i$, $\tilde{T}_{xi}$, $\tilde{T}_{yi}$, $\tilde{T}_{zi}$ and relevant calibration errors be $\triangle A_i$, $\triangle B_i$, $\triangle T_{xi}$, $\triangle T_{yi}$, $\triangle T_{zi}$. Therefore, equation (5) can be easily obtained.

$$\begin{aligned} \mathbf{N}_i &= \tilde{\mathbf{N}}_i + \Delta\mathbf{N}_i \\ \mathbf{T}_i &= \tilde{\mathbf{T}}_i + \Delta\mathbf{T}_i \end{aligned} \quad . \tag{5}$$

where $\tilde{\mathbf{N}}_i$ and $\tilde{\mathbf{T}}_i$ are calibration values; $\triangle \mathrm{N}_i$ and $\triangle \mathrm{T}_i$ are calibration errors.

Therefore, equation (3) can be represented as follows.

$$\left(\mathbf{R}_i\left(\tilde{\mathbf{N}}_i + \Delta\mathbf{N}_i\right)\right) \bullet \left(\mathbf{P} - \left(\tilde{\mathbf{T}}_i + \Delta\mathbf{T}_i\right)\right) = 0 \ . \tag{6}$$

The above equation can be expanded as shown in equation (7).

$$\begin{aligned} &\left(\mathbf{R}_i\tilde{\mathbf{N}}_i\right) \bullet \mathbf{P} - \left(\mathbf{R}_i\tilde{\mathbf{N}}_i\right) \bullet \tilde{\mathbf{T}}_i = \\ &\left(\mathbf{R}_i\tilde{\mathbf{N}}_i\right) \bullet \Delta\mathbf{T}_i - \left(\mathbf{R}_i\Delta\mathbf{N}_i\right) \bullet \mathbf{P} + \left(\mathbf{R}_i\Delta\mathbf{N}_i\right) \bullet \tilde{\mathbf{T}}_i + \left(\mathbf{R}_i\Delta\mathbf{N}_i\right) \bullet \Delta\mathbf{T}_i \end{aligned} \ . \tag{7}$$

To obtain the true coordinates of unknown points, it is necessary to eliminate or minimize the error terms on the right side of equation (7). In the following sections the method to compensate these terms will be discussed.

Suppose there is a known point C with coordinates $\boldsymbol{P}_c(x_c, y_c, z_c)$, and laser plane i rotates θ_c degrees as it passes through point C. Substitute the parameters of point C into equation (7).

$$\begin{aligned} &\left(\mathbf{R}_c\tilde{\mathbf{N}}_i\right) \bullet \mathbf{P}_c - \left(\mathbf{R}_c\tilde{\mathbf{N}}_i\right) \bullet \tilde{\mathbf{T}}_i = \\ &\left(\mathbf{R}_c\tilde{\mathbf{N}}_i\right) \bullet \Delta\mathbf{T}_i - \left(\mathbf{R}_c\Delta\mathbf{N}_i\right) \bullet \mathbf{P}_c + \left(\mathbf{R}_c\Delta\mathbf{N}_i\right) \bullet \tilde{\mathbf{T}}_i + \left(\mathbf{R}_c\Delta\mathbf{N}_i\right) \bullet \Delta\mathbf{T}_i \end{aligned} \ . \tag{8}$$

Comparing equation (8) with equation (7), it may be practicable to utilize right side of equation (8) to compensate that of equation (7).

From equation (7) and (8), it is observed that, for one laser plane, both equations have the same calibration parameters and calibration errors with the exception of point position and rotation angles. Error terms $(\mathbf{R}_i\tilde{\mathbf{N}}_i) \bullet \Delta\mathbf{T}_i$, $(\mathbf{R}_i\Delta\mathbf{N}_i) \bullet \tilde{\mathbf{T}}_i$, $(\mathbf{R}_i\Delta\mathbf{N}_i) \bullet \Delta\mathbf{T}_i$ can be eliminated with $\mathbf{R}_i$. For these three terms, only the compensation of $\mathbf{R}_i$ need to be considered.

$$\mathbf{R}_i = \begin{bmatrix} \cos\theta_i & -\sin\theta_i & 0 \\ \sin\theta_i & \cos\theta_i & 0 \\ 0 & 0 & 1 \end{bmatrix} . \tag{9}$$

From equation (9), it is shown that to compensate $\mathbf{R}_i$, $\cos\theta_i$ and $\sin\theta_i$ need to be compensated.

Expand the term $(\mathbf{R}_i \Delta \mathbf{N}_i)\cdot\mathbf{P}$ of equation (7) as shown in formula (10).

$$(\cos\theta_i x+\sin\theta_i y)\Delta A_i+(\cos\theta_i y-\sin\theta_i x)\Delta B_i+1 \ . \tag{10}$$

To eliminated the terms ΔA_i、ΔB_i, it is essential to eliminate the coefficients $(\cos\theta_i x+\sin\theta_i y)$、$(\cos\theta_i y-\sin\theta_i x)$ and 1. Therefore , the final compensated error terms are *cosθ*$\cos\theta_i$, $\sin\theta_i$, $(\cos\theta_i x+\sin\theta_i y)$, $(\cos\theta_i y-\sin\theta_i x)$ and 1. Thus, a number of known points are needed as base points for compensating the five terms. The compensation coefficients can be calculated with the method of undetermined coefficients. Considering the number of the compensated terms, there should be 5 base points.

Let base points be $C_1(x_1,y_1,z_1,\theta_1)$, $C_2(x_2,y_2,z_2,\theta_2)$, $C_3(x_3,y_3,z_3,\theta_3)$, $C_4(x_4,y_4,z_4,\theta_4)$, $C_5(x_5,y_5,z_5,\theta_5)$. The compensation coefficients equation is derived as shown in equation (11).

$$\begin{cases} \sum_{k=1}^{5} c_k \cos\theta_k = \cos\theta_i \\ \sum_{k=1}^{5} c_k \sin\theta_k = \sin\theta_i \\ \sum_{k=1}^{5} c_k (\cos\theta_k x_k+\sin\theta_k y_k) = \cos\theta_i x+\sin\theta_i y \\ \sum_{k=1}^{5} c_k (\cos\theta_k y_k-\sin\theta_k x_k) = \cos\theta_i y+\sin\theta_i x \\ \sum_{k=1}^{5} c_k = 1 \end{cases} . \tag{11}$$

where $c_k (k=1,2,3,4,5)$ are undetermined compensation coefficients.

After the compensation coefficients are determined, the following equation can be derived.

$$\begin{cases} \sum_{k=1}^{5} c_k (\mathbf{R}_{ck}\tilde{\mathbf{N}}_i)\bullet\Delta\mathbf{T}_i = (\mathbf{R}_i\tilde{\mathbf{N}}_i)\bullet\Delta\mathbf{T}_i \\ \sum_{k=1}^{5} c_k (\mathbf{R}_{ck}\Delta\tilde{\mathbf{N}}_i)\bullet\mathbf{P}_{ck} = (\mathbf{R}_i\Delta\tilde{\mathbf{N}}_i)\bullet\mathbf{P}_i \\ \sum_{k=1}^{5} c_k (\mathbf{R}_{ck}\Delta\mathbf{N}_i)\bullet\tilde{\mathbf{T}}_i = (\mathbf{R}_i\Delta\mathbf{N}_i)\bullet\tilde{\mathbf{T}}_i \\ \sum_{k=1}^{5} c_k (\mathbf{R}_{ck}\Delta\mathbf{N}_i)\bullet\Delta\mathbf{T}_i = (\mathbf{R}_i\Delta\mathbf{N}_i)\bullet\Delta\mathbf{T}_i \end{cases} . \tag{12}$$

From equation (8), equation (13) is obtained.

$$\begin{aligned}&\sum_{k=1}^{5} c_k\left(\left(\mathbf{R}_{ck}\tilde{\mathbf{N}}_i\right)\cdot\mathbf{P}_{ck}-\left(\mathbf{R}_{ck}\tilde{\mathbf{N}}_i\right)\cdot\tilde{\mathbf{T}}_i\right)=\\&\sum_{k=1}^{5} c_k\left(\left(\mathbf{R}_{ck}\tilde{\mathbf{N}}_i\right)\cdot\Delta\mathbf{T}_i-\left(\mathbf{R}_{ck}\Delta\mathbf{N}_i\right)\cdot\mathbf{P}_{ck}+\left(\mathbf{R}_{ck}\Delta\mathbf{N}_i\right)\cdot\tilde{\mathbf{T}}_i+\left(\mathbf{R}_{ck}\Delta\mathbf{N}_i\right)\cdot\Delta\mathbf{T}_i\right)\end{aligned} . \quad (13)$$

where $\mathbf{R}_{ck}$ is the rotation matrix of the ith laser plane as it passes through point C_k ;

$\mathbf{P}_{ck}=\left(x_k, y_k, z_k\right)^T$.

From equation (8), (12) and (13), the final compensation equation is derived as follows.

$$\begin{aligned}&\left(\mathbf{R}_i\tilde{\mathbf{N}}_i\right)\cdot\Delta\mathbf{T}_i-\left(\mathbf{R}_i\Delta\mathbf{N}_i\right)\cdot\mathbf{P}+\left(\mathbf{R}_i\Delta\mathbf{N}_i\right)\cdot\tilde{\mathbf{T}}_i+\left(\mathbf{R}_i\Delta\mathbf{N}_i\right)\cdot\Delta\mathbf{T}_i=\\&\sum_{k=1}^{5} c_k\left(\left(\mathbf{R}_{ck}\tilde{\mathbf{N}}_i\right)\cdot\mathbf{P}_{ck}-\left(\mathbf{R}_{ck}\tilde{\mathbf{N}}_i\right)\cdot\tilde{\mathbf{T}}_i\right)\end{aligned} . \quad (14)$$

Through equation (11) and (14), the error terms of one laser plane measurement equation could be eliminated, and then the coordinates of unknown points are calculated by solving the compensated equations. However, in actual measurement it is impossible to use the true coordinates of one measured point as x and y in equation (11). However, it is practicable to use the non-compensating measured values x_u and y_u to substitute for x and y. Because of errors, after compensation the calculated coordinates are more close to true values but probably still have biases.

After the first compensation, if the calculated coordinates still have non-negligible errors, the second compensation can be performed by substituting the first compensated coordinates into equation (11). Repeat this until satisfactory results are obtained. In general, after 3～5 iterations, there is no obvious effect on error compensation.

5 Simulations

To verity the error compensation method, the simulation experiments are performed using matlab. In the simulation, two laser transmitters with parameters known, that is, four laser planes, are utilized for verification of measured points. There are 15 verification points with known coordinates and the rotation angles of relevant laser plane are also known. The points are more than 10m far away from transmitters.

5.1 Simulation with No Angle Error

Suppose there is no angle measurement error. Some errors are introduced into the laser plane parameters. The results with/without compensation are shown in Fig. 2.

Without compensation, the mean error is 34.1248mm, compared with the mean error 0.2648mm with compensation. There is a great improvement on the result after

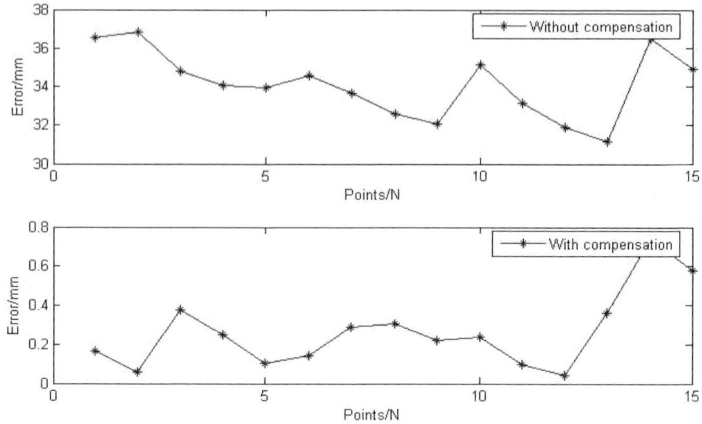

Fig. 2. Results with/without compensation without angle errors

compensation. The simulation results also show that it is easy to control the errors below 1mm with no angle error.

5.2 Simulation with Angle Errors

Now, it is not so difficult to measure angles with high accuracy. Constellation^{3Di} of Metris obtains horizontal angle measuring accuracy of less than 10″ and vertical angle measuring accuracy of less than 1″. Considering the actual angle measuring accuracy in our laboratory, the angle error range for the simulation is set at ±10″. Referring to Constellation^{3Di}, a series of random numbers is generated by matlab as random errors of angle measurement. The calibration errors are the same as that in the former simulation. The results are shown in Fig. 3

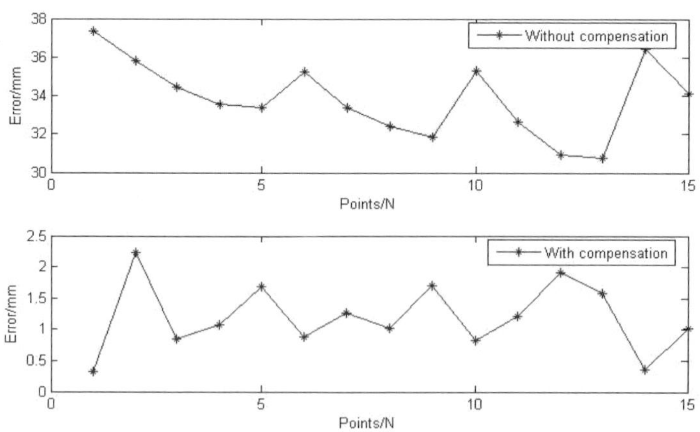

Fig. 3. Results with/without compensation with angle errors

Without compensation, the mean error is 33.8504mm, while the mean error with compensation is 1.1971mm. Compared with the non-compensating errors in Fig. 2, the errors in Fig. 3 change little, which shows that the effect of angle errors is limited for the results without compensation. In contrast, the compensated results in Fig. 3 change almost four times than that in Fig. 2. The reason is that the angle errors are random errors which can not be compensated with the previous method. As a result, the errors of final results will increase along with angle errors increase.

6 Conclusions

In this paper, a simple method based on the model of Indoor GPS measurement14 system to compensate system errors is proposed. Through computer simulation, the following conclusions can be drawn.

1. With this method, the compensation can be performed with accuracy approximately 1mm.

2. It is simple to use, as only five base points and a few iterations are involved to compensate the systematic errors effectively.

Acknowledgements

The work described in this paper was supported by a grant from the National Natural Science Foundation of China (Projects No.50575177 and 50305027).

References

1. Liu, W., Qu, X., Yan, Y.: Calibration and Error Compensation of Portable Coordinate Measuring Arm. J. Chinese Journal of Scientific Instrument 28, 81–84 (2007)
2. Wu, X., Zhang, G.: Indoor GPS Measuring System and Application in Aircraft Assembly. J. Aviation Precision Manufacturing Technology 42, 1–5 (2006)
3. Wang, H.: Principles and Applications of GPS Navigation. Science Press, Beijing (2003)
4. Arc Second, Inc: Constellation-3D Indoor GPS for Metrology. White paper 071502, 1–11 (2002)
5. Wu, X., Zhang, G.: Modern Large-Scale Space Measuring Techniques. J. Aviation Manufacturing Technology 10, 68–70 (2006)
6. Arc Second, Inc: Constellation-3D Error Budget and Specification. White paper 063102, 1–10 (2002)

A Method for Calibrating Camera Lens Distortion with Cross-Ratio Invariability in Welding Seam System

Guangtao Zhao and Hong Qiao*

Institute of Automation, Chinese Academy of Sciences, Beijing, China
zhaogt1979@163.com, hong.qiao@ia.ac.cn

Abstract. Wide-Angle lenses have broad applications in lots of fields for their larger fields of view. However, image deformation is its main backward. Thus, calibration of distortion parameters of wide-angle lens is an essential procedure for 3D information recovering from 2D images in applications. Based on our 3D welding seam extraction system, we propose a nonlinear calibration method by using calibration grid. This simple method only considers the distortion parameters so that the coupling between internal and external parameters of the camera is avoided. Moreover, it needs only feature point series which satisfy cross-ratio invariability, and need not know the exact position coordinates of the points. The nonlinear optimization is fast since the initial value of the distortion parameters can be obtained with cross-ratio invariability. Experiments show the efficiency and practicality of our method directly.

Keywords: camera calibration, radial distortion, decentering distortion, cross-ratio invariability, wide-angle lens.

1 Introduction

Wide-angle lens has a much larger field of view than common cameras, and is able to capture more information from the environment. Thus, it plays an important role in kinds of applications which desire more information with fewer cameras, such as supervisory systems, visions of mobile robots, visions in manufacturing systems, etc. In our 3D welding seam extraction system, a wide-angle lens is adopted to capture the welding seam information. However, the sever image distortion brought in by the wide-angle lens should be tackled in order to meet the reconstruction precision as high as 0.2mm. The real-time ability of the welding seam system puts forward another requirement. Therefore, a simple and efficient method for calibrating camera lens distortion should be proposed.

Camera calibration constructs the mapping between the camera plane and the 3D space, and indicates the accuracy of the 3D information a camera system can give. The mapping includes two different transformations which form the internal and external calibration parameters. Camera calibration is to recover these parameters in order to construct the relationship between the 2D computer image plane and the 3D space. Therefore, it is very meaningful to investigate the nonlinear distortion model.

* Corresponding author.

C. Xiong et al. (Eds.): ICIRA 2008, Part II, LNAI 5315, pp. 620–629, 2008.

1.1 Related Researches

In related calibration approaches of nonlinear model, the basic ones are those using a calibration grid with feature points whose 3D coordinates are known. Tsai [1] presented the simple radial alignment principle and created the two-stage technique which was aimed at efficient computation of camera external parameters and internal parameters. Compared with Tsai, Weng [2] considered both radial and decentering distortion parameters. Other methods depending on either 2D calibration objects [3 & 4] or 1D calibration objects [5] have the same key technology as the above methods. However, all these methods compute both the internal and external parameters together. This raises a problem that coupling between external parameters and internal parameters leads to high errors in the camera internal parameters [6].

Recently, R. Hartly and S. Kang [7] presented a non-iterative method which does not rely on any distortion model. This method can obtain radial distortion parameters of even term and odd term, the distributions of principal point and distortion center. G. P. Stein [8], S. Thirthala and M. Pollefeys [9] proposed calibration methods relying on the trilinear tensor of multiple images respectively. A method to calibrate the radial distortion only was proposed by G. J. Zhang [10]. Compared with traditional methods, these new calibration methods performed much better, but they neglected the decentering distortion of camera.

Another family of calibration methods is called self-calibration method which does not require exact position coordinates of calibration points. One of the most important methods, called self-calibration technique, is suitable for active vision systems. In this method, the vision system is positioned on a platform which can be accurately controlled, and the motion information of the platform is known. During calibration process, the platform is moved to different positions in order to get multiple images from which the calibration parameters can be obtained. In [11], Ma pointed out that (1) the external parameters can be computed by a sequence of three pure translational motions if the camera intrinsic parameters are known in advance; (2) two sequences of the three pure translational motions are necessary to recover the camera orientation parameters and intrinsic parameters. However, the method had two drawbacks: the parameters of the camera may be unstable if they are all unknown [12]; it is very difficult to get three pure translational motions orthogonally [11].

1.2 Overview of Our Method

Taking both the calibration methods presented by other researchers and the practical requirement of the welding seam system into account, we proposed a novel calibration technique for tackling the radial and decentering distortion. In the process of calibration, the known feature points, which were on a calibration grid and had some inner relationship with each other, were projected on the undistorted image. For each point, the undistorted coordinate is in accord with the distorted coordinate, the objective functions of the distorted coordinates can be established based on the relationship of the feature points. Then, the distortion parameters could be obtained by means of nonlinear optimization of the objective functions. It is noted that not only the radial parameters but also the decentering distortion parameters could be obtained by our method. Furthermore, an initial guess of the distortion parameters relying on the cross-ratio invariability was introduced to speed up the optimization.

1.3 Organization of This Paper

This paper is organized as follows. In section II we first introduce our welding seam extraction system. Section III describes the camera distortion model. In section IV a distortion measure that transforms the distorted image into undistorted image is derived. Following that, we design a method to minimize the distortion and present the calibration algorithm. Some experimental results are reported in Section V, followed by our concluding remarks in section VI.

2 The Welding Seam Extraction System

In this section, we first introduce our welding seam extraction system. As showed in Fig. 1, the welding seam extraction system consists of two CCD cameras and a workpiece with a welding seam waiting for constructed in 3D world space.

In this system, the stereo vision is utilized to reconstruct the welding seam in 3D world space. Thus, two CCD industrial cameras with wide-angle lens are used to capture the welding seam. The welding seam is on the smooth surface of a 3D workpiece. Its width is between 0.1mm to 3mm. Based on the pictures of the two cameras, we try to extract the seam and reconstruct with the precision of 0.1mm.

In order to achieve high precision, we must calibrate the camera precisely. Meanwhile, it is well known that the image captured from the wide-angle lens has severe distortion. Therefore, the image distortion must be dealt with also. Hence, by investigation, we proposed a method utilizing cross-ratio invariability for calibrating the camera lens distortion.

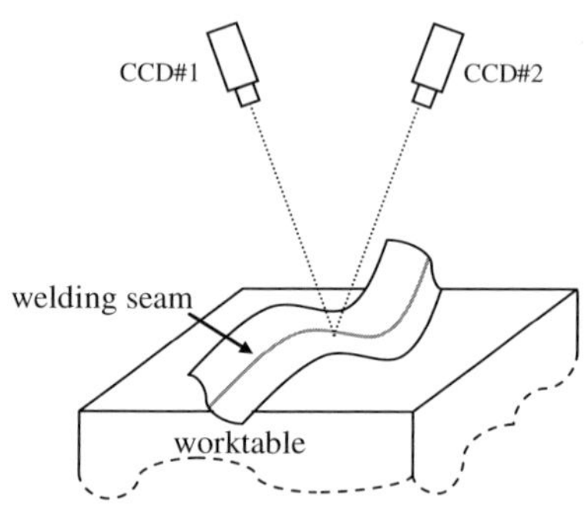

Fig. 1. Welding Seam Extraction System

3 Lens Distortion Model

The choice of the lens distortion model is the foundation of the camera calibration. For different applications, different camera model and different distortion parameters are choosen. The camera models can be classified into linear model and nonlinear model [13]. For linear model, the camera distortion is neglected. Consequently, the geometrical distortion of the lens can't be removed and it will bring in more errors, especially for wide angle lenses and low cost lenses.

In this paper, we principally consider two types of distortion: radial distortion and decentering distortion. The two forms are caused by improper lens and camera assembly and they bring in both radial and tangential errors in point positions. The standard nonlinear model is mapping from the distorted image coordinates (x_d, y_d) that are measurable, to the undistorted image coordinates (x_u, y_u), which can't be physically measured [14]. The relationship between (x_d, y_d) and (x_u, y_u) can be represented by

$$x_u = x_d + \overline{x}_d (K_1 r_d^2 + K_2 r_d^4 + K_2 r_d^6 + \ldots) + [P_1 (r_d^2 + 2\overline{x}_d^2) + 2P_2 \overline{x_d y_d}][1 + P_3 r_d^2] \qquad (1(a))$$

$$y_u = y_d + \overline{y}_d (K_1 r_d^2 + K_2 r_d^4 + K_2 r_d^6 + \ldots) + [P_2 (r_d^2 + 2\overline{x}_d^2) + 2P_1 \overline{x_d y_d}][1 + P_3 r_d^2] \qquad (1(b))$$

Where $\overline{x}_d = x_d - c_x$, $\overline{y}_d = y_d - c_y$, $r_d^2 = \overline{x}_d^2 + \overline{y}_d^2$ and K_1, K_2, K_3 are the radial distortion parameters and P_1, P_2, P_3 are the decentering distortion parameters. r_d is the radius of an image point from the distortion center (c_x, c_y).

Normally, it is enough to model one or two order distortion parameters because the higher order terms are comparatively small and may generate numerical instability [1]. On the other hand, wide angle lenses bring a significant distortion which is introduced on purpose. It is not sufficient to use radial distortion parameters only. Therefore, it is necessary to apply more terms in Equation (1), especially decentering distortion parameters [14]. According to the above discussions, we will calibrate the radial distortion parameters (K_1 and K_2) and the decentering distortion parameters (P_1 and P_2).

4 Proposed Approach

The proposed calibration method is based on the following hypothesis: the camera model is the perspective model, and the projection of the calibration grid on the image plane corresponds with the cross-ratio invariability. In this technique, the point series whose cross-ratio is known are projected on the distorted image; and the corresponding coordinates in the image can be obtained by image processing, followed by constructing nonlinear objective functions in order to find the best distortion parameters.

In the following segments, we describe both the proposed technique and the optimization process in detail.

4.1 Line Straightness Method

Supposing there is a line l on the calibration object plane. Through the transformation, a line l' can be obtained in the undistorted image plane. Given four random points α, β, μ, η on the line l, we can get the cross-ratio r about these four points like $f(\alpha,\beta,\mu,\eta)=\left(\frac{\alpha-\mu}{\beta-\mu}\right)\Big/\left(\frac{\alpha-\eta}{\beta-\eta}\right)=r$ .According to projective transformation, the points α,β,μ,η are related to the points $\alpha^u,\beta^u,\mu^u,\eta^u$ in the undistorted image plane. Based on the invariance of cross-ratio, we can conclude that $f(\alpha^u,\beta^u,\mu^u,\eta^u)=\left(\frac{\alpha^u-\mu^u}{\beta^u-\mu^u}\right)\Big/\left(\frac{\alpha^u-\eta^u}{\beta^u-\eta^u}\right)=r$.

Because of the camera lens distortion, the points in the distorted image are away from their ideal position. We can have the mapping between the points α,β,μ,η and the points $\alpha^d,\beta^d,\mu^d,\eta^d$ (here $\alpha^u=g(\alpha^d)$)

$$s=f(g(\alpha^d),g(\beta^d),g(\mu^d),g(\eta^d))-\left(\frac{\alpha-\mu}{\beta-\mu}\right)\Big/\left(\frac{\alpha-\eta}{\beta-\eta}\right)=0 \tag{2}$$

In Equation (2), the cross-ratio of the points along the line l can be physically measured and the coordinates of the points in the distorted image can be obtained by image processing. Therefore, it is possible to calibrate the camera lens distortion parameters by using Equation (2). On the other hand, in the distorted image we usually acquire the coordinates in two orientations which are x direction and y direction, and the two relations about the point series can be constructed by projecting Equation (2) on x and y axis of coordinates respectively by reason that such projection has advantage of reducing the calibration errors. The expressions about the projection are written as

$$s(x)=f(g_x(\alpha_x^d),g_x(\beta_x^d),g_x(\mu_x^d),g_x(\eta_x^d))-\left(\frac{\alpha-\mu}{\beta-\mu}\right)\Big/\left(\frac{\alpha-\eta}{\beta-\eta}\right)=0 \tag{3}$$

In the problem of distortion calibration, we usually get lots of point series which satisfy the relation Equation (3). What's more, we can get hold of two functions in the direction of x axis and y axis according to Equation (3). Under the correct values of the distortion parameters, the cross-ratio computed from Equation (2) should be the same, namely, both sides in expressions (3) are equal. But in fact, it is not avoidable for us to bring in the errors in measuring and computing process. Thereby, we can recover the distortion parameters by using the error relations $s_i(x)$ and $s_i(y)$ ($i=1,2\cdots,N$). Finally, we define the following total error function

$$E=\sum_{i=1}^{N}\left[\left(s_i(x)^2\right)+s_i(y)^2\right] \tag{4}$$

To improve the accuracy, more point series in accordance with Equation (3) ought to be used. Finally, the sum of the error in Equation (4) for all the segments is used in our calibration method.

4.2 Root-Finding Solution

In order to calibrate the distortion parameters exactly, it is necessary to make use of nonlinear optimization algorithm. However, the algorithm is iterative and it will take much time to optimize the objective function. In this paper, we adopt the Levenberg-Marquardt algorithm for its high speed and simplicity. Otherwise, it is very important to choose an appropriate initial guess. Because it can result in local minima and instability which may result in a false solution if the initial guess is not available.

The initial guess includes the distortion center and distortion parameters. In selecting the initial guess about distortion center, the article [15] proves two lemmas and reaches the conclusion that the uncertainty of the distortion center can be compensated by adjusting the distortion parameters P_1 and P_2. Thus, it is efficient to select a rational initial guess for the distortion center without considering the true position of the distortion center. In existing works, the center of the image is usually chosen as an appropriate initial guess [8 & 14]. Meanwhile, in some works [1 & 2], the distortion center is presumed to be coincided with the camera principal point.

The starting guess of the distortion parameters is often set to zero [1] or a value which satisfies some relation [1, 8 & 14] (e.g. $K1\times r^3 \le 0.1$, r is the distance between the image center and the adjacent corner). In camera calibration, the radial distortion is the main distortion and is more important than the decentering distortion. So in our method, we abandon the decentering distortion parameters at first and only compute the coefficients of the radial distortion, then place the decentering distortion parameters in an appropriate initial guess, followed by computing and optimizing all the distortion parameters.

In the radial distortion computation, the coefficients of the decentering distortion P_1 and P_2 are set to be zero. In this case, Equation (1) can be rewritten as the following:

$$x_u = x_d + K_1(x_d - c_x)\left[(x_d - c_x)^2 + (y_d - c_y)^2\right] + K_2(x_d - c_x)\left[(x_d - c_x)^2 + (y_d - c_y)^2\right]^2 \quad (5(a))$$

$$y_u = y_d + K_1(y_d - c_y)\left[(x_d - c_x)^2 + (y_d - c_y)^2\right] + K_2(y_d - c_y)\left[(x_d - c_x)^2 + (y_d - c_y)^2\right]^2 \quad (5(b))$$

Substituting (5) into (3), we can get the values of the parameters K_1 and K_2. At each point series extracted from the distorted image, the error equations Equation (4) can be constructed. Following that, all the equations according to the above point series are stacked in the form $Ax = b$ where x is the radial parameter K_1 and K_2. This over-determined set of equations can be efficiently solved by using the least square method. The computing result can be refined further by using the Levenberg-Marquardt algorithm in order to minimize the distortion errors. To improve the accuracy, more point series which scatter on the whole image should be chosen. Moreover, there should be more directions formed by these point series.

4.3 Computing Difficulties and Solutions

Theoretically, it is sufficient to gain the distortion parameter K_1 and K_2 by substituting (5) into (3) and the least square method. But in fact, Equation (3) is constructed on the basis of the cross-ratio of the point series. In computing and optimizing procession, there is a symbol problem in the use of cross ratio results. For instance, in Equation (3) for a given point series the cross-ratio of x axis is not equal to the one of y axis but equal in absolute value. The common way to deal with it is to move one term to another side of the equation and then square both sides. But this method does little work to this problem. In order to overcome the difficulties, we analyze the Equation (3) deeply and come to the conclusion that while $x_d > c_x$ and $y_d > c_y$, x_u and y_u monotonously increase with the increase of x_d and y_d (where (c_x, c_y) is the center of the distortion image). Therefore, if the parameters x_d and y_d selected satisfy Equation (3) and (5), the cross-ratio of x axis is equal to the one of y axis for a given point series. Using this method, we can directly compute the distortion parameters K_1 and K_2.

In addition, we found out in the experiments that the selected point series ought to be far away from the center of the distorted image in order to acquire better results.

4.4 The Algorithm

According to the above analysis, we bring up the calibration algorithm. In this algorithm, the input is a distorted image. However, in order to improve the calibration result, one can choose several images about the calibration grid.

1. Do subpixel edge detection to generate chains of corners in the calibration grid.
2. Group the corners of calibration block according to Eq(5).
3. Set the distortion center to an appropriate location (here is image center).
4. According to (3) and (5), compute the distortion parameters K_1 and K_2.
5. Optimize the parameters K_1, K_2 and the distortion center (c_x, c_y) using Levenberg-Marquardt algorithm.
6. Set the decentering distortion parameter P_1 and P_2 to zero and optimize all the distortion parameters.

5 Experiments

In this part, we give experiments to show the results of distortion removal for a known planar calibration grid.

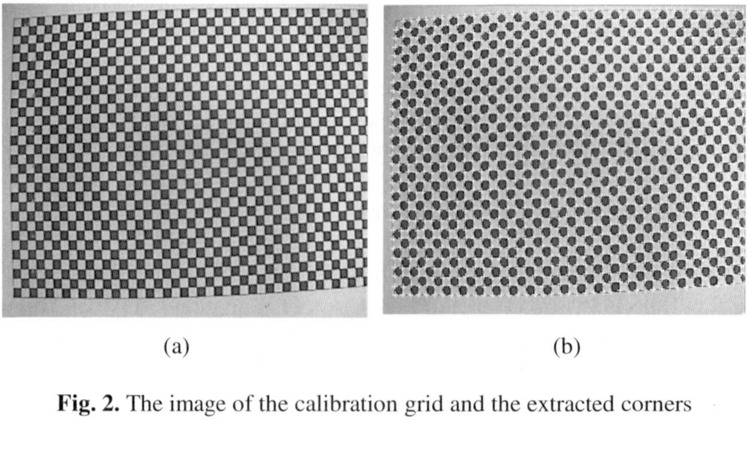

(a) (b)

Fig. 2. The image of the calibration grid and the extracted corners

Table 1. The claibration results of camera distortion parameters.

Distorted Image Center	c_x	c_y
Results	344.452795	293.584274
Radial Distortion Parameters	K_1	K_2
Results	1.280739e-007	-2.366564e-012
Decentering Parameters	P_1	P_2
Results	-6.021139e-007	-1.391637e-006

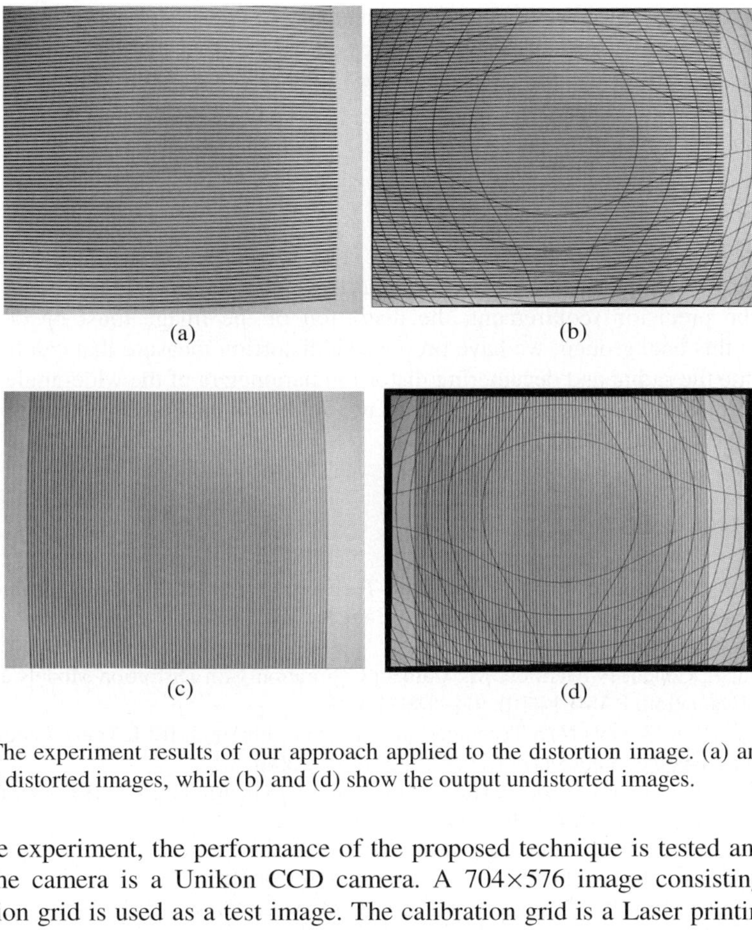

Fig. 3. The experiment results of our approach applied to the distortion image. (a) and (c) are the input distorted images, while (b) and (d) show the output undistorted images.

In the experiment, the performance of the proposed technique is tested and evaluated. The camera is a Unikon CCD camera. A 704×576 image consisting of the calibration grid is used as a test image. The calibration grid is a Laser printing paper which is drawn using AutoCAD. The distance between the adjacent corners is 2mm.

To improve accuracy, we do subpixel edge detection of the calibration grid, and the position of each point is perturbed by a distance governed by a Gaussian distribution with zero-mean and standard deviation 0.8 (The gauss width is 5). The adopted point series is in a line and the distance of adjacent point in a series is equal, therefore the cross ratio of point series is $4/3$. The camera parameters will be calculated using a nonlinear optimization program based on the subroutine LMDIF from the software package MINPACK. The subroutine uses a modified Levenberg-Marquart algorithm. The calibration pattern is a calibration grid with black and white squares (Fig. 2 (a)). The corners of the calibration grid are extracted by finding edges and computing intersection points. The results are shown in Fig. 2 (b).

After applying our technique as described in Sections 4.1--4.4, we get the calibration results. Table 1 is the calibration results of the radial distortion parameters K_1 and K_2, decentering parameters P_1 and P_2, and the center of the distorted image (c_x, c_y).

The results of the Table1 have been tested with the images with severe lens distortion. On one paper, we drew tens of lines and obtain two images (Fig. 3 (a) and (c)) from two different directions. From the images, we can find that the lines are curved due to the camera distortion. The undistorted images are shown in Fig. 3 (b) and (d) by applying above results.

6 Conclusion and Future Works

In this paper, we introduced our welding seam extraction system which aimed to extract the welding seam from two CCD cameras with wide-angle lenses. In order to satisfy the precision requirement, the distortion of the image must be dealt with. Based on this background, we have proposed a distortion measure that can be utilized to calibrate the radial and decentering distortion parameters of the wide-angle lens.

In future, we will consider the effect of the noise and analyze the robustness of the algorithm.

References

1. Tsai, R.: A Versatile Camera Calibration Technique for High-Accuracy 3D Machine Vision Metrology Using Off-the-Shelf TV Cameras and Lenses. IEEE J. Robotics Automation 3(4), 323–344 (1987)
2. Weng, J., Cohen, P., Herniou, M.: Camera Calibration with Distortion Models and Accuracy Evaluation. PAMI 14(10), 965–980 (1992)
3. Zhang, Z.: A Flexible New Technique for Camera Calibration. IEEE Trans. Pattern Analysis and Machine Intelligence 22(11), 1330–1334 (2000)
4. Cao, X., Foroosh, H.: Camera Calibration Using Symmetric Objects. IEEE Trans. Image Procession 15(11), 3614–3619 (2006)
5. Zhang, Z.: Camera Calibration with One-Dimensional Objects. IEEE Trans. Pattern Analysis and Machine Intelligence 26(7), 892–899 (2004)
6. Weng, J., Cohen, P., Herniou, M.: Calibration of Stereo Cameras Using a Non-Linear Distorton Model. In: Proc. International Conference on Pattern Recognation, pp. 246–253 (1990)
7. Hartley, R., Kang, S.B.: Parameter-Free Radial Distortion Correction with Centre of Distortion Estimation. IEEE Trans. Pattern Analysis and Machine Intelligence 29(8), 1309–1321 (2007)

8. Stein, G.P.: Lens Distortion Calibration Using Point Correspondences. In: CVPR, Cambridge, MA, pp. 602–608 (1997)
9. Thirthala, S., Pollefeys, M.: The Radial Trifocal Tensor: A Tool for Calibrating the Radial Distortion of Wide-Angle Cameras. In: CVPR, San Diego (2005)
10. Zhang, G.J., He, J.J., Yang, X.M.: Calibrating Camera Radial Distortion with Cross-Ratio Invariability. Optics and Laser Technology 35, 457–461 (2003)
11. Ma, S.D.: A Self-Calibration Technique for Active Vision System. IEEE Trans. Robot Automation 12(1), 114–120 (1996)
12. Devernay, F., Faugeras, O.: Straight Lines Have to Be Straight. Machine Vision and Applications 13(1), 14–24 (2001)
13. Ma, S.D., Zhang, Z.Y.: Computer Vision–Theory and Algorithm. Science Press, M. Beijing (1998)
14. Ahmed, M., Farag, A.: Nonmetric Calibration of Camera Lens Distortion: Differential Methods and Robust Estimation. IEEE Trans. Image Procession 14(8), 1215–1230 (2005)
15. Ahmed, M., Farag, A.: Differential Methods for Nonmetric Calibration of Camera Lens Distortion. In: Proc. CVPR, Hawaii (2001)

Analysis of Stable Grasping for One-Parameter Four-Pin Gripper

Zhicai Ou and Hong Qiao*

Institute of Automation, Chinese Academy of Sciences, Beijing, China
No.95, Zhongguancun East Road, Beijing, 100190, P.R. China
Tel.: +861062573736
{zhicai.ou,hong.qiao}@ia.ac.cn

Abstract. Locate and move the object from a region of initial state to a final stable state (form closure) is a guarantee of successful grasping. However, most previous grasping works only focus on how to keep a grasped object in a static state. Very few work concerns on the whole process to achieve stable grasping state and give the conditions of initial region by taking the objects shape into account. In this paper, dynamic grasping is analyzed by utilize attractive region [10]. Meanwhile, a one-parameter four-pin gripper, which can remove all the uncertainties of a planar object, is adopted as grasping tool. The graspable object set of the gripper is given; and the initial state region of the object for the gripper is presented. At last, simulations are given to show the validity of the grasping process analysis and the initial region respectively.

Keywords: Four-Pin Gripper, Form Closure, Grasp, Attractive Region.

1 Introduction

The static stability of a grasp can be characterized by form-closure and force-closure properties ([1], [4], etc). The necessary and sufficient condition for a form-closure grasp is that the entire wrench space can be positively spanned by the primitive contact wrenches generated by the contact forces at the contact points [1].

Lots of previous works focused on analysis of static grasping related to form/force closure, and on test methods for form/force closure ([11], [14] etc.). For example: (1) Nguyen [2] presented an algorithm for computing a subset of all form closure configurations which consists of all quadruples of independent edge regions. (2) Bicchi [4] investigated the form/force closure properties deeply, proved the equivalence between force closure and the ordinary differential equation, and presented a algorithm for force closure test by applying Lyapunov's direct method. (3) Brost and Goldberg [6] gave an algorithm for finding all the form closure configurations of a given polygonal part with n edges and a maximum diameter. However, all the above work did not analyze the dynamic grasping process, the grasp mode and the initial state of the object.

From the other point of view, even if there are stable states for given objects and gripper, it is necessary to give the initial region of the object state and the grasping

* Corresponding author.

C. Xiong et al. (Eds.): ICIRA 2008, Part II, LNAI 5315, pp. 630–639, 2008.

mode for handling error tolerance, position uncertainty and grasping tactics. Therefore, it is necessary to investigate the grasping process and the states of the objects during the whole process. Rimon and Blake [5] introduced the notion of the caging set of a gripper with one degree of freedom, and proposed the caging set for their one-parameter two-fingered gripper. Another similar notion capture region in robotic system was presented by Kriegman [3]; later Sudsang and his co-workers utilized this notion for some capturing researches [14]. A review on grasping and capturing works can be found in Bicchi and Kumar's paper [8].

The notion attractive region which concerns on every possible configuration of the object during the whole grasping process was proposed in our previous work [10] [11]. Attractive region is defined as the set of object configurations where there is a sensor-less input which guarantees the object move to a pre-defined stable state from any initial state in the set. Different from the above notions, attractive region describes the object's dynamic motion configurations related to the gripper.

Although the parallel-jaw is one of the most widely used grippers in practice, it can not eliminate the uncertainties completely. Qian and Shen [7] proposed a four-pin gripper as a RISC gripper and use the gripper to position and identify planar parts. Then, Qian, Qiao and Tso [12] investigated grasping properties, formulated and analyzed polygonal grasping, and presented a method of identifying the parts by using the gripper. We select the four-pin gripper as our grasping tool for its advantages such as simple mechanism, achieving form closure and versatile to grasp different parts.

In this paper, we present an object set in which the grasped object is form closure with a four-pin gripper. Different from most previous works which concerned on the static grasping conditions, our work focuses on the dynamic grasping process. We present the initial region in which an object can be grasped to be form closure. By investigating we find that whether an object is form closure depends on the gripper parameter and the object's geometric shape. Thus, we will show this relationship, and propose the algorithm how to adjust the gripper parameter to achieve form closure for some objects which do not achieve form closure with some gripper parameter. The validity of analysis is demonstrated by giving the initial region and choosing the gripper region parameter of the four-pin gripper according to a given rectangle and a specified object respectively.

The rest of the paper is arranged as follow. Section II illustrates the design of the one-parameter four-pin gripper and gives the expression of the gripper diameter. Next in section III, we present the relationship between the attractive region and form closure. In section IV, the object set in which the object can be grasped by the four-pin gripper is proposed. The initial region expression and simulation are given in Section V. Simulations and experiments for valid of the proposed analysis are given in section VI. At last, a conclusion of this paper is given to summarize this paper.

2 Gripper Illustration and Grasping Formulation

2.1 Gripper Illustration

Showed in Fig. 1 (a), we introduce a modified four-pin gripper as our grasping tool for orientating and grasping. The novel design in this gripper is the slots, with which the gripper span (the distance between the two pins on the same palm) can be adjusted according to different objects. Similar to our previous work [12], we installed rolling bearing on each finger to reduce the unfavorable friction on the grasping plane and keep the favorable friction perpendicular to the grasping plane.

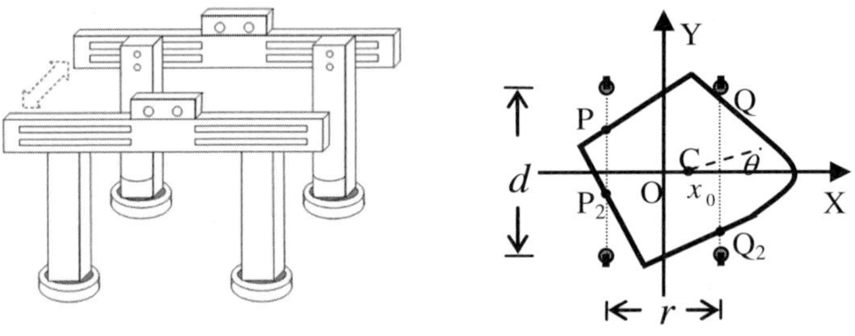

Fig. 1. (a) Shows the designed gripper with adjustable slots. (b) shows the reference frame.

2.2 Grasping Formulatioin

The reference frame related to the gripper is built up as showed in Fig. 1 (b). It is assumed that the origin of the coordinates O in the reference frame coincides with the gripper centre C. Let the X axis be along with the pipeline direction. It is assumed that the object can only move along the X axis. We use r to denote the gripper span, and d for the gripper squeeze. The position deviation of the object denoted by x_0, and θ is used to denote the rotation deviation.

The deviations along y direction during the conveying and grasping stage are small and transient, so the achievement of the final stable state will not be affected.

The four points P_1, P_2, Q_1, Q_2 is the virtual points which the fingers would touch the object possibly if the gripper squeezes. The virtual contacted edges are:
In such a reference frame, the gripper squeeze d can be formulated as:

$$\begin{aligned} d = \{ \ 2 * \max\{ \ \|y_i\| \ \} \mid & E_1(-\frac{r}{2}, y_1) = 0, E_2(-\frac{r}{2}, y_2) = 0, \\ & E_3(\frac{r}{2}, y_3) = 0, E_4(\frac{r}{2}, y_4) = 0, i = 1,2,3,4 \} \end{aligned} \quad . \tag{1}$$

Where $E_i(\bullet), i = 1, \cdots, 4$ are the edge expressions, y_1 is y coordinate for point P_1, y_2 is for P_2, y_3 is for Q_1 and y_4 is for Q_2. Since $y_i, i = 1,2,3,4$ are all related to x_0 and θ during the grasping process, it is obviously that the gripper squeeze d is the function of x_0 and θ.

3 Relationship between Attractive Region and Form Closure

The object state during grasping process is denoted by $\mathbf{X}=(x_0,\theta)$. Assumed that the object grasping can be described by $\frac{d\mathbf{X}}{dt}=f(\mathbf{X},F,t)$, where F represents the squeezing force of the gripper. We define that $g(\mathbf{X})=d$ in which d is the gripper squeeze and can be expressed by equation (1).

During the grasping process, the gripper squeeze d decreases under the force F. Thus, it can be inferred that $\frac{dg(\mathbf{X})}{dt}\le 0$. The grasping process will terminate as the gripper stably grasp the object. This stable state of the object is denoted by $\mathbf{X}_s$. Therefore, there should be a local minimum for the gripper squeeze. What's more, $g(\mathbf{X})$ is continuous since the state of the object can not change momentarily. Therefore, $g(\mathbf{X})=d$ is an specified attractive region within the neighborhood of $\mathbf{X}_s$.

Fig. 2 shows the simulation of $g(\mathbf{X})=d$ for a normal hexagon. Some bowl-like figures are formed in the configuration space, and these figures in the simulation are specified attractive regions. Each point on the curve indicates a pose of the object and the related gripper squeeze. We can identify that the bottom the bowl is the local minimum of the gripper squeeze d. The following proposition gives the relationship between the bottom of attractive region and form closure.

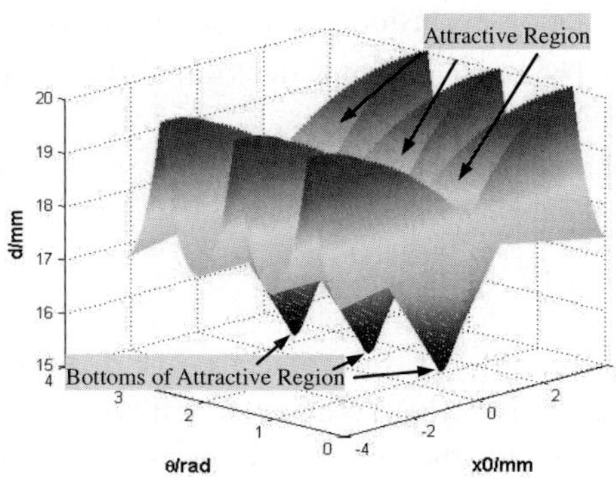

Fig. 2. Attractive Region Simulation of Normal Hexagon

Proposition 1: If an attractive region has an acute bottom, the bottom of the bowl-like attractive region indicates form closure of the grasped object.

Proof: If the object's state is on the bottom of the attractive region, that is $\mathbf{X}=\mathbf{X}_s=(x_{0s},\theta_s)$. In the case, the gripper squeeze reaches its local minimum $d_{\min}$. All the states of object in this attractive region will converge to the state $\mathbf{X}_s$ under the squeeze force F. Since the attractive region has an acute bottom, there is only one state of the object $\mathbf{X}_s$ corresponding to this situation. Thus, the object achieves form closure.

If the object achieves form closure, it means that the object can be at only one state while the gripper squeezes firmly. It is obvious that the acute bottom of the attractive region corresponds to this.

Thus, the acute bottom of the attractive region indicates form closure of the grasped object.

4 Graspable Objects

In this section, we investigate the set of object which can be grasped to a form closure state with the four-pin gripper.

4.1 Normal Relationship for Form Closure

While the four fingers of the gripper grasp the object, four normals located at the contact points are generated. The locations and directions of the normals determine whether the grasped object achieves form closure.

Showed in Fig. 3 (a), four normals, whose locations are not constrained, intersect each other on the plane. Assumed that an object are constrained by the fingers whose corresponding normals are $\mathbf{n}_1, \mathbf{n}_2, \mathbf{n}_3, \mathbf{n}_4$. It is intuitive that the object achieves form closure if the normals satisfy that: (A) the intersection point T_1 is in the rotation-exclusion sector formed by the supporting lines of $\mathbf{n}_3$ and $\mathbf{n}_4$; and (B) the intersection point T_2 is in the rotation-exclusion sector formed by the supporting lines of $\mathbf{n}_1$ and $\mathbf{n}_2$ simultaneously. The two conditions for form closure can be formulated by the following expression:

$$\begin{cases} \operatorname{sgn}\left(\overrightarrow{\mathrm{T}_1\mathrm{T}_2} \times \mathbf{n}_1\right) = -\operatorname{sgn}\left(\overrightarrow{\mathrm{T}_1\mathrm{T}_2} \times \mathbf{n}_2\right) \\ \operatorname{sgn}\left(\overrightarrow{\mathrm{T}_2\mathrm{T}_1} \times \mathbf{n}_3\right) = -\operatorname{sgn}\left(\overrightarrow{\mathrm{T}_2\mathrm{T}_1} \times \mathbf{n}_4\right) \end{cases} \tag{2}$$

For our specific four-pin gripper, the contact points between the gripper and the object form a rectangle (Fig. 3 (b)). While the gripper span r is r^*, the gripper squeeze d should be adjusted to the following range so as to satisfy expression (2):

$$d \in \begin{cases} \left(\max\{d_1, d_2\}, +\infty\right), & \text{if } \gamma_1 \le \gamma_2 \\ \left(\max\{d_3, d_4\}, +\infty\right), & \text{if } \gamma_1 > \gamma_2 \end{cases} \tag{3}$$

Where,

$$d_1 = r^* \frac{\tan\gamma_3(\tan\gamma_2 + \tan\gamma_4)}{\tan\gamma_3 + \tan\gamma_4}, d_2 = r^* \frac{\tan\gamma_2(\tan\gamma_1 + \tan\gamma_3)}{\tan\gamma_1 + \tan\gamma_2}$$

$$d_3 = r^* \frac{\tan\gamma_4(\tan\gamma_1 + \tan\gamma_3)}{\tan\gamma_3 + \tan\gamma_4}, d_4 = r^* \frac{\tan\gamma_1(\tan\gamma_2 + \tan\gamma_4)}{\tan\gamma_1 + \tan\gamma_3}$$

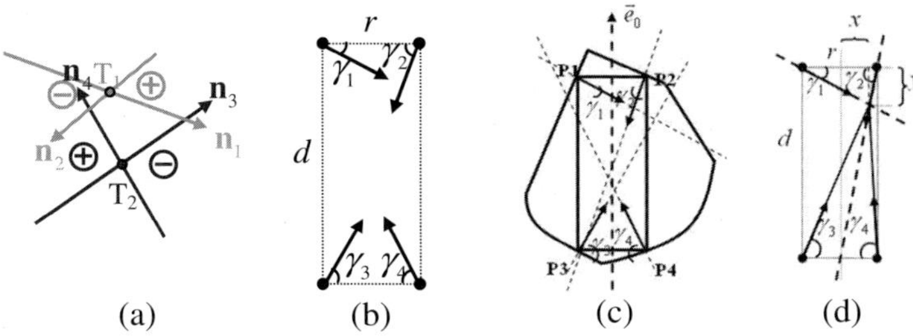

Fig. 3. Normal Relationship and Form Closure Condition Analysis

Equation (2) gives the general condition of form closure for grasping with four unlimited finger locations. Meanwhile, equation (3) presents the special condition of form closure for grasping with our one-parameter four-pin gripper.

4.2 Graspable Objects with Four-Pin Gripper

Before giving the graspable object set, we introduce some symbols first. As showed in Fig. 3(c), for any arbitrary direction, denoted by $\vec{e}$, we can draw a series of lines which are perpendicular to $\vec{e}$ and intersect the object. Assumed that the intersection points of each perpendicular line are $\vec{w}_1$ and $\vec{w}_2$. Then the length of the transversal line L can be presented as $L(\vec{e},\vec{w}_1,\vec{w}_2)$.

Theorem 1: A 2D object achieves stable state under the grasping of a four-pin gripper if there is at least one direction $\vec{e}_0$ satisfies that:

(1) Related to $\vec{e}_0$, the transversal line length $L(\vec{e}_0,\vec{w}_1,\vec{w}_2)$ is a function with only one peak in its domain.

(2) While two different transversal line lengths are equal: $L'\left(\overrightarrow{e_0},\overrightarrow{w_1'},\overrightarrow{w_2'}\right)=L''\left(\overrightarrow{e_0},\overrightarrow{w_1''},\overrightarrow{w_2''}\right)$, we get that $\overrightarrow{w_1'w_2'}\cdot\overrightarrow{w_1'w_1''}=0$.

(3) Assumed that the gripper squeeze is d, the gripper fingers are placed on the points w_1', w_2', w_1'' and w_2''. If the gripper span is r, when $\left\|\overrightarrow{w_1'w_2'}\right\|=\left\|\overrightarrow{w_1''w_2''}\right\|=r$ and specifically donated the four contact points by $P_1(w_1')$, $P_2(w_2')$, $P_3(w_1'')$ and $P_4(w_2'')$ (Fig.3(d)), the directions of the four normals at the contact points satisfy:

$$\begin{gathered}\gamma_1\in(0,\arctan C_1),\gamma_2\in(0,\arctan C_2)\\ \gamma_3\in(0,\arctan C_3),\gamma_4\in(0,\arctan C_4)\end{gathered}. \tag{4(a)}$$

or

$$\begin{gathered}\gamma_1\in\left(\arctan C_1,\frac{\pi}{2}\right),\gamma_2\in\left(\arctan C_2,\frac{\pi}{2}\right)\\ \gamma_3\in\left(\arctan C_3,\frac{\pi}{2}\right),\gamma_4\in\left(\arctan C_4,\frac{\pi}{2}\right)\end{gathered}. \tag{4(b)}$$

Where,

$$C_1 = \frac{d(\tan\gamma_3 + \tan\gamma_4) - r\cdot\tan\gamma_3\tan\gamma_4}{r\cdot\tan\gamma_4}, C_2 = \frac{d(\tan\gamma_3 + \tan\gamma_4) - r\cdot\tan\gamma_3\tan\gamma_4}{r\cdot\tan\gamma_3}$$

$$C_3 = \frac{d(\tan\gamma_1 + \tan\gamma_2) - r\cdot\tan\gamma_1\tan\gamma_2}{r\cdot\tan\gamma_2}, C_4 = \frac{d(\tan\gamma_1 + \tan\gamma_2) - r\cdot\tan\gamma_1\tan\gamma_2}{r\cdot\tan\gamma_1}.$$

Proof

When there are two different transversal lines with the same length and the intersection points satisfy $\overrightarrow{w_1'w_2'}\cdot\overrightarrow{w_1'w_1''}=0$, it can be deduced that a rectangle is formed by these points. Thus, that the four pin-fingers of the gripper touch the object simultaneously can be guaranteed. What is more, this kind of finger placement can restrict the translational movement of the object completely.

The gripper squeeze from the initial stage that the object is among the four pin-fingers; and two fingers move along $\vec{e}_0$, the other two move along the opposite of $\vec{e}_0$. Since $L(\vec{e}_0,\vec{w}_1,\vec{w}_2)$ has only one peak in its domain and $\left\|\overrightarrow{w_1'w_2'}\right\| = \left\|\overrightarrow{w_1''w_2''}\right\| = r$, the four pin-gripper will touch w_1', w_2', w_1'' and w_2'' finally.

As showed in Fig. 3(d), given $\mathbf{n}_1$ and $\mathbf{n}_2$ denoted by γ_1 and γ_2, it is the critic situation for $\mathbf{n}_3$ and $\mathbf{n}_4$ for achieving form closure. Easily, we can get that:

$$\gamma_3 = \arctan\frac{d(\tan\gamma_1 + \tan\gamma_2) - r\tan\gamma_1\tan\gamma_2}{r\tan\gamma_2}$$

$$\gamma_4 = \arctan\frac{d(\tan\gamma_1 + \tan\gamma_2) - r\tan\gamma_1\tan\gamma_2}{r\tan\gamma_1}$$

These are the two critical values for the directions of $\mathbf{n}_3$ and $\mathbf{n}_4$. In order to satisfy the condition proposed in equation (2), we get two different ranges for $\mathbf{n}_3$ and $\mathbf{n}_4$ just as equation (4) showed.

Since the derivation above can be reversed, the grasped object achieves form closure.

5 Initial Region

Fig. 4 shows the simulations of attractive region boundaries in attractive regions of the two example polygons. Intuitively, it is better to get a larger initial region. To give the general initial region expression, we must first find out the desirable form closure state which is the bottom of the attractive region.

We take a polygon to illustrate the formulation of the initial region. Showed in the left figure of Fig. 5, a polygon achieves form closure. If we translate the polygon along X axis or rotate the polygon about its centre C, the gripper squeeze parameter d will increase, and the finger constraints will be broken. Supposed that the four pins

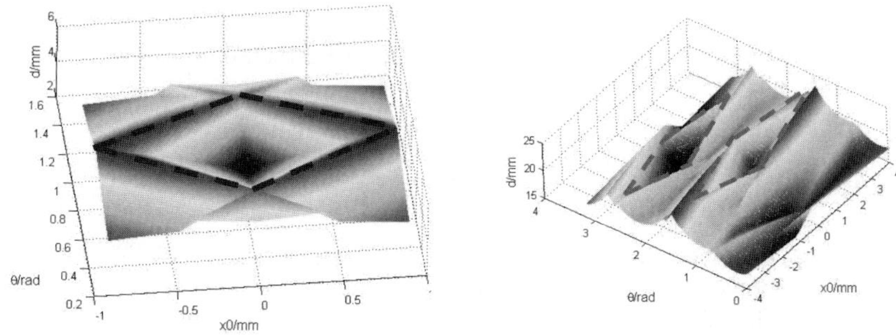

(a) (b)

Fig. 4. Initial Region. (a) shows the boundary of the attractive region (blue dashed line) of a square. (b) shows the boundary of the attractive region (pink dashed line) of the hexagon.

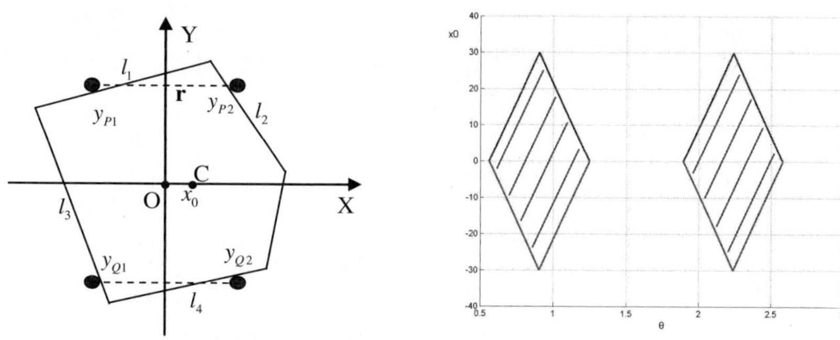

Fig. 5. The left figure is Initial Region Formulation Illustration. The right figure is Initial Region Simulation of a Rectangle. In this simulation, the edges of the rectangle are 140mm and 110mm respectively, the gripper span is 60mm.

contact on four edges $l_i, i=1,2,3,4$, and that the endpoints of the edges are denoted by P_{il} and P_{ir}, where the subscribe l and r stand for the left and the right endpoint of the edge respectively. The projection vertical to X axis of each pin should be kept on the edge which the pin contact in the initial form closure state. If the initial equations of the contacted four edges are:

$$\cos\theta_{i0}\cdot x+\sin\theta_{i0}\cdot y+d_i=0, i=1,2,3,4\,. \tag{5}$$

Then the initial region can be presented as:

$$\begin{aligned}\mathbf{S}_{\text{initial region}} &= \Big\{(x_0,\theta)\;\Big|\; x_{il}\le -\frac{r}{2}, x_{ir}\ge -\frac{r}{2}, x_{jl}\le \frac{r}{2}, x_{jr}\ge \frac{r}{2},\\ &\cos(\theta_{p0}+\theta)\cdot x+\sin(\theta_{p0}+\theta)\cdot y+(d_p-x_0\cdot\cos(\theta_{p0}+\theta))=0,\\ &i=1,3, j=2,4, p=i,j\Big\}\end{aligned} \tag{6}$$

By simulation and analysis, we can find that the initial region will be larger with a larger gripper span r. The initial region simulation of a rectangle is showed in Fig. 5 (the right figure).

6 Simulation

Showed in Fig. 6, these are two simulations for a general quadrangle and a planar part. Given the object to be grasped, we adjust the gripper span r so as to ensure form closure achievement. Although the planar objects have position and rotation deviations, the objects will be grasped to form closure ever since their initial states are located at the Initial Region.

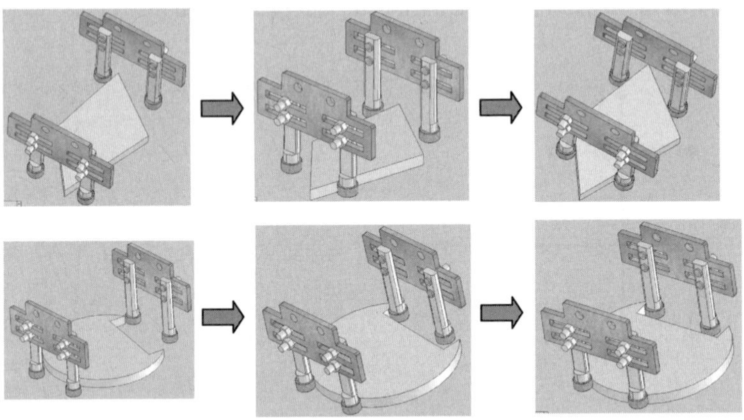

Fig. 6. Simulations for two planar objects

7 Conclusion

In this paper, we analyzed the dynamic grasping process by utilizing the notion attractive region; and proposed the relationship between form closure and attractive region. The one-parameter four-pin gripper, which is simply, universal and efficient, was introduced to complement the grasping action. Deep investigation of objects that can be grasped with the four-pin gripper was presented. Furthermore, the initial region, ensuring successful grasping, related to the planar object's shape, was also analyzed. At last, Some simulations for our proposed theory were given.

References

1. Salisbury, J.K., Roth, B.: Kinematic and Force Analysis of Articulated Hands. ASME J. Mech., Trans., Automat., Design 105, 34–41 (1982)
2. Nguyen, V.D.: Constructing Force-Closure Grasps. In: ICRA, vol. 3, pp. 1368–1373 (1986)

3. Kriegman, D.J.: Let Them Fall Where They May: Capture Regions of Curved 3D Objects. In: ICRA, vol. 1, pp. 595–601 (1994)
4. Bicchi, A.: On the Closure Properties of Robotics Grasping. Int. J. Robot. Res. 14(4), 319–334 (1995)
5. Rimon, E., Blake, A.: Caging 2D Bodies By 1-Parameter Two-Fingered Gripping Systems. In: ICRA, vol. 2, pp. 1458–1464 (1996)
6. Brost, R.C., Goldberg, K.Y.: A Complete Algorithm for Designing Planar Fixtures Using Modular Components. IEEE Trans. on Robotics and Automation 12(1), 31–46 (1996)
7. Qian, W.H., Shen, H.C.: Identifying and Positioning Parts Using RISC Sensors and RISC Grippers Together. In: Proc. IEEE Int. Symp. Assembly Task Planning, pp. 66–71 (1997)
8. Bicchi, A., Kumar, V.: Robotic Arasping and Contact: A Review. In: ICRA, vol. 1, pp. 348–353 (2000)
9. Qiao, H.: Attractive Regions in the Environment. In: ICRA, vol. 2, pp. 1420–1427 (2000)
10. Qiao, H.: Attractive Regions Formed by Constraints in Configuration Space - Attractive Regions in Motion Region of a Polygonal or a Polyhedral Part with a Flat Environment. In: ICRA, vol. 2, pp. 1071–1078 (2001)
11. Ding, D., Lee, Y.H., Wang, S.G.: Computation of 3-D Form-Closure Grasps. IEEE Trans. Robot. and Aut. 17(4), 515–522 (2001)
12. Qian, W.H., Qiao, H., Tso, S.K.: Synthesizing Two-Fingered Grippers for Positioning and Identifying Objects. IEEE Trans. Systems, Man and Cybernetics, Part B 31(4), 602–615 (2001)
13. Sudsang, A.: A Sufficient Condition for Capturing an Object in the Plane With Disc-Shaped Robots. In: ICRA, vol. 1, pp. 682–687 (2002)
14. Vahedi, M., van der Stappen, A.F.: Geometric Properties and Computation of Three-Finger Caging Grasps of Convex Polygons. In: Proc. IEEE Conf. on Aut. Sci. and Eng., pp. 404–411 (2007)

A Method for Evaluation of Coning Error Based on Adaptive Cone

Baoqing Liu and Huimin Dong

School of Mechanical Engineering Dalian University of Technology, Liaoning, Dalian, 116024, China
LBQ9905@yahoo.com.cn

Abstract. An approach to the coning error evaluation is presented in this paper. Firstly the initial point is calculated based on semi-cone angle and fitting cone axis obtained from fitting circle. Then, this paper puts forward a concise and visual model based on adaptive cone and proposes a solution of coning error base on sequential quadratic programming. Finally, the result of calculation based on many examples indicates that the initial point improves the evaluation of coning error.

Keywords: sequential quadratic programming; adaptive; saddle point programming; initial point.

1 Introduction

Due to the quickness and accuracy of the installation and orientation of conical parts and its reliability and tightness of parts combination, conical parts are widely applied in machinery industry and aerospace industry. However, it's not easy to measure and appraise the shape error of conical parts[1]. The special instruments for precise measurement of the conicity, radius, shape and dimensions of cone are not available, so usually three coordinates measuring machine is employed for the acquisition of cone data points, with the least square or adaptive method for the fitting of conicoid. The least square method is employed in reference [2] for the evaluation on coning errors, although the calculation process is very simple, which is inconsistent with the "least condition principle" for shape and position error evaluation, therefore, the adaptive cone method is employed in the paper to perform evaluation.

The adaptive cone is a kind of fitting cone acquired in accordance with the property of fitted point of trajectory and, meanwhile, under the principle of minimizing maximum normal fitting errors[3] . The solution of minimizing in maximum is vividly called saddle point in mathematics[4]. The solving of such problems are saddle point programming. The POWLL method is repeatedly and regularly utilized in reference [5] to seek the different partial optimal solutions, from which the best solution is picked up, but the searching with this method is too random. Therefore, under many circumstances, the optimized results obtained are far deviated from the global optimal solutions. Consequently the sequential quadratic programming (SQP) method is employed in the paper for optimal calculations. Same as the POWLL method, this method is a linear search in iteration process. However, the search could be performed

C. Xiong et al. (Eds.): ICIRA 2008, Part II, LNAI 5315, pp. 640–649, 2008.

toward the direction of optimizing the target functions through modifying Hessian matrix, thus the randomness of the searching direction in POWLL method is overcame, and the calculation results are closer to the global optimal solutions. Meanwhile, as for the complicated saddle point programming, the selection of initial point is very important to the calculation results. The multistep fitting method is employed in the paper to calculate an perfect initial point through analyzing the geometric relation between the measurement model and the ideal cone, and the superiority of the initial point selection method is verified through the examples.

2 Measurement of Cone Surface

The shapes and dimensions of the cone-axis parts can not be directly measured, the three coordinates measuring machine must be employed to measure the surface, which will be acquired through cone fitting. The acquisition methods of data points change with the cone fitting methods employed. Regular sampling methods are employed in this paper, through which have 5 sections with equal interval on part surfaces as the measurement surfaces. Position coordinates are acquired every 9° by surrounding its measurement axis from the position of the same generatrix with the probe on each measurement section. As shown in diagram Figure 1, the drive system and control system control the movement of the probe through collaboration. The probe touches the part surfaces, and their position coordinates are stored in the computer by the sampling system.

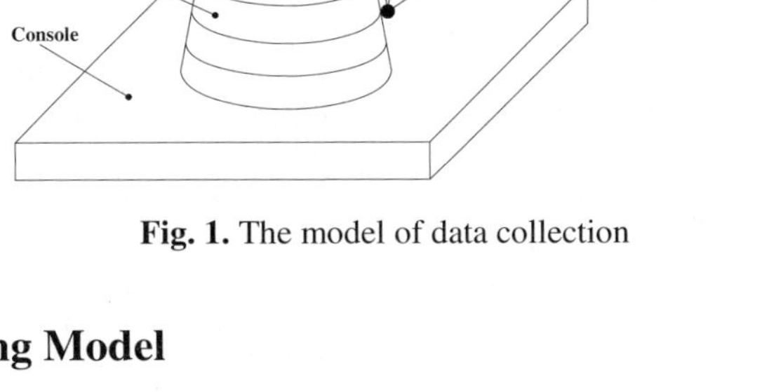

Fig. 1. The model of data collection

3 Cone Fitting Model

The purpose of evaluation on coning error is to find an ideal cone, the range of the distance from each data point to the ideal cone surface is the cone shape error. According to the different methods of ideal cone acquisitions, which are classified into least square fitting and adaptive cone fitting. The adaptive cone is a fitting cone acquired under principle of minimizing maximum normal fitting errors in accordance with the nature of the fitted point of trajectory, which is consistent with the "least condition principle" of the shape and position error evaluation.

In the process of data acquisition with the three coordinates measuring machine, attributed to the part machining or clamping problems, the part axis may deviate from the measurement axis. In order to make the coning error evaluation model visual and concise as well as convenient calculation, the measurement data points must be transformed into the standard calculation coordinate system from the measurement coordinate system.

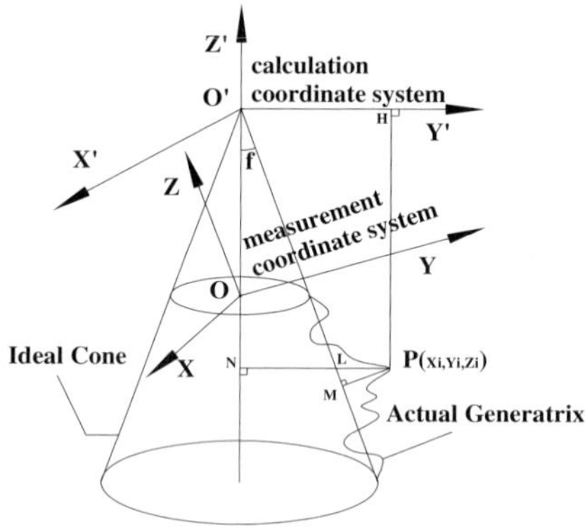

Fig. 2. The model of cone fitting

$$T_x = \begin{pmatrix} 1 & 0 & 0 & 0 \\ 0 & \cos\alpha & \sin\alpha & 0 \\ 0 & -\sin\alpha & \cos\alpha & 0 \\ 0 & 0 & 0 & 1 \end{pmatrix} \tag{1}$$

$$T_y = \begin{pmatrix} \cos\beta & 0 & -\sin\beta & 0 \\ 0 & 1 & 0 & 0 \\ \sin\beta & 0 & \cos\beta & 0 \\ 0 & 0 & 0 & 1 \end{pmatrix} \tag{2}$$

$$T_p = \begin{pmatrix} 1 & 0 & 0 & 0 \\ 0 & 1 & 0 & 0 \\ 0 & 0 & 1 & 0 \\ c & d & e & 1 \end{pmatrix} \tag{3}$$

In the formula: T_x is the matrix rotating surrounding axis X; T_y is the matrix rotating surrounding axis *X*; T_p is the translation matrix; a and b are respectively the rotating angles of the coordinate system surrounding axis *X* and axis *Y*; c, d and e are respectively the motion quantities of the coordinate system alongside axis *X*, axis *Y* and axis *Z*.

Total transformation matrix:

$$T = T_p T_x T_y \tag{4}$$

Then the transformation equation is:

$$\begin{pmatrix} x & y & z & 1 \end{pmatrix} = \begin{pmatrix} X & Y & Z & 1 \end{pmatrix} T \tag{5}$$

In the formula, $\begin{pmatrix} x & y & z & 1 \end{pmatrix}$ is the coordinate value in the calculation coordinate system, and $\begin{pmatrix} X & Y & Z & 1 \end{pmatrix}$ is the coordinate value in the measurement coordinate system. Then the target function is:

$$|PM| = \left(\sqrt{x^2 + y^2} - |z| \times \tan f\right) \times \cos f \tag{6}$$

There are 6 parameters to be optimized in the target function, which are a, b, c, d, e and f respectively.

After determining the target function, function fminimax in the optimization tool box of MATLAB is employed to solve the saddle point programming through direct programming and calculation, this function is based on sequential quadratic programming (SQP) method [6].

Currently, the sequential quadratic programming (SQP) method is one of the most efficient methods acknowledged in treating non-linear programming problem [7]. In fact, it is to perform iteration calculation by employing the non-linear equation formed by Kuhn-Tucker optimization condition, and the iteration process could be substituted by solving a corresponding quadratic programming problem. Therefore, the process of solving the former problem is transformed into a sequence of solving a quadratic programming[8].

The selection of initial point is very important for the above-mentioned multi-parameter non-linear optimization problem to obtain a better “global” optimal solution.

4 Calculation of Initial Point

As for the solving of complicated optimization problem, the ideal instance is the given initial point approaching the global optimal solution. After analyzing the difference between the measurement model and the ideal cone model, it’s found that the deflexion of axis is the key to the problem. Based on this, the multi-step fitting method is employed to calculate the initial point in the paper.

First, each measurement circle section is fitted to obtain the center and radius of the measurement position; then the axis equation is obtained through the coordinate of the circle center with the spatial linear fitting method; and then all the measurement data are transformed into a plane coordinate system and the generatrix is fitted through the coordinate transformation. The angle between the axis and the generatrix is semi-cone angle. Finally, the transformation matrix is calculated.

4.1 Fitting of the Measured Circle Surface

Figure 3 is the measurement section, the broken line indicates the line of the measurement point, and the center and radius of the ideal circle is fitted and obtained with the adaptive method.

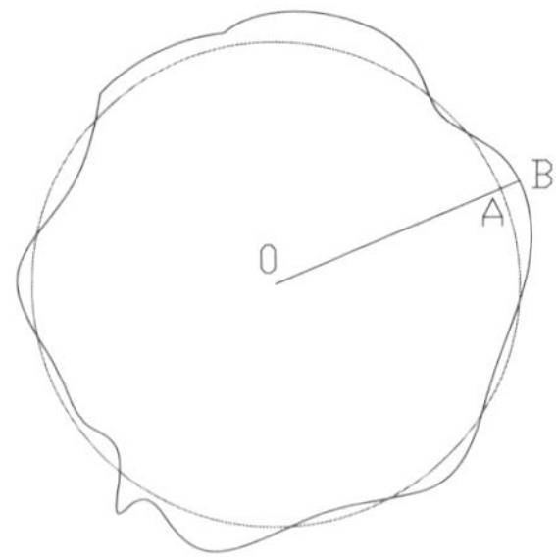

Fig. 3. The circular section

To suppose the circle equation is:

$$\left(X-O_x\right)^2-\left(Y-O_y\right)^2=R^2 \tag{7}$$

Then the mathematical model of the optimization problem is:

$$\min\left(\max|AB|\right) \tag{8}$$

Optimization target function:

$$|AB|=|OB|-|OA|=\sqrt{\left(X-O_x\right)^2+\left(Y-O_y\right)^2}-R \tag{9}$$

There are 3 optimization parameters in the target function, and the ideal optimal solution, fitted center and radius of each section could be obtained by selecting the design dimension of the axis as the initial point of optimization. As indicated by Figure 4, the broken line is the actual contour; the outermost circle is a maximum radius circle; the innermost broken line circle is a minimum radius circle, and the middle broken line circle is a adaptive circle.

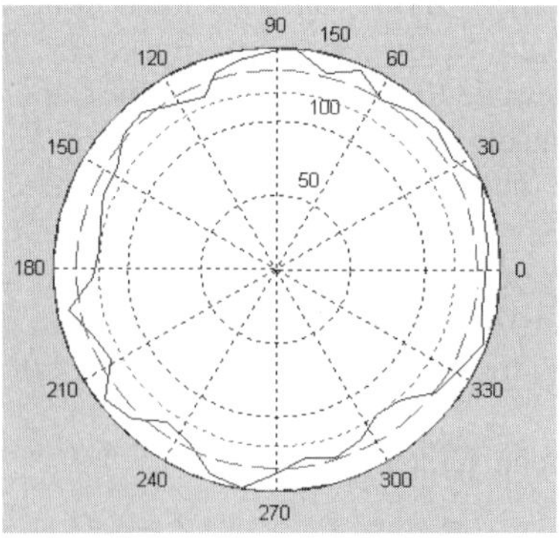

Fig. 4. The fitting of circular section

4.2 Fitting of Cone Axis

The cone axis equation could be obtained through fitting the 5 circle center coordinates fitted in the first step.

To suppose the equation of spatial axis is:

$$\frac{(X-x_0)}{l}=\frac{(Y-y_0)}{m}=\frac{(Z-z_0)}{n} \tag{10}$$

Formula for the distance from the spatial point to the straight line:

$$d=\frac{\left\|\begin{matrix}\vec{i} & \vec{j} & \vec{k} \\ x_0-x_1 & y_0-y_1 & z_0-z_1 \\ l & m & n\end{matrix}\right\|}{\sqrt{l^2+m^2+n^2}} \tag{11}$$

Perform axis fitting with the least square method, then the mathematical model is:

$$\min\left(\sum_{i=1}^{n} d_i^2\right) \tag{12}$$

The target function $f(x)$ is the square sum of the distance from each circle center coordinate to the fitting axis. Take the spatial straight line determined by the center of the first section and the center of the fifth section as the fitting initial value.

4.3 Calculation of Semi Cone Angle

The semi-cone angle is the angle between the axis and the generatrix. Therefore, the generatrix fitting shall be performed firstly.

The measurement data are transformed into a plane by surrounding the fitting axis in a certain mapping rules, then straight line fitting is performed, and the straight line is the generatrix.

The axis equation obtained from the previous section:

$$\frac{(X-x_0)}{l}=\frac{(Y-y_0)}{m}=\frac{(Z-z_0)}{n}$$

The distance from each measurement point to the axis could be obtained through formula (11), which is indicated as d_i.

Through the mapping equation:

$$\begin{cases} X'=d_i \\ Y'=z \end{cases} \tag{13}$$

The spatial measurement point is mapped into the same plane.

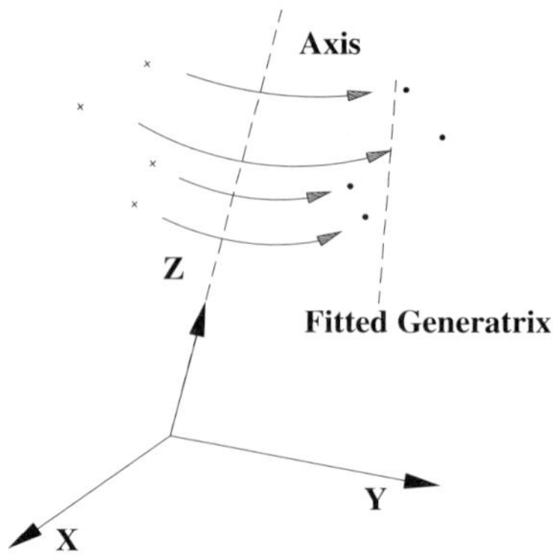

Fig. 5. Mapping the data to same planes

To suppose the fitting generatrix equation is:

$$Y' = k_1 X' + k_2 \tag{14}$$

In the formula:

$$k_1 = \frac{\sum_{i=1}^{n} X_i' Y_i' - n\bar{X}'\bar{Y}'}{\sum_{i=1}^{n} X_i'^2 - n\left(\bar{X}'\right)^2} \tag{15}$$

$$k_2 = \bar{Y}' - k_1 \bar{X}' \tag{16}$$

On this plane, the axis equation is:

$$X = 0 \tag{17}$$

Then semi-cone angle:

$$f = \arctan k_1 \cdot \tag{18}$$

4.4 Calculation of Transformation Matrix

As indicated by Figure 6, $\tan f = \frac{r1}{|e| + |Zz|}$, then $|e| = \frac{r1}{\tan f} - |Zz|$ ($r1$ is the fitting radius of the measurement surface on the topside of the axis), because Zz is negative in the testing data, therefore, $|e| = \frac{r1}{\tan f} + |Zz|$, that is, the Z coordinate at the cone apex is $\frac{r1}{\tan f} + Zz$, therefore, the translation amount alongside axis Z is $e = -\left(\frac{r1}{\tan f} + Zz\right)$.

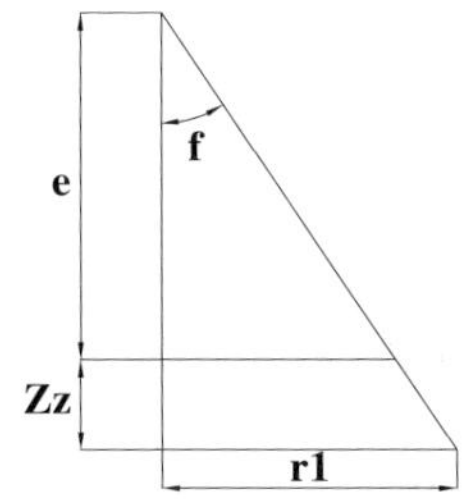

Fig. 6. The model of Z-Axis translation

As for the spatial axis equation: $\frac{(X-x_0)}{l}=\frac{(Y-y_0)}{m}=\frac{(Z-z_0)}{n}$,to suppose $Z=-e$, then $X=x_0+\frac{l(-e-z_0)}{n}$ $Y=y_0+\frac{m(-e-z_0)}{n}$.$c=-X=-x_0+\frac{l(e+z_0)}{n}$ is the translation amount alongside axis *X*, and $d=-y_0+\frac{m(e+z_0)}{n}$ is the translation amount alongside axis *Y*. Obtaining the unit vector form the direction vector of axis, suppose $\begin{bmatrix} l & m & n\end{bmatrix}^T$, because the vector of axis *Z'* is $\begin{bmatrix}0 & 0 & 1\end{bmatrix}^T$, and according to the following equation:

$$[0 \quad 0 \quad 1]=[l \quad m \quad n]\begin{pmatrix}1 & 0 & 0\\ 0 & \cos a & \sin a\\ 0 & -\sin a & \cos a\end{pmatrix}\begin{pmatrix}\cos b & 0 & -\sin b\\ 0 & 1 & 0\\ \sin b & 0 & \cos b\end{pmatrix} \tag{19}$$

Parameters a and b are obtained after solving the equation. By far, all the initial points required for cone fitting have been calculated, and then the optimal calculation of the coning error could be performed.

5 Calculation Example

To design 15 axial parts with the pitch diameter of 35.45mm and the conicity of 1□50 and measure the surface data with the three coordinates measuring machine according to the method mentioned above. As for the first one, the parameter of the initial point obtained from the design dimension is used for coning error evaluation, which is marked as C1; as for the second one, the initial point is fitted with the method mentioned in the paper and then the coning error evaluation is performed and is marked as C2, and then the two evaluation results are compared.

The data in Table 1 show that the result of the coning error evaluation performed through fitting the given initial point is averagely smaller by 13.9% than the evaluation result in accordance with the initial point directly calculated by the design dimension.

Table 1. The compare of results

Id	C1	C2	(C1- C2) / C1
1	0.021317	0.017004	20.2%
2	0.026757	0.01783	33.3%
3	0.012794	0.012648	1.1%
4	0.023057	0.022418	2.8%
5	0.016986	0.015684	7.7%
6	0.016802	0.013684	18.6%
7	0.015983	0.015054	5.8%
8	0.014398	0.014318	0.6%
9	0.025879	0.01735	33.0%
10	0.020069	0.019802	1.3%
11	0.016111	0.013954	13.4%
12	0.017838	0.011964	32.9%
13	0.015904	0.015672	1.5%
14	0.014426	0.01375	4.7%
15	0.021409	0.014584	31.9%

6 Conclusions

(1) The cone surface data measured by the three coordinates measuring machine are directly employed in the paper; concise and visual geometric models for cone shape errors are set up with the coordinate transformation method; the adaptive cone method is employed in performing error evaluation, which is consistent with the "least condition principle" of form and position error evaluation.

(2) As for the saddle point programming, SQP is employed for search calculation, and the partial optimal solution obtained is closer to the global optimal solution. After being proved by several calculation examples, the selection of initial point has very important influences to the result, and the cone shape error could be averagely reduced by 13.9% with the initial point calculation method illustrated in the paper.

(3) The method mentioned in the paper is for the evaluation of the cone contourerrors, and as for the column contour, its generatrix is parallel to the axis, then the semi-cone apex angle is 0°. Therefore, this method is still applicable, and the only difference is the shortage of 1 optimization parameter.

References

1. Yu, H., Zhiwen, Y.: Measurement and evaluation of conicity tolerance in arbitrary position and orientation. Modern Measurement and Test (4), 16–19 (1996)
2. Duping, T.: Least Square Evaluation Method on Contour Error of cone. Measurement Technique (3), 25–27 (2005)
3. Delun, W., Shufen, W., Tao, L.: New approach for mechanisms synthesis by adaptive saddle-fitting. Chinese Journal of Mechanical Engineering 37(12), 21–26 (2001)

4. Minghai, Q., Hongji, W., Libang, A., Jian, L.: Research on saddlepoint programming and geometric error evaluation. Journal of Dalian University of Technology 33(1) (1993)
5. Yuhua, W., Yanbin, F.: The minimal area method for the error evaluating of cone-type profile. Journal of Test and Measurement Technology 18(2), 147–150 (2004)
6. Hongsheng, C., Zengji, D., Jinhua, Y.: Guidance of optimal design examples for MATLAB7.2. China Machine Press (2007)
7. Shihuai, W., Yifang, X., Fu, S.: Research and progress on reduced hessian SQP methods for largescale nonlinear programming of process system. Journal of the university of petroleum 21(4), 101–106 (2007)
8. Guohua, L., Weiping, C., Guanjun, H.: Application study of successive quadratic programming in optimal schedule of multi-souses water distribution network. Journal of Hydraulic Engineering (2), 48–54 (2003)

Numerical Simulations of Open-Die Forging Process for Manipulator Design

Wen Chen, Xiaoxun Zhang, and Zhenshan Cui*

National Die and Mold CAD Engineering Research Center, Shanghai Jiao Tong University, Shanghai 200030, China
Tel.: +86-21-62827605; Fax: +86-21-62827605
{calvin,zhangxiaoxun,cuizs}@sjtu.edu.cn

Abstract. Numerical simulations for open-die forging process are conducted with different values of manipulator kinematic stiffness and press velocity. The influences of manipulator kinematic stiffness and press velocity on acceleration of jaw end are investigated. In contact and separation stages of a forging operation, acceleration of jaw end is nearly proportional to acceleration of the contact surface between upper die and workpiece; in deformation stage, acceleration of jaw end does not decrease as manipulator kinematic stiffness increases and it increases with press velocity. The ideal kinematic stiffness of manipulator should be close to zero, which leads to minimized forces exerted on the manipulator during deformation stage. The conclusion in this paper can be a reference for the design of manipulator.

Keywords: Open-die forging; Numerical simulation; Manipulator design; Kinematic stiffness.

1 Introduction

Open-die forging is commonly used in the production of medium and large forgings. In this process, a workpiece is locally squeezed between two opposite dies in each forging step and is finally formed to the desired shape by repeated and incremental steps. The uniformity of inner qualities (grain size, mechanical properties, etc.) is also actualized. In order to make the control of open-die forging process more accurate and efficient, robot manipulator has been used to grip workpiece at the jaw end and moves according to the movement of the jaw end during forging (Fig. 1).

In order to avoid damage to the manipulator mechanism, forces exerted on the manipulator during forging must be minimized [1]. When a workpiece is placed upon the lower die and squeezed by the upper die with its jaw end gripped by the manipulator, two kinds of forces are produced on the manipulator: static forces and dynamic forces. Static forces are related with mass of the workpiece, displacement of the jaw end and kinematic stiffness of the manipulator, while dynamic forces are related with acceleration of the jaw end and mass of the manipulator components. In this paper, open-die forging operations are simulated using the commercial finite element code

* Corresponding author.

C. Xiong et al. (Eds.): ICIRA 2008, Part II, LNAI 5315, pp. 650–658, 2008.

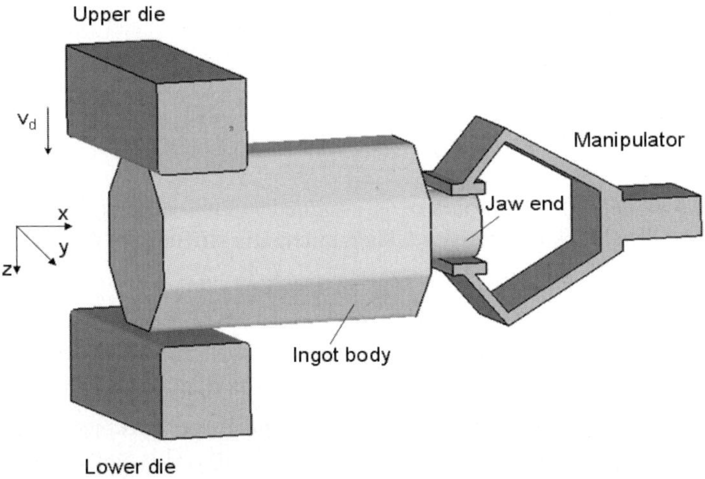

Fig. 1. A sketch for an open-die forging process

DEFORM-3D V6.1, with the aim to investigate influence factors of forces exerted on the manipulator. The influence of manipulator kinematic stiffness on dynamic forces is given special concerns.

2 Numerical Simulation

A sketch for an open-die forging process is shown in Fig.1, where v_d denotes velocity of the contact surface between workpiece and upper die. In the finite element models of this process:

(1) The workpiece is an octagonal ingot weighting 35 tons made of DIN42CrMo4 steel. Its temperature is 1150℃. Heat transfer is not considered.
(2) Length of the ingot body is 2400mm, and distance of the opposed sides of the octagonal cross section is 1500mm.
(3) Length of the jaw end is 600mm, and diameter is 600mm.
(4) Length of the ingot formed between the upper die and the lower die is 600mm.

It is assumed that velocity of the side surface of the jaw end is

$$\mathbf{v} = \begin{pmatrix} v_x & v_y & v_z \end{pmatrix}^T \tag{1}$$

and acceleration is

$$\mathbf{a} = \frac{\partial \mathbf{v}}{\partial t} = \begin{pmatrix} a_x & a_y & a_z \end{pmatrix}^T . \tag{2}$$

Because the jaw end can be considered to be rigid and it moves only in x and z direction during forging, v_y and a_y are considered to be zero. It means

$$\mathbf{v} = \begin{pmatrix} v_x & 0 & v_z \end{pmatrix}^T \tag{3}$$

and

$$\mathbf{a} = \begin{pmatrix} a_x & 0 & a_z \end{pmatrix}^T . \tag{4}$$

In present models, the manipulator is assumed as two springs exerted on the jaw end in x and z directions respectively. Then kinematic stiffness of the manipulator is

$$\mathbf{k} = \begin{pmatrix} k_x & 0 & k_z \end{pmatrix}^T . \tag{5}$$

A forging operation can be divided into three stages according to velocity of the contact surface between workpiece and upper die, which are:

(1) Contact stage, where the upper die starts to contact the workpiece and velocity of the contact surface increases from zero to press velocity. This stage is very short and acceleration of the contact surface is large.
(2) Deformation stage, where the workpiece is forged between upper and lower dies with a steady velocity (the press velocity) of the contact surface. This is the main stage of a forging operation.
(3) Separation stage, where the deformation has been finished and the upper die separates from the workpiece. Velocity of the contact surface decreases rapidly from the press velocity to zero in this stage.

In contact and separation stages during forging, displacement of the jaw end is very small, and static forces on the manipulator can be considered to be unrelated with manipulator kinematic stiffness. However, acceleration of the jaw end and dynamic forces on the manipulator may be large, because acceleration amount of the contact surface is very large. It means

$$k_x = k_z = 0 , \tag{6}$$

$$a_d = \frac{\partial v_d}{\partial t} \neq 0 , \tag{7}$$

and

$$\mathbf{a} = \frac{\partial \mathbf{v}}{\partial t} = \frac{\partial \mathbf{v}}{\partial v_d} \cdot \frac{\partial v_d}{\partial t} = \frac{\partial \mathbf{v}}{\partial v_d} \cdot a_d . \tag{8}$$

In order to investigate the relationship between acceleration of the jaw end **a** and acceleration of the contact surface a_d , velocities of the jaw end are calculated with contact surface velocities varying from 0 to 100mm/s.

In the deformation stage, velocity of the contact surface is constant and equals the press velocity, which means

$$a_d = \frac{\partial v_d}{\partial t} = 0 . \tag{9}$$

In order to investigate the relationships between **a** and **k** , v_d , a number of simulations are conducted with different values of manipulator kinematic stiffness and different press velocities.

3 Results and Discussion

Fig. 2 shows the relationships between $v_i (i = x, z)$ and v_d during the contact and separation stages of forging. $\frac{\partial v_x}{\partial v_d}$ and $\frac{\partial v_z}{\partial v_d}$ are both positive and nearly constant. It can be concluded from Eq. (8) that a_x and a_z will both increase when a_d increases. So in these two stages, dynamic forces exerted on the manipulator are well correlated with the amount of a_d . In order to minimize forces on the manipulator, a smaller amount of a_d is better. On the other hand, when the amount of a_d is greater during contact and separation stages, the manipulator will suffer more intensive dynamic forces and strength of the manipulator components must be designed to be greater.

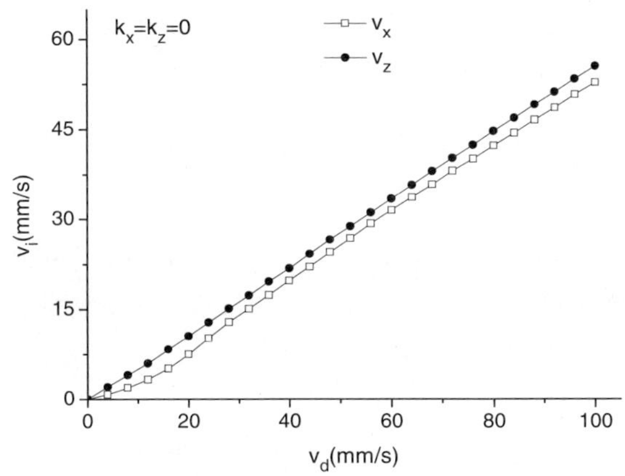

Fig. 2. Relationships between $v_i (i = x, z)$ and v_d

Fig. 3-6 show variations of $v_i (i = x, z)$ with stroke during the deformation stage of forging with different values of v_d and $k_i (i = x, z)$. It is notable that spiking behavior of v_i occurs in simulation results of some forging operations, as shown in Fig. 3(e) and Fig. 4(e). That is because the finite element solver accumulates computational error of nonlinear iteration in time steps. Despite the occasional spiking behavior, the variations of v_i with stroke have shown significant smoothness. $a_i (i = x, z)$ are then calculated with forward differencing, which means

$$a_{i,t} = (v_{i,t+\Delta t} - v_{i,t}) / \Delta t . \tag{10}$$

The discrete values of a_i imply computational errors in finite element simulations for v_i and in forward differencing for a_i. FFT filter is used for smoothing the original data of a_i. Relationships between a_i and v_d, k_i can be revealed by the smoothed curves.

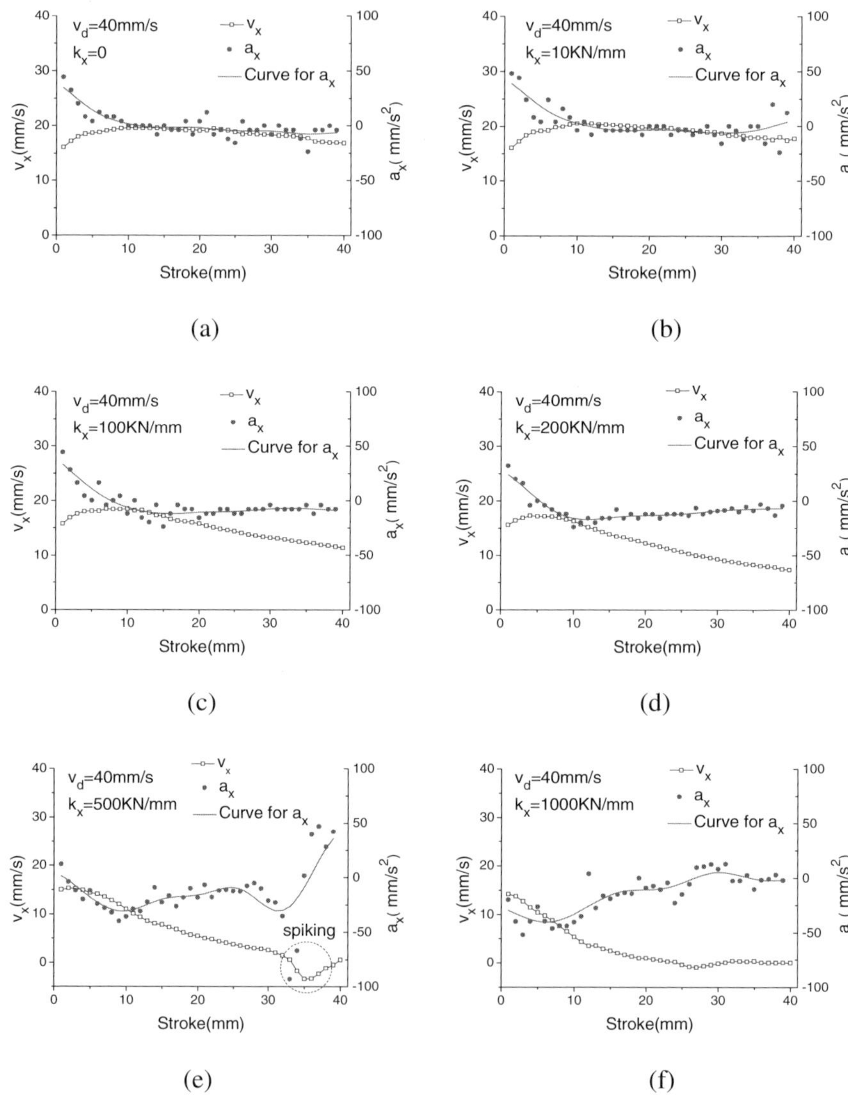

Fig. 3. Variations of v_x, a_x with stroke (v_d =40mm/s, k_x =0~1000KN/mm)

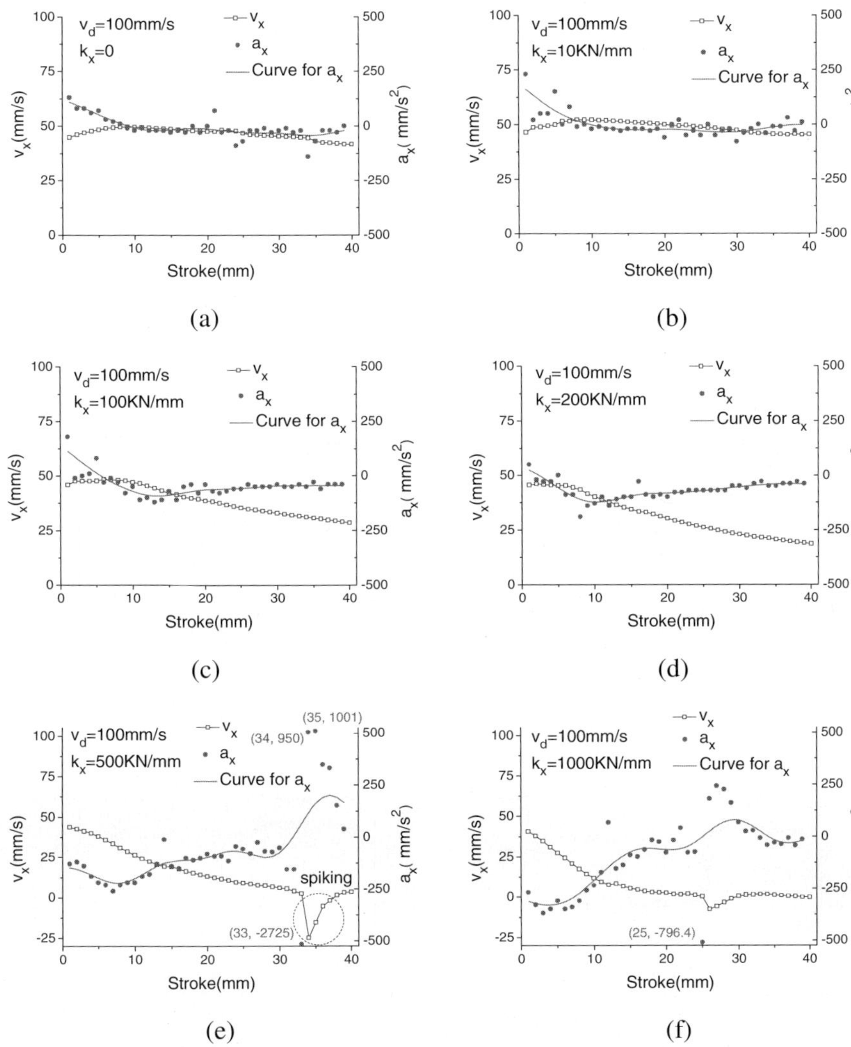

Fig. 4. Variations of v_x, a_x with stroke (v_d =100mm/s, k_x =0~1000KN/mm)

It is concluded from Fig. 3 and Fig. 4 that during the deformation stage of forging, when k_x increases, v_x decreases significantly, but a_x does not decrease. The same effect of k_z on v_z and a_z can be seen in Fig. 5 and Fig. 6. In addition, with k_x and k_z increase, static forces exerted on the manipulator will increase for the same amount of stroke. So in order to minimize static and dynamic forces on the manipulator during deformation stage, the ideal kinematic stiffness of manipulator should be close to zero.

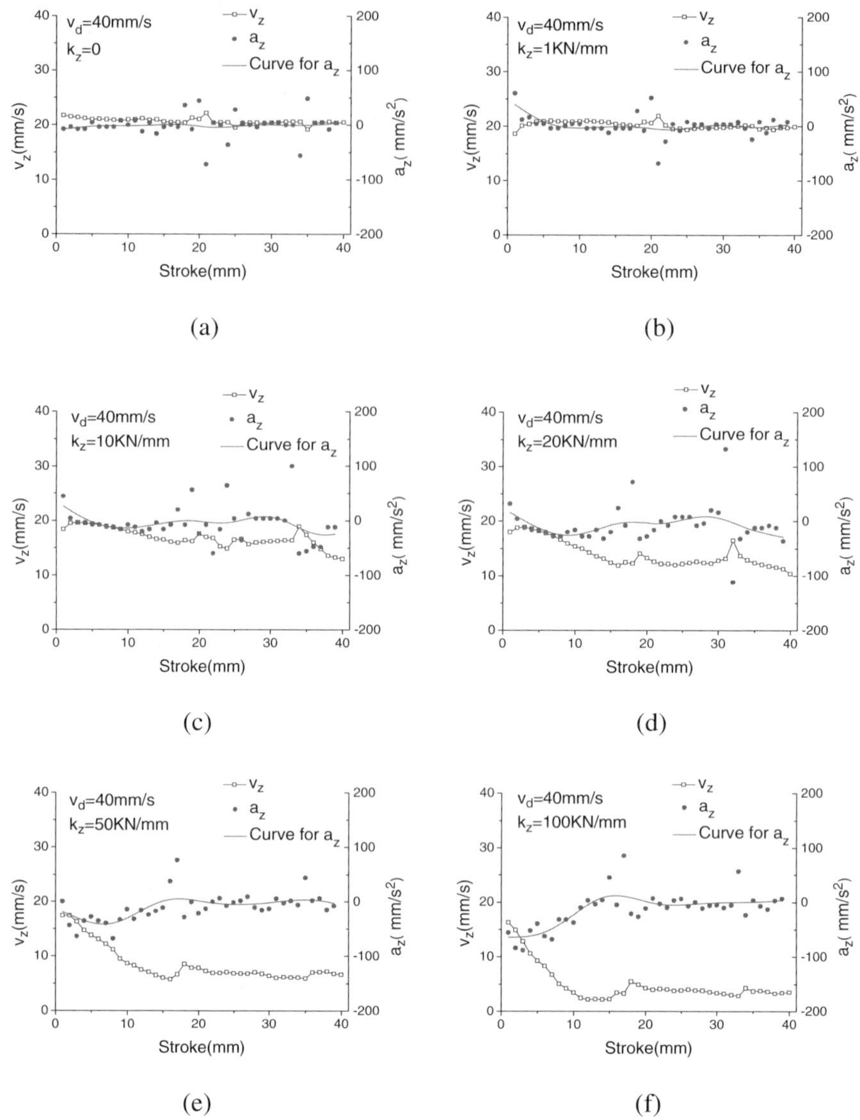

Fig. 5. Variations of v_z , a_z with stroke (v_d =40mm/s, k_z =0~100KN/mm)

It is also shown in Fig. 3-6 that when v_d increases, a_x and a_z will both increase significantly. So a smaller press velocity is better for reducing dynamic forces on the manipulator. On the other hand, in the deformation stage of forging, when the amount of press velocity is larger, strength of the manipulator components must be designed to be greater.

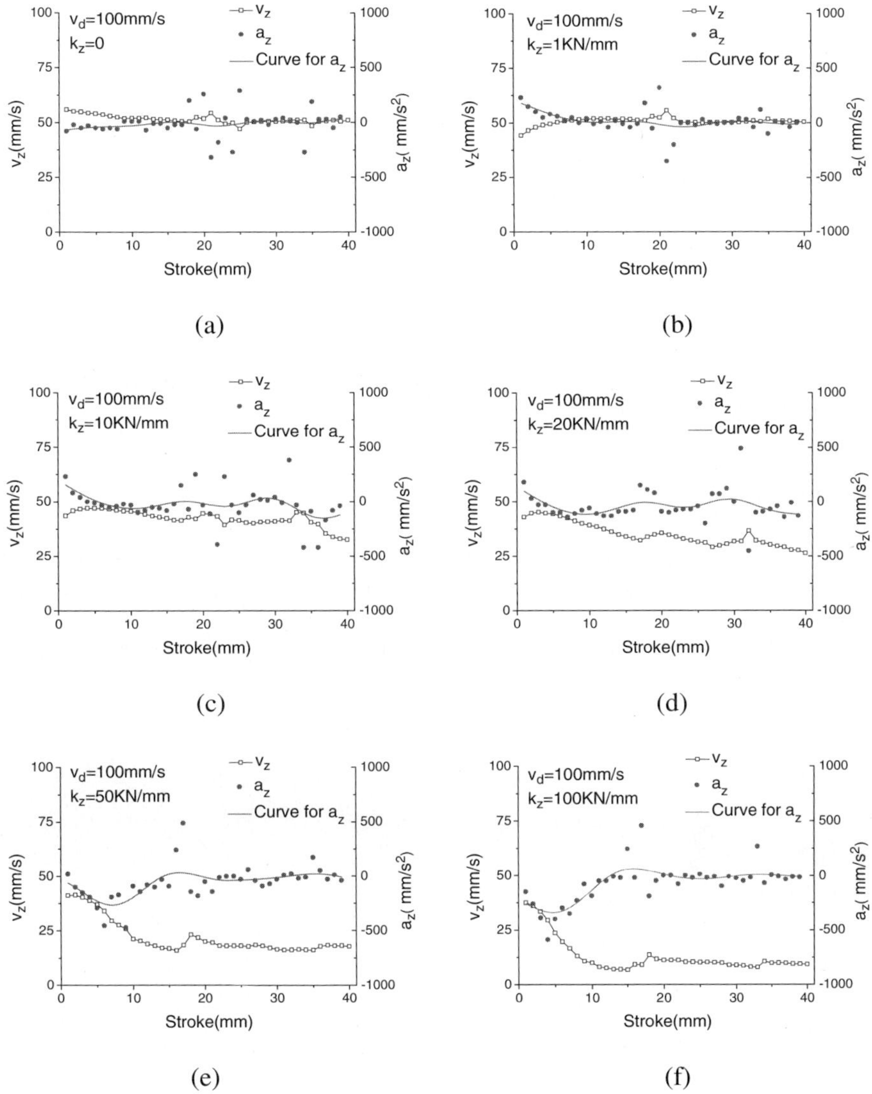

Fig. 6. Variations of v_z, a_z with stroke (v_d =100mm/s, k_z =0~100KN/mm)

4 Conclusion

A series of numerical simulations for an open-die forging process have been conducted with different values of press velocity and manipulator kinematic stiffness. The simulation results indicate that:

(1) In contact and separation stages, acceleration components of the jaw end are nearly proportional to acceleration of the contact surface. In order to minimize

dynamic forces exerted on the manipulator, a smaller acceleration of the contact surface is better. On the other hand, strength of manipulator components must be designed to be greater when acceleration of the contact surface during contact or separation is larger.
(2) In deformation stage, acceleration components of the jaw end do not decrease as the manipulator kinematic stiffness increases, and static forces exerted on the manipulator increases as the kinematic stiffness increases. So the ideal manipulator kinematic stiffness should be close to zero. In addition, strength of manipulator components must be designed to be greater when press velocity in this stage is larger.

Acknowledgments

This work was supported by the National Basic Research Program of China under Grant No. 2006CB705401.

References

1. Lilly, K.W., Melligeri, A.S.: Dynamic Simulation and Neural Network Compliance Control of an Intelligent Forging Center. Journal of Intelligent and Robotic Systems 17, 81–89 (1996)
2. DEFORM-3D V6.1 User's Manual, Scientific Forming Technology Corporation (2007)

A New, Simple and Universal Four-Finger Gripper for 3D Objects Grasping

Jianhua Su, Chuankai Liu, and Hong Qiao

Institute of Automation, Chinese Academy of Sciences, 100080, Beijing, P.R.China
hong.qiao@ia.ac.cn

Abstract. In manufacturing, it is common to handle objects with different geometries and weights. For example, there are more than ten types of objects required to assemble together in the automotive product line. The parallel-jaw gripper in wide use is inflexible and inefficient to meet the requirements. In this paper, a new, simple and flexible four-finger gripper, called CBF (Cross Bar Four-Finger) gripper, is designed to grasp various objects. The gripper with 8 degrees of freedom has compact architectures and can be easily built. It can perform both enveloping grasps and fingertip grasps. We present some properties of 3D objects that can be enveloping grasped. A sufficient condition is given for selecting the stable fingertip grasping points. Two strategies are proposed to select the contact points in two grasp modes respectively. Some examples are presented to validate our approach.

Keywords: Four-finger gripper, enveloping grasps, fingertip grasps, grasp planning.

1 Introduction

In order to perform various tasks in the automatic assembly system, it is necessary to supply numerous grippers and intelligent tool-changers as the part with different types and poses. However, the cost of grippers and their switch mechanism, and the time-consuming process of replacement limit the application of fixed-shaped gripper [1]. For example, it requires various special grippers and costs lots of time to assemble peg, rod, and piston, engine cylinder together. Therefore, manufacturers are eager for a simple, flexible and universal gripper to accomplish different tasks (grasping, handling and inserting) in the manufacturing process.

There are two main philosophies in the mechanical gripper design [2]: Anthropomorphic method, which attempts to imitate the appearance and performance of human hands, responses to the efforts on dexterous hands. Minimalistic method, which tries to partial imitation of the performance and mechanical architecture of human hands, leads to lots of works on reduced-complexity grippers in manufactories.

1.1 Dexterous Hands

The dexterous hands, such as the Shadow hand [4] and the DLR hand [5] etc., have complex mechanical and control architecture, and can perform dexterous manipulations. But

C. Xiong et al. (Eds.): ICIRA 2008, Part II, LNAI 5315, pp. 659–668, 2008.

these expensive hands with lots of actuators and sensors can not be built and controlled easily. Most of them are still in the laboratory stage and have not been used in the industrial practice.

1.2 Reduced-Complexity Gripper

The gripper with medium complex mechanical systems and control architecture is defined as "Reduced Complexity Gripper". Efforts for this kind of gripper include:

a. Improved parallel-jaw gripper. For example, Nagata et al. [6] developed a non-articulated parallel-jaw gripper with a turntable at each fingertip for regrasping, rotating or sliding the object on the low pair. But it could not be used to grasp or handle the 3D parts in assembly system. Sudsang et al. [7] presented a reconfigurable parallel-jaw gripper with actuated pins on the top plate to immobilize the objects placed on the gripper.

b. Underactuated hands, which use the passive elements such as springs or mechanical limits, can obtain good grasping performance with shape adaptation. The efforts include: the SARAH (Self Adaptive Robotic Auxilary Hand) hand by Birglen and Gosselin [8] and the RTR II hand by Carrozza et al. [9] etc. However, very few underactuated hands have been applied to practical applications, because they would lead to slightly non-intuitive behaviors and produce non-stable grasping [10].

c. Multi-purpose grippers, driven by the actuators, are developed for some expecting tasks in manufactories. They are less complex than dexterous hands but more flexible than parallel-jaw gripper. Examples of this kind of gripper include: A six DOFs reconfigurable gripper, designed by Benny and James [11], can pick and place thin-wall panels in automotive body assembly industries. A suction-based reconfigurable gripper, developed by Kolluru [12], can reliably handle and fold limp material without distortion and deformation. These two grippers were designed for the special applications of grasping panels [11] or apparels [12], not for other demands (such as handling engine or inserting peg). On the other side, Barrett hand, designed by Barrett Company [13], was a 3-finger with 8-DOFs gripper and could securely grasp different parts with whole palm or fingertips. But the operation and maintenance cost were high for industrial application. A four-pin gripper, presented by Qian and Qiao [14], could be used to identify and pose planar polygons as well as other curved object.

1.3 Organization of the Paper

In this paper, a simple, flexible and universal four fingers gripper with 8-DOFs is developed to grasp, handle and manipulate different parts in the process of automotive assembly.

The rest of this paper is arranged as following: The part 2 gives the design methods of the gripper. The part 3 presents the properties of objects can be grasped by enveloping or fingertip of the gripper. Then, we give some examples for grasp planning. Finally, a conclusion is given for summary of the paper.

2 Design Methodologies

2.1 Our Previous Works

In our previous works, two special parallel-jaw grippers have been designed for grasping, handling and inserting the parts of automotive engine (such as peg, bolt and rod), shown as Fig.1.

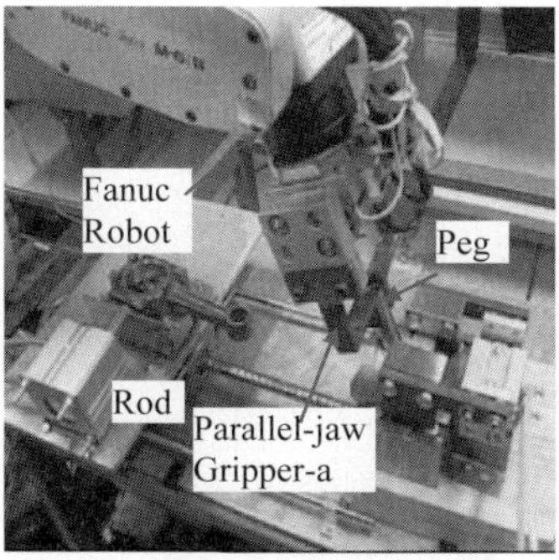

(a) Grasp and Insert the Peg into the hole of the Peg and Rod

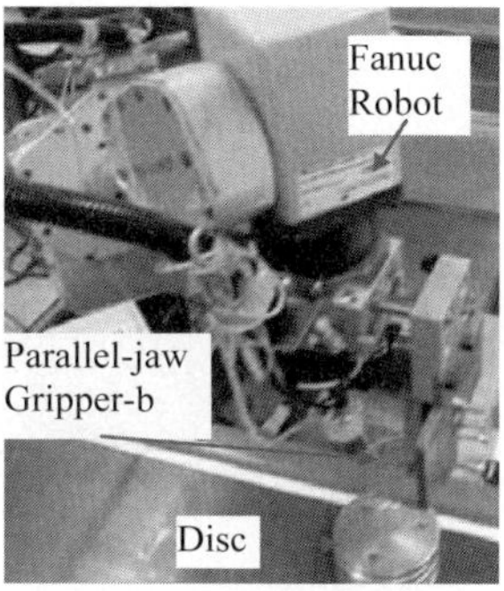

(b) Grasp the Disc to other worktable

Fig. 1. (a) We used one gripper to operate the piston, peg and rod. (b) But we have to use another gripper for picking the disc.

2.2 Design Methods

In order to grasp, handle and assemble objects in the hazardous industrial circumstances, the design philosophy of our gripper is medium-complexity mechanism and simple control architecture. Our gripper is not developed for the maximum flexibility and performance, but for massively reducing the complexity and cost. Here are the design principles:

- The gripper is simple for operating reliably and safely in the hazardous conditions. It is required to be easier built, operated and maintained.
- The gripper is flexible and universal for manipulating parts with different weights and geometries. It has enough workspace and degrees of freedom to operate various objects.
- The gripper has powerful grasping force for handling heavy parts firmly. The rigid actuators of the joints can output big torque.
- The gripper is cheap enough for the manufacturers. The sensors, actors and other electronics components of gripper are commercially available.

Based on the above principles, the CBF gripper is designed with compact mechanism and control architecture. Four fingers have the same mechanism and open control architectures, and can move along two cross-bar linear guides. This mechanism makes gripper to be more easily built. Each finger has two moveable joints that are driven by powerful servomotor built into the palm. Therefore, the gripper has large workspace and big output torque for firmly holding heavy and large size parts.

As shown in Fig. 2, the CBF gripper consists of three parts: disc-shape palm, four fingers with 2-DOFs, and two cross-bar linear guides. 1st-finger and 2nd-finger, driven by two actuators, can move along the linear guide 1. Similarly, 3rd-finger and 4th-finger can move along the linear guide 2. The phalanx 2 of each finger can adduct or abduct 180 degree. All the actors, electronics and other drive units are built in the palm.

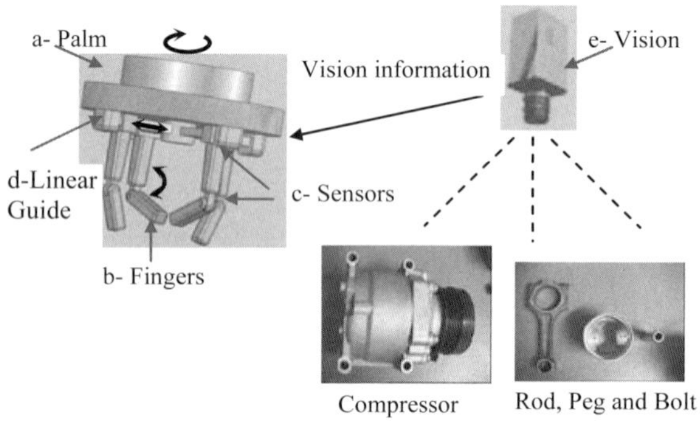

Fig. 2. An overview of CBF gripper grasps system

a. Palm unit

Different from human hands, the actuators and drivers of gripper are built in palm. The palm consists of two disc-geometries, the upper disc is mounted to the robot, while the lower one is equipped with the actuators, electronic components and so on. The wires between the servomotor and driver circuit are built in the palm, which can improve the performance of anti-electromagnetic.

b. Finger units

a) Numbers of joints: The four-finger gripper with eight joints ensure that it can finely manipulate objects with four fingertips, or firmly restrain objects by more than seven contact points among the palm, the fingers and the object.

b) Actuation: Four servomotors with good rigidity and big power are used to actuate fingers.

c) Architecture: The same mechanism and open control architectures of finger make the gripper be easily built.

c. Sensors

a) Position sensor: The position sensor that fixed on the linear slide is used to get the position phalanx 1; and the rotation degree of phalanx 2 can be measured by the angular sensor.

b) Force sensor: Each finger of the gripper is equipped with a force sensor for detecting the contact force between the fingertip and the object.

d. Linear guide

The linear guide has many good performances: precise linear motion, low rolling friction force, perfect following dynamic characteristic, extra load-bearing ability, adjustable rigidity, and simple mechanism features.

e. Vision unit

The vision unit is used to identify the type and pose of the parts in the worktable. Guided by the visual signal, the gripper can grasp, move and manipulate the real parts.

2.3 Architecture of Gripper

The gripper consists of two layers: upper layers and finger devices. The upper layer is designed to interface with the robot and vision unit. The geometries information, which is extracted by the vision unit, is used to guide the operation of gripper. The grasp synthesis is finished in the upper modular. The signal of position and angle of the finger is transferred by the serial bus to the finger control modular. Actuated by the servomotor, four fingers can stably grasp the objects.

3 Grasp Planning

In the industry applications, grippers are usually used to restrain objects firmly or grasp objects finely. In general, one can obtain two grasping modes [2]:

Enveloping grasps, which has multiple contacting points between the phalanges of the fingers, palm and object, can be applied to grasp the part firmly. It can get better robustness performance than fingertip grasps in term of restraining objects.

Fingertip grasps, which has contacting points among the distal phalanges, the fingertip and the objects, can be applied to grasp the object finely. It can provide precise high accessibility performance in term of manipulation.

The planar grasping planning has been studied by many researchers. For 3D grasping planning, most algorithms, which assumed having known the geometry information of part, find the stable graspable region on the whole surface.

In this section, a simple approach is given to select the stable grasping region on the edges of parts. Based on the projection of space part in three orthogonal planes, the problem of closure grasps a space part is reduced to a test of three subproblems of planar projection closure properties. Then a space part can be grasped by the four fingers with the guidance of the image information.

Considering the geometry constraints of the four finger gripper, the enveloping and fingertip grasps planning are given in part 3.1 and 3.2 respectively.

3.1 Enveloping Grasps

In this part, we address the problem of enveloping grasps of CBF gripper. When grasp a slippery or heavy object (such as the compressor and engine cylinder), it is necessary to prevent the slippage of the object, or hold the object firmly in the operating process. Whole palm grasps can achieve good performance of restraining.

a. The properties of enveloping grasps

In this subsection, we discuss the properties of objects that can be restrained by whole palm of CBF gripper in frictionless case.

Form closure, which related to the ability to prevent the motion of grasped object [2, 15], should be guaranteed for restraining objects.

Definition 1: A set of contact constraints are defined as planar form closure, if any motions of the 3D object on a plane can be restrained by the contact points.

Lemma 1: A set of contact constraint is spatial form closure if the set of the contact restraints can achieve planar form closure on three mutually orthogonal planes.

Proof: Let the three orthogonal planes be xoy, xoz and yoz planes. The constraints of object on space can be written as [2]

$$n_i^T c_i' \geq 0. \tag{1}$$

where $n_i = (n_{ix}, n_{iy}, n_{iz})$ is the inward normal of object at the point $c_i = (c_{ix}, c_{iy}, c_{iz})$. c_i' is the velocity of c_i.

The constrains of projection of the object on the three coordinate planes can be expressed as

$$(n_{ix}, n_{iy})^T (c_{ix}', c_{iy}') \geq 0. \ (n_{ix}, n_{iz})^T (c_{ix}', c_{iz}') \geq 0. \ (n_{iy}, n_{iz})^T (c_{iy}', c_{iz}') \geq 0. \tag{2}$$

If the projection contact constraints can achieve planar form closure on three orthogonal planes, any motion of the projection on the relating planes will violated the equation (2).

Suppose the object has a motion $\Delta c_i' = (\Delta c_{ix}', \Delta c_{iy}', \Delta c_{iz}')$ on the space. Then the projection also has a motion $\Delta c_i' = (\Delta c_{ix}', \Delta c_{iy}')$ on xoy plane. It is contradict to the planar form closure.

Thus the contact constraints can achieve space form closure. □

When CBF gripper grasps the object with palm and phalanges, the contact points are on the edge of object. Thus, the form closure grasps points can be searched along the edges of the object.

b. Enveloping grasps planning

In this subsection, the grasp regions of 3D parts are presented as three planar form closure problems. On each plane, we can decompose the planer form closure problem into two subproblems [14]: translational constraint and rotational constraint.

We now propose an approach to search the contact points on the edges of the 3D object. We assume that the edges of object can be obtained from the sensors.

Suppose the contacting points between the object and the four finger grippers are Ci (i=1,…,9). The problem of 3D form closure grasps can be divided into planar subproblems.

The approach includes three consecutive steps. We first select the planar projection constraint points on the xoy-plane, and then find the projection contact constraints on the other two planes.

Step 1: Project the object on the xoy-plane, and select four projection points c_{11}, c_{21}, c_{31}, c_{41} that satisfy

a1) $c_{11}c_{21} \perp c_{31}c_{41}$;

a2) and can achieve translational and rotational constraints on xoy-plane.

Step 2: The plane passing through c_{11}, c_{21} and perpendicular to xoy-plane is denoted by xoz-plane. Denote the contact points among 1st-finger, 2nd-finger and the edges of object are C_1, C_2, C_5, and C6. The contact point between palm and the object is C_9.

The five points satisfy
a3) they can achieve translational and rotational constraints on xoz-plane.

If not satisfaction, return to the step 1 and select another four contact points on the projection of object on xoy-plane.

Step 3: The plane passing through c_{31}, c_{41} and perpendicular to xoy-plane is denoted by yoz-plane. Denote the contact points among 3rd-finger, 4th-finger and the edges of object are C_3, C_4, C_7, and C_8. The five contact points C_3, C_4, C_7, C_8, and C_9 satisfy:
a4) they can achieve translational and rotational constraints on yoz-plane..

If not satisfy, return to the step 1.

If conditions a1)-a4) are satisfied, we can get the nine contact points $C_i(i=1,\ldots,9)$ that can achieve space form closure.

3.2 Fingertip Grasps

In this part, we will address the problem of fingertip grasps. When the gripper is required to pick a peg from the assembly line, or insert a peg, the fingertip operation can provide the precise performance.

Consider a rigid body in 3D space, we assume that:

- There are Coulomb frictions on contact points;
- There is no deformation on the contact points.

When grasps an object on frictional case, the force closure properties of grasping should be investigated. Force closure implies that all motions of the grasped object are completely constrained by the suitable contact wrenches [15,16]. The problem of computing stable grasps of object is equivalent to a test for the ability for restraining external wrenches by a system of contact wrenches (3-dimension wrench in 2D case, 6-dimension wrench in 3D case).

Definition 3: A system of 6D contact wrenches $W_1, W_2, \ldots W_m$ is defined as planar projection force closure, if the set of projections of wrenches balance a external planar force.

Suppose $\Pi_i(i = xoy, xoz, yoz)$ are three orthogonal planes, w_i is the projection of contact wrench on plane Π_i.

A contact wrench is denoted as $W_i = (F_i, M_i)^T$, where $f_i = (f_{ix}, f_{iy}, f_{iz})$ is the contact force applied by ith-finger. $M_i = r_i \times f_i$ is the moment vector of the wrench, where $r_i = (r_{ix}, r_{iy}, r_{iz})$ is the vector of the contact point.

Theorem 2: A set of contact wrenches achieves 3D force closure if the projections of the contact wrenches achieve planar force closure on three orthogonal planes.

Proof: Let the three orthogonal planes be the xoy, xoz and yoz plane. The projection of the external wrench $W_{ext} = (F_{ext}, M_{ext})^T$ on coordinate plane can be expressed as

$$w_{xoy} = (F_x, F_y, M_z)^T.\ w_{xoz} = (F_x, F_z, M_y)^T\ .\ w_{yoz} = (F_y, F_z, M_x)^T \tag{3}$$

Suppose the projection of wrenches on three coordinate planes can achieve planar projection force closure. One obtains

$$F_x = \sum f_{ix},\ F_y = \sum f_{iy},\ M_z = \sum(r_{ix} f_{iy} - r_{iy} f_{ix}). \tag{4}$$

$$F_x = \sum f_{ix},\ F_z = \sum f_{iz},\ M_y = \sum(R_z F_x - R_x F_z) \tag{5}$$

$$F_y = \sum f_{iy},\ F_z = \sum f_{iz},\ M_x = \sum(R_z F_x - R_x F_z) \tag{6}$$

Equations (3)-(6) show that

$$W_{ext} = (\sum f_{ix},\ \sum f_{iy},\ \sum(r_{ix} f_{iy} - r_{iy} f_{ix}),\ \sum(R_z F_x - R_x F_z),\ \sum(R_z F_x - R_x F_z))^T$$

Thus the contact wrenches can achieve space force closure. □

Thus the fingertip grasp of 3D parts are presented as three planar force closure problems.

4 Example

In this part we give an example of the enveloping grasps. Suppose a compressor is grasped by the CBF gripper. As shown in Fig 3. E_1, E_2, E_3 are the three edges on different sides of object, the set of contact points consists of C_1, C_2, C_3, C_4, C_5, C_6, C_7, C_8, C_9. It is obvious that contact points C_1, C_2 , C_5, C_6 are on xoy plane and C_3, C_4, C_7, C_8 are on yoz plane

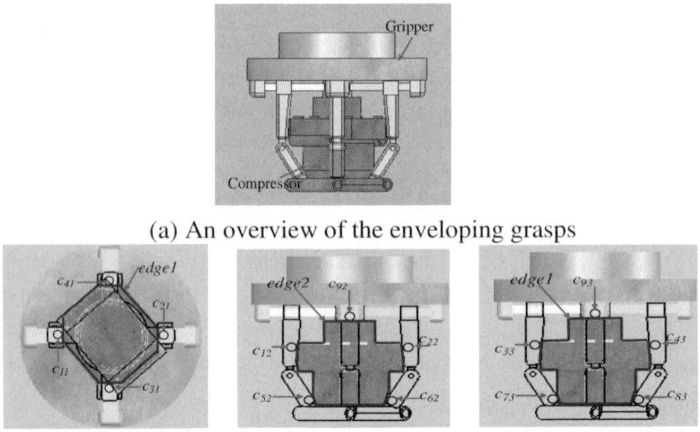

(a) An overview of the enveloping grasps

(b) Top view (c) Front view (d) Right side view

Fig. 3. The projection of contact constraints between the CBF gripper and the object

Step1: As shown in Fig.3 (b), searching the planar form closure contact points on the edge1 of compressor along the top direction. We can obtain four points c_{i1} (i=1,2,3,4).

Step2: As shown in Fig.3 (c), the edge2 of the object is on the front direction. Searching the planar form closure contact points on edge2, we can obtain five points c_{i2} (i=1,2,5,6,9).

Step3: As shown in Fig.3 (d), the edge3 of the object is on the right side direction. Searching the planar form closure contact points on edge3, we can obtain five points c_{i3} (i=3,4,7,8,9).

As shown in Fig.3 (a), the compressor can be grasping firmly by the CBF gripper in enveloping mode.

5 Conclusion

The development of a simple, universal and flexible gripper is necessary to grasp different geometric bodies in the practical assembly system. In this work, a new four-finger gripper, with compact mechanism and control architecture powerful actors and commercial available electronics components is designed. We present the design methods of our four-finger gripper a) simple enough for operating reliably and safely in the hazardous conditions, and b) flexible and universal for manipulating parts with different weights and geometries, and c) having sufficient grasping force for firmly handling heavy parts, d) cheap enough.

We address the problem of searching the stable grasping points on the object by some image information of objects. The problem of grasping a 3D body firmly is reduced to three subproblems of testing for the planar projection closure properties, which decreases the computational complexity of grasps.

As a future work, contours of object should be extracted from the image of the object for selecting the optimal grasping points. At last, the operations of gripper should be guided by the vision information.

References

1. William, T.T.: The Barrett Hand Grasper-Programmable Flexible Part Handling and Assembly. Industrial Robot 27(3), 181–188 (2000)
2. Bicchi, A., Kumar, V.: Robotic Grasping and Manipulation. Articulated and Mobile Robots for Services and Technology 270, 55–74 (2001)
3. Salisbury, J.K., Craig, J.J.: Articulated Hands: Force Control and Kinematics Issues. The International Journal of Robotics Research 1(1), 4–17 (1982)
4. Shadow Dextrous Hand - Technical Specification, `http://www.shadowrobot.com/hand/`
5. Liu, H., Butterfass, J.: A New Control Strategy for DLR'S Multisensory Articulated Hand. IEEE Control Systems 19(2), 47–54 (1999)
6. Nagata, K.: Manipulation by a Parallel-Jaw Gripper Having a Turntable at Each Fingertip. In: Proc. IEEE ICRA, vol. 2, pp. 1663–1670 (1994)
7. Sudsang, A., Srinivasa, N., Ponce, J.: On Planning Immobilizing Grasps for a Reconfigurable Gripper. In: Proc. IEEE IROS, vol. 1, pp. 106–113 (1997)
8. Birglen, L., Gosselin, C.M.: Kinetostatic Analysis of Underactuated Fingers. IEEE Transactions on Robotics and Automation 20(2), 211–221 (2004)
9. Carrozza, M.C., Massa, B., et al.: The Development of a Novel Prosthetic Hand-Ongoing Research and Preliminary Results. IEEE/ASME Transactions on Mechatronics 7(2), 108–114 (2002)
10. Bégoc, V., Durand, C., et al.: On the Form-Closure Capability of Robotic Underactuated Hands. In: Proc. ICARCV, pp. 1–8 (2006)
11. Yeung, B.H.B., Mills, J.K.: Design of a Six DOF Reconfigurable Gripper for Flexible Fixtureless Assembly. IEEE Trans. On Systems, Man, and Cybernetics, Part C 34(2), 226–235 (2004)

12. Kolluru, R., Valvanis, K.P., et al.: Design Fundamentals of a Reconfigurable Robotic Gripper System. IEEE Trans. on Systems, Man, and Cybernetics, Part A 30(2), 181–187 (2000)
13. Barrett BH8-262 Data Sheet, http://www.barrett.com
14. Qian, W.H., Qiao, H., Tso, S.K.: Synthesizing Two-Fingered Grippers for Positioning and Identifying Objects. IEEE Trans. On Systems, Man, and Cybernetics, Part B 31(4), 602–615 (2001)
15. Bicchi, A.: On the Closure Properties of robotic grasping. Int. J. of Robotics Research 14(4), 319–334 (1995)
16. Ponce, J., et al.: On Computing Four-Finger Equilibrium and Force-Closure Grasps of Polyhedral Objects. Int. J. Robot. Res. 16(1), 11–35 (1997)

Reliability Assessment of Machining Accuracy on Support Vector Machine

Chao Deng, Jun Wu, and Xinyu Shao

State Key Lab of Digital Manufacturing Equipment & Technology,
Huazhong University of Science & Technology, Wuhan, China 430074
dengchao@mail.hust.edu.cn

Abstract. In order to establish the reliability model of limited samples, a kind of support vector machine (SVM) tools LSSVM.M is used to process reliability assessment data. The choice of parameters is the key factor to affect the forecasting accuracy. To improve the accuracy, a method of advanced parameters choice is proposed, which consists of two steps. First step is to optimize the scope of parameters, gradually narrowing the initial large scope. The next step is to find out the optimal parameters. Finally, the reliability model of NC machining accuracy was established, and the prediction result in NC machining accuracy case proves that this method is valid and effective.

Keywords: support vector machine (SVM); radial basis function (RBF); parameters optimization; reliability assessment.

1 Introduction

The number of Large NC equipments is small and their life-cycle lengths are long. Currently, the research results based on normal NC equipment can not be fully applicable to the large NC equipment. Therefore, reliability analyzing on large NC equipment is meaningful to develop and enhance reliability technology. In this paper, we take the example of large NC equipment's machining ability to establish the reliability assessment model by using the method of support vector machines.

Support vector machine (SVM), which based on the structural risk minimization (SRM) principle, can get the decision-making rules from limited samples. It can obtain small error for independent test sets, and solve the learning problems effectively. The least squares support vector machines (LS_SVM), developed from the standard SVM method, has a better resistance impatient capacity and a faster operation speed. Same as other learning algorithm, its performance is greatly affected by the selection of parameters.

It has carried out a feasibility study on the application of attempting to use the theory of support vector machine in the machinery's state prediction[1]. At the same time, it has obtained the result that the nuclear radial basis function's generalization ability is the best, and the selection of parameters is important to forecasting accuracy. In general, to ascertain the connectivity of the network, it requires data from the cut sets or path sets of the system and uses a depth-first procedure[2-3]. Several approaches have been presented to address the definition of these approximated

C. Xiong et al. (Eds.): ICIRA 2008, Part II, LNAI 5315, pp. 669–678, 2008.

algorithms[4-8]. The literature focus on the study of radial parameter selection and it determines the optimal parameters in a good area where $\gamma\sigma^2 = C$ (constant) [9-12]. But at present, there is no promotion of a universal approach. In this paper, an empirical model built by training a support vector machine is proposed. In order to achieve accurate predicting result, it improves the method of parameters selection of LSSVM.M by analyzing specific data.

2 SVM Modeling Theory

The nonlinear modeling problem based on measurable data essentially is a nonlinear regression problem. The LS_SVM regression model employs the following linear representation in a so-called higher dimensional feature space:

$$H \subseteq R^{nh};\ y(x) = w^T \varphi(x) + b \tag{1}$$

Where $x \in R^n$ is an input vector, $y \in R$ is an output value, and $w \in H$ is a feature vector. $\varphi(\cdot): R^n \to R^{nh}$ means that a nonlinear regression in the input space is converted to linear regression in the feature space.

Given a training set $\{x_i, y_i\}_{i=1}^N$, the LS_SVM method considers the regression problem as the following optimization problem:

$$\begin{aligned} &\min_{w.b.e} J = \frac{1}{2} w^T w + \frac{1}{2} \gamma \sum_{i=1}^{l} e_i^2 \\ &s.t. y_i = w^T \phi(x_i) + b + e_i, i = 1, \ldots l \end{aligned} \tag{2}$$

Where γ is the regularization parameter, e_i is the prediction error for data point i.

By applying the Lagrange multiplier method, the solution to above optimization problem is obtained as the following linear equations:

$$\begin{aligned} &L = J - \sum_{i=1}^{l} \alpha_i \left[w^T \bullet \phi(x_i) + b + e_i - y_i \right] \\ &i = 1, \cdots, l \end{aligned} \tag{3}$$

Where $\alpha = [\alpha_1, \ldots, \alpha_N]^T$ is the Lagrange multiplier vector. The solution to the above optimization problem is given by the saddle point of the Lagrange. It means that, by minimizing L(w, b, e_i, α_i) with respect to w and b, and by maximizing L(w, b, e_i, α_i) with respect to α, it obtains:

$$\begin{pmatrix} 0 & 1^T \\ 1 & \Omega + \gamma^{-1} I \end{pmatrix} \begin{pmatrix} b \\ \alpha \end{pmatrix} = \begin{pmatrix} 0 \\ y \end{pmatrix} \tag{4}$$

$$\Omega_{ij} = \phi(x_i)^T \bullet \phi(x_j) = K(x_i, x_j) \tag{5}$$

$y = [y_1, ..., y_N]^T$, $1 = [1, ..., 1]^T \in R^N$, and Ω is an $N \times N$ kernel matrix. By using the kernel trick[10], the resulting LS_SVM regression model becomes:

$$y(x) = \sum_{i=1}^{l} \alpha_i K(x, x_i) + b \tag{6}$$

Where α_i and b are the solution to Eq.(4).

Given a training set, the training of an LS_SVM is equal to solving a set of linear equations as Eq.(4). This greatly simplifies the regression problem.

The chosen kernel function must satisfy the Mercer's condition. The linear, polynomial and radial basis functions kernel are the commonly used kernel functions. In this paper, the popular Radial Basis Function (RBF) kernel is used of the form $K(x, x_i) = e^{\{-(x-x_i)^2 / \sigma^2\}}$. Then we will study the regression performance of SVM on RBF kernel function.

3 The Optimization of RBF Kernel's Parameters

In LSSVM.M, the selection of kernel functions is not important for a same data set. Taking the example of RBF, parameters' selection is the key factor impacting the training result, such as γ and σ^2 must be input before training. γ is the adjustable parameter, which aims to control the right-wrong-classify sample's punishment level. σ^2 is a parameter of RBF kernel.

There is not a good method to find the best parameters at present. The tool LSSVM.M applies the gird-search and cross-validation approach (Fig. 1) to select the best set of parameters (γ, σ^2) with $\gamma = [0.1, 0.2, ..., 1]$ and $\sigma^2 = [0.1, 0.2, ..., 1]$. Different pairs ($\gamma, \sigma^2$) are used to select the best cross-validation accuracy. However, the accuracy is not good by training the specific data set with the optimal γ and σ^2.

For example, data set of 25 pairs: $x = (1, 2, ..., 25)$ and $y = \exp(x)$ are specified. The first 20 pairs are trained and the last 5 pairs are used to test the trained accuracy. Supposing the original searching boundaries are $\gamma \in [1, 10^{20}]$ and $\sigma \in [10^{-10}, 10^{10}]$, the transformed index are [0, 46] and [-23, 23]. In the process of optimizing parameters with the total of 100 lines (shown in Table 1), the second row is γ (searching between 0 and 46), the third row is σ^2 (searching between -23 and 23), and the last row is training error. The smallest error is obtained at the 56 time, and the corresponding parameter set is (5.584, 2.5584).

The second time of searching is shown in Table 2. The searching step is the 1/10 of the last time, and the smallest error is obtained in the 91st searching. Using the optimized parameters γ and σ^2 to train the data set, 5 groups of predicted value are obtained, in which the error between predicted value and the true value is 2.4. It is obvious that the result is not satisfactory (Fig. 2).

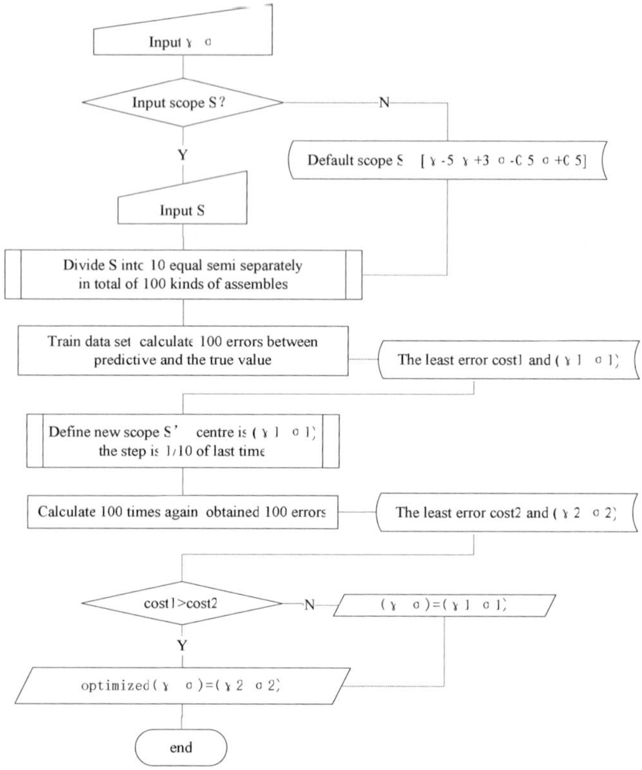

Fig. 1. Parameter optimization on grid-searching

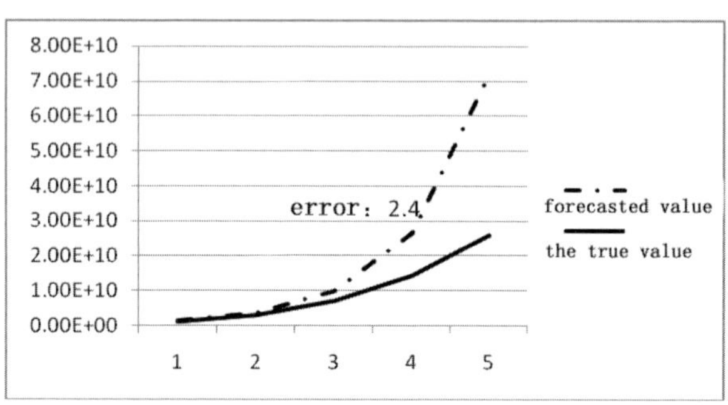

Fig. 2. Forecasted result of $y = \exp(x)$

As shown in Fig. 2, if the selected scope is too big, the searching step is big. Therefore some good parameters may be missed. It means that the scope and step of searching are the key factors to affect prediction accuracy in parameter (such as γ and σ^2) optimization.

Table 1. First time of searching

node	γ	σ^2	error
51	25.584	-23.026	5.82E-05
52	25.584	-17.909	5.82E-05
53	25.584	-12.792	5.82E-05
54	25.584	-7.6753	5.82E-05
55	25.584	-2.5584	7.02E-06
56	**25.584**	**2.5584**	**3.79E-06**
57	25.584	7.6753	3.45E-05
58	25.584	12.792	4.61E-05
59	25.584	17.909	5.47E-05
60	25.584	23.026	5.47E-05
61	30.701	-23.026	5.82E-05
62	30.701	-17.909	5.82E-05
63	30.701	-12.792	5.82E-05
64	30.701	-7.6753	5.82E-05
65	30.701	-2.5584	7.02E-06
66	30.701	2.5584	0.024966
67	30.701	7.6753	5.42E+06
68	30.701	12.792	5.19E+06
69	30.701	17.909	9.14E+34
70	30.701	23.026	9.89E+33

Table 2. Second time of searching

node	γ	σ^2	error
81	28.673	0.31085	1.13E-07
82	28.665	0.82091	2.21E-07
83	28.657	1.331	5.05E-07
84	28.649	1.841	9.80E-07
85	28.641	2.3511	1.90E-06
86	28.633	2.8611	3.44E-06
87	28.625	3.3712	5.20E-06
88	28.617	3.8813	7.26E-06
89	28.609	4.3913	1.06E-05
90	28.601	4.9014	1.34E-05
91	**29.545**	**0.32448**	**9.16E-08**
92	29.537	0.83453	1.80E-07
93	29.529	1.3446	4.39E-07
94	29.521	1.8546	8.97E-07
95	29.513	2.3647	1.78E-06
96	29.505	2.8748	3.07E-06
97	29.497	3.3848	4.39E-06
98	29.489	3.8949	7.08E-06
99	29.481	4.4049	9.14E-06
100	29.473	4.915	1.30E-05

4 The Improved Method of Searching Parameters

The selection of original searching scope of the parameter is depended on experiences greatly. If the scope is too small, the optimal parameters may not be included inside and it will be missed. On the other hand, if the searching scope and step are both too big, the optimal parameters will be missed also. Therefore, the search method has obvious limitations. We could optimize the scope firstly, and select the parameter with the good scope. It means that the good scope, in which the optimal parameter will be found, is not too big, and the searching efficiency is high.

From this idea, we try to improve the original parameter searching method of LSSVM.M. The first step is to normalize the data set using grid-search and cross-validation method. The next step is to fit the specified data set with a defined original scope: $\gamma \in [10, 10^{20}], \sigma^2 \in [10^{-10}, 10]$. The scope is so big that the good parameters are not missed, and the narrow margin of the scope is reduced. The process of scope optimization is shown as Fig. 3. The last step is to define the new scope whose centre is the optimal values of γ and σ^2 in last time of optimization, and the new searching step is 2/3 searching step in the last time. When the scope is smaller, the result will be more satisfied (shown at Fig. 4). This process is called parameter optimization. Although the computing amount is great, it is suitable for searching optimal parameter.

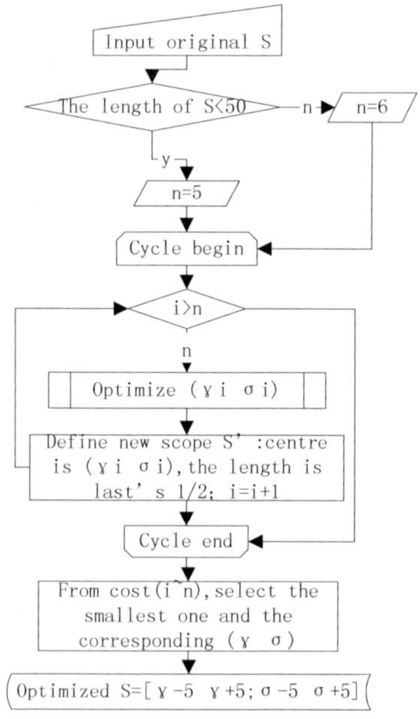

Fig. 3. Process of scope optimization

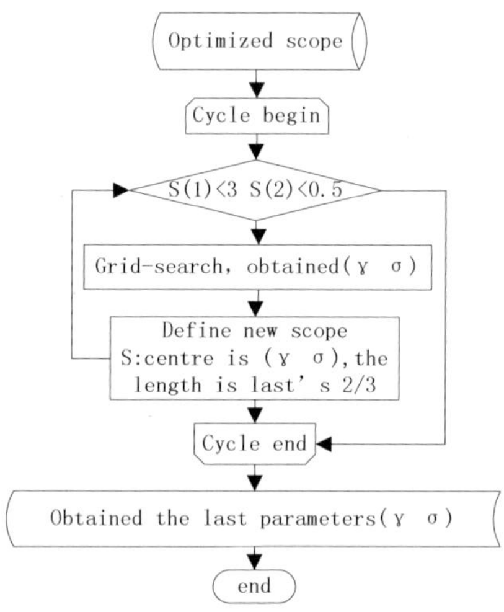

Fig. 4. Process of parameter optimization

5 Verification of Forecasting Performance

It takes an example of Reliability data for a simulating NC's performance failure model to compare the forecasting performance. Table 3 lists the data for the failure model of NC machining accuracy, which corresponding the value of time. In the data set, the values of time and accuracy have already been dealt with the total of 5 data sample. Each simple contains 25 groups data.

We use the first sample to test the forecasting performance. Data 1st to 20th are used as the modeling data set, and those data 21st to 25th are used as the testing data set. The first method's result error is 0.0172 without optimizing parameters. The

Table 3. Degraded data of machining accuracy

t×100/h	sample1	sample 2	sample 3	sample 4	sample 5
0.1	1.389	1.4136	1.4098	1.323	1.4754
0.11611	1.3728	1.396	1.3924	1.3065	1.4574
0.13481	1.3543	1.3759	1.3725	1.2876	1.4369
0.15652	1.3331	1.3529	1.3497	1.2661	1.4134
0.18173	1.309	1.3267	1.3237	1.2414	1.3865
0.211	1.2814	1.2969	1.2942	1.2135	1.3561
0.24498	1.2502	1.2632	1.2607	1.1818	1.3215
0.28444	1.2149	1.225	1.2229	1.146	1.2825
0.33025	1.1752	1.1823	1.1805	1.1058	1.2386
0.38344	1.1307	1.1344	1.1331	1.061	1.1895
0.4452	1.0811	1.0813	1.0804	1.0111	1.135
0.51691	1.0263	1.0228	1.0223	0.95623	1.0748
0.60016	0.96611	0.95879	0.95873	0.89619	1.0089
0.69682	0.90066	0.88948	0.88988	0.8312	0.9375
0.80906	0.8302	0.81527	0.81613	0.76164	0.86087
0.93937	0.75528	0.73684	0.73813	0.68814	0.77973
1.0907	0.67673	0.65519	0.65686	0.61165	0.69505
1.2663	0.59572	0.57168	0.57367	0.53344	0.60821
1.4703	0.51375	0.48797	0.4902	0.4551	0.5209
1.7071	0.43262	0.40604	0.40841	0.37845	0.43513
1.982	0.35435	0.328	0.3304	0.3055	0.3531
2.3013	0.28106	0.25601	0.25832	0.23826	0.27705
2.6719	0.21477	0.19201	0.19412	0.17852	0.20905
3.1023	0.15715	0.13748	0.13931	0.12768	0.15075
3.6019	0.10935	0.093282	0.094776	0.086523	0.10313

second method's result error is 0.0802 with LSSVM.M optimizing parameters. The last result error is 0.00082 with improved method. The result shows that the improved parameter optimization method can improve the accuracy of forecasting performance (shown as Fig.5).

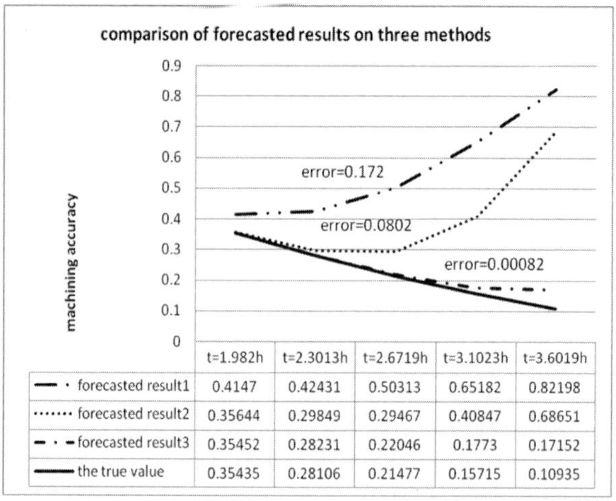

Fig. 5. Comparison of forecasted results with three methods

6 Reliability Assessment Model

The data set samples listed in the Table 3 is subject to exponential distribution. It is fail when the accuracy is equal to or less than 0.05. The function model is established after training the 5 groups data set with support vector machine. Each group of data is modeled with LSSVM.M toolbox based on the Eq.(6), called function model.

Table 4. Forecasted results of 5 samples

t	sample1		sample 2		sample 3		sample 4		sample 5	
	True value	Forecasted value	True value	Forecasted value	True value	Forecasted value	True value	Forecasted value	True value	Forecasted value
1.98	0.3544	0.3545	0.328	0.3277	0.3304	0.3302	0.3055	0.3050	0.3531	0.3528
2.30	0.2811	0.2823	0.2560	0.2536	0.2583	0.2566	0.2383	0.2349	0.2770	0.2753
2.67	0.2148	0.2205	0.1920	0.1812	0.1941	0.1860	0.1785	0.1664	0.2090	0.2051
3.10	0.1572	0.1773	0.1375	0.1007	0.1393	0.1088	0.1277	0.0972	0.1508	0.1520
3.60	0.1094	0.1715	0.0933	0.0873	0.0948	0.0865	0.0865	0.0367	0.1031	0.1509
	error=0.00082		error =0.00064		error =0.00085		error =0.00071		error =0.00046	

From the function model established, we can obtain the value of the time when every group is fail. Take the example of the first training result:

α = (2.1498e+006; 1.4658e+006; -9.4994e+005; -69929; -4.0484e+006; -1.5393e+006;-1.2321e+006;86500;2.2794e+006;2.3802e+006;3.9039e+006; -5.825e+005;-3.899e+006;12987;3.0971e+006;2.1718e+006;1.1881e+006; 2.4562e+006;-3.7323e+006;2.3531e+005;1.5319e+006;-9.09e+005;2.1919e+005; -20667;-22.033);

$b = 3.2511$; $\sigma^2 = 7.5266$.

When the three values are obtained, function model is successfully establish. Then get the value of the failed time: t (1)=146(h), t (2)=235(h),t (3)=800(h), failed times r=3, samples times n=5. So the total time is $T_{r,n}$ =146+235+800+800×2=2781(h).

Failure rate is $\hat{\theta} = \frac{2781}{5} = 566.2$; $\hat{\lambda} = \frac{1}{\hat{\theta}} = 0.001766(h^{-1})$.

In 50h, $\hat{R}(50) = e^{-t_0/\hat{\theta}} = e^{-50/566.2} = 0.9155$.

When $R_0 = 0.9$, $\hat{t}(0.9) = \hat{\theta}\ln\frac{1}{R_0} = 566.2 \cdot \ln\frac{1}{0.9} = 59.6651(h)$;

$$R(50) \geq e^{\frac{t_0\chi^2_{1-\alpha}(2r)}{2T_{r,n}}} = 0.8093\,; \quad t(0.9) \geq \frac{2T_{r,n}\ln\frac{1}{R_0}}{\chi^2_{1-\alpha}(2r)} = 52.2165(h).$$

Table 5. Reliability assessment result

Parameter	Point estimation	L estimation
R(50)	0.9155	0.8093
T(0.9)	59.6651(h)	52.2165(h)

7 Conclusions

The regression performance of the least square support vector tool box LSSVM.M is suitable for fitting the small samples of data sets, but is not good for forecasting. The optimization parameters obtained from grid-searching is the key factor of effecting the result's accuracy. This paper tries to improve the optimized method for forecasting performance. Finally, the prediction result in NC machining accuracy case proves that the improved method was valid and effective.

Acknowledgment

The authors would like to thank the National Basic Research Program, China (No. 2005CB724107), the National Natural Science Foundation, China (No. 50705032), and the National High-Tech. R&D Program, China (No. 2006AA04Z407) for the supporting.

References

1. Smith, T.F., Waterman, M.S.: Identification of Common Molecular Subsequences. J. Mol. Biol. 147, 195–197 (1981)
2. Jun, L.L., Suo, Z.Z., Jia, H.Z.: Research on Machinery State trend's prediction based on Support vector machines. Xi'an Jiaotong University Journal 38, 230–234 (2004)
3. Billinton, R., Allan, R.N.: Reliability Evaluation of Engineering Systems, Concepts and Techniques, 2nd edn. Plenum Press (1992)

4. Reingold, E., Nievergelt, J., Deo, N.: Combinatorial Algorithms: Theory and Practice. Prentice Hall, New Jersey (1977)
5. Marseguerra, M., Masine, R., Zio, E., Cojazzi, G.: Using Neural Networks as Nonlinear Model Interpolators in Variance Decomposition-Based Sensitivity Analysis. In: Third International Symposium on Sensitivity Analysis of Model Output, Madrid (2001)
6. Merrill, H., Schweppe, F.C.: Energy Strategic Planning for Electric Utilities Part I and Part II, Smarte Methodology. IEEE Transactions on Power Apparatus and Systems. PAS 2, 90–101 (1982)
7. Sapio, B.: SEARCH (Scenario Evaluation and Analysis through Repeated Cross- impact Handling). A new method for scenario analysis with an application to the Videotel service in Italy. International Journal of Forecasting 11, 113–131 (1995)
8. Mukerji, R., Lovell, B.: Creating Data Bases for Power Systems Planning Using High Order Linear Interpolation. IEEE Transactions on Power Systems 3, 441–467 (1988)
9. Rahman, S., Shrestha, G.: Analysis of Inconsistent Data in Power Planning. IEEE Transactions on Power Systems 6, 82–95 (1991)
10. Rocco, C.M., Moreno, J.: Fast Monte Carlo reliability evaluation using support vector machine. Reliability Engineer and System Safety 76, 237–243 (2002)
11. Suykens, J.A.K., Branbanter, J.K., Lukas, L.: Weighted least squares support vector machines: robustness and spare approximation[J]. Neurocomputing 48, 85–105 (2002)
12. Burges, J.C.: A tutorial on support vector machines for pattern recognition. Data Mining and Knowledge Discovery 2, 121–167 (2002)

A Multi-aspect Simulation System for Flexible Aircraft Wing Assembly

Jihong Liu and Cheng Zou

School of Mechanical Engineering and Automation, Beihang University,
No.37, Xueyuan Road, Haidian District, Beijing, 100083, China
ryukeiko@buaa.edu.cn, chaferzealot@163.com

Abstract. The utilization of automatic machines controlled numerically is significant for achieving flexible aircraft wing assembly. This paper presents an off-line programming and simulation system for flexible aircraft wing assembly, which is composed of two modules. The off-line programming module generates tool path of drills according to the 3D solid model designed in advance and the accurate position of each part which is provided by optical measuring machine, and then translates it to NC code with taking the process parameters into consideration. This paper details the second module, the visualized simulation module, which validates and optimizes the related assembly process. The scope of simulation covers three aspects, those are, the tool path simulation, NC code simulation and assembly environment simulation. The system is developed based on CATIA and DELMIA. An example of an aircraft wing assembly process is used to illustrate the detail and advantage of the system.

Keywords: Flexible assembly, Visualized simulation, Aircraft wing.

1 Introduction

Aircraft assembly is considered to be the most time-consuming process in aircraft manufacturing because of the labor work and the dedicated fixtures. So the developed countries are dedicated to develop flexible aircraft assembly technology, e.g. JAM (Jigless Aerospace Manufacture) and AWBA (Automated Wing Box Assembly) [1] projects, to reduce the use of the dedicated fixtures and increase the automation.

Automated drilling is a significant part of flexible aircraft assembly. According to the requirements of large aircraft assembly, in order to drill and rivet the huge fuselage of C-17, which is 28×5.5×3.8m in size, Brotje has spent 18 months to design, build and test a new huge riveting robot with ten degrees of freedom for the Boeing Company[2]. Due to the complexity of this robot, programming it manually to finish the riveting has become impossible. Off-line programming for the complex automated machinery becomes critical. To achieve the goal of automatic control, Deneb/IGRIP of Dassault Systems is used to program and incorporate the real-world robotic, peripheral equipment, motion attributes, kinematics, dynamics and I/O logic. In addition, Virtual Numerical Control (Virtual NC) is used to simulate and validate the program generated.

More precise and strict demands are given for drilling of aircraft wings that should be durable, with high quality and realization of the aerodynamic requirements. At the

C. Xiong et al. (Eds.): ICIRA 2008, Part II, LNAI 5315, pp. 679–687, 2008.

same time, the use of composite materials and titanium alloy gives special demands as well [3]. To satisfy these demands, drilling for aircraft wing assembly should be more complex and precise. To improve the correctness of the programming, minimize the risk of failures in machining, and optimize the process planning, simulations are involved to validate the details of automatic assembly processes. However, it is also noted that due to the complexity of aircraft assembly and its process, to simulate all process details in any simple manner is impractical.

This paper presents an off-line programming and simulation system for flexible aircraft wing assembly, which has two modules. The off-line programming module generates tool paths of drills according to the 3D solid model designed in advance and the accurate position of each part which is provided by optical measuring machine, and then translates them to NC codes with taking the process parameters into consideration. The second module, the visualized simulation module, is the main topic of this current paper, which validates and optimizes related assembly process. A multi-aspect simulation strategy is proposed and detailed in this paper.

2 A Brief of Off-Line Programming and Simulation System

The off-line programming and simulation system for aircraft wing assembly realizes two main functions: (1) the off-line programming, and (2) the visualized simulation. Fig. 1 shows the framework of this system.

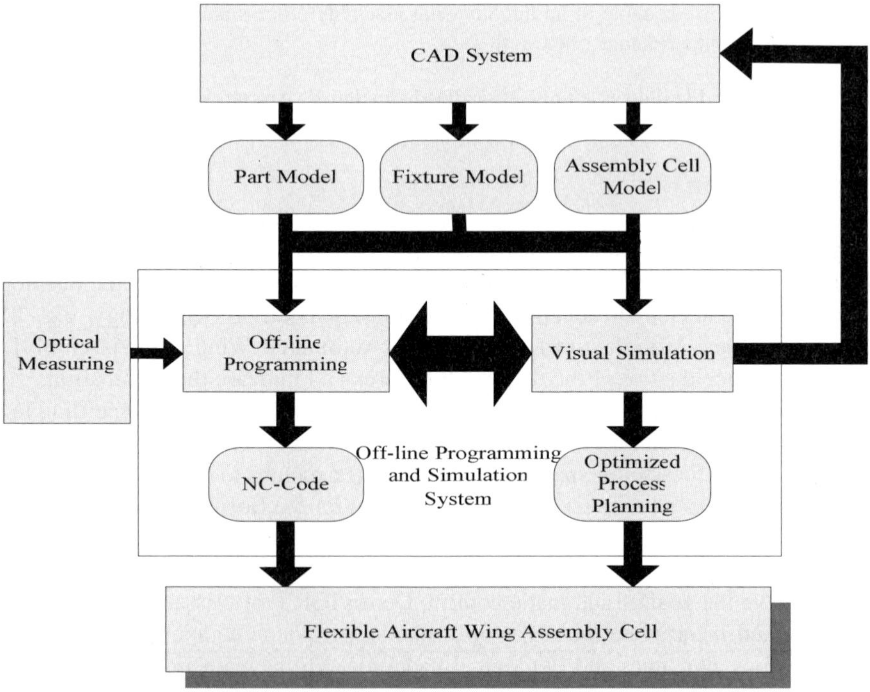

Fig. 1. The framework of off-line programming and simulation system for flexible aircraft wing assembly

In the off-line programming, an optical measuring machine is used to adjust the actual positions of wing parts to accord with their ideal positions. The optical machine provides the coordinates of some key points in the wing parts to modify the CAD models of the wing parts, from which more precise tool path can be gotten. With post-processing, the NC code for flexible aircraft wing assembly is finally obtained with high precision. The generation of tool path and post-processing can be realized with the secondary development of the commercial CAD/CAM software, CATIA.

The off-line programming module can program the NC machine, keep the programmer away from potentially dangerous environment, and generate more reusable and more precise NC code rapidly [4]. Fig. 2 provides the flowchart of the off-line programming module.

In the visualized simulation, the generated tool path is validated and optimized for the off-line programming. By using NC code to drive the movements of drill tool and machines, potential collisions can be detected, and the NC code can be validated. The whole assembly environment composed of the flexible tooling, aircraft wing and drilling machine is also simulated to evaluate and improve the feasibility, rationality and efficiency of the assembly process. The detail of the visualized simulation module is explored in the next section.

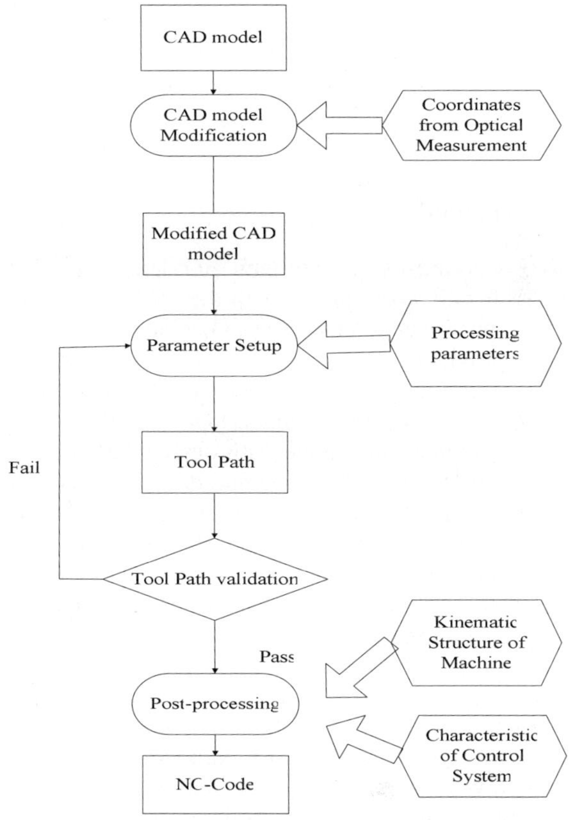

Fig. 2. Flowchart of the off-line programming module

3 Multi-aspect Visualized Simulation

The visualized simulation provides validation and optimization for both NC programming and assembly process planning. Three aspects of visualized simulation are considered in the system, i.e., the tool path simulation, the NC code simulation and the environment simulation. Fig. 3 shows the relationship between the multiple aspects of simulations.

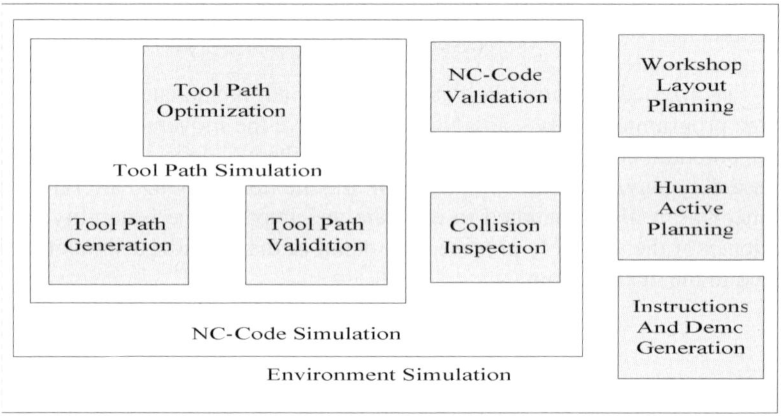

Fig. 3. The relationship between the three aspects of aircraft wing assembly visualized simulation

3.1 Tool Path Simulation

Tool path simulation optimizes the tool path and detects the collision between tools and workpieces [5]. It fully corresponds with the off-line programming, so the errors can be fed back to parameters setup for immediate correction. CATIA Advanced Machining function provides the environment for tool path simulation.

To generate tool path, the machined objects should be selected first. As the holes on aircraft airfoil surface parts are abundant, to choose the machined holes manually is low efficiency and often accompanied with objects missing. Selecting object holes by feature can solve this problem. This method does not only help to setup machined object rapidly but also provide an interface for tool path optimization [6].

The translation, rotation, and changing of tools may cause much additional time in machining, so to generate the tool path with less changes and moves of tools is significant. The tool path optimization is a typical discrete optimization problem, and with optimization algorithms such as genetic algorithm and others, the problem can be settled well. An optimized tool path is shown in Fig.4. The holes with same diameter are selected and the shortest tool path can be chosen automatically.

After all parameters have been set up and features are selected, CATIA Advanced Machining function can generate tool path automatically, which is written in APT format. In order to prevent collisions, overcuts and undercuts in this tool path, CATIA Advanced Machining can simulate drilling process and analyze potential collisions.

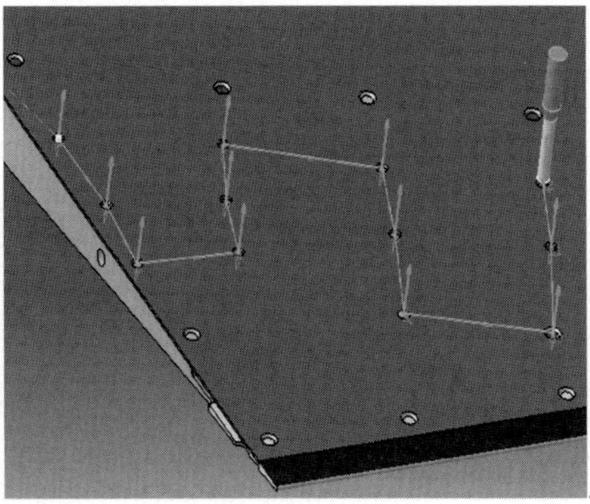

Fig. 4. Optimized tool path and its simulation

3.2 NC Code Simulation

NC code simulation for aircraft assembly is based on construction of NC code simulation model and visualization of drilling process. The simulation model is defined in three parts: geometrical model, kinematic model and collision model.

The geometrical model presents the geometrical performance of machines, tools and fixtures which are involved in the assembly process. It can be gotten from CATIA, but some changes should be made for building the kinematic models. The NC machine dealt with in this paper has a mechanism with five degrees of freedom controlled by SINUMERIK 840Di system.

The kinematic model presents the relationship between the kinematic parts and their kinematic attributes. It is built by five steps: (1) Associate parts with their movements according to the structure of the mechanism. (2) Setup the range of each part, such as displacement type and range, max speed and acceleration. (3) Establish all coordinates cornered with the NC machine. (4) Define accessorial parameters such as initial position. (5) Establish the relationship between NC code and geometrical model's movements by programming the configuration files for simulation. Virtual NC [7] can partially support the visualized simulation in our work. Its configuration files are used to translate the NC code into mechanism movements.

The collision model records collision relationship between parts. It is built by collision chains. According to the process needed, there can be one or more collision chains to bring the parts which may have collisions in the same collision chain for certain checks. The collided or colliding parts will be highlighted with special color as defined when the collision or near-by situation is happening. The collision chain mechanism makes all collision check in one simulation possible. Certain mistakes can be detected by NC code simulation such as out-range or collision, as shown in Fig. 5. These mistakes may be caused by improper layout of the machines, or error of NC code. They will prompt the off-line programming or process redesign.

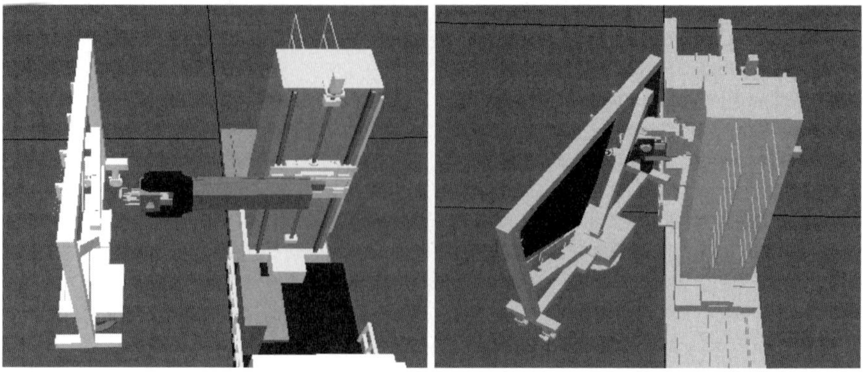

Fig. 5. The left figure shows an out-range error occurring in the machine, and the right one shows a collision between the fixture and the machine. The related parts are highlighted.

3.3 Environment Simulation

The assembly environment simulation is to simulate all the steps of assembly, including the installation of the workpieces, the machine layouts, human actions and so on. The assembly environment simulation can validate the detail of the wing assembly, plan the safety zone for human activity, and correspond to the movements of the machines. Furthermore, with the help of Ergonomics and IGRIP of DELMIA, better environment for workers and control programs for robots can be designed [8].

Based on PPR (product, process, resource) model, DPM (Digital Process Manufacture) in DELMIA V5 provides a platform to simulate the assembly environment. Human, machine, and fixture are defined as Resources. Their actions can be virtualized as Process, and the Product is made after the final process. [9]

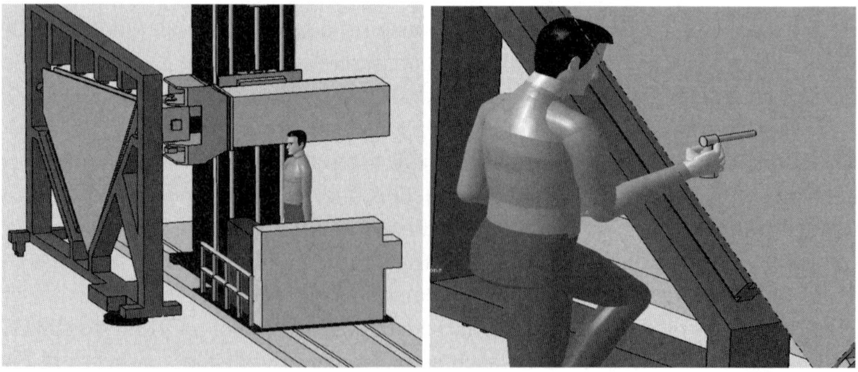

Fig. 6. The general view of the whole wing assembly process. The left one shows the drilling process, and the right one shows the riveting process.

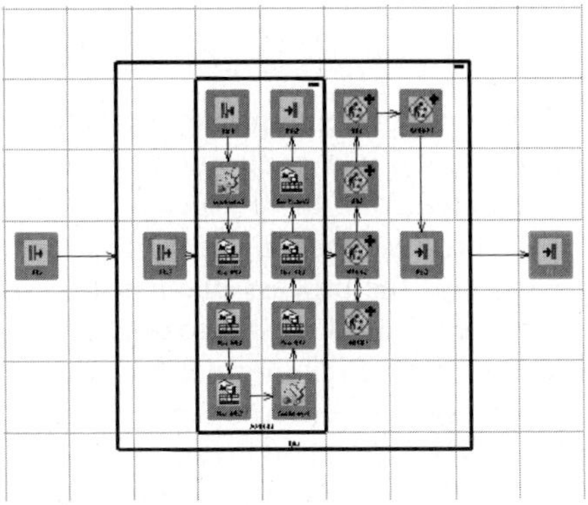

Fig. 7. The PERT chart shows the relationship of the procedures and the activities

Each procedure is defined as Process separately in the PPR tree. All the resources being used are added to the procedure. Each procedure is divided into several activities. Each activity performs certain movements of resources. In this case, design of the process is facility, as the changing the sequence of procedures and process can be separate. The PERT chart can manage these procedures and activities, and the Gantt chart can provide a schedule of the whole process. Fig. 6 is a general view of the whole process. Fig. 7 shows the PERT chart of the process.

In the environment simulation, the ergonomics is involved. There is still some manually work involved, such as machine control, and clamping checking. Simulating human work before real work can provide a demonstration for the workers so that there can be a general idea before work goes on. On the other hand, the safety zone of the workshop can be found by analyzing the comfort of human operators. Fig. 8 shows an optimization of the vision of machine controller.

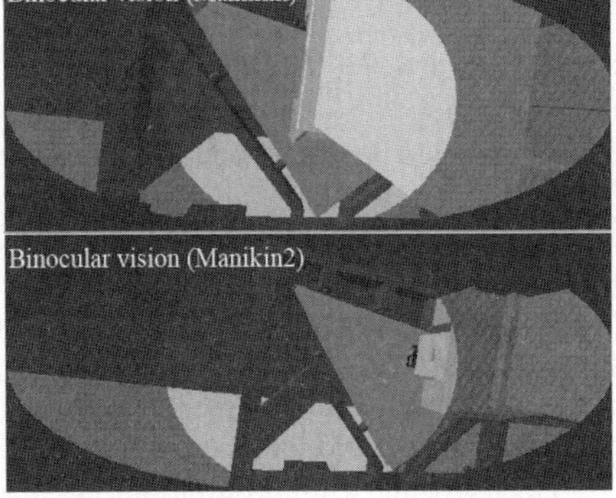

Fig. 8. The poorer visual angle for machine controller (manikin1) as the control platform designed is too close to the drill. A better visual angle (mankin2) design of the control platform changed 50cm further from the drill.

4 Conclusions

This paper presents an off-line programming and simulation system for flexible aircraft wing assembly, with a detailed introduction on multi-aspect simulation strategy. The assembly process is simulated from three aspects for different purposes. The tool path simulation facilitates the process planning on parameters setup level. It generates the optimized tool path, and helps the process planner to know the result of their parameters setup directly so they can select the processing parameters correctly. The NC code simulation fully simulates the machining details. This simulation can provide a correct NC code for machining. The environment simulation concentrates on the whole assembly process level. The workshop layout, human activity and other process details are planned and validated in this simulation. This simulation can give the process planners a full concept of the assembly process and generate the assembly instruction for the assembly operators.

For ordinary products, single-aspect simulation for the whole process may be sufficient. However, for complex products, especially for aircraft, to validate all process details in one simulation is difficult to manipulate because the details to be validated are numerous. The proposed three-aspects of simulation strategy can divide these works into certain levels so the engineers and process planners can dedicate themselves to the current level and error occurrence can be settled immediately.

The machining simulation is widely used in nowadays manufacturing planning, but it is not considered in a systematic way. The multi-aspect simulation can be used in most automated manufacturing especially for the complex product process planning.

Acknowledgments

The authors gratefully acknowledge the fund support from the National High-Tech Research and Development Program of China (863 program), Grant No.2006AA04Z138.

References

1. Jayaweera, N., Webb, P.: Automated Assembly of Fuselage Skin Panels. Assembly Automation 27(4), 343–355 (2007)
2. Robert, D.: Offline Programming and Simulation Help Boeing Use Gant Automated Riveter on C-17 Aircraft. Industrial Robot 28(6), 478–482 (2001)
3. Frederic, L., Robert, P., Francis, C., Laurent, S.: Drilling of Composite Structures. Composite Structures 52(3), 511–516 (2001)
4. Carvalho, G.C., Siqueira, M.L., Absi-Alfaro, S.C.: Off-line Programming of Flexible Welding Manufacturing Cells. Journal of Materials Processing Technology 78(1), 24–28 (1998)
5. Li, J.G., Zhao, H., Yao, Y.X.: Off-line Optimization on NC Machining Based on Virtual Machining. International Journal of Advanced Manufacturing Technology 36(9-10), 908–917 (2008)
6. Sheng, W.H., Xi, N., Song, M.M., Chen, Y.F.: Robot Path Planning for Dimensional Measurement in Automotive Manufacturing. Journal of Computing and Information Science in Engineering 127(2), 420–428 (2005)

7. Liu, H.X., Wang, X., Wu, B., Cai, L.: Virtual NC Laser Cutting Machine Tool and Cutting Process Simulation. In: 4th International Conference on Virtual Reality and Its Application in Industry, pp. 345–350. SPIE Press, Bellingham (2004)
8. Edward, S.P., Christian, B.: Digital Manufacturing: The Virtual Shipyard. Whitepaper. An IBM / Dassault Systems (2003)
9. Butterfield, J., Crosby, S., Curran, R., Price, M., Armstrong, C.G., Raghunathan, S., McAleenan, D., Gibson, C.: Optimization of Aircraft Fuselage Assembly Process Using Digital Manufacturing. Journal of Computing and Information Science in Engineering 7(3), 269–275 (2007)

Design of an RFID-Based Manufacturing Data Tracking System in Plant Production

Guanghui Zhou, Pingyu Jiang, and Mei Zheng

State Key Laboratory for Manufacturing Systems Engineering,
Xi'an Jiaotong University, Xi'an, Shaanxi 710049, China
{ghzhou,pjiang,zhengmei}@mail.xjtu.edu.cn

Abstract. In the past, the manufacturing data related to workpieces and equipment in plants acquired was not real time which has heavily hampered the optimal decision-making on plant production. In this paper, an RFID-based manufacturing data tracking system (RFID-MDTS) is designed to help users to collect the all kinds of data and further track them in real time. Through retrieving and analyzing the useful data, all kinds of users in the plants can guarantee to execute their operations in both time saving and cost effective manner. In this manufacturing data tracking system, the Radio Frequency Identification (RFID) technology is utilized to acquire the data derived from the plant in real time. In order to provide the correspondent data for different users, a time-dependent instantiated template (TIT) model is built to visually describe and supply the concrete data. For demonstrating the validity of the proposed system, a snapshot of running procedure of the prototype is presented which following some concluding remarks.

Keywords: RFID, Data-tracking, Template, Multiple views, Real-time, Plant production.

1 Introduction

To be worldwide competitive, manufacturing systems for enterprises must be flexible, collaborative, and responsive to meet the changing needs of markets so that quality products and services can be delivered in a timely manner [1]. To arrive at this goal, the production control in plants plays an important role. General speaking, the plant production control mainly refers to adopt some new or advanced methods or means to assure that all activities related to the plant production can be executed efficiently and effectively [2][3]. The contents of plant production control mainly contain production planning and scheduling, quality control, and material tracking and decision-making, and so on. In order to implement the validity of plant production control, the real-time acquirement of manufacturing data and further transmission to related users to help them make decisions in a timely manner is becoming the key issue. However, in the traditional plant, there exists a gap between the bottom-level manufacturing sites and the top-level control systems because of lacking the feasible real-time data acquiring and bidirectional transmitting methods and ways, and especially for bottom-level manufacturing data, this problem is expressly serious. The gap heavily influences on

C. Xiong et al. (Eds.): ICIRA 2008, Part II, LNAI 5315, pp. 688–696, 2008.

the efficiency and accuracy of plant production. Though a number of enterprises have introduced and adopted Enterprise Resource Planning (ERP) systems and Materials Resource Planning II (MRP II) systems to help the information transmitting and sharing between the top-level control systems and bottom-level manufacturing sites, the above problem does not be dealt with successfully yet.

Noting this shortcoming, in this paper, an RFID-based manufacturing data tracking system (RFID-MDTS) is presented. This is a real-time manufacturing data acquiring and tracking system incorporating the wireless mobile technology and RFID technology to explore the requirements of users. Using this system, the manufacturing data related to concrete manufacturing sites can be obtained and tracked in the real-time manner. With the help of RFID technology, a flexible and timely manufacturing data accessing and collection framework for the system is achieved. In addition, through adopting the TIT model, the multiple views of manufacturing data correspondent to different users' requirements in the plant are produced. The aim of this system is to maximize both the real-time collection and productive views of manufacturing data which establish the data source for optimal decision-making on plant production control.

2 RFID Technology and Its Applications

RFID is a technology which allows remote interrogation of objects using radio waves to read data from RFID tags which are at some distance from an RFID reader. This has several advantages over manual scanning using optical barcodes, since many tagged items could be simultaneously identified in an automated manner, very quickly and without the need for line-of-sight to each item [4][5].

Generally speaking, an RFID system typically comprises the following three components [6]:

- An RFID device (tag);
- A tag reader with an antenna and transceiver; and
- A host system or connection to an enterprise control system.

Fig. 1 illustrates the relationship of three components and working mechanism in an RFID system.

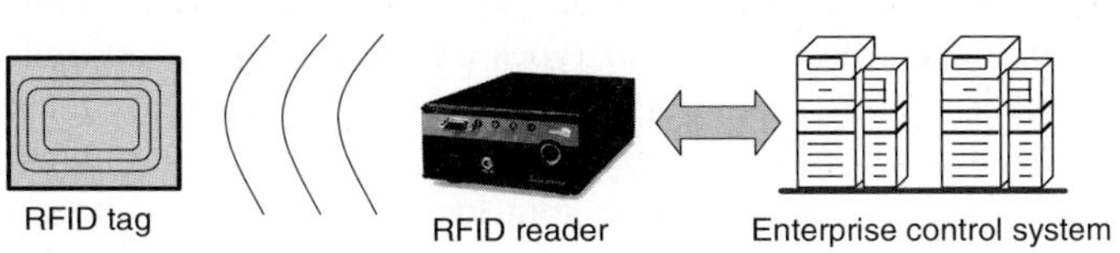

Fig. 1. A typical RFID system

Currently, the RFID technology and systems has been widely applied in numerous areas including logistics and supply chain management, product manufacture and assembly, aero baggage transaction, post/giggited package transaction, library management, and roadway automatic charge, etc. which has gained the notable effects. In the product manufacture and assembly area, Huang et al presented an affordable solution to the walking-worker fixed-position flexible assembly line by using wireless manufacturing (WM) and RFID technology. Through deploying the WM and RFID technology to implement the real-time manufacturing information visibility and traceability, the concept of Just-In-Time (JIT) manufacturing to reduce the plant work-in-progress (WIP) inventories and smoothening their flows was realized well[7]. Thiesse et al. we investigated the value of real-time location systems (RTLSs) information on the locations of physical objects in complex manufacturing processes to the problem of efficient job scheduling and proposed a simplified simulation model that captures the main characteristics and information of the real manufacturing process[8]. In order to implement the integration of factory systems efficiently and effectively, Qiu proposed an RFID-based method to bridge the gap between shop floor automation and factory information systems[1]. The above research provides the methods and implementing techniques for our study.

3 Overall Architecture of RFID-MDTS

The proposed system in this paper is used for manufacturing controllers in plants to enhance their correspondent operations by means of collecting and tracking the manufacturing information utilization. RFID-MDTS takes advantages of the wireless mobile technology and a multi-view information retrieval engine to precisely collect, track, and manage the manufacturing data in the plant. The overall architecture of RFID-MDTS is illustrated in Fig. 2 which is composed by two basic modules i.e. front-end module and back-end module.

3.1 Front-End Module

The front-end module mainly answers for manufacturing data collection and transfer which provides functional applications on radio frequency signal transferring, data filtering and processing. In the manufacturing plant, the types of manufacturing data mainly include the workpiece-related data such as workpiece's name, current status, location, batch, and quality, machine-related data liking machine's name, status, task sequence, loading, and so on, and resource-related data such as materials, WIP, cutting tools, measures and clamps, and so on which are the base for plant control. In order to implement the collection of all types of data, in this front-end module, we take advantage of low-power radio signals to exchange the data wirelessly between the passive tags and readers. The passive tags are attached on the items like pallets, workpieces, shelf or operators to record item identity. The tag readers, on the other hand, are integrated to fix positioned antenna that are mounted on objects such as machine entrance and export, dock door, forklift or other facilities. The received signals and data will be decoded and passed through a data connection device to the application server that runs the production control logic. The function of the connection device is to exchange data between the readers and manufacturing data management engine via the wireless LAN.

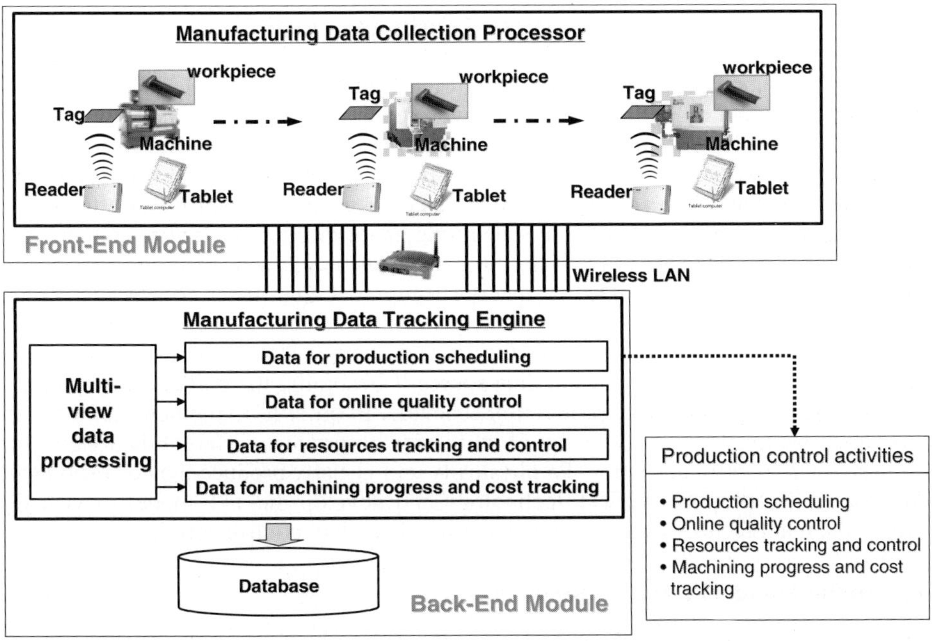

Fig. 2. Overall architecture of RFID-MDTS

3.2 Back-End Module

The back end of RFID-MDTS is used for manufacturing data filtering, processing and management. It acts as a server that stores all tags data and provides an executive environment for the data manipulation software to manage, filter and transmit all the useful data to the manufacturing data tracking engine for supporting the all kinds of plant control activities and making decisions. It is the foundation for manufacturing data tracking engine to perform the plant control activities like production scheduling, online quality control, resources tracking and control and machining progress and cost tracking. Because different plant control activities require the supports of different kinds of manufacturing data, in order to satisfy the requirement, the back-end module should have the capability of translating the tags data into the acceptable formats related to the correspondent plant control activities. To arrive at this objective, the time-dependent instantiated template (TIT) model is built to visually produce the multi-view manufacturing data whose working mechanism and logic is described in detail in the next section.

In the back-end module, the database is used to store all data from different internal systems as well as from external sources. The internal data source contains workpiece data, equipment data, material data and operator data that come from the manufacturing data tracking engine. In contrast, the external data mainly relates to orders and control instructions interfaced from the plant's or enterprise's business logic. In general, the database manages and exchanges all data between different internal and external systems.

4 TIT Model for Manufacturing Data Tracking

As described above, different plant control activities require different formats of manufacturing data to make decision. However, the manufacturing data obtained by the RFID system in real time always is isomerous and is not classified for specific plant control activities. Therefore, it is difficult to filter and organize the useful data to help correspondent plant control activities make decisions efficiently and effectively. For example, concerning production scheduling, the useful manufacturing data mainly refers to workpieces' name, due date, process plans, equipment loading, staring and finishing machining time related to specific equipment, and material data, etc. which serves as a data source for supporting the production schedule decision, but actually they are stored in the whole manufacturing data source. Thus, how to retrieve these data from the whole manufacturing data source is becoming the bottleneck to guarantee the efficient and effective production schedule. In order to implement this goal, in this paper, we introduce the concept of multi-view to produce different data views for different plant control activities. To physically and visually produce the correspondent data views, we propose the TIT technology and develop the TIT model to visually supply the manufacturing data for the correspondent plant control activities.

4.1 Definition of TIT and Its Structure

TIT is defined as a container of manufacturing data. Just like the concept of class in computer programming, a TIT only contains the names of manufacturing data but not contains the concrete content. In order to supply different manufacturing data to different plant control activities, the different specific TITs have to be designed and developed. As described above, for the plant control, there exist a number of activities such as production schedule, quality control, material tracking and cost tracking and each activities may contains a series of sub-activities which emerge as a complicated networked diagram, therefore, the TITs corresponding to the plant control activities also emerge as the networked diagram. Fig. 3 illustrates the structure of the TITs networked diagram.

When the plant control activities require the correspondent manufacturing data to make decisions, they correspondent TITs are transferred and instantiated by the real-time manufacturing data. During the plant control activities execution, the manufacturing data in the instantiated TIT is continually filled out or updated automatically.

4.2 Mathematical Description of TIT Selection for Plant Control Activities

Because each TIT is the set of manufacturing data and each plant control activity only corresponds to the definite accessible data, how to select the usable TIT for each activity is becoming the important issue.

In order to describe the relationship between the TITs and plant control activities, we design a series of matrix to arrive at the goal which are expressed in the following:

- **The relationship matrix of plant control activities:** to describe the accessible manufacturing data for plant control activities shown as follows

$$M_{UM} = \begin{bmatrix} 1 & 1 & 0 & 0 & 0 & \cdots & 0 \\ 0 & 0 & 0 & 1 & 1 & \cdots & \\ 0 & 0 & 0 & 0 & 0 & \cdots & 1 \end{bmatrix} \tag{1}$$

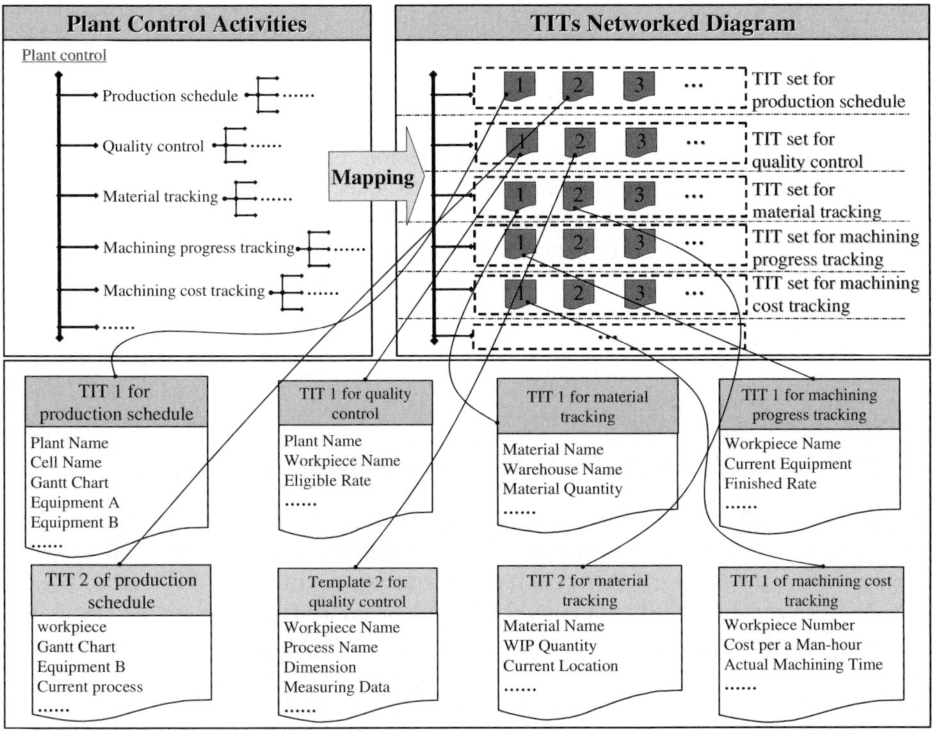

Fig. 3. Structure of TITs networked diagram

Where the rows represent the plant control activities and the columns represent the accessible manufacturing data for each correspondent plant control activities. In this matrix, "1" represents there exists the accessible manufacturing data for plant control activities whilst "0" represents no manufacturing data for plant control activities.

- **The relationship matrix of TITs:** to describe the accessible manufacturing data the correspondent TITs contain described in the following:

$$M_{TM} = \begin{bmatrix} 1 & 1 & 1 & \cdots & 1 \\ 1 & 1 & 0 & \cdots & 1 \\ 1 & 1 & 1 & \cdots & 0 \\ \cdots & \cdots & \cdots & \cdots & \cdots \\ 1 & 0 & 0 & \cdots & 0 \end{bmatrix} \tag{2}$$

Where rows represent the TITs and columns represent the manufacturing data that each TIT contains.

- **The relationship matrix of plant control activities and TITs:** to describe the relationship between the plant control activities and TITs which are described in the following:

$$M_{UT} = \begin{bmatrix} 1 & 0 & 0 & \cdots & 0 \\ 0 & 0 & 1 & \cdots & 0 \\ 0 & 0 & 0 & \cdots & 1 \end{bmatrix} \tag{3}$$

Where the rows represent the plant control activities and the columns represents the correspondent TIT for each plant control activity. This relationship matrix is deduced by matrix (1) and (2). The deducing logic is described as follows:

Firstly, compare the accessible manufacturing data of plant control activities in matrix (1) with manufacturing data related to correspondent TITs in matrix (2) and obtain the accessible TITs for each plant control activities; and then, for each plant control activities, select the TIT which contains the maximum data items as its final TIT. On the basis of this deducing logic, each plant control activity only has a optimal TIT which is shown in matrix (3).

4.3 pcXML-Based Manufacturing Data Description and Tracking

The designed TITs provide the organizational model of manufacturing data for plant control activities. In order to implement the standardized description of all kinds of manufacturing data and effective exchange them among different TITs or activities, pcXML ((eXtensible Markup Language for plant control) is devised to act as the uniform describing language for manufacturing data. pcXML is the special-purpose language devised in this paper for defining the manufacturing data in TITs which is based on XML. The TIT definition encompasses two aspects: general TIT description information and defining the manufacturing data structure and contents.

In pcXML, each TIT component is defined by the "TIT" tag – the pair of brackets ""<Targent …> … </Targent>". Each TIT is defined with several key attributes including "id" and "name". The "id" attribute is unique to the TIT and must not be the same between any two TITs. Fig. 4 illustrates a snapshot of TIT description based on pcXML. Based on this method, the manufacturing data contained in TITs can be described in the standard manner which provides the way for the convenient and effective manufacturing data tracking and sharing in plant control.

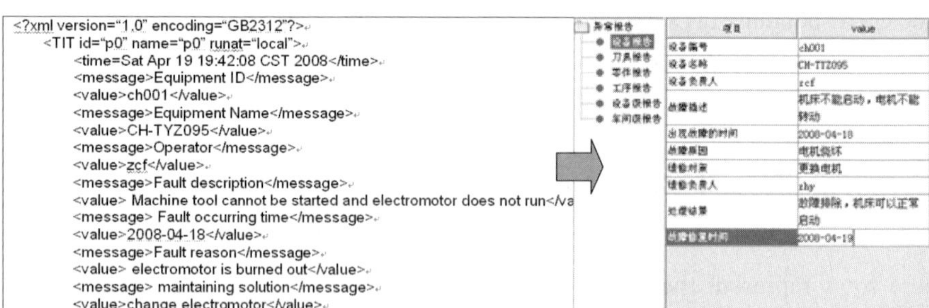

Fig. 4. The snapshot of TIT description based on pcXML

5 Case Study

Based on the above methods and technologies, we develop a prototype of RFID-based manufacturing data tracking system. In this prototype, through taking advantage of RFID system and TIT model, we implement the manufacturing data collection, filtering, transmitting and sharing which provides the real-time manufacturing data for intelligent plant control decisions. Fig. 5 is the snapshot of manufacturing data tracking in the plant control. In this figure, the decisions on production scheduling, online quality control, material tracking and control, machining progress tracking and machining cost tracking are implemented well.

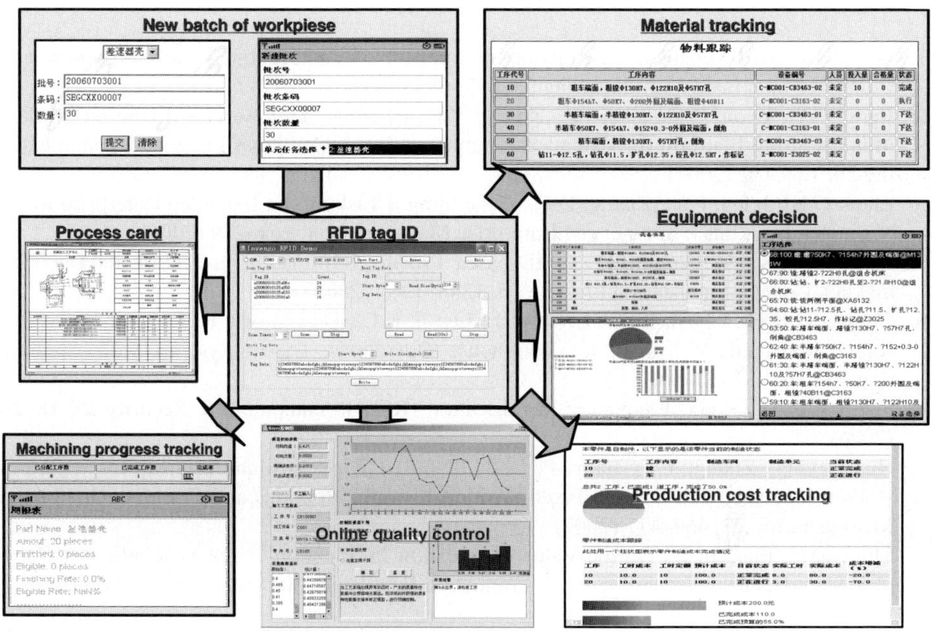

Fig. 5. The snapshot of manufacturing data tracking in the plant control

6 Concluding Remarks

This paper mainly has discussed the manufacturing data real-time acquiring and tracking methods and technologies in the plant production control. In general, plant production control is a complicated systematical engineering, which relates to all kinds of activities and has a lot of intelligent deciding behaviors. Because of lacking the methods and means of acquiring the manufacturing data in real time, the traditional production control methods cannot satisfy the real plant production control requirement well. To deal with this problem, in this paper, we have introduced the RFID technology and developed an RFID-based manufacturing data tracking system. The presented system can implement the acquiring, filtering, transmitting and sharing of manufacturing data in real time produced at the correspondent sites which can fully provides the specific manufacturing data for the correspondent plant production control activities to make decisions. The presented methods and technologies and developed prototype establish the base for the study of intelligent plant production control.

Acknowledgments

Gratitude is extended to National Natural Science Foundation of China (Grant No.: 50605050 and Grant No.: 50575174) for the financial support.

References

1. Qiu, R.G.: RFID-enabled Automation in Support of Factory Integration. Robotics and Computer-Integrated Manufacturing 23, 677–683 (2007)
2. Jiang, P.Y., Zhou, G.H., Zhao, G., Zhang, Y.F.: e2-MES: An e-Service-driven Networked Manufacturing Platform for Extended Enterprises. Int. J. Computer Integrated Manufacturing 20, 127–142 (2007)
3. Zhou, G.H., Jiang, P.Y., Zhang, D.H.: Generating a Task-driven Extended Enterprise for e-Manufacturing. Int. J. Internet and Enterprise Management 3, 264–279 (2005)
4. Parlikad, A.K., McFarlane, D.: RFID-based Product Information in End-of-life Decision making. Control Engineering Practice 15, 1348–1363 (2007)
5. Chowa, H.K.H., Choya, K.L., Lee, W.B., Lee, L.K.C.: Design of a RFID Case-based Resource Management System for Warehouse Operations. Expert Systems with Applications 30, 561–576 (2006)
6. Roberts, C.M.: Radio Frequency Identification (RFID). Computers & Security 25, 18–26 (2006)
7. Huang, G.Q., Zhang, Y.F., Jiang, P.Y.: RFID-based Wireless Manufacturing for Walking-worker Assembly Islands with Fixed-position Layouts. Robotics and Computer-Integrated Manufacturing 23, 469–477 (2007)
8. Thiesse, F., Fleisch, E.: On the Value of Location Information to Lot Scheduling in Complex Manufacturing Processes. Int. J. Production Economics 30, 1321–1335 (2008)

A Visual Servoing System for the Torch Alignment to Initial Welding Position

Zhiguo Yan[1,2], De Xu[1], and Yuan Li[3]

[1] Key Laboratory of Complex System and Intelligent Sciences, Institute of Automation, Chinese Academy of Sciences, Beijing, 100190

[2] Graduate University of Chinese Academy of Science, Beijing, 100049

[3] Department of Information Science and Technology, Beijing Institute of Technology, Beijing, 100081

zhgyanchn@yahoo.com, sdxude@yahoo.com, liyuan@compsys.ia.ac.cn

Abstract. It is an important aspect to locate the initial welding position automatically. In this paper, a visual servoing system is proposed. Two CCD cameras are employed as the senseors to get the information of the welding seam. The designed visual servoing controller, which is based on Takigi-Sugeno (T-S) fuzzy model, is applied to the stepper motors to adjust the welding torch in the up-down and left-right direction. Experimental results are provided to demonstrate the validity of the proposed system.

Keywords: welding automation, initial welding position, visual servoing, T-S fuzzy model.

1 Introduction

Arc welding is the most common method of permanently joining metallic pieces together. It plays an important role in machinery manufacture. Over the last thirty years, welding automation has received considerable interest because of its merits, such as higher quality and higher productivity.

One of the tasks of the welding automation is to align the welding torch to the initial welding position automatically. At present, industrial welding vehicles are the most widely used welding tools in the field. Generally, the welding torch is adjusted manually to the initial welding position before welding. However, under some situations, the method of locating the initial welding position automatically is needed. Some efforts have been made in automated welding community to deal with this problem. In Ref [1], the guiding of initial welding position was researched, but it cannot meet the requirements of practical production because of the big deviation. Chen [2] presented a vision-based system to guide the welding robot to the initial welding position of the weld seam. In his system, calibration is needed.

Guiding a robotic system using the information obtained from cameras has been studied for decades(Ref [3], [4]). visual servoing is classified into three groups such as position-based visual servoing (Ref [5]), image-based visual servoing (Ref [6]), and hybrid visual servoing (Ref [7]). Here, a vision system, which is based on image-based visual servoing and T-S fuzzy model (Ref [8], [9]), is designed to locate the

C. Xiong et al. (Eds.): ICIRA 2008, Part II, LNAI 5315, pp. 697–706, 2008.

initial welding position. Two un-calibrated CCD cameras are exploited to get the information of the welding seam.

The remainder of this paper is structured as follows. Section 2 introduces the structure of the system. The image features selection and errors detection are given in section 3. In Section 4, the visual servoing strategy is given in detail. Experiments are provided to verify the effectiveness of the algorithm in section 5. Finally, the paper is concluded in Section 6.

2 The Structure and Principle of the System

The overall vision system is composed of an industrial welding vehicle, an industrial control computer, two CCD mini cameras, and an image grabber card. The two cameras are mounted behind the welding torch where the torch tip can be seen.

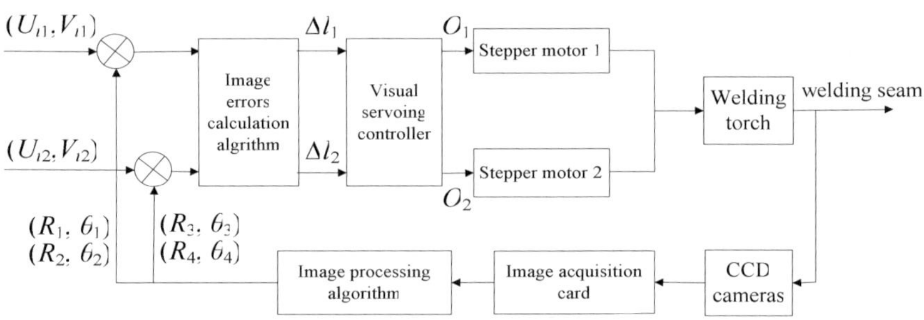

Fig. 1. Block diagram of the system

Fig. 1 is the block diagram of the system. (U_{t1}, V_{t1}) and (U_{t2}, V_{t2}) are the image coordinates of the welding torch tip in images captured by camera 1 and camera 2, respectively. They are invariable because the relation between the welding torch and two cameras are fixed. The symbols in Fig. 1 are explained as follows. The reference image coordinates (U_{t1}, V_{t1}) and (U_{t2}, V_{t2}) are obtained manually before the working process. (R_1, θ_1) and (R_2, θ_2) are the parameters of the two feature lines of the welding seam in images captured by camera 1. (R_3, θ_3) and (R_4, θ_4) are these parameters in images captured by camera 2. Δl_1 and Δl_2 are the image errors and the input of the visual sevoing controller. O_1 and O_2 are the output of the controller to the stepper motors. The welding torch is adjusted in two directions. Stepper motor 1 and 2 adjust the welding torch in left-right and up-down direction, respectively.

Before the working process, the industrial welding torch is adjusted to the initial welding position in front-back direction. When the working process starts, the two cameras take pictures of the welding seam, and then the image grabber transfers them to the computer. The image processing algorithm detects the features of the seam. The errors are calculated directly in image space. According to the image errors, the movements of the torch are determined by the visual servoing controller.

3 The Image Features Selection and Errors Detection

In a vision system, the selection of the image features is very important. Fig. 2 gives an example of the captured welding seam picture, where FL_1 and FL_2 are the two feature lines. T denotes the welding torch tip. The image processing task is to detect FL_1 and FL_2 reliably.

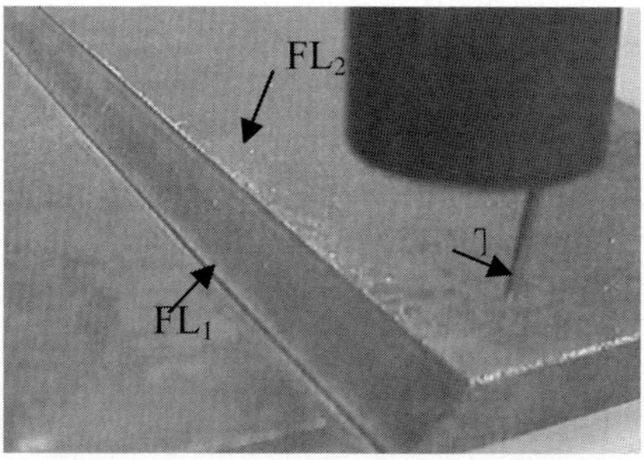

Fig. 2. The captured welding seam picture

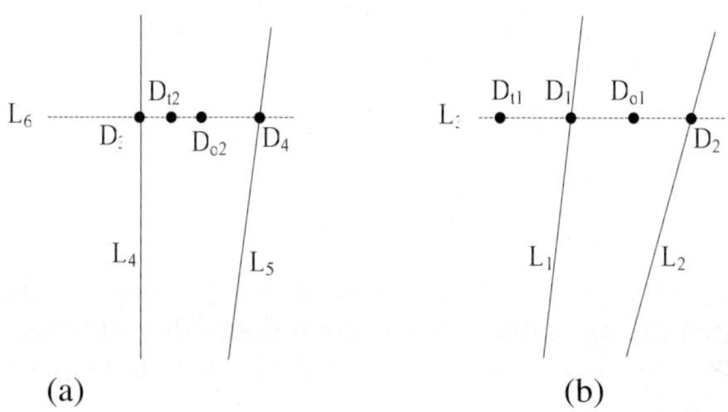

Fig. 3. The calculation of image errors. (a) The feature lines extracted from images captured by camera 1; (b) The feature lines extracted from images captured by camera 2.

$$\begin{cases} U_{o1} = \dfrac{U_{i1} + U_{i2}}{2} \\ V_{o1} = \dfrac{V_{i1} + V_{i2}}{2} \end{cases} \tag{1}$$

After the straight feature lines are tracked out by the image processing algorithm (Ref [10]), the image errors are calculated. Fig. 3 demonstrates the calculation of the image errors. Fig. 3(a) and 3(b) represent the feature lines extracted from images captured by camera 1 and camera 2, separately. L_1 and L_2 are the two feature lines in the image captured by camera 1. Point D_{t1} denotes the welding torch tip, whose image coordinate is (U_{t1}, V_{t1}). Line L_3 is the line $V = V_{t1}$. Point D_1 and D_2 are the intersections of L_3 with L_1 and L_2, respectively. And (U_{i1}, V_{i1}), (U_{i2}, V_{i2}) are the image coordinates of D_1 and D_2. Point D_{o1} is the midpoint of line segment D_1D_2, its image coordinate (U_{o1}, V_{o1}) is given by equation (1). The definitions of L_4, L_5, L_6, D_3, D_4, D_{t2}, and D_{o2} are similar to those of L_1, L_2, L_3, D_1, D_2, D_{t1}, and D_{o1}.

The distance between D_t and D_o is selected as the image error Δl_1. The other image error Δl_2 is calculated in the same way, as shown in equation (2).

$$\begin{cases} \Delta l_1 = U_{t1} - U_{o1} \\ \Delta l_2 = U_{t2} - U_{o2} \end{cases} \quad (2)$$

4 The Visual Servoing Strategy

In this section, the visual servoing strategy is given in detail. The controller is designed according to the distribution of Δl_1 and Δl_2. The four distribution situations are shown in Fig. 4 - Fig. 7. Fig. 4(a), 5(a), 6(a) and 7(a) show the relations among the cameras, welding torch and welding seam in different situations, respectively. In these figures, point C_1 and C_2 are the optical centres of camera 1 and camera 2. Point T is the welding torch tip. T_1 is the intersection of line C_1T with the surface of the work-piece and T_2 is the intersection of line C_2T with the surface of the work-piece. Fig. 4(b), 5(b), 6(b) and 7(b) show the feature lines extracted from the images captured by camera 1 in different situations. Fig. 4(c), 5(c), 6(c) and 7(c) show the feature lines extracted from the images captured by camera 2. The symbols in these figures have the same meaning as they are in Fig. 3(a) and 3(b). It should be noticed that only in Fig. 4, D_{o1} and D_{o2} represent the same point in Cartesian space. In Fig.5 – Fig. 7, they represent different point in Cartesian space. Based on equation (2) and Fig. 4 - Fig. 7, the distributions of image errors, the relations between the welding torch and the welding seam, and the corresponding adjustments are concluded as follows.

(1) Situation 1: $\Delta l_1 = 0$ and $\Delta l_2 = 0$. The welding torch is at the welding seam centre. There is no need to adjust the welding torch under this situation. Actually, in the propose system, adjustments are not needed too if $|\Delta l_1|$=Δt and $|\Delta l_2|<\Delta t$. Here, Δt is a preset threshold.
(2) Situation 2: Fig. 5(b) and 5(c) demonstrate that $\Delta l_1 < 0$ and $\Delta l_2 < 0$. From Fig. 5(a), it can be seen that the welding torch is at the left of the centre of the welding seam. The welding torch should be adjusted to right under this situation.
(3) Situation 3: In Fig. 6, the image errors $\Delta l_1 > 0$ and $\Delta l_2 > 0$. The welding torch is at the right of the centre of the welding seam. And the welding torch should be adjusted to left under this situation.
(4) Situation 4: Under this situation, $\Delta l_1 > 0$ and $\Delta l_2 < 0$. Fig. 7 demonstrates that the welding torch should be adjusted downwards. Similarly, the torch should be adjusted in the same way if $\Delta l_1 < 0$ and $\Delta l_2 > 0$. Particularly; when $\Delta l_1\Delta l_2$=0, and Δl_1+Δl_2≠0, Downward adjustment is also conducted to the welding torch.

Based on above conclusions, two T-S fuzzy systems are designed to control the welding torch in the left-right direction and up-down direction. Δl_1 and Δl_2 are the two inputs. The outputs are pulse numbers for the two stepper motors. In the two fuzzy systems, most of the fuzzy rules have the expression shown as below.

R_1^m: IF Δl_1 is $\Delta\tilde{l}_1$ and Δl_2 is $\Delta\tilde{l}_2$ THEN

$$p_1^m = a_1^m \Delta l_1 + a_2^m \Delta l_2$$

R_2^m: IF Δl_1 is $\Delta\tilde{l}_1$ and Δl_2 is $\Delta\tilde{l}_2$ THEN

$$p_2^m = b_1^m \Delta l_1 + b_2^m \Delta l_2$$

where R_1^m and R_2^m denote the m-th fuzzy rule of the two systems, and m=1, 2, … , 25. p_1^m and p_2^m are the m-th output. a_1^m, a_2^m, b_1^m, b_2^m are the model parameters of the fuzzy system.

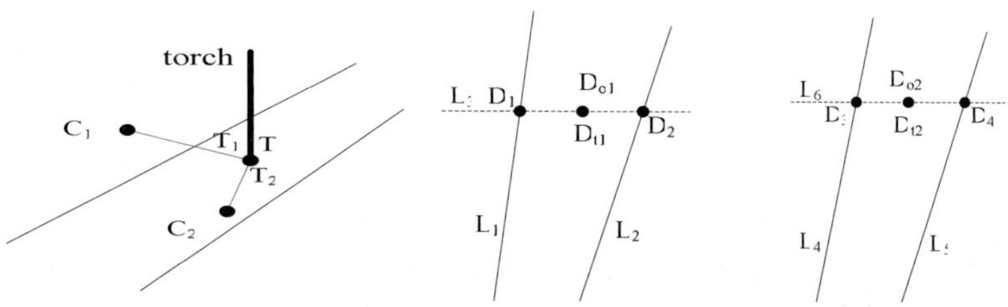

(a) (b) (c)

Fig. 4. Situation 1: the welding torch is at the seam centre. (a) The relations among the cameras, welding torch and welding seam; (b) The feature lines extracted from the images captured by camera 1; (c) The feature lines extracted from the images captured by camera 2.

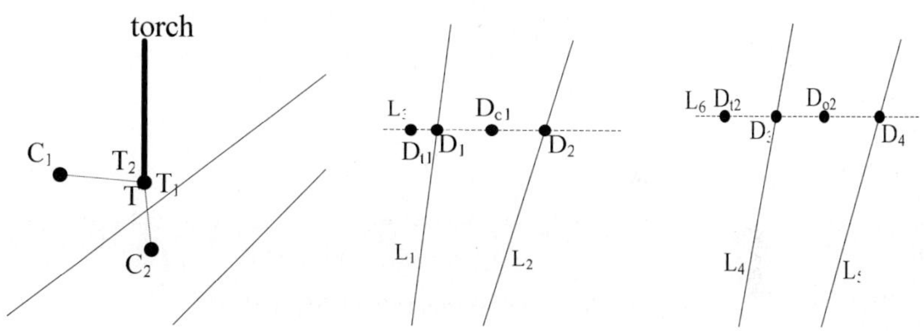

(a) (b) (c)

Fig. 5. Situation 2: the welding torch is at the left of the seam centre. (a) The relations among the cameras, welding torch and welding seam; (b) The feature lines extracted from the images captured by camera 1; (c) The feature lines extracted from the images captured by camera 2.

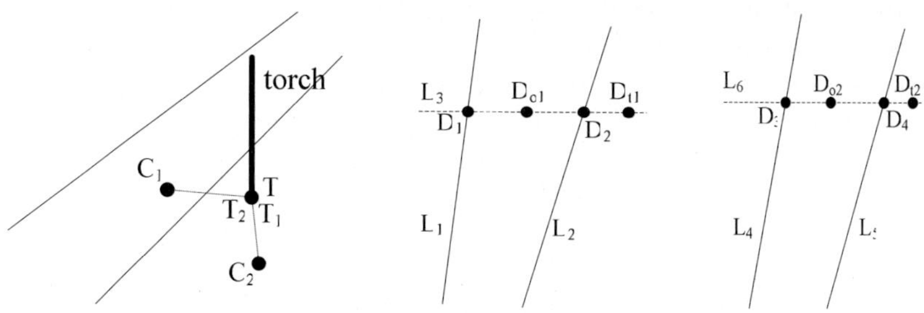

(a) (b) (c)

Fig. 6. Situation 3: the welding torch is at the right of the seam centre. (a) The relations among the cameras, welding torch and welding seam; (b) The feature lines extracted from the images captured by camera 1; (c) The feature lines extracted from the images captured by camera 2.

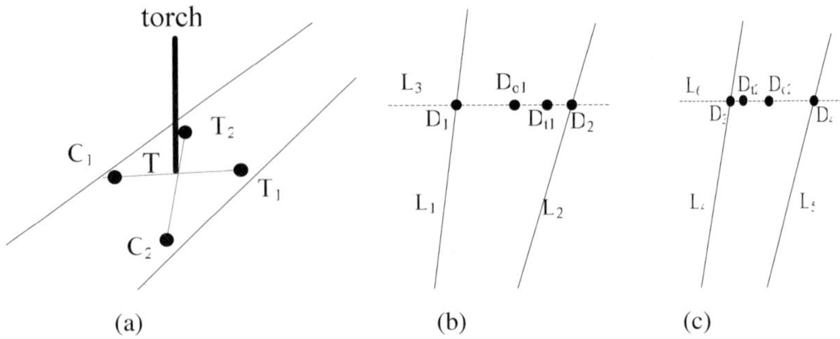

Fig. 7. Situation 4: the welding torch is above the seam centre. (a) The relations among the cameras, welding torch and welding seam; (b) The feature lines extracted from the images captured by camera 1; (c) The feature lines extracted from the images captured by camera 2.

$\Delta\tilde{l}_1$ and $\Delta\tilde{l}_2$ denote the fuzzy sets of Δl_1 and Δl_2. $\Delta\tilde{l}_1$, $\Delta\tilde{l}_2 \in \{$NB, NS, Z, PS, PB$\}$. Here, fuzzy sets NB, NS, Z, PS and PB denote negative big, negative small, zero, positive small and positive big, respectively. Fig. 8 shows the membership function. Where, $\mu(\Delta l_1)$ and $\mu(\Delta l_2)$ are the memberships of the input variables Δl_1 and Δl_2.

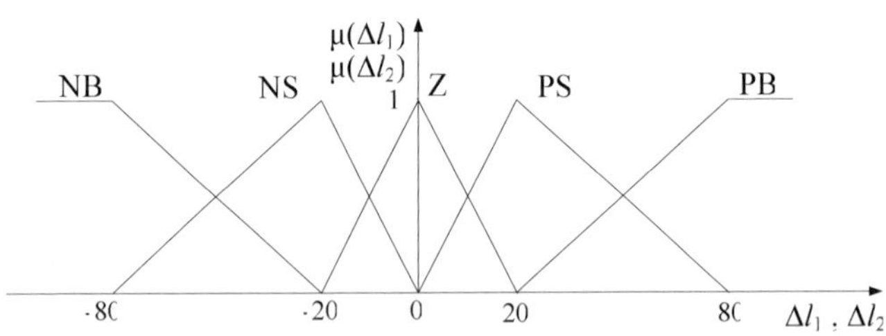

Fig. 8. Membership function of Δl_1 and Δl_2

Not all the fuzzy rules have the same expression. Both of the two fuzzy systems have eight specific rules. These rules are shown as follows.

R_1^3: IF Δl_1 is NB and Δl_2 is Z, THEN
$p_1^3 = -\text{sgn}(\Delta l_2)\,[1-\text{sgn}(\Delta l_2)]\,(a_1^3\Delta l_1+a_2^3\Delta l_2)$

R_1^8: IF Δl_1 is NS and Δl_2 is Z, THEN
$p_1^8 = -\text{sgn}(\Delta l_2)\,[1-\text{sgn}(\Delta l_2)]\,(a_1^8\Delta l_1+a_2^8\Delta l_2)$

R_1^{11}: IF Δl_1 is Z and Δl_2 is NB, THEN
$p_1^{11} = -\text{sgn}(\Delta l_1)\,[1-\text{sgn}(\Delta l_1)]\,(a_1^{11}\Delta l_1+a_2^{11}\Delta l_2)$

R_1^{12}: IF Δl_1 is Z and Δl_2 is NS, THEN
$p_1^{12} = -\text{sgn}(\Delta l_1)\,[1-\text{sgn}(\Delta l_1)]\,(a_1^{12}\Delta l_1+a_2^{12}\Delta l_2)$

R_1^{14}: IF Δl_1 is Z and Δl_2 is PB, THEN
$p_1^{14} = \text{sgn}(\Delta l_1)\,[1+\text{sgn}(\Delta l_1)]\,(a_1^{14}\Delta l_1+a_2^{14}\Delta l_2)$

R_1^{15}: IF Δl_1 is Z and Δl_2 is PS, THEN
$p_1^{15} = \text{sgn}(\Delta l_1)\,[1+\text{sgn}(\Delta l_1)]\,(a_1^{15}\Delta l_1+a_2^{15}\Delta l_2)$

R_1^{18}: IF Δl_1 is PS and Δl_2 is Z, THEN
$p_1^{18} = \text{sgn}(\Delta l_2)\,[1+\text{sgn}(\Delta l_2)]\,(a_1^{18}\Delta l_1 + a_2^{18}\Delta l_2)$
R_1^{23}: IF Δl_1 is PB and Δl_2 is Z, THEN
$p_1^{23} = \text{sgn}(\Delta l_2)\,[1+\text{sgn}(\Delta l_2)]\,(a_1^{23}\Delta l_1 + a_2^{23}\Delta l_2)$
R_2^{3}: IF Δl_1 is NB and Δl_2 is Z, THEN
$p_2^{3} = [1+\text{sgn}(\Delta l_2)]\,(b_1^{3}\Delta l_1 + b_2^{3}\Delta l_2)$
R_2^{8}: IF Δl_1 is NS and Δl_2 is Z, THEN
$p_2^{8} = [1+\text{sgn}(\Delta l_2)]\,(b_1^{8}\Delta l_1 + b_2^{8}\Delta l_2)$
R_2^{11}: IF Δl_1 is Z and Δl_2 is NB, THEN
$p_2^{11} = [1+\text{sgn}(\Delta l_1)]\,(b_1^{11}\Delta l_1 + b_2^{11}\Delta l_2)$
R_2^{12}: IF Δl_1 is Z and Δl_2 is NS, THEN
$p_2^{12} = [1+\text{sgn}(\Delta l_1)]\,(b_1^{12}\Delta l_1 + b_2^{12}\Delta l_2)$
R_2^{14}: IF Δl_1 is Z and Δl_2 is PB, THEN
$p_2^{14} = [1-\text{sgn}(\Delta l_1)]\,(b_1^{14}\Delta l_1 + b_2^{14}\Delta l_2)$
R_2^{15}: IF Δl_1 is Z and Δl_2 is PS, THEN
$p_2^{15} = [1-\text{sgn}(\Delta l_1)]\,(b_1^{15}\Delta l_1 + b_2^{15}\Delta l_2)$
R_2^{18}: IF Δl_1 is PS and Δl_2 is Z, THEN
$p_2^{18} = [1-\text{sgn}(\Delta l_2)]\,(b_1^{18}\Delta l_1 + b_2^{18}\Delta l_2)$
R_2^{23}: IF Δl_1 is PB and Δl_2 is Z, THEN
$p_2^{23} = [1-\text{sgn}(\Delta l_2)]\,(b_1^{23}\Delta l_1 + b_2^{23}\Delta l_2)$

p_1 and p_2 are the numbers of pulses for the left-right and up-down adjusting stepper motors. And they are calculated as shown in equation (3).

$$p_1 = \frac{\sum_{m=1}^{25} \omega^m p_1^m}{\sum_{m=1}^{25} \omega^m} \qquad p_2 = \frac{\sum_{m=1}^{25} \omega^m p_2^m}{\sum_{m=1}^{25} \omega^m} \tag{3}$$

where ω^m is the firing strength of the m-th rule and it is given in equation (4).

$$\omega^m = \mu^m{}_{\Delta\tilde{l}_1}(\Delta l_1)\,\mu^m{}_{\Delta\tilde{l}_2}(\Delta l_2) \tag{4}$$

where $\mu^m{}_{\Delta\tilde{l}_1}(\Delta l_1)$ is the membership of Δl_1 belonging to $\Delta\tilde{l}_1$ in the m-th rule, and $\mu^m{}_{\Delta\tilde{l}_2}(\Delta l_2)$ is the membership of Δl_2 belonging to $\Delta\tilde{l}_2$ in the m-th rule.

5 Experiments

In this section, experiments are introduced. Fig. 9 shows the experimental system. Two stepper motors were mounted on the welding vehicle. Stepper motor 1 and 2 adjusted the welding torch in up-down and left-right direction, respectively. Two mini cameras were employed to capture the pictures of the welding seam. The size of the captured pictures was 640×480 in pixel. A V-shaped straight welding seam, whose width, depth, and length were 10mm, 16mm, and 400mm, was used. A Pentium(R) IV, 1.8GHz, and 512M memory computer was employed to carry out the experiments.

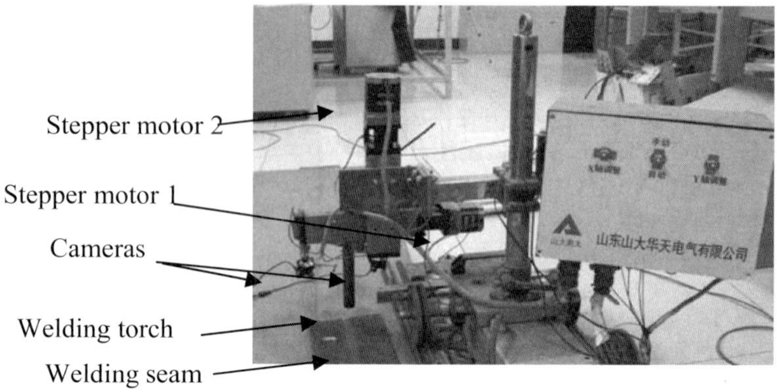

Fig. 9. The experimental system

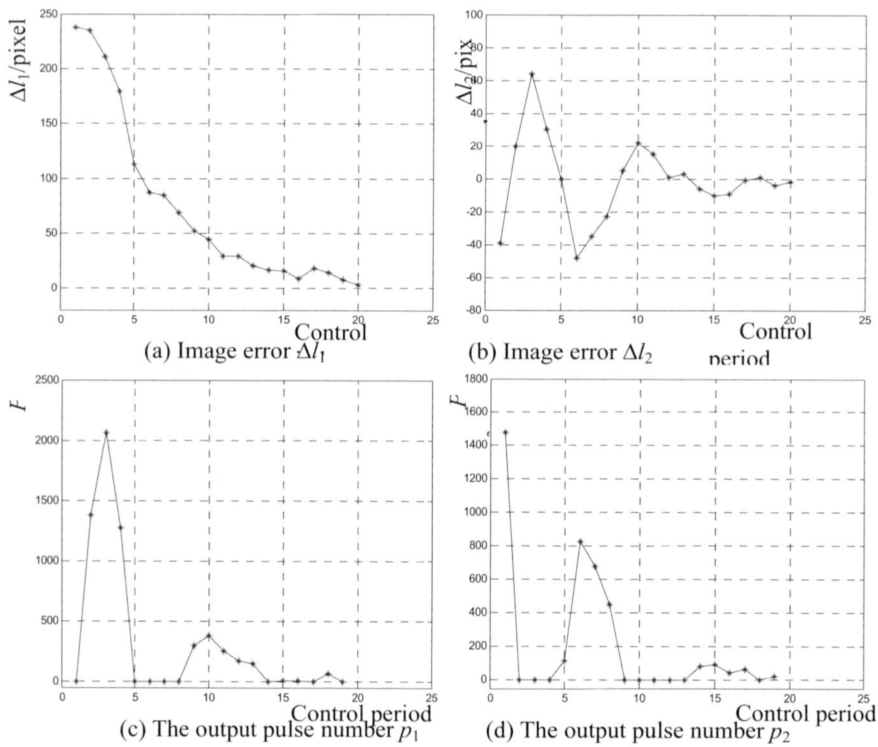

(a) Image error Δl_1 (b) Image error Δl_2

(c) The output pulse number p_1 (d) The output pulse number p_2

Fig. 10. Experimental results

In the experiment, Δt was set to 5. The control period was 250ms.The model parameters a_1^m, a_2^m, b_1^m and b_2^m were given in Table 1 and Table 2. Before the experiment, the welding torch was adjusted to the initial welding position in front-back direction manually. At the moment, welding torch was at the upper-right of the welding seam. During the experiments, the adjustments to left and downwards were carried out by turns. After 20 control periods, when Δl_1=3 and Δl_2=-2, the adjusting task was fulfilled. Fig. 10 gave the experimental results. The image errors Δl_1 and Δl_2 were shown in Fig. 10(a) and (b), and the pulse number p_1 and p_2 were shown in Fig. 10(c) and (d).

Table 1. The model parameters a_1 and a_2

a_1, Δl	NB	NS	Z	PS	PB
NB	8, 8	10, 5	4, 2	0, 0	0, 0
NS	5, 10	5, 5	5, 3	0, 0	0, 0
Z	2, 4	3, 5	0, 0	3, 5	2, 4
PS	0, 0	0, 0	5, 3	5, 5	5, 10
PB	0, 0	0, 0	4, 2	10, 5	8, 8

Table 2. The model parameters b_1 and b_2

b_1, Δl	NB	NS	Z	PS	PB
NB	0, 0	0, 0	2, -1	8, -4	7, -7
NS	0, 0	0, 0	3, -2	4, -4	4, -8
Z	-1, 2	-2, 3	0, 0	2, -3	1, -2
PS	-4, 8	-4, 4	-3, 2	0, 0	0, 0
PB	-7, 7	-8, 4	-2, 1	0, 0	0, 0

The calibration result showed that a pixel around the welding torch in image space of the system was about 0.09mm in horizontal direction and 0.07mm in vertical direction in Cartesian space. Without considering the image processing errors, the system error was less than 0.45mm ×0.35mm in the two directions. Conclusion can be made that the system meets the requirement of the applications.

6 Conclusions

In this paper, a vision based welding system, which has the initial welding position guiding function, is proposed. The system can be applied to straight welding and pipe welding. Two cameras are employed as the sensors. The selection of the image features and the calculation of the image errors are introduced. Based on the analysis of the relations between the welding torch and the welding seam, a T-S fuzzy controller is designed. A straight welding seam is used to do the experiment. And the experimental results demonstrate that the system can perform its task successfully.

Acknowledgement

This work is supported by the National High Technology Research and Development Program of China under grant 2006AA04Z213.

Reference

1. Guo, Z.M., Chen, S.B., Tao, Q., Lin, W.: A method of initial welding position guiding for arc welding robot based on visual servo control. China Weld. 12(1), 29–33 (2003)
2. Chen, S.B., Lin, T., Yu, C.: Practical method to locate the initial weld position using visual technology. The International Journal of Advanced Manufacturing Technology 30(7-8), 663–668 (2006)
3. Mahony, R., Hamel, T.: Image based visual servo control of aerial robotic systems using linear image features. IEEE Transactions on Robotics 21(2), 227–239 (2005)
4. Zhang, H., Ding, X.L., Chen, M.H., Da, B.Q., Zou, C.H.: The seam tracking system for submerged arc welding. In: Proceedings of Robotic Welding, Intelligence and Automation. LNCIS, vol. 299, pp. 144–151. Springer, Heidelberg (2004)
5. Wilson, W.J., Hulls, C.C.W., Bell, G.S.: Relative end-effector control using Cartesian position-based visual servoing. IEEE Transactions on Robot and Automat 12(5), 684–696 (1996)
6. Mahony, R., Hamel, T.: Image-based visual servo control of aerial robotic systems using linear image features. IEEE Transactions on Robotics 21(2), 227–239 (2005)
7. Malis, E., Chaumette, F., Boudet, S.: 2-1/2-D Visual Servoing. IEEE Transactions on Robotics and Automation 15(2), 238–250 (1999)
8. Tseng, C.S., Chen, B.S., Uang, H.J.: Fuzzy tracking control design for nonlinear dynamic systems via T-S fuzzy model. IEEE Transactions on fuzzy system 9(3), 381–392 (2001)
9. Gang, F.: A survey on analysis and design of modelbased fuzzy control systems. IEEE Transactions on fuzzy system 14(5), 676–697 (2006)
10. Yan, Z.G., Xu, D., Li, Y.: An adaptive binary threshold based method for extracting edge features of welding seam. Transactions of the China Welding Institution (in press)

Design of Motion Controlling System Based on Structured Grating 3D Measuring Machine

Junting Cheng, Wantao He, and Can Zhao

College of Mechanical Engineering, Heilongjiang University of Science & Technology, Harbin Heilongjiang 150027, China

Abstract. A method of the open motion controlling system based on PC and motion card was introduced to improve the corresponding system of a self-developed structured grating 3D measuring machine. PC was used as the core operation unit of the system, and the whole motion controlling was manipulated by the motion card in this method. In addition, the motion controlling software was developed using Microsft Visual C++ as a tool. After combined adjustment of the 3D measuring machine equipped with the above mentioned motion controlling system, the result shows that the mothod of PC and motion control card provides a higher positioning accuracy and quicker response speed, which is benefit for the further research.

Keywards: Measuring system; Motion control; Motion control card; PC.

1 Introduction

Motion control system is an important part of structured grating 3D measuring system. The measuring precision and efficiency of 3D measuring equipment is directly affected by the orientation precision and speed of the motion system. A method of the open motion control is proposed under the consideration of the measuring precision, speed, cost and structure of structured grating 3D measuring system in this work. SCM system, professional motion control PLC, special control system and “PC+ motion control card” are used in this method[1,2]. There are several methods except for “PC+ motion control card”, SCM is used to achieve motion control and is lower cost, but it developed difficultly and time-consuming; PLC is generally employed to control the equipment that have relatively simple motion process and fixed track; dedicated control system is usually used for special equipment or special Industry; While "PC + Motion Control Card" can make full use of computer resources to control complicated motion process, mechanical track and a strong flexible equipment. At present, popular open CNC system relies largely on the use of this programme. "PC + Motion Control Card" is adopted in this work to achieve the structured grating 3D measuring instrument of movement control system[1~3].

C. Xiong et al. (Eds.): ICIRA 2008, Part II, LNAI 5315, pp. 707–712, 2008.

2 Hardware Composition of the Motion Controlling System and Control Implementation

2.1 Hardware Composition and Controlling Principle

Main function of motion control system of measuring equipment is to bring the grating to move in accordance with a certain requirements. And the system is consisted of a motion control card, a driver, a stepper motor and a device which can bring grating movement horizontal. The fig.1 shows the structured of system. The system uses PC as the core of the control system, motion control card is responsible for the completion of the entire control details. In the design of the control system, a master-slave control structure is composed of PC and motion control card. The motion control card send out synchronization pulse control signal which is magnified by the driver to drive the stepper motor according to corresponding operating frequency and angle. Pulse signal comes back from optical encoder and enters the driver component steep ring. While displacement signal enter the motion control component location ring. Displacement signal plus is sent the counter to count, the value is currently actual location[4~5].

2.1.1 Motion Control Card

In this work, the card is a high-powered motion control card which is based on PCI bus and control four stepper motors simultaneously. It has many advance functions such as plug and play, ultimate 400KHZ pulse frequency, S curve, and momentarily change speed. Its location instruction can be single plush (plush + direct) or double plush (CW plus + CCW plush) output. The signal mode can be difference or single-end. The output of the card can be synchronously plush and direct signal in its four axes to control motor at the same time. it can also connect signal such as origin, speed-down, and limit switch to realize back origin and protection. Those signals can be detected automatically and response simutanously. In addition, it is also have 12 outputs and 15 inputs which are insulated to provide using for consumer.

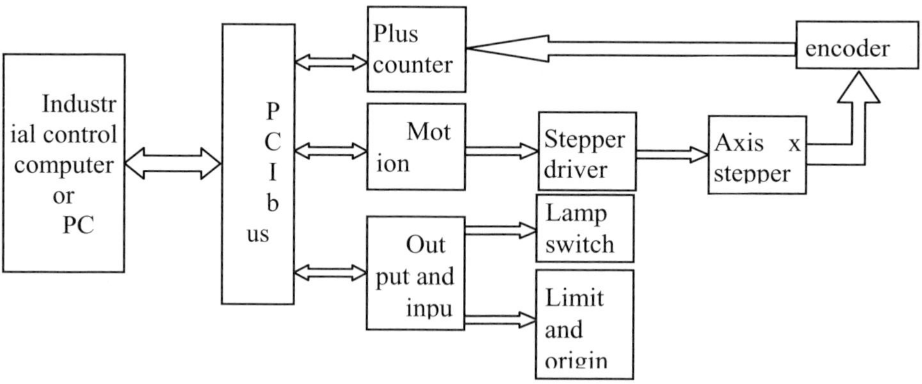

Fig. 1. Composition of motion control system

2.1.2 Step Motor Driver

For improving measuring efficiency and precision, the stepper motor must move highly and precisely in measuring machine working. This needs the stepper motor driver not only can output higher speed, higher power and reduce the motor and itself generating heat but also have higher subdivision precision. Driver performance determines the performance of the whole implementing agencies at a large extent, so it is very important to select a suited driver. In this work, the selected driver has the following characters:

(1) It adopts the technology of bipolar constant current chopped wave to output higher speed and power.

(2) It has little current wave and auto halve when at rest to reduce motor and itself generating heat.

(3) It uses photoisolator input and alternative subdivision precision. The highest subdivision precision is 64*200 step/circle.

In fact, the highest subdivision driver is selected and the plush loses is less than 1/1000 and does not increase with the augment of plush number. As the pitch of lead screw is 0.5 mm/r to calculate, the precision of control system is 0.5 μm which can meet the system demands.

2.2 Selection of Controlling Mode

2.2.1 Plus Output Mode

As the selected driver needs a long wire to transmit the signal in the measuring system, single-end plush and difference mode is taken as output signal in order to reduce the signal attenuation in the procession of transmission.

2.2.2 Motion Mode

The motion control card has four motion control modes:

(1) Trapeziform velocity motion mode: it is impossible to reach the designated speed instantly for the inertia of the motor axis and drove object. Losing step and vibrating of the motor can be avoided if there is a little time before it accelerates because of the shortage of time. Velocity curve is shown in fig.2.

(2) Continuous motion mode: this mode accelerates after it start and reach the designated speed to work continuously. It is similar to the trapezoidal motion mode at the start time. The difference between continuous mode and trapezoidal mode dwell on the stopping speed. The continuous mode is zero while the trapezoidal mode is the muzzle velocity. Velocity curve is shown in fig.3.

(3) S curve mode: this mode makes the process of acceleration become “S” which makes the motion more smooth, and reduces the concussion, noise and abrasion. These characters are obviously advantageous over the trapezoidal mode. Fig.4 shows the velocity curve.

(4) Back to origin mode: this mode starts at a lower speed, then accelerates to the high speed until it receives the back-to-original signal. It will stop after it reaches the original signal. Velocity curve is shown in fig.5.

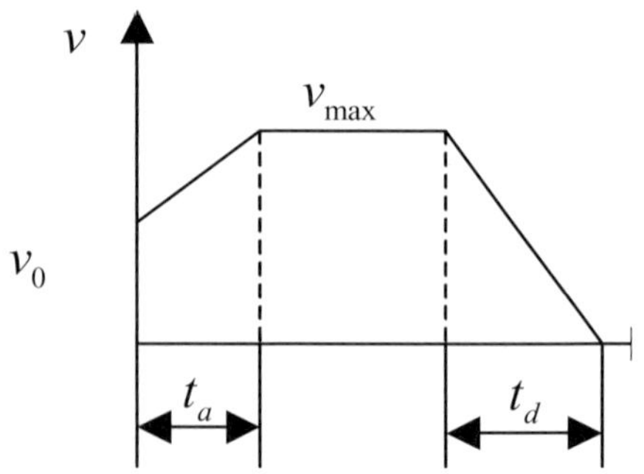

Fig. 2. Velocity curve diagram of trapeziform motion modes

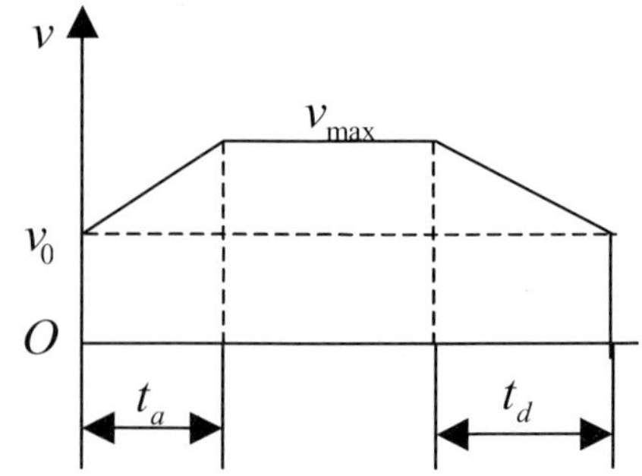

Fig. 3. Velocity curve diagram of continuous motion modes

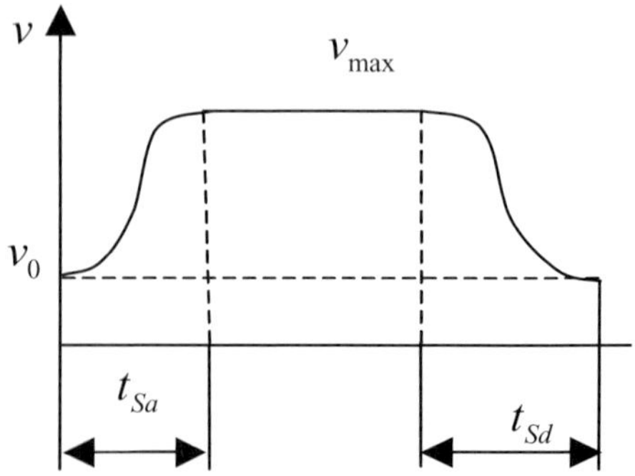

Fig. 4. Velocity curve diagram of S curve modes

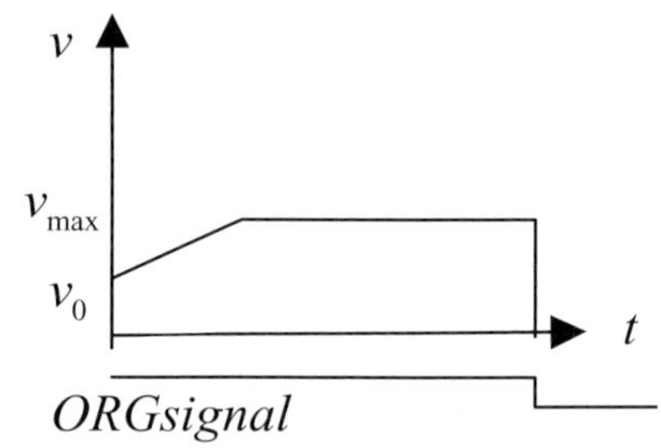

Fig. 5. Velocity curve diagram of back origin

Trapezoidal motion mode is a constant acceleration mode, and it will produce a great impact while operating at high-speed, get the noise of the machine and transmit mechanism of wear and tear easily. So usually, it is adopted when the acceleration is not high. Acceleration can reach to the largest in some way in the "S" mode. The motor will prolong the time of acceleration to reach the set speed in the same high-speed. "S" mode is chosen in this work to decrease the vibration and noise of the motion device, prolong the life of mechanical drive. Furthermore, the precision of motion controlling and velocity is satisfied either.

3 Software Design

Measuring machine drives grating to move according a certain demand through motion control system and projects grating stripe on the surface of measured object. Then the image capture system captures the image and stores the image in the computer. So when the control system controls the motion, it should send the control signal to the image capture system to make it capture the image. Therefore, it is necessary to solve the correspond problems between the control system and the capture system.

Windows is a multithreading and multi-process operation system. When an executable program is executed, windows will create a process. It has independent memory space, file handles and other system resources. A process have multiple threads, one of which is dominated thread, others are auxiliary threads. All the code and data space of the process are used by its thread which is the basic unit of the operation system. So we can solve the problems between communication systems by using communication between threads[6~8].

Communication control between threads can be achieved through the programs that are developed using Microsoft Visual C++. First, the system initializes the card which includes opening the card and setting the motion control parameter (setting plush output mode and velocity control mode). When the control motion system receives the control plush, the motor will run a constant angle through ball screw to make it move in a line. When the motion control system receives the message that the image acquisition system has finished the capture of the image, it will begin the next step. Furthermore, the system also assumes to control the lame using the I/O port. The whole flow process chart is shown in fig.6.

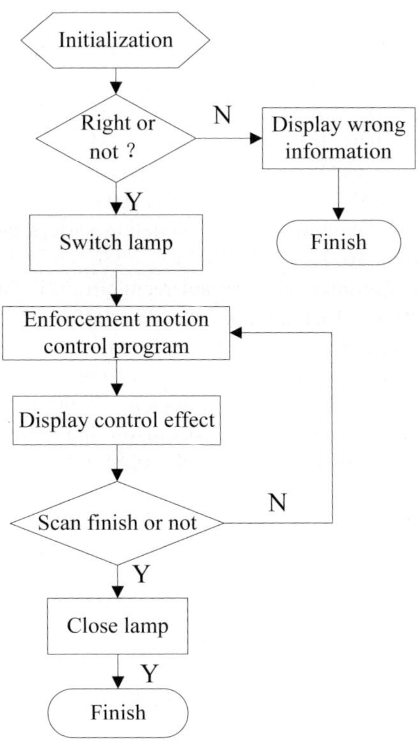

Fig. 6. Software flow

4 Conclusions

Measurement system takes the dedicated motion control card as its core. It adopts the mode of motion control card +PC, so the structure is sample and easy to actualize. It is a good solution for the motion control systems of the measurement system with high precision and fast response requirements. Besides, it reduces the research and development cycle of measuring machine control system significantly. The practice indicates that this method is feasible and obtains perfect effect.

Acknowledgements

The authors are grateful for the support provided by foundation of Heilongjiang Education Department in China (No. 1152G036 and No.1055G042).

References

1. Cheng, J.-T., Wang, C.-J., Zhao, C., Mo, J.-H.: Design of a servo motion system and an image sampling and processing system on a 3D laser scanner. J. Int. J. Adv. Manuf. Technol. 33, 1143–1148 (2007)
2. Missaoui, R., Sarifuddin, M., Vaillancourt, J.: Similarity measures for efficient content-based image retrieval. J. IEE Proc. Vis. Image Process 152, 875–887 (2005)
3. Ghosh, S., Moorthy, S.: Three dimensional Voronoi cell finite element model for microstructures with ellipsoidal heterogeneities. J. Comput. Mech. 34, 510–531 (2004)
4. Dankers, A., Zelinsky, A.: CeDAR: a real-world vision system—mechanism, control and visual processing. J. Mach. Vis. Appl. 16, 47–58 (2004)
5. Park, S.-Y., Subbarao, M.: A multiview 3D modeling system based on stereo vision techniques. J. Mach. Vis. Appl. 16, 148–156 (2005)
6. Yang, J., Al-Rawi, M.: Illumination invariant recognition of three-dimensional texture in color images. J. Comput. Sci. Technol. 20, 378–388 (2005)
7. Tsai, R.Y.: An efficient and accurate camera calibration technique for 3D machine vision. In: Proceedings of the IEEE Conference on Computer Vision and Pattern Recognition (CVPR 1996), pp. 364–374. IEEE Press, San Francisco (1996)
8. Van De Weijer, J., Den, V.: Boomgaard Least squares and robust estimation of local image structure. J. Int. J. Comput. Vis. R. 64, 143–155 (2005)

Dynamic Analysis and Control of the MJR Robot Palletizer

Fengyan Ning, Chao Yun, and Xinyi Chen

School of Mechanical Engineering and Automation, Beihang University,
100083, Beijing, P.R. China
nfy198@tom.com

Abstract. The MJR120 palletizer is researched and manufactured by the paper. Using the Second Lagrangian kinetics, the author analyses the dynamical features of the robot, derives the generated driving torque of the arms, and sets up its inverse dynamical equations. To improve its performance of the system, a new controller is designed with a self-adaptive fuzzy PID control algorithm, which makes use of the merits both of the fuzzy control and the self-adaptive control algorithm. The effectiveness of the proposed control method is verified by simulation based on Matlab. The controller has better performance and robustness than the conventional PID controller in the Palletizer system.

Keywords: palletizer; dynamical features; self-adaptive fuzzy PID control.

1 Introduction

In the past few years, Palletizing technology, especially robotic Palletizing technology, had been developed rapidly, the throughput of on-line palletizers had been increasing and the flexibility, processing velocity, and payload of robotic palltizers had been upgrading [1]. Among the palletizers, their links are either revolving with the R-joint, or moving by a geodetic coordinate system; By heavy coupling, the kinematical and dynamical analysis of the forth are very complex; and the latter overcomes coupling, and is easy to control, but it covers much space and has very bad flexibility. In the current situation, after a great deal of analysis, computation and optimized design, the MJR120 palletizer has been researched and manufactured by the Robot Research of Beihang University for the Wenzhou Hualian Package Ltd., to transfer and palletize materials on the packing production line. The robot's maximum gripping load is 120*kg*, the maximum rotation velocity is 1400r/h, and the maximum rotation angle of the waist is 330^0. The palletizer has been manufactured and equipped well, and now is being debugged and test run. The whole structure is show in the Fig. 1. The links of the palletizer consist of a closed parallel four-bar linkage, couples two groups of little paralle four-bar linkages. Each link may revolve by driving of the level and vertical sliders to control the spread and pitch of the wrist in the level and vertical direction, respectively. The mechanism can make the actuators of the two arms and their reducing mechanism be be installed into the waist to improve its dynamic features. By chosing the adaptive parameters, its kinematics may be decoupling, thus it is easy to control by kinematics, but with the partical closed links, some constraint forces act on

C. Xiong et al. (Eds.): ICIRA 2008, Part II, LNAI 5315, pp. 713–722, 2008.

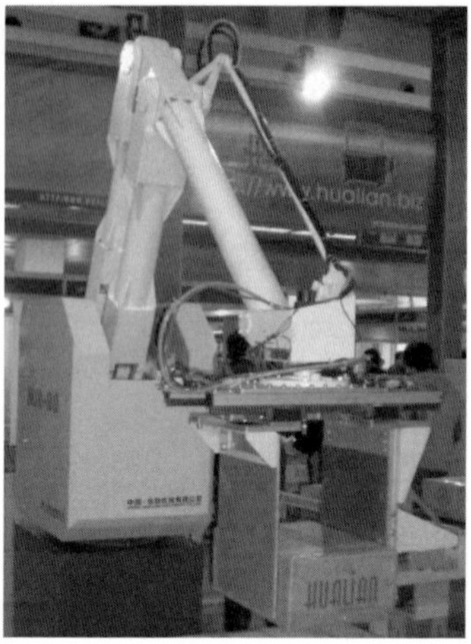

Fig. 1. MJR120 palletizer

the corresponding the links so that the robot is coupling in dynamics, thus it is very difficult to analysis their dynamics.

Using the Second Lagrangian, the paper completes its analysis and derivation of its dynamical model. The system is very uncertain, time-varying and nonlinear, so it is difficult for the conventional PID to adjust automatically its parameters. However, the fuzzy PID controller can not only satisfy the needs but also improves the capacity of eliminating system's steady-state error. In this paper, the self-adaptive fuzzy PID method is used in the pallizater. The simulation results verify the feasibility of the scheme presented in the paper.

2 Dynamic Analysis of the MJR120 Robot Palletizer Model

2.1 Simplied Model of the Robot

The main structure of the palletizer is a closed paralle four-bar linkage, and couples two groups of little paralle four-bar linkages. Four motors are used to drive the revolving and moving of the wrist, the level slider and the vertical slider, respectively. For simplicity, we only consider the dynamics of its waist and paralle four-bar linkages, and neglect the others. Thus, we can obtain the robot's simplied structure, and set up its coordinate system, shown in the Fig. 2. Now, denote the length of the front arm *AE*, connection-rod *AB*, rear arm *CD* and the little arm *DP* by l_2, l_3, l_5 and l_6, respectively; denote the distance between their mass centers and their rotating axis by l_{2c}, l_{3c}, l_{5c} and l_{6c} respectively; and the length of *BC*, the length between the mass center of the connection-rod and the B point, the length between the mass center of the rear arm and its *C* point, between the mass center of the little arm and the *E* point, and its end *P* point denoted by l_0, r_3, r_5, $r_6$and rr_6; denote the level distance between O_1 point and the vertical slider; θ_1, θ_2 and θ_3 are the revolving angle of the waist, front arm and little arm respectively, as shown in the Fig. 2.

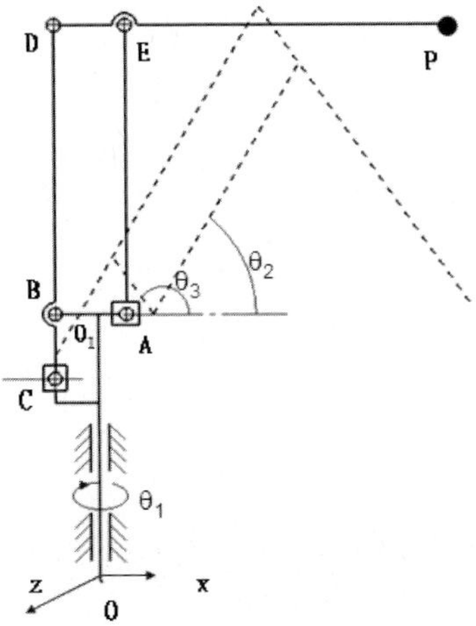

Fig. 2. MJR robot's simplied model

Here, we analyse and derive the dynamical equations of the robot by the Second Lagrangian kinetics, which is the difference of the kinetic and potential energy of the system [2-4].

2.2 Generalized Coordinate of the System

To simplied computation, we neglect the movment of the wrist, thus, the system becomes a three-dimensional model with three free-degrees. We can transform the position coordination x_1 and y_4 of the two sliders into angle variety θ_2 and θ_3 in the *XOY*. Therefore, taking the θ_1, θ_2 and θ_3 as the generalized coordination of the system.

2.3 Dynamical Model of the Robot

Because of the parallel four-bar mechanism, great constrait forces exit among the links. To simply, we first derive Lagrangian equations of the system.

Supposing that the vector radius of every link in the coordinates *OXYZ* is r_i (i=1,2,...7). Referring to their geometrical relation [5] , yields

$$\mathbf{r}_1 = \begin{bmatrix} (l_0c_2 - l_3c_3 - l)c_1 \\ (l_0c_2 - l_3c_3 - l)s_1 \\ 0 \end{bmatrix} \tag{1}$$

$$\mathbf{r}_2 = \begin{bmatrix} (l_0c_2 - l_3c_3 + l_{2c}c_2 - l)c_1 \\ (l_0c_2 - l_3c_3 + l_{2c}c_2 - l)s_1 \\ l_{2c}s_2 \end{bmatrix} \tag{2}$$

$$\mathbf{r}_3 = \begin{bmatrix} (l_0 c_2 - r_3 c_3 - l)c_1 \\ (l_0 c_2 - r_3 c_3 - l)s_1 \\ l_{3c} s_3 \end{bmatrix} \tag{3}$$

$$\mathbf{r}_4 = \begin{bmatrix} -lc_1 \\ -ls_1 \\ l_3 s_3 - l_0 s_2 \end{bmatrix} \tag{4}$$

$$\mathbf{r}_5 = \begin{bmatrix} (l_{5c} c_2 - l)c_1 \\ (l_{5c} c_2 - l)s_1 \\ l_3 s_3 + r_5 s_2 \end{bmatrix} \tag{5}$$

$$\mathbf{r}_6 = \begin{bmatrix} (l_5 c_2 - l_{6c} c_3 - l)c_1 \\ (l_5 c_2 - l_{6c} c_3 - l)s_1 \\ l_2 s_2 - r_6 s_3 \end{bmatrix} \tag{6}$$

$$\mathbf{r}_7 = \begin{bmatrix} (l_5 c_2 - l_6 c_3)c_1 \\ (l_5 c_2 - l_6 c_3)s_1 \\ l_2 s_2 - r_6' s_2 \end{bmatrix} \tag{7}$$

where s_1=sinθ_1, c_1=cosθ_1, s_2=sinθ_2, c_2=cosθ_2, s_3=sinθ_3, and c_3=cosθ_3, the following is as so.

Differenttiating the expressions of (1) to (7), we can have the velocity expression of every link $\boldsymbol{v}_i$ (i=1,2,…7).

Now differentiating (1)~(7), the kinetic energy of the system can be given by

$$T = \sum_{i=1}^{7} \left(\frac{1}{2} m_i \mathbf{v}_i^2 + \frac{1}{2} I_i \dot{\theta}_i^2 \right) \tag{8}$$

where I_2, I_3, I_5 and I_6 are the rotational inertias of the link 2, 3, 5 and 6, respectively; m_i (i=1,2,...,7) denote the mass of the level slider, front arm, connection-rod, vertical slider, rear arm, little arm and wrist, respectively.

Turning now to the potential energy, we have that

$$U = \sum_{i=1}^{7} m_i g y_{ci} \tag{9}$$

where, y_{ci} is the vertical coordiation of the link i.

The non-conservative forces of the robot are the joint troques τ_1, τ_2 and τ_3, which are the output torque of the motors of waist, level slider and vertical slider, respectively [6] :

$$\tau = [\tau_1, \tau_2, \tau_3]^T \tag{10}$$

The virtual workof the robot is

$$\delta Q = \tau^T \delta\theta = \tau_1 \delta\theta_1 + \tau_2 \delta x_1 + \tau_3 \delta y_4 \tag{11}$$

Referring to the Fig. 2, we can derive the following geometry relation

$$\begin{cases} x_1 = l_0 c_2 - l_3 c_3 \\ y_4 = l_3 s_3 - l_0 s_2 \end{cases} \tag{12}$$

Differenttiating the above expression gives

$$\begin{cases} \delta x_1 = -l_0 s_2 \delta\theta_2 + l_3 s_3 \delta\theta_3 \\ \delta y_4 = l_3 c_3 \delta\theta_3 - l_0 c_2 \delta\theta_2 \end{cases} \tag{13}$$

Therefore, with the virtual work principle, we have

$$\delta Q = \tau_1^* \delta\theta_1 + \tau_2^* \delta\theta_2 + \tau_3^* \delta\theta_3 \tag{14}$$

Thus, the generalited force of the system is

$$\tau^* = D\tau \tag{15}$$

After substituting Lagrange function and generalized force into the Lagrange, those nonlinear dynamic equations of the robot can be written in matrix form as

$$M(\theta)\ddot{\theta} + C(\theta,\dot{\theta})\dot{\theta} = D\tau \tag{16}$$

where the matrix M is a 3×3 positive definite, symmetry and time-varying generalized quality matrix, $M_{12}= M_{13}= M_{21}=M_{31}=0$, $M_{23}=M_{32}$, $C_{12}= C_{13}=0$, $G_1=0$

$$\begin{aligned} C_{11} = {} & 2m_1 (l_0 c_2 - l_3 c_3 - l)\left(l_3 s_3 \dot{\theta}_3 - l_0 s_2 \dot{\theta}_2 \right) \\ & + 2m_2 (l_0 c_2 + l_{2c} c_2 - l_3 c_3 - l)\left(-l_0 s_2 \dot{\theta}_2 - l_{2c} s_2 \dot{\theta}_2 + l_3 s_3 \dot{\theta}_3 \right) \\ & + 2m_3 (l_0 c_2 - r_3 c_3 - l)\left(-l_0 s_2 \dot{\theta}_2 + r_3 s_3 \dot{\theta}_3 \right) + 2m_5 \left(l_{5c} l s_2 \dot{\theta}_2 - l_{5c}^2 s_2 c_2 \dot{\theta}_2 \right) \\ & + 2m_6 (l_5 c_2 - l_{6c} c_3 - l)\left(-l_5 s_2 \dot{\theta}_2 + l_{6c} s_3 \dot{\theta}_3 \right) + 2m_7 (l_5 c_2 - l_6 c_3 - l)\left(-l_5 s_2 \dot{\theta}_2 + l_6 s_3 \dot{\theta}_3 \right) \end{aligned}$$

$$C_{21} = m_1 (l_0^2 s_2 - l_0 l s_2 - l_0 l_3 s_2 c_3)\dot{\theta}_1 + m_2 (l_0 c_2 + l_{2c} c_2 - l_3 c_3 - l)\left(-l_0 s_2 \dot{\theta}_2 - l_{2c} s_2 \dot{\theta}_2 \right)\dot{\theta}_1$$

$$+m_3\left(l_0^2 s_2 c_2 - l_0 l s_2 - l_0 r_3 s_2 c_3\right)\dot{\theta}_1 + m_5\left(l_{5c}^2 c_2 s_2 - l_{5c} l s_2\right)\dot{\theta}_1$$

$$+m_6\left(l_0 l_5 s_2 + l_5 l_{6c} s_2 c_2 - l_5^2 s_2 c_2\right)\dot{\theta}_2\dot{\theta}_1 + m_7\left(l_0 l_5 s_2 + l_5 l_6 s_2 c_2 - l_5^2 s_2 c_2\right)\dot{\theta}_2\dot{\theta}_1$$

$$C_{22} = s_2 c_2 \dot{\theta}_2 (m_1 l_0^2 + m_2 r_2^2 - m_2 l_{2c}^2 + m_3 l_0^2 + m_5 l_{5c}^2$$
$$- m_5 r_5^2 - m_4 l_0^2 + m_6 l_5^2 - m_6 l_2^2 + m_7 l_5^2 - m_7 l_2^2)$$

$$C_{23} = s_2 c_3 \dot{\theta}_3 \left(-m_1 l_0 l_3 - m_2 l_3 r_2 - m_3 l_0 r_3 - m_6 l_5 l_{6c} - m_7 l_5 l_6\right)$$
$$+ c_2 s_3 \dot{\theta}_3 \left(-m_5 l_3 r_5 + m_4 l_0 l_3 + m_6 l_2 r_6 + m_7 r_1 r_6'\right)$$

$$C_{31} = m_1\left(l l_3 s_3 + l_3^2 s_2 c_3 - l_0 l_3 c_2 s_2\right)\dot{\theta}_1 + m_6\left(l l_{6c} s_3 - l_{6c}^2 c_3 s_3 + l_5 l_{6c} c_2 s_3\right)\dot{\theta}_3\dot{\theta}_1$$
$$+ m_7\left(l l_6 s_3 - l_6^2 c_3 s_3 + l_5 l_6 c_2 s_3\right)\dot{\theta}_3\dot{\theta}_1$$
$$+m_2\left(l_3^2 s_3 c_3 + l l_3 s_3 - l_{2c} l_3 c_2 s_3 - l_0 l_3 c_2 s_3\right)\dot{\theta}_1 + m_3\left(r_3^2 s_3 c_3 + l r_3 s_3 - l_0 r_3 c_2 s_3\right)\dot{\theta}_1$$

$$C_{32} = c_2 s_3 \dot{\theta}_2 \left(-m_1 l_0 l_3 - m_2 l_3 r_2 - m_3 l_0 r_3 - m_6 l_5 l_{6c} - m_7 l_5 l_6\right)$$
$$+ s_2 c_3 \dot{\theta}_2 \left(-m_5 r_5 l_3 + m_4 l_3 l_0 + m_6 l_{6c}^2 + m_7 r_6'^2\right)$$

$$C_{33} = s_3 c_3 \dot{\theta}_3 (m_1 l_3^2 + m_2 l_3^2 + m_3 r_3^2 - m_3 l_{3c}^2 - m_4 l_0^2$$
$$- m_5 l_3^2 + m_6 l_{6c}^2 - m_6 r_6^2 + m_7 l_6^2 - m_7 r_6'^2)$$

$$G_2 = g c_2 \left(m_2 l_{2c} - m_4 l_0 + m_5 r_5 + m_6 l_2 + m_7 l_2\right)$$

$$G_3 = g c_3 \left(m_3 l_{3c} + m_4 l_3 + m_5 l_3 - m_6 r_6 - m_7 r_6'\right)$$

The other elements of the matrixes have been derived out, but they are ommitted here because of their long expressions.

3 Design of the Self-adaptive Fuzzy PID Control

The parameters of PID can be adjusted on-line, which can be changed through the inquiry to the fuzzy control rules table saved aforehand in the computer [7-10].

The conventional PID controller can be described as :

$$u(t) = K_P e(t) + K_I \int e(t)dt + K_D \frac{de(t)}{dt} \tag{19}$$

where, K_P, K_I and K_D are the proportional, integral and derivative gains respectively, $u(t)$ is the output of controller; $e(t)$ is the error signal. The control performance can become better through adjusting the K_P, K_I and K_D according to the changing control parameters condition. The design algorithm in this paper is to adjust the K_P, K_I and K_D parameters on line trough fzzy inference based on the current e and $de(t)/dt$ to make the controlled object attain good performances. The block diagram of self-adaptive fuzzy PID controller is shown in Fig. 3 [12-13].

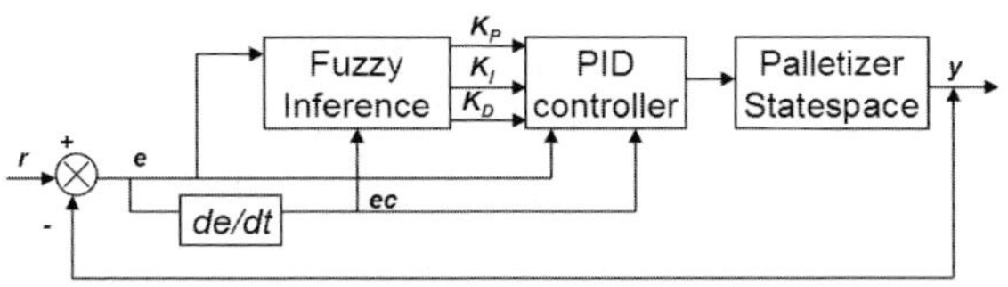

Fig. 3. Block diagram of self-adaptive fuzzy PID controller

The design process of controller is divided into four aspects:

The input variables and output variables. In the design, speed error *e* and error change rate *ec* are used as fuzzy input and the proportional factor K_I , the integral factor K_P, and the differential factor K_D are used as fuzzy output.

Fuzzy language of input and output variables. The fuzzy variable of input variable is *e* and *ec*, the fuzzy variable of output variable is K_P, K_I and K_D. Firstly, it must be confirmed the universe of discourse, quantum rank and quantum factor (K_e, K_{ec}, K_{Up}, K_{Ui}, *and* K_{Ud}) of the input variables *e, ec* and output variable K_P, K_I and K_D. Here, quantum rank of *e, ec* is chosen as thirteen ranks {-6, -5, -4, -3, -2, -1, 0, 1, 2, 3, 4, 5, 6,}. The fuzzy sets of *e* and *ec* are all defined as {*NB, NS, ZO, PS, PB*}. The quantum rank of K_P, K_I and K_D is chosen as ten ranks {0, 1, 2, 3, 4, 5, 6, 7, 8, 9}. The fuzzy sets of *KP, KI, and KD* are all defined as {Z, S, M, B}. The membership function of *E, EC, KP, KI, and KD* is the triangle distrbution function. The suitable quantum factor of each variable is adopted by considering the experiment and simulation results of the Palletizer. The quantum factor of *e* is K_e=10; The quantum factor *ec* is K_{ec}=100; The quantum factor of K_P, K_I and K_D is K_{Up}=2.5; K_{Ui}=0.6; K_{Ud}=0.4 [11-12].

Fuzzy rules regulation. The principle of designed fuzzy rules is that the output of controller can optimize the output response of the system. The fuzzy rules are generalized as table I, table II and table III according to the expert experiment in the pallizer and simulation analysis of the system [13-14].

PID parameters regulation. *KP, KI, and KD* can be regulated after completing the fuzzy rule table of *KP, KI, and KD.*

Table 1. The control rulers of *KP*

ec e	NB	NS	ZO	PS	PB
NB	B	B	B	B	B
NS	M	B	S	S	S
ZO	M	B	Z	S	B
PS	S	S	S	S	S
PB	B	B	B	M	B

Table 2. The control rulers of *KI*

ec e	NB	NS	ZO	PS	PB
NB	Z	M	B	M	Z
NS	S	M	B	B	S
ZO	S	B	B	M	Z
PS	S	B	M	M	S
PB	Z	S	M	S	Z

Table 3. The control rulers of *KD*

ec e	NB	NS	ZO	PS	PB
NB	B	B	B	B	B
NS	M	B	S	S	S
ZO	M	B	Z	S	B
PS	S	S	S	S	S
PB	B	B	B	M	B

4 Simulation Results

To demonstrate the effectiveness of the designed controller, the MATLAB is used to the whole system simulation. With the block diagram in the Fig. 3 and the fuzzy control rules in the table I, II and III, the simulation results are shown in the Fig. 4. Here, we only show the controls of the waist, the others are ommited. From the figure, we can see when its input angle is 1 radian, the ascending time is 50ms, the adjusting time is 10ms, and the error of the steady state is 1.3% with the self-adaptive fuzzy PID control, while the tranditional PID control has the defects of lower response rate, longer delay and regulating time, so the forth has much obvious advantage than the later in response for the nonlinear system, and have no overshoot which is easy to occur in the fuzzy control. Therefore, the controller can satisfy the performance requirement of the palletizer system.

With frequently changing of the load, the controller is required to posses good robustness. The Fig. 5 shows the system's response when there is disturbance from the external world. We can see that the self-adaptive fuzzy PID controller can suspress the disturbance much quickly than the tranditional one, and let the robot have small fluctation and its restoring time is relatively short, hence the controller have strong robustness.

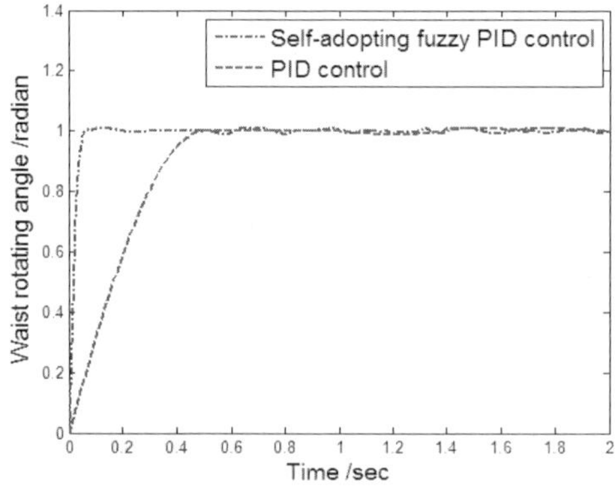

Fig. 4. Comparison of the step response results for traditional PID controller and self-adoptive fuzzy PID controller

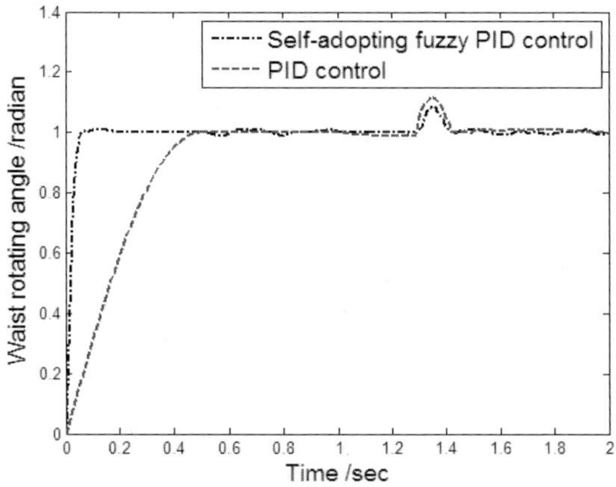

Fig. 5. Comparison of the response curve of the waist under the disturbance of 1.4s

5 Conclusion

The MJR120 palletizer can satisfy the requirement of high-speed and heavy load for material handling, whose mechanism can improve its dynamic features. By the method of Lagrangian, this paper analyses its dynamical performance, derives the generated driving torque of the arms, and sets up its inverse dynamic model. The paper introduces the self-adaptive fuzzy PID control algorithm into the control system of the palletizer. From the simulation results, we can see that the self-adaptive fuzzy PID control has more obvious advantage than the traditional PID control, and the designed controller can eliminate overshoot and posses strong robustness.

References

1. Hu, H.G., Gao, J.H., Yang, R.Q.: The development of palletizing technology. Modular Machine Tool & Automatic Manufacturing Technique 6, 54–59 (2000)
2. Zhu, Z.X., Zhou, Q.H., Yin, J.S.: Theoretical Mechanics, pp. 315–325. Beijing University Press (1997)
3. Fei, X.: Advanced Dynamics, pp. 27–42. Zhejiang University Press (1993)
4. Fei, R.Y., Zhang, H.H.: Mechabical design and analysis of robots, pp. 123–128. Beijing Industry University Press (1998)
5. Tang, X.Y., Li, W.: Effect of parallel four-bar mechanism on spotwelding robot. Journal of China Agricultural University 8(4), 36–40 (2003)
6. Ma, X.F.: Robot Mechanisms, pp. 233–239. Medical Industry Press (1991)
7. Spong, M.W., Vidyasagar, M.: Robot Dynamics and control, United States of America, pp. 234–245 (1989)
8. Terano, T., Asai, K., Sugeno, M.: Applied Fuzzy Systems. AP Professional 1994, p. 302 (1994)
9. Tanaka, K., Sugeno, M.: Stability Analysis and Design of Fuzzy Control Systems. Fuzzy Sets and Systems 45(2), 135–156 (1992)

10. Adachi, G., Horikawa, S., Furuhashi, T., Uchikawa, Y.: A New Linguistic Design Method of Fuzzy Controller Using a Description of Dynamical Behavior of Fuzzy Control Systems. In: Proceedings of ACC 1995, pp. 2282–2286 (1995)
11. Tao, Y.H., Yin, Y.X., Ge, L.S.: The control and application of late-model PID, pp. 211–219. China Machine Press, Beijing (1999)
12. Buja, G.S., Todesco, F.: Neural network implementation of fuzzy logic controller. IEEE Trans. Ind. Rlectron. 41, 663–667 (1994)
13. Zhang, J.H.: Study and compare for PID control system and fuzzy self-adaptive PID control system. Journal of Wuhan University of Technology 27, 286–290 (2005)
14. Liu, J.K.: Advanced PID control and Matlab simulink, pp. 125–190. Publishing House of Electronics Industry, Beijing (2004)

Isotropic Design of Stewart Platform-Based Force Sensor

Jiantao Yao, Yulei Hou, Hang Wang, and Yongsheng Zhao

College of Mechanical Engineering, Yanshan University,
066004, Qinhuangdao, China
yszhao@ysu.edu.cn, ysuyjt@Gmail.com

Abstract. The modified isotropy indices of Stewart platform-based force sensor are proposed by introducing the orthogonality condition, the physical meanings of the modified isotropy indices, the orthogonality condition and the concept of full isotropy are given. The isotropy performance of the general 6-6 Stewart platform-based force sensor is studied in detail based on the modified isotropy indices, the result indicates that it is impossible to realize full isotropy in theory, and the best comprehensive isotropy performance is obtained by compromising the isotropy indices. A novel 6/3-3 Stewart platform-based force sensor which can achieve full isotropy is proposed and a numeric example is given. The research results are useful for structure design of the six-axis force sensor.

Keywords: Stewart platform, Force sensor, Full isotropy, Modified indices.

1 Introduction

Stewart[1] platform structure possesses the distinguishing advantages of good stiffness, symmetric and compact design, and concise mapping expression[2] between the wrenches applied on the upper platform and the leg reacting forces. These advantages make it particularly suitable for certain applications in six-axis force sensors.

The force/toque sensor based on Stewart platform has attracted great interest and been extensively studied by many authors. Gaillet and Reboulet[3] proposed an isostatic six-axis force sensor based on the octahedral structure of Stewart platform. Kerr[4] suggested that the Stewart platform with instrumented elastic legs be used as a six-axis force sensor and enumerated a few design criteria for the sensor structure. Nguyen et al.[5] reported the development of a Stewart platform-based sensor with LVDT (linear voltage different transforms) mounted along the legs for force/torque measurement in the presence of passive compliance. Dwarakanath et al.[6] reported the design of a Stewart platform-based force sensor obtained by considering maximization signal to noise ratio and satisfying the dual objective of isotropy and sensitivity. Zhao[7] developed a pre-stressed six-axis force sensor based on the Stewart platform. Gao et al.[8] developed a six-axis controller based on six-axis force sensor based on Stewart platform, and introduced the elastic joints to replace the real spherical joints which made the micromation of the sensor possible.

Structural design is particularly important since the improvements of its performance can be achieved with the aid of the proper design. Design indices for Stewart platform-based force sensor include isotropy, sensitivity, stiffness and so on. Among

C. Xiong et al. (Eds.): ICIRA 2008, Part II, LNAI 5315, pp. 723–732, 2008.

them, isotropy is of special importance for the structural design of force sensor, isotropy leads to the minimum relative error in the force mapping[9]. Uchiyama et al.[9,10] proposed an index of condition number for the evaluation of a structural isotropy of the force sensor body. Xiong[11] presented the concept of isotropy on the basis of Fisher's information matrix. Rreference [12] studied the force and torque isotropy indices, and defined the force and torque sensitivity isotropy indices. Rreference [13] presented the forward and inverse force/torque isotropy indices, and presented the concept of complete isotropy.

This paper proposed the modified isotropy indices by introducing the orthogonality condition and conducts isotropic design of parallel 6-axis force sensor based on Stewart platform.

2 The Modified Isotropy Indices and the Physical Meanings

The forces and moments applied to the Stewart platform-based force sensor can be evaluated from measuring the axial forces of the six elastic legs. The relation between the six-dimension external force and the six axial forces can be expressed as

$$\boldsymbol{F}_{\mathrm{o}} = \boldsymbol{G}\,\boldsymbol{f}\,. \tag{1}$$

where, $\boldsymbol{f}$ is a vector composed of the axial forces of the six legs, $\boldsymbol{F}_{\mathrm{o}}=\{F_{\mathrm{x}}\ F_{\mathrm{Y}}\ F_{\mathrm{Z}}\ M_{\mathrm{X}}\ M_{\mathrm{Y}}\ M_{\mathrm{Z}}\}^{\mathrm{T}}$ is a six-dimensional vector composed of the external forces and moments, $\boldsymbol{G}$ is the force mapping matrix, the characteristics of matrix $\boldsymbol{G}$ will directly impact the performance of the sensor, which is the basis of the isotropic design.

2.1 The Modified Force and Torque Isotropy Indices

The first three rows of the force mapping matrix $\boldsymbol{G}$ are corresponding to force vectors, while the last three rows are corresponding to torque vectors, these two parts of matrix $\boldsymbol{G}$ have different dimensional unit. So we discuss the force isotropy and moment isotropy respectively, then matrix $\boldsymbol{G}$ can be rewritten as

$$\boldsymbol{G} = \begin{bmatrix} \boldsymbol{G}_{\mathrm{F}} \\ \boldsymbol{G}_{\mathrm{M}} \end{bmatrix}. \tag{2}$$

where, $\boldsymbol{G}_{\mathrm{F}}$ is the force mapping matrix, $\boldsymbol{G}_{\mathrm{M}}$ is the torque mapping matrix.

Some literatures[12,13] studied isotropy indices of Stewart platform-based force sensor, but they didn't consider the effect of the following orthogonality condition.

$$\boldsymbol{\Omega} = \boldsymbol{G}_{\mathrm{F}}\boldsymbol{G}_{\mathrm{M}}^{\mathrm{T}} = -\boldsymbol{G}_{\mathrm{M}}\boldsymbol{G}_{\mathrm{F}}^{\mathrm{T}} = \boldsymbol{O}\,. \tag{3}$$

where, $\boldsymbol{O}$ is a 3×3 zeros matrix.

The isotropy indices based on the premise that the orthogonality condition are called modified isotropy indices, which are defined as follows:

1. Force isotropy index ξ_{F}:

$$\xi_{\mathrm{F}} = 1/cond(\boldsymbol{G}_{\mathrm{F}}) = [\lambda_{\min}(\boldsymbol{G}_{\mathrm{F}}\boldsymbol{G}_{\mathrm{F}}^{\mathrm{T}})]^{1/2}/[\lambda_{\max}(\boldsymbol{G}_{\mathrm{F}}\boldsymbol{G}_{\mathrm{F}}^{\mathrm{T}})]^{1/2}\,. \tag{4}$$

2. Torque isotropy index ξ_{M} :

$$\xi_{M} = 1/cond(\boldsymbol{G}_{\mathrm{M}}) = [\lambda_{\min}(\boldsymbol{G}_{\mathrm{M}}\boldsymbol{G}_{\mathrm{M}}^{\mathrm{T}})]^{1/2} / [\lambda_{\max}(\boldsymbol{G}_{\mathrm{M}}\boldsymbol{G}_{\mathrm{M}}^{\mathrm{T}})]^{1/2} . \tag{5}$$

where, *cond*(·) is the condition number of the matrix, $\lambda_{\min}(\cdot)$ and $\lambda_{\max}(\cdot)$ are the minimum and maximum of matrix eigenvalue respectively.

A sensor is said to be force isotropic, when both $\boldsymbol{\Omega}=\boldsymbol{O}$ and $\xi_{\mathrm{F}}=1$ are satisfied.

A sensor is said to be torque isotropic, when both $\boldsymbol{\Omega}=\boldsymbol{O}$ and $\xi_{\mathrm{M}}=1$ are satisfied.

A sensor is said to be fully isotropic, when all the three conditions $\boldsymbol{\Omega}=\boldsymbol{O}$, $\xi_{\mathrm{F}}=1$ and $\xi_{\mathrm{M}}=1$ are satisfied.

Rreference [13] defined the forward and inverse isotropy indices and proposed the concept of complete isotropy, but it is worth mentioning that the concept of full isotropy here is different from the concept of complete isotropy. Complete isotropy only means that the isotropy indices in reference [13] all equal 1, which didn't consider the effect of the orthogonality between $\boldsymbol{G}_{\mathrm{F}}$ and $\boldsymbol{G}_{\mathrm{M}}$. The orthogonality condition is the precondition to achieve the best isotropy performance.

2.2 The Physical Meanings

The external force $\boldsymbol{F}_{\mathrm{o}}$ will produce the infinitesimal changes of the platform, we write the infinitesimal changes $\Delta\boldsymbol{D}$ in the form of

$$\Delta\boldsymbol{D} = \left[\Delta\boldsymbol{d}^{\mathrm{T}}, \Delta\boldsymbol{\theta}^{\mathrm{T}}\right]^{\mathrm{T}} = [\Delta x, \Delta y, \Delta z, \Delta\alpha, \Delta\beta, \Delta\gamma]^{\mathrm{T}} . \tag{6}$$

where, $\Delta\boldsymbol{d}$ is the resulting linear displacement, $\Delta\boldsymbol{\theta}$ is the resulting rotational displacement.

And the external force $\boldsymbol{F}_{\mathrm{o}}$ will produce axial elastic deformation of the elastic legs, relating the reacting force $\boldsymbol{f}$ with the axial elastic deformation $\Delta\boldsymbol{l}$, we have

$$\boldsymbol{f} = k_l \Delta\boldsymbol{l} . \tag{7}$$

where, $\Delta\boldsymbol{l}=\{\Delta l_1\ \Delta l_2\ \Delta l_3\ \Delta l_4\ \Delta l_5\ \Delta l_6\}$ is a vector composed of the elastic deformation of the six legs; k_l is the axial stiffness coefficient, we set the six legs have same stiffness. To relate $\Delta\boldsymbol{l}$ with $\Delta\boldsymbol{D}$, we have

$$\Delta\boldsymbol{l} = \boldsymbol{G}^{\mathrm{T}}\Delta\boldsymbol{D} . \tag{8}$$

Combining equation (1) with equations (7) and (8), we have

$$\boldsymbol{F}_{\mathrm{o}} = k_l \boldsymbol{G}\boldsymbol{G}^{\mathrm{T}}\Delta\boldsymbol{D} = k_l \begin{bmatrix} \boldsymbol{G}_{\mathrm{F}}\boldsymbol{G}_{\mathrm{F}}^{\mathrm{T}} & \boldsymbol{G}_{\mathrm{F}}\boldsymbol{G}_{\mathrm{M}}^{\mathrm{T}} \\ \boldsymbol{G}_{\mathrm{M}}\boldsymbol{G}_{\mathrm{F}}^{\mathrm{T}} & \boldsymbol{G}_{\mathrm{M}}\boldsymbol{G}_{\mathrm{M}}^{\mathrm{T}} \end{bmatrix} \begin{bmatrix} \Delta\boldsymbol{d} \\ \Delta\boldsymbol{\theta} \end{bmatrix} . \tag{9}$$

where, the matrix $\boldsymbol{G}\boldsymbol{G}^{\mathrm{T}}$ is the stiffness matrix[2].

Due to the structure symmetry of the Stewart platform-based force sensor, the matrices $\boldsymbol{G}_{\mathrm{F}}\boldsymbol{G}_{\mathrm{F}}^{\mathrm{T}}$, $\boldsymbol{G}_{\mathrm{M}}\boldsymbol{G}_{\mathrm{M}}^{\mathrm{T}}$ are diagonal matrices, which can be written in the following form.

$$\boldsymbol{G}_{\mathrm{F}}\boldsymbol{G}_{\mathrm{F}}^{\mathrm{T}} = diag(\Lambda_{\mathrm{F1}}, \Lambda_{\mathrm{F2}}, \Lambda_{\mathrm{F3}}); \boldsymbol{G}_{\mathrm{M}}\boldsymbol{G}_{\mathrm{M}}^{\mathrm{T}} = diag(\Lambda_{\mathrm{M1}}, \Lambda_{\mathrm{M2}}, \Lambda_{\mathrm{M3}}). \tag{10}$$

where, Λ_{F1}, Λ_{F2}, Λ_{F3}, Λ_{M1}, Λ_{M2}, Λ_{M3} are the diagonal elements.

Adding the orthogonality condition $\boldsymbol{\Omega}=\boldsymbol{O}$, we can obtain

$$\boldsymbol{F}_{\mathrm{o}} = \begin{bmatrix} F_{\mathrm{x}} \\ F_{\mathrm{y}} \\ F_{\mathrm{z}} \\ M_{\mathrm{x}} \\ M_{\mathrm{y}} \\ M_{\mathrm{z}} \end{bmatrix} = k_l \begin{bmatrix} \Lambda_{\mathrm{F1}} & 0 & 0 & 0 & 0 & 0 \\ 0 & \Lambda_{\mathrm{F2}} & 0 & 0 & 0 & 0 \\ 0 & 0 & \Lambda_{\mathrm{F3}} & 0 & 0 & 0 \\ 0 & 0 & 0 & \Lambda_{\mathrm{M1}} & 0 & 0 \\ 0 & 0 & 0 & 0 & \Lambda_{\mathrm{M2}} & 0 \\ 0 & 0 & 0 & 0 & 0 & \Lambda_{\mathrm{M3}} \end{bmatrix} \begin{bmatrix} \Delta x \\ \Delta y \\ \Delta z \\ \Delta \alpha \\ \Delta \beta \\ \Delta \gamma \end{bmatrix}. \tag{11}$$

By expression (11), it is easily seen that, the orthogonality condition means that the stiffness of the sensor in all the directions are decoupling.

Especially, when the full isotropy is satisfied, we have $\Lambda_{\mathrm{F1}} = \Lambda_{\mathrm{F2}} = \Lambda_{\mathrm{F3}}$ and $\Lambda_{\mathrm{M1}} = \Lambda_{\mathrm{M2}} = \Lambda_{\mathrm{M3}}$.

Then, we can conclude that full isotropy means that the sensor exhibits a homogeneous stiffness characteristic in all the directions, the isotropy indices show how far the sensor is from being fully isotropic.

3 The General 6-6 Stewart Platform-Based Force Sensor

The 6-6 Stewart platform-based force sensor is shown in Fig.1. It is composed of an upper platform, a lower platform and six elastic legs connecting the two platforms with spherical joints; $u_i(i=1,2\ldots,6)$ and $U_i(i=1,2\ldots,6)$ are the center of i-th spherical joint of the upper platform and lower platform respectively; the Cartesian coordinate O_c-XYZ, called frame $\{\Omega_c\}$, is set up with its origin located at the geometrical center of the upper platform, the X axis is perpendicular to the line connecting U_1 and U_6; the central angles between u_1 and u_3, u_3 and u_5 are $2\pi/3$, and the central angles between U_1 and U_3, U_3 and U_5 are $2\pi/3$ too; φ_1 denotes the central angle between U_6 and

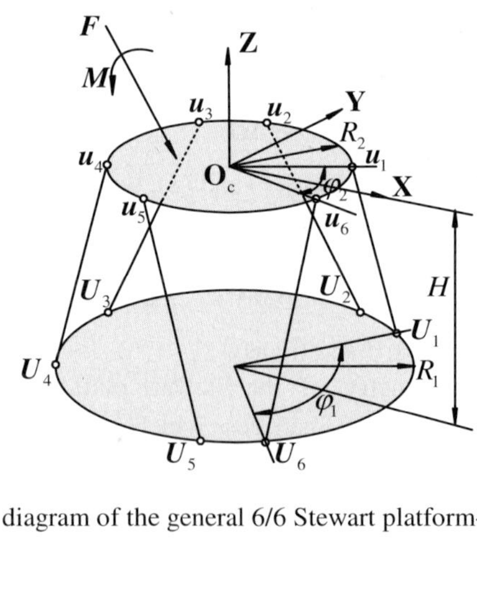

Fig. 1. Schematic diagram of the general 6/6 Stewart platform-based force sensor

U_1; φ_2 denotes the central angle between u_6 and u_1; R_1 denotes the radius of the lower platform; R_2 denotes the radius of and the upper platform.; H denotes the distance between the upper and lower platform.

For the 6/6 Stewart platform-based force sensor, the force mapping matrix $\boldsymbol{G}_c$ [14] can be expressed as

$$\boldsymbol{G}_c = \begin{bmatrix} \boldsymbol{S}_1 & \boldsymbol{S}_2 & \boldsymbol{S}_3 & \boldsymbol{S}_4 & \boldsymbol{S}_5 & \boldsymbol{S}_6 \\ \boldsymbol{S}_{01} & \boldsymbol{S}_{02} & \boldsymbol{S}_{03} & \boldsymbol{S}_{04} & \boldsymbol{S}_{05} & \boldsymbol{S}_{06} \end{bmatrix}. \quad (12)$$

where, $\boldsymbol{S}_i=(\boldsymbol{u}_i-\boldsymbol{U}_i)/|\boldsymbol{u}_i-\boldsymbol{U}_i|$, $\boldsymbol{S}_{0i}=(\boldsymbol{U}_i\times\boldsymbol{u}_i)/|\boldsymbol{u}_i-\boldsymbol{U}_i|$, $\boldsymbol{u}_i$ and $\boldsymbol{U}_i$ denote the position vectors of the center of the i-th spherical joints u_i and U_i with respect to frame $\{\Omega_c\}$ respectively.

3.1 Isotropic Performance of General 6/6 Stewart Platform-Based Force Sensor

The matrices $[\boldsymbol{G}_c]_F[\boldsymbol{G}_c]_F^T$, $[\boldsymbol{G}_c]_M[\boldsymbol{G}_c]_M^T$, $[\boldsymbol{G}_c]_F[\boldsymbol{G}_c]_M^T$, $[\boldsymbol{G}_c]_M[\boldsymbol{G}_c]_F^T$ can be expressed as

$$[\boldsymbol{G}_c]_F[\boldsymbol{G}_c]_F^T = diag(\Lambda'_{F1},\Lambda'_{F2},\Lambda'_{F3});\ [\boldsymbol{G}_c]_M[\boldsymbol{G}_c]_M^T = diag(\Lambda'_{M1},\Lambda'_{M2},\Lambda'_{M3}). \quad (13)$$

$$[\boldsymbol{G}_c]_F[\boldsymbol{G}_c]_M^T = [\boldsymbol{G}_c]_M[\boldsymbol{G}_c]_F^T = \begin{bmatrix} 0 & \Gamma & 0 \\ -\Gamma & 0 & 0 \\ 0 & 0 & 0 \end{bmatrix}. \quad (14)$$

where $\Lambda'_{F1}=\Lambda'_{F2}=\dfrac{3m}{L^2}$, $\Lambda'_{F3}=\dfrac{6H^2}{L^2}$; $\Lambda'_{M1}=\Lambda'_{M2}=\dfrac{3H^2R_2^2}{L^2}$, $\Lambda'_{M3}=\dfrac{3R_2^2\,n}{L^2}$;

$L=\sqrt{R_1^2+R_2^2-2R_1R_2\cos((\alpha_1-\alpha_2)/2)+H^2}$; $m=R_1^2+R_2^2-2R_1R_2\cos((\alpha_1-\alpha_2)/2)$;

$n=2R_1^2\sin^2((\alpha_1-\alpha_2)/2)$; $\Gamma=\dfrac{3HR_2(R_1\cos((\varphi_1-\varphi_2)/2)-R_2)}{L^2}$.

The modified isotropy indices require the orthogonality condition must be satisfied, then we have

$$\Gamma=0 \Rightarrow R_1\cos((\varphi_1-\varphi_2)/2)-R_2=0 \Rightarrow R_2=R_1\cos((\varphi_1-\varphi_2)/2). \quad (15)$$

Substituting expression (15) into the expression m we have

$$m=R_1^2\sin^2((\alpha_1-\alpha_2)/2)=n/2. \quad (16)$$

By the definition of the modified isotropy indices, we can obtain

$$\begin{cases} \xi_F=(\Lambda'_{F1}/\Lambda'_{F3})^{1/2}=(n/4H^2)^{1/2}, (n\le 4H^2); \\ \xi_F=(\Lambda'_{F3}/\Lambda'_{F1})^{1/2}=(4H^2/n)^{1/2}, (n\ge 4H^2); \\ \xi_M=(\Lambda'_{M1}/\Lambda'_{M3})^{1/2}=(H^2/n)^{1/2}, (n\ge H^2); \\ \xi_M=(\Lambda'_{M3}/\Lambda'_{M1})^{1/2}=(n/H^2)^{1/2}, (n\le H^2). \end{cases} \quad (17)$$

Make a summary of all the cases above, it is found that there are special mathematical relationships between force and torque isotropy indices as follow.

$$\begin{cases} \xi_{\mathrm{F}}\xi_{\mathrm{M}} = 1/2, \left(H^2 \le n \le 4H^2\right); \\ \xi_{\mathrm{F}}\xi_{\mathrm{M}} = \left(n^2/4H^4\right)^{1/2} < 1/2, \left(n < H^2\right); \\ \xi_{\mathrm{F}}\xi_{\mathrm{M}} = \left(4H^4/n^2\right)^{1/2} < 1/2, \left(n > 4H^2\right). \end{cases} \tag{18}$$

From equation (17), it can be seen that the sensor can achieve the force isotropy when $n=H^2$, and the torque isotropy is realized when $n=4H^2$.

To achieve the full isotropy for the sensor, both $\xi_{\mathrm{F}}=1$ and $\xi_{\mathrm{M}}=1$ must be satisfied, it can be easily seen that the two equations can't be satisfied simultaneously. Then it can be concluded that it is impossible for the general 6/6 Stewart platform-based force sensor to realize the full isotropy.

3.2 The Best Comprehensive Isotropic Performance

To make sure the sensor has the comprehensive isotropy performance, we must optimize the structure parameters by compromising the two isotropy indices. We know the sensor achieves the best force and torque isotropy performances indices when the condition number of $\boldsymbol{G}_{\mathrm{F}},\boldsymbol{G}_{\mathrm{M}}$ reach the minimum respectively, then the objective function of comprehensive performance can be defined as follow.

$$\boldsymbol{g} = k_1 \cdot cond(\boldsymbol{G}_{\mathrm{F}}) + k_2 \cdot cond(\boldsymbol{G}_{\mathrm{M}}) = \frac{k_1}{\xi_{\mathrm{F}}} + \frac{k_2}{\xi_{\mathrm{M}}} . \tag{19}$$

where, k_1, k_2 are the weight coefficients of the related performance indices, we set $k_1=1$, $k_2=1$.

In order to achieve the best comprehensive performance, it is easily seen that, from equation (18), the condition $\xi_{\mathrm{F}}\xi_M=1$ must be satisfied. And we know the sensor achieves the best comprehensive performance when the objective function $\boldsymbol{g}$ reaches the minimum, then the comprehensive performance optimization problem can be formu-lated as an extremum problem of multi-variable object functions of with constraint equation $\xi_F\xi_M=1$.

By solving the conditional extremum of function $\boldsymbol{g}$, it is found that the sensor obtains the best comprehensive performance when the following equation is satisfied.

$$\xi_{\mathrm{F}} = \xi_{\mathrm{M}} = \sqrt{2}/2 \approx 0.707 . \tag{20}$$

The related analytic expressions of the key structural parameters are obtained as follow when the sensor achieves the best comprehensive performance.

$$H = R_1 \left|\sin((\varphi_1 - \varphi_2)/2)\right| . \tag{21}$$

The expressions (15) and (21) are the analytic expressions of the key structural parameters when the sensor achieves the best comprehensive performance. Reference [15] obtained the best comprehensive performances by a numeric method, but its structural parameters are just one numerical example of expressions (15) and (21).

4 A Novel 6/3-3 Stewart Platform-Based Force sensor

It is impossible to realize full isotropy for the general 6/6 Stewart platform-based force sensor, then a novel 6/3-3 configuration of Stewart platform-based force sensor is proposed here, which is shown in Fig.2. The Cartesian coordinate O_c-XYZ, called frame $\{\Omega_n\}$, is located at the geometrical center of the upper platform; R_b denotes the radius of the circle on the upper platform, with which the centers of six spherical joints located; R_{a1} and R_{a2} denote the outer and inner radii of the circles, with which the centers of spherical joint located, on the lower platform respectively; $A_i(i=1,2\ldots,6)$ and $b_i(i=1,2\ldots,6)$ are the center of i-th spherical joint respectively; A_1,A_2,A_3 are placed symmetrically on the circle of radius R_{a1}, A_4,A_5,A_6 are placed symmetrically on the circle of radius R_{a2}; b_1,b_2,b_3 are placed symmetrically on the circle of radius R_b, b_4,b_5,b_6 are also placed symmetrically on the circle of R_b; h denotes the distance between the upper and lower platform; α_1,β_1 denote the twist angles of the first spherical joint of the lower platform and upper platform with respect to X axis respectively; α_2,β_2 denote the twist angles of the fourth spherical joints of the lower platform and upper platform with respect to X axis respectively.

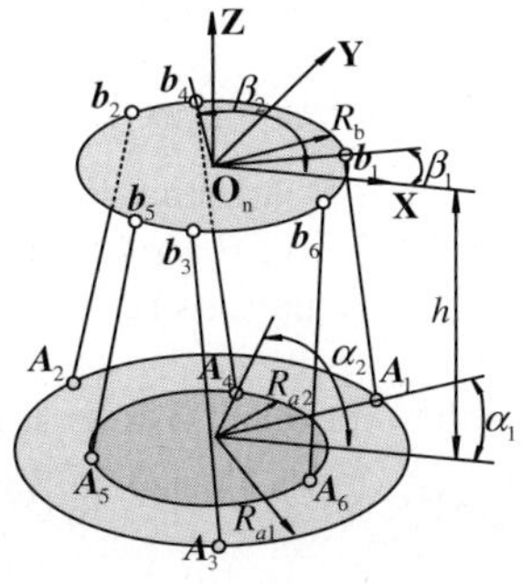

Fig. 2. Schematic diagram of the novel 6/3-3 Stewart platform-based force/torque sensor

For the 6/3-3 Stewart platform-based force sensor, the force mapping matrix can be expressed as

$$G_n = \begin{bmatrix} \frac{b_1 - A_1}{|b_1 - A_1|} & \frac{b_2 - A_2}{|b_2 - A_2|} & \frac{b_3 - A_3}{|b_3 - A_3|} & \frac{b_4 - A_4}{|b_4 - A_4|} & \frac{b_5 - A_5}{|b_5 - A_5|} & \frac{b_6 - A_6}{|b_6 - A_6|} \\ \frac{A_1 \times b_1}{|b_1 - A_1|} & \frac{A_2 \times b_2}{|b_2 - A_2|} & \frac{A_3 \times b_3}{|b_3 - A_3|} & \frac{A_4 \times b_4}{|b_4 - A_4|} & \frac{A_5 \times b_5}{|b_5 - A_5|} & \frac{A_6 \times b_6}{|b_6 - A_6|} \end{bmatrix}. \quad (22)$$

where, $\boldsymbol{b}_i$ and $\boldsymbol{A}_i$ (i=1,2…,6) denote the position vectors of the center of i-th spherical joints b_i and A_i with respect to frame $\{\Omega_n\}$ respectively.

For the 6/3-3 Stewart platform based force/torque sensor, the matrix $[G_n]_F [G_n]_F^T$, $[G_n]_M [G_n]_M^T$, $[G_n]_F [G_n]_M^T$, $[G_n]_M [G_n]_F^T$ can be expressed as

$$[\boldsymbol{G}_{\mathrm{n}}]_{\mathrm{F}}[\boldsymbol{G}_{\mathrm{n}}]_{\mathrm{F}}^{\mathrm{T}} = diag(\Lambda''_{\mathrm{F1}},\Lambda''_{\mathrm{F2}},\Lambda''_{\mathrm{F3}});\ [\boldsymbol{G}_{\mathrm{n}}]_{\mathrm{M}}[\boldsymbol{G}_{\mathrm{n}}]_{\mathrm{M}}^{\mathrm{T}} = diag(\Lambda''_{\mathrm{M1}},\Lambda''_{\mathrm{M2}},\Lambda''_{\mathrm{M3}})\,. \tag{23}$$

$$[\boldsymbol{G}_{\mathrm{n}}]_{\mathrm{F}}[\boldsymbol{G}_{\mathrm{n}}]_{\mathrm{M}}^{\mathrm{T}} = -[\boldsymbol{G}_{\mathrm{n}}]_{\mathrm{M}}[\boldsymbol{G}_{\mathrm{n}}]_{\mathrm{F}}^{\mathrm{T}} = \begin{bmatrix} \Gamma_1 & \Gamma_2 & 0 \\ -\Gamma_2 & \Gamma_1 & 0 \\ 0 & 0 & -2\Gamma_1 \end{bmatrix}. \tag{24}$$

where $\Lambda''_{\mathrm{F1}} = \left(-3R_{\mathrm{b}}(R_{a1}\cos\theta_1 + R_{a2}\cos\theta_2) + 3R_{\mathrm{b}}^2 + 3/2(R_{a1}^2 + R_{a2}^2)\right)/L_{\mathrm{n}}^2$; $\Lambda''_{\mathrm{F3}} = 6h^2/L_{\mathrm{n}}^2$; $\Lambda''_{\mathrm{M1}} = 3h^2R_b^2/L_{\mathrm{n}}^2$; $\Lambda''_{\mathrm{M3}} = 3R_b^2(R_{a1}^2\sin^2\theta_1 + R_{a2}^2\sin^2\theta_2)/L_{\mathrm{n}}^2$; $\Lambda''_{\mathrm{F1}} = \Lambda''_{\mathrm{F2}}$; $\Lambda''_{\mathrm{M1}} = \Lambda''_{\mathrm{M2}}$;
$\Gamma_2 = \frac{3}{2}hR_{\mathrm{b}}\left(R_{a1}\cos\theta_1 + R_{a2}\cos\theta_2 - 2R_{\mathrm{b}}\right)/L_{\mathrm{n}}^2$; $L_n = \sqrt{R_{a1}^2 + R_{\mathrm{b}}^2 - 2R_{a1}R_{\mathrm{b}}\cos\theta_1 + h^2}$;
$\Gamma_1 = -\frac{3}{2}hR_{\mathrm{b}}\left(R_{a1}\sin\theta_1 + R_{a2}\sin\theta_2\right)/L_{\mathrm{n}}^2$; $\theta_1 = \beta_1 - \alpha_1$; $\theta_2 = \beta_2 - \alpha_2$.

From the concept of full isotropy and the expressions (23) and (24), we know the isotropy performance of the sensor is determined by six parameters R_{a1}, R_{a2}, R_b, h, θ_1, θ_2. For the 6/3-3 Stewart platform-based force sensor to be full isotropy, the following four equations should be satisfied simultaneously.

$$\Lambda''_{\mathrm{F1}} = \Lambda''_{\mathrm{F2}} = \Lambda''_{\mathrm{F3}};\ \Lambda''_{\mathrm{M1}} = \Lambda''_{\mathrm{M2}} = \Lambda''_{\mathrm{M3}};\Gamma_1 = 0;\ \Gamma_2 = 0. \tag{25}$$

We suppose the parameters R_{b} and θ_2 are known, which can be determined by the design requirement, here we set $R_{\mathrm{b}}=1$ and $\theta_2=\pi/4$. Then the other parameters can be obtained by solving the simultaneous equations (25), there are four solutions are given in Table 1.

It is found that only the fourth solution in Table 1. has the practical meaning, the matrix $[\boldsymbol{G}_{\mathrm{n}}]_{\mathrm{F}}[\boldsymbol{G}_{\mathrm{n}}]_{\mathrm{F}}^{\mathrm{T}}, [\boldsymbol{G}_{\mathrm{n}}]_{\mathrm{M}}[\boldsymbol{G}_{\mathrm{n}}]_{\mathrm{M}}^{\mathrm{T}}, [\boldsymbol{G}_{\mathrm{n}}]_{\mathrm{F}}[\boldsymbol{G}_{\mathrm{n}}]_{\mathrm{M}}^{\mathrm{T}}, [\boldsymbol{G}_{\mathrm{n}}]_{\mathrm{M}}[\boldsymbol{G}_{\mathrm{n}}]_{\mathrm{F}}^{\mathrm{T}}$ at the configuration of the fourth solution are as follow.

Table 1. The values of the parameters θ_1, h, R_{a1}, R_{a2} when the sensor satisfies full isotropy

Solution No.	θ_1	h	R_{a1}	R_{a2}
1	0.3855	1.9319	3.6327	-1.9319
2	-2.7561	1.9319	-3.6327	-1.9319
3	2.9212	0.5176	-1.6745	0.5176
4	-0.2204	0.5176	1.6745	0.5176

$$[\boldsymbol{G}_{\mathrm{n}}]_{\mathrm{F}}[\boldsymbol{G}_{\mathrm{n}}]_{M}^{\mathrm{T}} = -[\boldsymbol{G}_{\mathrm{n}}]_{M}[\boldsymbol{G}_{\mathrm{n}}]_{\mathrm{F}}^{\mathrm{T}} = \begin{bmatrix} 0.0000 & -0.0000 & -0.0000 \\ 0.0000 & 0.0000 & 0.0000 \\ 0.0000 & 0.0000 & -0.0000 \end{bmatrix}. \tag{26}$$

$$[\boldsymbol{G}_{\mathrm{n}}]_{F}[\boldsymbol{G}_{\mathrm{n}}]_{F}^{\mathrm{T}} = diag(2.0001, 2.0001, 2.0000)\,. \tag{27}$$

$$[\boldsymbol{G}_{\mathrm{n}}]_M [\boldsymbol{G}_n]_M^{\mathrm{T}} = diag(1.0000, 1.0000, 1.0001)\,. \tag{28}$$

From equations (26)~(28) we know, all the three conditions $\boldsymbol{\Omega}=\boldsymbol{O}$, $\xi_{\mathrm{F}}=1$ and $\xi_{\mathrm{M}}=1$ are satisfied, namely the sensor at the configuration achieves full isotropy.

5 Conclusions

This paper has conducted the isotropic design of the Stewart platform-based force sensor based on the proposed modified isotropy indices. A novel 6/3-3 configuration of Stewart paltform-based force sensor is proposed, which can realize full isotropy. The isotropy performance of the general 6/6 Stewart platform-based force sensor is analyzed in detail, we found that it is impossible to realize the full isotropy in theory, and the best comprehensive isotropic performance is obtained by solving the extremum of the objective function. The contents of this paper should be useful for the further research and practical application of the six-axis force/torque sensor.

Acknowledgments

This research is financially supported by the National Natural Science Foundation of China under Grant No. 50575192 and the Natural Science Foundation of Hebei Province, China under Grant No. E2007000349.

References

1. Stewart, D.: A Platform with Six Degrees of Freedom. Proc. Inst. Mech. Eng. 180, 371–378 (1965)
2. Merlet, J.-P.: Parallel Robots, 2nd edn. Springer, Heidelberg (2006)
3. Gaillet, A., Reboulet, C.: An Isostatic Six Component Force and Torque Sensor. In: Proceedings of the 13th International Symposium on Industrial Robotics, pp. 102–111 (1983)
4. Kerr, D.R.: Analysis, Properties and Design of a Stewart-Platform Transducer. ASME, Design Engineering Division (Publication) DE, Trends and Developments in Mechanisms, Machines and Robotics 15(3), 139–145 (1988)
5. Nguyen, C.C., Antrazi, S.S., Zhou, Z.L.: Analysis and Implementation of a 6-dof Stewart Platform-based Force Sensor for Passive Compliant Robotic Assembly. In: IEEE Proc. of the Southeast Conf., Williamsburg, VA, pp. 880–884 (2001)
6. Dwarakanath, T.A., Dasgupta, B., Mruthyunjaya, T.S.: Design and Development of a Stewart platform Based Force-Torque Sensor. Mechatronics 11(7), 793–809 (2001)
7. Zhao, Y.S., Hou, Y.L., Yan, Z.W., Yuan, H.L., Gao, J.: Research and Design of a Pre-Stressed Six-Component Force/Torque Sensor Based on the Stewart Platform. In: Proceedings of the ASME International Design Engineering Technical Conferences DETC 2005, USA, California, vol. 7 B, pp. 573–581 (2005)
8. Gao, F., Zhang, Y., Zhao, X.C., Guo, W.Z.: The Design and Applications of F/T Sensor Based on Stewart Platform. In: Proceedings of the 12th IFToMM World Congress, France, Besancon (2007)

9. Uchiyama, M., Hakomori, K.: A Few Considerations on Structure Design of Force Sensor. In: Proceedings of the Third Annual Conference Japan Robotics Society, pp. 17–18 (1985)
10. Uchiyama, M., Nakarnura, Y., Hakomori, K.: Evaluation of Robot Force Sensor Structure Using Singular Value Decomposition. Journal of the Robotics Society of Japan 5(1), 4–10 (1987) (in Japanese)
11. Xiong, Y.L.: On isotropy of robot's force sensors. Acta Automatica Sinica 22(1), 10–18 (1996) (in Chinese)
12. Jin, Z.L., Gao, F.: Optimal Design of a 6-Axis Force transducer Based on Stewart platform related to sensitivity isotropy. Chinese Journal of Mechanical Engineering 16(2), 146–149 (2003)
13. Hou, Y.L., Yao, J.T., Lu, L., Zhao, Y.S.: Performance Analysis and Comprehensive Index Optimization of a New Configuration of Stewart Six-component Force Sensor. Mech. Mach. Theory (2008)
14. Huang, Z., Zhao, Y.S., Zhao, T.S.: Advanced Spatial Mechanism, pp. 195–201. Higher Education Press, Beijing (2006) (in Chinese)
15. Zhao, Y.Z., Zhao, T.S., Wen, R.: Performance Analysis and Optimal Design of Parallel 6-axis Force Sensor. China Mechanical Engineering 17, 299–302 (2006) (in Chinese)

Service Design for Product Lifecycle in Service Oriented Manufacturing

Liping Zhao, Jun Wan, Pingyu Jiang, and Yongtao Qin

State Key Laboratory for Manufacturing Systems Engineering,
Xi'an Jiaotong University, 710049, China

Abstract. In order to provide value-added service for products during product lifecycle and service support for manufacturing enterprises in global range, based on the production mode of service oriented manufacturing(SOM), the development flow of service design based on product lifecycle and Six Sigma is established. In the base of each stage information of product lifecycle, the development flow is divided into service requirement analysis, service design, service machining and service maintenance four stages. According to requirements of SOM, the family of methods and development tool of service design are provided based on Six Sigma concept, a service design for product lifecycle development system framework in SOM is constructed, which is with service requirement as service object, by means of product lifecycle management (PLM) managing product data in entire product lifecycle, transforming information from service manufacturing and equipment e-maintenance into service design information. Finally, a product lifecycle oriented information model of service design is studied, by which data on product design, process and crafts, quality, cost, sale and maintenance could be contacted and feedback manufacturing and maintenance information to service design process, for laying a foundation for satisfying requirements of service oriented manufacturing.

Keywords: Product lifecycle, Service oriented manufacturing, Service design, Six Sigma, PLM, e-maintenance.

1 Introduction

With the development of economy globalization, service becomes more important in product value chain. Service oriented manufacturing (SOM) is such a new advanced manufacturing mode that combines manufacturing with service, to achieve value-added of various stakeholders in manufacturing value chain. Through the introduction of service value-added, SOM can create greater value in product lifecycle to enable enterprises to obtain high returns. During each stage of product lifecycle, as 80% of the cost is used for design, in order to shift from disorderly passive service to orderly active service, under the mode of SOM, new demands are put forward for product design, which consist of product function, service ability, service design ability, service flow management, and service demand for sharing of product information. Based on it, service design for product lifecycle in SOM is proposed, which can meet the need of product performance guarantee, service flow management and service ability

C. Xiong et al. (Eds.): ICIRA 2008, Part II, LNAI 5315, pp. 733–742, 2008.

of cross-enterprise, to provide value-added service for product lifecycle, as well as service support in manufacturing enterprise on global scale.

With the demand of SOM, service design is taken as the core, based on information of product lifecycle, the development flow of service design oriented to product lifecycle and Six Sigma is established. The flow is divided into service requirement analysis, service design, service machining and service maintenance four stages. Based on the family of methods and the development tool of service design, by means of PLM managing, product data of design, manufacturing, quality, after-sale service and maintenance are carried out service management. Based on Six Sigma concept, a service design for product lifecycle development system framework in SOM is constructed. Based on it, product lifecycle oriented information model of service design is studied.

2 Related Work

At present, research of SOM mode from domestic and foreign scholars are more limited to issues of enterprise-class, including how to construct the corresponding service oriented architecture and grid service etc. Liu Min, Yan Junwei[1] presents a Grid Manufacturing mode based on the Service Oriented Architecture and Networked Manufacturing to integrate and share the dynamic manufacturing resources effectively. Yang zhonghua [2] proposes a SOM environment based on semantic modeling for various resources to realize real-time discovery of manufacturing resources in web environment. Ruyue [3] presents SOM grid environment using web-services technology for the manufacture of different resources for the package to realize dynamic allocation of distributed manufacturing resources with specific tasks.

At the same time, many further researches have been done on product lifecycle management. Shu Qilin and Wang Cheng'en [4] divided product lifecycle into different stages and built model in each stage, then studied methods which make stage models transform to product service model. Cui Jian et al. [5] built requirement information flow chart and constructed a customer requirement information management model using structure diagram.

Recently, more and more people begin to pay attention to service design and also have some preliminary researches. Zhang Wei et al. [6] started with the definition of service design and found out the indexes which customers apperceive service design quality, built a preliminary evaluation model on service design. Basem El-haik and David M.Roy [7] brought forward that service design itself was a structured and data-driven approach, and designed service using Six Sigma tools. Khan, M.H., Madisetti, V.K. [8] presented a multiple-field simulation structure and applied integrated multiple-network simulation methodology in solving advanced distributed service design problem. However, how to make service design in product lifecycle much well need further research.

3 Service Design for Product Lifecycle Development System Framework in Service Oriented Manufacturing

With the demand of SOM, in order to solve the situation that information among different enterprises cooperate hard and lack of effectively management for entire product lifecycle, a service design for product lifecycle development system framework in service oriented manufacturing is constructed. Based on the framework, the development flow of service design is divided into four stages according to product lifecycle. By means of family of methods and development tool of service design, information from service manufacturing and equipment e-maintenance are transformed into service design information. In the service design stage, based on Six Sigma concept of process improvement and optimization, the specific form and details of product service information created by product lifecycle can be expressed and analyzed.

3.1 Service Design for Product Lifecycle Development Framework in Service Oriented Manufacturing

With service requirement as service object, the product lifecycle oriented development framework of service design is constructed, as is shown in Fig.1.

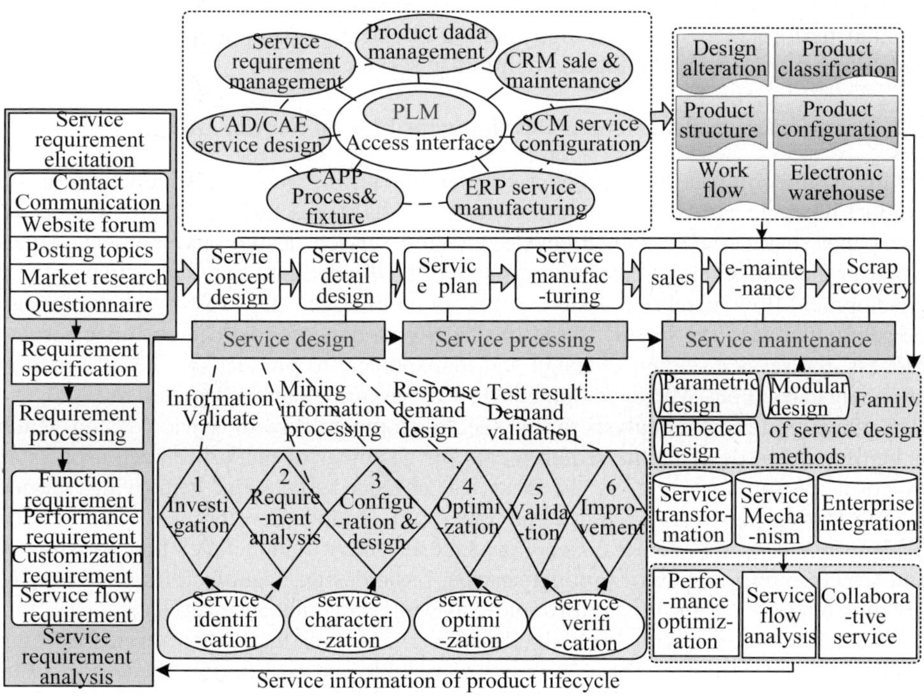

Fig. 1. Product lifecycle oriented development framework of service design

To product information in every stage of product lifecycle, to meet service demand under the mode of SOM, the service design development flow can be divided into service requirement analysis, service design, service processing and service maintenance. Based on Six Sigma concept of process improvement and optimization, service design can be subdivided into service investigate, service requirement analysis, service configuration and design, configuration optimization, service improvement as well. The personnel, organization, process design, and service information can be integrated and shared by PLM. Combined with CAD/CAE/CAM, PDM, ERP, and so on, the product geometric structure information with CAD,CAE,CAM files as core, and data, conceptual expression relationship, resources files with PDM/ERP as object can complete multiple term data processing including service configuration management, product service structure management, and service performance optimization etc.. In six stages of service design stage, the specific form and details of product service information created by product lifecycle of cross-enterprise can be expressed and analyzed by means of service design development tools. Depending on family of service design methods of e-maintenance, which consist of embedded design, parametric design and modular design. Information from service manufacturing and equipment e-maintenance are transformed into service design information. Combined with service information form other stages of product lifecycle, the service design stage can construct an integrated and organic product lifecycle service design development flow. The flow can make full use of service design information to be created, managed, integrated in all stages of product lifecycle, and information resource across the entire product lifecycle to extend the service design field, besides; it can acquire optimal performance service design method by means of key process characteristic and other optimizing technologies, to optimize service process.

3.2 Product Lifecycle Oriented Development Flow of Service Design

Owing to the complexity of product's development, it's getting difficult to describe product lifecycle as a whole, should be described by stages and from many aspects. In this paper, based on product lifecycle oriented service design development framework, product lifecycle of cross-enterprise will be divided into four stages to complete development flow of service design. At the same time, the stage of service design can be subdivided into six stages. Based on Six Sigma concept that can optimize service process, the service sequence design and management to product service information are being carried out. The development flow of service design is depicted as Fig.2.

Service requirement analysis during the development flow of service design which is being used to describe the requirements for customer or market to such aspects as function, performance etc. is the basis of product innovation, improving service manufacturing satisfaction, and achieving rapid product development. The service design stage is used to depict concept product service, which includes function, theory and structure information of product service, basic design, manufacturing and assembly information of parts, cost information, as well as maintenance service.

The service requirement is obtained with service investigate, then service is being configured and designed. Through function, reliable and cost design, the service configuration can be optimized. Then by means of requirement test, function comparison and service simulation, the service is validated. Finally, the service is improved. Service processing is depicted with emphasis on information required in manufacturing process on the basis of product service design. Service maintenance is significantly described information such as delivery state, installation, and maintenance service of product service. Service is provided for after-manufacturing stage according to maintenance, to realize value-added of product lifecycle of cross-enterprise. Meanwhile, through feedback mechanism, information from service manufacturing and equipment

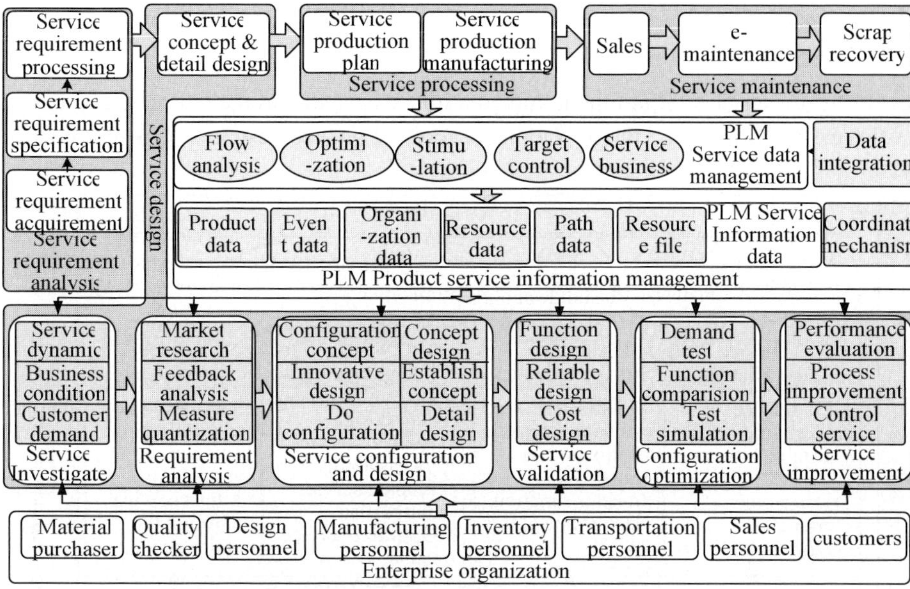

Fig. 2. Product lifecycle oriented development flow of service design

e-maintenance can be transformed into service design information, and then service information of product lifecycle can be designed.

In the stages of service processing and service maintenance, personnel, organization, design management activity, and service information of product lifecycle are being integrated and shared by PLM. By coordinating service flow management with product development environment, enterprises alliance, the relational data and resource file can be carried out multi data processing that contains service flow analysis, service performance evaluation, and service dynamic simulation etc.. Meanwhile, in the stage of service design, based on the Six Sigma concept that subdivides and improves process, by means of service development tools and family of methods for service design, particular form and content of product information in each stage of product lifecycle can be expressed and analyzed. Product is depicted by quantitative language to evaluate and validate satisfaction of service manufacturing and adaptability between developing product and object market. In manufacturing enterprise, personnel can obtain roles of various organizations in accordance with the organizational structure. Product dada is processed by various information systems. By means of feedback mechanism, it is transferred to the service design-stage in order to carry out detail design of new product on the premise of meeting service manufacturing requirement. The flow is not isolated, but constitutes a complete organic integrated product lifecycle oriented development flow of service design together with other stages of product, in order to improve actual effect of following stages which are product design, manufacturing sales, and maintenance, to enhance satisfaction of service manufacturing maximally.

3.3 Product Lifecycle Oriented Family of Methods and Development Tools of Service Design

According to service requirement information, based on product lifecycle oriented development framework, the development tools of service design is shown in Fig.3.

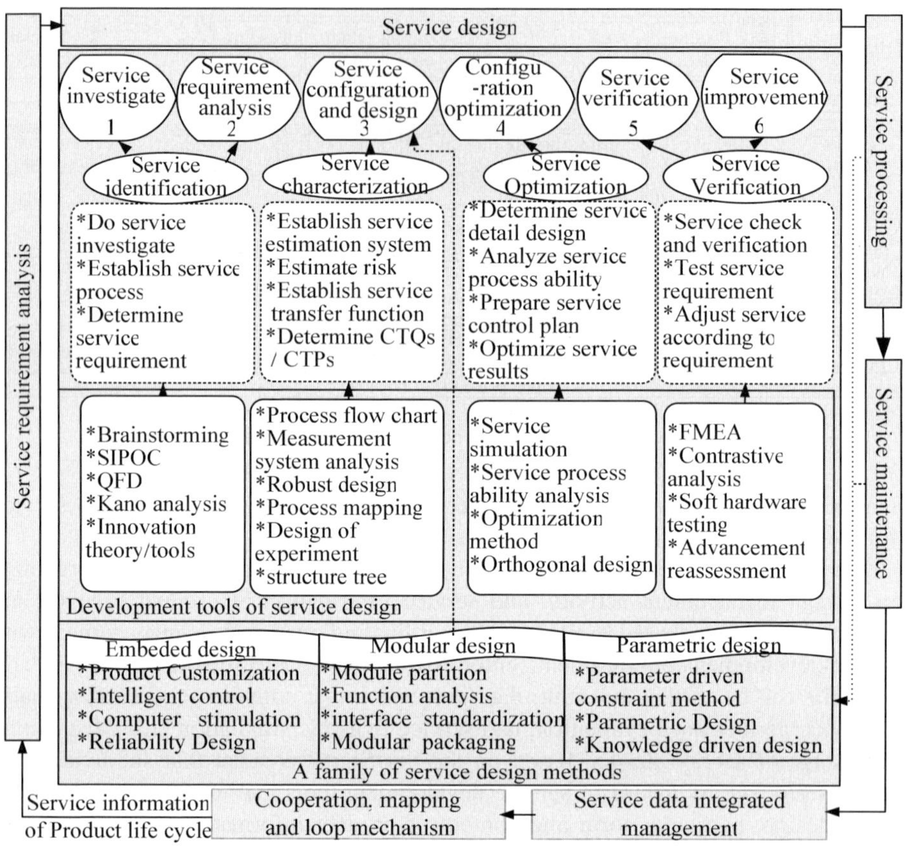

Fig. 3. Product lifecycle Oriented family of methods and development tools of Service Design

In order to express and analyze particular form and detail requirements, the development tools of service design based on Six Sigma which outspreads as the flow of service identification- service characterization- service optimization- service verification is established as above. By providing family of e-maintenance service design methods in service design stage, service is being designed after configuration. Service processing and maintenance is supported with the family of service design methods.

In service identification stage, service information resources are confirmed first, service is investigated and then the process of it is established. Resource information is acquired by using of questioning technology to collect and survey design content.

Brainstorming, QFD, SIPOC diagram, Kano analysis etc. information and data processing and analysis tools are adopted to guarantee to obtain necessary and critical requirement and data of service. Simultaneously, critical data information is supplied for concept design. In service identification stage, concept design and preliminary design stage, service requirement can be specified. The data/information obtained from identification stage is used to conceive product lifecycle service design and establish service evaluation system. FMEA and reliability-verification-analysis tools are usually used to discover failure fault model in product manufacturing and application processes, then potential quality problem could be avoided and application risk could be reduced, thus the safety reliability of product and service is guaranteed. Then into service optimization stage, cause of potential problem is analyzed, computer simulation, experiment design etc. design optimization methods and tools are utilized to perfect service object. Computer simulation, soft and hardware test etc. are employed to test the development results and to check whether the new product could satisfy service requirement. As a result, the design of service design stage could be completed. Meanwhile, in service maintenance stage, by using of parametric design, modular design and embedded design, Service information of other lifecycle stages could be feedback into service requirement analysis via collaboration, mapping and loop mechanism for product lifecycle. With the feedback information, the level service design oriented to product lifecycle could be improved and more perfect gradually.

4 Product Lifecycle Oriented Information Model of Service Design

In order to offer outsourcing for service information of entire product lifecycle, to realize information sharing and collaboration of cross-enterprise, the product lifecycle oriented information model of service design is constructed. Based on product lifecycle oriented development framework of service design, by means of family of methods and the development tool of service design, dada of product design, technology, quality, cost, sales and operating maintenance are linked organically. Based on Six Sigma concept of process improvement and optimization, service is designed according to the development flow. Information from service manufacturing and equipment e-maintenance are transformed into service design information. So the cycle is repeated to improve product service ability. The model can be shown in Fig. 4.

During the product manufacturing process of cross-enterprise, first is begin with service requirement analysis. Customer interaction is realized with some service research methods such as contact communication, website or forum, and market research. Then, information of customer service requirement which consists of product function, performance, customization frame information can be acquired by some means such as explanation, treatment, analysis and feedback. Service requirement information is transferred into design information after being analyzed. The service requirement information can definite product design objects, structure, characteristic, and improve design satisfaction degree.

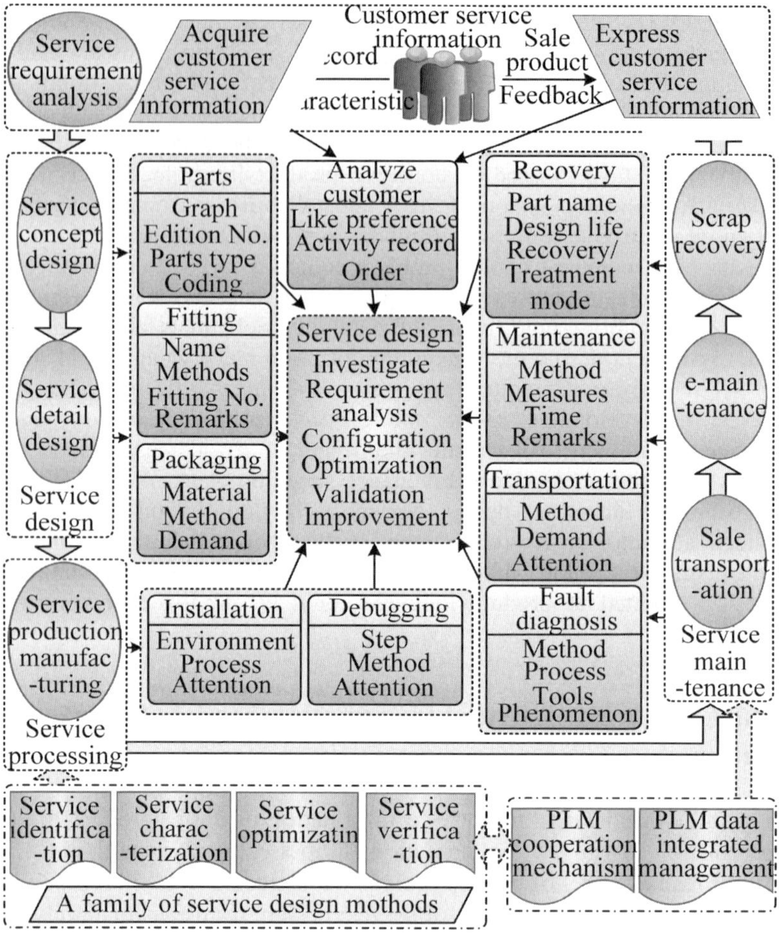

Fig. 4. Product lifecycle oriented information model of service design

In product information model of cross-enterprise, in order to realize information sharing and collaboration, it is not only need to consider information from product design stage, but also information from other stages which is feed-backed to design stage and then transformed into service design information. For the product service information of service design, service processing and service maintenance, by the integrated data management and collaboration mechanism of PLM, the product information of different stages in product lifecycle can realize service performance evaluation, service flow analysis, and service dynamic simulation. In six stages of service design, based on Six Sigma concept, service information of product lifecycle is carried out flow management, making full use of the service design information by created, managed and integrated in entire product lifecycle, the specific form and details of product service information can analyzed and expressed. The service design stage and other stages of product lifecycle can construct an integrated and organic product lifecycle service design development. In the model, service design information includes packaging information, installation requirement, installation instruction, debugging instruction, performance parameter, fault diagnosis, maintenance information, sales information and so on. The service design information can embody in product design development process by means of electronic documents, graphs(two-dimensional or three-dimensional), multimedia files, and so on.

5 Conclusion

In this paper, the development flow of service design is divided into service requirement analysis, service design, service processing and service maintenance four stages according to product lifecycle, based on family of methods and the development tool of service design, design data, manufacturing data, quality data and service maintenance data are being managed by PLM. On the basis of Six Sigma concept, a service design for product lifecycle development framework in service oriented manufacturing is constructed. Based on this framework, a product lifecycle oriented information model of service design is established, by which data on product design, process, crafts, quality, cost, sales and maintenance can be connected and feedback information of manufacturing and equipment e-maintenance into service design process. Product information of development flow can be designed for service by Six Sigma concept. Service design based on PLM and design for Six Sigma can be made full use for product information resource crossing different stages of the lifecycle of product of cross-enterprise, can achieve product innovation maximization, increase product development efficiency, and improve the capacity of product customization in order to meet service manufacturing requirement maximally.

Acknowledgement

This research was supported by the National High-Tech. R&D Program for contemporary manufacturing integrated technology, China (No. 2006AA04Z149).

References

1. Liu, M., Yan, J.W.: Study on SOA Based Grid Manufacturing and Its Architecture. J. Journal of Tongji University(Natural Science) 35(2), 239–243 (2007)
2. Yang, Z.H., Zhang, J.B.: Building a semantic-rich service-oriented manufacturing environment. In: 6th International Conference on Web Information Systems Engineering, WISE, New York, NY, United States, November 20-22 (2005)
3. Ma, R.Y., Wu, L., Zhang, S.H.: Design and implementation of a service-oriented manufacturing grid system. In: APWeb 2006 International Workshops: XRA, IWSN, MEGA, and ICSE, Harbin, China, January 16-18 (2006)
4. Shu, Q.L., Wang, C.E.: Customer-Oriented Product Service Model within the Product Lifecycle. China Mechanical Engineering 16(15), 1358–1362 (2005)

5. Cui, J., Qi, G.N., Ji, Y.J., Gu, Q.X., Si, S.H., Hu, H.: Management model on requirement information oriented to product lifecycle. Computer Integrated Manufacturing Systems 13(12), 2406–2414 (2007)
6. Zhang, W., Zhang, J.C.: Customer Perceived service quality and evaluation system. 12, 189–191 (2004)
7. Melhalk, B., Mroy, D.: Service Design for Six Sigma. Wiley-Inter Science Publication, Chichester (2005)
8. Khan, M.H., Madisetti, V.K.: A Multidomain Modeling and Simulation for Advanced Services Design.Communication System Software and Middleware (2006)
9. Shirwaiker, R.A., Okudan, G.E.: TRIZ and Axiomatic Design: A Review of Manufacturing Case-Studies & Their Compatibility. Technology Management for the Global Future 7(6), 2510–2520 (2006)
10. Bian, X.H.: Quality Function Deployment(QFD): an Extended Framework for Hotel Service Quality Management. Journal of Guilin Institute of Tourism 18(4), 558–563 (2007)
11. Li, G.H.: The Product-the line Approach and Empowerment Approach Discussion on the Design of Library Service Model. Library Tribune 20(3), 80–82 (2000)
12. Ji, Z.Y., Xu, M.: Ervice Blueprinting-An Effective Technique for Service Design. Journal of Donghua University, Natural Science 25(5), 77–79 (1999)
13. Bakrir, R.: Towards a New Service Design Approach Assisted by Computer Tools:A typology of services and a post sale service case study in the automotive industry. In: IEEE International Conference Systems, Man and Cybernetics, 2003, vol. 4, pp. 3899–3904 (2003)
14. Sawatani, Y.: Value Oriented Service Design.Computer society. In: The 9th IEEE International Conference on E-Commerce 2007, pp. 495–496 (2007)
15. Xie, S.I., Zhang, J.C., Zhou, S.Z.: QFD and Design of Aerial Transport Service. Policymaking Reference 14(5), 18–43 (2001)
16. Liu, L.W.: The Design of Service Package and Service Delivery System. Journal of Tsinghua University 17(2), 39–45 (2002)

Look-Ahead Scheme for High Speed Consecutive Micro Line Interpolation Based on Dynamics of Machine Tool

Fangyu Peng, Xubin Chen, Yong Zhou, Li Li, and Bin Li

National Numerical Control System Engineering Research Center,
Huazhong University of Science and Technology, Wuhan 430074, China
zwm8917@263.net

Abstract. This paper presents a new look-ahead Scheme with adaptability of dynamics of machine tool for high speed consecutive micro-line interpolation. A backtracking arithmetic is used to calculate the speeds in the link points of consecutive micro-lines. Moreover, the speed limitations in the link points are analyzed in detail and the compound constraint conditions of the motion axes is introduced based the dynamic characteristics of machine tool. The case studies indicate that, using the scheme presented by this paper, the actual interpolation speed is closer to the command speed and the shock that results from the sharp fluctuate of feed speed is depressed, which will improve the machining efficiency and quality.

Keywords: Micro-line, Interpolation, Look-ahead, Machine Tool Dynamics.

1 Introduction

With the development of high speed machining (HSM) in modern industry, CNC machine tools ask for high speed interpolation technology. At present, small lines generated from CAM software are used to approximat the complicated surface in machining. In order to get accurate and smooth contours, the lengths of the small lines usually are limited less than 1mm, which means that there will have ten thousands even hundred thousands of program segments in machining a part. However, HSM requires that the feed drive has high speed and high acceleration to ensure high machining efficiency. Therefore, the consecutive micro-line interpolation technique that maintains a high speed in the link point between adjoining line blocks is required to avoid the frequent stop and startup of the feed motors.

Many researchers have presented their works in realizing the consecutive micro-line interpolation. Zhong[1] regarded smooth adjoining line blocks without inflexion as a whole and used curve perimeter approximating trace length to estimate acceleration/ deceleration area in interpolation. Ye[2] presented a consecutive interpolation method that reduced the precision of the link point becomingly. Moreover, in the process of the continuous interpolation, the control information, such as the optimal speed in passing the link point, should be acquired ahead to ensure that the CNC system could tune the feed speed to avoid the over-cutting. Therefore, some commercial CNC controllers adapt various kind of look-ahead algorithm as an optional function[3]. Han[4] presented an efficient look-ahead algorithm that improves interpolation speed in the machining of

C. Xiong et al. (Eds.): ICIRA 2008, Part II, LNAI 5315, pp. 743–753, 2008.

small line blocks by adding a moving buffer. Xu[5] presented an adaptive method to decide the numbers of look-ahead path segments according to the actual conditions of the current machining path. The methods presented by them adapted a forward arithmetic to calculate the speeds of the start point and end point in a path segment, where the speed of the next point was calculated in terms of the information of the previous point. If the results could not satisfy the setting conditions, they would be modified from the contrary direction.

The interpolation arithmetic mentioned above only analyzes the geometrical characteristics of the interpolated objects. However, in the feed process of machine tool, especially in the corner of the motion, the speed and the acceleration will be limited by the dynamics of machine tool. Some researchers have considered the effect of the machining dynamics. Geel[6] indicated that the main factor to ensure the surface quality in machining was the constant cutting force and proposed curve interpolation arithmetic with constant cutting force. Tikhon[7] considered the cutting speed as a programming aim in NURBS curve interpolation. Liu[8] considered machining dynamics in NURBS curve interpolation for three aspects: sharp corners or feedrate sensitive corners on the curves, components with high frequencies or frequencies matching machine natural ones and high jerks. Yong[9] researched the limitation conditions of the corner error and acceleration/deceleration in parameter curve interpolation. Chen[10] proposed a drive force constrain of the motor in the interpolation speed programming to limit the load torque under the capacity of the machine tool. However, these investigations are considered only for free curve. Because of the continuous changing of the direction vector in consecutive micro-line interpolation, the dynamic constrains are more complex.

This paper presents a look-ahead scheme for high speed consecutive small line blocks interpolation based on dynamics of machine tool. A backtracking arithmetic that calculates the speed of the link point from opposite direction in a buffer of N segments is used in the look-ahead scheme, which simplifies the calculation process comparing with the forward arithmetic. Moreover, the geometric characteristics of the machined contour are combined with the dynamic characteristics of the machine tool to calculate the speed constrain conditions in the end of small lines, which maintains smooth speed in the corner of the lines allowed by the capacity of the machine tool.

2 Look-Ahead Interpolation Based on Backtracking Arithmetic

Although the speed of the end point of the small line relates to the former motion segments, its speed limitation is decided by the angle of the corner and the latter segments. In the backtracking arithmetic, the speed in the end of the buffer is set to be zero, then the speed in the end point of the former segment, which is calculated in terms of certain accelerating/decelerating rule, will be compared with the other limiting conditions to get a limitation value. This process will be carried though iteratively using the acquired limitation value as a preliminary value, until the speed limitation value is obtained in current interpolation segment, namely in the first segment of the buffer. Because every limitation value only need be calculated one time in the course of backing, the calculated capacity is reduced.

The look-ahead interpolation module adapted by this paper need not operate in real time environment, but keep the First IN First OUT (FIFO) buffer to be not emptied. Firstly, the data of certain segments are read ahead according to setting up FIFO buffer. When the buffer is full, the limiting speed in every inflexion will be calculated from the back to the front. The section 3 will analyze the speed limitation conditions in detail. The steps of the algorithm are as follows, shown in Fig. 1.

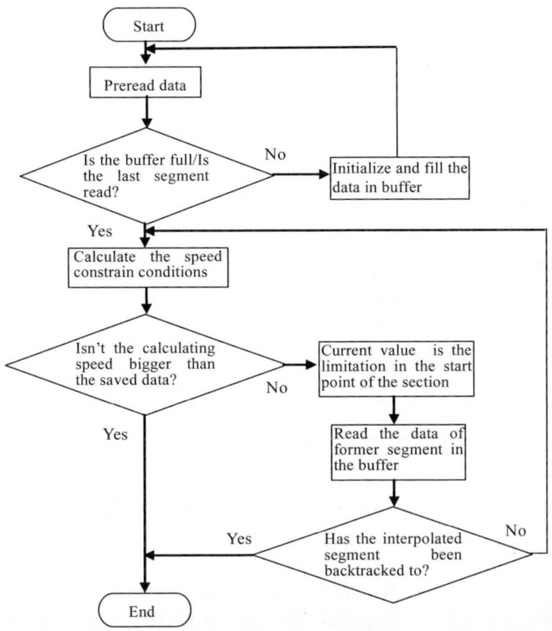

Fig. 1. Shows the Flow chart of the backtracking arithmetic

1) The buffer whose size is set to be the same as that of the maximal backtracking segments is initialized before interpolation.

2) The data are sent into the buffer to calculate the angle of corner and the error, if the buffer has vacancies

3) The maximal speed in every inflexion is calculated starting from the end of the segments. If a calculated speed is below or equal to the speed that is saved in the buffer in the last backtracking, the backtracking process is stopped. Therefore, the speed limitations of the former inflexions would not be affected by the following segments and the backtracking process can be stopped.

4) If the buffer is full or the data of the machined segments is written into the buffer, a segment can be taken out from the buffer to be interpolated and a backtracking step is over.

3 Dynamic Constrains for the Speed of the End Point

If the machining speed is beyond the accelerating/decelerating capacity of the motors in feed drives, a resulting oscillation appears to depress the machining quality. Therefore, the geometric characteristics of the contour and the dynamic characteristics of machine tools should be considered synthetically. This paper analyzes the motion constrain conditions based on the geometric relationship of the consecutive micro-line blocks, the error of the corner and the dynamic characteristics of machine tools, respectively [11-12]. These conditions are used to calculate the speed limitation in backtracking arithmetic.

3.1 Geometric Constrain Based on Accelerating/Decelerating Characteristic

In the backtracking algorithm, the geometric constrain is just to calculate the start speed according to the accelerating/decelerating capacity of the machine tool, knowing speed of the end point and length of the segment. Take *s* accelerating/decelerating curve method as an example. Let the speed of the end point be v_e, the length of the segment be L, the start speed be v_s, the maximal acceleration be a_{max}, the jerk be j, the time in jerk phase be t_1, the time in acceleration phase be t_2, and the time in deceleration phase be t_3, then v_s can be calculated by

$$v_s = v_e - jt_1^2 - a_{\max} t_2 \tag{1}$$

where, the calculation is simplified by introducing $t_1=t_3$.

3.2 Motion Constrain Based on the Transition Error between the Segments

Because the consecutive small line blocks are used to fit the surface, it is insignificant only to keep the precision of the start point and the end point of every line block. Here, a transition fragment is inserted into the transition area between the segments when the machining time of a line segment is not the integer multiple of the interpolation period. The transition fragment length is the distance in one interpolation period. The sketch map of the transition error is shown in Fig. 2.

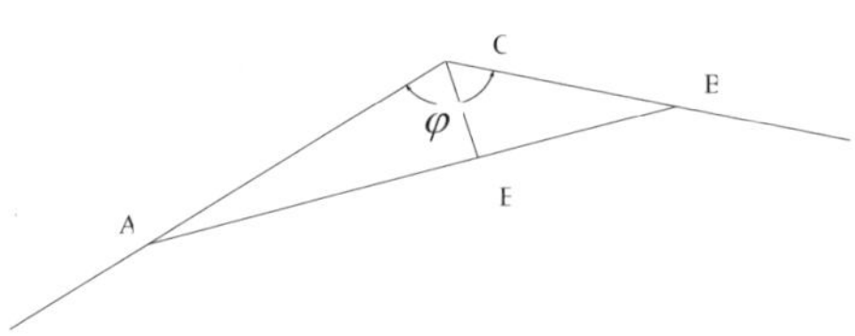

Fig. 2. Sketch map of the transition error

In Fig. 2, AC is the distance of the remaining segment, and AB is the travel in an interpolation period, namely the inserted transition fragment. Then the error is CE, the distance from point C to the line AB. Let the lengths of AC, CB and AB be s_1、s_2 and s, respectively, the angle between AC and CB be φ, the speed of the transition area be

v, the interpolation period be T, the interpolation error be ℓ, and the permissive error in the corner be ℓ_{lim}.

If $60° \leq \varphi \leq 180°$, the error will achieve the biggest value when $s_1=s_2$, then

$$\ell = \frac{s}{2\tan(\frac{1}{2}\varphi)} = \frac{vT(1+\cos\varphi)}{2\sin\varphi} \leq \ell_{\text{lim}} \tag{2}$$

If $\varphi<60°$, because $s_1<s$ and $s_2<2\, s\cos\varphi$, one can get

$$\ell = \frac{s_1 s_2 \sin\varphi}{s} < s_2 \sin\varphi < 2vT\cos\varphi\sin\varphi < \ell_{\text{lim}} \tag{3}$$

Therefore, the speed limitation value v_ℓ can be expressed by

$$v_\ell = \begin{cases} \dfrac{2\ell_{\text{lim}}\sin\varphi}{T(1+\cos\varphi)}, & 60° \leq \varphi < 180° \\ \dfrac{\ell_{\text{lim}}}{2T\cos\varphi\sin\varphi}, & \varphi < 60° \end{cases} \tag{4}$$

3.3 Motion Constrain in the Corner Based on the Maximal Acceleration

Let the angles between the current line and the coordinate axes are α^i_n ($i = x,y,z$), and the angles between the next line and the coordinate axes are α^i_{n+1} ($i = x,y,z$), then

$$V^i_{n,e} \leq \left| \frac{Ta_{mi}}{\cos\alpha^i_n - \cos\alpha^i_{n+1}} \right|, i = x, y, z \tag{5}$$

And

$$V_n = \min\{V^x_{n,e}, V^y_{n,e}, V^z_{n,e}\} \tag{6}$$

where, $V^x_{n,e}$, $V^y_{n,e}$ and $V^z_{n,e}$ are the speed maximums of the three axes in the corner, respectively, and V_n is the speed limitation.

3.4 Motion Constrains Based on the Dynamic Characteristics of Machine Tool

Commonly, AC servo motor has powerful instantaneous over loading capacity to carry out the high speed and high acceleration motion command. However, the capacity is limited by the torque and power of the motor. Commonly, the output torque is in inverse proportion to the rotate speed, namely higher speed corresponding to smaller torque.

Therefore, under the rated rotate speed, a torque constrain can be taken:

$$|M_i| \leq M_{mi}, \qquad i = x, y, z \tag{7}$$

where, M_i is the actual motor torque and M_{mi} is the rated motor torque.

Upon the rated rotate speed, a power constrain can be taken:

$$|P_i| \le P_{mi}, \qquad i = x, y, z \tag{8}$$

where, P_i is the actual motor power and P_{mi} is the rated motor power.

Let the dynamic friction coefficient of the rail in every axis be μ_i, the normal force to the rail be N_i, the component of cutting force in the direction of every axis be F_{ci}, the pitch of the ball screw in every axis be l_i, the mass of the translation components in every axis be m_i, the total inertia of rotation components in every axis be J_i, here, $i = x, y, z$.

Considering the constrain conditions and dynamic functions based on Kane method, then the motion constrain functions of every axis under the rated rotate speed are as follows:

$$\begin{cases} \left|(\mu_x N_x \operatorname{sgn}(\dot{x}) + F_{cx})\dfrac{l_x}{2\pi} + k_{vx}\dot{x}\dfrac{l_x}{2\pi} + (m_x \dfrac{l_x}{2\pi} + \dfrac{2\pi J_x}{l_x})\ddot{x}\right| \le M_{mx} \\ \left|(\mu_y N_y \operatorname{sgn}(\dot{y}) + F_{cy})\dfrac{l_y}{2\pi} + k_{vy}\dot{y}\dfrac{l_y}{2\pi} + (m_y \dfrac{l_y}{2\pi} + \dfrac{2\pi J_y}{l_y})\ddot{y}\right| \le M_{my} \\ \left|(\mu_z N_z \operatorname{sgn}(\dot{z}) + F_{cz} + m_z g)\dfrac{l_z}{2\pi} + k_{vz}\dot{z}\dfrac{l_y}{2\pi} + (m_z \dfrac{l_z}{2\pi} + \dfrac{2\pi J_z}{l_z})\ddot{z}\right| \le M_{mz} \\ |\dot{x}| \le v_{mx}, |\dot{y}| \le v_{my}, |\dot{z}| \le v_{mz} \end{cases} \tag{9}$$

where, v_{mi} is the rated feed speed in every axis, $i = x, y, z$.

And the motion constrain functions of every axis upon the rated rotate speed is

$$\begin{cases} \left|(\mu_x N_x \operatorname{sgn}(\dot{x}) + F_{cx})\dot{x} + k_{vx}\dot{x}^2 + (m_x + \dfrac{4\pi^2 J_x}{l_x^2})\dot{x}\ddot{x}\right| \le P_{mx} \\ \left|(\mu_y N_y \operatorname{sgn}(\dot{y}) + F_{cy})\dot{y} + k_{vy}\dot{y}^2 + (m_y + \dfrac{4\pi^2 J_y}{l_y^2})\dot{y}\ddot{y}\right| \le P_{my} \\ \left|(\mu_z N_z \operatorname{sgn}(\dot{z}) + F_{cz} + m_z g)\dot{z} + k_{vz}\dot{z}^2 + (m_z + \dfrac{4\pi^2 J_z}{l_z^2})\dot{z}\ddot{z}\right| \le P_{mz} \\ v_{mx} \le |\dot{x}| \le v_{x\_\max}, v_{my} \le |\dot{y}| \le v_{y\_\max}, v_{mz} \le |\dot{z}| \le v_{z\_\max} \end{cases} \tag{10}$$

where, $v_{i\_\max}$ is the feed speed maximum in every axis, $i = x, y, z$.

3.5 Compound Constraint Conditions

Synthesizing the speed constrain conditions mentioned above, the final speed limitation can be gotten by

$$V_{\lim} = \min\{V_n, v_s, v_\ell, F\} \tag{11}$$

where, v_s and v_ℓ and V_n are obtained from the formula (1), (4) and (6), respectively, and F is the command feed speed. Because the real time acquisition for the parameters in the formula (9) and (10) is necessary, the current speed should be validated whether it satisfy the dynamic characteristics of the machine tool according to the formula (9) and (10).

4 Simulation Software and Experiment Platform

To test the interpolation algorithm, evaluation software and CNC experiment platform are developed.

The evaluation software is used to simulate the interpolator of CNC system and estimate the interpolation algorithm according to the changing of the interpolation parameters. The interpolation algorithm is independent executable program that can be programmed using arbitrary language, only input and output interface should be defined uniformly. The interface of the software is shown in Fig. 3.

The experiment platform includes the following equipments: one HNC-22MF CNC system, two HSV-16-020 servo drivers, two GK6040-6AC31-FE servo motors and CNC software platform based on real time Linux, shown in Fig. 4.

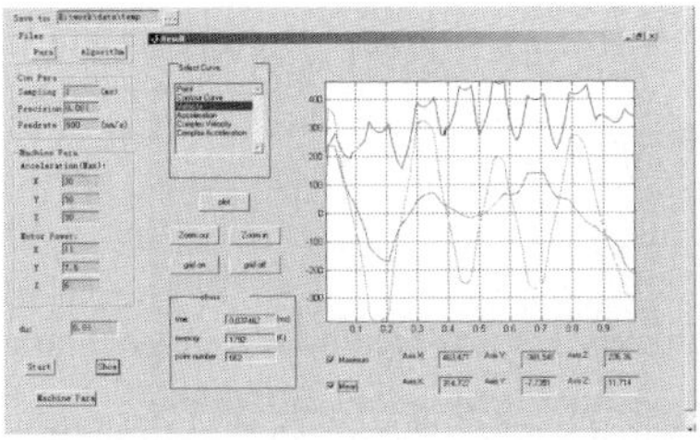

Fig. 3. Interface of the evaluation software

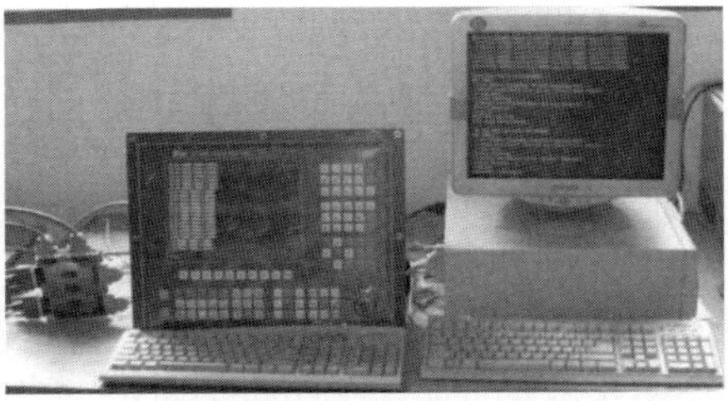

Fig. 4. Photos of the experiment platform

5 Case Studies

The backtracking algorithm is compared with the forward algorithm in look-ahead scheme. The curve taken from the surface of a screw propeller has 120 segments and 1mm length of every segment, shown in Fig. 5. In the experiment, the command feed speed 500mm/s, the precision of interpolation 0.001mm and the acceleration maximum in all axes $5m/s^2$ are adopted. Fig. 6 shows the feedback contour curve of the motors in the experiment platform, Fig. 7 shows the speed and acceleration curves of

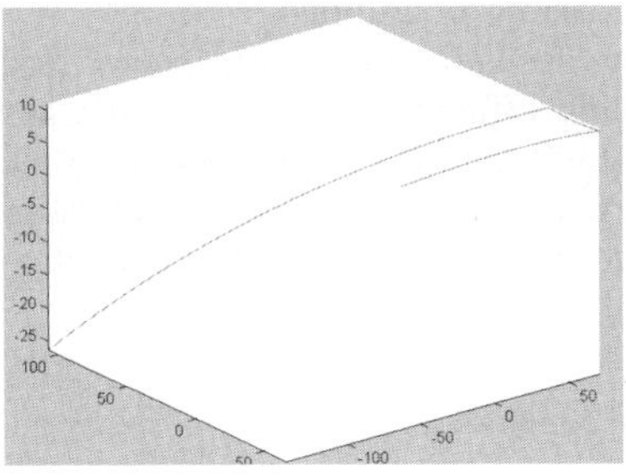

Fig. 5. Curve taken from the surface of a screw propeller

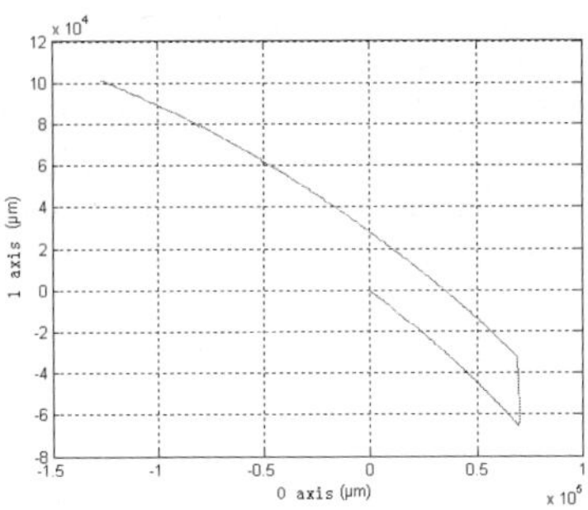

Fig. 6. Feedback contour curve of the motors in the experiment platform

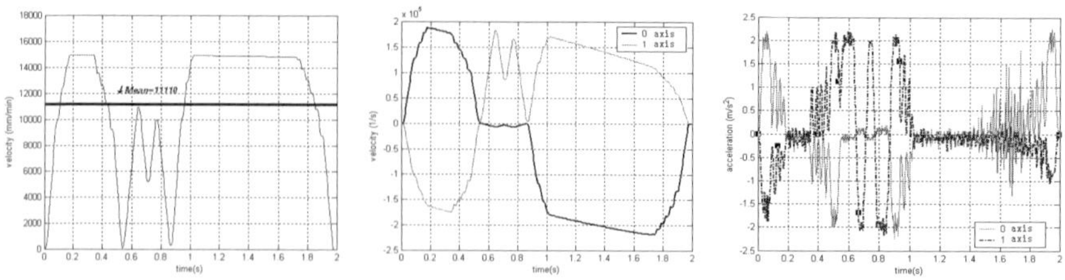

(a) compound speed (b) speed in each axis (c) acceleration in each axis

Fig. 7. Speed and acceleration curves of the feedback using the backtracking arithmetic

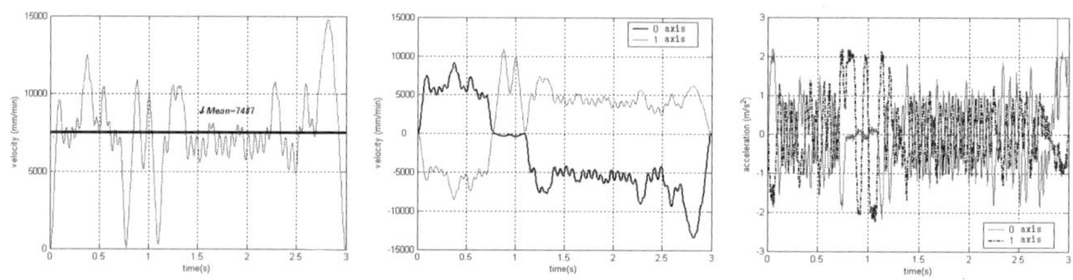

(a) compound speed (b) speed in each axis (c) acceleration in each axis

Fig. 8. Speed and acceleration curves of the feedback using the forward arithmetic

the feedback using the backtracking algorithm and Fig. 8 shows the speed and acceleration curves of the feedback using the forward algorithm.

Comparing Fig. 7 with Fig. 8, the actual interpolation speed using forward algorithm is far lower than the command speed, and that using backtracking algorithm is closer to the latter. Further more, the fluctuating of the speed and acceleration using backtracking algorithm is lesser than that using forward algorithm. The reason is that the backtracking algorithm considers synthetically the error limitations and the accelerating/decelerating constrains. Therefore, the backtracking algorithm can improve the machining efficiency and quality effectively. Moreover, the effects of the dynamic characteristics is researched. Take command speed be 3000mm/min and interpolation precision be 5μm, and other experimental conditions are listed in the Table 1. Fig. 9 ~12 are the measured feedback of the motors in various conditions.

From the figures shown above, the accelerating/deceleration performance of machine tool is the main factor in impacting the machining efficiency and precision when the angles of the fold lines are small, and the error limitation is a contradiction to the improvement of the speed when the angles are big. Anyhow, increasing the acceleration has an important effect on improvement of the average speed, but the higher acceleration and speed are limited by the dynamic characteristics of machine tool.

Table 1. Experimental conditions

	I	Π	III	IV
Line angle(deg)	150	150	5	5
Line length(mm)	2	2	1	1
Acceleration(m/s^2)	1	2	1	2

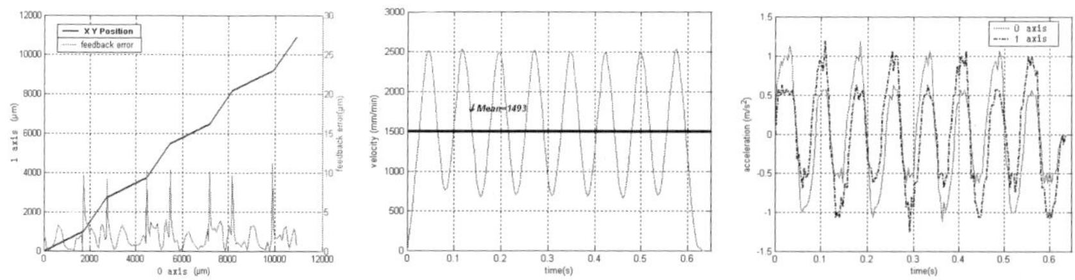

(a) error distribution (b) compound speed (c) acceleration in each axis

Fig. 9. Feedback of the motors in the I group condition

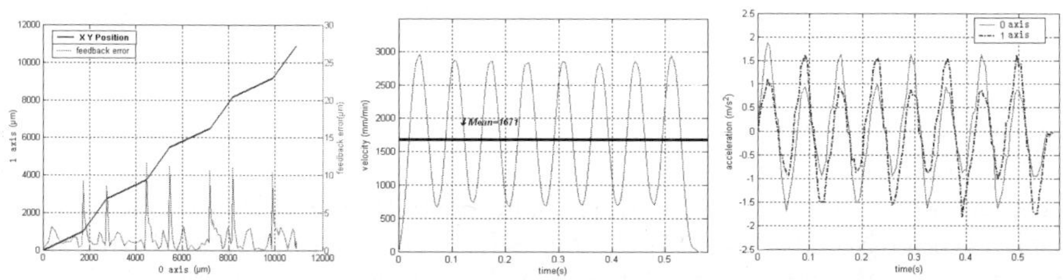

(a) error distribution (b) compound speed (c) acceleration in each axis

Fig. 10. Feedback of the motors in the Π group condition

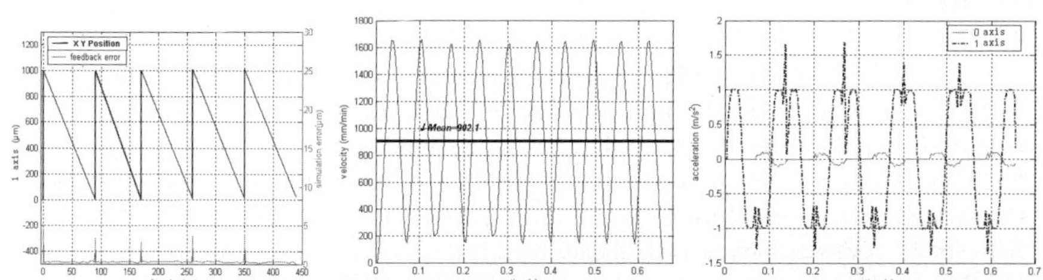

(a) error distribution (b) compound speed (c) acceleration in each axis

Fig. 11. Feedback of the motors in the III group condition

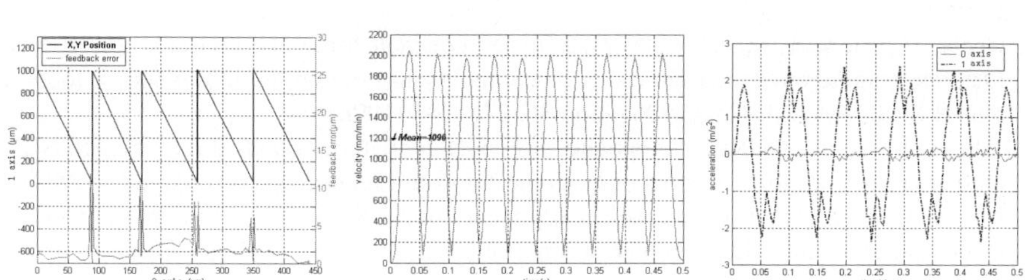

(a) errors distribution (b) compound speed (c) acceleration in each axis

Fig. 12. Feedback of the motors in the IV group condition

6 Conclusions

Case studies that take examples for the machining of screw propeller and the interpolation of various fold lines are adopted to validate the look-ahead scheme for high speed consecutive small line interpolation based on dynamics of machine tool presented by this paper. The results obtained demonstrate that the consecutive small line interpolation is improved in the two aspects as follows:

(1) The average interpolation speed is increased, so the actual speed is closer to the command speed.
(2) The fluctuating of feed speed is depressed to avoid shocking the axes of machine tool sharply.

Acknowledgements

This research is sponsored by the Major State Basic Research Development Program of China (Grant No. 2005CB724101), the NSFC (Grant No. 50335020) and the Key Items Program of International Science and Technology Cooperation (Grant No. 2003DF000021).

References

1. Zhong, Q., Li, J., Huang, S.H.: Interpolation of the micro-line at high continuum speed with high accuracy in RP System. Journal of Huazhong University of Science and Technology (Nature Science) 28(3), 39–41 (2000) (in Chinese)
2. Ye, P.Q., Zhao, S.L.: Study on control algorithm for micro-line continuous interpolation. China Mechanical Engineering 15(15), 1354–1356 (2004) (in Chinese)
3. Schuett, T.: A closer look at look-ahead, http://www.mmsonline.com
4. Han, G., et al.: A high speed machining algorithm for CNC machine tools. In: Proceedings of IEEE IECON 1999, San Jose, California, pp. 1493–1497. IEEE Press, San Jose (1999)
5. Xu, Z.M., et al.: High-speed adaptative look-ahead interpolation algorithm for continuous micro path sections. Manufacturing Technology & Machine Tool (12), 20–23 (2003) (in Chinese)
6. Geels, K., Ruckert, M.: Comparison between constant force and constant rate of feed in material graphic cut-off machines: Surface quality in relation to cutting speed, force, and rate of feed. Materials Characterization 36, 225–233 (1996)
7. Tikhon, M., et al.: NURBS interpolator for constant material removal rate in open NC machine tool. International Journal of Machine Tools & Manufacture 44, 237–245 (2004)
8. Liu, X.B., et al.: Adaptive interpolation scheme for NURBS curves with the integration of machining dynamics. International Journal of Machine Tools & Manufacture 45, 433–444 (2005)
9. Yong, T., Narayanaswami, R.: A parametric interpolator with confined chord errors, acceleration and deceleration for NC machining. Computer Aided Design 35, 1249–1259 (2003)

10. Chen, J.C., et al.: Analysing kinematic and dynamic properties of a machine tool path in high machining. Chinese Journal of Mechanical Engineering 38(1), 31–34 (2002) (in Chinese)
11. Peng, F.Y., He, Y., et al.: NURBS curve interpolation algorithm with the adaptation to machine tool kinetic character. Journal of Huazhong University of Science and Technology (Nature Science) 33(7), 80–83 (2005) (in Chinese)
12. Peng, F.Y., Li, L., et al.: Corner Constraint Conditions Based on Machining Dynamics in High Speed and High Precision Continuous Micro-Line Interpolation. Journal of Computer-Aided Design & Computer Graphics 18(12), 1812–1816 (2006) (in Chinese)

Robotic Digital Manufacturing of FGM Component

Haiou Zhang[1], Haiping Zou[2], Guilan Wang[2], and Weisheng Xia[2]

[1] State Key Laboratory of Digital Manufacturing Equipment and Technology
[2] State Key Laboratory of Material Processing and Die & Mould Technology, Huazhong University of Science and Technology, LuoYuRoad.1037, 430074 Wuhan, China
zholab@mail.hust.edu.cn, zouhaipinghust@gmail.com

Abstract. In this paper, a robotic digital manufacturing process for fabrication of FGM (Functionally Graded Materials) component was presented. Firstly, the construction procedure of robotic FGM digital manufacturing process was described. Then a method of transforming CL (cutter location) code trajectory into robotic trajectory instruction format was proposed. As the key apparatus for FGM component fabrication, a new flexible numerical synchronously controlled FGM powder feeder system and its superior computer control program was developed. Finally a functionally graded PEN (positive electrode/ electrolyte/ negative electrode) of SOFC (Solid Oxide Fuel Cell) was fabricated to evaluate the manufacturing process. The Scanning Electron Microscopy (SEM) observation indicated that the variation of PEN composition was continuous functionally gradient transition as expected

Keywords: robotic, FGM, digital manufacturing, powder feeder.

1 Introduction

Functionally graded materials (FGM) are a new generation of engineering materials with continuous changes of microstructures and properties across the material [1]. The unique characteristics in structure distribution make FGM offer great promising characteristics such as low residual and thermal stresses and improved bonding strength between dissimilar materials. Generally the manufacturing processes that can fabricate FGM objects are Laser Engineered Net-Shaping (LENS) [2], Directed Light Fabrication (DLF) [3], Electron Beam Freeform Fabrication (EBF) [4], Plasma Deposition Manufacturing (PDM) [5] which are termed as rapid prototyping (RP) or layered manufacturing (LM). Those fabrication techniques involve deposition of material to create objects, unlike conventional methods, where material is removed to obtain the final object [6]. The deposition of material can be explicitly controlled thereby providing unique opportunities to selectively deposit material. In other words, the material deposited can be varied continuously to yield a functionally graded material object with varying material distribution [7].

All those processes mentioned above have to employ customization RP machine which are not commonly used. In this study, we conducted developmental research of fabricating FGM component via robotic digital manufacturing process. With the

C. Xiong et al. (Eds.): ICIRA 2008, Part II, LNAI 5315, pp. 754–763, 2008.

employing of robot of versatility and flexibility, our developed robotic FGM digital manufacturing process only need to add a mix-flowing device, a superior computer, a powder supplying device and a deposition device to implement the FGM fabricating process.

Although lots of commercial RP software can generate computer numerically controlled (CNC) machine CL files from CAD model at present [8-9], until recently, there is still some lack of ready-made software that can generate suitable trajectory file of robot job file format (*.JBI) for the use of RP manufacturing process. Therefore it is of great significance to conduct a study on the robotic trajectory transformation method from CL file for robotic FGM digital manufacturing process.

Powder feeder is the key apparatus for FGM component fabricating. There are various powder feeders based on different principles having been developed at home and abroad. Screw feeder, turntable feeder and tub wheel feeder are used broadly in powder applications. But these feeders are not quite fit for the FGM component fabricating for the reason of blocking powders frequently, poor capability of deliver superfine powders, can not keep the powder flow continuous and steady especially in low feed speed. And most of all, these feeders can not realize numerical control to supply mixing powders with desired blend ratio at fabricating spot. So it is necessary to develop an apparatus which can well meet the requirement of FGM component fabricating process.

2 Outline of Manufacturing Process

Our robotic FGM component digital manufacturing process is based on the 6-DOF (Degree Of Freedom) industry robot and it mainly consists of two sub-processes: component geometry entity fabricating process and heterogeneous materials distribution realization process. Fig.1 shows flow chart of the robotic FGM component digital manufacturing process.

The component geometry entity fabricating process is the layered manufacturing process. Firstly, the 3-D model of the component is built up in CAD (computer aimed design) soft and transformed into STL file format. Then the STL format component model is input into RP software and sliced into serials certain thickness laminar along the Z-build direction to obtain the outline information of the processing section. Thirdly, after input process parameters, the RP software generates CNC codes which usually are CL files. Finally the CL files are transformed into robot executable instruction format and executed by robot with deposition device to form the component along building trajectory.

The heterogeneous materials distribution realization process is a different material powders synchronously controllable delivering process. Firstly, the materials gradient mode is built up in corresponding of the component model and the expression of materials distribution function is obtained. Then by comparing the geometry information of the CL file, we get the material quantity information in each fabricating spot on the robotic trajectory, thus we can generate powder feeder control codes .Finally, the control codes are sent into FGM powder feeder control program to control the powder feeder delivering proportion form of each powder into the deposition spot during the whole fabricating process.

The two sub-processes are converged in the robotic RP fabricating process which the component building trajectory is carried out by robot to form the component body while the powder feeder system feeding in heterogeneous material powders synchronously to realize the desired ingredient gradient distribution of the component.

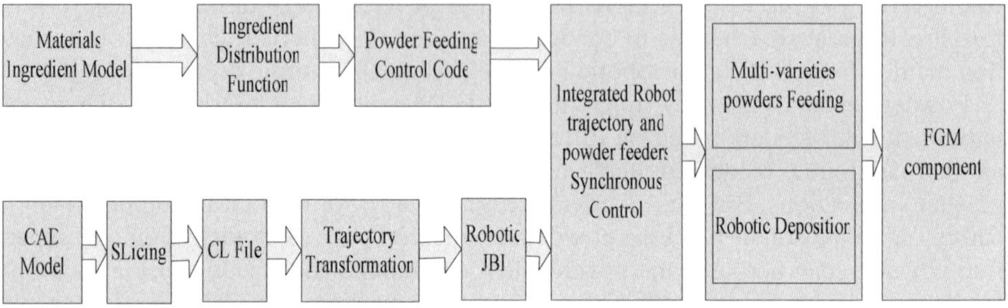

Fig. 1. Flow chart of the robotic FGM component digital manufacturing process

3 Trajectory Transformation

Generally, the output of RP software are computer numerically controlled (CNC) machine CL files. In our study, a type of UP20 industrial robot of MOTOMAN Company is employed for executing the trajectory of component digital manufacturing. The robot has 6 DOF and therefore the robot's posture must be determined by six values of (X, Y, Z, RX, RY, RZ). It is necessary to transforming CL file into the robot executable trajectory (*.JBI) format file.

The point data in CL file outputted by RP software is composed of six values. The first 3 values are coordinate figures of cutting tool control point inside manufacturing coordinate system. The latter 3 values are unit vector of cutting tool direction inside manufacturing coordinate system. As mentioned above, the robot posture was determined by 6 values, (X, Y, Z, RX, RY, RZ), the (X, Y, Z) values express the coordinate figure of robot execution point in its user coordinate system. (RX, RY, RZ) values express three axis rotation angle of the robot execution point around the three coordinate axis of its user coordinate system. So if we make the direction and origin of robot user coordinate coincide with the manufacturing coordinate's direction and origin defined in RP software, the trajectory point data's coordinate figure in CL file can be treated as coordinate figure of execute trajectory point in robot user coordinate. Then, as we transform the trajectory path direction vector into robot rotate angle, the CL file can be transformed into robot executed format file. The process of transforming CL file into robot executed format JBI file is shown as fig 3.

To transform the CL file into robot executable JBI format, we can transform the path direction vector into robot posture rotate angle using matrix transformation method.

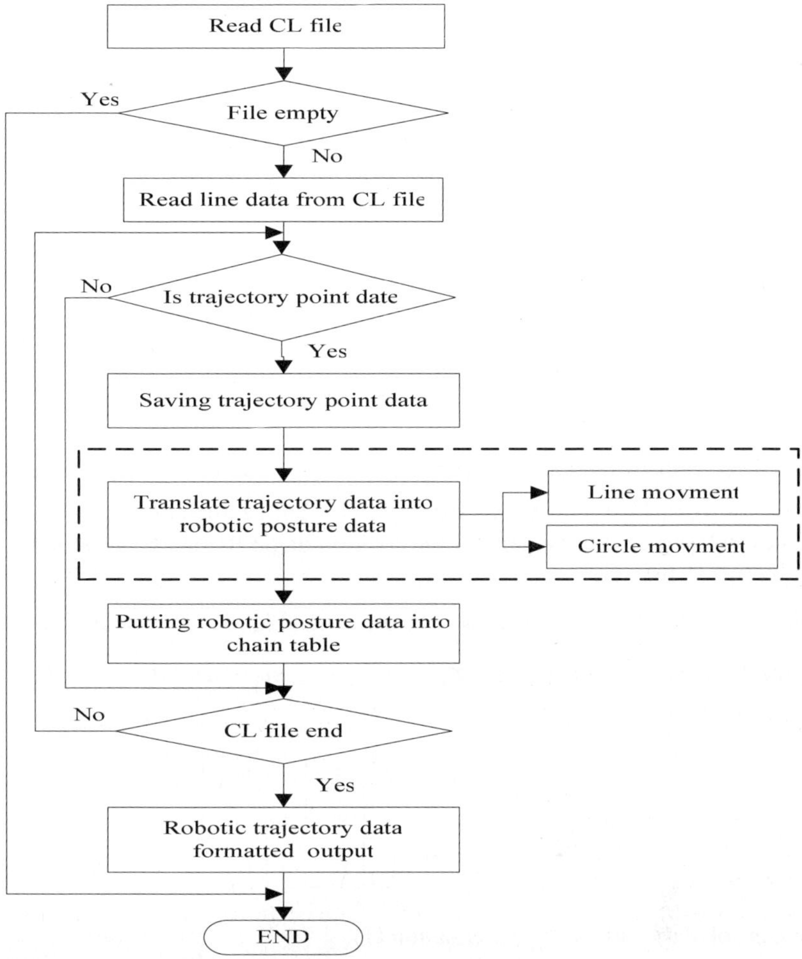

Fig. 3. Program flow diagram of transforming CL file into robot executed format JBI file

Consider the vector of random trajectory point in CL file (this vector is a unit vector) $\vec{\varepsilon}_{x,y,z}$ =(n_x , n_y , n_z), we can rotate the vector $\vec{\varepsilon}_{x,y,z}$ around Z axis for angle θ2 degree and make the vector arrive at the XOZ coordinate plane and obtains the vector $\vec{\varepsilon}_{x,z}$ = (n_{x1} , 0, n_{z1}), then rotate the vector $\vec{\varepsilon}_{x,z}$ around Y axis for angle θ1 degree, enable it coincided with the Z axis superposition, obtains the vector $\vec{\varepsilon}_z$ = (0,0,1), as shown in Fig.4. This position is also the robot tool execution initial point where its vector is vertical downward and the rotation angles around three coordinate axes are respectively (180, 0, 0).

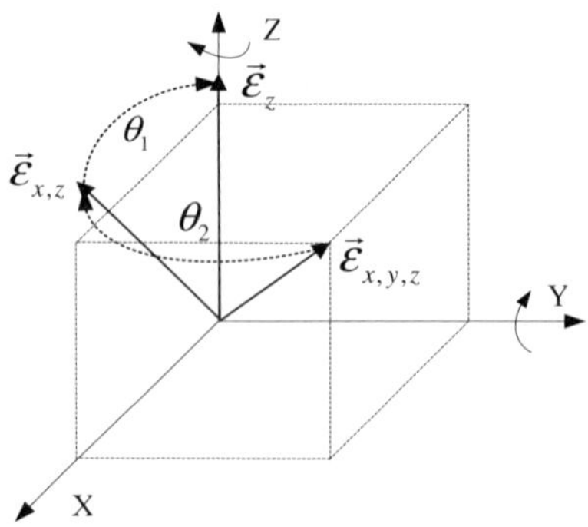

Fig. 4. Schematic drawing of vector and rotate angle

Therefore, to the arbitrary units vector (n_x, n_y, n_z), it can be obtained by rotating vector (0, 0, 1) around Y axis for angle - θ1 degree, then rerolls it around Z axis for angle - θ2 degree. So we can get the rotation angle θ1 and θ2 of arbitrary units' vector by two steps:

The First Step: make (n_x, n_y, n_z) rotate around Z axis for angle θ2 degree and reach the XOZ plane. Meanwhile (n_x, n_y, n_z) becomes (n_{x1}, 0, n_{z1}). It has the following linear relationship:

$$\begin{bmatrix} \cos\theta_2 & -\sin\theta_2 & 0 \\ \sin\theta_2 & \cos\theta_2 & 0 \\ 0 & 0 & 1 \end{bmatrix} \begin{bmatrix} n_x \\ n_y \\ n_z \end{bmatrix} = \begin{bmatrix} n_{x1} \\ 0 \\ n_{z1} \end{bmatrix} \tag{1}$$

We can solve θ_2, n_{x1}, n_{z1} by equation (1)

The Second Step: make (n_{x1}, 0, n_{z1}) rotate around Y axis for angle θ1 degree and vector (n_{x1}, 0, n_{z1}) becomes unit vector (0, 0, n_{z2}). It has the following linear relationship:

$$\begin{bmatrix} \cos\theta_1 & 0 & \sin\theta_1 \\ 0 & 1 & 0 \\ -\sin\theta_1 & 0 & \cos\theta_1 \end{bmatrix} \begin{bmatrix} n_{x1} \\ 0 \\ n_{z1} \end{bmatrix} = \begin{bmatrix} 0 \\ 0 \\ n_{z2} \end{bmatrix} \tag{2}$$

where: n_{z2} =1 in equation (2).

From equation (2), we can solve out angle θ1 and then we obtain robot rotation angle for (180, - θ1, - θ2). So each trajectory point data in CL file transformed into robot posture data is: (x, y, z, 180, -θ1, -θ2).

4 FGM Powder Feeder System

Fabricating FGM component via robotic digital manufacturing process not only need execute robotic trajectory to build the component geometry entity, but also need feed mixed material powders with desired ratio into deposition spot according to the FGM component ingredients distribution required. After planning the path of the FGM component in the RP software, we can generate materials feed control code by mapping CL code onto the 3-D materials distribution model of the component. Then the feed control code was input into our new developed FGM powder feeder system which drives the powder feeders send out proportion form of each powder into the deposition spot during the whole fabricating process until the components was generated finally.

4.1 Principle of Powder Feeder Unit

Powder feeder is a key apparatus for FGM component fabricating. There have been developed several kind of powder feeders based on different principles for various purposes. Screw feeder, turntable feeder and tub wheel feeder are commonly used powder feeders. But they are not quite fit the powder feeding requirements of FGM component digital manufacturing. In our study, a new flexible numerical synchronously controlled FGM powder feeder system was developed.

The flexible numerical control FGM powder feeder unit was based on the timing belt driving and Pneumatic conveying principle. It mainly consists of mechanism which can transport quantity powders accurately includes powder barrel, time belt, belt pulley, air vibrator, powder falling tube and its adjust device and so on; the powder feeder body; carrying gas channel; the step-motor and the control electro circuit. Fig.5 shows the schematic drawing and photograph of powder feeder unit.

During the powder delivering process, material powders fall from powder barrel onto the timing belt by the gravity function. An air vibrator installed near the powder barrel shakes in a Vibration frequency of 30000 vpm. The high frequency vibration of the powder barrel enhanced the flow ability of powders and avoided powders block as well as the powder bridging. The powder falling tube automatic adjust device eliminates the gap between powder falling tube and time belt, so the quantity measurement of delivered powders is decided by the through hole size at the bottom of falling tube which guarantees delivering the powders with accurate quantity. The time belt droved by belt pulley carries the material powders into the outlet channel at the one side of powder feeder body. The belt structure is able to ensure send the material powders on it to the powder outlet channel completely. The accelerated powder carrying gas is sent into the powder outlet channel through the gas inlet hole on the top of the powder feeder body. By using accelerated powder carrying gas, the material powders out of the feeder can keep good concentration after a long transportation distance

Compared with traditional powder feeders such as gravity type, scraper type, screw rod type and wheel hub type, our developed FGM powder feeder unit can easily keep deliver powders flow continuously and deliver the powder precisely with assigned feed quantity speed. Meanwhile, the whole powder deliver process is numerical controlled by the superior computer control program described below. By using several feeder units, it can realize two or three kinds of materials powder delivered into the fabricating spot synchronously to manufacturing function gradient components.

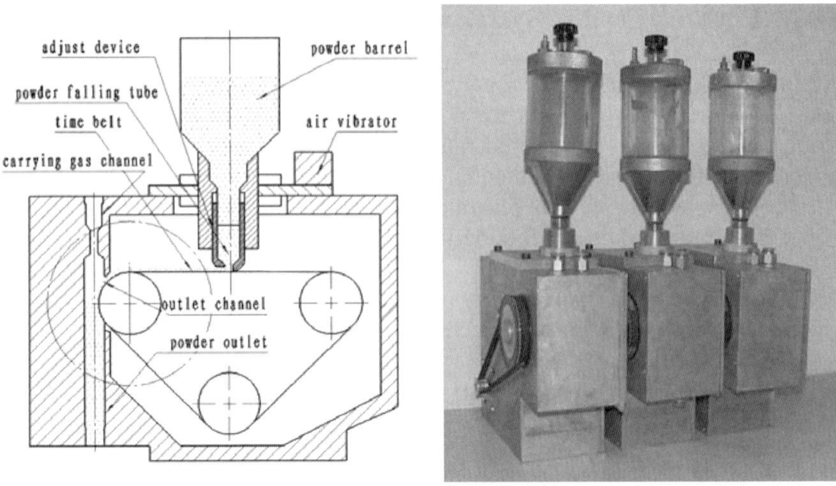

Fig. 5. (a) Schematic drawing of powder feeder unit (b) Photograph of powder feeder unit

4.2 Superior Computer Control Program of Powder Feeder

The superior computer control program of FGM powder feeder was developed based on lab windows/CVI program developing environment with good man-machine conversation interface Fig.6 shows the GUI of FGM powders feeder control system. The program realized communication between motors control circuit which installed in powder feeder control box and superior machine program through the serial port. By setting the figures of desired powder deliver quantity in the control program GUI (Graphical User Interface) panel, the computer control program sends out 3-ways electrical pulse signal unceasingly to the monolithic integrated circuit. The monolithic

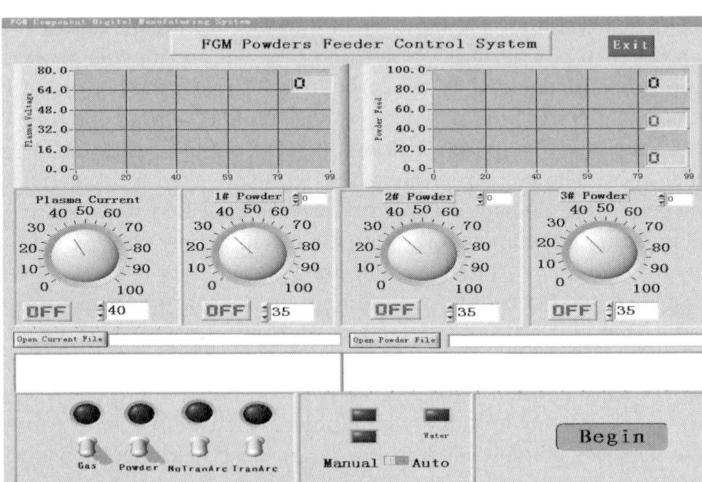

Fig. 6. GUI of FGM powders feeder control system

integrated circuit then actuates the step-motor to rotate at certain speed thus makes the time belt of powder feeder unit move in corresponding velocity and the material powders are sent out with the quantity as expected. The superior computer control program can also realize control of the powder feeders in both manual and automatic mode. It realizes two or three material gradient changes synchronously by adjusting the 3-ways output electrical pulse signal in the pre-defined mode corresponding to the materials gradient distribution.

5 Experiment

Solid Oxide Fuel Cell (SOFC) is a new generation fuel cell. The contact resistance between electrode and electrolyte has great influence on the battery output, and the thermal-expansion coefficient difference between electrode and electrolyte is easy to cause fuel cell failure in their services because of electrode detaching within the warm cycle operation. Researches indicate that fabricating the PEN (positive electrode/ electrolyte/ negative electrode) of SOFC using Functionally Gradient Materials (FGM) may improve the contact condition between electrode and electrolyte and cause the PEN part's thermal-expansion coefficient to increase SOFC service life.

In our experiment, the functionally gradient material PEN was fabricated using the robotic digital manufacturing process. Fig.7a shows the picture of fabricating PEN process. During the fabricating process, we used the YSZ powders (8YSZ) as electrolyte material, Ni/YSZ cermets (45%Ni+55%YSZ, volume percent) as the anode material, and La0.8Sr0.2Co0.5Fe0.5O3 (LSCF) powders as the negative pole material. Between electrolyte layer and positive electrode layer, electrolyte layer and negative electrode layer, we set up transitional layer that the material powders feed from one kind of powders 50g/min to 0, simultaneously another kind of powders from 0 transits 50g/min, the materials gradient realized by the superior computer control program of FGM powder feeder.

Then the fabricated PEN test specimen was observed .The overall cross section appearance and its elemental composition line scanning graph of SEM is shown in Fig.7b. We can see 3 layers structures which can be testified by power spectrum analysis method to be the anode layer, the electrolyte layer and the negative pole layer and two thin transitional layers between the electrode layer and electrolyte layer. The elemental composition line scanning of SEM is along the ingredient gradient direction of the transitional layer. It was found that between the anode and the electrolyte layer, the element of Sr and Zr increased gradually which presents materials gradient and the transition section width was approximately 60μm. Between the electrolyte layer and the negative pole layer, the element of Sr and Zr decreased gradually and the transition section width was approximately 20μm. The transitional layer ingredient gradient change was mainly realized by change the powder quantity feeding into the fabricating process which testified the new flexible numerical synchronously controlled FGM powder feeder system and the robotic SOFC PEN process were feasible.

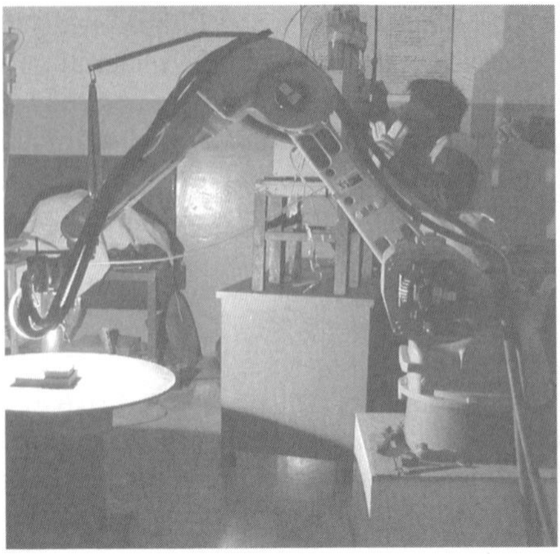

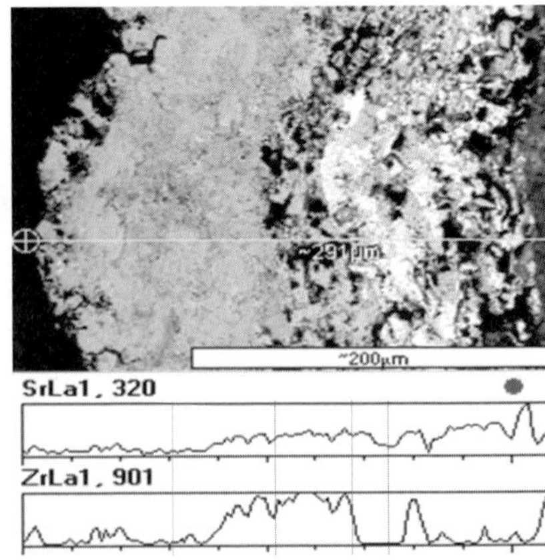

Fig. 7. (a).Process of fabricating SOFC PEN (b). SEM graph of fabricated SOFC PEN

6 Conclusions

In this paper, a robotic digital manufacturing process for fabrication of Functionally Graded Materials (FGM) component was introduced. Firstly, the construction procedure of robotic FGM digital manufacturing process was described. Then while robot-based system can only execute trajectory code in robotic instruction format (*.JBI), a method of transforming CL file trajectory into robotic trajectory instruction format was presented. As the key apparatus for FGM component fabrication, a new developed flexible numerical synchronously controlled FGM powder feeder system and its superior computer control program was described in details.

To verify the proposed fabrication system of FGM component, a functionally graded PEN of SOFC was successfully fabricated. The composition changed from Ni/YSZ cermets powder to YSZ powder in the transitional layer between positive electrode layer and electrolyte layer in width of 60μm. Meanwhile, the composition changed from YSZ powder to LSCF powder in the transitional layer between electrolyte layer and negative electrode layer in width of 20μm.With the ease of delivering the constituent materials and available process control, the robotic digital manufacturing process can be used for the fabrication of FGM components.

Acknowledgments

The research described in this paper was supported by the National Nature Science Foundation of China under project No. 50475134 and the State High-Technology Development Program of China under project No. 2007AA04Z142. The authors would like to acknowledge Mr. Guangchao Han and Yandong Zhang for the helping in the performance of the experiment.

References

1. Banks, L., Eliasi, R., Berlin, Y.: Modeling of functionally graded materials in dynamic analyses. J. Composites Part B: Engineering 33, 7–15 (2002)
2. Griffith, M., Keicher, D.M., Atwood, C.L.: Freeform fabrication of metallic components using laser engineered net shaping (LENS). In: Proceedings of the Solid Freeform Fabrication Symposium, University of Texas at Austin, pp. 125–131 (1996)
3. Lewis, G., Milewski, J., Thoma, D.: Properties of near-net shape metallic components made by the direct light fabrication process. In: Proceedings of the Solid Freeform Fabrication Symposium, University of Texas at Austin, pp. 513–520 (1997)
4. Karen, M.B., Taminger, R.: A electron beam freeform fabrication a rapid metal deposition process: A rapid metal deposition process. In: Proceedings of the 3rd Annual Automotive Composites Conference, pp. 9–10 (2003)
5. Zhang, H., Xu, J., Wang, G.: Fundamental study on plasma deposition manufacturing. Surf. Coat 171, 112–118 (2003)
6. Karapatis, N.P., Griethuysen, J.P., Glardon, R.: Direct rapid tooling: a review of current research. Rap. Proto. J. 4, 77–89 (1998)
7. Zhou, M.Y., Xi, J.T., Yan, J.Q.: Modeling and processing of functionally graded materials for rapid prototyping. J. Mater PR. 146(3), 396–402 (2004)
8. Lacalle, L.L., Lamikiz, A.: Tool path selection based on the minimum deflection cutting forces in the programming of complex surfaces milling. Int. J. Mach. 47, 388–400 (2007)
9. Xu, X.W., He, Q.: Striving for a total integration of CAD, CAPP, CAM and CNC. Robot Cim 20, 101–109 (2004)

Dual-Core Embedded Real-Time Inspection and Analysis Platform for Field Quality Control and Application

Yiyong Yao[1,2], Liping Zhao[1], Xin Li[1,2], and Damin Xu[1]

[1] State Key Laboratory for Manufacturing Systems Engineering, Xi'an Jiaotong University, 710049, China
[2] School of Mechanical Engineering, Xi'an Jiaotong University, 710049, China

Abstract. Under the demands of powerful performance for field data measuring and controlling, an embedded data acquisition frame based on ARM+HPI+DSP is presented in this paper, by adopting HPI driver technology, the two cores are seamless connected in WinCE system frame. A method for manufacturing process oriented field quality data real-time acquisition and analysis is established by adopting event driven and multi-thread dispatch strategy. With this framework, a real-time acquisition and analysis system platform of field quality data is realized to meet the demands of processing quality control. The ability of real-time acquisition and analysis for field dynamic data is improved effectively.

Keywords: ARM+HPI+DSP, Inspection, Quality Control.

1 Introduction

With the change of enterprise manufacturing mode, relationship between enterprises becomes more and more complex, which leads the product quality management and quality control technology to focus on the field data acquisition and real-time quality control. Meanwhile, in order to meet the demand of management and control in field manufacturing process, extended enterprises constantly strengthen the analysis of real-time data processing capacity for each production link. The traditional data acquisition system "sampling device + digital signal processing device + PC computer" has some disadvantages in field data acquisition and processing [1-2]. Nowadays, embedded computer technology, very-large-scale integrated circuit technology, real-time acquisition and processing of field data are becoming possible and will provide a better platform for technology development.

At present, data processing operation ability of digital signal processor (DSP) is becoming stronger and stronger. However, as a sort of hardware, DSP lacks of friendly user interface and can only be used as a black box; ARM has not only a rich on-chip resource, but also it has a humanized man-machine interface, perfect task management and coordination strategy, as well as good network support by means of embedded operating system. Data processing operation ability of ARM is not as strong as DSP. This system combines the both sides' advantages to achieve data

C. Xiong et al. (Eds.): ICIRA 2008, Part II, LNAI 5315, pp. 764–772, 2008.

display, coordination of two processors, data remote communication, partial data processing and storage.

In modern ARM+DSP system, the typical structure mostly adopted is ARM + FIFO (or dual-port RAM) + DSP, serial or parallel communication is adopted between the two processors. Its shortcoming is that serial communication can not meet the high-speed data transmission requirement, and there are difficulties of speed matching and programming in parallel communication [3-4].

As stated above, data acquisition and analysis architecture based on ARM + HPI + DSP is adopted by the system, dual-processor is connected seamlessly with HPI bus, to guarantee data transmission of real-time and effective among processors. In order to meet real-time requirement of field control and service, an embedded system frame of field control and service is proposed. Based on this, the results and objectives of quality control can be shared among enterprises through network.

2 System Frame of Measurement and Control Platform Based on ARM+HPI+DSP

In this part, a system frame of measurement and control platform is established for real-time management and control, the function of the platform is analyzed subsequently.

2.1 System Frame of Measurement and Control Platform

Based on ARM+HPI+DSP, a system frame of embedded data acquisition and analysis platform oriented to real-time management and control of field data for inter-enterprise is established. The frame is shown in Fig.1.

This system is divided into three layers: application layer of field control, network service layer of field measurement and control, and remote service layer. Remote data measurement and control output are realized in application layer. Client application request and agent client application are responded to realize process management, function call and task scheduling etc in network service layer. Remote analysis, evaluation, monitoring and scheduling are achieved in remote service layer.

In measurement and control platform based on ARM+DSP, ARM9 core processor is adopted to use rich on-chip resources of ARM9-2440 system, which main processor has a humanized man-machine interface, perfect task management and coordination strategy, good network support, as well as multi-thread distribution scheduling strategy. On the other hand, based on DSP5509's computing speed and ability for data processing functions, data dynamic acquisition and real-time processing are implemented in various environments.

Exterior of ARM is extended with a variety of peripherals as storage for kernel mirror image file and quality data of operating system, such as FLASH, SDRAM and permanent storage device; Through TCP / IP protocol, Ethernet controller transmits quality data, control result and quality state collected by acquisition system to the network-monitoring, which can realize the remote monitoring and control.

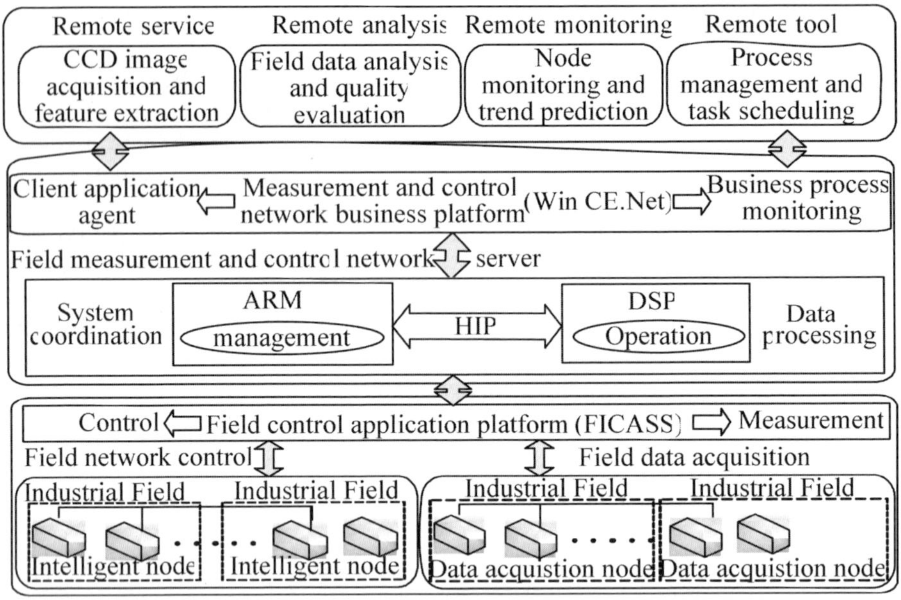

Fig. 1. System frame of measurement and control platform

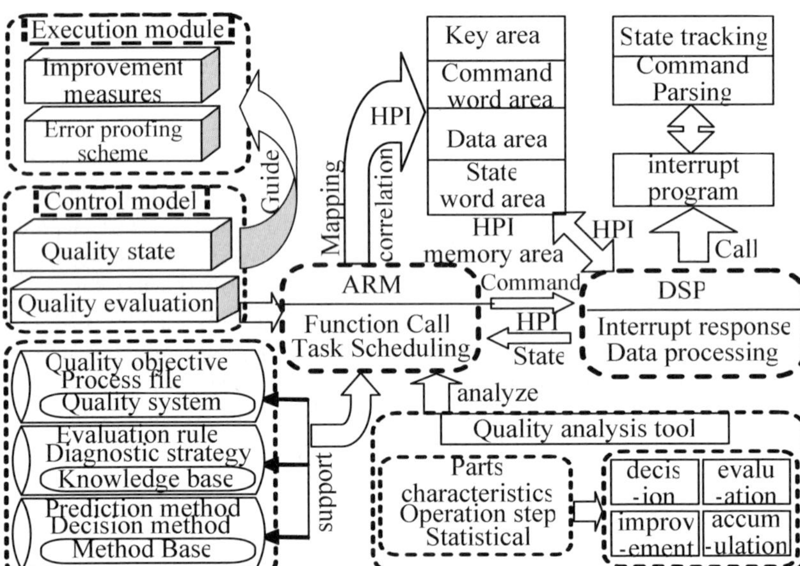

Fig. 2. Function frame of measurement and control platform

2.2 Function Analysis of Measurement and Control Platform

Based on the field's real-time characteristics of product manufacturing and quality control process, a function frame of measurement and control platform is constructed. There are two parts in the function frame. One part is physical supporting layer which consists of key area, command area, state area and data area. The other part is tool layer of field analysis and control, which is mainly in charge of field quality analysis, quality evaluation, state measurement and control, quality trend prediction as well. The frame is shown in Fig.2.

With HPI interface, the physical supporting layer can be used by DSP, ARM and remote server together. ARM is mainly in charge of command distributing, state monitoring and task scheduling management. DSP makes response to the interrupt request of ARM. The task will be deposited in task chain table, in accordance with the priority order, DSP is in charge of a large amount of data processing, and then it sends the results back to the HPI memory. Meanwhile, aiming at different quality state, different improvement measures and correction schemes are adopted.

3 Implementation Methods of Measurement and Control Platform Based on ARM+HPI+DSP

Some implementation methods of measurement and control platform are discussed, including communication methods with dual-core based on HPI interface, an approach for activity priority scheduling based on chain table, as well as driver program flow for HPI interface. Finally, the development of application program for the platform is introduced.

3.1 Communication Methods with Dual-Core Based on HPI Interface

To resolve bottleneck problem of data transmission speed between dual cores, to reduce complexity of system design, and to achieve real-time and effectiveness, the processors are connected by adopting Non_ multi_ plexed working model, as is shown in Fig.3.

The ARM and DSP are connected seamlessly by EHPI bus in the system. Data & address bus and control bus of ARM can be connected directly with DSP's, other control bus of DSP can be simulated through some GPI0 ports of ARM port; data is wrote into different registers across HPI bus timing sequence by ARM, and can be read and wrote to identify the access to HPI interface [7-9], the integration of sharing memory areas among processors is implemented through memory mapping technology.

Event-driven mechanism is used at ARM port with man-machine interface, through mapping of system kernel layer, command configuration files are associated with HPI drivers, then interruption is sent to DSP through the HPI bus of ARM port, DSP enters interrupt handling routine after receiving post trigger interruption, sets up flag bit, starts command analysis API function, and analyzes the command words.

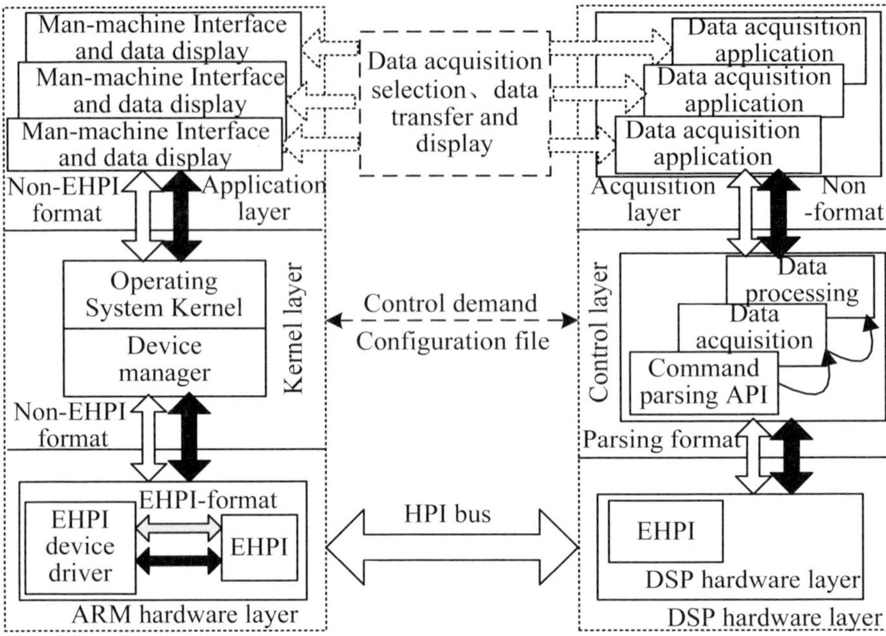

Fig. 3. HPI communication interface structure based on event driven

3.2 Activity Priority Scheduling Approach Based on Chain Table

In order to accomplish real-time data processing and transmission, approaches for measurement classification and priority partition are adopted to create a priority chain table of data acquisition. According to the sampling frequency, the acquisition data is first classified as rapidly varying signal and slowly varying signal. It is also classified as control signal and state signal based on different functions, finally the priority chain table of data acquisition is formed for query. Synchronous acquisition term is added at the same time.

On the basis of the priority in the priority chain table, area is queried firstly, and then other terms are searched. The flow of priority guarantee strategy on the basis of chain table is shown in Fig.4.

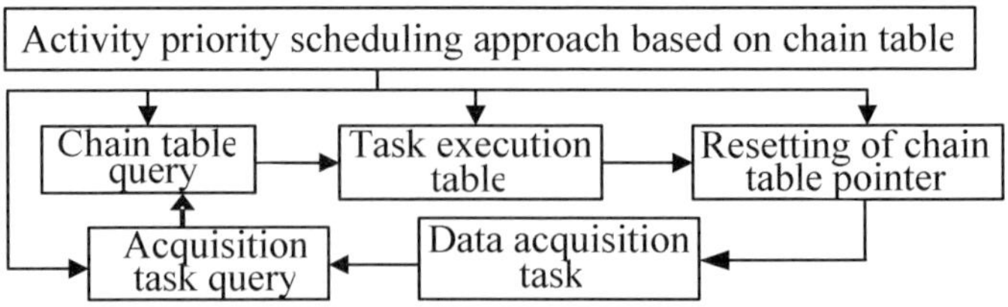

Fig. 4. Priority guarantee strategy based on chain table

3.3 Development of Application Program for Measurement and Control Platform

Take the complexity of dual-core application program into account, the system is divided into different modules. The application program frame of measurement and control platform is designed, as is shown in Fig.5.

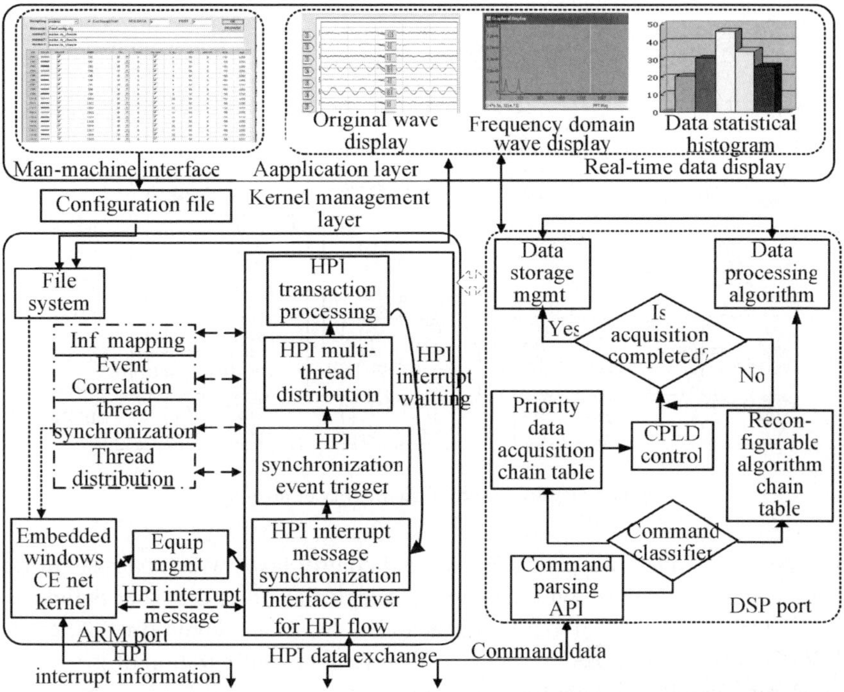

Fig. 5. Application program frame of measurement and control platform

On the aspect of function implementation, the design idea of modularization is adopted to exert the ARM+DSP dual-core processor's advantages of data management and data processing.

In the DSP port, data filtering and FFT etc. algorithms library for optimizing data processing are used and transplanted sufficiently. In the ARM port, coordination among processors, management of events, man-machine interface and real-time display of data etc. are accomplished and managed accurately. Driven software in base layer, system kernel, device driven interface, communication protocol, graphical interface, standard browser etc. correlatively with hardware are supported well [10-13].

4 Application

The measurement and control platform is applied to process dimension measurement and surface quality detection in a tile production line and the structure of tile quality control system is constructed, as is shown in Fig.6.

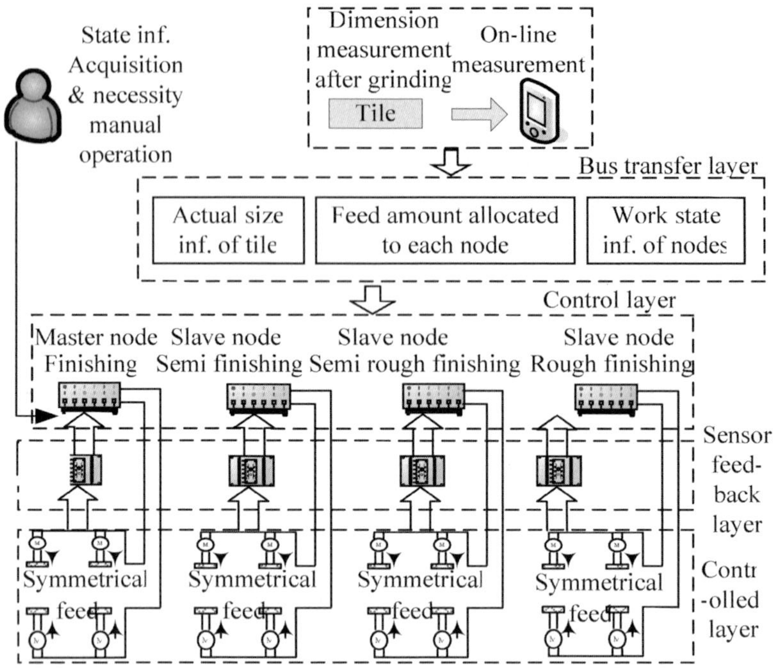

Fig. 6. Structure graph of tile quality control system

The system includes two parts. One is field control layer which consists of finishing, semi finishing, semi rough finishing and rough finishing; the other is field server layer which is composed of field data analysis and state monitoring. After power starts, the system is initialized firstly, and then related configuration of system clock, strapping pin function distribution, interrupt vector table and CAN communication etc. are finished in succession.

During the tile quality control process, the position and thickness of grinding wheel, as well as other measure information are detected. After master nodes receive tile outline dimension information sent out by measurement and control system for, correlation analysis is carried out, the feed of each grinding wheel is worked out and transferred to corresponding control nodes. After the slave nodes receive data, grinding wheel is adjusted to the specified position.

The operation instance of quality control system is shown in Fig.7.

CCD camera is used for field products' image acquisition and tile shape characteristics extraction, with which the overall dimension of tile is calculated. When the ARM port receives the dimension data via HPI interface, sent it to each control node by CAN network. In the next place, the multiplex quality data in field collected by DSP is used for frequency spectrum analysis and statistical analysis etc. Then the results are transmitted to ARM port application for data displaying. Simultaneously, the command is transmitted to inform field execution nodes for controlling field.

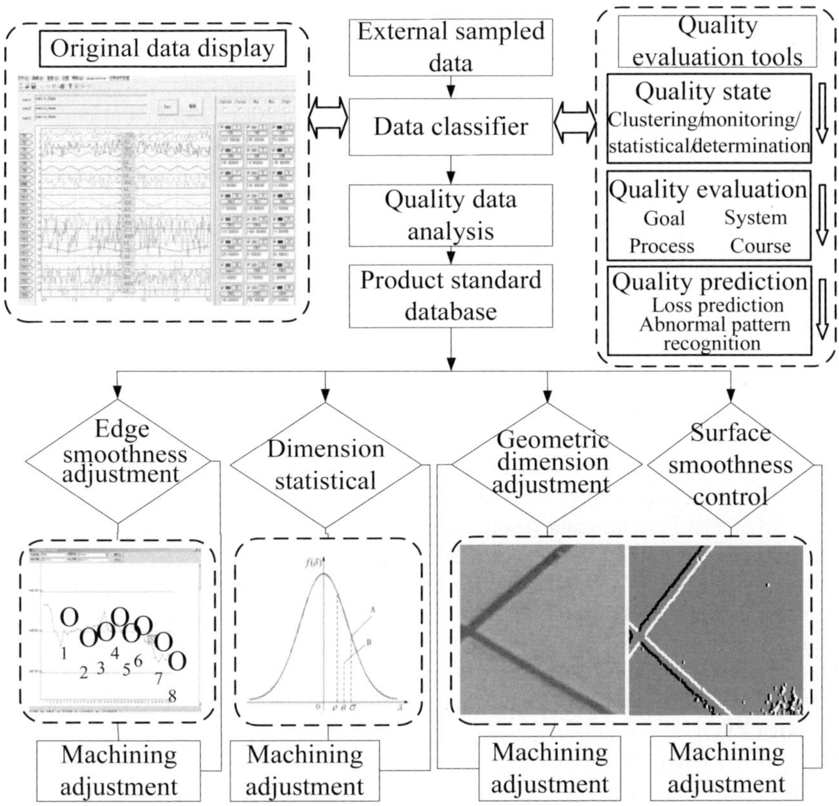

Fig. 7. Application instance of tile quality control system

5 Conclusions

By using the powerful data processing ability of DSP, WinCE organization management of ARM, friendly graphic interface, and good support of network functions, through HPI interface and memory mapping strategy, the seamless connection of ARM+DSP is realized, and the bottleneck problem of data transmission speed between dual cores is resolved. Meanwhile, making use of the activity priority control strategy based on chain table and external event-driven technology, real-time field data processing is achieved. Based on manufacturing process, all of above provides a good solution to real-time acquisition and analysis platform of the embedded quality data in inter-enterprise quality control.

Acknowledgement

This research was supported by the National High-Tech. R&D Program for contemporary manufacturing integrated technology, China (No. 2006AA04Z149).

References

1. Duan, G.J., Tang, X.Q., Wang, S.C.: The Model of Integrated Quality System in Modern Manufacturing Company. China Mechanical Engineering 10(3), 292–294 (1999)
2. Chen, B., Jiang, P.Y.: Research on Quality Data Require and Analyzing Technologies for Supporting Digital Manufacturing. Aviation Maintenance & Engineering 4, 38–42 (2006)
3. Zhu, F.Y., Zhang, G.B., Wang, G., Xie, R.C.: Research and Realization of Quality Management Control Chart on Embedded Terminal. Journal of Chongqing University(Natural Science Edition) 28(6), 23–25 (2005)
4. Ma, Y.W., Wu, J., Liu, D., Wang, S.W.: Design of Power Quality Monitoring in Wind Power Plant Based on Embedded System. Microcomputer Information 23(3-2), 17–19 (2007)
5. Wang, Y.H.: Real-time Data Collection System of Bridge with Fiber Sensor Based on DSP and ARM Technologies. Journal of Wuhan University of Technology 28(8), 108–109 (2006)
6. Wu, Y., Xiong, Z.H., Ding, H.: Data acquisition and control systembased on RTX and MFC packaging platform. Systems Engineering and Electronics 26(9), 1257–1261 (2004)
7. Sun, Y.Q.: The Principle and Application of Enhanced 8-bit Host Port Interface(HPI-8). Electronic & Computer Design World 22, 49–50 (2002)
8. Zhang, G., Zhang, J.T.: Application for HPI interface in multi-processor system. Application of Electronic Technique 7, 72–74 (2002)
9. Zhu, S.D., Zhang, D.X., Wu, X.P.: Application of HPI in Data Communication of Master-Slave System. Computer Technology and Development 16(12), 213–214 (2006)
10. Tang, Y.: Applied Guide to Real-Time Operating System. China Electric Power Press, BeiJing (2002)
11. Zhao, W.G., Wang, W.H., Fen, H.: Application of the Embedded System in Industrial Instrument. Automation and Instrumentation 4, 55–57 (2003)
12. Liu, G.M., Dai, Q.Y., Gao, M.G.: Application for Real-Time Operating System VxWorks in Tracking Radar System. Application of Electronic Technique 10, 47–49 (2002)
13. Dong, X.X.: Implementation of a Real Time Control System Based on QNX. Modern Radar. 6, 26–28 (2002)
14. Qu, Y.F., Pu, S.B., Wang, Y.A.: Contrast Study of Subpixel Edge Detections in Vision Measuring System. Chinese Journal of Scientific Instrument 24(4), 460–462 (2003)
15. Zhang, Y.H., Hu, D.J.: Gray moment operators for subpixel edge detection on CCD images. Optical Technique 30(6), 693–698 (2004)
16. Qu, Y.D., Cui, C.S.: Analysis of the influencing factors on subpixel Sobel-Zernike moments edge operator. Opto-electronic Engineering 37(7), 71–73 (2005)

Tension/Position Hybrid Control of a Web-Conveyed System

JianKui Chen, Yuhui Wang, and Zhouping Yin

State Key Laboratory of Digital Manufacturing Equipment and Technology, Huazhong University of Science and Technology, Wuhan, 430074, P.R. China

Abstract. Tension control and precise conveyance in web-handling machines are critical to ensure product quality. The focus of this paper is on actualizing tension/position hybrid control of a web-conveyed system. First, the reasonable algebraic dynamical velocity model of the unwind/rewind roller section and nip roller sections is presented, which plays an important role for the moving control of flexible web. Second, the hybrid control strategy with CCD vision position error feedback is exploited to implement precision conveying. Based on the new mathematical model and control strategy, an experiment platform is established. Several experiments have been performed to show the efficiency and feasibility of this established system.

Keywords: tension/position hybrid control, web-conveyed system, vision feedback.

1 Introduction

In the manufacture of continuous webs such as paper products, plastic films etc., it is significantly important to control the tension and the speed in the web feeding. The web-conveyed system typically consists of an unwind roller, draw rollers, leading section rollers, lateral guiding rollers, processing section, and a rewind roller. The reference values of the tension must be maintained between the consecutive pairs of drive rolls. A tension control system of moving web is inherently sensitive to external disturbances during operation, especially while the thickness of the web is less than 70 microns. A time-varying payload or torque of the driving motors can cause severe tension variation. A moving web under insufficient tension cannot track properly and may be wrinkled, while excess tension may result in web deformation or even a web break. At the same time, unacceptable levels of speed variation can also cause detrimental variation in tension.

In practice, the tension control system may be subjected to many uncertainties, such as a periodic disturbance from the eccentricity of the driving pulley, a torque variation caused by the torque ripple of the motor, or a time-varying radius of the unwinding/rewinding rollers. Thus, the tension control is extremely important for flexible web-conveyed system. Precise feeding position is particularly important in noncontinuous web lines, especially when the web has been printed some patterns. Steady tension control is the premiss for precise position control, but precise position has been the more urgent condition in those noncontinuous web-conveyed jobsite.

C. Xiong et al. (Eds.): ICIRA 2008, Part II, LNAI 5315, pp. 773–783, 2008.

Current trends in the development of electronics systems show that the roll-to-roll processes of web system may be the choice as a very economic production method and will most probably play an important part in the future. Electronic elements, like sensors, flexible batteries, displays, labels, or ICs are disposed on the web. The tension control and the position control of the web system must be implemented at the same time.

Considerable research has been conducted in order to solve the tension variation problem. A control technology was described for a VCR motor employing acceleration controller by Nagasawa et al. in [1]. The system had improved robustness and disturbance suppression, and can eliminate some irregular disturbance resulting from mass production. Sakamoto and Izumihara [2] presented the decentralized control concept to design a high gain adaptive control and an H-infinity control, and the latter formulated the weighting function for cooperation with a neighboring roll. Okada and Sakamoto [3] introduced a methodology for a self-fuzzy controller in which the control parameters can be altered so that the whole system has sufficient stability and performance in the presence of system parameter or structure uncertainty. An adaptive interstitial vibration control strategy was proposed in [4] for an axially moving string system under the assumption of constant axial velocity. Nagarkatti et al. [5] applied control torques to rollers at the boundaries of an axially moving system to regulate the web speed and tension using speed and tension sensors. The boundary control system stabilized the tension and speed at desired setpoints and stabilizes longitudinal vibration of an axially moving web. In [6], they presented a control strategy to regulates transverse vibration and ensure the web speed tracks a desired trajectory. This control method applied a standard torque-level controller to achieve axial speed tracking and a force-level Lyapunov-generated boundary controller to get vibration regulation. The authors in [7] aimed to reject the tension disturbances caused by unknown shapes of rolls. An adaptive eccentricity compensation method was proposed by decreasing the oscillation of the roll velocity. Carrasco and Valenzuela [8] developed two tension estimators for a two-drum electric braking generator production winder based on unwinding and rewinding variables to permit elimination of the load cell sensors. Kang and Lee [9] introduced a stability analysis of a linearized web-tension system of a high-speed gravure printing machine considering span-length variations due to dancer rollers. The nonlinear web-tension system considered span length variation due to dancer and used eigenvalue trajectories of the linearized model to analyze the plant stability. However, the mentioned works pay little attention on the study of conveying position control.

Noncontinuous convey has more strict requirements for tension and position than continuous convey. Frequent start-stop causes biggish tension disturbance and web deformation in noncontinuous web-conveyed system, which encumbers the tension stableness and position precision. Tension and position have been compactly coupled. Preconditioned the precise synchronized control, decentralized PID tension control and CCD vision position error feedback control, the reasonable conveying position precision and stable tension can be obtained in system proposed in this paper.

The primary goal of this paper is to actualize tension/position hybrid control in a web-conveyed system, which will support steady tension and low position error. This system is designed for Radio Frequency Identification (RFID) electronic-label integrated equipments. Some inerratic circuitry patterns have been printed or enchased on the web, which requires that the flexible web must be conveyed stably, accurately and intermittently. The dynamic mathematical model, the tension/position hybrid control strategy and implementing results will be spread out in the following three sections. The mathematical model for the emblematical web-fed structure in the experimental platform, such as the unwind/rewind roller and the nip rollers, will be developed firstly. Function relations of the variables, like tension, velocity, will be presented. Secondly, the tension/position control strategy will be described, including the decentralized PID control and position error feedback control. Finally, some experiment results are proposed to illustrate the performance and feasibility of this hybrid control web-conveyed system.

2 Mathematical Modeling

As shown in Fig.1, the web-conveyed system considered in this work is equipped with two automatic lateral web guides and two load cells. Each of the four active rollers is driven by a single-phase AC servomotor whose velocity or torque can be controlled. Angular velocity of each motor is measured by an encoder. The web system has more than 20 rollers over which the web passes; four rollers are driven and the remains are idlers with fixed inertia and radii. The unwind/rewind rollers release/accumulate material to/from the processing section of the web line. Thus, their radii and inertia are time-varying. The master nip rollers are used to set and maintain the web transport speed. The aim of the slave nip rollers is just to retain the web velocity dynamics. The two controlled lateral guides, near unwind and rewind sections, respectively, are used to maintain the lateral position of the web on the rollers during web transporting. The purpose of the two load cells is to detect the web tension's varying.

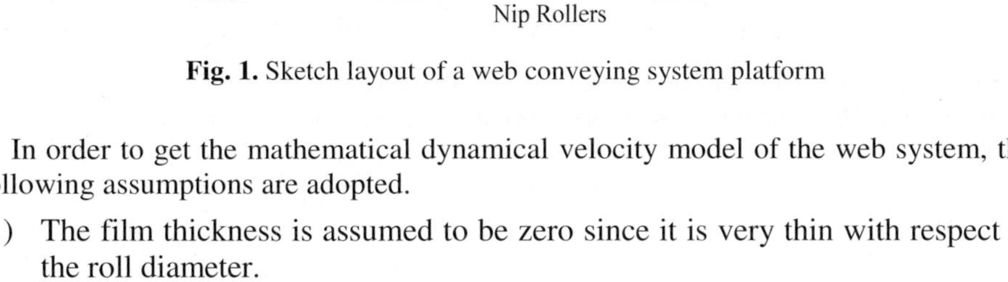

Fig. 1. Sketch layout of a web conveying system platform

In order to get the mathematical dynamical velocity model of the web system, the following assumptions are adopted.

(1) The film thickness is assumed to be zero since it is very thin with respect to the roll diameter.
(2) There is no slippage between the flexible web material and rollers.
(3) The strain and tension are uniform within a span.
(4) Variations of web properties due to temperature and humidity change do not considered.
(5) Web wrinkling is ignored.

2.1 Unwind/Rewind Roller Section

A cross-sectional view of the unwind/ rewind roller is shown in Fig. 2. The associated variables for this section are velocity v_0 and tension T_0. The n_0 is the gearing ratio of the reducer, which connects the motor shaft with the unwind/rewind roller shaft. The τ_0 presents the rated torque of the motor.

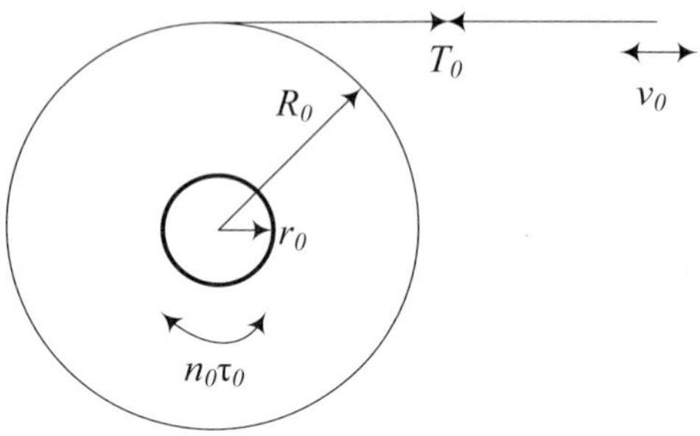

Fig. 2. Cross-sectional view of the unwind/rewind roller

At any instant of time t, the effective inertia $J_0(t)$ of unwind/rewind section is given by:

$$J_0(t)_0(t)=n_0^2 J_{m0}+J_{c0}+J_{\omega 0}(t) \tag{1}$$

where $J_{c0}J_{c0}$ is the inertia of the driven unwind/rewind roller, $J_{m0}\,J_{m0}$is the inertia of all the rotating elements on the motor side, including inertia of the motor armature, driving shafts of the motor and the reducer, driving gears of the reducer, etc., and $J_{\omega 0}(t)J_{\omega 0}(t)$ is the inertia of the rotating web material. Both $J_{c0}\,J_{c0}$and $J_{m0}J_{m0}$ are constants. But $J_{\omega 0}(t)J_{\omega 0}(t)$ is changing, which is given by:

$$J_{\omega 0}(t)=\pi W\rho(R_0^4(t)-r_0^4)/2 \tag{2}$$

where W is the web width, ρ is the density of the web material. $R_0\,(t)R_0(t)$ is the changing radius of the roller.

Synthesizing (1) and (2) gives:

$$J_0R_0\dot{v_0} = (J_0v_0 - 2\pi W\rho R_0^4 v_0)\dot{R_0} + T_0R_0^3 - n_0\tau_0R_0^2 - f_0R_0v_0 \tag{3}$$

In the section of unwind and rewind roller, equation (3) presents the function relation between the tension T_0 and the velocity v_{00} and the radii $R_0$and their rate of change.

2.2 Nip Roller Section

Nip rollers are special thin-film-driven components in many devices which transport dielectric webs or other materials in the form of sheets. Thus, it is important to understand the dynamical principle of the driven nip rollers. Fig. 3 shows the cross-sectional view of the two nip rollers, used in this web-conveyed system. In the RFID packaging equipment, the space between the master nip roller and the slave nip rollers is the work area. The two nip rollers are endowed with the same tangential velocity to keep precision web-conveyed. Both the nip rollers will be analyzed as one part.

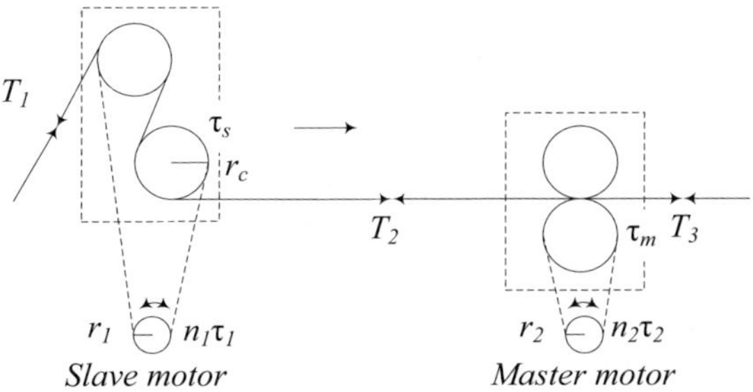

Fig. 3. Cross-sectional view of the nip rollers

It is assumed that the mass of the timing-belt is zero and that he transmitting efficiency is 100%. According to the Newton's law of motion and the law of energy conservation, the relation between the nip roller torque and the web tensions can be represented as:

$$\frac{J_1}{n_1 r_c}\dot{v_1} = (T_2 - T_1)r_c - 2\tau_s - \frac{f_1}{r_c}v_1 \tag{4}$$

$$\frac{J_2}{n_2 r_c}\dot{v_2} = (T_3 - T_2)r_c - \tau_m - \frac{f_2}{r_c}v_2 \tag{5}$$

where vv is the velocity of the motor and f is the viscous friction coefficient. Assuming n_1=$n_2$$n_1 = n_2$, f_1=$f_2$$f_1 = f_2$, r_1=$r_2$$r_1 = r_2$, and the dynamic equation for tangential velocity of the nip rollers can be written as:

$$\frac{J_1 + J_2}{n_1 r_c}(\dot{v_1} + \dot{v_2}) = (T_3 - T_1)r_c - \frac{n_1 r_1}{r_c}(\tau_1 + \tau_2) - \frac{f}{r_c}(v_1 + v_2) \tag{6}$$

Equation (6) can definitely present the function relation of the variables between the two nip roller systems.

2.3 Simplified Drive Model

Ignored the inertia of idlers, and synthesized the above-mentioned dynamics models of unwind/rewind roller and nip rollers, the simplified drive model of this web-conveyed system is shown in Fig. 4.

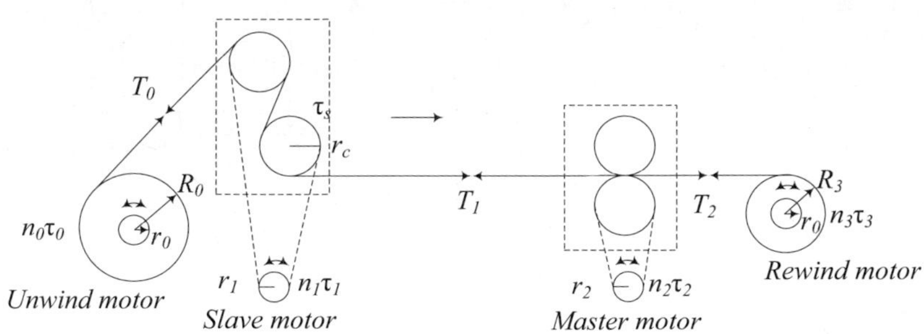

Fig. 4. Simplified drive model

The correlatively variables between unwind section, nip roller section and rewind section can be eliminated. Colligating equations (3) and (6), and simplifying the interim parameters gives:

$$\begin{aligned}\frac{J_1+J_2}{n_1 r_c^2}(\dot{v_1}+\dot{v_2})+\frac{J_0}{R_0^2}\dot{v_0}-\frac{J_3}{R_3^2}\dot{v_3} &= \frac{J_0 v_0-2\pi W\rho R_0^4 v_0}{R_0^3}\dot{R_0}-\frac{J_0 v_3-2\pi W\rho R_3^4 v_3}{R_3^3}\dot{R_0}-\frac{n_0}{R_0}\tau_0 \\ &\quad -\frac{n_1 r_1}{r_c^2}(\tau_1+\tau_2)+\frac{n_0}{R_3}\tau_3-\frac{f_0}{R_0^2}v_0-\frac{f_1}{r_c^2}(v_1+v_2)-\frac{f_0}{R_3^2}v_3\end{aligned} \tag{7}$$

In this simplified multi-input multi-output drive model, equation (7) illuminates the interaction between the constants and the variables in the conveying system. It can be seen that the unwind/rewind roller radii $R_0 R_0$ and $R_3 R_3$ directly correlated with web tension, and the speeds $v_0 v_0$, $v_1 v_1$, $v_2 v_2$, and $v_3 v_3$ are the main controlled variables. Considering the relationship between roll radii and tension difference due to the tangential velocity oscillation, special control must be made to eliminate the tension disturbance for the precision position conveyance. Using the proposed dynamic model, a suitable control strategy will be spread out in the following section to achieve both the steady tension and the precision position for the noncontinuous web-conveyed system.

3 Tension/Position Control Method

The sketch of the tension/position control strategy in this web-conveyed system is shown in Fig. 5. Turbo PMAC-PCI board provided by the Delta Tau Data Systems Inc. is used to implement the control system. This card makes it possible for users to compile individualized programs to the card directly and modify the control structure.

All operations for the tension control and position hybrid control are completed by the PMAC-PCI board, except that the two lateral guides have their own controllers. Special software programs for the web-fed are achieved to modify the control system.

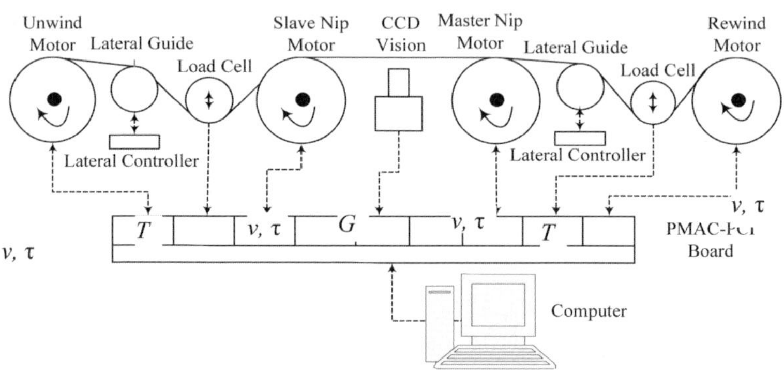

Fig. 5. Sketch of the tension/position hybrid control strategy

In the dynamic control system of the motors, decentralized PID control, provided by the PMAC, is used to endow the motors with excellent dynamical performances. The tension control and position control are coupled in this noncontinuous web-conveyed system. The tension/position hybrid control, which will be resolved in two dissevered part, should be conquered as one entire system. In this conveyance process, the synchronized control scheme is adopted to the slave and master nip motors to get the same tangential velocity, which implies that precise control must be implemented to overcome the synchronization error between the two drive axes.

In the experiment, the tension data are detected, analyzed and disposed to control the speed and torque of the unwind and rewind motors. The closed-loop tension control sub-system, composed by the load cell, the unwind (or rewind) motor and the PMAC, provides the moving web a condignly stable tension. Stable tension keeps the lateral guide system working well at the same time. The proposed decentralized PID tension control scheme is shown in Fig.6. The expression of the unwind/rewind roller dynamics is acquired from equation (3) based on the rated parameters in the experiment. The reference velocity in the block diagram may be seemed as a feedforward gain settled in the PMAC control card.

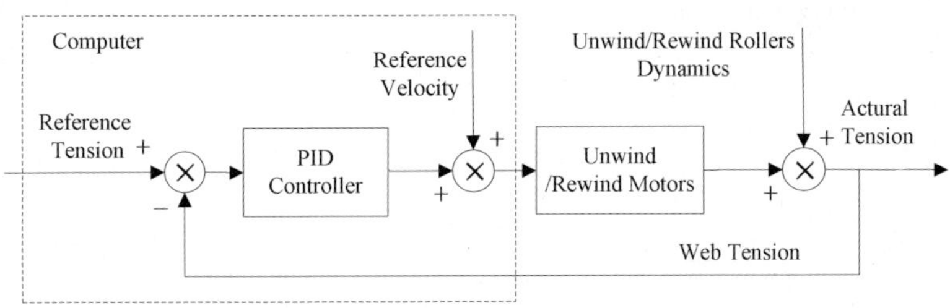

Fig. 6. Proposed decentralized PID tension control scheme

The decentralized position control scheme for an accurate feeding is shown in Fig. 7. The conveying position error can be gained by the CCD vision system. This position error is used as a feedback to control the feeding position and velocity of the master and slave nip motors. This closed-loop position control sub-system keeps the web moving with a high precision, which is our ultimate purpose. The nip rollers dynamics' expression in Fig. 7 can be got from equation (6), by the substitution of known quantity into parameters.

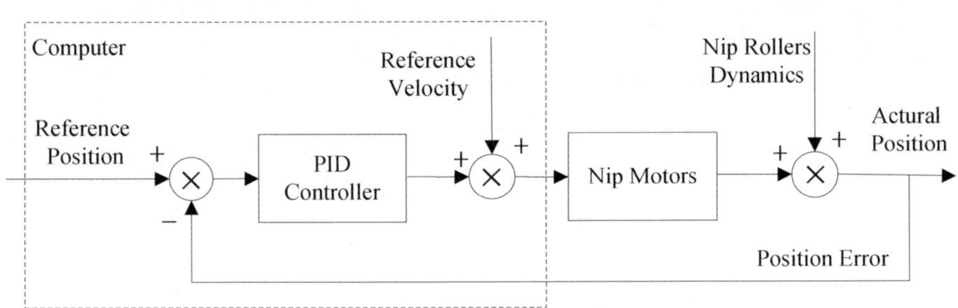

Fig. 7. Step move plot result of the unwind motor

The step move plot result of unwind motor is shown in Fig. 8. Regulated the PID parameters by the PMAC software, the unwind motor shows good reliable performance. The step move plot presents that the following error between the command position and the actual position is kept reasonable. The trapezoidal move plot result of the master nip motor is shown in Fig. 9. In the regulated process, the motors were endowed with the same parameters as in the real work process, including the velocity, the acceleration time, the dwell time. All the four motors' PID gains and velocity/acceleration/friction feedforward gains had been adjusted to keep the motors regaining quick response and stability performance.

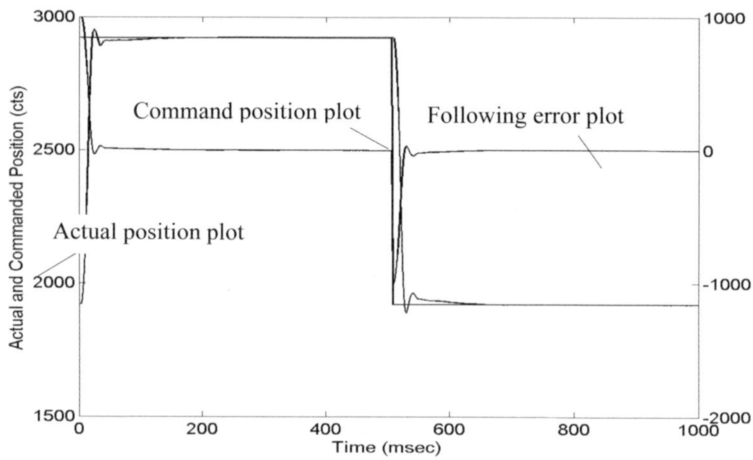

Fig. 8. Step move plot result of the unwind motor

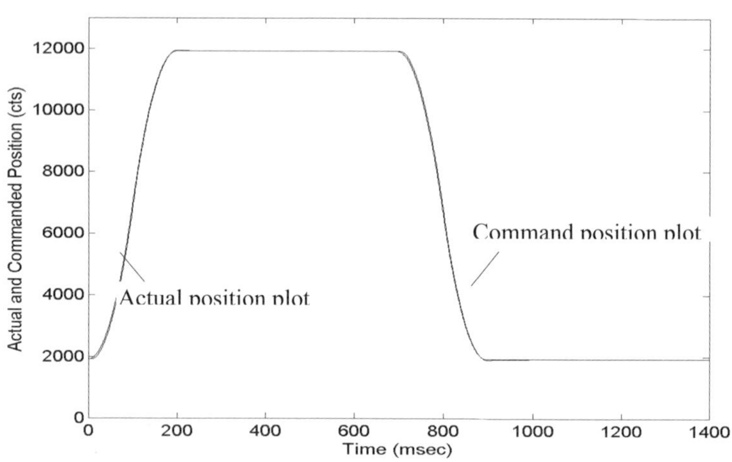

Fig. 9. Trapezoidal move plot result of the master nip motor

The main parameters of the four AC motor is shown in Table 1. The data is initial numerical value for the parameters. The value will be continually renewed in the conveying process by the control software.

Table 1. Initial value of the main parameters

	Unwind motor	Slave nip motor	Master nip motor	Rewind motor
Proportional Gain	7834	48000	22000	15000
Integral Gain	2000	1000	2000	1000
Derivative Gain	800	3500	1500	1380
Velocity Feedforward Gain	3500	5000	3900	4500

4 Implementing Results

Tension values, obtained in the implementing process, are shown in Fig.10. It can be seen that the tension keeps benignly steady in an acceptable confined scope. But when the displacement alters peremptorily, especially in the time of starting and stopping of the web conveying, the tension is affected slightly and has some confusing oscillations. The acceleration of the web generates positive damping but deceleration generates a negative or destabilizing damping. The plot of the conveying displacement is presented in Fig.11, which can be used to analyze the changing of the tension in the moving web.

The changing of tension value causes the distortion of the flexible web, especially in the process of accelerating and decelerating in the conveying. The hybrid control proposed in this paper make it possible to keep the conveying process stabilized and supply good position precision at the same time. The position errors in both the lateral and longitudinal directions are shown in Fig. 12 and Fig. 13 respectively. The data are captured by the vision system in the noncontinuous feeding process. Some special marks have been printed on the web for the CCD's graphics disposal system. The graph data indicates that this web-conveyed system works well on the performance of

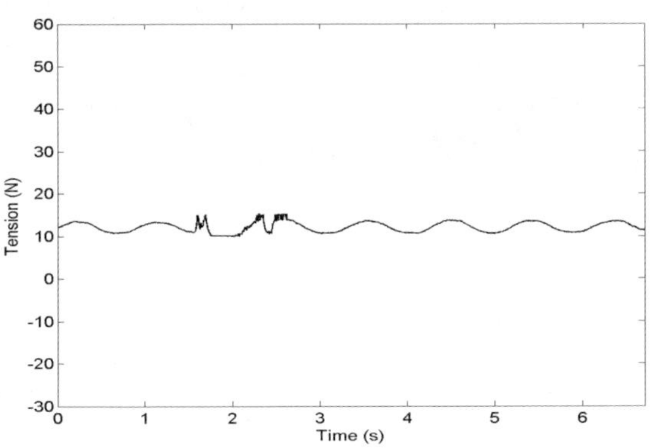

Fig. 10. Plot of tension value in the conveying process

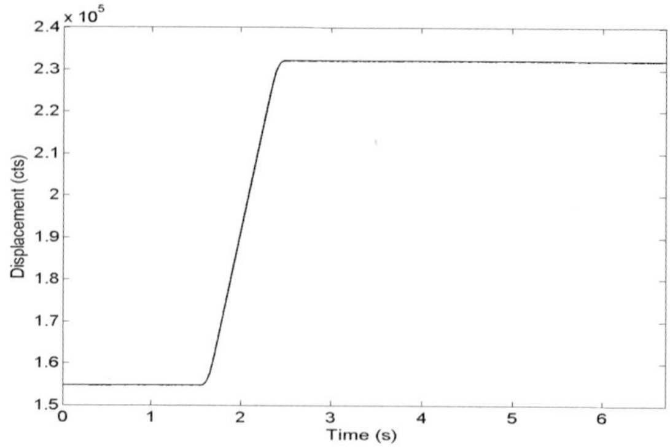

Fig. 11. Plot of the conveying displacement

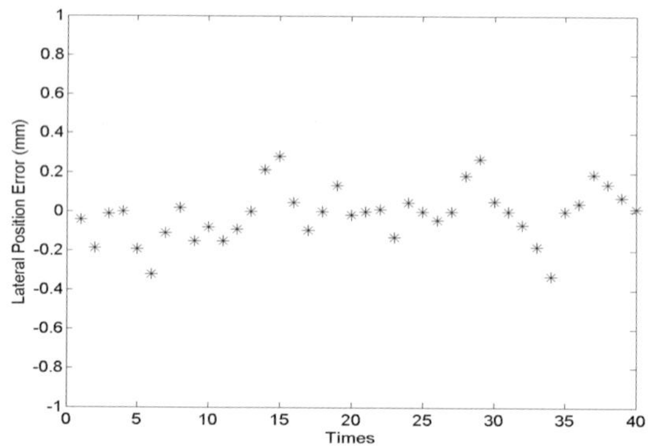

Fig. 12. Plot of the lateral position error

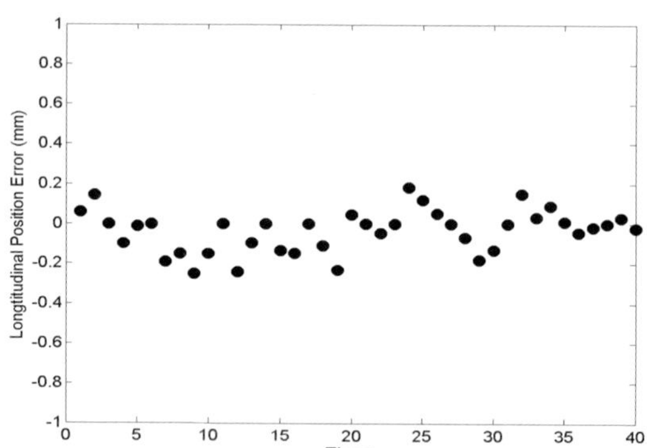

Fig. 13. Plot of the longitudinal position error

the precise feeding. The points, representing the value of position errors, were jumping in limited interspace, which implies that this system could fulfill flexible web's precise position requirements.

5 Conclusions

This paper outlined the design of a tension/position hybrid control strategy for a non-continuous web-conveyed system adapted to RFID integrated equipments. Not only the precise synchronized control and the decentralized PID control but also the vision position error compensation scheme is synthesized adopted in this system. The implementing results show that the system has highly tension stability and precise feeding position, which means the tension/position hybrid control strategy is a successful case in this web-conveyed system. It is important to note that there exists biggish tension fluctuation in the starting and stopping of feeding process, and that there is some uncertain steady error in the tension control. Future work will focus on solving these problems.

Acknowledgement

The work is supported by the Natural Science Fund of China (NSFC) (Project No 50625516), the National Fundamental Research Program (973) (Project No. 2003CB716207) and the 863 program of China under Grant No. 2006AA04A110.

References

1. Nagasawa, M., Yokoyama, E., Ishida, Y.: Precision motor control system for VCR using disturbance and velocity observer. IEEE Transactions on Consumer Electronics 38(4), 747–754 (1992)
2. Sakamoto, T., Izumihara, Y.: Decentralized control strategies for web tension control system. In: Proc. IEEE International Symposium on Industrial Electronics, pp. 1086–1089 (1997)
3. Okada, K., Sakamoto, T.: An adaptive fuzzy control for web tension control system. In: IEEE International Symposium on Industrial Electronics, pp. 1762–1767 (1998)
4. De Queiroz, M., Dawson, D., Rahn, C., Zhang, F.: Adaptive vibration control of an axially moving web. ASME Journal of Vibration and Acoustics 121, 41–49 (1999)
5. Nagarkatti, S., Zhang, F., Rahn, C., Dawsonv, D.: Tension and speed regulation for axially moving materials. Journal of Dynamic Systems, Measurement, and Control 122, 445–453 (2000)
6. Nagarkatti, S., Zhang, F., Costic, B., Dawsonv, D.: Speed tracking and transverse vibration control of an axially accelerating web. Mechanical Systems and Signal Processing 16(2-3), 337–356 (2002)
7. Shin, K., Jang, J., Kang, H., Song, S.: Compensation Method for Tension Disturbance Due to an Unknown Roll Shape in a Web Transport System. IEEE Transactions on Industry Applications 39(5), 1422–1428 (2003)
8. Carrasco, R., Valenzuela, M.: Tension Control of a Two-Drum Winder Using Paper Tension Estimation. IEEE Transactions on Industry Applications 42(2), 618–628 (2006)
9. Kang, C.-G., Lee, B.-J.: Stability Analysis for Design Parameters of a Roll-to-Roll Printing. In: Machine International Conference on Control, Automation and Systems, pp. 1460–1465 (2007)

Testing Technology of Torsional Vibration Spring Static Stiffness

Zhengfeng Jiang, Shaobo Xu, and Lei Chen

School of Mechanical and Electronic Engineering, Wuhan University of Technology, Wuhan 430070, China
Bobo379511@163.com

Abstract. The principle and method of testing static stiffness of torsional vibration spring are put forward based on the structure of dual-mass flywheel with torsional vibration spring, and the test bench is designed for these. The testing data is collected by using the PXI-6259 data collection card of National instrument and the data is processed by the LabVIEW software system. The elastic characteristic of the torsional vibration spring is obtained by analyzing the data.

Keyword: dual-mass flywheel; torsional vibration spring; static stiffness; LabVIEW.

1 Introduction

The driveline of automotive is a torsional vibration system of multi-DOF. The performance of automotive is greatly reduced by the torsional vibration and noise. Because of the restriction of space structure, the traditional torsional vibration damper of clutch is less effective in reducing vibration. So the traditional torsional vibration damper of clutch has been increasingly difficult to meet the requirement of vehicles' comfort. The dual-mass flywheel was invented as a new type damper in Europe in 1985. The torsional vibration spring is arranged in a long curved slide-way of the flywheel. The radius of this spring can be greater, so the spring's stiffness can be smaller and the reverse angle of relative can be greater. Then the effect of reducing vibration is much better than the traditional torsional vibration damper of clutch. Besides, the dual-mass flywheel's structure is simple and easy to implement. However, the dual-mass flywheel's requirement of design and processing is difficult and its performance indicator of technical also is strict. So it is still an advanced technology [1]. For a typical dual-mass flywheel of torsional vibration spring, this paper brought forward a method to test the static stiffness of torsional vibration spring, which is necessary to the mass production of the dual-mass flywheel.

The dual-mass flywheel, the tradition flywheel is divided into two parts along the direction of perpendicular to crank shaft, consists of primary flywheel and secondary flywheel. The two parts are connected by the torsional vibration spring. The function of the torsional vibration spring is to reduce vibration and noise. Therefore, it is the core component to dual-mass flywheel and its elastic characteristics impact directly on the performance of dual-mass flywheel [2].

C. Xiong et al. (Eds.): ICIRA 2008, Part II, LNAI 5315, pp. 784–793, 2008.

According to the difference of torsional vibration spring, the forms of dual-mass flywheel's structure are various. In this paper, the object of studying is the dual-mass flywheel of viscous oil damping and long arc spring. The dual-mass flywheel is shown in figure.1. It consists of primary flywheel, secondary flywheel and torsional vibration spring. Primary flywheel and secondary flywheel can rotate relatively. The two flywheels are connected by torsional vibration spring. During driving, secondary flywheel is driven by primary flywheel through torsional vibration spring. The torsional vibration spring's structure is that: the small arc spring is installed in the big arc spring and they consist of a group of springs. The two same groups of torsional springs are installed in the airtight chamber which consists of disc, covered and chute. The two group of spring are connected by rotation pan. Besides, each group of springs is consisting of two parallel arc springs of inside and outside and the two parallel arc springs' structure parameters and distribution radius are the same. So the two group springs are the same exactly.

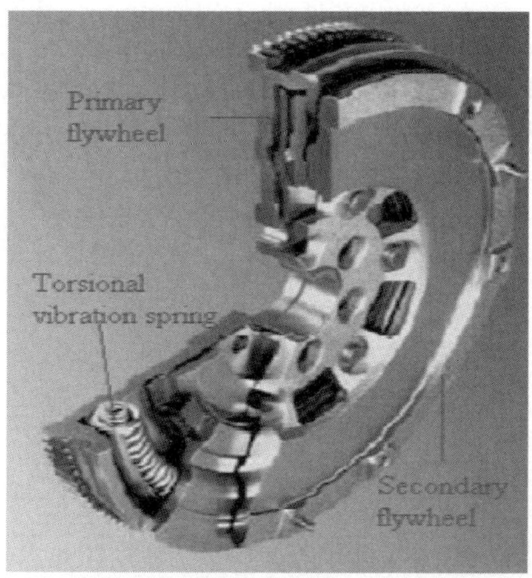

Fig. 1. The structure of dual-mass flywheel

2 The Principle and Method of Testing Static Stiffness of Torsional Vibration Spring

2.1 The Method of Testing Static Stiffness of Torsional Vibration Spring

Static stiffness of torsional vibration spring refers to the degree of deformation of the torsional vibration spring under a certain torque. The degree of deformation is equivalent to the relative rotational angle between the primary flywheel and the secondary flywheel. Therefore, the test data includes the torque transferred to the torsional vibration springs and the relative rotational angle between the primary flywheel and the secondary flywheel.

Because the torque transferred to the torsional vibration springs is difficult to test directly, we adopt technical method as follows: Because the torque on the transmission shaft of neighboring dual-mass flywheel is equivalent to the torque on the torsional vibration springs under the condition of loading slowly, we can test the torque on the transmission shaft of neighboring dual-mass flywheel to obtain the torque on the torsional vibration springs.

The degree of deformation of torsional vibration springs is also difficult to test directly. We adopt technical method as follows: the secondary flywheel is fixed and the rotational angle of the primary flywheel is the relative rotational angle between the two flywheels.

2.2 Principle of Test Bench

Static stiffness is tested, so the power of the test bench is loaded by manually driving worm and gear reducer. Using manual mode can make the measurement result more accurately and it is also easy to implement. The principle diagram of test bench is shown in figure 2. Torque is manually generated by the worm and gear reducer, and then the torque is transferred to primary flywheel by transmission shafts. During transmission of torque, torque and angle are real-time tested by a torque sensor and an angle sensor. The voltage signal generating from sensors is amplified by amplifying circuit and is converted into digital signal by A/D conversion. The signal is collected in use of PXI-6259 data collection card of National instrument and is processed by LabVIEW software system.

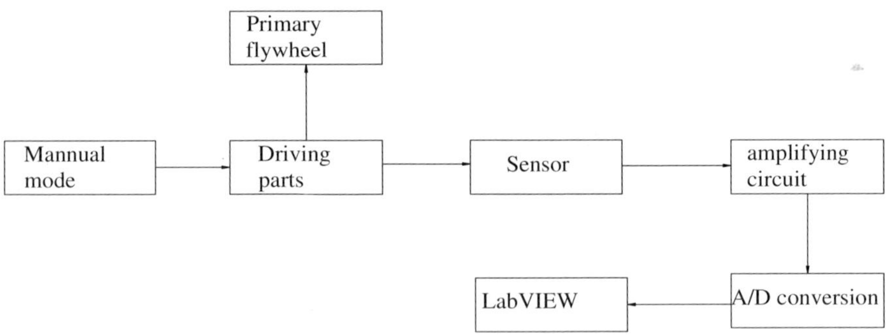

Fig. 2. Principle diagram of test bench

3 Design of Test Bench

3.1 Structural Design of Test Bench

Symmetry principle should be taken into the design of the test bench structure. Reducer as power-source and tested part are arranged on opposite sides of test bench, and torque sensor is arranged in the middle of teat bench. They are connected by shafts and couplings. Taking into account the shaft diameter of angle sensor is much smaller; the angle sensor is arranged at the end of test bench. Using the structure can avoid that the torque sensor had reading data before loading, and then it is helpful to improve the accuracy of test.

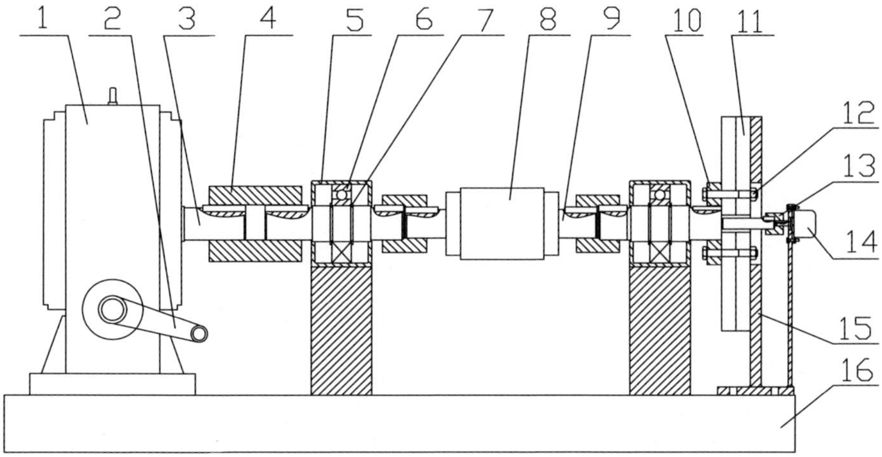

Fig. 3. Structural diagram of test bench / 1. Worm and gear reducer; 2. Handle; 3. The first shaft; 4. Coupling; 5. The first bearing seat; 6. The first bearing; 7. Shaft spring collar; 8. Torque sensor; 9. The second shaft; 10. Flange; 11. Dual-mass flywheel; 12. Bolt and nut; 13. Connecting bushing; 14. Angle sensor; 15. Support plate; 16. Bottom plate.

The test bench structure is shown in figure 3. The reducer is connected with torque sensor by the first shaft and two couplings. The other side of torque sensor is connected with the primary flywheel by the second shaft, coupling and flange. The secondary flywheel is fixed on the support plate by screws and it doesn't rotate with the primary flywheel. The shaft of angle sensor is connected with the other side of the second shaft by coupling and it rotates with the second shaft at real-time. Two bearings and bearing seats are arranged at both side of torque sensor, and they are not only used to support but also used to adjust the coaxiality of various components. Thus, torque is transferred to primary flywheel by reducer, shaft and coupling, and then generating relative rotation between primary flywheel and secondary flywheel. At the same time, torque and angle are tested by torque sensor and angle sensor.

3.2 Design of Test System

This test system includes software system, such as LabVIEW software, and hardware, such as sensors, signal conditioning and data acquisition module. Among them, sensor is the most basic element and its function is to convert physical quantity into electricity; the function of data acquisition is to convert analog signal into digital signal for computer; signal conditioning always is the bridge of them and its function is to connect output signal of sensor with other signal which can be accepted by data acquisition module [3]. The hardware structure diagram of test system is shown in figure 4. The test device of bench includes torque sensor, angle sensor, conversion card of data communication, PXI-6259 data acquisition card of National instrument, monitor, and so on.

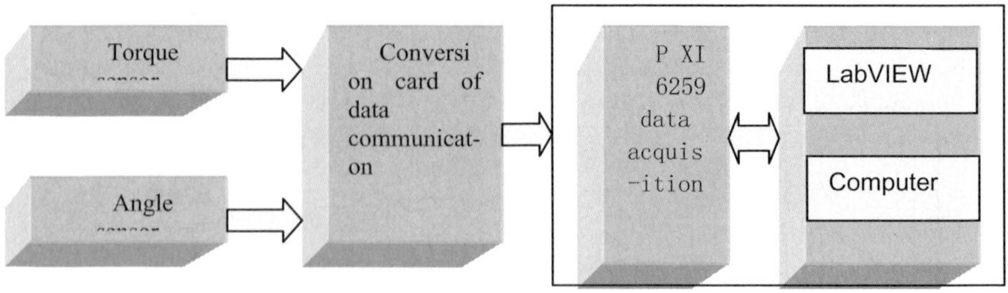

Fig. 4. Hardware structure diagram of test system

During testing of torque, the torque sensor, PS-T static torque sensor, is a resistance strain torque sensor. Measurement range of the sensor is 0-600 N.m and the range of output voltage is 1-10 V. The value of output torque and output voltage meets the linear relationship:

$$y = 0.007\ x + 5.505.$$

Where, y is the value of output voltage; x is the value of output torque.

During testing of angle, the angle sensor, DWQT non-contact angle sensor, is an angle sensor of potential. Measurement range of the sensor is 0°-90°and the range of output voltage is 0.5-5 V. The value of output angle and output voltage meets the linear relationship:

$$y = 0.045\ x + 0.476.$$

Where, y is the value of output voltage; x is the value of output angle.

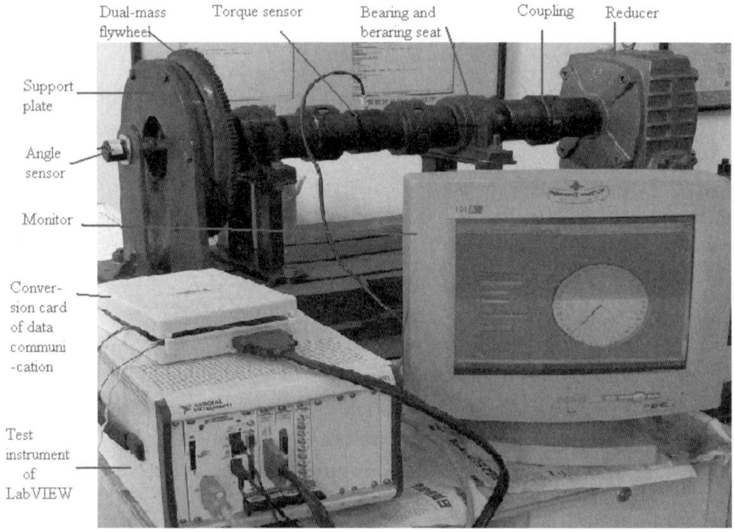

Fig. 5. Test bench and test system

The value of torque and angle are tested by torque sensor and angle sensor, and the form of output is voltage signal. Then, the voltage signal is transferred to the data acquisition card of LabVIEW measuring instrument, which converts analog signal into digital signal. Finally, the real value of torque and angle are shown on the monitor [4]. The test bench and test system are shown in figure 5.

3.3 Data Acquisition and Data Processing Based on LabVIEW

Data acquisition of analog includes two key components: data acquisition card and LabVIEW software. Analog signal of multi-channel is converted into digital signal by data acquisition card which includes multiplexer, A/D converter and data buffer. Then the digital signals are stored in data buffer. The data exchange between data acquisition card and computer is realized by a high speed bus [5]. Besides, the data acquisition VI compiled by LabVIEW controls the operation of data acquisition card. The type of data acquisition card is PXI-6259, which is provided by NI Company.

Step of data acquisition:

1) The Measurement & Automation Explorer is used to manage all hardware in the LabVIEW software system. This module can be implemented for detecting the data acquisition card, configuring properties of the card, and deleting properties.
2) Set up virtual channel to the data acquisition card.
3) Compiling data acquisition VI (figure 6) with LabVIEW.

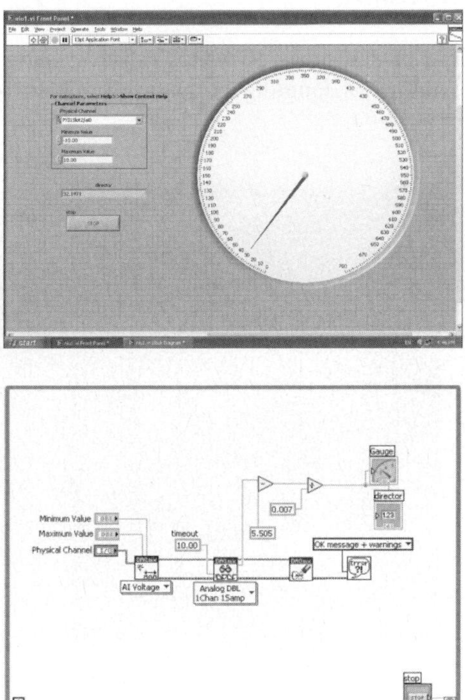

Fig. 6. Front panel and back panel of data acquisition VI

Method of data processing: use data-processing functions of LabVIEW and the linear relationships of every sensor to generate curve of torsional vibration spring static stiffness, and then these discrete data is linearly fitted with least-square algorithm to obtain static stiffness value of the springs of inside and outside. The program of data processing VI is shown in figure 7 [6].

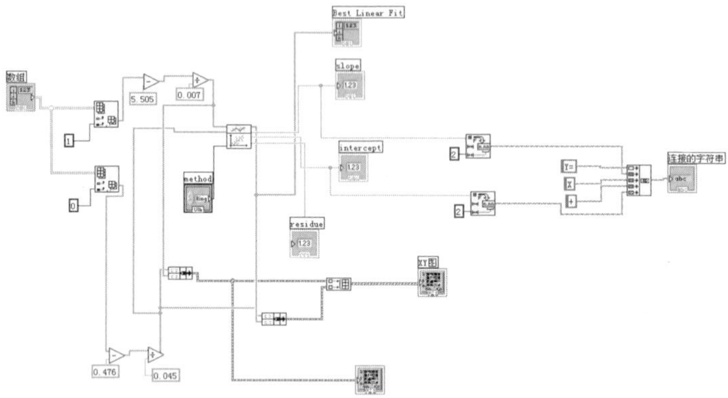

Fig. 7. Program of data processing VI

4 Analysis of Test Result

The static stiffness curve of dual-mass flywheel JMGE is shown in figure 8 that belongs to an automobile engine of Jangling Company. Static stiffness of springs at idle

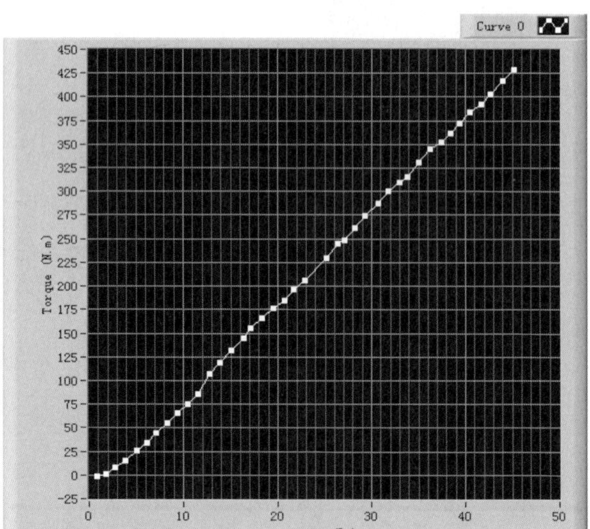

Fig. 8. Static stiffness curve of torsional vibration spring

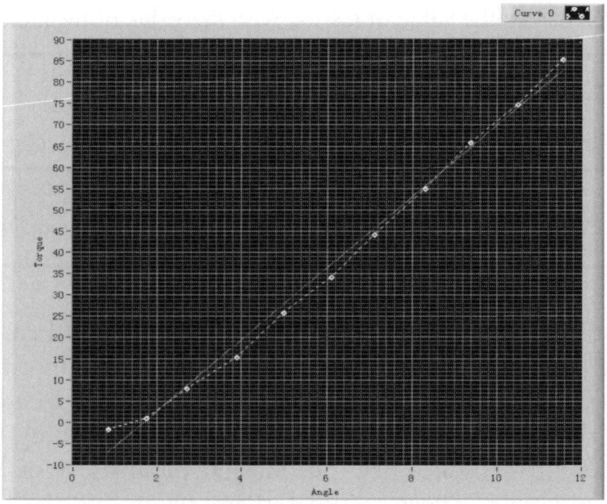

Fig. 9. The linear fitting of static stiffness curve at idle speed

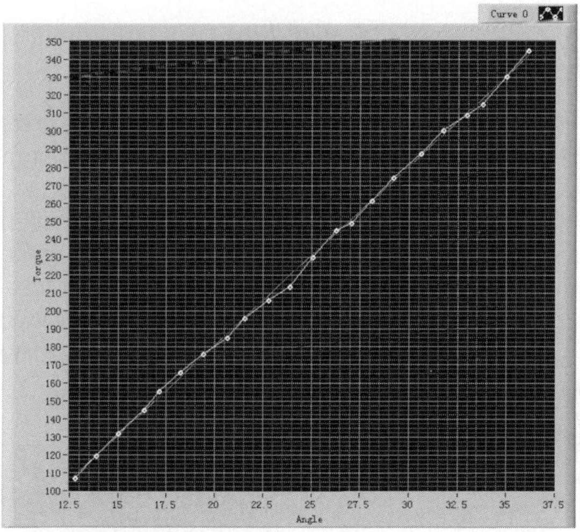

Fig. 10. The linear fitting of static stiffness curve at normally running speed

Table 1. Design parameters of torsional vibration spring

	Big arc spring	Small arc spring
Steel wire diameter (mm)	4	2
Pitch diameter (mm)	16	8
Number of active coils	33	31
Distribution diameter (mm)	220	220

Table 2. Comparing the value of testing with the value of formula calculation

Working state of automotive	Angle (°)	Static stiffness (N.m/rad)	
		Testing	Calculat-ion
Idle speed	0------12	246.13	224.87
Normal running speed	12-----45	323.89	344.56

speed and Static stiffness of springs at normally running speed can be obtained from the curve by using piecewise linear fitting with least-square algorithm. The degree of deformation, from 0°to 12°, is corresponding to the idle speed of automotive(figure 9) and the degree of deformation, from 12°to 45°, is corresponding to the normal running speed of automotive(figure 10). The design parameters of torsional vibration spring are shown in table 1. These parameters are taken into the formula calculation of arc spring stiffness [7] as follows, and then the value of formula calculation can be obtained.

$$K = \frac{Gd^4R^2}{8nD^3}$$

Where, K is the stiffness of spring; G is the shear modulus of spring; d is the diameter of spring wire; R is the radius of spring; n is the effective coil number of spring; D is the mean diameter of coil.

Comparing the value of test with the value of formula calculation, in the table 2, the data of them is similar and the error between them is within the scope of allowed. The result of test shows that the test method and the design of test bench provided by this paper are practicable. There are many reasons for the error, such as, processing precision error, test error of sensor, calculation error of grease damping, formula calculation error of static stiffness, and so on.

5 Conclusion

During designing the spring, various analytical methods can be used to obtain the curve of static stiffness. However, even if the calculation is very accurately and carefully, there is always the error between calculation value and actual value, which is caused by technical error, non-absolute uniformity of material, and so on. Therefore, the testing technology of torsional vibration spring static stiffness not only can test the result of analytical method, but also can guide the design and processing of torsional vibration spring.

Reference

1. Liu, W.X.: Automobile Design. Tsinghua University Press, M. Peking (2001) (in Chinese)
2. Zhou, J.Q.: Simulation Analysis of Dual-mass Flywheel. J. Mechanical Engineer. 4, 24–26 (2006) (in Chinese)

3. Shi, B.Q., Zhao, D.Y., Li, C.: Practical Handbook of LabVIEW 6.1 Programming. China Railway Publishing House, M. Peking (2002)
4. Shi, Y.C., Lang, H., Niu, C.H.: Test Technology of Sensor. Defense Industry Press, M. Peking (2007)
5. Deng, Y., Wang, L.: Test Technology and Instrument Application of LabVIEW 7.1. Machinery Industry Press, M. Peking (2004)
6. Ding, S.: Realization of Experimental Data Curve Fitting Based on LabVIEW. J. Journal of Liaoning Institute of Technology 27(6), 372–374 (2007)
7. Chen, T., Lu, Z.H., Su, C.Q.: Analysis Method for Elastic Characteristics of Arc Spring. J. China Mechanical Engineer 17(4), 493–495 (2006)

Research of Integrated Access Control Based on Task-Driven RBAC for Lifecycle Software Quality Management

Xiaogang Wang[1], Zhuoning Chen[1,2], and Junxiang Tu[1]

[1] School of Mechanical Science & Engineering, Huazhong University of Science & Technology, 430074 Wuhan, China
[2] Wuhan Kaimu Information Technology Ltd., 430223 Wuhan, China
Xiaogang Wang, victor.hust@gmail.com

Abstract. This paper presents a solution of integrated access control and user authentication by employing a software product lifecycle management relevant technology based on the research of user authentication and dynamic access in web-based software quality management and support platform (SQMSP). The used task-driven role-based on access control (T-RBAC) model is also constructed, which is a combination of RBAC and TBVC models to implement the dynamic access control of SQMSP by workflow engine. Meanwhile, single-sigh-on, hierarchical management are introduced in this paper in order to meet the requirements of security and ease-of-use, respectively.

Keywords: Task-driven role-based access control (T-RBAC), Software lifecycle management, Software Quality Management and Support Platform (SQMSP).

1 Introduction

The main aims for the software quality management and support platform (SQMSP), which should be consistent with the standards of ISO9001 and the requirements of SW-CMM/CMMI model level 3, are to satisfy with the requirements of software development lifecycle supporting. At the same time, the platform also provide some better supports for the software process management, software project management, software configuration management, software quality management, and organizational level software balance and control, in some degree.

With the expansion of an enterprise and the increasing projects it takes, the amount of software developing work and software developers are increasing very fast under the software life cycle management support collaborative environment. And the data security and confidentiality issues in SQMSP arise as time passes. The information security protection policies include the following aspects: user authentication, authorization and access control. This paper mainly describes user authentication, authorization and access control based on task-driven role based access control (T-RBAC) in SQMSP.

C. Xiong et al. (Eds.): ICIRA 2008, Part II, LNAI 5315, pp. 794–802, 2008.

Data access control is restrictions or methods to read data or make changes to data like inserting, updating or deleting. To achieve information sharing and collaborative software development are the two major goals that data access control under the software life cycle management should do and it has the following characteristics:

1) The simultaneous access of the same data by multiple users under the software concurrency permissions. All members of the project developing team can visit dynamic project data that others update it in time.
2) To protect the data security and confidentiality, policies of data access control should be taken dynamic adjustment as the changes of projects at various stages in the whole life cycle.

2 Requirements of Access Control in Software Development and the Solutions

2.1 Requirements of Access Control in Software Development and the Solutions

Several sub modules are required and collected in the SQMSP model in stratifying with the information collection, configuration management, process control and software testing management during the exploitation for the software. Moverover, for each module referred, they have their own independent management model during the user registration and access-rights. The SQMSP administrator must protect sets of gigantic and superfluous databases and set each user's access to each module while for the user various user names consistent with different sub-module must be remembered, which is very complicate and difficult once the number of sub-module is too large. According to the previous experience for the software integration projects, This user management mode presented herein is not only benefit to sub-modules coordinating work, but also restricts the users operating efficiency in SQMSP.

From the point of the software development life-cycle management, there is an urgent need of access control model using Single-Sign-On (SSO). By appling SSO method, the SQMSP can povide the same consistent login interface with different sub function modules. Users accessing authentication from the server can operate all authorized modules and resources. A basic Single-Sign-On schematic is shown in Fig. 1.

The mechanisms of SSO evidently reduce the time of logging in different sub applications [3]. At the same time, by integrating sub-modules into a unified authentication module, Administers can easily add/delete user accounts in a GUI Window.

Access control management module of the SQMSP system provides authentication and authorization for other functional modules in the platform. A user can access the right modules and data by the authority provides by access control management module. Once the security polices and access control mode is defined, the system can work safely. Therefore a reasonable rights management module should be designed to ensure the safety of the system. In this paper, an access control mode based on T-RBAC is introduced to provide a unified access control management module and to improve the security of business information.

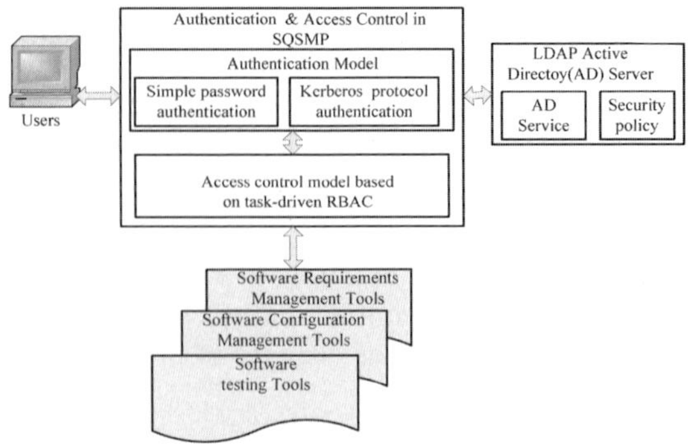

Fig. 1. Scheme of SSO and Access Control in SQMSP

2.2 Basic Features of the User Access Management Model in SQMSP

We introduce a solution of unified identity authentication control model based on RBAC (role-based access control) which has four remarkable features: Single-sigh-on (SSO), unified identity authentication, hierarchical authentication management and user-role authorization & mapping.

First of all, domain administrators can collect and control information scattered throughout the organization, giving each user with a unified account. Once the user logins in the domain with this account, he also gets the access to SQMSP by the unified identity authentication control module.

Secondly, the hierarchical authentication management is introduced in the SQMSP. Director of the Group or Department managers give the specific project manager his probable role and access permission. Then the project manager gives his team members their probable roles and access permission.

Finally, user-role configuration tool based on RBAC assigns permissions to users, with the aim of mapping users' identities to permissions and providing authorization and access control mechanisms.

On the hand, this mechanism not only protects the integrity of the SQMSP's database, but also is flexible and convenient to manage since it can separate users from permissions logically through the concept of role, consisting with actual work.

On the other hand, this mechanism works well with the original distributed access model and is suitable for monitoring the working state of sub-projects developed by outer software enterprise or group.

3 Framework of Unified Identity Authentication in SQMSP

3.1 Principles of the Framework Based on T-RBAC

As mentioned above, the SQMSP is a hierarchical structure platform. As shown in Fig. 2, the platform is between OS supporting layer and application layer and all function modules, which can only be assessed by the uniqie application interface, such as object management, project management, are packaged together. The basic function

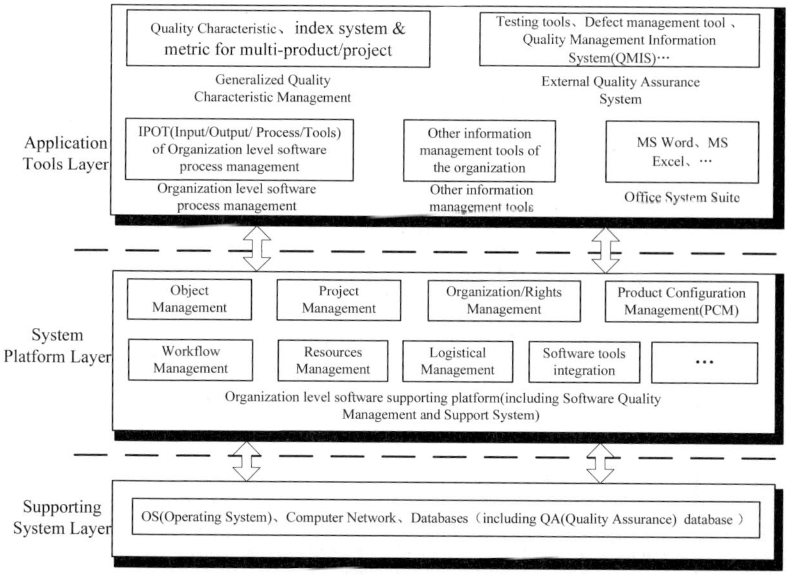

Fig. 2. Scheme of the SQMSP

modules such as process management and software quality characteristic management supporting by outer sub-function modules can be called and communicated by the unified interfaces of the platform.

The functions such as identity authentication and user's role and data access permission control included in this paper are achieved in the platform layer and can be deployed in the application servers which communicate with the Domain Server. The four main functional modules are user identity authentication, data access permission control, user-role configuration tool and common proxy module for application service [4]. Fig. 3 shows functional modules of the platform in detail.

Users in the software enterprise can log in to the platform by two methods: via Web browser or client software. Both of them are consistent with the unified identity authentication module for access authentication. This module is developed based on the LDAP protocol [5], obtaining the ability to directly access active directory database in Windows Domain Server. That is when the user logs in the client computer, he is be authenticated by SQMSP which can not only provide Single-Sigh-On mode, but also reduce the extra spending of user management. The result of the log info is stored in the log database in Domain Server and the Administrator can inquiries the log file at any time.

The administrator configures several templates of particular role and data access permission control. The particular users are mainly group headers or department managers and they gain the high class power of management. At the same time, they can configure their own team members' probable roles and access permission.

The application service module which is composed of application service driven engine is the proxy of sub functional modules and outer modules. The main function is information exchange and application proxy. User who gets the right authorization from the user-role configuration tool has access to the applications which is defined in the user-role configuration tool.

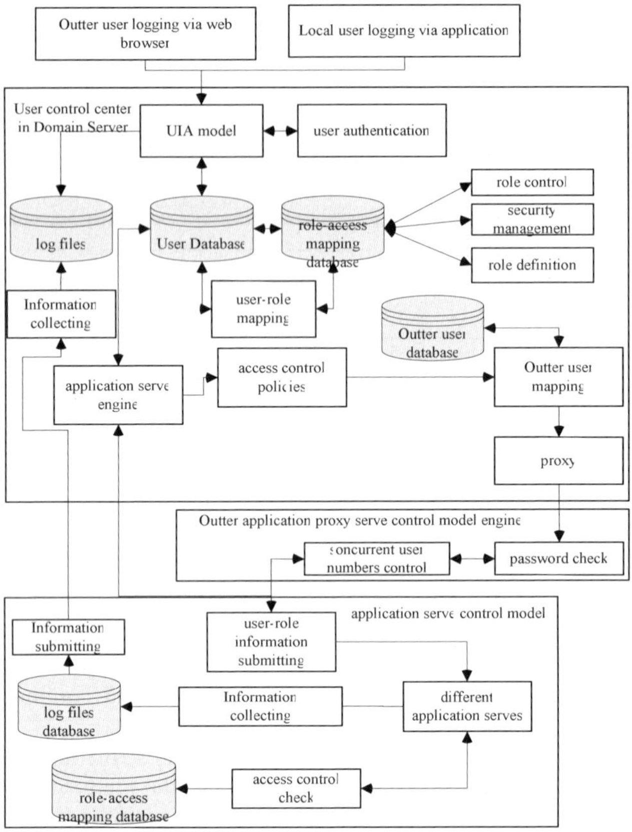

Fig. 3. Scheme of the framework using unified identity authentication based on RBAC

After logging in the platform, the user's operations are transferred in the real-time log files. It is easy for administrator to track and manage the system and is also very convenience for system maintenance.

3.2 Task-Driven RBAC Model

3.2.1 Basic Model of RBAC

Role-Based Access Control (role-based access control, RBAC) is a control mode that users are assigned to roles [6], permissions are assigned to roles and users acquire permissions by being members of roles. If users are part of an organization, permissions are assigned to their roles in particular project. The definition of the users' roles mainly depends on users' duty and qualifications. Permissions are assigned to roles and divided into groups according to the roles. Role-based Access Control (RBAC) model separates users from permissions logically through the concept of role. The structure and strategy is flexible, and the best advantages are its management support which can adapt to different security demands. So, RBAC model has been widely used.

The basic elements and their relationship of RBAC model are shown in shown in Fig. 4. As the conception of role in RBAC is correspond to the enterprise or department in real work, we can easily correspond role in RBAC to user's positions or responsibilities in real work. Therefore the RBAC model can easily be used from the perspective of the entire enterprise. But it has shortcomings not considering the workflow, and it does not support the dynamic changes of access control in the whole software lifecycle management.

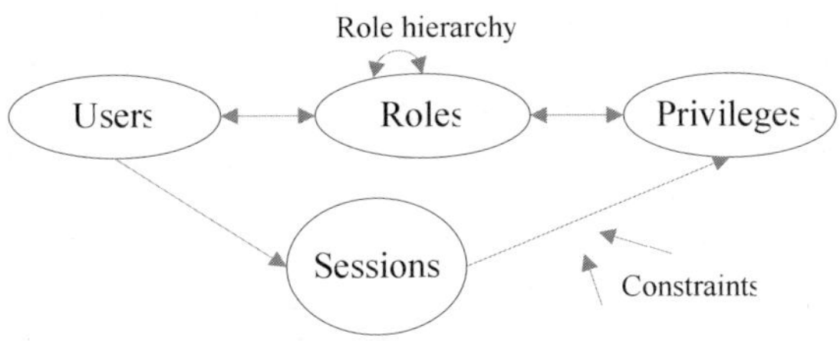

Fig. 4. Scheme of basic elements and their relationship of RBAC model

3.2.2 Task-Driven RBAC Model

To meet the requirements of the software lifecycle development quality management, this paper introduces a task-based RBAC model[7][8] that can effectively overcome the shortcomings of basic RBAC model. Figure 5 is the schematic of the task-driven RBAC model.

In this model, access control achieved by designating the specific data to the given user. Data object access control authority consists of static constraints and dynamic constraints. Static constraints in this model are inherited from the basic RBAC model, and the dynamic constraints are defined by the different roles in different projects that a user undertakes. Project managers can dynamic adjust the access or permission of a team memeber according his role's changes in the software development lifecycle. The status of software development lifecycle and workflows of defines the changes of access control, and the access control authority can be delegated to an organization or a role.

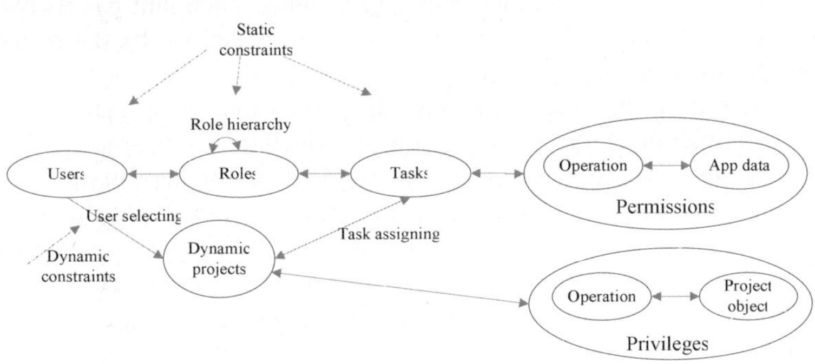

Fig. 5. Scheme of elements and their relationship of task-driven RBAC model

3.2.3 User-Role/Authentication Configuration Based on RBAC

The administrators at all levels define the roles according to the enterprise rules and the authority permissions are assigned to the roles. When a user logs in the client, he will get the permission defined by the role assigned in the particular project. He can directly operate the modules without logging since his authentication is mapped to the sub-modules in the SQMSP .

Fig. 6 shows the scheme of SQMSP's user-role access control mechanism. It is clear that when the user logs in the platform he will undertake the specific role and permission assigned by the project manager. The authority information is sent to the application module for validating through the APIs of the identity authentication module. Once the application module checks this information and proves its be successful, the user can call the application services function to complete his work successfully.

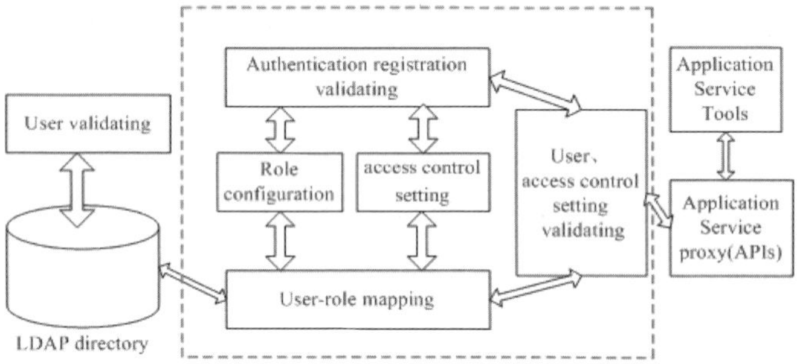

Fig. 6. Scheme of the SQMSP's user-role access control mechanism based on RBAC

4 Applications

The user-role unified identity authentication access mode based on RBAC has been applied in the SQMSP system in WAN environment.

By rationally planning the structure of directory in Domain server, R&D, testing and management users are classified into several units. Each unit has its own access permission to the directory. When the user's account is defined by the administrator, he can change his password immediately effortlessly. Moreover, his private information can be viewed by other users who have the permissions in the domain.

All the information of the software projects (including the projects which have been implemented) will be gathered by the SQMSP and be kept to update the database. According to the rules of hierarchical management, each project configuration admin can co-figurate and manage the information and tasks within his projects. Fig. 5 shows the snap of team members' roles definition and permissions configuration of a project running on the platform. All users will see the unified UI (user interface) of the platform, but the access to different modules is different by the permissions according to the role the user undertakes.

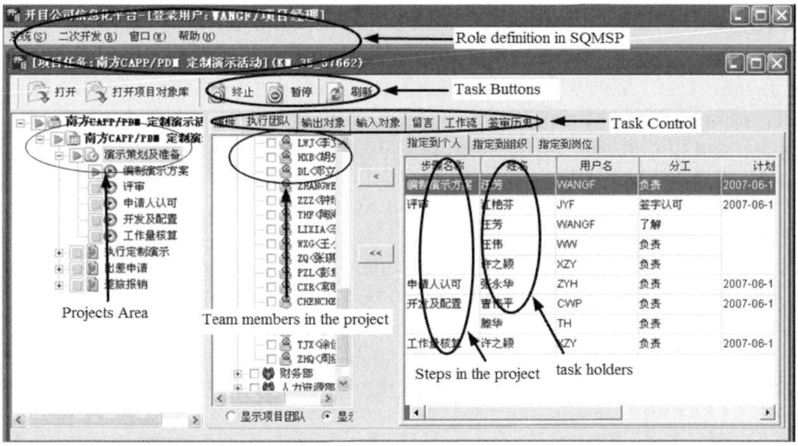

Fig. 7. Screenshot of the role definitions in SQMSP

This unified identity authentication control, permissions assigned by the role, and hierarchical authentication management mechanism can not only protects the consistency of the SQMSP's database data, but also has characteristics of high reliability and scalability [9].

5 Conclusions

The detail work process of users' access control privileges configuration and management in SQMSP is very complex. To obtain a unified identity authentication control mode, the SQMSP is presented, which is very effective for all users in improving their work, increasing productivity and efficiency and protecting the security, integrity and consistency of the software development.

In summary, users' access control privileges configuration and management in SQMSP is complex and effective, which is proved in this paper. To obtain a unified identity authentication control mode, the SQMSP is presented in this paper, which is very effective for all users in improving their work, increasing productivity and efficiency and protecting the security, integrity and consistency of the software development. We believe that the SQMSP presented herein will open many potential applications due to its advantages, such as simple, safe and effective.

Acknowledgment

We would like to thank our project partners for helpful comments. This work is done within the The National High Technology Research and Development Program of China (863 Program) which is supported by The Ministry of Science and Technology, The People's Republic of China, contract No. 2006AA01Z187 and No. 2007AA04060. The content of this publication is the sole responsibility of the authors.

References

1. Qiu, J., Ma, C.H., Yin, J.W., Dong, J.X.: Research and Implementation of Role-Based RBAC Administration Model. In: Proceedings of the The Fifth International Conference on Computer and Information Technology, pp. 746–750. IEEE Press, New York (2005)
2. Fredj, D., Björn, M., Günther, P.: Administration of an RBAC system. In: Proceedings of the 37th Hawaii International Conference on System Sciences, pp. 1–4. IEEE Press, New York (2004)
3. Li, X.W., Tang, L.P., Zhu, H., Li, X.J.: A Single Sign On Model Based On B/S Architecture. Journal of Sichuan University(Engineering Science Edition) 38(2), 132–135 (2005) (in Chinese)
4. Zhang, J., Chen, Y.J., Chen, Z.N.: Research on Transparent Integration of CAx/PDM Based on Agent. Mechanical Science and Technology for Aerospace Engineering 24(8), 969–973 (2005) (in Chinese)
5. Hu, L.C., Wu, Y.X., Zhang, Y., Jiang, X.D.: Research and implementation of unified user management system in environment of LDAP. Computer Engineering and Design 28(4), 823–825 (2007) (in Chinese)
6. Guo, H., Li, Y.M., Wang, L.F.: Design and Research of Access Control Model Based on Role and Task. Computer Engineering 32(16), 143–145 (2006) (in Chinese)
7. Wan, L., Zheng, X., Liu, Q.H.: Research and realization of integrated product development flow based on product lfecycle management. Computer aided engineering 14(2), 68–74 (2005) (in Chinese)
8. Sejong, O., Seong, P.: Task-role-based access control model. Information Systems 28(6), 533–562 (2003)
9. Zhang, J., Wang, X.G., Chen, Z.N.: Research on Application Integration of PDM System Based on C/S Mode in Network-distributed Environment. Machine Tool & Hydraulics 9, 202–205 (2006) (in Chinese)

Adaptive Notch Filter Control for the Torsion Vibration in Lead-Screw Feed Drive System Based on Neural Network

Yong Zhou[1,2], Fangyu Peng[2], and Bin Li[2]

[1] School of Logistics Engineering ,Wuhan University of Technology, Wuhan 430063, Hubei Province, China
[2] National NC System Engineering Research Center, Huazhong University of Science and Technology, Wuhan 430074, Hubei Province, China
zwm8917@263.net

Abstract. In the machining process, the nature vibration characteristics of feed drive frames are in time-varying. The nature frequencies of the torsion vibration in the lead-screw feed drives are notably changed with the table position, which further influences the stability of servo control. Building the model of servo drive system under consideration of torsion vibration of rotor-screw system, this paper analyzes the effect of changing torsion vibration modes on the notch filter control. The results display that the compensation using the conventional notch filter cannot suppress those disturbances induced by the time-varying vibration modes. Therefore, an adaptive notch filter control method is presented based on an improved BP neural network in this paper. A case study demonstrates that the parameters of the notch filter can be adjusted rightly according to the different table position. Consequently, the torsion vibration modes are compensated efficiently for the time-varying table positions.

Keywords: Feed drive; Lead-screw; Torsion vibration; Neural network; Adaptive notch filter.

1 Introduction

The high speed machining (HSM) in the high speed machine tools requires that its feed drives have high speed and high acceleration as well as that the feed drives remain high location accuracy. In the typical researches, the designs of control systems for high speed machines are based on ideal rigid bodies to the transmission elements of feed drive system [1-5], i.e., the existing resonance in the system or deformable behavior of the structural components is neglected in the design, which is one of the main concentrations to design a high precision machine. To compensate this influence, Chen and Tlusty [6] proposed various compensation strategies for the cancellation of vibrations of lowly damped structural modes that limit bandwidth. Smith [7] studied characteristic of the torsion and axial dynamics of lead-screw feed drives to design a compensation for filtering the first two natural modes of torsion vibration using notch filtering inside the feedback loop. Poignet et al. [8] considered the feed

C. Xiong et al. (Eds.): ICIRA 2008, Part II, LNAI 5315, pp. 803–812, 2008.

drive model with lumped springs and lumped masses. Erkorkmaz [9] identified the structural dynamics of lead-screw mechanism and compensated the first natural mode of torsion vibration using notch filter. Zaeh and Oertli [10] established the whole FEM model of ball screw feed drive systems and simulated the axis control system. Varanasi and Nayfeh [11] developed a model of lead-screw system dynamics that accounts for the distributed inertia of the screw, the compliance, damping of the thrust bearings, nut, and coupling. Whalley et al. derived lumped, finite element and hybrid, distributed-lumped models for torsional shaft–rotor–bearing systems [12].

Although these researches are recently considered to be efficient in compensating the vibration models, they all are on the status to select the practical moving table in a specified fixed position, usually, such as the middle of lead-screw. Actually, the natural frequencies of the first three orders in lead-screw feed drives are notably changed with the position change of the table movement and the compensation using the conventional notch filter cannot suppress those disturbances induced by the vibrations associated with the changing table position [13].

Here, based on an improved BP neural network, an adaptive notch filter control method is presented to compensate the first two torsion vibration modes that are changed with the position change of the table movement in lead-screw feed drive system.

2 Analysis of Notch Filter Control in Servo Drive System

2.1 Model of Servo System under Consideration of Torsion Vibration Modes

A full-digital permanent magnet synchronous motor (PMSM) and its AC servo drive system are adopted in this paper. Fig. 1 illustrates the block diagram of the servo drive system.

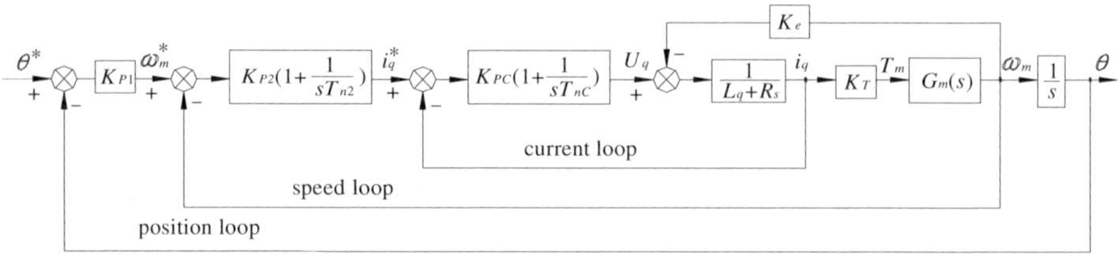

Fig. 1. Block diagram of servo drive system

Here, K_{P1}, K_{P2} and K_{PC} are the proportion gains of position loop, speed loop and current loop, respectively; T_{n2} and T_{nC} are the integral time constants of speed loop and current loop, respectively; ω_m and θ are the mechanical rotor angle velocity and angle, respectively ; i_q^*, ω_m^* and θ^* are the command current, the command angle velocity and the command angle, respectively; U_q is the equivalent winding voltage; i_q is the equivalent winding current; L_q is the equivalent winding inductance; R_s is the stator phase resistance; K_T is the motor torque constant; K_e is the back electromotive force constant; T_m is the electromagnetic torque; $G_m(s)$ is the mechanical transfer function; s is the Laplace operator.

In actual digital servo control system, the whole system can be regarded as a discrete time system to be modeled. Let the sampling time be T_s, and then the discrete mathematic model of the servo control system is acquired as shown in Fig. 2.

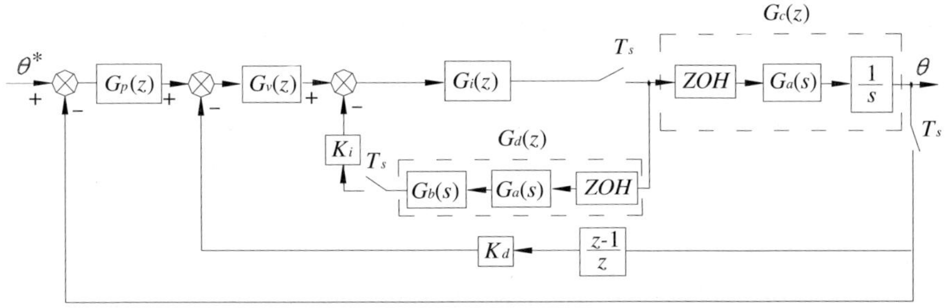

Fig. 2. Discrete mathematic model of the servo control system

where,

$$G_p(z) = K_{P1} \tag{1}$$

$$G_v(z) = K_{P2}\left[1 + \frac{z}{T_{n2}(z-1)}\right] \tag{2}$$

$$G_i(z) = K_{PC}\left[1 + \frac{z}{T_{nC}(z-1)}\right] \tag{3}$$

$$G_a(s) = \frac{K_T G_m(s)}{L_q s + R_s + K_e K_T G_m(s)} \tag{4}$$

$$G_b(s) = \frac{1}{K_T G_m(s)} \tag{5}$$

$$G_c(z) = (1 - z^{-1}) Z\left[\frac{G_a(s)}{s^2}\right] \tag{6}$$

$$G_d(z) = (1 - z^{-1}) Z\left[\frac{G_a(s) \cdot G_b(s)}{s}\right] \tag{7}$$

K_i and K_d are the feedback gains of the current loop and speed loop, respectively.

For the simple model that only takes mechanical rotational inertia into account, one can get $G_m(s)=1/(Js)$ (J is the equivalent rotational inertia of mechanical system converted into the motor rotor). Apparently, because the long slender assembly of the lead-screw, coupling, and rotor creates torsion vibration modes which can cause instability of servo control loop, the simple mechanical system model is insufficient for the exact analysis of feed drive system.

Divide the rotor-screw system into n torsion elements along its length. Using mode analysis method for the system, the transfer function between the motor torque and the angle speed that considers the first two torsion modes can be expressed by

$$G_m(s)=\frac{\dot{\theta}_1(s)}{T_1(s)}=\frac{1}{\sum_{j=1}^{n}J_j s}+\frac{1/\sum_{j=1}^{n}\left(\frac{A_j^{(1)}}{A_1^{(1)}}\right)^2 J_j\cdot s}{s^2+2\xi^{(1)}\omega^{(1)}s+(\omega^{(1)})^2}+\frac{1/\sum_{j=1}^{n}\left(\frac{A_j^{(2)}}{A_1^{(2)}}\right)^2 J_j\cdot s}{s^2+2\xi^{(2)}\omega^{(2)}s+(\omega^{(2)})^2} \tag{8}$$

Where, $\omega^{(1)}$, $\xi^{(1)}$, $\omega^{(2)}$ and $\xi^{(2)}$ are the first two nature frequency and the corresponding damping ratio of the torsion vibration, respectively, J_j is the rotational inertia of the jth element (j=1,2, …,n), and $A_j^{(i)}$ is the vibration amplitude of the jth element in the ith mode (i=1,2).

2.2 Analysis of Notch Filter Control for Torsion Vibration

Because the transfer function of the mechanical system considers the first two torsion modes which may induce the instability of the control system, the IIR notch filter can be employed in the speed loop to eliminate the first two torsion modes. The notch filter can be mathematically formulated in the following equation,

$$H_v(z)=\prod_{i=1}^{2}\frac{1-(2r_{zi}\cos\theta_{zi})z^{-1}+r_{zi}^2 z^{-2}}{1-(2r_{pi}\cos\theta_{pi})z^{-1}+r_{pi}^2 z^{-2}} \tag{9}$$

Where, r_{zi} and r_{pi} are the radii from the centre; θ_{zi} and θ_{pi} are the angles in z-plane, respectively; and K_N is an adjustment factor. Here, the subscripts "p" and "z" indicate pole and zero, respectively.

However, the dynamic characteristic including free torsion vibration in the machine system should be in time-varying with the machining process and influenced by the position of moving table, which further influences the quality of the control. Here, we check the influence of the changeable position of moving table on the control system with the conventional notch filter. Fig. 3 illustrates the simulation results of frequency responses of the closed position loop of the servo drive system when the table locates in 0.2L, 0.5 L, and 0.8 L, respectively. From this figure, it is found that the notch filter has a good compensation to disturbance of the first two order vibrations, and when the table locates at the position either 0.2 L or 0.8 L, the notch filter loses its validity due to the change of dynamic behavior of the torsion vibrations. These results suggest us that a new adaptive compensation filter for the lead-screw feed drives should be designed to compensate the disturbance.

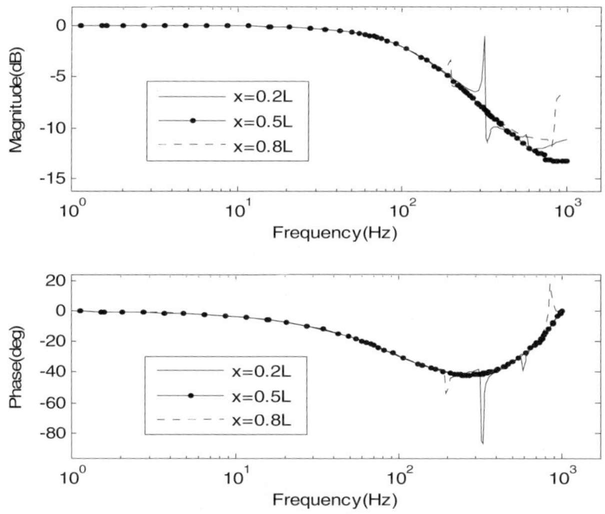

Fig. 3. Numerical results of frequency responses of the closed position loop of the servo drive system designed by the conventional notch filter on the basis of fixed position of table (i.e., x=0.5L) to the practical dynamic system with moving position of the table

3 Adaptive Notch Filter Based on Neural Network

3.1 Design Scheme

The design idea of adaptive notch filter based on neural network is that the parameters of the filter are changed according to neural network inspecting the operation conditions of the controlled object. The block diagram of servo control system with notch filter based on neural network is shown in Fig. 4.

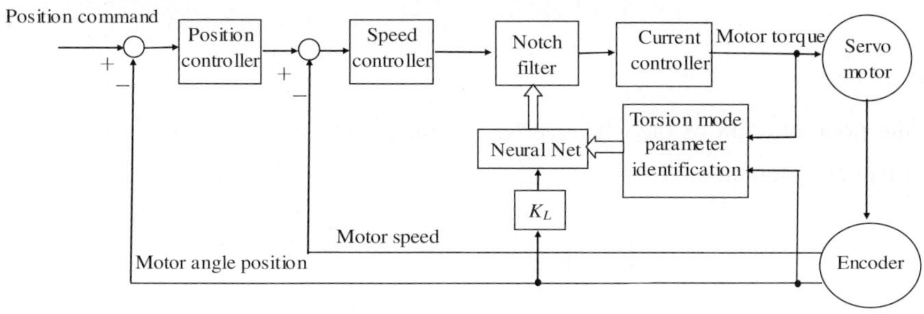

Fig. 4. Block diagram of servo control system with notch filter based on neural network

In Fig. 4, the table position and the corresponding adjusted parameters of the notch filter that are acquired according to measurement or calculation are used as the input and output samples of a neural network, respectively, then these samples are trained off line by the neural in terms of certain precision. After the training achieves a convergence, an optimized control model will be acquired to adjust the parameters of the notch filter on line.

3.2 BP Neural Network Model

This paper adapts BP network to build the neural network control model of adaptive notch filter. The notch filter of the Eq. (9) is actually two cascade controllers that compensate the first and second torsion modes respectively. Therefore, the parameters of the notch filter can be adjusted by two parallel neural nets apart. The structure of the designed neural network is shown in Fig. 5.

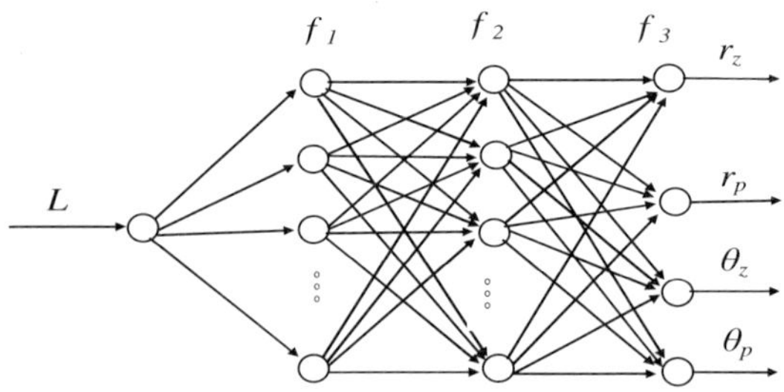

Fig. 5. Structure of the neural network

In Fig. 5, the table position L is the input of the neural network and the parameters of the notch filter, r_z, r_p, θ_z and θ_p are the corresponding outputs. This neural network has three layers (not including input layer), in which the first and the second layers are the hidden layers where the S-type transfer function is used and the third layer is the output layer where the linear transfer function is used. The transfer functions are explicitly formulated by

$$\begin{cases} f_{1,2}(x) = \dfrac{1}{1+e^{-x}} \\ f_3(x) = x \end{cases} \tag{10}$$

Let the node amount of the l layer be n_l. Then, the output $y_k^{(l)}$ of the node k in the l layer can be calculated by

$$\begin{cases} \bar{y}_k^{(l)} = \left\{W_k^{(l)}\right\}^T \cdot \left\{y^{(l-1)}\right\} = \sum_{j=1}^{n_{l-1}} w_{kj}^{(l)} y_j^{(l-1)} \\ y_k^{(l)} = f_l(\bar{y}_k^{(l)}), k = 1, 2, \cdots n_l \end{cases} \tag{11}$$

In which $\{W_k^{(l)}\}$ is the weight vector that links the node of the l-1 layer and the node k of the l layer and $\{y^{(l-1)}\}$ is the output vector of the l-1 layer where $\{y^{(0)}\} = \{L\}$.

Giving the sample mode $(\{X\},\{Y\})$, the weight values of the neural network will be adjusted to minimize the following criterion function

$$E(W)=\frac{1}{2}\left\|\{Y\}-\{\hat{Y}\}\right\|^2=\frac{1}{2}\sum_{k=1}^{n_3}(Y_k-\hat{Y}_k)^2 \tag{12}$$

Where $\hat{Y}_k$ is the output of the network, and $\hat{Y}_k = y_k^{(3)}$.

According to the gradient descent method, the correction of the weight vector $E(W)$ can be calculated to modify the weight values, which is formulated as

$$\left\{\Delta W_i^{(l)}\right\}=-\alpha\frac{\partial E}{\partial\left\{W_i^{(l)}\right\}}=\alpha\delta_i^{(l)}\left\{y^{(l-1)}\right\} \tag{13}$$

Where α is the learning rate. For the third layer, namely output layer, one can get

$$\delta_i^{(3)}=(Y_i-y_i^{(3)})f_3'(\overline{y}_i^{(3)}) \tag{14}$$

For the other layers, we have

$$\delta_i^{(l)}=\sum_{j=1}^{n_{l+1}}W_{ij}^{(l+1)}\delta_j^{(l+1)}f_l'(\overline{y}_i^{(l)})\,,\quad l=1,2 \tag{15}$$

3.3 Improvement of BP Neural Net

The hidden layers of the neural network model designed by this paper all adapt the S-type transfer function. But very small gradient may be brought when the multi-layer BP neural network with S-type nerve cell is trained, which results in the small changes of weight values and threshold values that depress the training speed. The resilient BP algorithm that can eliminate the effect of the gradient modulus value on the net training is adapted by this paper. In the resilient BP algorithm, the sign of the gradient decides the changing directions of the weight values and the threshold values, but the modulus value does not influence the changes. Here, independent parameters are used to update the weight values and the threshold values. When the differentials of performance function of the network to certain weight coefficient in two consecutive training periods have the same sign, the change rate of the weight value will increase according to an increasing parameter, or else decrease according to a decreasing parameter. If the differential is zero, the changing rate will be kept invariable. The iterative process to modify the weight values can be formulated by

$$W_{ij}^{(l)}(m+1)=\begin{cases}W_{ij}^{(l)}(m)+\Delta i & ,K_s>0\\ W_{ij}^{(l)}(m) & ,K_s=0\\ W_{ij}^{(l)}(m)-\Delta d & ,K_s<0\end{cases} \tag{16}$$

In which $K_s=\frac{\partial E}{\partial W_{ij}^{(l)}(m)}\times\frac{\partial E}{\partial W_{ij}^{(l)}(m-1)}$, Δi and Δd that are all greater than zero are the increasing parameter and decreasing parameter respectively, and m is the amount of iteration.

4 Case Study

Using the finite element method, the mode parameters in changing table position can be calculated [13], thus corresponding parameters of notch filter are acquired. Table 1 lists the table position and corresponding parameters of notch filter that compensates the first torsion vibration mode.

Table 1. Table position and corresponding parameters of notch filter

Table position L (mm)	r_{z1}	r_{p1}	θ_{z1} (rad)	θ_{p1} (rad)
40	0.972183	0.986584	1.410298	0.994707
80	0.971925	0.989584	1.423533	0.868920
120	0.972347	0.989745	1.401840	0.847165
160	0.973468	0.988242	1.344228	0.885345
200	0.974874	0.986832	1.272087	0.906022
240	0.976250	0.986419	1.201601	0.890441
280	0.977492	0.986630	1.138030	0.858729
320	0.978589	0.987063	1.081971	0.823857
360	0.979554	0.987542	1.032689	0.790504
400	0.980406	0.988005	0.989206	0.759975
440	0.981164	0.988429	0.950616	0.732438
480	0.981840	0.988807	0.916149	0.707815
520	0.982449	0.989069	0.885173	0.687796
560	0.982999	0.988956	0.857173	0.679656
600	0.983500	0.989245	0.831730	0.660144
640	0.983957	0.989607	0.808498	0.639928
680	0.984360	0.989951	0.788013	0.621942

The neural network toolbox of the MATLAB is used to achieve a simulation analysis. The parameters in Table 1 are adapted as the input and output samples of the neural network. Let the learning rate of α=0.02 and the minimal expectation error of e_g=0.00001. Using the resilient BP algorithm, the training achieves a convergence after 411 cycles. The input and output relation of the neural network obtained is shown in Fig. 6 where the symbol "+" represents the sample points. From Fig. 6, it is found that the neural network trained approaches the sample points accurately and the control curve of the network is smooth.

Moreover, using the adaptive notch filter based on neural network, the frequency responses of the closed position loop of the servo drive system are simulated numerically when the table locates in 0.2L, 0.5 L, and 0.8 L, respectively, which are exhibited in Fig. 7. The results display that the frequency response curves of the closed position loop in different table positions are all smooth, which indicates that the vibration modes are compensated efficiently for the time-varying table positions.

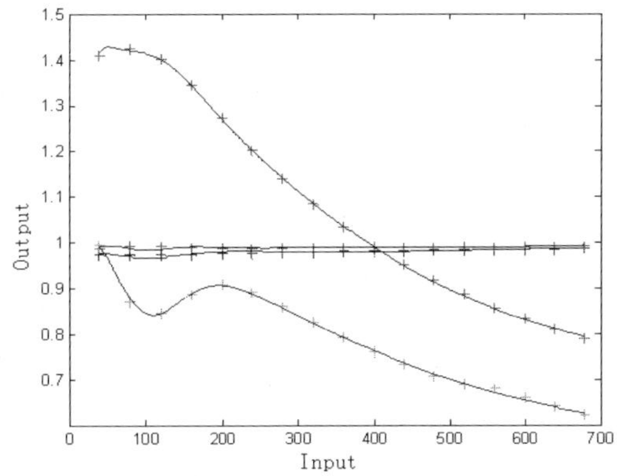

Fig. 6. Input and output relation of the neural network obtained

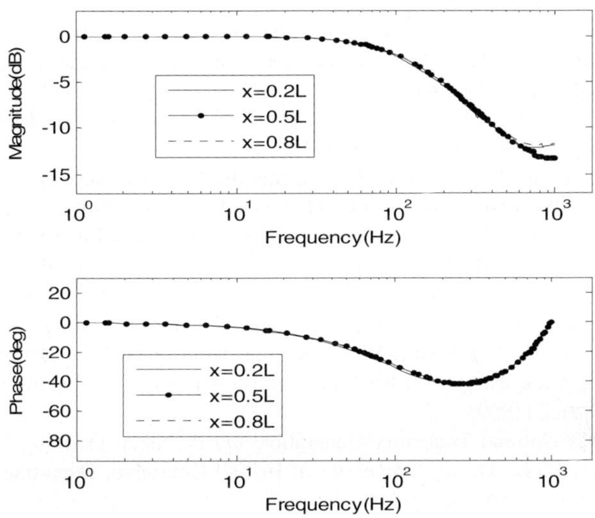

Fig. 7. Numerical results of frequency responses of the closed position loop of the servo drive system designed by the adaptive notch filter based on neural network to the practical dynamic system with moving position of the table

5 Conclusions

The effect of the changeable torsion vibration modes on the notch filter control in the lead-screw feed drives is analyzed. The results obtained display that the compensation using the conventional notch filter cannot suppress those disturbances induced by the time-varying vibration modes. Therefore, this paper presents an adaptive notch filter control method based on the resilient BP neural network. A case study demonstrates that the parameters of the notch filter can be adjusted rightly according to the different table position. Consequently, the torsion vibration modes are compensated efficiently for the time-varying table positions.

Acknowledgements

The authors gratefully acknowledge the supports of the Major State Basic Research Development Program of China (2005CB724101) and the Key Items Program of International Science and Technology Cooperation (2003DF000021).

References

1. Tomizuka, M.: Zero Phase Error Tracking Algorithm for Digital Control. ASME J. Dyn. Syst., Meas., Control 109, 65–68 (1987)
2. Weck, M., Ye, G.: Sharp Corner Tracking Using the IKF Control Strategy. Annals of CIRP 39(1), 437–441 (1990)
3. Pritschow, G., Kosiedowski, U.: Optimization Strategies for Adaptive Feedforward Control. Production Engineering Research and Development in Germany; Annals of the German Academic Society for Production Engineering 4(2), 69–72 (1997)
4. Van Brussel, H., Van den Braembussche, P.: Robust Control of Feed Drives with Linear Motors. Annals of CIRP 47(1), 325–328 (1998)
5. Boucher, P., Dumur, D., Rahmani, K.F.: Generalized Predictive Cascade Control(GPCC) for Machine Tools Drives. Annals of CIRP 39(1), 357–360 (1990)
6. Chen, Y.C., Tlusty, J.: Effect of Low-Friction Guideways and Lead-Screw Flexibility Dynamics of High-Speed Machines. Annals of CIRP 44(1), 353–356 (1995)
7. Smith, D.A.: Wide Bandwidth Control of High-Speed Milling Machine Feed Drives. Ph.D. Thesis, University of Florida, Department of Mechanical Engineering, Florida (1999)
8. Poignet, P., Gautier, M., Khalil, W.: Modeling, Control and Simulation of High Speed Machine Tool Axes. In: 1999 IEEE Int. Conf. on Advanced Intelligent Mechatronics, Atlanta, pp. 617–622 (1999)
9. Erkorkmaz, K.: Optimal Trajectory Generation and Precision Tracking Control for Multi-axis Machines. Ph.D. Thesis, University of British Columbia, Department of Mechanical Engineering, Vancouver (2004)
10. Zaeh, M.F., Oertli, T.: Finite Element Modeling of Ball Screw Feed Drive System. Annals of CIRP 53(1), 289–292 (2004)
11. Varanasi, K.K., Nayfeh, S.A.: The Dynamics of Lead-Screw Drives: Low-Order Modeling and Experiments. ASME J. Dyn. Syst., Meas., Control 26, 388–396 (2004)
12. Whalley, R., Ebrahimi, M., Jamil, Z.: The Torsional Response of Rotor Systems. Proc. Instn Mech. Engrs, Part C: J. Mechanical Engineering Science 219, 357–380 (2005)
13. Zhou, Y., Peng, F.Y., Chen, J.H.: Torsion Vibration Analysis of Lead-screw Feed Drives with Changeable Table Position and Work-piece Mass. In: Proc. 2007 IEEE Int. Conf. on Mechatronics and Automation, Harbin, vol. 3, pp. 2194–2199 (2007)

Fusion of Data and Expert Judgments with Imprecise Probabilities for Decision Making

Junxiang Tu[1], Jin Zhang[1,2], Zhuoning Chen[1,2], and Xiaogang Wang[1]

[1] School of Mechanical Science and Engineering,
Huazhong University of Science and Technology, Wuhan 430074, P.R. China
[2] Kaimu Information Technology Ltd., Wuhan 430223, P.R. China
junxiangtu@yahoo.com.cn

Abstract. Bayesian approaches to decision analysis are geared towards determining the optimal alternative by combining expert knowledge and data in small sample situations. However, Traditional Bayesian decision models assume that all probabilities are precise. In practical applications the probabilities of the states of nature are often under uncertainty due to the imprecision in the experts' judgments. In this paper, we present a decision support model that uses interval-valued probabilities to represent experts' uncertain beliefs. The model performs reasoning and decision making by integrating expert uncertain information and historical statistical data for Bayesian analysis. An example concerning risk assessment is given to demonstrate the applicability of the model in a real-world domain.

Keywords: decision making; interval-valued probabilities; Bayesian analysis; uncertain beliefs.

1 Introduction

In the field of decision making it is good practice to combine domain expert knowledge and data from experimental studies. This is particularly true in cases where the sample data is sparse due to the expense or difficulty of experimental trials. Bayesian theory has attracted much attention in the literature for its proper way to make formal use of subjective information such as expert opinion in such situations [1], [2], [3]. Consider a finite set of states $\{\theta_1, \theta_2, ..., \theta_n\}$. A decision a is assigned a utility value by a utility function $f_a(\theta)$ for each possible state of the world. Bayesian theory postulates that the decision a is evaluated through its expected value $E_p[f_a]$ with respect to a posterior probability distribution $P(\theta \mid x)$ computed from the prior and the likelihood:

$$E_p[f_a] = \sum_i f_a(\theta_i) P(\theta_i \mid x) \ . \tag{1}$$

A key assumption made by conventional Bayesian theory, however, is that all probabilities (including the prior, the posterior and the likelihood) are precise. This

C. Xiong et al. (Eds.): ICIRA 2008, Part II, LNAI 5315, pp. 813–819, 2008.

constraint can be problematic in practical application if the probability of an event is defined by a group of disagreeing experts who provide different values of the probability. For example, two experts are asked the subjective probability, $P(E)$, to assign to an event E. The first expert says that $P(E)=0.5$. The second expert states that $P(E)=0.8$. Does $P(E)=0.5$ or does $P(E)=0.8$? Maybe the best characterization of the experts' judgments is to say that $P(E)=[0.5, 0.8]$. Therefore, we need to extend the traditional Bayesian theory by accepting imprecise probabilities such as interval-valued probabilities to overcome the limitation of the precise probability. Previous studies have demonstrated the successful applications of imprecise probabilities. In Walley's theory of imprecise probability, one of the most complete frameworks for imprecise probability, Walley defined upper and lower probabilities as special cases of upper and lower previsions [4]. Coolen and Newby [5] applied lower and upper conjugate density families to model prior beliefs of experts. Cano and Moral [6] provided an approximate algorithm to obtain a posteriori intervals of probability when prior information was available at given intervals. In this paper, we use interval-valued probabilities to clearly quantify experts' uncertain beliefs and incorporate them into Bayesian decision analysis to support better decision making.

2 Interval Expression of Bayesian Rule

In Bayesian decision analysis the states of nature $\{\theta_1, \theta_2, ..., \theta_n\}$ are assigned prior probabilities by the analyst. The prior probabilities are built on the analyst's belief, which may also stem from experts' judgments. Let $\boldsymbol{\theta}$ denote the set of states $\{\theta_1, \theta_2, ..., \theta_n\}$. As soon as experimental data are available, they should be used to update the assumed prior probabilities of $\boldsymbol{\theta}$ by calculating the conditional probabilities of $\boldsymbol{\theta}$ given the observed data. According to Bayesian rule this is

$$P(\theta_k \mid x) = \frac{P(\theta_k)P(x \mid \theta_k)}{\sum_{j=1}^{n} P(\theta_j)P(x \mid \theta_j)}, \ k = 1, ..., n, \tag{2}$$

where $P(\theta_k)$ is the prior probability for the state θ_k and $P(x \mid \theta_k)$ is the likelihood function of observation x. It can easily be seen that both the prior probabilities and the likelihood functions are used for obtaining the posterior probabilities $P(\theta_k \mid x), k = 1, 2, ...n$. Therefore, the updated belief about the elements of $\boldsymbol{\theta}$ is a compromise between the initial expert assessments and the evidence of the collected data from experimental trials.

In practical application it would be preferable to use interval-valued prior probabilities to represent subjective information of experts' judgments when experts are asked to provide their beliefs on the elements of $\boldsymbol{\theta}$ under uncertainty due to sparse statistical data. In such situation $P(\theta_k)$ and $P(\theta_j)$ in Eq.(2) are now intervals rather than point values. Because both $P(\theta_k)$ and $P(\theta_j)$ appear multiple times in Eq.(2), ordinary interval analysis cannot reliably be used to compute with this formulation. It would be preferable to use a linear program to simplify Eq.(2) [7], [8]. Denote $\boldsymbol{P} = (P(\theta_1), P(\theta_2), ..., P(\theta_n))$. Suppose that experts assess interval-valued prior probabilities as follows:

$$l_k \leq P(\theta_k) \leq u_k, k = 1, ..., n, \tag{3}$$

where

$$0 \leq l_k \leq u_k \leq 1, \tag{4}$$

$$\sum_{k=1}^{n} l_k \leq 1 \leq \sum_{k=1}^{n} u_k. \tag{5}$$

The constraints (4) and (5) ensure the experts' assessments meeting the condition of avoidance of sure loss that is a necessary condition for imprecise probability analysis. As Walley states, "failure to avoid sure loss reflects a fundamental irrationality or error in judgment." Denote the row vector $\boldsymbol{B} = (-l_1, -l_2, ..., -l_n, u_1, u_2, ..., u_n)$. The constraint (3) can be rewritten as: $\boldsymbol{AP}^T \leq \boldsymbol{B}^T$, where A is a $2n \times n$ matrix. Define a new matrix as follows: $\boldsymbol{C} = \boldsymbol{A} - \boldsymbol{B}^T \boldsymbol{H}$, where $\boldsymbol{H}$ is a row vector of n ones. The linear programming formulation for calculating the lower and upper posterior probabilities of the elements of $\boldsymbol{\theta}$ can be written as:

$$\underline{P}(\theta_k \mid x) = \min\left(P(x \mid \theta_k)\gamma(\theta_k)\right), \ \overline{P}(\theta_k \mid x) = \max\left(P(x \mid \theta_k)\gamma(\theta_k)\right) \tag{6}$$

subject to

$$\boldsymbol{C\gamma}^T \leq 0, \tag{7}$$

$$\gamma(\theta_j) \geq 0, \tag{8}$$

$$\sum_{j=1}^{n} P(x \mid \theta_j)\gamma(\theta_j) = 1, \tag{9}$$

where $\gamma(\theta_k) = P(\theta_k) / \sum_{j=1}^{n} P(x \mid \theta_j) P(\theta_j)$, $\boldsymbol{\gamma} = (\gamma(\theta_1), \gamma(\theta_2), ..., \gamma(\theta_n))$, $k = 1, 2, ..., n$.

3 Decision Making

Suppose that a decision a is assigned a utility value by a utility function $f_a(\boldsymbol{\theta})$. Given the interval-valued posterior probabilities of the elements of $\boldsymbol{\theta}$, the decision a is evaluated through its expected value $E_p[f_a]$ that can be computed as follows:

$$\underline{E}[f_a] = \min\left(\sum_{k=1}^{n} f_a(\theta_k) P(\theta_k \mid x)\right), \ \overline{E}[f_a] = \max\left(\sum_{k=1}^{n} f_a(\theta_k) P(\theta_k \mid x)\right) \tag{10}$$

subject to

$$\underline{P}(\theta_k \mid x) \le P(\theta_k \mid x) \le \overline{P}(\theta_k \mid x),\ k = 1, 2, ..., n, \tag{11}$$

$$\sum_{k=1}^{n} P(\theta_k \mid x) = 1. \tag{12}$$

Because the expected utility is now an interval, a decision maker cannot choose a decision alternative that maximize the expected utility in the traditional sense. Consider the intervals of expected utility for two decision alternatives (a and b) shown in Fig. 1(a). Because the intervals do not overlap, alternative a is clearly better than b . In the example in Fig. 1(b), the intervals overlap. Notice that $\overline{E}[f_a]$ is greater than $\overline{E}[f_b]$, but $\underline{E}[f_a]$ is less than $\overline{E}[f_b]$. Because the true expected utility of a can be either better or worse than that of b , the decision maker cannot determine which alternative is the most preferred. In order to make decisions in such situations, different methods are needed.

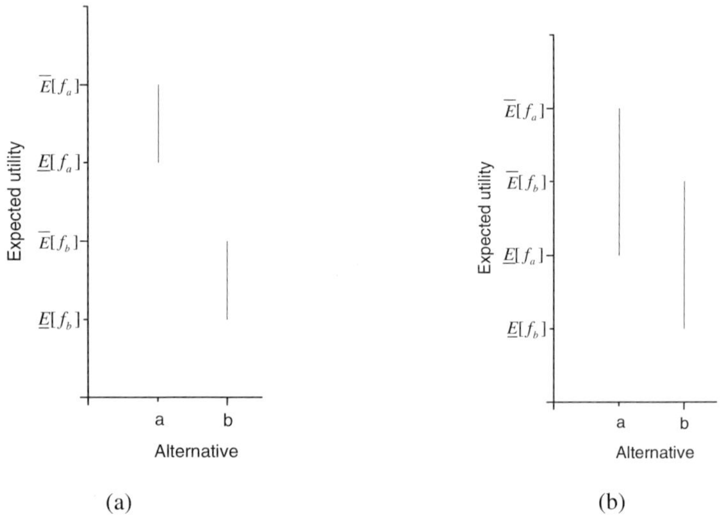

Fig. 1. Intervals of expected utility for two alternatives

In this paper, a conservative Γ-maximin policy is used. We choose the decision alternative a^* that has the highest lower bound $\underline{E}[f]$ on the expected utility. The optimal decision alternative a^* can be expressed as follows under Γ-maximin policy:

$$a^* = \arg\max(\underline{E}[f]) . \tag{13}$$

It should be noted that the approach of this paper is also applicable to other possible policies such as maximality and E-admissibility for managing interval-based decisions. Detailed description of interval-based decision policies can be found in [9].

4 Application to Risk Analysis

In order to increase productivity, a company brought forward a plan of production process improvement. The results from cost-benefit analysis of the plan revealed that the qualification rate of the product must be above 85% to ensure profitability after rebuilding the production process. Let θ denote the qualification rate of the product. Domain experts' assessments for the qualification rate for the new production process were: $\theta_1 = 0.7$, $\theta_2 = 0.8$ and $\theta_3 = 0.9$. The experts also assigned the lower and upper prior probabilities on the values of θ indicated in Table 1.

Table 1. Lower and upper prior probabilities assigned by experts

Parameter θ	Lower prior probability $\underline{P}(\theta)$	Upper prior probability $\overline{P}(\theta)$
0.7	0.1	0.4
0.8	0.3	0.5
0.9	0.4	0.7

To making decision by way of precaution, the decision maker of the company experimented by manufacturing 25 trial products in accordance with the new production process. The results showed that two of them were unqualified. The likelihood function for this experiment is

$$P(x \mid m, \theta) = \binom{m}{x} \theta^x (1-\theta)^{m-x}, \tag{14}$$

where the total number of trial products $m = 25$, the number of qualified products among trial products $x = 23$. We used Eqs.(6-9) to update the experts' prior beliefs to obtain the interval-valued posterior probabilities of the assessed values. Table 2 contains the normalized likelihoods and the lower and upper posterior probabilities of all assessed values of θ.

Table 2. Normalized likelihoods and lower and upper posterior probabilities

Parameter θ	$P(x \mid m, \theta)$	$\underline{P}(\theta \mid x)$	$\overline{P}(\theta \mid x)$
0.7	0.021	0.004	0.017
0.8	0.206	0.117	0.249
0.9	0.773	0.746	0.879

From the perspective of decision making, the assessed values of θ are decision alternatives. In such situation, the utility function $f_{\theta_k}(\theta)$ for alternative θ_k can be expressed as an indicator function:

$$f_{\theta_k}(\theta) = \begin{cases} 1 & if\ \theta = \theta_k \\ 0 & if\ \theta \neq \theta_k \end{cases}. \tag{15}$$

By substituting Eq.(15) into Eqs.(10-12), we obtain $\underline{E}[f_{\theta_k}] = \underline{P}(\theta_k \mid x)$ and $\overline{E}[f_{\theta_k}] = \overline{P}(\theta_k \mid x)$. The resultant intervals of the expected utilities are plotted in Fig. 2, which shows that θ_3 is the optimal decision alternative.

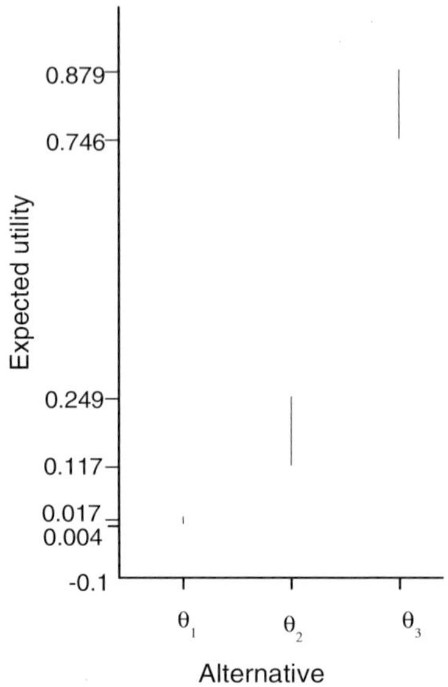

Fig. 2. Expected utilities of decision alternatives

5 Conclusions

Interval-valued probabilities are more appropriate for representing the imprecision in the experts' judgments than precise probabilities used in existing Bayesian decision models. The present model uses interval-valued probabilities to clearly quantify uncertain judgments from domain experts and combines them with the actual sample data to support better decision making.

Acknowledgement

The authors would like to thank the National High Technology Research and Development Program of China for financial support (No: 2007AA040605).

References

1. Berger, J.O.: Statistical Decision Theory and Bayesian Analysis. Springer, New York (1985)
2. Zhukovskaya, O.A., Fainzilberg, L.S.: Interval Generalization of the Bayesian Model of Collective Decision-making in Conflict Situations. Cybern. Syst. Anal. 41, 427–436 (2005)

3. Anandalingam, G., Chatterjee, K., Gangolly, J.S.: Information, Incentives and Decentralized Decision-making in a Bayesian Framework. J. Oper. Res. Soc. 38, 499–508 (1987)
4. Walley, P.: Statistical Reasoning with Imprecise Probabilities. Chapman & Hall, London (1991)
5. Coolen, F.P.A., Newby, M.J.: Bayesian Reliability Analysis with Imprecise Prior Probabilities. Reliab. Eng. Syst. Safety. 43, 75–85 (1994)
6. Cano, A., Moral, S.: Using Probability Trees to Compute Marginals with Imprecise Probabilities. Int. J. Approx. Reason. 29, 1–46 (2002)
7. Cozman, F.G.: Computing Posterior Upper Expectations. Int. J. Approx. Reason. 24, 191–205 (2000)
8. Snow, P.: Improved Posterior Probability Estimates from Prior and Conditional Linear Constraint Systems. IEEE Trans. Syst. Man Cybern. 21, 464–469 (1991)
9. Troffaes, M.C.M.: Decision Making under Uncertainty Using Imprecise Probabilities. Int. J. Approx. Reason 45, 17–29 (2007)

MIMO Probability Density Function Control Using Simple LOG-MLP Neural Networks

Wen Wang[1], You Lun Xiong[1], Hong Wang[2], and Hong Yue[3]

[1] Huazhong University of Science & Technology, China
[2] University of Manchester, UK
[3] Institute of Automation, Chinese Academy of Sciences, China
hughwwang@gmail.com

Abstract. This paper presents a new model for the control of multivariable output probability density function (PDF). Firstly, a Multi-Layer Perceptron (MLP) neural network is adopted to approximate the static output PDF of the MIMO systems. Nonlinear principal component analysis (NLPCA) is then used to reduce the order of the obtained static neural network model and the dynamics of the system is considered based on the lower-order model. After this, an integrated solution is provided to set up the system with lower-order dynamics for the purpose of stochastic distribution control. The controller design is then presented in detail. Finally, a simulation example is given to demonstrate the effectiveness of the method and encouraging results have been obtained.

Keywords: Stochastic systems, combined probability density function, MLP neural networks, nonlinear principal component analysis.

1 Introduction

Research on the control of stochastic systems in the past several decades has been mainly focused on the following four methods: minimum variance control, self-tuning control, stochastic control for systems with Markovian jump parameters and linear quadratic Gaussian (LQG) control etc[1]. In these methods, based on the assumption that the random variables in the system are subjected to Gaussian processes, the mean and variance of the output are the purpose of control. Then control characteristics and rules of the system are studied.

In fact, there is a new control problem in this area called stochastic distribution control, in which the shape of the output probability density function is the aim of control. Typical industrial processes are as follows[2]: i) formation control in paper industry; ii) molecular weight distribution control and particle size distribution control in polymerisation processes; and iii) grey-level distribution control of combustion flame systems.

The method that the PDF is selected as the purpose of control was proposed in 1996[3]. Since then two groups of methods have been developed: i) closed loop probability density function control; and ii) output probability density function control. The first method was developed by Kárný in 1996[3], in which the closed loop probability density function is formed as a joint probability density function between the system

C. Xiong et al. (Eds.): ICIRA 2008, Part II, LNAI 5315, pp. 820–828, 2008.

and a randomized controller that is also characterized by a probability density function. A recursive algorithm has been established for the generation of the probability density function of the controller.

In the second groups of approaches[4][5], the shape control of the output probability density function (not the closed loop probability density function) is addressed. The purpose of controller design is to select a crisp control input so that the shape of the output probability density function of the stochastic system is made as close as possible to a given distribution function. Different from the work of Kárný, in these approaches, the control inputs of stochastic systems are taken as deterministic variables, and the outputs are the measured probability density functions of the system output.

Different forms of B-spline neural networks[6] have been used to approximate the probability density function of the system output[5], which enables the transform from the original PDF control problem into the weights control of B-spline models. These approximations prove to be successful for single-input and single-output stochastic systems because the number of weights necessary for B-spline modelling is within a acceptable range for further controller design[7]. However, for a system with multivariable outputs, using B-spline neural networks to approximate the multiple PDFs would require a large number of basis functions, which results in complicated modelling and controller design. To overcome this limitation, a square root model based on an MLP neural network is proposed by Wang[8] for the modelling of output PDFs of an MIMO system, in which strict constraint is imposed on the weights in the output layer. In this paper, a new modelling method based on an improved MLP neural network and nonlinear principle component analysis (NLPCA) is proposed which can be used for PDF modelling of MIMO stochastic systems and has no constraints on weights at all.

The paper is organized as follows. In section 2, an MLP neural network model is proposed to approximate the combined output probability density function. Nonlinear principal component analysis is then used in section 3 to reduce the order of the static neural network model. At the same time, an integrated solution is provided in section 3 to set up the lower-order dynamic model for the purpose of stochastic distribution control. In section 4, the method for controller design is developed and a detailed control algorithm for the proposed model is given. A simulation example is given to illustrate the presented algorithm in section 5, which is followed by the concluding remarks in section 6.

2 System Description

In this paper, without loss of generality, the following combined probability density function $\gamma(\mathbf{y}, \mathbf{u}(t))$ is considered:

$$P(\mathbf{a} \leqslant \mathbf{v}(t) \leqslant \xi, \mathbf{u}(t)) = \int_{\mathbf{y}\in[a,\xi]^n} \gamma(\mathbf{y}, \mathbf{u}(t)) d\mathbf{y}, \tag{1}$$

where

$$\mathbf{a}=\begin{bmatrix}a_1\\a_2\\\vdots\\a_n\end{bmatrix},\mathbf{v}=\begin{bmatrix}v_1\\v_2\\\vdots\\v_n\end{bmatrix},\xi=\begin{bmatrix}\xi_1\\\xi_2\\\vdots\\\xi_n\end{bmatrix},\mathbf{b}=\begin{bmatrix}b_1\\b_2\\\vdots\\b_n\end{bmatrix}.$$

In (1) **a** and **b** are known, and $a_1=a_2=\cdots=a_n=a$, $b_1=b_2=\cdots=b_n=b$. $\mathbf{v}(t)\in\mathbb{R}^n$ is a uniformly bounded random vector which denotes the output of a dynamic stochastic system, $\mathbf{u}(t)\in\mathbb{R}^m$ is the control input vector which controls the distribution of $\mathbf{v}(t)$, $\mathbf{y}=[y_1,y_2,...,y_n]^T$ is a definite vector whose components are defined on the following product space

$$\Omega=[a_1,b_2]\times[a_2,b_2]\times...\times[a_n,b_n]=[a,b]^n$$

and all the variables in **v** are independent, therefore

$$P(\mathbf{a}\leqslant\mathbf{v}(t)\leqslant\xi,\mathbf{u}(t))=\prod_{i=1}^{n}P(a_i\leqslant v_i(t)\leqslant\xi_i,\mathbf{u}(t))\qquad(2)$$

represents the combined probability of each output component $v_i(t)$ lying inside the known interval $[a_i,\xi_i)$ when $\mathbf{u}(t)$ is applied to the system. In (1), $\xi\in[\mathbf{a},\mathbf{b}]$, and

$$d\mathbf{y}=dy_1dy_2...dy_n.$$

The integration is an n-fold one. The combined probability density function $\gamma(\mathbf{y},\mathbf{u}(t))$ of the output vector $\mathbf{v}(t)$ is controlled by $\mathbf{u}(t)$.

It is well known that an MLP neural network with at least a single hidden layer has an inherent ability to learn and approximate a nonlinear continuous function to an arbitrary precision[6]. Therefore, it has been used widely in modelling complex nonlinear processes. This property of neural networks is referred to as the universal approximation property. Using such a property, the following MLP neural network approximation can be obtained

$$\gamma(\mathbf{y},\mathbf{u}(t)) = poslin\left(\mathbf{W}(\mathbf{u}(t))\,logsig\left(\Theta(\mathbf{u}(t))\,\mathbf{y}+\mathbf{b}(\mathbf{u}(t))\right)+d(\mathbf{u}(t))\right)+e_0\qquad(3)$$

where $\mathbf{W}(\mathbf{u}(t))\in\mathbb{R}^{1\times p}$ and $\Theta(\mathbf{u}(t))\in\mathbb{R}^{p\times n}$ are the weights of the neural network, $\mathbf{b}(\mathbf{u}(t))\in\mathbb{R}^p$ and $d(\mathbf{u}(t))\in R$ are the biases of the neural network, and e_0 is the approximation error. Transfer functions $poslin(\cdot)$ and $logsig(\cdot)$ are defined as follows:

$$poslin(x)=\begin{cases}x, & x\geqslant 0\\0, & x<0\end{cases}\qquad(4)$$

and

$$logsig(x)=\frac{1}{1+e^{-x}},\quad\forall x\in\mathbb{R}\qquad(5)$$

In this paper, a single hidden MLP neural network is applied to approximate the given combined probability density function. Hence the shape of the output PDF can be controlled by adjusting the elements of the set $\{\mathbf{W}(\mathbf{u}(t)),\Theta(\mathbf{u}(t)),\mathbf{b}(\mathbf{u}(t)),d(\mathbf{u}(t))\}$.

To simplify the formulation, it is assumed that $e_0 = 0$. This means that the following expression

$$\gamma(\mathbf{y},\mathbf{u}(t)) \quad = \quad poslin\left(\mathbf{W}\left(\mathbf{u}(t)\right) logsig\left(\Theta\left(\mathbf{u}(t)\right)\mathbf{y}+\mathbf{b}\left(\mathbf{u}(t)\right)\right)+d\left(\mathbf{u}(t)\right)\right) \quad (6)$$

will be used for the approximation of the combined PDF of the system outputs. In (6), the two transfer functions of the MLP neural network, $poslin(\cdot)$ and $logsig(\cdot)$ have positiveness characteristics, therefore in (6)

$$\gamma(\mathbf{y},\mathbf{u}(t)) \geqslant 0, \forall \mathbf{y} \in [a,b]^n \quad (7)$$

can be automatically guaranteed. Since $\gamma(\mathbf{y},\mathbf{u}(t))$ is a combined probability density function, the following equality should be satisfied

$$\int_{\mathbf{y}\in[a,b]^n} \gamma(\mathbf{y},\mathbf{u}(t))d\mathbf{y} = 1, \forall \mathbf{u}(t) \in \mathbb{R}^m \quad (8)$$

By substituting (6) into (8), and considering the characteristics of the functions $poslin(\cdot)$ and $logsig(\cdot)$, the following equation can be obtained

$$\int_{\mathbf{y}\in[a,b]^n} poslin(\eta(\mathbf{y},\mathbf{u}(t))+d(\mathbf{u}(t)))d\mathbf{y} = 1 \quad (9)$$

where

$$\eta(\mathbf{y},\mathbf{u}(t)) = \mathbf{W}(\mathbf{u}(t))logsig(\Theta(\mathbf{u}(t))\mathbf{y}+\mathbf{b}(\mathbf{u}(t)))$$

This leads to when $\eta(\mathbf{y},\mathbf{u})+d(\mathbf{u}) \geqslant 0$

$$d(\mathbf{u}(t)) = \frac{1}{(b-a)^n}\left(1-\int_{\mathbf{y}\in\Omega}\eta(\mathbf{y},\mathbf{u}(t))d\mathbf{y}\right) \quad (10)$$

and when $\eta(\mathbf{y},\mathbf{u})+d(\mathbf{u}) < 0$

$$d(\mathbf{u}(t)) = -\eta(\mathbf{y},\mathbf{u}(t)) \quad (11)$$

To summurize, at each time instant t, the combined PDF $\gamma(\mathbf{y},\mathbf{u}(t))$ can be approximated by (6) subject to the constraint in (10) and (11). This completes the mathematical formulation for the output PDF.

Compared with the MLP based square root PDF model proposed in paper[8], this model takes the advantages of no constraint on weights. For comparison, the MLP based square root PDF model developed in [8] is rewritten as follows,

$$\begin{aligned}\sqrt{\gamma(\mathbf{y},\mathbf{u}(t))} = \mathbf{W}\left(\mathbf{u}(t)\right) tansig\left(\Theta\left(\mathbf{u}(t)\right)\mathbf{y}+\right.\\ \left.\mathbf{b}\left(\mathbf{u}(t)\right)\right)+d\left(\mathbf{u}(t)\right)\end{aligned} \quad (12)$$

$$d(\mathbf{u}) = \frac{-\sigma_1 \pm \sqrt{\sigma_1^2-4\sigma_2(b-a)^n}}{2(b-a)^n} \quad (13)$$

$$\sigma_1 = 2\int_{\mathbf{y}\in\Omega}\zeta(\mathbf{y},\mathbf{u})d\mathbf{y} \quad (14)$$

$$\sigma_2 = \int_{\mathbf{y}\in\Omega}\zeta(\mathbf{y},\mathbf{u})^2d\mathbf{y}-1 \quad (15)$$

$$\sum_{i=1}^{n} |\omega_i(\mathbf{u})| \leqslant \frac{1}{(b-a)^{\frac{n}{2}}} \tag{16}$$

where

$$\zeta(\mathbf{y},\mathbf{u}(t)) = \mathbf{W}(\mathbf{u}(t))tansig(\Theta(\mathbf{u}(t))\mathbf{y}+\mathbf{b}(\mathbf{u}(t))). \tag{17}$$

Equation (16) of the above model is very strict in practice. In fact, the more the number of weights $\omega_i(\mathbf{u})$ is in the left-hand side of (16), the more strict constraint (16) is. And the bigger the interval $[a,b]$ is in the right-hand side of (16), the more strict constraint (16) is too. It can be seen that there is no such a constraint using model (6), therefore the advantages of the model proposed in this paper is shown.

3 Using Low-Order Dynamic Systems to Approximate High-Order Static Systems

In this paper, only the static model is considered. The static model of the output PDFs of the system is described as (6) subject to (10) and (11)

By grouping vectors $\mathbf{W}(\mathbf{u})$, $\Theta(\mathbf{u})$, and $\mathbf{b}(\mathbf{u})$ to a vector $\mathbf{x}$ as follows

$$\mathbf{x} = [\mathbf{W},\Theta^T,\mathbf{b}^T]^T \tag{18}$$

where $\mathbf{x} \in \mathbb{R}^{p(n+2)\times 1}$, the static model between $\mathbf{x}$ and $\mathbf{u}$ can be expressed as follows,

$$\gamma(\mathbf{y},\mathbf{u}) = \mathbf{f}(\mathbf{x},\mathbf{u}) \tag{19}$$

where $\mathbf{f}(\cdot,\cdot)$ is a nonlinear function as specified in (6), (10) and (11).

The static system described in (19) is a high-order static system with input dimension $p(n+2)$. For such a high-order static system, it is difficult to apply control methods to the system directly. Hence the model reduction is implemented in the following.

It is well known that the MLP neural networks is not only an effective approximation method but also provides an effective technique for dimensionality reduction. In this paper, the following MLP neural network as shown in Figure 1 is to be used for model reduction. This kind of MLP neural network is composed of one input layer (layer $\mathbf{x}$), three hidden layers (layer $\mathbf{h}(\mathbf{x})$, $\mathbf{z}$, and $\mathbf{h}(\mathbf{z})$), and one output layer (layer $\underline{\mathbf{x}}$)[9][10]. For convenience, from left to right, each layer is marked by 1, 2, 3, 4, and 5 respectively as shown in Figure 1. The number of neurons in each layer are denoted by l_1, l_2, l_3, l_4, and l_5 respectively. Since nonlinear functions, *sigmoid* transfer function for example, are often used in layers between 1 and 2, and layers between 3 and 4, this kind of MLP neural network is usually called nonlinear principal component analysis.

In Figure 1, next to the input layer 1 is the encoding layer 2. Encoding layer 2 maps data from the high dimension input space to a low dimension space. The transfer functions of the first three layers are as follows,

$$\mathbf{h}(\mathbf{x}) = \mathbf{f}^1(\mathbf{W}^1\mathbf{x}+\mathbf{b}^1) \tag{20}$$

$$\mathbf{z} = \mathbf{f}^2(\mathbf{W}^2\mathbf{h}(\mathbf{x})+\mathbf{b}^2) \tag{21}$$

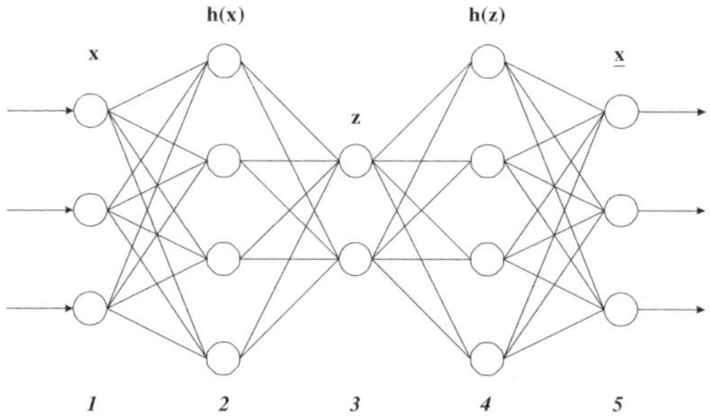

Fig. 1. NN model for NLPCA

where $\mathbf{W}^1 \in \mathbb{R}^{l_2 \times l_1}$, $\mathbf{b}^1 \in \mathbb{R}^{l_2 \times 1}$, $\mathbf{h}(\mathbf{x}) \in \mathbb{R}^{l_2 \times 1}$, $\mathbf{W}^2 \in \mathbb{R}^{l_3 \times l_2}$, $\mathbf{b}^2 \in \mathbb{R}^{l_3 \times 1}$ and $\mathbf{z} \in \mathbb{R}^{l_3 \times 1}$. Combining the above two functions, the following function can be obtained

$$\mathbf{z} = \mathbf{f}^2(\mathbf{W}^2\mathbf{f}^1(\mathbf{W}^1\mathbf{x}+\mathbf{b}^1)+\mathbf{b}^2) \tag{22}$$

Next to the layer 3 is the decoding layer 4 which maps data from the low dimension space to the output high dimension space. The input high dimension space and the output high dimension space are the same in the NLPCA model. In fact, decoding layer is an inverse transformation of encoding layer. The two transfer functions between layer 3 and 4 and between layer 4 and 5 are as follows,

$$\mathbf{h}(\mathbf{z}) = \mathbf{f}^3(\mathbf{W}^3\mathbf{z}+\mathbf{b}^3) \tag{23}$$

$$\underline{\mathbf{x}} = \mathbf{f}^4(\mathbf{W}^4\mathbf{h}(\mathbf{z})+\mathbf{b}^4) \tag{24}$$

where $\mathbf{W}^3 \in \mathbb{R}^{l_4 \times l_3}$, $\mathbf{b}^3 \in \mathbb{R}^{l_4 \times 1}$, $\mathbf{h}(\mathbf{z}) \in \mathbb{R}^{l_4 \times 1}$,$\mathbf{W}^4 \in \mathbb{R}^{l_5 \times l_4}$, $\mathbf{b}^4 \in \mathbb{R}^{l_5 \times 1}$ and $\underline{\mathbf{x}} \in \mathbb{R}^{l_5 \times 1}$. By substituting (23) into (24), the following function can be obtained,

$$\underline{\mathbf{x}} = \mathbf{f}^4\left(\mathbf{W}^4\mathbf{f}^3\left(\mathbf{W}^3\mathbf{z}+\mathbf{b}^3\right)+\mathbf{b}^4\right. \tag{25}$$

In (22) and (25), $\mathbf{f}^2(\cdot) = \mathbf{f}^4(\cdot) = \mathbf{x}$, $\mathbf{f}^1(\cdot) = \mathbf{f}^3(\cdot) = (e^{\mathbf{x}} - e^{-\mathbf{x}})/(e^{\mathbf{x}} + e^{-\mathbf{x}})$, and $l_1 = l_5 > l_3$, $l_2 = l_4 > l_3$.

In this NLPCA model, the values of the output neurons should be trained as closely as possible to that of the inputs. This means the optimal values of $\mathbf{W}^1$, $\mathbf{W}^2$, $\mathbf{W}^3$, $\mathbf{W}^4$, $\mathbf{b}^1$, $\mathbf{b}^2$, $\mathbf{b}^3$ and $\mathbf{b}^4$ should be found such that the cost function

$$J = E\left(\|\mathbf{x} - \underline{\mathbf{x}}\|^2\right) \tag{26}$$

is minimized, where $E(\cdot)$ means expectation.

Applying the above NLPCA method to the high-order system expressed by (6), a low-order system can be obtained. The relationship between the state vector $\mathbf{z}$ and the input vector $\mathbf{u}$ can be expressed as the following nonlinear differential equation

$$\dot{\mathbf{z}} = \mathbf{g}(\mathbf{z}, \mathbf{u}) \tag{27}$$

where $\mathbf{g}(\cdot,\cdot)$ is a nonlinear function.

In order to simplify the controller design, a linearization model

$$\mathbf{z}_{k+1} = \mathbf{A}\mathbf{z}_k + \mathbf{B}\mathbf{u}_k \tag{28}$$

can be used to approximate the dynamic model (27), where $A \in \mathbb{R}^{m\times m}$ and $B \in \mathbb{R}^{m\times n}$. In practice, $\mathbf{A}$ and $\mathbf{B}$ in (28) can be obtained via multi-variables linear regression method. For a given PDF,

- Changing the input vector $\mathbf{u}$ in its definition area from lower limit to upper limit with a fixed step, a series of PDFs can be obtained.
- Using the model described in section 2, training the neural networks which approximates the PDF obtained from the above step, one gets $\mathbf{x}_k(k = 1,\cdots,n)$ expressed in (18).
- Applying NLPCA model, $\mathbf{x}_k(k = 1,\cdots,n)$ which are in the high dimension space can be mapped to the low dimension space as $\mathbf{z}_k(k = 1,\cdots,n)$.
- After getting a series of $\mathbf{z}_k$, apply multivariable linear regression method to estimate $\mathbf{A}$ and $\mathbf{B}$.

This means that the high-order original static system can be approximated by a low-order dynamic system. For the low-order system expressed by (28), conventional controller design method can be applied.

Applying the decoding transformation given by (25) to the low-order state vector $\mathbf{z}$ obtained from (28), $p(n+2)$ independent weights and biases can be obtained. That is to say, the weights such as $\mathbf{W}(\mathbf{u})$ and $\Theta(\mathbf{u})$ and biases such as $\mathbf{b}(\mathbf{u})$ used to express the output PDF can be obtained. With these weights and biases, $d(\mathbf{u})$ can be calculated via (10) or (11). Thus, the model using low-order dynamic system to approximate the high-order static system can be obtained.

The above modelling procedures can be rewritten in a compact form as

$$\begin{cases} \mathbf{z} = \mathbf{f}^2(\mathbf{W}^2\mathbf{f}^1(\mathbf{W}^1\mathbf{x}+\mathbf{b}^1)+\mathbf{b}^2) \\ \mathbf{z}_{k+1} = \mathbf{A}\mathbf{z}_k + \mathbf{B}\mathbf{u}_k \\ \underline{\mathbf{x}} = \mathbf{f}^4\left(\mathbf{W}^4\mathbf{f}^3\left(\mathbf{W}^3\mathbf{z}+\mathbf{b}^3\right)+\mathbf{b}^4\right) \\ [\mathbf{W},\Theta^T,\mathbf{b}^T]^T = \underline{\mathbf{x}} \\ \gamma(\mathbf{y},\mathbf{u}) = \mathbf{W}(\mathbf{u})\mathbf{logsig}(\Theta(\mathbf{u})\mathbf{y}+\mathbf{b}(\mathbf{u}))+d(\mathbf{u}) \\ d(\mathbf{u}) = \left(1-\int_{\mathbf{y}\in[a,b]^n}\eta(\mathbf{y},\mathbf{u})\,d\mathbf{y}\right)\Big/(b-a)^n \\ \qquad\qquad\qquad\qquad : \ \eta(\mathbf{y},\mathbf{u})+d(\mathbf{u}) \geqslant 0 \\ d(\mathbf{u}) = -\eta(\mathbf{y},\mathbf{u}) \qquad : \ \eta(\mathbf{y},\mathbf{u})+d(\mathbf{u}) < 0 \\ \eta(\mathbf{y},\mathbf{u}) = \mathbf{W}(\mathbf{u})logsig(\Theta(\mathbf{u})\mathbf{y}+\mathbf{b}(\mathbf{u})) \end{cases} \tag{29}$$

To summarize, using low-order dynamic systems to approximate high-order static systems includes the following four steps,

- Firstly, apply (22) to the obtained high-order static system, a low-order dynamic system can be obtained.

– Secondly, for the obtained low-order system, it can be expressed in the standard state space function as (28). Applying traditional controller design method to the low-order system, it is not difficult to get the state vector $\mathbf{z}$ which can track target.
– Thirdly, map the state vector $\mathbf{z}$ in low-order space back into the high-order model by using (25), the weights and biases used to express the output PDF can be obtained ((18), (10) and (11)).
– The high order system to express the output PDF can be obtained via (6).

4 Controller Design for the Low-Order Dynamic System

The purpose of controller design is to choose a control input $\mathbf{u}(t)$ such that the actual combined probability density function of the system output is made as close as possible to a pre-specified continuous density function $\gamma(\mathbf{y})$, which is independent of $\mathbf{u}(t)$ and defined on $[a,b]^n$.

Applying NLPCA to reduce the system order, a low-order system with the same dimensions of input and output, an l-inputs and l-outputs system for example, can be obtained. The dimensions of matrices $\mathbf{A}$, and $\mathbf{B}$ will be reduced from $p(n+2)\times p(n+2)$, and $p(n+2)\times m$ to $l\times l$, and $l\times l$ respectively. The PDF control problem is then transformed into the tracking of the state $\mathbf{z}_k$ to its targeting value. For the low-order dynamic system, conventional state feedback law can be used. Let

$$\mathbf{u}_k = -\mathbf{K}\mathbf{z}_k + \mathbf{L}\mathbf{z}_r \tag{30}$$

where $\mathbf{z}_r$, which corresponds to the target combined PDF in the high-order system expressed by (6), is the target value for the state $\mathbf{z}_k$ and can be obtained by the same modelling procedures when the target PDF is given; $\mathbf{K}$ and $\mathbf{L}$ are two matrices need be designed in this section. $\mathbf{K}$ can be designed by pole-assignment method. As for $\mathbf{L}$, it should be solved from (28). By substituting (30) into (28), the following closed loop formulation can be obtained

$$\mathbf{z}_{k+1} = (\mathbf{A}-\mathbf{B}\mathbf{K})\mathbf{z}_k + \mathbf{B}\mathbf{L}\mathbf{z}_r \tag{31}$$

whose solution is expressed as

$$\mathbf{z}_k = \mathbf{C}^k\mathbf{z}_0 + \sum_{i=1}^{k}\mathbf{C}^{i-1}\mathbf{D}\mathbf{z}_r \tag{32}$$

where $\mathbf{C}=\mathbf{A}-\mathbf{B}\mathbf{K}$, and $\mathbf{D}=\mathbf{B}\mathbf{L}$.

For $\|\mathbf{C}\|_2 < 1$, when k tends to infinity, the first item of the right-hand side of (32) is equal to 0. $\mathbf{z}_k$, which is $\mathbf{z}_\infty$ now, should track the given input vector $\mathbf{z}_r$. That means $\mathbf{z}_\infty = \mathbf{z}_r$. Then the following expression is obtained

$$\mathbf{z}_r = (\mathbf{I}-\mathbf{C})^{-1}\mathbf{D}\mathbf{z}_r$$

where $\mathbf{I}$ is the identity matrix. This leads to

$$\mathbf{L} = \mathbf{B}^{-1}(\mathbf{I}-\mathbf{A}+\mathbf{B}\mathbf{K}) \tag{33}$$

5 Conclusions

In this paper, an MLP neural network model for MIMO stochastic PDF control is presented. The model takes advantages of no constraint on weights and biases, which makes it more easy to be used in practice. For high-order static systems the NLPCA model reduction method is used to reduce the model order. It enables transform from the high-order static systems into the low-order dynamic systems. Therefore, the controller design is mostly simplified.

Acknowledgements

The authors would like to thank the financial support from the National Fundamental Research Program of China under Grants 2007CB714005 and 2005CB724100.

References

1. Aström, K.J.: Introduction to stochastic control theory. Academic Press, New York (1970)
2. Yue, H., Wang, H.: Recent developments in stochastic distribution control: a review. Journal of Measurement and Control 36(7), 209–215 (2003)
3. Kárný, M.: Towards fully probabilistic control design. Automatica 32(12), 1719–1722 (1996)
4. Wang, H.: Bounded dynamic stochastic distributions: modelling and control. Springer, London (2000)
5. Wang, H., Zhang, J.H.: Bounded stochastic distribution control for pseudo ARMAX systems. IEEE Trans. on Automatic control 46(3), 486–490 (2001)
6. Girosi, F., Poggio, T.: Networks and the best approximation property Biol. Cybern. 63, 169–176 (1990)
7. Wang, H.: Robust control of the output probability density functions for multivariable stochastic systems with guaranteed stability. IEEE Trans. on Automatic Control 44(11), 2103–2107 (1999)
8. Wang, H.: Multivariable output probability density function control for non-Gaussian stochastic systems using simple MLP neural networks. In: Proc. IFAC Int. Conf. on Intelligent Control Systems and Signal Processing Algarve, Portugal (2003)
9. Kramer, M.A.: Nonlinear principal component analysis using autoassociative neural networks. AIChE Journal 37(2), 233–243 (1991)
10. William, W.H.: Nonlinear principal component analysis by neural networks. Tellus 53A, 599–615 (2001)

Research on Intelligent Manufacturing System Based on Multi-Agent

Qinglin Guo[1,2] and Ming Zhang[2]

[1] School of Computer Science and Technology, North China Electric Power University, Beijing 102206, China
[2] Department of Computer Science and Technology, Peking University, Beijing 100871, China
{qlguo,mz88}@pku.edu.cn

Abstract. Agent and Multi-Agent system is one of the main research directions in distributed artificial intelligence. It has been considered that the Agent technology is an important method to build the model of distributed industrial system, the most natural way to design and implement the distributed Intelligent Manufacturing environment, and one of the significant technologies to construct the manufacturing system of next generation. The manufacturing system based on Agent is the specific application of the theory and method of multi-Agent system in manufacturing domain. On the basis of briefly summarizing the technology of Agent and Multi-Agent system, the architecture of Intelligent Manufacturing System based on Multi-Agent is put forward, among which, agent represents the basic processing entity. The scheduling optimization algorithm of Intelligent Manufacturing is provided, which is feasible proved by the result of stimulation experiment. Compared with the traditional artificial scheduling, it has distinct advantages. Finally, the model of communication and negotiation between Agents in the Intelligent Manufacturing System is studied, which utilizes the features of Agent such as autonomy, social interaction, response capability, preliminary capability, etc so that Intelligent Manufacturing System could make distributed decisions. The cooperation of system is completed by communication and negotiation. During the process of interaction, Agent is endowed with a role to meet the demand of flexibility of building models in the complicated process of Intelligent Manufacturing, as well as to construct an extended frame for reusable components.

Keywords: Multi-Agent; Petri net; Intelligent Manufacturing; scheduling optimization; model.

1 Introduction

With the fast development of information technology and intensified economic globalization trend, manufacturing business has to face the increasingly fierce market competition. Shorter products life cycles, faster updating speeds, and individual and diversified demands of customers for products, all of which make the producing modes and manufacturing organization methods of companies gradually turn from product-oriented to customers, demands and services oriented. In order to succeed in

C. Xiong et al. (Eds.): ICIRA 2008, Part II, LNAI 5315, pp. 829–838, 2008.

the competition, companies are in urgent need of distributed net cooperation producing and manufacturing system complete with good flexibility, quick response and fault tolerant ability. The manufacturing system shall fast adapt to the turn of the market in the situation of possessing certain cost benefit, construct manufacturing process quickly and economically based on different products demands, and carry out self adaptive, self organizing, self studying, liberalization and self maintaining for the whole manufacturing process dynamically. The research results of distributed artificial intelligence domain indicate that, the Intelligent Manufacturing System built with Agent technology is the most potential development direction.

Intelligent Manufacturing System (IMS) shall be considered as a complicated large system organically integrating various intelligent subsystems that complete the distributed solution procedure on the basis of exchanging large quantities of materials, energies and information [1]. The Multi-Agent system theory in distributed artificial intelligence (DAI) provides feasible technical support for modeling and realization of Intelligent Manufacturing System, which becomes one of the research hot points in manufacturing domain. Manufacturing process is a typical Multi-Agent questions solution process, and every department (or segment) in manufacturing system is equal to an Agent in the process. Every sub-mission or unit equipment in manufacturing system could be acted and realized by single Agent or well-organized Agent group, and complete the manufacturing tasks together through their interaction and mutual coordination and cooperation. The manufacturing system shall be stimulated as the Multi-Agent system, which makes the system easier to design, reduces the complexity of the system, intensifies the recombination, expandability and reliability of the system, and improves the flexibility, adaptability and dexterity of the system.

The Intelligent Manufacturing System model based on Agent presented in the thesis adopts Agent as the basic processing entity. Agent is mainly related with transition, the feature of which is described by Petri net. In the end, a method based on dialogue mode is put forward to design the communication between Agents, which is checked by coloring Petri net.

2 Agent and Multi-Agent System

So far, there is no unified definition on Agent [2]. We consider that Agent is the object which could finish the given task independently without people's interference. Now the more common view is that Agent should possess three important features, i.e. autonomy, adaptability and coordination. Autonomy means that the agent shall complete the related tasks actively without external interference (human or other software); adaptability refers to that Agent has the abilities of perceiving and adapting to the external environment and self studying. Coordination is an important feature of Multi-Agent system, in which Agents coordinate and complete a task together. Therefore, the capability of Multi-Agent system is not determined by that of single Agent, but by the intelligence showed by mutual coordination between Agents [3]. Agent possesses the basic attributes such as object, knowledge, label, etc, which is composed of functional units like communication module, business processing module, inference module, study module, information transmission, etc. Agent has the feature of Object-Oriented technology, e.g. inheritance, packaging, information transfer, etc, so the Object-Oriented technology could be used to realize the function of Agent [4].

The specific composition structure of Agent is as follows:

(1) Label: a property feature that one Agent differentiates from others in Multi-Agent system, including name, address of Agent;

(2) Object: Agent consistently operates the pursued specific objects that determine the responsibility and obligation of Agent ;

(3) Knowledge: it includes facts and rules stored in the knowledge base of Agent

(4) Communication module: it is responsible for the communication, information receiving and sending and could transfer tasks, operate results and realize knowledge share.

(5) Inference module: it infers and makes decision based on the object, knowledge, ability and latest information of Agent, and affects on information processing and business procession modules. The decisions it makes must be helpful for the realization of the objects.

(6) Business processing module: processes business. As the main body of Agent realizing objects, it is composed by business processing method.

(7) Study module: summarizes the experiences from the operating process of Agent, increases new knowledge for knowledge base, and improves the capability of adapting to the changeable environment.

Multi-Agent system is composed of a group of Agents distributed in logical or physical positions [5]. The Agents share resources through network, and compose an organized group to complete common task. It is generally considered that Multi-Agent system is especially suitable for the applications based on space, time or function to disintegrate and divide. Adopting Multi-Agent system in these applications will bring the following advantages: (1) the operating speed will be faster due to the parallelization of processing; (2) the demand for communication band width is low because the processing for information is carried out near information source; (3) the error of one Agent will not affect the operation of the whole system, so the system has higher reliability; (4) since the close connection of sense, processing and action, the system has higher response speed.

3 The Structure of Intelligent Manufacturing

Manufacturing industry has experienced all the changes, i.e. manual operation, mechanization, automatization, informatization, integration and intelligence. Industrialization realizes the liberation of human manual labor, informatization further realizes the liberation of human mental work, and intelligent manufacturing has been developed since the recent years. Intelligent Manufacturing, IM for short, is a man-machine integrated intelligent system composed by intelligent machine and human experts, which can carry out intelligent activities such as analysis, inference, judgment, conception and decision-making during the process of manufacturing. The cooperation between human and intelligent machine will expand, extend and partially replace the mental work of human experts during the process of manufacturing [6]. At the same time, it will collect, store, perfect, share, inherit and develop the manufacturing intelligence of human experts [7].

The main types of Intelligent Manufacturing System are: Intelligent Manufacturing System that takes improving manufacturing system intelligence as the object and intelligent robot and Agent as the tool; Intelligent Manufacturing System that integrates the modeling, processing, measuring and operating of corporations through Internet; biological Intelligent Manufacturing System that adopts solution procedure for biological problems. At present, the distributed network IMS model based on Agent is mainly adopted [8], the architecture of which is illustrated in Figure 1. On the one hand, each manufacturing unit is endowed autonomy by Agent to become the entity with perfect functions and autonomy independence; on the other hand, the system is endowed with self organization capacity through the coordination and cooperation between Agents.

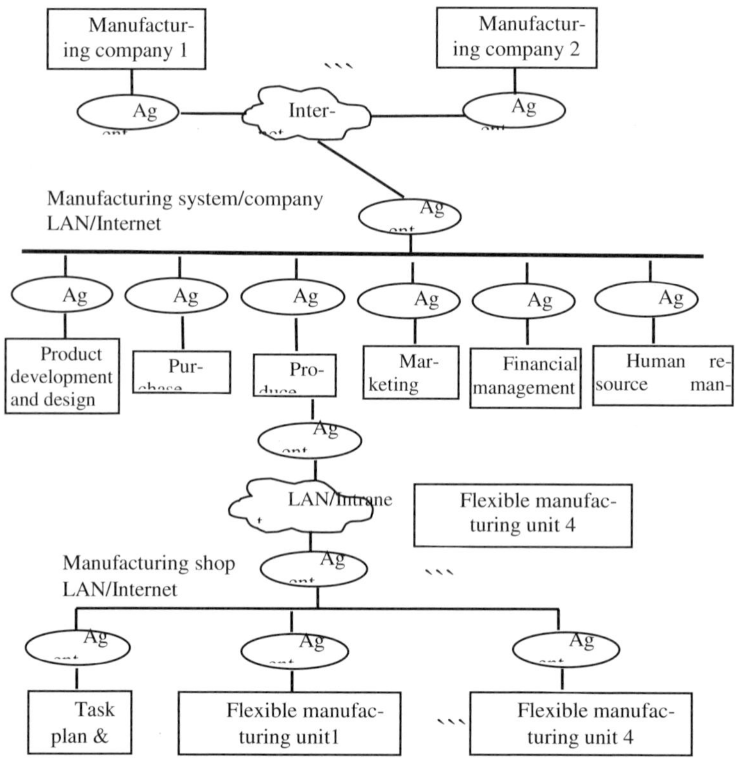

Fig. 1. Network model block graph

When Intelligent Manufacturing System integrates the intelligent machine and human on production site, it shall use all knowledge activities, and flexibly centralizes all activities such as order, design, produce and sales of the company through knowledge base, database, computers and communication network in order to improve the overall efficiency. View from the whole manufacturing process, the segments of order, design, produce and sales are functional independent from each other, and their solution procedures are quite different. The functional subsystems of each segment independently complete manufacturing sub-tasks as well as coordinate with each other. Therefore, inside the manufacturing company, the whole manufacturing process from design to sale is a typical solution procedure for Multi-Agent questions. In order to improve the adaptability of manufacturing system to the state changes from inside to outside, the general structure design of Intelligent Manufacturing System shall obey the open principles, which are showed as: ① openness of the task: the task could be input and processed at any time; ②openness of the system: the system shall hold the changes from interior system (e.g. Malfunction), and accept the interference from outside (e.g. the configuration that changes physical equipments); ③openness of solution procedure: the solution procedure shall accept the changes of information and knowledge.

In order to realize the openness of the above three aspects, distributed structure is resorted to in the Intelligent Manufacturing System, which endows every component entity and subsystem of the system with larger autonomy to form the intelligent autonomous agent. Intelligent autonomous agent is connected with computer communication network by means of intelligent nodes, which are equal in logic (no direction control relations between each other), dispersive in physic and independent in function. The nodes have the loosely coupled relations [9], which contact each other by transferring messages. Based on the common communication language, they coordinate and cooperate to complete the manufacturing tasks.

4 Scheduling Optimization of Intelligent Manufacturing

The scheduling model of the research is: production workshop needs to process multiple components, each of which has many processing methods; a production plan shall be made not only to decide a processing method for each component, but also to ensure the shortest production cycle of the whole shop. During the modeling process, in order to meet the scheduling objects, some complements are made on the basis of the standard hypothesis of the previous scheduling:

(1) Processing in advance is not allowed for any components.

(2) All components could be processed at zero time [10].

(3) Every procedure has specified working contents and processing time.

(4) When a component is finished processing in one machine tool, it will be sent to next machine tool in the processing method immediately. The time for delivery shall be omitted.

(5) The mechanical processing auxiliary time for different procedures is different, which is included in mechanical processing time.

(6) The delay time of workers and robots shall be neglected [11].

Scheduling object:

$$\text{Minimize } Z$$

Constraint condition:

The last procedure in h processing method of component i,

$$T_{ihjk} - H(1 - X_{ih}) \le Z \tag{1}$$

Not the last procedure in h processing method of component i,

$$T_{ihjk} - T_{ih(j-1)g} + H(1 - X_{ih}) \ge t_{ihjk} \; \forall i, j, k, h, g, \quad j \ne 1 \tag{2}$$

The first procedure in h processing method of component i (j=1),

$$T_{ihjk} + H(1 - X_{ih}) \ge t_{ihjk} \qquad \forall i, j, k, h, \tag{3}$$

There are procedures in h processing method of component i and q processing method of component p processed on the machine tool equipment k,

$$T_{ihjk} - T_{pqjk} + HY_{ihjpqsk} + H(1 - X_{ih}) + H(1 - X_{pq}) \ge t_{ihjk} \tag{4}$$

$$T_{pqsk} - T_{ihjk} + H(1 - Y_{ihjpqsk}) + H(1 - X_{ih}) + H(1 - X_{pq}) \ge t_{pqsk} \tag{5}$$

For all components, only one processing method is chosen,

$$\sum_h x_{ih} = 1 \tag{6}$$

Any processing method of component i and component p need to use machine tool equipment k,

$$-x_{ih} + \sum_q Y_{ihjpqsk} \le 0 \tag{7}$$

$$-x_{pq} + \sum_h Y_{ihjpqsk} \le 0 \tag{8}$$

Any procedure in h processing method of component i,

$$T_{ihjk} \ge 0 \tag{9}$$

There are procedures in h processing method of component i and q processing method of component p processed by worker w,

$$T_{ihjk} - T_{pqjk} + HY_{ihjpqsk} + H(1 - X_{ih}) + H(1 - X_{pq}) \ge t_{ihjk} \tag{10}$$

$$T_{pqsk} - T_{ihjk} + H(1 - Y_{ihjpqsk}) + H(1 - X_{ih}) + H(1 - X_{pq}) \ge t_{pqsk} \tag{11}$$

me robot in different working time slice should meet,

$$[b_k, b_{k+i}] \cap [b_e, b_{e+i}] = \Phi \tag{12}$$

If the h processing method of component i is chosen under the constraint conditions (formula 1 and formula 6), the objective equation in formula (1) will be used to confine the completion time of the last procedure in the processing method; constraint condition (formula 6) ensures that only one processing method of each component is selected; constraint conditions (formula 2 and formula 3) make sure that for one designated component, the procedure j-1 processed on machine tool g is prior to the next procedure j processed on machine tool k, meanwhile, it explains the working sequence of robots; constraint conditions (formula 4 and formula 5) guarantee that two different procedures cannot be processed on the same machine tool at the same time, and any machine tool cannot process more than one procedures at any time; constraint condition (formula 4) indicates that the s procedure in q processing method of component p is processed prior to the j procedure in h processing method of component i on the machine tool k, and constraint condition (formula 5) shows the opposite processing sequence; in the meantime, when only one processing method of each component is chosen, this precedence is ensured by constraint conditions (formula 7 and formula 8). Constraint conditions (formula 10 and formula 11) guarantee that two different procedures cannot be processed by one worker at the same time and any worker cannot process more than one procedure at any time; constraint condition (formula 12) ensures that the working time of any one robot cannot be intersected [12].

The scheduling algorithm is showed as follow:

Step 1: Calculate the ideal start time of processing for all procedures
Suppose a_k=0, P_w=0, R_r=(0,0), r_n=0
$R_u = L_{i(j-1)} + r_{i(j-1)} + t_{i(j-1)k} + U_{i(j-1)}$ (i=1, 2,…,n and j=2,…,J_i)
Step 2: If there are non-scheduling procedures in procedure set, the non-scheduling procedure ranked the first shall be taken out from the set, and then turn to step 3
If not, suppose makespan = max (F_i) (i = 1,2,…,n)
Step 3: $L(k,1) = \max\{a_h, P_{w,} r_{ij}\}$
$L(k,2) = L(k,1) + L_{ij}$
If ($L(k,1)$, $L(k,2)$)$\in R_R$, adjust $L(k,1)$ and $L(k,2)$
$U(k,1) = L(k,2) + t_{ijk}$
$U(k,2) = U(k,1) + U_{ij}$
If ($U(k,1)$, $U(k,2)$) $\in R_R$, adjust $U(k,1)$ and $U(k,2)$
$f_{ijk} = U(k,2)$
Step 4: Suppose $C_{ij} = \min(f_{ijk})$
If $j = J_i$, $F_i = C_{ij}$
If not, calculate $r_{i(j+h)} = r_{i(j+h)} + (C_{ij} - r_{i(j+1)})$, ($h$ = 1,2,…,(J_i - j))
Step 5: Suppose $a_k = E_{ij}$, $P_w = C_{ij}$
Combine ($L(k,1)$, $L(k,2)$) and ($U(k,1)$, $U(k,2)$) into corresponding set R_r
Step 6: Check if there are non-scheduling procedures in set S; if there is, turn to step 2.
If not, makespan = max (F_i)

In each generation, the algorithm distributes machine tools and workers to every procedure, and ensures no interference with the working time of robots.

5 Experimental Results and Analysis

We conduct experiment on our scheduling optimization algorithm of Intelligent Manufacturing. Figure 2 is the convergence process of scheduling algorithm in multi-resources workshop; figure 3 is tasks distribution of workers.

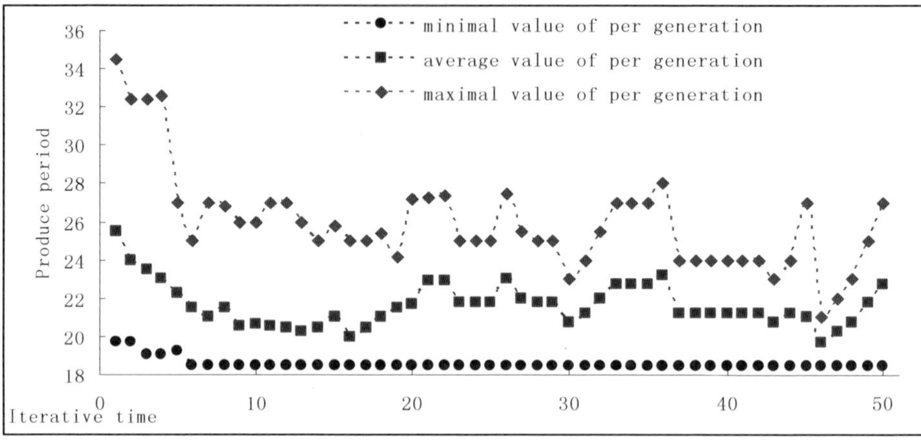

Fig. 2. Convergence process of scheduling algorithm in multi-resources shop

Figure 2 illustrates the convergence process of the algorithm. We can see that, the minimum value of function is decreasing with the evolution of group, and finally, the speed of convergence to extreme value is fast. The average value of objective function in the group is also decreasing with the evolution of group, and tends to the minimum value of the objective function.

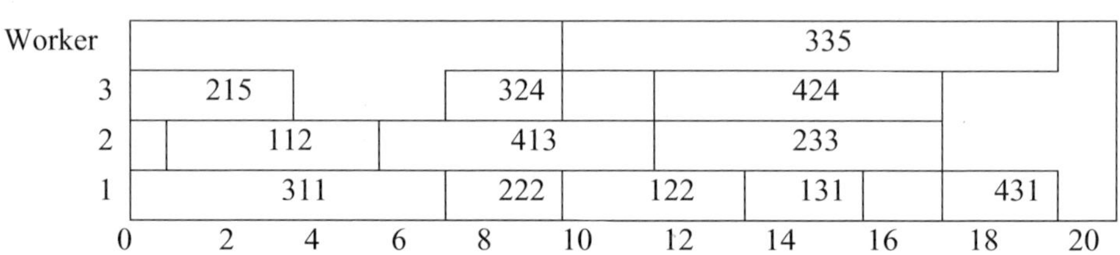

Fig. 3. Tasks distribution of workers

Figure 3 illustrates the corresponding relation among components, workers and machine tools. The abscissa in the figure shows the time of components processing, while ordinate indicates workers. A square with three characters stands for one procedure: the first character is the number of component, the second is the number of procedure, and the third is the number of machine tool. For example, worker 3 with the first work "215" means he processes the first procedure of component 2 on the fifth machine tool, and the man-hour shall be obtained from abscissa. The time from processing start to finish shall be checked from abscissa, in the same way, the final completion time of each component shall be obtained. From this figure, it is easy to count workload of each worker.

6 Conclusion

The thesis makes thorough research on Intelligent Manufacturing System. Considering the features of manufacturing system, we conclude the definition and structure of Agent and discuss the applications of Agent technology in manufacturing system. On the basis of multi-technique scheduling problem, we study the constraint of machine tools, workers and robots in production workshop scheduling problem for the first time. The thesis also studies the production workshop scheduling problem and gives the algorithm and results of scheduling. The stimulation result proves the algorithm is feasible. Compared with traditional artificial scheduling, it has distinct advantages.

In the thesis, the manufacturing system modeling and processing model based on Agent have the following features: compared with general Petri net model, the processing entity Agent has the features of autonomy, response capacity and activity. The cooperation is completed through the interaction and negotiation between Agents, thus the consistency of functions could be guaranteed. Meanwhile, the distributed feature of processing entity Agent can meet the geographic distribution in supply chain of virtual companies. In addition, because of the close connection with Petri net, it can stimulate and evaluate the performance of system, as well as carry out consistency inspection on associated rule in knowledge base.

The future focal point of the research should be on this basis and in accordance with the purpose of the research to reasonably divide the granularity of Agent in manufacturing system, establish the deep relation between Agents, and realize high-precision coordinating work of Multi-Agent. In the course of research, Internet and Intranet technology shall be fully used, especially the inherent distributed computing environment such as Web, distributed object technology, XML, etc. The combination of Agent technology and computer network is the fundamental way to realize network Intelligent Manufacturing and global manufacturing.

Acknowledgments

We would like to acknowledge the support from the Foundation of Post-Doctor in China, the National Natural Science Foundation of China (90412010, 60573166), the Specialized Research Fund for the Doctoral Program of Higher Education （SRFDP No. 20070001073） , the HP University Collaborative Foundation of China (HLCFY08-001) , the National High Technology Research and Development Program (863 Program in china: 2004AA1Z2450).

References

1. He, Y.L., He, W.P., Yang, H.C.: Towards an Agent and Knowledge Enacted Dynamic Workflow Management System for Intelligent Manufacturing Grid. In: Luo, Y. (ed.) CDVE 2006. LNCS, vol. 4101, pp. 75–82. Springer, Heidelberg (2006)
2. Martinez, J.L., Colombo, A.W.: Engineering framework for agent-based manufacturing control. Int. J. Engineering Applications of Artificial Intelligence 19, 625–640 (2006)
3. Ilariam, B., Giuseppe, C., Giuseppe, S.: Development of a Multi-Agent Model for Production Scheduling in Innovative Flexible Manufacturing System. In: Manufacturing Systems and Technologies for the New Frontier, The 41st CIRP Conference on Manufacturing Systems, pp. 279–283 (2008)
4. Hou, J.L., Sun, M.T., Chuo, H.C.: An Intelligent Knowledge Management Model for Construction and Reuse of Automobile Manufacturing Intellectual Properties. The International Journal of Advanced Manufacturing Technology 26(1), 99–102 (2005)
5. Paul, A., Buhler, J.: Towards adaptive workflow enactment using multi agent systems. Int. J. Information technology and management 6, 61–87 (2005)
6. Raffaello, L.: Advanced human–machine system for intelligent manufacturing. Journal of Intelligent Manufacturing 17(6), 653–666 (2006)
7. Shaw, C.: Preliminary design and manufacturing planning integration using web-based intelligent agents. Journal of Intelligent Manufacturing 16(4), 423–437 (2005)
8. Yang, P., Liao, N.B.: A mixed isomorphism approach for kinematic structure enumeration graphs based on intelligent design and manufacturing. The International Journal of Advanced Manufacturing Technology 31(9), 841–845 (2007)
9. Indira, M.: Fuzzy-based methodology for multi-objective scheduling in a robot-centered flexible manufacturing cell. Journal of Intelligent Manufacturing 19(2), 93–97 (2008)
10. Han, Y., Xin, B., Dan, C.: Workflow management and resource discovery for an intelligent grid. Int. J. Parallel computing 31(7), 797–811 (2005)
11. Wei, T.: Integration of Process Planning and scheduling–a review. Journal of Intelligent Manufacturing 11, 51–63 (2000)
12. Lee, Y.G., Malone, M.F.: Batch Process schedule Optimization under Parameter volatility. International Journal of Production Research 4, 603–623 (2001)

Influence of Contact Forces on Stable Gripping for Large-Scale Heavy Manipulator

Qunming Li, Dan Gao, and Hua Deng

College of Mechanical and Electrical Engineering
Central South University, Changsha, China
liqm@mail.csu.edu.cn

Abstract. Stably and safely gripping work-piece during the forging process is very important for large-scale heavy manipulators. Among various factors that influence stably gripping, the contact status between grippers and work-piece plays a significant role. In order to achieve stable gripping, a three-dimension gripping-contact model based on the assumption of point contact with friction is presented to calculate closed-form solutions of contact forces. Moreover, force equilibrium conditions are analyzed qualitatively. Relations between joint space, contact forces space and work piece space are derived by exponential map in terms of spatial manipulator Jacobian matrix and griping matrix. Adams' simulation results based on a large-scale heavy forging manipulator is used to determine the position and change of different contact points while moving. The influence of contact forces on stable gripping is analyzed by academic calculation and computer simulation. The work is helpful for the optimal design of the grippers and the stable gripping analysis for large-scale heavy manipulators.

Keywords: Large-scale heavy manipulator, gripper, contact force, stabile gripping.

1 Introduction

A forging manipulator plays a very important role in achieving mechanization and automation of forging [1]. Stably and safely gripping work-piece during the forging process is very important to large-scale heavy manipulators. Whether the gripper of a forging manipulator can achieve stable gripping depends mainly on the position and constraint pattern of contact points. Thus the analysis of contact status between the gripper and work piece is essential for the design of a large-scale heavy forging manipulator.

Contact is a complex phenomenon, which occurs when two or more bodies undergo a collision. Contact dynamics is an active research area in robotics [2-5]. The gripping in large-scale heavy manipulators is achieved by two four-link mechanisms with only one active driver. The contact status is more complex than that of dexterous robotic hands because of the varying of the positions and the number of the contact points for large-scale heavy grippers. In this paper, the contact problem is simplified to solve the force/torque closure and form closure by the assumption of

C. Xiong et al. (Eds.): ICIRA 2008, Part II, LNAI 5315, pp. 839–847, 2008.

point contact with friction, and the three-dimension gripping-contact model is established based on space decomposition method[6], which can be used to calculate closed-form solutions of contact forces and force equilibrium conditions. With the ADAMS' dynamic simulation results for a large-scale heavy forging manipulator loading work-piece of 250 tons, the influence of contact forces on stable gripping is analyzed.

2 Gripping-Contact Modeling

2.1 Gripping-Contact Force

Fig.1 shows the simplified structure of the large-scale heavy gripper that can grasp an object more than 250tons. The coordinate system and the locations and directions of the contact forces are shown in the figure. Assume that the system is rigid and point contact with friction on the contact surface. The sufficient condition of stable gripping to balance the gravity of the forging piece and external forces is force-closure gripping. The contact forces between the gripper and work piece have the relation to the external wrench and the joint torque of grippers, which are determined by equilibrium equations as follows [6].

$$Gf = \mathbf{w}\,, \tag{1}$$

$$J^T f = \tau\,. \tag{2}$$

where G is the grasp matrix, J is the Jacobian matrix of the gripper joints, $w \in R^6$ is 6D external wrench on work piece, $\tau \in R^m$ is joint torque on gripper with m being the number of joints, $f \in R^n$ is the contact force on work piece with n being the number of contact constraints.

After the manipulator is designed and work piece is given, the external wrench w is known, however, the joint torque τ and the contact force f are unknown which are expected to be calculated from equations (1)-(2). Consider the contact status shown in Fig.1, where the contact points c_1 and c_2 have the same contact force, and so do the contact point c_3 and c_4. For point contact with friction between the gripper and work-piece, Coulomb friction model is used to ensure that the contact forces f_i are in friction cone which are satisfied by constraint inequation as follows [7-11].

$$\begin{cases} \sqrt{f_1^2 + f_2^2} \le \mu f_3^2 \\ f_3 \ge 0 \end{cases}. \tag{3}$$

where f_1, f_2, f_3 are vectors of contact forces on the contact surface, f_1 and f_2 are tangent forces, and f_3 is the normal force.

Contact forces are determined by substituting equation (1) into equation (3). Generally, when the number of contact points is more than two, root of contact forces are not unique. Thus contact forces must be given by finding an optimal root.

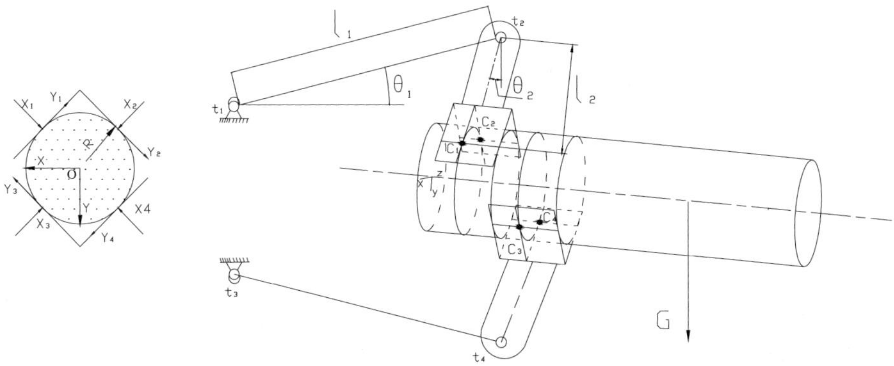

Fig. 1. Gripping-contact model

2.2 Calculation Model

The parameters of the gripping contact model are given in **table 1**. For the gripping mechanism shown in **Fig.1**, the Jacobian matrix and grasp matrix can be given as follows.

$$J^T = \begin{pmatrix} a_1 & -a_1 & a_2 & a_1 & a_1 & a_2 & 0 & 0 & 0 & 0 & 0 & 0 \\ a_3 & -a_3 & a_4 & a_3 & a_3 & a_4 & 0 & 0 & 0 & 0 & 0 & 0 \\ 0 & 0 & 0 & 0 & 0 & 0 & a_1 & -a_1 & a_2 & a_1 & a_1 & a_2 \\ 0 & 0 & 0 & 0 & 0 & 0 & a_3 & -a_3 & a_4 & a_3 & a_3 & a_4 \end{pmatrix}, \tag{4}$$

where $a_1 = -\frac{\sqrt{2}}{2}(l_1 \cos\theta_1 - l_2 tg\theta_2)$, $a_2 = l_2 - l_1 \sin\theta_1$, $a_3 = \frac{\sqrt{2}}{2} l_2 tg\theta_2$, $a_4 = l_2$, and the definitions of l_1, l_2, θ_1, and θ_2 are illustrated in **Fig.1.**

Table 1. Parameters of Gripping-Contact Model

Joints number	Contact constraints	contact points
m=4	n=12	4

$$G = (\mathbf{G}_1 \quad \mathbf{G}_2 \quad \mathbf{G}_3 \quad \mathbf{G}_4), \tag{5}$$

$$G_1=\begin{pmatrix} -\frac{\sqrt{2}}{2} & -\frac{\sqrt{2}}{2} & 0 \\ \frac{\sqrt{2}}{2} & -\frac{\sqrt{2}}{2} & 0 \\ 0 & 0 & 1 \\ -\frac{\sqrt{2}}{2}z_1 & \frac{\sqrt{2}}{2}z_1 & -\frac{\sqrt{2}}{2}R \\ -\frac{\sqrt{2}}{2}z_1 & -\frac{\sqrt{2}}{2}z1 & -\frac{\sqrt{2}}{2}R \\ 0 & -R & 0 \end{pmatrix} \qquad G_2=\begin{pmatrix} \frac{\sqrt{2}}{2} & -\frac{\sqrt{2}}{2} & 0 \\ \frac{\sqrt{2}}{2} & \frac{\sqrt{2}}{2} & 0 \\ 0 & 0 & 1 \\ -\frac{\sqrt{2}}{2}z_1 & -\frac{\sqrt{2}}{2}z_1 & -\frac{\sqrt{2}}{2}R \\ \frac{\sqrt{2}}{2}z_1 & -\frac{\sqrt{2}}{2}z_1 & \frac{\sqrt{2}}{2}R \\ 0 & -R & 0 \end{pmatrix}$$

$$G_3=\begin{pmatrix} -\frac{\sqrt{2}}{2} & \frac{\sqrt{2}}{2} & 0 \\ -\frac{\sqrt{2}}{2} & -\frac{\sqrt{2}}{2} & 0 \\ 0 & 0 & 1 \\ \frac{\sqrt{2}}{2}z_2 & \frac{\sqrt{2}}{2}z_1 & \frac{\sqrt{2}}{2}R \\ -\frac{\sqrt{2}}{2}z_2 & \frac{\sqrt{2}}{2}z_2 & -\frac{\sqrt{2}}{2}R \\ 0 & -R & 0 \end{pmatrix} \qquad G_4=\begin{pmatrix} \frac{\sqrt{2}}{2} & \frac{\sqrt{2}}{2} & 0 \\ -\frac{\sqrt{2}}{2} & \frac{\sqrt{2}}{2} & 0 \\ 0 & 0 & 1 \\ \frac{\sqrt{2}}{2}z_2 & -\frac{\sqrt{2}}{2}z_2 & \frac{\sqrt{2}}{2}R \\ \frac{\sqrt{2}}{2}z_2 & \frac{\sqrt{2}}{2}z_2 & \frac{\sqrt{2}}{2}R \\ 0 & -R & 0 \end{pmatrix}$$

where z_1 and z_2 are the axial position of contact points on grippers in terms of coordinates of the work piece, and R is the radius of the work piece.

Assume that contact forces $f=(f_{x1},f_{y1},f_{z,},\ldots\ldots f_{x4},f_{y4},f_{z4})^T$ have identical friction constraints. Then contact force f can be determined by the following equations:

$$\begin{cases} Gf = w \\ \sqrt{f_{yi}^2 + f_{zi}^2} \le \mu f_{xi}^2 \\ f_{xi} \ge 0 \\ f_1 = f_2,\ f_3 = f_4 \end{cases} \quad \text{Where} \quad \begin{array}{l} f_i = \left(f_{xi} \quad f_{yi} \quad f_{zi}\right) \\ i = 1,2,3,4 \end{array} \tag{6}$$

In terms of equations (5) and (6), the optimal roots of contact forces can be obtained. Then joint torque τ which is controlled by active joints to satisfy stable gripping can be determined by substituting the optimal root of contact forces and equation (4) into equation (2).

From the calculation model, the grasp matrix G and the joint Jacobian matrix J, which are determined by the positions of contact points, mainly affect contact forces and the required joint torque. Either the changes of contact status or movements of contact points as in process of rotation are displayed as jaws' rotation around their link pins, which cause the value of variables θ_2, z_1 and z_2 of equation (4) and equation (5) to vary. Accordingly, the grasp matrix G and Jacobian matrix J change which result in changes of the contact forces and joint force according to equation (1) and equation (2), which are identical with the dynamic simulation results by ADAMS.

Usually, jaws of the gripper can rotate freely around their link joints within limited angles in order to be easier grasped and better positioned, which is obviously different from multi-fingered hands. Therefore reactive force on the gripper will cause rotation around the fixed pins, resulting in that the work piece is away from its horizontal axis and the sliding of contact points happens. Then the gripping stability and dynamic performance decreased. Thus, the study of the change of contact points while moving is important for the analysis of stable gripping.

3 Dynamic Simulation

The above gripping-contact model is based on that the contact points are known in advance while the manipulator is moving during the forging process. Contact constraints are complex especially when sliding exists between the work piece and the grippers. Thus dynamic simulation tool ADAMS is used to study the contact status between the gripper and work piece.

3.1 Dynamic Modeling

Fig.2 shows the mechanism principle and the three-dimensional model of the forging manipulator which is created in ADAMS/VIEW. The operations of the manipulator include tilting, gripping, horizontal moving; vertical lifting and gripper rotating, All of the operations are driven by hydraulic system. Dynamic simulation parameters are given in **Table 2**.

The dynamic simulation process is set as follows, gripping work piece (0s~1s), lifting work piece (1s~3s), manipulator moving (5s~20s), the grippers rotating 360 degrees (20s~40s). By set relative motion parameters and external forces, ADAMS software can simulate the dynamic feature of each links and the magnitude and position of contact forces [12].

Table 2. Parameters of Dynamic Simulation

material	steel	Penetration depth	0.1
Mass (work piece)	250t	Damping coefficient	50
Length(work piece)	15m	Static coefficient of friction	0.3
Stiffness coefficient	1.0×10^5	Dynamic coefficient of friction	0.25
Stiffness force exponent	1.5		

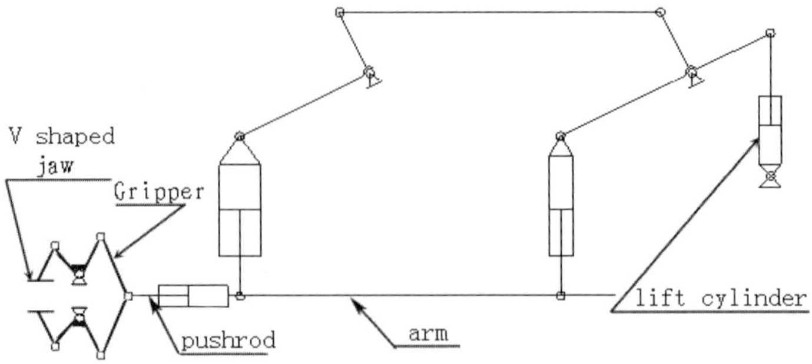

(a) Simplified mechanism

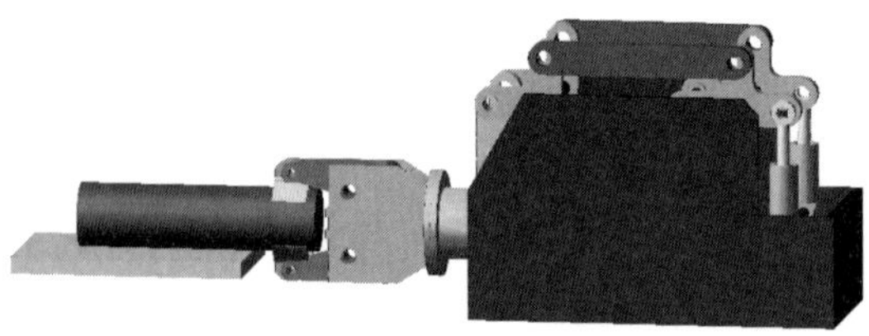

(b) 3D model of the forging manipulator

Fig. 2. Sketch drawing and three-dimension model of forging manipulator

3.2 Result Analysis

Fig.3 shows five different kinds of contact status and the force direction of each contact point between grippers and work-piece during gripping, lifting and moving in simulations. The relative joint force curve from the push rod of the gripping hydraulic cylinder is given in **Fig.4**.

Fig.3 and Fig.4 show that joint force changes a lot if contact points slide. Among the five different cases, the stable gripping of status (A) requires the biggest joint force, and the status (E) requires the smallest. The nearer the positions of contact points are from the revolute joint of jaw, the smaller the joint force of the pushrod is. Even if the contact points slide tens of millimeters, the joint force would increase hundreds of thousands of Newton. For example, from status (C) to status (B), the upper contact points move about forty millimeters, the joint force of pushrod increases to 2.7E7 Newton from 2.25E7 Newton.

Obviously in Fig. 4, the gripping is stable during the process of gripping, lifting and moving except the moment(0.9s) when the jaws first contact the work-piece and the moment(2.8s) when the work-piece first leave the block.

Fig.5 shows that the joint forces shift during the rotation process in case (E). The joint force is fluctuating while rotating. Equation (2) shows that the change of joint forces refers to the change of contact forces, which is reflected by the positions of contact points through gripping matrix G and Jacobian matrix J.

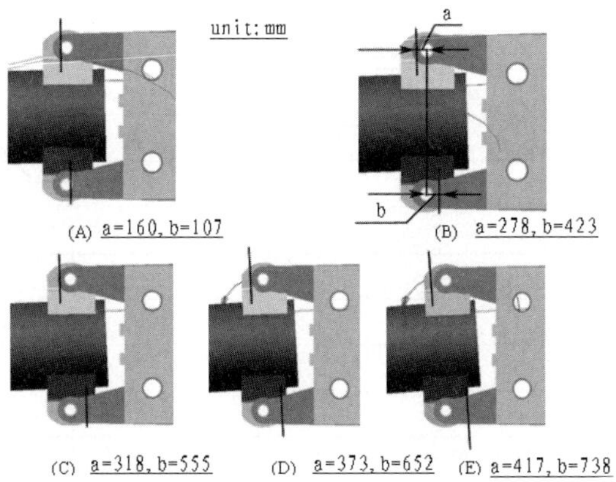

Fig. 3. Positions of contact points for different contact status

(Definitions of a and b are as shown in (B))

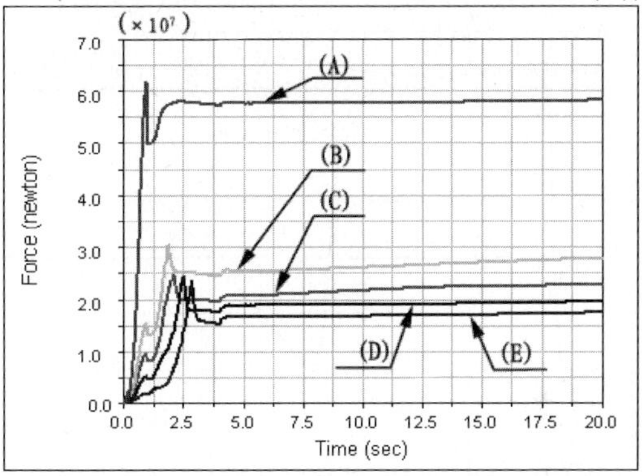

Fig. 4. Joint forces for different contact status

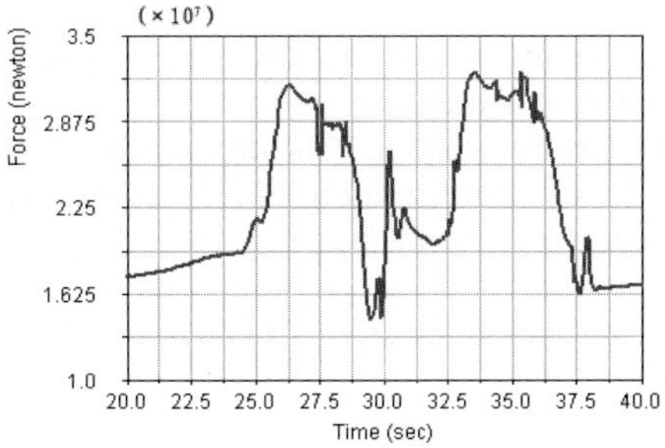

Fig. 5. Joint forces curve in rotation process of status (E)

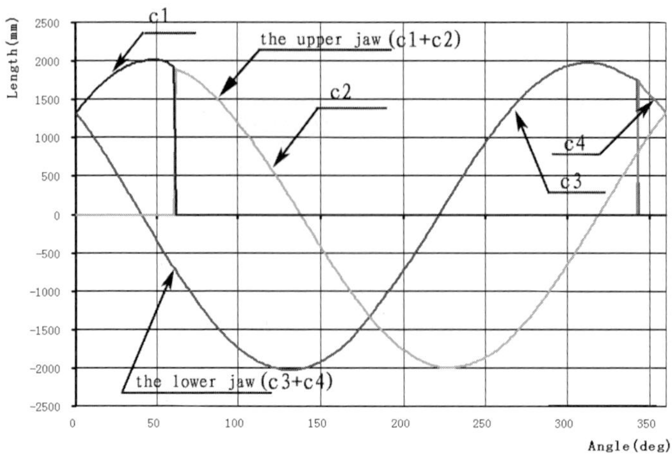

Fig. 6. Circumferential position of contact points during rotation (c_i means the contact point i)

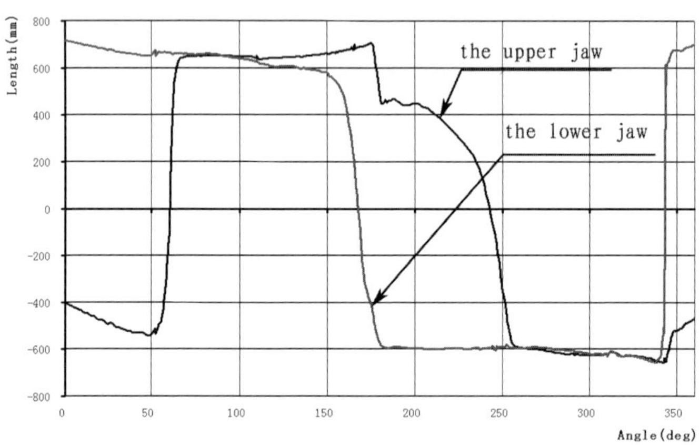

Fig. 7. Axial position of contact points during rotation

There are eight contact points during rotating 360 degrees. Take one face of each jaw for example; the other side is the same.

Fig.6 shows the contact status changes during rotating. On the upper jaw the contact point c_1 is replaced by c_2 while rotating 60.35 degree, and on the lower jaw the contact point c_3 is replaced by c_4 while rotating 342.59degree. This means that there are three different contact statuses during rotating due to sliding. In case of a certain contact status, the position of contact points changes due to rotation of grippers as shown in Fig.6 and Fig.7.

From the dynamic simulation results with the gripping-contact model, it can be seen that contact status including position of both gripper and contact points is the main factor affecting stale gripping. Contact forces are sensitive to the change of contact points. Minor sliding of contact points will lead to great fluctuation of contact forces and joint force. Large-scale change of force is bad for the control of stable gripping. The rotating process is a period in which unstable gripping is easy to occur due to the change of the positions of gripper's. During forging operations, the position change of grippers is unavoidable whereas the change of contact points should be reduced to improve stable gripping.

4 Conclusions

Contact status between the jaws of grippers and the work piece is the main factor influencing stable gripping during forging operations for large-scale heavy manipulators. The issue of stable gripping is studied in terms of the contact forces between the gripper and work piece, which are calculated by force-closure gripping. The influence of contact points on contact forces and joint force is analyzed by dynamic simulations. Contact forces during gripping, lifting, moving and rotating are analyzed by academic calculation and computer simulation. The above analyses provide a good foundation for the optimal design of the grippe, and are helpful for the control system design of large-scale heavy forging manipulators.

Acknowledgments

This work is from "973"project (2006CB705400) supported by National Basic Research Program of China.

References

1. Wan, S.D., Wang, Y.G.: Mechanization and automation of Forging. China machine press, Beijing (1983)
2. Vukobratovic, M.K., Potkonjak, V.: Dynamics of contact tasks in robotics Part I: General model of robot interacting with environment. J. Mechanism and Machine Theory 34, 923–942 (1999)
3. Vukobratovic, M.K., Potkonjak, V.: Dynamics of contact tasks in robotics Part II: Case study in dynamics of contact motion. J. Mechanism and Machine Theory 34, 943–972 (1999)
4. Buss, M., Hashimoto, H., Moore, J.B.: Dextrous hand grasping force optimization. J. IEEE Trans Robot Automat. 12(3), 406–418 (1996)
5. Al-Gallaf, E.A.: Multi-fingered robot hand optimal task force distribution neural inverse kinematics approach. J. Robotics and Autonomous Systems 54, 34–51 (2006)
6. Li, J.T., Zhang, Y.R., Zhang, Q.X.: Calculation of Contact Forces in Grasping by Space Decomposition. J. Chinese Journal of Aeronautics 14(2), 112–117 (2001)
7. Muway, R.M., Li, Z.X., Sastry, S.S.: A Mathematical Introduction to Robotic Manipulation. CRC Press, Inc., Florida (1994)
8. Zhang, Y.R., Li, J.T., Li, J.F.: Robot Arms. China machine press, Beijing (2007)
9. Johnson, K.L.: Contact mechanics. Cambridge University Press, Cambridge (1985)
10. Eberhard, P., Hu, B.: Advanced contact dynamics. Southeast university press, Nanjing (2003)
11. Chen, J.P., Wei, Z.Y.: Grasping force optimize of multi-fingers. J. Journal of Nanjing Engineering Institute 13(2), 34–41 (1998)
12. Fan, C.J., Xiong, G.M., Zhou, M.F.: Application and Advance of Virtual Prototype Software MSC.ADAMS. China machine press, Beijing (2006)

Macro-micro Driven Ultra-Precision Positioning Stage for Conventional Grinder

Jialiang Zhang, Beizhi Li, Yuan Xu, and Jianguo Yang

College of Mechanical Engineering, Donghua University, Shanghai 201620, China
zjili@dhu.edu.cn

Abstract. Precision positioning stage is the key part of precision feed system of a machine. To compensate for the effect of processing precision affected by the vibration of wheelhead of precision grinder, a micro-feed worktable using piezoelectric actuators, which serves as an auxiliary feeding device, has been introduced for common cylindrical grinders. The stiffness of its support-oriented mechanism is modeled and analyzed by PRO/E and FEA. A close-loop control system based on special algorithm is presented and the prototype of a macro-micro driven ultra-precision positioning stage on grinder is developed. The experimental results show that the positioning accuracy of the stage is 0.1±0.02 μm, its average stiffness is 207 N/μm and the cylindricity of machined parts is less than 2 μm.

Keywords: Macro-micro driven; precision grinder; micro feed; piezoelectric actuator; flexible hinge.

1 Introduction

Nowadays, there are a growing number of motion control applications that require ultra precision positioning accuracy. Piezoelectric actuators, with their indefinite resolution and high stiffness, have been increasingly applied in many areas where ultra precision positioning is needed, such as optics, electronics, aviation, biologic engineering and robotics [1, 2].

The positioning accuracy of the precision stage is one of the key factors constraining the machining accuracy of machine tools. The macro-micro driven ultra-precision positioning stage divides the system into two parts, macro positioning stage and micro positioning one. The macro positioning stage completes the movement with high speed, large travel range and low resolution. The micro positioning stage compensates macro positioning error, and restrains vibration suppression. Therefore, the whole system gains many advantages, such as large travel range, high speed, high resolution and high frequency response. The macro-micro driven ultra-precision positioning stage is a new way to resolve the contradiction between long travel range and high resolution in the positioning of machine system [3-7].

In this paper, we develop the micro positioning stage by piezoelectric ceramic and flexible hinges for common grinders, so as to obtain higher resolution and faster response speed. The positioning system uses precise detecting system as the feedback element of the closed-loop system to ensure global precision.

C. Xiong et al. (Eds.): ICIRA 2008, Part II, LNAI 5315, pp. 848–857, 2008.

2 System Constitution

Because wheelhead feed system of traditional grinder is heavy and there is friction and heat distortion among guideways, the positioning precision of grinding wheel worktable fixed on ball screw shaft is low. The feed error of wheelhead is notable, so it is hard to guarantee the requirements of ultra-precision process. If piezoelectric actuators driving flexible worktable and closed loop feedback control technology are adopted, it becomes easier to realize the ultra-precision positioning of nano scale. However, the maximum operation range of piezoelectric actuator is scores of microns, so only adopting micro system still cannot satisfy long travel requirements [8-10].

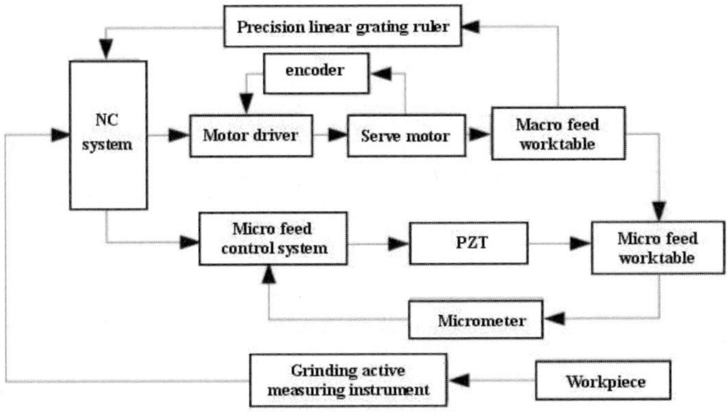

Fig. 1. The schematic diagram of the ultra-precision positioning stage

The general construction of the macro-micro driven ultra-precision feed system is designed as shown in Fig. 1. It includes a macro feed positioning system and a micro one. The micro system consists of a micro displacement worktable driven by piezoelectric actuators, power supply, control system and micro displacement transducer. On-line measurements on external dimension of the machining part are made by an active measuring instrument to get the displacement of whole system. The macro and micro driven ultra-precision positioning stage is finally controlled by NC system to achieve full closed loop control of position. Its work principle is as follows:

(1) Input movement information to micro feed control system. NC system and micro feed control system are communicated through driving interrupted signals.

(2) According to input movement information, NC system controls the movement of macro feed worktable, to realize macro positioning requirements of ultra-precision positioning stage based on scheduled control algorithm.

(3) Precision grating ruler feeds back signals to NC system and checks the movement situations of macro feed worktable while the macro drive part is moving.

(4) When macro drive part moves to threshold range that micro feed system can compensate, NC system sends movement signals to micro feed control system. Start

micro feed positioning worktable and control micro feed system to realize micro feed according to requirements of the micro feed system and actual process.

(5) When macro-micro positioning stage achieves positioning requirement by active measuring instrument, the system finishes precision positioning control.

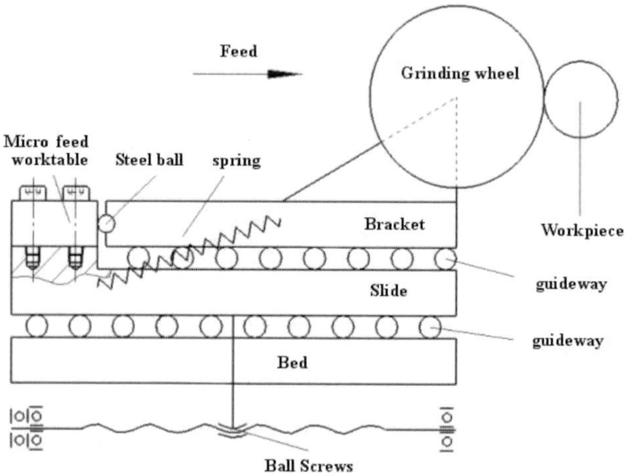

Fig. 2. The connecting sketch between micro feed worktable and the grinder

As shown in Fig. 2, connect micro feed worktable and micrometer with first level worktable by bolts in the horizontal installation plane instead of its side vertical plane. The installation position of the head of micrometer should be in the same plane of the axial central plane of grinding wheel, so as to reduce the possible error occurred by the twist of second level worktable. Constant force springs are adopted between two worktables to make sure that the second level worktable can stick to ultra-precision feed worktable when the micro feed worktable works, and the micro feed system can reset timely when the system returns to zero. With this connection method, the cantilever mode of micro feed worktable is avoided, the integrate stiffness of the system is greatly improved, and intermediary paths and the influence of connection to feed precision is reduced to the minimum level.

3 Micro Feed Worktable Structure

The requirements of ultra-precision micro-feed function realized on common grinders are as follows.

(1) The location precision of the micro feed system is less than±0.05 μm.
(2) The static stiffness of the micro feed system is 200 N/μm or more.
(3) The travel range of the micro feed system is no less than 25 μm.
(4) The micro feed system is modularized to fit variable grinders.
(5) The micro feed system has advantages such as lower cost and higher reliability.

Based on the work character of piezoelectric actuator, a right-circular flexible hinge group is selected to make the support-oriented mechanism of the micro displacement worktable according to the lever principle. The simplified model is shown as Fig. 3. The piezoelectric ceramics are set in the parallelogram to produce a force F and point O is the force point of micro feed worktable. A definite preload force is commonly put on the mechanism to prevent overloading damage [11, 12].

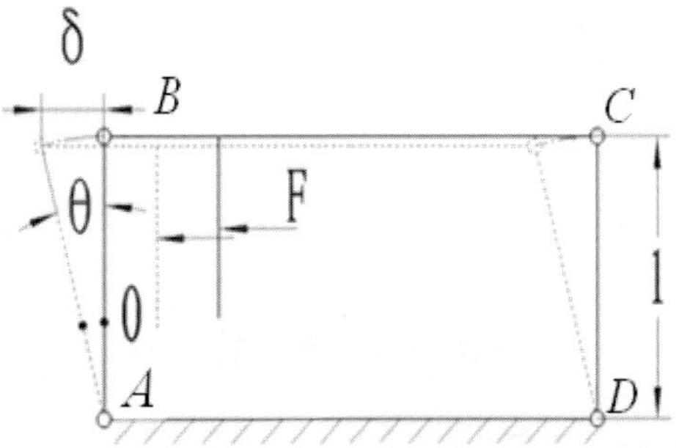

Fig. 3. Simplified model of the support-oriented mechanism

3.1 Stiffness Analysis

In the preload phase, if we let the force of the piezoelectric actuator and flexible hinge be F_0 and $F_0^{'}$, we get

$$F_0 = K_p \cdot L_0 . \quad (1)$$

$$F_0^{'} = K_f \cdot L_0^{'} . \quad (2)$$

where K_p is the stiffness of piezoelectric actuator, K_f is the oriented stiffness of flexible hinge, L_0 is the compressed displacement of piezoelectric actuator and $L_0^{'}$ is the distortion quantity of flexible hinge in the function of preload. From equilibrium equation, we can get

$$L_0 = \frac{K_f \cdot L_0^{'}}{K_p} . \quad (3)$$

In the voltage loading phase, if the distortion of piezoelectric actuator is $L^{'}$, the final output displacement $Y^{'}$ and elastic counterforce $P^{'}$ can be expressed as follows.

$$Y^{'} = L + L_{\max} - (L - L_0) - L^{'} = L_{\max} + L_0 - L^{'} . \quad (4)$$

$$P^{'} = K_P \cdot [L + L_{\max} - (L - L_0) - L^{'}] = K_P \cdot (L_{\max} + L_0 - L^{'}) . \quad (5)$$

where L is the static length of piezoelectric actuator, and $L_{\max}$ is the maximum output displacement of piezoelectric actuator.

According to force analysis of the mechanism, the overall output displacement δ and counterforce P of point B are

$$\delta = \frac{K_P}{K_P + K_f} L' \quad . \tag{6}$$

$$P = K_f \cdot Y = K_f \cdot (\frac{K_P}{K_P + K_f} L' + L_0') \quad . \tag{7}$$

Here, if the system has a load F_0, $A0 = l_1$, $AB = l$, then

$$Fl + \sum_{i=1}^{4} M_i = F_0 l_1 \cdot \tag{8}$$

Let the corner stiffness of flexible hinge be K_θ, so the torque of piezoelectric actuator M_i is

$$M_i = K_\theta \cdot \theta = K_\theta \frac{\delta}{l} \cdot \tag{9}$$

The system stiffness can be described as

$$K_s = \frac{Fl_1^2}{yl^2} + 4\frac{K_\theta^2}{l_1^2} \approx \frac{K_p}{T_f^2} + 4\frac{K_\theta^2}{l_1^2} \cdot \tag{10}$$

The system output displacement can be described as

$$Y = \frac{K_P}{K_P + K_f} L_{\max} \cdot T_f \cdot \tag{11}$$

where $T_f = \frac{l_1}{l}$.

According to actual demands, let preload force is 150 N, $T_f = 0.3434$, then $K_s = \frac{K_p}{T_f^2} + 4\frac{K_\theta^2}{l_1^2} > \frac{35}{0.3434^2} = 296 > 200$ N/μm, $K_f = 5.20$ N/μm, $\delta = \frac{K_p}{K_p + K_f} L_{\max}$ = 87.06 N/μm.

The output displacement of the micro feed system is

$$Y = T_f \cdot \delta = 0.3434 \times 87.06 = 30 \ \mu\text{m}$$

3.2 FEA Checking

If the flexible support-oriented mechanism is loaded and restricted as Fig. 4, the displacement at x direction can be analyzed by the FEA module of PRO/E. We let the material of the mechanism be 45 steel and the force on screw A be 100 N and restrict all freedoms of fixing screws. Then, the maximum displacement of the crossbeam is 18.04 μm. According to $K_f = F/\delta$, its oriented stiffness is about 5.54 N/μm. The displacements at y and z direction are 1.743 μm and 8.843×10^{-2} μm respectively, much less than the displacement at x direction and therefore can be neglected.

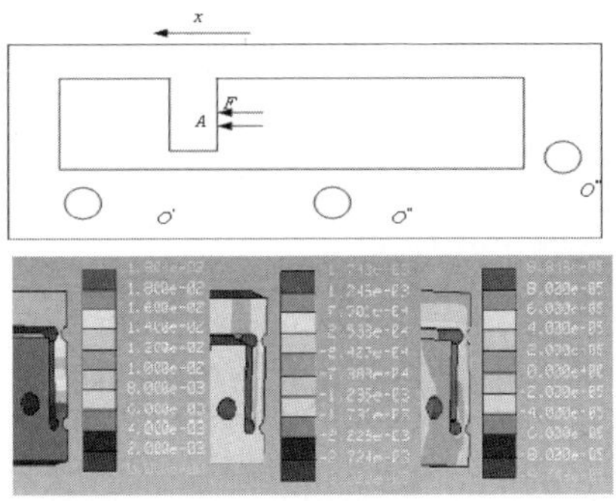

Fig. 4. FEA of the flexible support-oriented mechanism

3.3 Structure Fatigue Life Analysis

Based on the basic theory of the structure fatigue life analysis and the finite element method, the flexible hinge structure fatigue life is analyzed by Fatigue Advisor module of PRO/E. The result shows that the fatigue life of flexible hinge is $10^{6.314}$, which meets use requirements of high-cycle fatigue life.

4 Micro Displacement Control System

Piezoelectric ceramics strain in the external electric field, the level of strain is proportional to electrical field intensity, the direction of strain is dependent on the direction of electrical field. However, the nonlinear effect of PZT brought by its lag and creep makes the control of the piezoelectric ceramic difficult [13, 14].

4.1 Overall Design of Micro Displacement Control System

To improve the nonlinearity of PZT, the closed-loop control mode is applied in the micro-feed system. The stage is fed back by a displacement transducer and thus obtains higher resolution and better dynamic stiffness. The positioning error of the system can be compensated by using software algorithms.

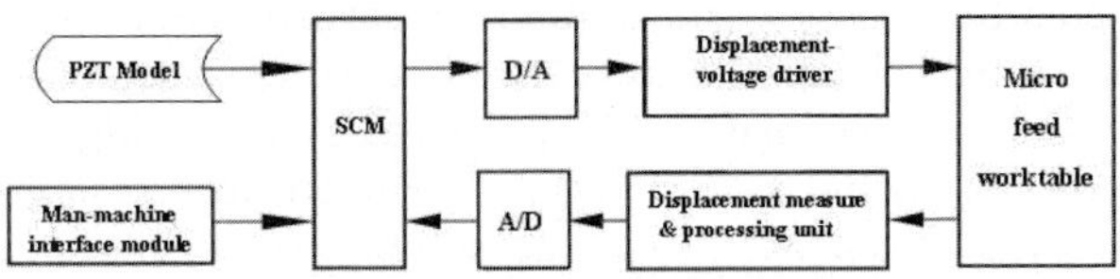

Fig. 5. The schematic diagram of the close-loop control system

The schematic diagram of the close-loop control system is shown as Fig. 5. The system is advantaged with quick response velocity, small overshoot, as well as relatively high positioning accuracy. The accuracy is 0.03μm and the resolution is 0.01μm, measured by the high-accuracy inductive micro-displacement transducer. For the sampling module, we use the 12-bit A/D module, which is with high accuracy and high responsivity. The signal is transacted by 8-bit high-speed SCM.

4.2 The Control Process of Software

To enable the micro-feed system to communicate with NC grinding machine in the processing, we add a signal processing program, which can communicate with the NC grinding machine, into the main program. The signals are sent out by CNC system except the workpiece-dimension-reached signal, which depends on the measured dimension of the workpiece. By implementing emergency stop control for the micro-feed system, we efficiently prevent the accidents in the processing and protect the operators, the micro-feed system and workpiece machined.

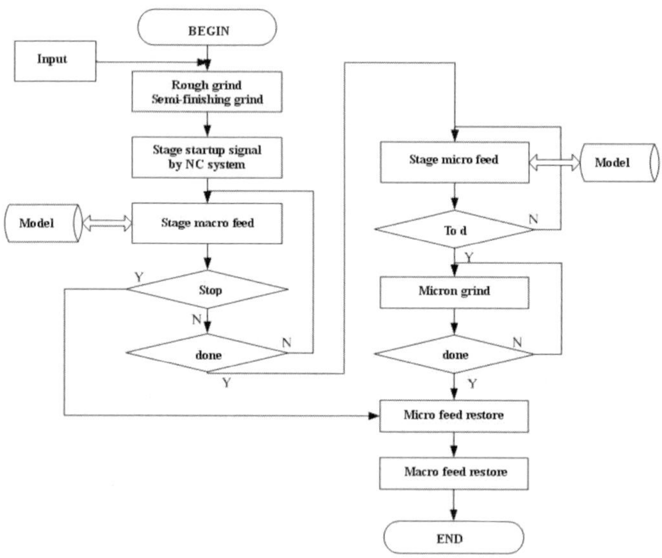

Fig. 6. The software control process

The software control process is shown in Fig. 6. The system is on standby when we input the parameters that process needs, such as micro-feed step size, feed times and feeding interval, through the man-machine interface. When digital control system sends startup signals to the micro-feed system, the micro-feed system begins to work. Based on input displacement parameter, the system uses displacement-voltage data model to get the digital volt and then the piezoelectric ceramic is made to drive the power supply by D/A, and thus to drive the micro-feed stage. Conversed by A/D, the precision measurement system feed the instant displacement back to the MPU of the feeding system. The system tries to compensate until the processing completes. In the while, if the main CNC system sends out the emergency stop signal, the micro-feed system stops, and the micro-feed stage restores.

5 Experiments

Working surroundings will greatly influence the system precision. The temperature is set to 20±2℃ in the lab, and workbench is fixed on marble vibration isolation mount to decrease the effect from outside vibrancy to minimum.

5.1 Static Performance Test of the Micro Feed System

One endpoint of the flexible support-oriented mechanism is forced by an ergometer SKN-2, and the output displacement is measured at the other corresponding endpoint by an inductive micrometer DGS-6C. The average stiffness of the micro feed system in variable powered voltages and forces is shown in Table 1. The average stiffness of the micro feed system is 207.112 N/μm and the travel range of the micro feed system is 30.3 μm.

Table 1. The stiffness of the micro feed system (N/μm)

Voltage/V / Force/N	0	30	60	90	120
50	207.430	199.020	206.612	198.473	203.542
100	204.082	201.535	199.024	207.469	221.853
120	202.102	213.694	206.992	223.388	211.466

5.2 Dynamic Performance Test of the Micro Feed System

Connect micro feed worktable and micrometer with the wheelhead, as shown in Fig. 2. The feed processes are displayed in the computer with a data acquisition card and data acquisition system developed by software Labview. The parameters are set as follows: the sampling frequency is 1000 Hz, the measure range, corresponding output voltage and resolution of the micrometer is 0~10 μm, 0~5 V and 0.01 μm. The positioning accuracy of the system is as shown in Table 2. It is 0.1±0.02 μm, and maximum response time is 70~80 ms.

Table 2. The positioning accuracy of the micro feed system (μm)

Positioning value	1	2	3	4	5	Average value	Average error
0.10	0.08	0.08	1.01	0.08	0.09	0.08	0.02
0.60	0.60	0.60	0.58	0.60	0.59	0.594	0.006
0.90	0.89	0.89	0.91	0.90	0.88	0.894	0.006
2.00	2.00	1.98	1.99	2.01	1.98	1.992	0.008
4.00	4.01	3.99	4.00	3.98	3.97	3.936	0.064
5.00	5.02	4.98	4.99	5.01	5.00	5.00	0

5.3 Machining Experiments

We perform real machining experiments on a CNC cylindrical grinder with the developed micro-feed system. The experiment equipments are shown in Fig. 7. The primary machine tool can be equipped with radial measuring instrument and axial measuring instrument, and the sizes for diameters of parts can actually be controlled within 3 μm.

We process on the cylindrical surfaces of 50 parts in the experiment, and then use the microkator to measure the dimensions at their upper, middle and lower plane. The results show that the cylindricity is less than 2 μm, and the external roundness and surface roughness of parts are all improved. The system has lower cost, smaller cubage, higher reliability, better capacity of resisting disturbance and easiness in application.

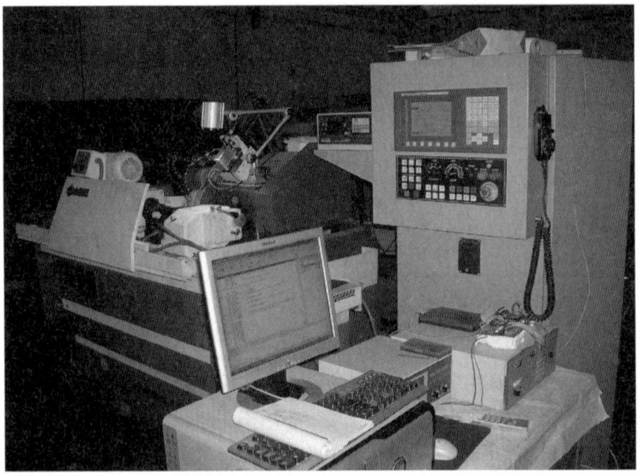

Fig. 7. The machining and measuring scene

6 Conclusions

The macro-micro driven ultra-precision positioning stage is a new way to resolve the contradiction between long travel range and high resolution in the positioning of machine system. This paper presents a macro-micro driven ultra-precision positioning stage for common grinders. The micro system consists of a micro displacement worktable driven by piezoelectric actuators, power supply, control system and micro displacement transducer. The right-circular flexible hinge group is selected to make the support-oriented mechanism of the micro displacement worktable according to the lever principle. The stiffness of the support-oriented mechanism is modeled and analyzed by PRO/E and FEA, and a close-loop control system based on special algorithm is presented. The prototype has been developed and experimented. The results show that the average stiffness and travel range of the micro feed system is 207.112 N/μm and 30.3 μm respectively; the positioning accuracy of the stage is 0.1±0.02 μm, max. response time is less than 80 ms; the cylindricity of machined parts is less than 2 μm, and the external roundness and surface roughness are all improved. The stage meets the requirements of ultra-precision machining on common grinder with lower cost and higher reliability.

Acknowledgment

This research was supported by Shanghai Leading Academic Discipline Project, project number B602, and Shanghai Science foundation and Technology Innovation Fund of Shanghai Science and Technology Committee, fund number 041111007.

References

1. Owen, R.B., Maggiore, M., Apkarian, J.: A High-Precision, Magnetically Levitated Positioning Stage: Toward Contactless Actuation for Industrial Manufacturing. IEEE Control Systems Magazine 26, 82–95 (2006)
2. Choi, Y., Sreenivasan, S.V., Choi, B.J.: Kinematic Design of Large Displacement Precision XY Positioning Stage by Using Cross Strip Flexure Joints and Over-Constrained Mechanism. Mechanism and Machine Theory 43, 724–737 (2008)
3. Okazaki, Y.: A Micro-Positioning Tool Post Using a Piezoelectric Actuator for Diamond Turning Machines. Journal of the America Society of Precision Engineering 12, 151–156 (1990)
4. Agathe, H., Roland, S.: End-Point Control of a Fast and Precise Macro/Micro-Manipulator. IEEE Trans. on Neural Networks 5, 26–38 (1994)
5. Tal, J.: Servomotors Take Piezoceramic Transducers for a Ride. Machine Design 9, 1–3 (1999)
6. Pahk, H.J., Lee, D.S., Park, J.H.: Ultra Precision Positioning System for Servo Motor-Piezo Actuator Using the Dual Loop and Digital Filter Implementation. Machine Tools & Manufacture 4, 51–63 (2000)
7. Woronko, A., Huang, J., Altintas, Y.: Piezoelectric Tool Actuator for Precision Machining on Conventional CNC Turning Centers. Precision Engineering 27, 335–345 (2003)
8. Kim, J.D., Nam, S.R.: Development of a Micro-position Grinding Table Using Piezoelectric Voltage Feedback. Journal Engineering Manufacture 209, 469–474 (1995)
9. Stephenson, D.J., Corbett, J., Hedge, J.: Ultra Precision Grinding Using the Tetraform Concept. Abrasives, February/March 12–16 (2002)
10. Wang, L.F., Li, B.Z., Yang, J.G., Wang, H.L.: A Study on Micro-Position System Based on PZT. Piezoelectrics and Acoustooptics 29, 240–242 (2007)
11. Yang, R., Jouaneh, M.: Design and Analysis of a Low Profile Micro-Positioning Stage. Precision Engineering 15, 131–142 (1993)
12. Gang, X., Mei, D., Chen, Z.: A Micro-Feed Actuator for Ultraprecision. Grinding of Brittle Materials 6, 259–260 (2004)
13. Ge, P., Jouaneh, M.: Tracking Control of a Piezoceramic Actuator. IEEE Transactions on Control Systems Technology 4, 209–216 (1996)
14. Yan, R.Z., Li, B.Z., Yang, J.G., Du, D.C.: Research on Micro-Feed System in Ultra-Precision Grinder. In: Proceedings of ICAL, Jinan, pp. 304–308 (2007)

Hierarchical Reasoning Model of Tolerance Information and Its Using in Reasoning Technique of Geometric Tolerance Types

Yi Zhang, Zongbin Li, and Jikong Wang

State Key Laboratory for Manufacturing Systems Engineering of China
School of Mechanical Engineering, Xi'an Jiaotong University, Xi'an 710049, China
zhangyi.jd@stu.xjtu.edu.cn, lzb9910@mail.xjtu.edu.cn

Abstract. On the basis of study of variational geometric constraints, a kind of hierarchical representation model of tolerance information reasoning is presented. Using the polychromatic sets, the feature tier and variational geometric constraint tier of this model are described. Then, using the reasoning relation matrix between unified colours and individual colours of the polychromatic sets, the reasoning of the feature tier and variational geometric constraint tier is realized, and the method and process of the reasoning are presented. Finally, its using in the generation of tolerance network for assembly is introduced.

Keywords: Tolerance information, Reasoning model, Polychromatic sets, Tolerance types.

1 Introduction

Computer aided tolerance design (CAT) is one of key technology in CAD/CAM integration. A general CAT system can be divided into two major parts [1]: determining tolerance types and constructing dimension chains based on parts and assembly information of CAD system, and designing tolerances based on the above-mentioned tolerance chains.

The current research mainly focuses on dimension tolerance design based on two-dimensional (2D) dimension chain. With the development of three-dimensional (3D) CAD system, it has become an urgent problem to be settled that how to construct 3D dimension chain and to design dimension and geometric tolerance. Reference [2] put forward variational geometric constraint (VGC) theory which effectively solved the comprehensive design of dimension and geometric tolerance, but in which a large quantity of existing rules brought certain difficulties in computer programming. Reference [3] only researched the problem for generating 2D dimension chains.

On the basis of the above-mentioned studies, this paper introduces the polychromatic sets theory[4,5] into CAT based on VGC theory, develops hierarchical reasoning model of tolerance information, uses the polychromatic sets theory to describe this model, optimizes computer-aided generation of tolerance types, and provides basis for developing tolerance network and designing tolerance. Eventually, this paper

C. Xiong et al. (Eds.): ICIRA 2008, Part II, LNAI 5315, pp. 858–868, 2008.

introduces the application of hierarchical reasoning model as well as its reasoning method on assembly-oriented tolerance generation.

2 Establishment of Reasoning Model of Hierarchical Tolerance Information

In order to comprehensively deal with dimension and geometric tolerance, tolerance can be divided into two types [2]: self-referenced tolerance and cross-referenced tolerance. Self-referenced tolerance standardizes self-referenced variational geometric constraint (SVGC), which includes: size dimension tolerance and form tolerance, and cross-referenced tolerance standardizes cross-referenced variational geometric constraint (CVGC), which includes: location dimension tolerance and position tolerance.

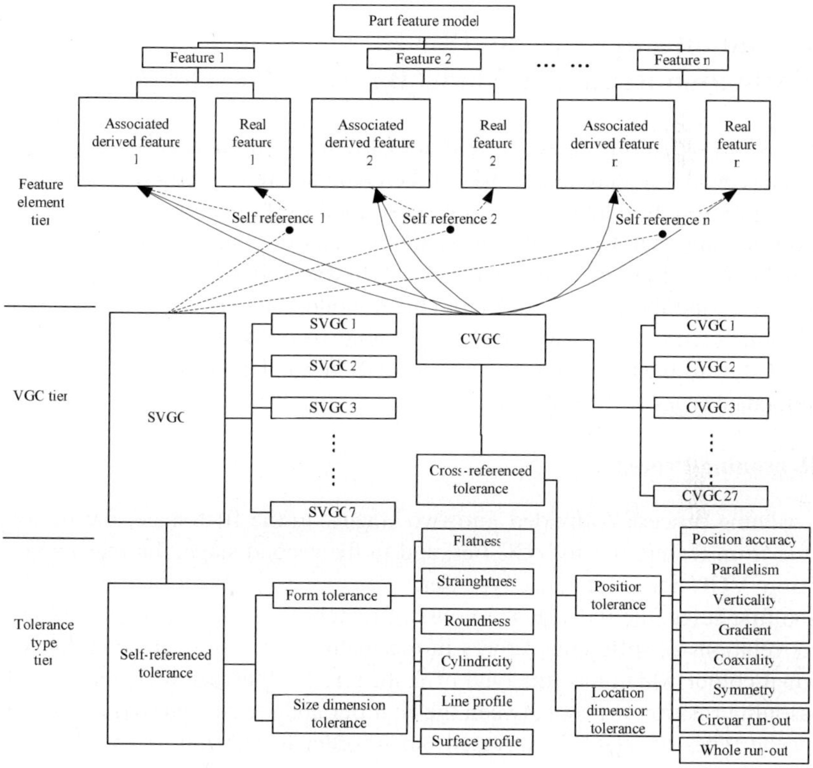

Fig. 1. Reasoning model for hierarchical tolerance information

This paper divides dimension tolerance into size dimension tolerance and location dimension tolerance, in which the tolerance feature of size dimension tolerance is its real feature, the referenced feature is associated derived feature of this real feature, and the other types of dimension tolerances are location dimension tolerances. This kind of division method is beneficial to comprehensive design for dimension tolerance and geometric tolerance.

According to the above classification method of tolerance and the related theory of VGC, this paper presents a kind of hierarchical reasoning model for tolerance information used to deduce tolerance information.

Hierarchical reasoning model of tolerance information is a hierarchical tree structure which consists of three tiers. The relations among different tiers are that: at first, the first tier (namely feature element tier) is constructed through part feature, then the second tier (namely VGC) is reasoned out using the first tier, and finally by means of second tier, the third tier (namely tolerance type tier) can be reasoned out so as to obtain concrete tolerance types.

In the synthesis of the above contents, the hierarchical reasoning model of tolerance information is established as Fig.1.

3 Description and Reasoning for Hierarchical Tolerance Information Reasoning Model Based on Polychromatic Sets

The theory of polychromatic sets is a kind of extended set theory. As long as a model has a hierarchical structure and in which the elements among different tiers have certain logical reasoning relations, it can be described using polychromatic sets and reasoned out among each tier based on reasoning relation matrix of unified colour and individual colour of polychromatic sets [6, 7]. In the sections that follow, on the foundation of realizing the first tier of hierarchical model, namely obtaining the types and interrelations of different features, the reasoning from the first tier to VGC tier and from VGC tier to the tier of tolerance types will be implemented, and finally the concrete tolerance types will be obtained.

3.1 Reasoning Process

The reasoning process is divided into two stages. In the first stage, the reasoning is executed from feature tier to VGC tier, and in the second stage, the reasoning is executed from VGC tier to tolerance type tier.

In the first stage, the individual colours of feature tier can be obtained by means of the interrelations of different features in the feature tier. The corresponding value of individual colour which has this type of feature is 1, otherwise 0. Then, according to the reasoning relation matrix between the first tier and the second tier, the second tier, namely the types of VGC, is reasoned out in order to generate the well-constrained VGCN and make it easy to reason in the next stage.

In the second stage, using the types of VGC generated above, the colours of the second tier are obtained. Then according to the reasoning relation matrix between the second tier and the third tier, the third tier, namely the concrete types of tolerance, can be achieved, which facilitates to generate well-constrained tolerance network. In the reasoning matrix, if there is reasoning relation between upper tier and lower tier, the corresponding value is 1, otherwise 0.

3.2 Reasoning Relation Matrix

According to hierarchical method, the meanings of different tiers and the related data, the colours of each tier and reasoning relation matrices are established. The reasoning relation matrix between individual colours and unified colours in polychromatic sets should be determined based on the knowledge of the related fields. Therefore, if individual colour affects the existence of unified colour, the corresponding value of reasoning relation matrix is 1, otherwise 0. In this paper, referring to the theory of VGC [2] and the related knowledge of tolerance types, the reasoning matrices are constructed as followings.

1) The First Stage

1.1) Generator Matrix of SVGCs (See Fig. 2)

In the first tier, (S, C, P1, H, R, P, E): (spherical surface, cylindrical surface, plane, helicoids, rotation surface, prismatic surface, complex surface).

In the second tier, (F1.1~F1.7): (SVGC1~SVGC7).

1.2) Generator Matrix of CVGCs (See Fig. 3-5)

	S	C	P_1	H	R	P	E
$F_{1.1}$	●						
$F_{1.2}$		●					
$F_{1.3}$			●				
$F_{1.4}$				●			
$F_{1.5}$					●		
$F_{1.6}$						●	
$F_{1.7}$							●

Fig. 2. Generator matrix of SVGCs

	$F_{0.1}$	$F_{0.2}$	$F_{0.3}$	$F_{0.4}$	$F_{0.5}$	$F_{0.6}$	$F_{0.7}$	$F_{0.8}$
$F_{3.1}$	●			●				
$F_{3.2}$	●							●
$F_{3.3}$		●		●				
$F_{3.4}$		●						●
$F_{3.5}$			●	●				
$F_{3.6}$			●					●

Fig. 3. Generator matrix of CVGCs taking-point as referenced feature

	$F_{0.1}$	$F_{0.2}$	$F_{0.3}$	$F_{0.4}$	$F_{0.5}$	$F_{0.6}$	$F_{0.7}$	$F_{0.8}$
$F_{3.7}$	●			●				
$F_{3.8}$	●							●
$F_{3.9}$		●		●				
$F_{3.10}$		●			●			
$F_{3.11}$		●				●		
$F_{3.12}$		●					●	
$F_{3.13}$		●						●
$F_{3.14}$			●	●				
$F_{3.15}$			●		●			
$F_{3.16}$			●			●		
$F_{3.17}$			●				●	

Fig. 4. Generator matrix of CVGCs referenced feature

	$F_{0.1}$	$F_{0.2}$	$F_{0.3}$	$F_{0.4}$	$F_{0.5}$	$F_{0.6}$	$F_{0.7}$	$F_{0.8}$
$F_{3.18}$	●			●				
$F_{3.19}$	●							●
$F_{3.20}$		●		●				
$F_{3.21}$		●			●			
$F_{3.22}$		●				●		
$F_{3.23}$		●					●	
$F_{3.24}$			●	●				
$F_{3.25}$			●		●			
$F_{3.26}$			●			●		
$F_{3.27}$			●				●	

Fig. 5. Generator matrix of CVGCs taking line as taking plane as referenced feature

In the first tier, F0.1: point, F0.2: line, F0.3: plane, F0.4: inclusion relationship ($\in$), F0.5: parallel relationship ($\parallel$), F0.6: vertical relationship ($\perp$), F0.7: plane intersection relationship, F0.8: space intersection relationship ($\times$).

Note: if a point doesn't coincide with another point, a point doesn't lie on a line or a point doesn't lie in a plane, they are all defined as space intersection relationships. The types of constrained feature are expressed as F0.1, F0.2 and F0.3. The relationships between referenced feature and constrained feature are represented by F0.4～F0.8.

In the second tier, (F3.1～F3.27): (CVGC1～CVGC27).

2) The Second Stage

2.1) Generator Matrix of Self-reference Tolerance (See Fig. 6)

In the second tier, (F1.1～F1.7): (SVGC1～SVGC7).

In the third tier, F2.1: straightness, F2.2: flatness, F2.3: roundness, F2.4: cylindricity, F2.5: line profile, F2.6: surface profile, F2.7: size dimension tolerance.

2.2) Generator Matrix of Cross-referenced Tolerance (See Fig. 7-9)

	$F_{1.1}$	$F_{1.2}$	$F_{1.3}$	$F_{1.4}$	$F_{1.5}$	$F_{1.6}$	$F_{1.7}$
$F_{2.1}$		●	●		●	●	
$F_{2.2}$			●				
$F_{2.3}$	●	●			●		
$F_{2.4}$		●					
$F_{2.5}$					●	●	●
$F_{2.6}$					●	●	●
$F_{2.7}$	●	●					

Fig. 6. Generator matrix of self-reference tolerance

	$F_{3.1}$	$F_{3.2}$	$F_{3.3}$	$F_{3.4}$	$F_{3.5}$	$F_{3.6}$
$F_{4.1}$						
$F_{4.2}$						
$F_{4.3}$						
$F_{4.4}$	●					
$F_{4.5}$						
$F_{4.6}$		●	●	●	●	●
$F_{4.7}$						
$F_{4.8}$						
$F_{4.9}$		●		●		●
$F_{4.10}$						

Fig. 7. Generator matrix of cross-referenced tolerance taking point as referenced feature

	$F_{3.7}$	$F_{3.8}$	$F_{3.9}$	$F_{3.10}$	$F_{3.11}$	$F_{3.12}$	$F_{3.13}$	$F_{3.14}$	$F_{3.15}$	$F_{3.16}$	$F_{3.17}$
$F_{4.1}$				●					●		
$F_{4.2}$					●					●	
$F_{4.3}$						●					●
$F_{4.4}$			●								
$F_{4.5}$								●			
$F_{4.6}$	●	●		●			●	●	●		
$F_{4.7}$			●							●	
$F_{4.8}$			●							●	
$F_{4.9}$		●					●		●		
$F_{4.10}$						●					●

Fig. 8. Generator matrix of cross-referenced tolerance taking line as referenced feature

	$F_{3.18}$	$F_{3.19}$	$F_{3.20}$	$F_{3.21}$	$F_{3.22}$	$F_{3.23}$	$F_{3.24}$	$F_{3.25}$	$F_{3.26}$	$F_{3.27}$
$F_{4.1}$				●				●		
$F_{4.2}$					●				●	
$F_{4.3}$						●				●
$F_{4.4}$										
$F_{4.5}$			●				●			
$F_{4.6}$	●	●	●	●			●	●		
$F_{4.7}$										
$F_{4.8}$										
$F_{4.9}$		●		●				●		
$F_{4.10}$						●				●

Fig. 9. Generator matrix of cross-referenced tolerance taking plane as referenced feature

In the second tier, (F3.1～ F3.27): (CVGC1～CVGC27).

In the third tier, F4.1: parallelism, F4.2: verticality, F4.3: gradient, F4.4: coaxiality, F4.5: symmetry, F4.6: position accuracy, F4.7: circular run-out, F4.8: whole run-out, F4.9: location dimension tolerance, F4.10: location angle tolerance.

4 Application of Hierarchical Model of Tolerance Information Reasoning in the Process of Tolerance Network Generation for Assembly

The known conditions are as follows:

1) The production is divided into two parts: Part A and Part B (See Fig. 10).

2) There are two pairs of mating relations: the mating between Face A4 and Face B4, and the mating between Face A5 and Face B5.

3) The datum planes of Part A are Face A1, Face A2 and Face A3, and the datum planes of Part B are B1, B2 and B3.

4) The assembly sequence is that: On the orientation of the mating between Face A4 of Part A and Face B4 of Part B, Face A5 and Face B5 have a good mating in the end. As a result, Part A can be assembled with Part B.

The solution procedure is shown as follows:

1) The first stage: the VGCs of complete constraint are generated.

Step 1: the mate tree is generated. The feature recognition of the parts is topologically carried out and its result is shown as Fig. 10. In order to construct the well-constrained VGCN, the uniquely determined SVGC and the mating variational geometric constraints (MVGC) are combined into the mate tree. Taking mate tree as node, the loop circuit can be searched. According to the second known condition, the two pairs of mating relations determine the two mate trees (MT): MT (A4, B4) → MT1 and MT (A5, B5) → MT2.

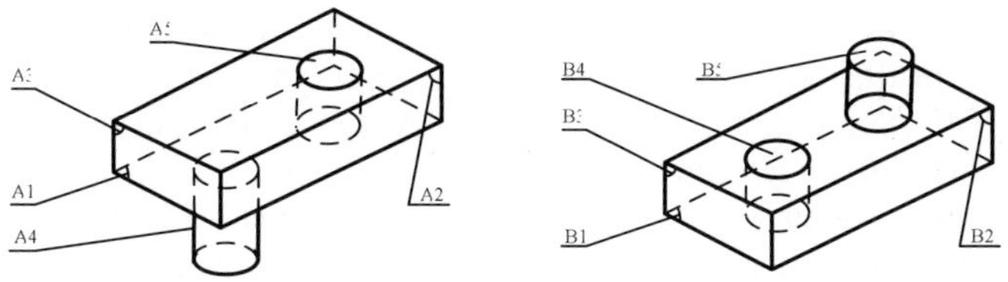

Fig. 10. Feature recognition of the assembly parts

Step 2: assembly function requirement and datum reference frame are determined. The assembly sequence is that: On the orientation of the major axis A4's face of Part A and the hole B4's face of Part B, the face of the hole A5 is mated with the face of the minor axis B5, then Part A and Part B is assembled. So, in the fourth known condition, assembly function requirement is the mating between Face A5 and B5, namely MT2 is a closed mate matrix. According to the third known condition, the datum reference frames of Part A and Part B are respectively that: DRF1: (A1, A2, A3) and DRF2: (B1,B2,B3) .

Step 3: loop circuit is generated. Based on Reference [2], only one loop circuit exists. The same kinds of mate trees among all the mate trees need to be determined. At first, it starts to search from closed mate tree MT2. Because the datum reference frame related with MT2 is DRF1 and DRF2, and according to the properties of mate tree, the kindred mate tree of MT2 is MT1, the next node searched by MT2 is DRF1, DRF2 or MT1. Using the related rules, the next node selected by MT2 is DRF1 or DRF2. The start node and end node of loop circuit both are MT2. Eventually, the loop circuit determined is as follows:

$$MT2 \rightarrow DRF1 \rightarrow MT1 \rightarrow DRF2 \rightarrow MT2$$

The MT of loop circuit is further divided into the loop circuit in which feature is used as node. It's shown as follows:

$$B5\_RF \xleftrightarrow{VGC0} A5\_RF \xleftarrow{VGC1} A5\_ADF \xleftarrow{VGC2,\ VGC3,\ VGC4} (A1\_ADF, A2\_ADF, A3\_ADF) \xrightarrow{VGC5,\ VGC6,\ VGC7} A4\_ADF \xrightarrow{VGC8} A4\_RF \xleftrightarrow{VGC9} B4\_RF \xleftarrow{VGC10} B4\_ADF \xleftarrow{VGC11,\ VGC12,\ VGC13} (B1\_ADF, B2\_ADF, B3\_ADF) \xrightarrow{VGC14,\ VGC15,\ VGC16} B5\_ADF \xrightarrow{VGC17} B5\_RF$$

in which ADF is associated derived feature, RF is real feature, → represents the path from referenced feature to constrained feature, ↔ represents that the two features connected by this path are referenced feature and constrained feature of each other.

In the following sections, based on polychromatic sets, the relations among the features in the above-mentioned loop circuits are reasoned so as to obtain VGC types between different features.

A5_RF ↔ A5_ADF: both are the real feature and associated derived feature of the same feature A5. So firstly they are judged to be SVGC, further more Feature A5 is cylindrical surface, so the colour of this feature tier is (0100000). Then using the generator matrix of SVGC (See Fig. 2), the colour of VGC tier can be obtained as (0100000), which represents that the feature is SVGC2.

A5_ADF ←A1_ADF: both are the associated derived feature of different features of the same part. So firstly they are judged as CVGC. By means of feature recognition, the colour of this feature tier is obtained as (0100000). Then using the generator matrix of CVGC (See Fig. 5), the colour of VGC tier can be achieved as (0100000), which represents that the feature is CVGC22.

In the same way, other VGC types also can be reasoned out. The VGC types and their degrees of freedom are added into loop circuit as follows:

$$B5\_RF \xleftrightarrow[Tx,\ Ty,\ Rx,\ Ry]{MVGC2} A5\_RF \xleftarrow[Tx,\ Ty,\ Rx,\ Ry]{SVGC2} A5\_ADF \xleftarrow[Tx,\ Ty,\ Rx,\ Ry]{CVGC21,\ CVGC21,\ CVGC22} (A1\_ADF, A2\_ADF, A3\_ADF) \xrightarrow[Tx,\ Ty,\ Rx,\ Ry]{CVGC21,\ CVGC21,\ CVGC22} A4\_ADF \xrightarrow[Tx,\ Ty,\ Rx,\ Ry]{SVGC2}$$

$$A4\_RF \xleftrightarrow[Tx,\ Ty,\ Rx,\ Ry]{MVGC2} B4\_RF \xleftarrow[Tx,\ Ty,\ Rx,\ Ry]{SVGC2} B4\_ADF \xleftarrow[Tx,\ Ty,\ Rx,\ Ry]{CVGC21,\ CVGC21,\ CVGC22} (B1\_ADF, B2\_ADF, B3\_ADF) \xrightarrow[Tx,\ Ty,\ Rx,\ Ry]{CVGC21,\ CVGC21,\ CVGC22} B5\_ADF \xrightarrow[Tx,\ Ty,\ Rx,\ Ry]{SVGC2} B5\_RF$$

in which Tx, Ty are the translational DOFs, and Rx, Ry are the rotational DOFs respectively.

Step 4: complete constraint is evaluated. The path of loop circuit in Step 3 can be further decomposed. For example, the following path:

$$A5\_ADF \xleftarrow[Tx,\ Ty,\ Rx,\ Ry]{CVGC21,\ CVGC21,\ CVGC22} (A1\_ADF, A2\_ADF, A3\_ADF)$$

which is divided shown in Fig. 11.

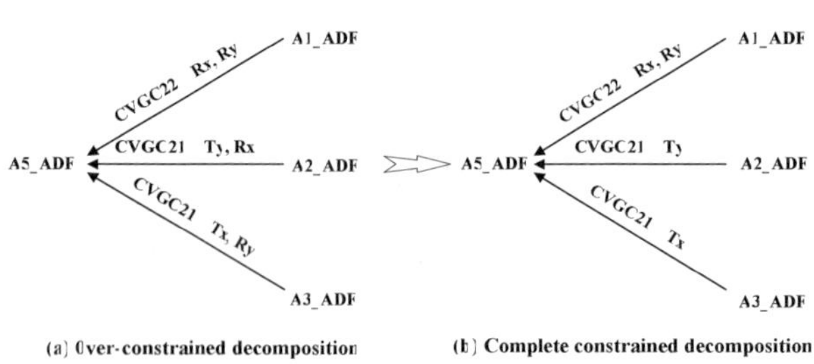

Fig. 11. Evaluation for complete constraint

According to the corresponding rules, A5_ADF in Fig. 11 (a) has over constraints, because for the degree of freedom Ry, there are two different connections between referenced feature and constrained feature. Based on judgement rules, the decomposed figure (See Fig. 11 (b)) reduced over constraints has been completely constrained. Similarly, other paths can also be decomposed. Eventually, loop circuit is divided into two components, in which one along the translational directions of X-axis and Y-axis aiming at controlling the translational DOFs, namely Tx and Ty required by assembly function, is shown as follows:

$$\mathrm{B5\_RF} \xleftrightarrow[\mathrm{Tx,\ Ty}]{\mathrm{MVGC2}} \mathrm{A5\_RF} \xleftarrow[\mathrm{Tx,\ Ty}]{\mathrm{SVGC2}} \mathrm{A5\_ADF} \xleftarrow[\mathrm{Tx,\ Ty}]{\mathrm{CVGC21,\ CVGC21}}$$

$$(\mathrm{A2\_ADF,A3\_ADF}) \xrightarrow[\mathrm{Tx,\ Ty}]{\mathrm{CVGC21,\ CVGC21}} \mathrm{A4\_ADF} \xrightarrow[\mathrm{Tx,\ Ty}]{\mathrm{SVGC2}} \mathrm{A4\_RF}$$

$$\xleftrightarrow[\mathrm{Tx,\ Ty}]{\mathrm{MVGC2}} \mathrm{B4\_RF} \xleftarrow[\mathrm{Tx,\ Ty}]{\mathrm{SVGC2}} \mathrm{B4\_ADF} \xleftarrow[\mathrm{Tx,\ Ty}]{\mathrm{CVGC21,\ CVGC21}}$$

$$(\mathrm{B2\_ADF,B3\_ADF}) \xrightarrow[\mathrm{Tx,\ Ty}]{\mathrm{CVGC21,\ CVGC21}} \mathrm{B5\_ADF} \xrightarrow[\mathrm{Tx,\ Ty}]{\mathrm{SVGC2}} \mathrm{B5\_RF}$$

and another along the rotational directions of X-axis and Y-axis aiming at controlling the rotational DOFs, namely Rx and Ry required by assembly function, is shown as follows:

$$B5\_RF \xleftrightarrow[Rx,\ Ry]{MVGC2} A5\_RF \xleftarrow[Rx,\ Ry]{SVGC2} A5\_ADF$$

$$\xleftarrow[Rx,\ Ry]{CVGC22} (A1\_ADF) \xrightarrow[Rx,\ Ry]{CVGC22} A4\_ADF$$

$$\xrightarrow[Rx,\ Ry]{SVGC2} A4\_RF \xleftrightarrow[Rx,\ Ry]{MVGC2} B4\_RF \xleftarrow[Rx,\ Ry]{SVGC2}$$

$$B4\_ADF \xleftarrow[Rx,\ Ry]{CVGC21,\ CVGC21,\ CVGC22} (B1\_ADF)$$

$$\xrightarrow[Rx,\ Ry]{CVGC22} B5\_ADF \xrightarrow[Rx,\ Ry]{SVGC2} B5\_RF$$

The components of loop circuit respectively along the translational directions of X-axis and Y-axis and the rotational directions of X-axis and Y-axis can be integrated into a loop circuit. The above loop circuit constitutes VGCN because there is only one assembly functional requirement.

To summarize and compare the above contents , it can be found that all the constrained features in VGCN which has been eventually generated in the first stage are well constrained.

2) The second stage: generating the tolerance types and constructing the tolerance network.

Step 1: the information of VGCs is extracted. All the types of VGC, constrained features and referenced features are extracted from the well-constrained VGCN generated in the first stage.

Step 2: the tolerance types are determined. Each constrained feature is regarded as the tolerance feature. Using the reasoning matrix, each tolerance type of VGCs is determined and standardized.

For example, the component's path of loop circuit along the rotational direction of X-axis and Y-axis is shown as follows:

$$A5\_ADF \xleftarrow[Rx,\ Ry]{CVGC22} (A1\_ADF)\ ,$$

in which the CVGC belongs to the twenty-second type of CVGC, namely CVGC22, so the colour of its second tier is (0 0 0 0 1 0 0 0 0 0). According to the generator matrix of CVGC (See Fig. 9), it can be known that the colour of its third tier is (0 1 0 0 0 0 0 0 0 0), and it represents that squareness tolerance needs to be marked. Thereupon, squareness tolerance is added to the following path:

$$A5\_ADF \xleftarrow[Rx,\ Ry\ \perp]{CVGC\,22} (A1\_ADF)\ .$$

The component's path of loop circuit along the translational direction of X-axis and Y-axis is shown as follows:

$$A5\_ADF \xleftarrow[Tx,\ Ty]{CVGC\,21} (A1\_ADF)\ ,$$

in which the CVGC belongs to the twenty-first type of CVGC, namely CVG21, so the colour of its second tier is (0 0 0 1 0 0 0 0 0 0). According to the generator matrix of CVGC (See Fig. 9), it can be known that the colour of its third tier is (1 0 0 0 0 1 0 0 1 0), and it represents that the following tolerances are required to be marked: parallelism tolerance, position tolerance or location dimension tolerance. Since assembly function has a requirement for the translational directions along X-axis and Y-axis, position tolerances are selected to control position variation along the direction of X-axis and Y-axis.

$$B5\_RF \xleftrightarrow[Tx,\ Ty]{MVGC\,2} A5\_RF \xleftarrow[Tx,\ Ty\ \pm]{SVGC\,2} A5\_ADF$$
$$\xleftarrow[Tx,\ Ty\ \oplus]{CVGC\,21,\ CVGC\,21} (A2\_ADF, A3\_ADF)$$
$$\xrightarrow[Tx,\ Ty\ \oplus]{CVGC\,21,\ CVGC\,21} A4\_ADF \xrightarrow[Tx,\ Ty\ \pm]{SVGC\,2} A4\_RF$$
$$\xleftrightarrow[Tx,\ Ty]{MVGC\,2} B4\_RF \xleftarrow[Tx,\ Ty\ \pm]{SVGC\,2} B4\_ADF$$
$$\xleftarrow[Tx,\ Ty\ \oplus]{CVGC\,21,\ CVGC\,21} (B2\_ADF, B3\_ADF)$$
$$\xrightarrow[Tx,\ Ty\ \oplus]{CVGC\,21,\ CVGC\,21} B5\_ADF \xrightarrow[Tx,\ Ty\ \pm]{SVGC\,2} B5\_RF$$

(a)

$$B5\_RF \xleftrightarrow[Rx,\ Ry]{MVGC\,2} A5\_RF \xleftarrow[Rx,\ Ry]{SVGC\,2} A5\_ADF$$
$$\xleftarrow[Rx,\ Ry\ \perp]{CVGC\,22} (A1\_ADF) \xrightarrow[Rx,\ Ry\ \perp]{CVGC\,22} A4\_ADF$$
$$\xrightarrow[Rx,\ Ry]{SVGC\,2} A4\_RF \xleftrightarrow[Rx,\ Ry]{MVGC\,2} B4\_RF \xleftarrow[Rx,\ Ry]{SVGC\,2}$$
$$B4\_ADF \xleftarrow[Rx,\ Ry\ \perp]{CVGC\,21,\ CVGC\,21,\ CVGC\,22} (B1\_ADF)$$
$$\xrightarrow[Rx,\ Ry\ \perp]{CVGC\,22} B5\_ADF \xrightarrow[Rx,\ Ry]{SVGC\,2} B5\_RF$$

(b)

Fig. 12. The tolerance network components

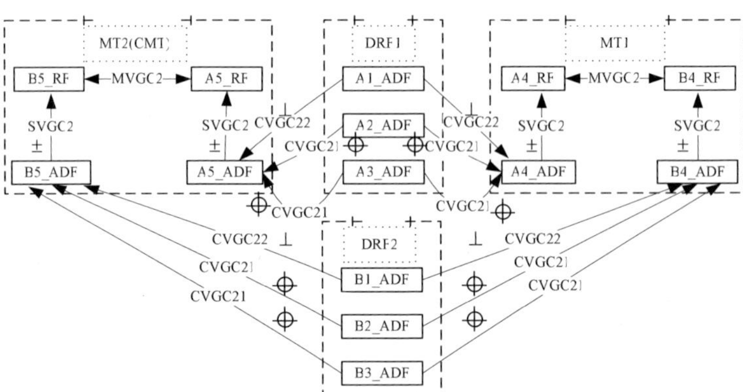

Fig. 13. Well-constrained tolerance network

The position tolerance information is added to the path:

$$A5\_ADF \xleftarrow[Tx,\ Ty\ \oplus]{CVGC\,21} (A1\_ADF)$$

In the same way, the other types of tolerance can be reasoned out.

Step 3: the tolerance network is constructed.

All the tolerances generated in Step 2 are respectively added to the loop circuit constructed in the first stage to form the tolerance network components. The component along the translation direction of X-axis and Y-axis is shown in Fig. 12 (a) and another one along the direction of rotation of X-axis and Y-axis is shown in Fig. 12 (b). The well-constrained tolerance network finally generated is shown in Fig. 13.

5 Conclusions

In this paper, the main research works are as follows:

1) A hierarchical representation model of tolerance information reasoning was presented.

2) Using the polychromatic sets theory, the feature tier and the VGC tier were described. By means of the reasoning matrix between the unified colours and individual colours of the polychromatic sets, the reasoning of tolerance types was realized. At the same time, the method and process of the reasoning were presented.

3) Using the hierarchical reasoning model of tolerance information and the reasoning method, the reasoning of tolerance types was achieved in the process of generating tolerance network for assembly.

Compared with previous studies, the hierarchical model of tolerance reasoning and the reasoning omitted reasoning rules in the reasoning process, realized automatic generation of tolerance types and provided a basis for further formalization of tolerance information reasoning.

Acknowledgements

The authors are grateful to the National Natural Science Foundation of China (NSFC) for supporting this research under Grant Number 60773117. The research conditions are provided by State Key Laboratory for Manufacturing Systems Engineering, Xi'an, China.

References

1. Hu, J., Wu, Z.T.: Methods for generation of variational geometric constraints network for assembly. J. Journal of Computer-aided Design & Computer Graphics 14(1), 79–82 (2002)
2. Hu, J.: Study on theories and methods of geometric tolerance design based on variational geometric constraints network: [A dissertation for the degree of doctor of philosophy]. Zhejiang University, Zhejiang (2001)
3. Zhang, B., Li, Z.B.: Modeling of tolerance information and reasoning technique study using polychromatic sets. J. Chinese Journal of Mechanical Engineering 41(10), 111–116 (2005)
4. Pavlov, V.V.: Mathematics simulation of discrete production system. J. Information Technology 0, 15–19 (1995)

5. Pavlov, V.V.: Polychromatic sets and graphs for CALS technology. STANKIN Press, Moscow (2000)
6. Tong, Y.G., Li, Z.B., Li, S.C.: Formalized solution of conceptual design based on polychromatic sets. J. Journal of Xi'an Jiaotong University 38(1), 68–72 (2004)
7. Pavlov, V.V.: Polychromatic sets and graphs for CALS in machine building. Science Press, Moscow (2006)

Role Identification and Reallocation of a Distributed Sensor Network in Manufacturing Floor

Bo Tao, Han Ding, and Youlun Xiong

National Key Lab. of Digital Equipment and Tech., Huazhong University of Sci. and Tech., Wuhan, Hubei, China
{taobo,dinghan,famt}@mail.hust.edu.cn

Abstract. Modern manufacturing plants have a desperate need for large amounts of sensor information, to refine and improve their production. A device description sheet mechanism for distributed sensor network is presented in this paper to continue the previous research of the IP sensor. In the new proposal, two key problems, including the self-identification and the dynamic reallocation of each sensor's role at *run-time* for a large sensor network, are efficiently settled. Also, a virtual mapping mechanism, named transducer domain name server, is also presented, with the help of which, the reallocation of each sensor's role at *run-time* is achieved by performing a dynamic binding between the devices monitored and the IP sensors. All of the methods presented will be an important step to seek for a practical use at the production floor.

Keywords: Manufacturing Automation, Distributed Sensor Network, IP Sensor, Device Description Sheet.

1 Introduction

Sensors and actuators have been widely used for decades in production situations to monitor and control critical industrial processes or equipments [1-3]. It has been a necessity to gather complete and detailed information to ensure operation security in today's modern productions. However, due to the limited sensing range, the information obtained by each sensor only includes a very small portion of the production. Evidently, only a few sensors cannot achieve such a mission with the accuracy and efficiency required. In fact, this problem will be further enlarged with the improvement of automation of the manufacturing process, where more and more production information need be available to ensure the productivity and quality. To overcome this problem, many sensors are networked together to co-gather the information needed, bringing the birth of distributed sensor network (DSN), where many spatially dispersed sensors, mounted on or near the production machines, are connected together according to some rules or protocols to collaboratively perform some tasks, such as collecting the necessary equipment status information.

However, difficulties arise when creating a sensor network. Among them, several key obstacles must be overcome firstly when seeking for a practical use at the factory floor. First is the establishment of network connection. This problem is equal to how to connect numerous sensors to each other and how to connect the sensors to network.

C. Xiong et al. (Eds.): ICIRA 2008, Part II, LNAI 5315, pp. 869–878, 2008.

Establishing connections between sensor nodes is easy while the number of sensor nodes is small. However, the number of connections will increase exponentially with the increment of sensors participated. The second problem is the identification of heterogeneous sensors. In a sensor network, the functions and types of sensors may differ greatly from each other if the roles of sensors differ. It is unimaginable to deal with this problem without an automatic processing mechanism, especially for a large sensor network. Another problem is the reallocation of sensors' role at *run-time*. Information to be collected is usually situation dependent and application specific. In some case, several sensors are cooperated for a same purpose while in another case they may work independently. Therefore, it was preferable if each sensor's role could be reallocated during *run-time*. Unfortunately, no sufficient publications have been found in the literature to solve these problems.

To overcome these problems aforementioned, a novel web-enabled networked sensor model namely IP sensor, conforming to the well-known IEEE 1451 transducer standard [4, 5], has been presented in our previous research [6], where numerous sensors equipped with TCP/IP protocols can be networked together via Ethernet and direct communication is allowable among sensors without the participation of a central server. In this way the obstacle to establish network connection for a sensor network disappears. In this paper, a device description sheet mechanism for distributed sensor network is presented, by which, the two problems left, i.e. the self-identification and the reallocation of each sensor's role at *run-time* for a large sensor network, are efficiently settled. Also, a virtual mapping mechanism, named transducer domain name server, is also presented, with the help of which, the reallocation of each sensor's role at *run-time* is achieved by performing a dynamic binding between the devices monitored and the sensors. Doubtlessly, sensors are the core and the soul of a sensor network and dominate the development of the sensor network. Therefore, before describing the work of this paper, it is necessary to digress for a brief introduction of the IP sensor firstly.

2 Architecture of IP Sensors

Generally speaking, the IP sensor model is mainly composed of two functional blocks, namely IP module (IPM) and smart transducer interface module (STIM), which are connected to each other using a well-defined dual-port buffered interface (DPBI). For expansion purpose, physical link between more STIMs and one IPM is enabled by DPBI and one-to-more data transfer mechanism is achieved. Among them, the STIM is used to achieve the sensing activities of a sensor and provides all the needed functions to transform a simple sensor into a smart one, while the IPM, which provides an interaction mechanism based on TCP/IP protocol to support client-server communication, is exclusively responsible to deal with the accesses of the sensor to the Internet. A further description about the IP sensor model is omitted herein, which can be found in reference [6]. In return, one typical working prototype of an IP sensor achieved is shown in Fig.1.

Comparing to the IEEE 1451 standard, a thin-server/fat-client networking model is presented in IP sensor, where the virtual peripheral and component techniques of window 2000 are used. In return, the complex network-independent information model, defined in IEEE 1451.1, can be implemented using a web-enabled ActiveX or Java Applet method, which will be downloaded and run on the local computer during the working phase, instead of the sensor itself. It cancels the excessive need of high performance microprocessor when designing a smart sensor. IP sensor model provides an application interaction mechanism based on TCP/IP protocol to support peer-to-peer communication. If an IP sensor wants to transfer data with other IP sensor (called interesting sensor), it will first create a logical port and then bind itself to this active port. After the address parsing procedure to find the interesting sensor is achieved, the two sensors are bound logically through a port-specific pair. Once bound, data transfer starts. This procedure is similar to the standardized socket-based programming method, where a socket is created and bound with an application specific port number and IP address. It should be mentioned that to achieve the purpose mentioned above, each IP sensor must be assigned a network address like a PC does for a unique identifier, by which an IP sensor can be accessible by any other IP sensor or computer located in the Intranet. Possessing the distinguished characteristics to enable direct communication among sensors, IP sensors open a charming chance for distributed measurement system in manufacturing floor. However, two key obstacles, i.e. identification and reallocation, must be overcome firstly before they are put into use. In the next section, a device description sheet mechanism is presented, by which the two problems aforementioned are solved.

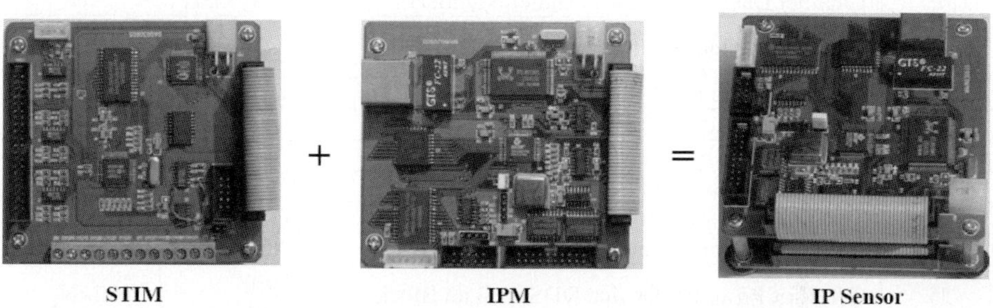

Fig. 1. A working prototype of a typical IP sensor

3 Device Description Sheet Mechanism

Sensors have been used for manufacturing automation for decades. Usually these sensors are heterogeneous and have various functions and types for different sensing purpose, such as temperature sensor, pressure sensor, etc. In fact, even for same type sensors, their output may differ. Hence, how to describe these various sensors using a standardized mechanism, which can ease the identification of sensors, is an important issue. In a sensor network, the functions and types of sensors may differ greatly from each other if the roles of sensors participated differ. It is hard imaginable to deal with the identification without an automatic processing mechanism, especially for a large sensor network. Electronic Description Sheet (EDS) is a feasible choice to achieve equipment self-description. EDS is not a new concept, which contains fields that could fully describe the type, operations, and attributes of the equipments. It makes system easier to implement. In fact, companies have been embedding data structure in memory associated with their products for many years. Among them, USB standard is the most famous one. USB standard provides a standardized and machine-readable attribute definition for each USB enabled equipment, which can be identified by most main-dream operating systems and makes USB equipment driver-free. In our opinion, TEDS is one of the most important innovations introduced by IEEE 1451 standard, which presents a general model for transducer to support a wide variety of sensors and actuators. However, for a generalization purpose, no sufficient concerns for application-specific purpose are involved. In this paper, an EDS for networked sensors, namely device description sheet (DDS), is presented stemming from TEDS.

Table 1. Data structure of device-related DDS data block

Field No.	Description	Type	Bytes
1	Device DDS Length	U32L	4
2	Number of Language of Device DDS = L	U8C	1
3	String Language Code List	Array U8E	L
Field 4-27 are repeated L times, once for each supported language			
4	Language Sub-Block Length	U16L	2
5	String Specification of Sub-Block	STRING	3
6	Terminal Type (0 is IP Sensor, 1 is EmAgent)	U8C	1
7	Channel Data Type (N is Channel Number)	Array U8C	N
8	Terminal Channel Buffer Length List	Array U32C	4×N
9	Global Unique Identifier of Terminal	UUID	10
10	Terminal IP Address	Array U8C	4
11	Terminal Port Number	U16C	2
12	Terminal Description Length	U16L	2
13	Terminal Description	STRING	≤65536
14	Device Number Bound with Terminal = N_1	U8C	1
15	Offset of Primitive Device DDS in Data Block	Array U16C	$2\times N_1$
Field No. 16-24 are repeated N_1 times, once for each primitive device DDS			
16	Unique Identifier of Device Bound	U16C	2
17	Name of Device Bound with Terminal	STRING	≤255
18	Device Description Length	U16L	2
19	Device Description	STRING	≤65536
20	Object Number of Device Bound = N_2	U8C	1
Field No. 21-24 are repeated N_2 times, once for each object of primitive devices			
21	Object Description Length	U16L	2
22	Object Description	STRING	≤65536
23	Upper Range Limit List	Array F64	$8\times N_2$
24	Lower Range Limit List	Array F64	$8\times N_2$
25	Number of Group Broadcast Participated = N_3	U8C	1
26	Group Broadcast Address List	Array U32C	$4\times N_3$
27	Checksum for Language Sub-Block	U16C	2
28	Checkup for Device DDS	U16C	2

In a DDS, eight different DDS sections are defined, where Meta DDS, Channel DDS, Device DDS, Service DDS are mandatory and must remain with the STIM for the duration of its lifetime. The other four, namely Calibration DDS, Meta identification DDS, Channel identification DDS, and Calibration identification DDS, are optional. The Meta TEDS, one for each sensor, contains data that describe the sensor as a whole, including revision levels, extensions, worst-case timing values, and channel grouping information. The Channel TEDS, one for each sensor channel, defines the functional model, calibration model, upper and lower limits, timing restrictions, and any other data needed to describe the functionality of each sensor channel. Among the eight sections, except for Device DDS and Service DDS, the other six sections are stemming from TEDS based on a customization for IP sensor purpose. The detailed data format is omitted herein. Device DDS and Service DDS are two new-added sections, defined for application-specific purpose for IP sensors. Their data frames are shown in Table 1 and 2 respectively.

Table 2. Data structure of service-related DDS data block

Field No.	Description	Type	Bytes
1	Service DDS Length	U32L	4
2	Number of Languages of Service DDS = L	U8C	1
3	String Language Code List	Array U8E	L
Field No. 4-18 are repeated L times, once for each supported language			
4	Language Sub-Block Length	U16L	2
5	String Specification of Sub-Block	STRING	3
6	Terminal Description Length	U16L	2
7	Terminal Description	STRING	≤65536
8	Number of Services Supported = N	U8C	1
9	Offset of Primitive Service DDS in Data Block	Array U16C	2×N
Field No. 10-17 are repeated N times, once for each supported primitive service			
10	Global Unique Identifier of Primitive Service	UUID	10
11	Primitive Service Description Length	U16L	2
12	Primitive Service Description	STRING	≤65536
13	Entry Address of Primitive Service	U8C	1
14	Number of Input Parameters = N_1	U8C	1
15	Input Parameters Type List	Array U8E	N_1
16	Number of Output Parameters = N_2	U8C	1
17	Output Parameters Type List	Array U8E	N_2
18	Checksum of Language Sub-Block	U16C	2
19	Checksum of Service DDS Block	U16C	2

4 Identification and Reallocation of DSN

An IP sensor is much different from the traditional sensor. It is more than a sensor simply but an Internet intelligent node with sensing capability. Adopting the unified TCP/IP communication protocols, the sensor network based on the IP sensors will benefit from all of the advantages of Ethernet technology, such as integration, plug and play, and the cross platform interoperability. All of these will bring the IP sensor distinguished characteristics and open new challenge for the creation of a distributed sensor network.

4.1 Identification of IP Sensors in DSN

With the increment of the sensor number in a sensor network, the administration to so many sensors become very complicate and become another new challenge. In addition, the functions of IP sensors are also different from each other due to the role difference of IP sensors. So it is unimaginable to deal with sensor identification without an automatic processing mechanism, especially for a large sensor network. Fortunately, DDS can be used to solve this problem. As stated above, a DDS provides a permanent repository of information related to the sensor, including fields that could fully describe the type, operation, and attributes of the sensor. Equipped with a DDS, an IP sensor could tell the network what it is and what it can do. In a real application, a DDS is written as a formatted electronic document and stored in a non-volatile memory, including the channel number, sensing type, calibration model with the corresponding coefficients, and any other necessary information used to fully describe the functionality of an IP sensor. During the sensor identification phase, the DDS data is sent to the central server, either automatically at power up or upon a request, to report what kind of sensors are being connected to the sensor network. In this way, it is very convenient for users to manage and update the sensor related information. In a distributed sensor network, all of the DDS data from each IP sensor in the local network is organized into a sensor information database, and a computer is usually assigned as the central server, responsible to maintain and update such a database. If a sensor node requests some function that may be implemented in another sensor node, the central server can lookup the database and redirect the request to the right destination. A program to implement the identification has been developed, and an identification procedure is shown in Fig.2.

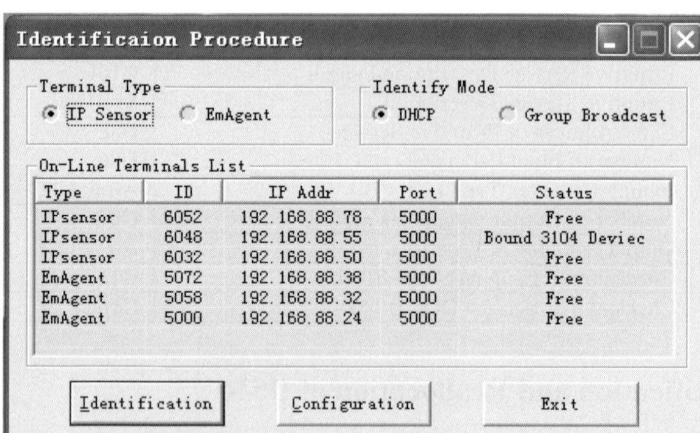

Fig. 2. Identification procedure of IP sensor in a DSN

To support web-enabled accessing, the DDS data has been formatted in a XML document in our solution, conforming to the web service description language. The lookup procedure is probably very complicated and is a large workload for a resource-limited sensor node, but fortunately, the mechanism proposed only needs the central server to handle the lookup procedure in one sensor network. Hence, this method will not bring extra burdens to the resource-limited sensor nodes. Each IP sensor possesses its own DDS that is written after the IP sensor is manufactured ahead the first use.

4.2 Reallocation of IP Sensors in DSN

In a distributed networking sensing and control system, all the operations or manipulations are achieved through various transducers. However, it is neither convenient nor according with the operation custom to ask the end-user to remember a task or a device by use of a sensor ID. This is boring similar to ask a person to remember a PC through its network address. In fact, in some cases, several sensors are used for a same purpose. Evidently, the way to achieve an operation based on the task name or the device name is preferable. For example, the end-user would like to remember the words such as "lathe" or "current output" in a workshop application. Moreover, to meet the reconfiguration of a production line, the sensors' roles are usually changing due to the change of the application purpose. For example, in one case, several sensors are cooperated to monitor a machine's status while in another case they may work independently. Therefore, it is preferable if each sensor's role can be reallocated at *run-time*. In our solution, a virtual mapping mechanism, called TDNS, is presented based on DDS method to solve these two problems mentioned above and described below.

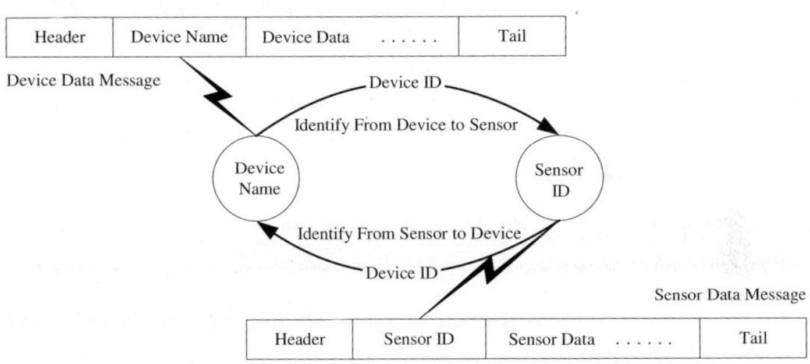

Fig. 3. Data identify between IP sensors and the device bound based on TDNS

A full DDS includes two classes of device attributes of each IP sensor, i.e. static attributes and dynamic attributes. For a brief writing, in this section only the attributes necessary for TDNS are mentioned. There are three important device attributes necessary for TDNS. Among them, sensor ID is a static attribute that is written to each IP sensor ahead its first use and cannot be modified during its lifetime. However, device ID and device name are dynamic attributes, which are configured by the end-user before each use according to the correlation of an IP sensor and a device. Dynamic attributes keep unchanged until the end-use modifies them explicitly. It should be noticed that in one system, the two dynamic attributes of two IP sensors must keep different, while they can keep identical if the two sensors are located in two systems respectively. During the system configuration phase, an Attribute-Mapping Table

(AMT) is built up by the central server based on the DDS information of each IP sensor. An AMT records all the correlations of each device and the corresponding sensors, which is the reference of the later operations. During the data identify phase, based on the mapping correlations between a device ID and a sensor ID, the system can understand exactly which device the data published by an IP sensor belongs to, or which sensor the command subscribed by a device belongs to. Fig.3 depicts the principle for data identify between IP sensors and the device bound, which has been achieved, as shown in Fig.4.

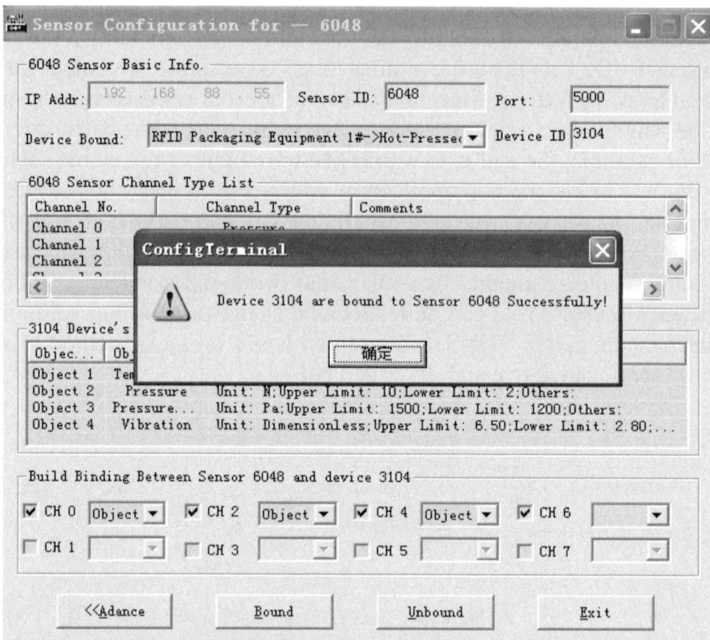

Fig. 4. Data identify between IP sensors and the device bound based on TDNS

4.3 Peer-to-Peer DSN Architecture

As well known, Ethernet is a peer-to-peer network, widely accepted all over the world as a de facto standard for many years. Adopting the Ethernet with TCP/IP protocols, it is very natural and simple to create a peer-to-peer DSN, similar to the creation of a computer network via Ethernet. Herein, the so-called peer-to-peer sensor network architecture means that direct communication is allowable between any two sensors in such a DSN without the interaction of a central server. This is very useful in a highly autonomous monitoring and control system. For example, within the DSN of a production line, if a sensor wants to know whether the previous process step has been performed successfully, it can inquire the previous sensor node directly, not the central server. This will reduce the amount of information on the network greatly. All the information will come directly from the source.

A peer-to-peer DSN architecture based on IP sensors is depicted in Fig.5 (b). For comparison, a typical Fieldbus based solution is also given in Fig.5 (a). It can be found from Fig.5 (a) that adopting Fieldbus, the workshop control network is usually a master-slave architecture, where many sensors are connected to a central server using a star-link. This means only the central server can poll all the sensors, and direct communication between two sensors is unallowable. Moreover, workshop networks are separated not only from each other but also from the office LAN. To enable the information flow between device level and management level, a gateway is needed for protocol translating between control network and information network. Such a solution always has a pyramidal architecture. Evidently, it is not only inefficient but also resulting in data transfer bottleneck. All of the deficiencies disappear with the new proposal of Fig.5 (b), where Ethernet with TCP/IP protocols is the common backbone of workshop network and office LAN. In the new proposal the control network and information network are integrated seamlessly into a unified enterprise information network. All the nodes, either computers or sensors, are autonomous and coequal to each other in the Intranet. Cross system interoperability is feasible. That means all the information either from management level or from device level can be shared by each other. Moreover, with the support of web-enabled capability, any authorized administrator can access the built-in web pages to brow the information obtained by an IP sensor by use of the Internet Explorer or Netscape widely used by the office automation.

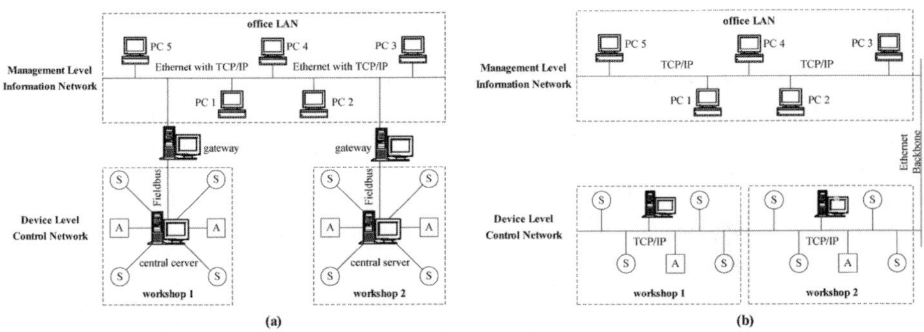

Fig. 5. Comparison of two kind of sensor network architecture: (a) Traditional with a pyramidal architecture, and (b) New proposal. A represents an actuator, and S represents a sensor.

5 Conclusions

Modern manufacturing plants have a desperate need for large amounts of sensor information, to refine and improve their production. As the amount of sensors grows, the sensor network grows rapidly. How to solve the connection establishment of a large sensor network as well as the reallocation of each sensor's role at *run-time* becomes new challenge. Continuing the previous research of the IP sensor, a device description sheet mechanism, stemming from the TEDS format of IEEE 1451 standard, is presented to achieve the self-identification and self-description of each IP sensor in a DSN environment. Moreover, a virtual mapping mechanism named TDNS is also presented to perform the dynamic binding between the devices monitored and the IP sensors, which can be used to achieve the reallocation of each sensor's role at *run-time*. All of the efforts in this paper will provide a strong support for distributed measurement system in manufacturing floor.

Acknowledgments

This work is partially supported by National Fundamental Research Program of China under Grant 2007CB714005, the National Science Foundation of China under Grant No. 50625516 and the China Postdoctoral Fund under the grant of 20070420173.

References

1. Baer, W.G., Lally, R.W.: An open-standard smart sensor architecture and system for industrial automation. In: IEEE Aerospace Conference Proceedings, Big Sky, MT, USA, March 18-25 (2000)
2. Seveda, M., Vrba, R.: Integrated Smart Sensor Networking Framework for Sensor-Based Appliances. IEEE Sensors Journal 3, 579–586 (2003)
3. Lee, K.B., Schneeman, R.D.: Distributed Measurement and Control Based on the IEEE 1451 Smart Transducer Interface Standards. In: Proceedings of the Instrumentation Measurement Conference (IMTC 1999), Venice, Italy, May 24-28 (1999)
4. The Institute of Electrical and Electronics Engineers. IEEE Standard for a Smart Transducer Interface for Sensors and Actuators – Transducer to Microprocessor Communication Protocols and Transducer Electronic Data Sheet (TEDS) Formats. IEEE Std. 1451.2-1997 (1997)
5. The Institute of Electrical and Electronics Engineers: IEEE Standard for a Smart Transducer Interface for Sensors and Actuators – Network Capable Application Processor (NCAP) Information Model. IEEE Std. 1451.1-1999 (1999)
6. Tao, B., Ding, H., Xiong, Y.L.: Design and Implementation of an Embedded IP Sensor for Distributed Networking Sensing. Sensors and Actuators A 119, 567–575 (2005)

Dynamic Modeling of Large Scale Heavy Duty Grippers Based on the Response Dead Zone of Counteracting Force

Jingfei He, Yan Chen, Hua Deng, and Rongguang Nie

College of Mechanical & Electrical Engineering, Central South University, Changsha 410083, China
chenyanchenzhou@126.com

Abstract. This paper presents the concept of the response dead zone of counteracting force through dividing the mechanism operation into forward movement state and reverse micro-movement state for the large scale gripper of heavy duty forging manipulators. All the gravity effect as well as the Coulomb friction at the joints is considered. It is shown that the Coulomb friction has a significant effect on the gripping force. Dynamic simulations by using ADAMS software shows that stable gripping can be achieved if the gripping force is within the response dead zone of counteracting force. The findings provide a theory basis for the operation and control of the large scale heavy duty grippers.

Keywords: Response Dead Zone of Counteracting Force, Gripper, Dynamic, Modeling.

1 Introduction

The dynamic effect of friction on the motion of light duty grippers is generally neglected. But for the large scale heavy duty gripper, the surge of friction coefficient at joints result from insufficient lubricant oil film to form dynamic pressure has significant effect on dynamics properties of gripper during alternating heavy load and non-consecutive etc work condition. Zhang Jingfu and Xu [1] found that the joint driven torque (or force) is much different when friction is considered. Bhaskar Dasgupta and Mruthyunjaya T.S. [2] modeled the viscous friction for the joint of the Steward platform and implemented the formulation. Many authors [3-7] have studied the friction model and its effects on mechanism, their researches pointed out the dynamic properties of mechanism can be much different if friction was included in the model. In this paper, the concept of the response dead zone of counteracting force was proposed by dividing the mechanism operation into forward movement state and reverse micro-movement state. Then the dynamic model of a typical gripper of forging manipulators was established with friction .The influence of the response dead zone of counteracting force on the dynamic properties of the gripper has been studied. Finally, influence of the response dead zone of counteracting force are validated through dynamic simulations.

C. Xiong et al. (Eds.): ICIRA 2008, Part II, LNAI 5315, pp. 879–886, 2008.

2 The Response Dead Zone of Counteracting Force

Under the impact or dynamic load, mechanical systems will have a reverse micro-movement tendency till the reverse micro-movement happens. Then, the mechanism dynamics changes from forward movement state (Fig.1) to reverse micro-movement state (Fig. 2):

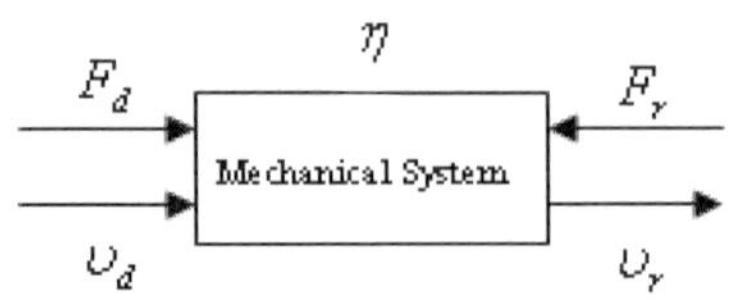

Fig. 1. Mechanical model of forward movement state

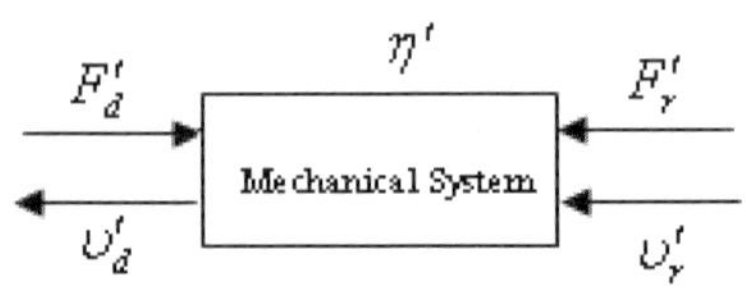

Fig. 2. Mechanical model of reverse micro-movement state

Fig. 1and Fig. 2 indicate that the driving force F_d has the same direction with its speed v_d when the system is in the forward movement state, while the direction of resistance F_r and its speed v_r are reverse. However, during the reverse micro-movement state, the input force becomes resistance force F_d' and has the reverse direction with its speed v_d' while the output force F_r' becomes driving force and has the same direction with its speed v_r'. The role of driving component and follower component was changed.

The mechanical efficiency in the forward movement state and in the reverse micro-movement state can be expressed as follows:

$$\eta = \frac{F_r \cdot v_r}{F_d \cdot v_d} \qquad \eta' = \frac{F_d' \cdot v_d'}{F_r' \cdot v_r'} \quad . \tag{1}$$

When the impact load or dynamic load is less than F_r', only reverse micro-movement tendency exists and impact load or dynamic load will not result in the change of input force because of joint friction effect, that is, $F_d' = F_d$. Consider that the instantaneous transmission ratio is unchanged, that is, $\frac{v_r}{v_d} = \frac{v_r'}{v_d'}$. Substituting the ration into (1) yields:

$$\eta\eta' = \frac{F_r}{F_r'} \ . \tag{2}$$

According to (2), one has $F_r' = \frac{F_r}{\eta\eta'} > F_r$. The input force F_d will not increase as work resistance force F_r increases until the impact load or dynamic load is larger than F_r'. Then reverse movement happens as the impact load or dynamic load is larger than F_r'. Thus, the response dead zone of counteracting force is defined as:

$$\mathrm{K} \in (F_r, F_r') \ . \tag{3}$$

3 Dynamic Modeling of Grippers

A typical gripper [8, 9] is composed of putting 1, link 2, gripper arm 3, jaw 4, bracket 5(see Fig. 3). During gripping F_0 is the driven force and the system is in forward movement state with its force model as shown in Fig. 3. During lifting and rotating, the system is in reverse micro-movement state and the gripper will have the tendency of reverse movement due to the counteracting force of forging on the jaw. The direction of the pair counteracting force will change as the friction circle from shearing to tangency and the force model is shown in Fig. 4.

Mechanical Model of mechanism established by Newton equation [2, 10, 11] is as follows:

$$\begin{cases} F_{ix} + F_{(i+1)x} = 0 \\ F_{iy} + F_{(i+1)y} - m_i g \cos\varphi = m_i \omega^2 R_{ic} \\ F_{iz} + F_{(i+1)z} - m_i g \sin\varphi = m_i R_{ic} a \\ M_{ix} + M_{(i+1)x} + F_{iz} r_{icy} + F_{(i+1)z} r_{(i+1)cy} = 0 \\ M_{iy} + M_{(i+1)y} + F_{iz} r_{icx} + F_{(i+1)z} r_{(i+1)cx} = 0 \\ M_{iz} + M_{(i+1)z} + F_{ix} r_{icy} + F_{(i+1)x} r_{(i+1)cy} - F_{iy} r_{icx} + F_{(i+1)y} r_{icx} + M_{fi} + M_{f(i+1)} = 0 \\ M_{fi} = r_i \bullet \kappa \sqrt{F_{ix}^2 + F_{iy}^2} \\ M_{f(i+1)} = r_{(i+1)} \bullet \kappa \sqrt{F_{(i+1)x}^2 + F_{(i+1)y}^2} \end{cases} \ . \tag{4}$$

where $i = 1,2,3,4$; $-F_i$ and $-M_i$ are the force and moment of the part i-1 exerted on the part i respectively, F_{i+1} and M_{i+1} are the force and moment of the part i+1 exerted on the part i respectively, ω and α are the angle velocity and acceleration of rotation respectively, R_{ic} is rotation radial of part i, r_{ic} is the distance from joint i to the mass center of part i, M_{fi} and $M_{f(i+1)}$ are the friction moment of pair i and i+1 respectively. r_i is the friction circle of joint i, κ is the tangent coefficient of constraint reaction at joint with friction circle with $\kappa \in (-1,1)$ .When κ =-1, constraint reaction tangent with friction circle is in clockwise and the mechanism is in forward movement state. When $\kappa = 1$, constraint reaction tangent with friction circle is in counterclockwise and the system is in reverse micro-movement state. The zone between this two critical forces F_r (named pre-gripping force) and F_r' (named critical-gripping force) is the response dead zone of counteracting force.

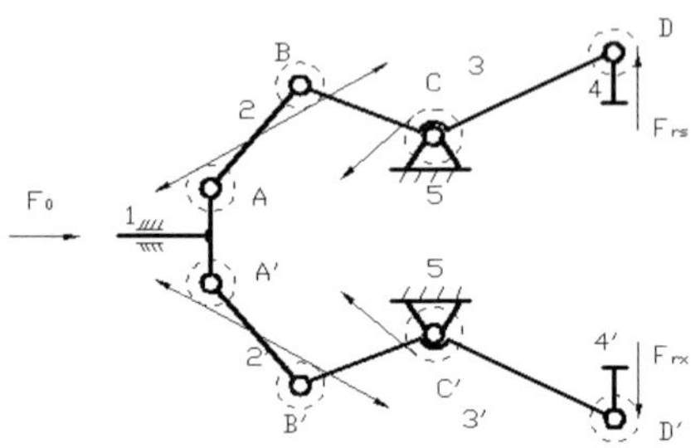

Fig. 3. Forward movement state

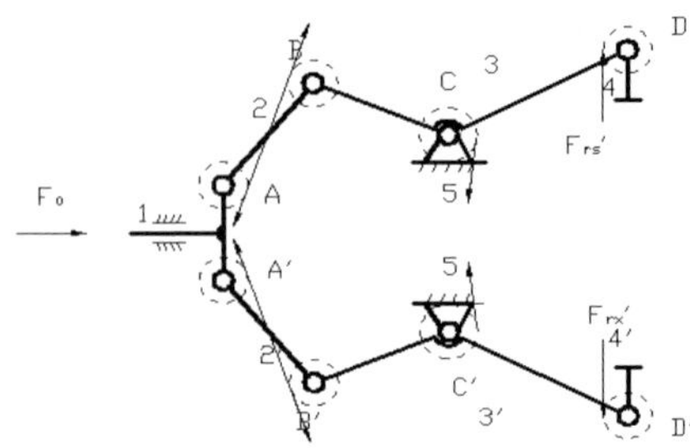

Fig. 4. Reverse micro-movement state

4 Example

The geometry parameters of the gripper are given as follows: L_2 =2.8m, L_{3B} =2.4m and L_{3F} =3.6m. h' =1.5m is the distance of joint A and A', h =2.7m is the distance of joint C and C'. The angle of forward and back gripper arm is θ =120.8°. Each joint friction circle r_A =0.06m、 r_B =0.09m、 r_C =0.06m and r_D =0.06m. The sliding coefficient of friction between jaw and work piece is 0.3. The performance parameters are as follows: Diameter and length of work piece is 2.26m and 8m. The driving force is F_0 =1000T. Initial position is in vertical direction. The pre-gripping force and critical-gripping force with respect to angle calculated by MATLAB [12] are shown in Fig. 5 and Fig.6, respectively.

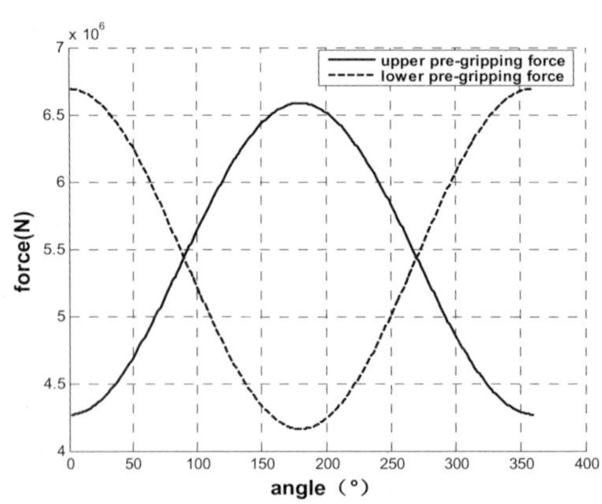

Fig. 5. Pre-gripping force

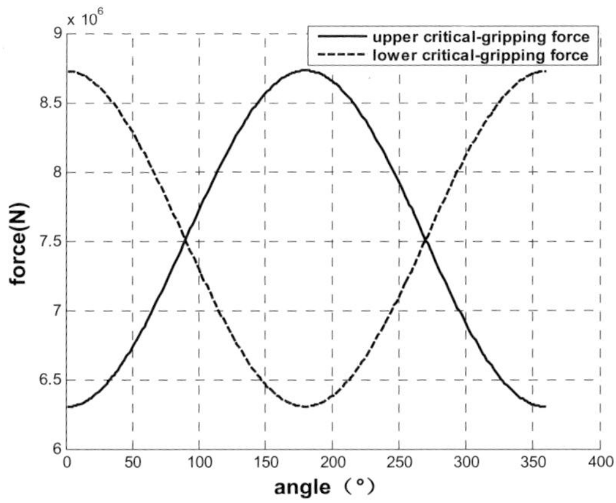

Fig. 6. Critical-gripping force

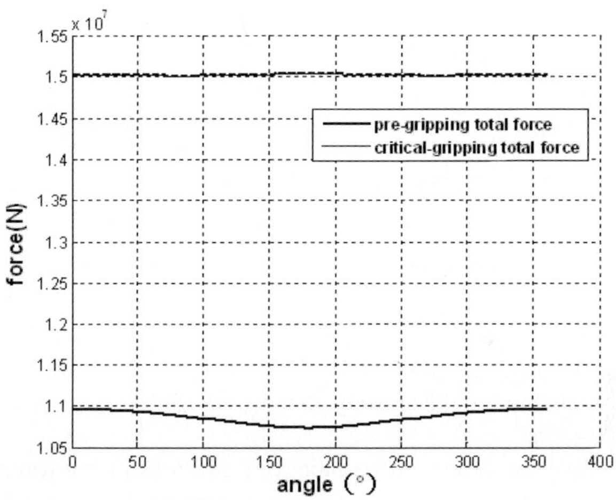

Fig. 7. Response dead zone of counteracting force

Fig.5 shows that, during forward movement state, the gripping force ranged from 4.25×10^6 N in upper position to 6.75×10^6 N in lower position. The difference of these two forces is the Y component of the gravity of the work-piece.

However, during reverse micro-movement state, the gripping force, as shown in Fig. 6, ranged from 6.3×10^6 N in upper position to 8.75×10^6 N in lower position and it is much larger than that in forward movement state with the same driven force.

The difference between the total pre-gripping force and the total critical-gripping force is the response dead zone of counteracting force, as shown in Fig. 7.

Fig.7 shows that the response dead zone of counteracting force is wide. If the practical gripping force is between these zones, stable gripping can be achieved. In this case, there is no need to increase the driven force to resist the dynamic force of mechanism rotating as the direction of friction force changes, which can increase the gripping capacity of the gripper.

5 Simulations by ADAMS

Dynamic simulations of mechanism during rotating by using ADAMS have been done and the gripping force is recorded as shown in Fig. 8.

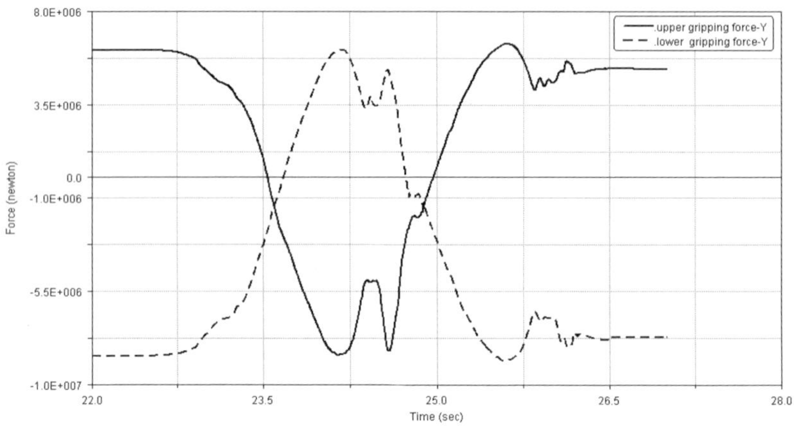

Fig. 8. Gripping force recorded in ADAMS.

The gripping force change is consistent with that calculated in MATLAB except a few fluctuations after rotating about 180 degrees. This is because the work-piece has no upward movement under the gravity during 90-180 degrees and it falls suddenly during 180-270 degrees.

In order to validate the effect of the pair friction on gripping force, the simulations of gripping force with and without pair friction are presented as Fig. 9.

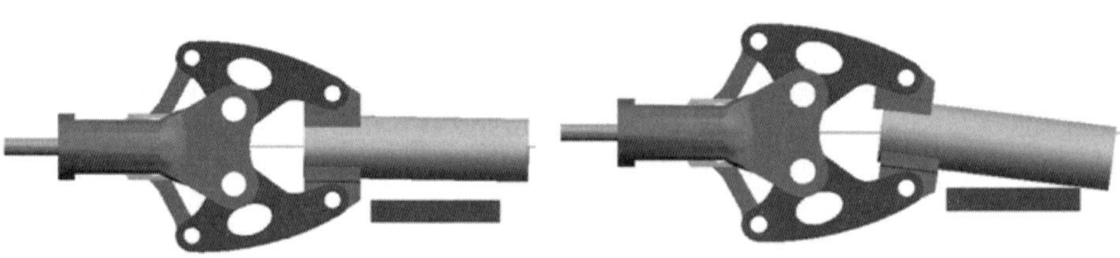

(a) With pair friction (b) Without pair friction

Fig. 9. Gripping effect

Fig.9(a) shows the deflection angle of the work-piece with the pair friction, Fig.10(b) shows the deflection angle of work-piece without the pair friction. The gripping force between the work-piece and the jaw is given in table 1.

Table 1. Data comparison of gripping force

Force/N	with friction	without friction
Maximum upper gripping force Y component	6.44×10^6	5.01×10^6
Maximum lower gripping force Y component	8.83×10^6	7.23×10^6
Maximum total gripping force Y component	1.527×10^7	1.224×10^7

The recorded gripping force with friction in ADAMS, as shown in table.1, are almost the same as that in micro-movement state calculated by MATLAB, which indicates that the model with joint friction is reasonable. In addition, gripping force with friction is larger than that without friction, which means that the joint friction is helpful to increasing the gripping force.

6 Conclusion

The concept of the response dead zone of counteracting force was proposed in this paper, and then the gripper has been established. Calculation and simulation results show that the response dead zone of counteracting force has significant effect on the dynamic properties of gripper. Therefore, the impact of the pair friction should be considered for the design and performance analysis of the large scale heavy duty grippers.

Acknowledgments

This work was supported by a grant from the National Basic Research Program of China(2006CB705400).

References

1. Zhang, J.F., Xu, Q.Y.: Inverse dynamic problem of manipulators with friction. J. Eng. Mech. 19(4), 104–108 (2004)
2. Bhaskar, D., Mruthyunjaya, T.S.: A Newton-Euler formulation for the inverse dynamics of the stewart platform manipulator. Mech. Mach. Theory 33(8), 1135–1152 (1998)
3. Fan, S.C., Ding, W.J.: Effects of friction on the motion of a manipulator. J. Eng. Mech. 2, 64–67 (2002)
4. Ryu, J.H., Song, J., Kwon, D.: A nonlinear friction compensation method using adaptive control and its practical application to an in-parallel actuated 6-DOF manipulator. J. Control Eng. Pract. 9, 159–167 (2001)
5. Shang, W.W., Cong, S., Zhang, Y.X.: Nonlinear friction compensation of a 2-DOF planar parallel manipulator. J. Mechatronics 1, 1–6 (2008)
6. Armstrong, B., Dupont, P., Wit, C.C.: A survey of models, analysis tools and compensation methods for the control of machines with friction. Automatica 30, 1083–1138 (1994)

7. Olsson, H., Astrom, K.J., Wit, C.C., Gafvert, M., Lischinsky, P.: Friction models and friction compensation. Eur. J. Control 4, 176–185 (1998)
8. Wang, F.X.: Recent development of forging manipulators technology. J. Heav. Mach. 6, 13–17 (1994)
9. Wan, S.D., Wan, Y.G.: Forging Mechanization and Automation, pp. 169–241. China machine press, Beijing (1983)
10. Huang, Z.: Spatial Mechanisms. China machine press, Beijing (1991)
11. Chen, M.W., Zalzala, A.M.S.: Dynamic modeling and genetic-based trajectory generation for non-holonomic mobile manipulators. Control Eng. Pract. 5(1), 39–48 (1997)
12. Gardner, J.F.: Simulation of machines using MATLAB and SIMULINK. Jiaotong University Press, Xi'an (2002)

Toolpath Generation for Four-Axis Rough Milling of Sculptured Surface Turbine Blade

Ming Luo, Baohai Wu, Dinghua Zhang, Shan Li, and Ying Zhang

Key Laboratory of Contemporary Design and Integrated Manufacturing Technology (Northwestern Polytechnical University), Ministry of Education, 710072, Xi'an, PR China
mingluonpu@gmail.com

Abstract. Presented in this paper is a method for four-axis rough milling of sculptured surface turbine blade. The proposed method consists of two steps, cutter-contact (CC) points generation and tool orientation planning. In the first stage, CC points for trimmed blade surface are generated in the parametric domain and then they are converted into the physical domain to get flow line toolpaths. In the second stage, optimized representative tool orientations are generated first, and then interpolation algorithm is employed to determine all tool orientations. With this method, smooth tool orientations can be obtained. Finally, computational examples were implemented to generate symmetrical spiral four-axis rough milling toolpath for the turbine blade disk. Simulation results show that the proposed method is efficient and it can improve the utilization of four-axis machine tools in the milling of turbine blade.

Keywords: Toolpath generation, turbine blade, rough milling, sculptured surface.

1 Introduction

Turbine blade disk is a typical kind of thin-walled sculptured surface part. The majority of these parts are produced by multi-axis milling, where multi-axis machine tools play an important role. In order to improve the utilization of four-axis machine tools in the milling of turbine blade and reduce the machining cost, Four-axis rough milling method is studied in this paper.

Turbine blade surfaces are highly sculptured surface, many studies have been carried out to investigate the toolpath generation methods for turbine blade surface[1-2]. Since the blade surface is trimmed surface, Ding[3] presented a detailed method of flow line toolpath generation for trimmed blade surface. Similar studies on machining of turbine blades and impellers made of ruled surfaces have also been studied by Monies[4] and Young[5].

Owning to the narrow space between neighbouring blades, difficulties in tool orientation determination have posed a long-standing problem, much research has been carried out in the CAM field to investigate more efficient methods. Jun[6] studied configuration-space search method to optimize tool orientations. Ho[7] introduced the quaternion interpolation algorithm to get smooth tool orientation, which can reduce

C. Xiong et al. (Eds.): ICIRA 2008, Part II, LNAI 5315, pp. 887–895, 2008.

machining errors. In this study, we also introduced the quaternion interpolation algorithm to get smooth tool orientation in four-axis rough milling of turbine blade.

Focused on four-axis rough milling of turbine blade, we presented an efficient method in this study. While generating toolpaths for turbine blade, two steps are presented in this paper: cutter-contact points generation and tool orientation planning. Section 2 discussed the generation of cutter-contact points, and section 3 discussed the optimized representative tool orientation generation and interpolation algorithm. Finally, computational examples are presented in section 4 with conclusion in section 5.

2 Four-Axis Rough Milling of Turbine Blades

2.1 Structure of Turbine Blade

As shown in figure 1, each turbine blade consists of two working surfaces on opposite sides, one is suction surface and the other is pressure surface. Both surfaces are sculptured surfaces designed in accordance with aero-dynamic principles. Surfaces that connecting the suction surface and pressure surface at the front and back edge are termed as leading edge and trailing edge. All blades intersect with the hub surface at the bottom. Space between two neighboring blades is referred to as the blade disk channel.

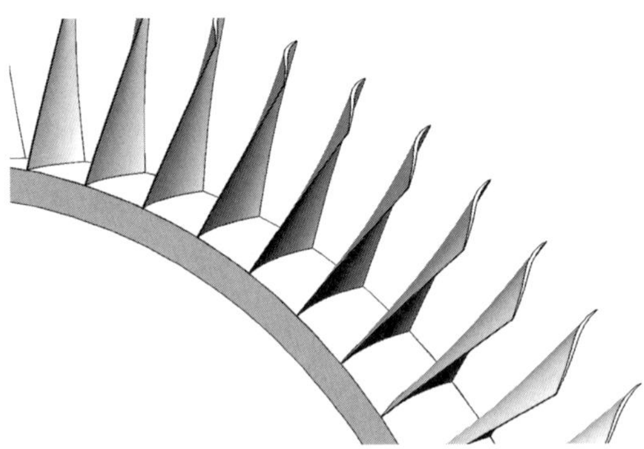

Fig. 1. Structure of turbine blade

Owning to the highly sculptured shape of the suction surface and pressure surface as well as the narrow blade disk channel, collision and interference between the cutter and the blade disk are prone to occur. For tool orientation doesn't change in three-axis milling, collision and interference will certainly happen, it cannot be used in the milling of turbine blades. In this research, four-axis milling approach is used to get collision-free and interference-free toolpath. In four-axis milling process, the blade disk can rotate about its axis to reach a position where no collision or interference will happen.

Besides the highly sculptured shape, turbine blades are thin-walled parts, deformation due to residual stress in the milling process is prone to occur. To achieve better surface finish and higher machining accuracy, symmetrical spiral milling approach is employed. The basic idea of symmetrical spiral milling approach is: the suction surface and the pressure surface of the blade will be machined in the same circle, the toolpath is a spiral curve around the turbine blade. With this approach, residual stress of both sides inside the turbine blade will release in the same circle, deformation will be suppressed at a certain extent.

2.2 Toolpath Generation Strategies

There are three steps for generating four-axis milling toolpaths, the first step is to calculate the initial toolpaths and corresponding cutter-contact (CC) points. In the second step, representative tool orientation for representative CC points are generated. In the last step, tool orientation for every CC point will be interpolated by the representative tool orientation, further modifications of tool orientations are also performed to adjust the cutter to an optimized and collision-free and interference-free orientation. Algorithm for CC points generation will be discussed in this section, algorithms for the second and last steps will be discussed detailedly in the following section.

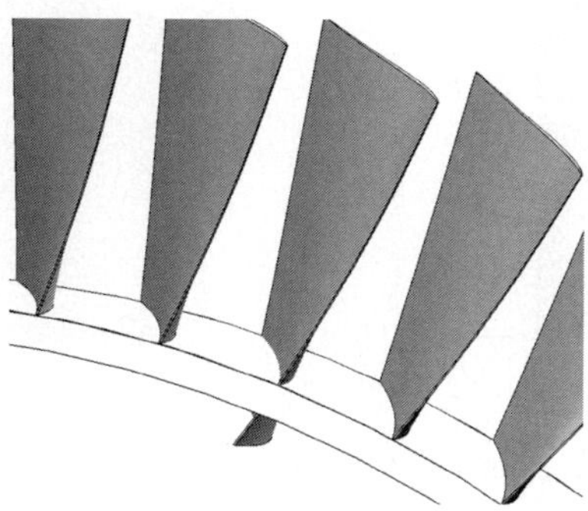

Fig. 2. The intersection between turbine blade and hub-surface

As shown in figure 2, surfaces of the blade are trimmed surfaces, while generating initial toolpaths, two steps are needed to get flow line toolpaths. The first step is to convert the trimmed surfaces in the physical domain into the parametric domain. In the second step, CC points in the parametric domain will be generated first, after that, they will be converted into the physical domain to get flow line toolpaths.

- Step1: Convert the trimmed surfaces in the physical domain into the parametric domain. As shown in figure 3, the original designed blade surface is a whole surface that its parametrical *uv* domain is a unit square in the parametric domain. In the CAD modeling of the blade disk, the unwanted portion of the blade surface is trimmed off by the hub-surface. Therefore, its *uv* domain is no longer a unit square again. In the parametric domain, the right boundary corresponds to the top edge of the blade, while the left boundary corresponds to the intersection curve between the blade surface and the hub-surface.
- Step2: Generate CC points in the parametric domain and converted them into the physical domain.

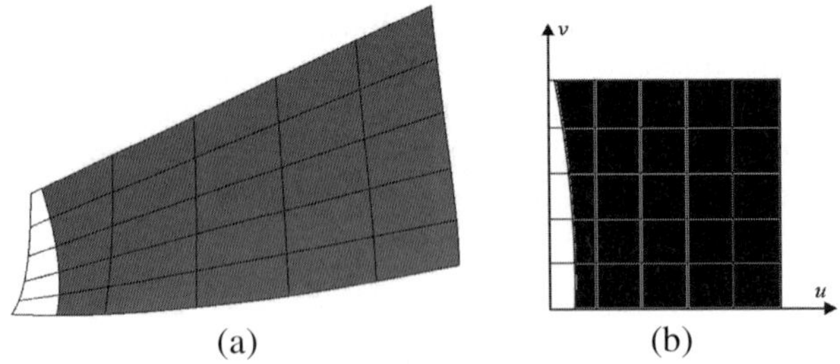

Fig. 3. Trimmed blade surface in the physical domain and the corresponding area in the parametric domain. (a) Trimmed blade surface in the physical domain; (b) Trimmed blade surface in the parametric domain.

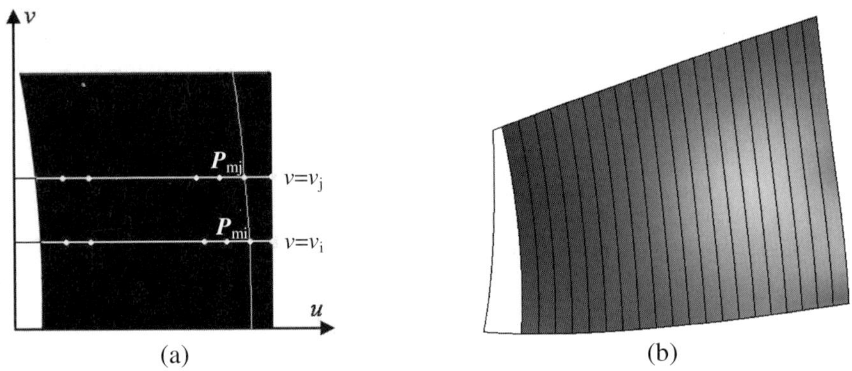

Fig. 4. (a) Generation of CC points in the parametric domain; (b) Flow line toolpath in the physical domain

To get flow line toolpath, CC points will be generated with the following method in the parametric domain. As shown in figure 4(a), in the parametric domain, divide v iso-parametric curves into n segments with equal parameter increment for each v iso-parametric curve. For example, iso-parametric curve $v=v_i$ begins at $u=u_i$ and ends at $u=1.0$ in the trimmed blade surface, it can be divided into n segments with equal parameter increment Δu_i between $u=u_i$ and $u=1.0$. As for iso-parametric curve $v=v_j$, it can also be divided into n segments with equal parameter increment Δu_j between $u=u_j$ and $u=1.0$. For every division point in the same iso-parametric curve, they are numbered one by one from 1 to n. All points with the same number on every iso-parametric curve from $v=0.0$ to $v=1.0$ form a single cutter-contact curve in the parametric domain, then it is converted into the physical domain. Figure 4(b) shows the cutter-contact curves on the trimmed blade surface in the physical domain.

3 Tool Orientation Planning

One major problem in the milling of turbine blade is the determination of tool orientation in the channel of blade disk. Optimized tool orientation should first guarantee collision-free and interference-free between the cutter and the workpiece. Moreover, researches show that if the tool orientations vary considerably in a cutting step, grooves may exist and interferences will easily happen, and cutting errors will be large in this case. To solve this problem, the tool orientation interpolation algorithm is employed to get smooth tool orientation variation. In this section, representation tool orientation generation method is first discussed, followed by the tool orientation interpolation algorithm and interference detection.

3.1 Generation of Representative Tool Orientation

At the top edge of the blade, there is broad space for the cutter to vary its orientation, it's easy to determine the optimized tool orientation. At the bottom of the blade, the tool orientation variation space is narrow, collision and interference are prone to occur, it's more difficult to determine the optimized tool orientation.

Each blade of the disk has a stack-up axis through the center of the disk, it is in the plane perpendicular to the rotary axis. As shown in figure 5, the vector sum of the two neighbouring stack-up axis vectors can be used as the initial tool orientation in the blade disk channel.

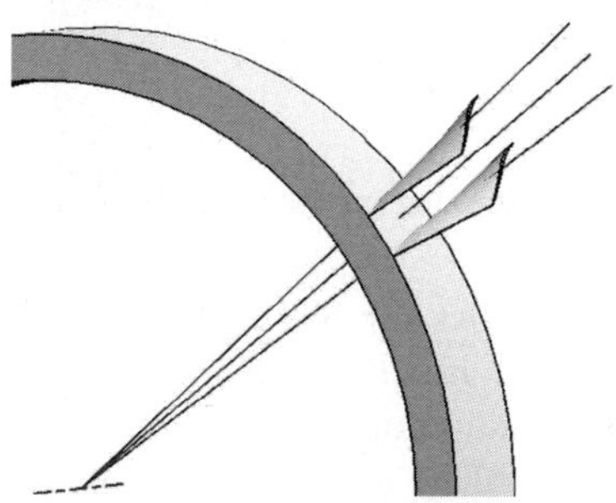

Fig. 5. Initial tool orientation for representative position

From the top edge to the bottom edge of the blade, some representative tool orientations are determined. The basic two steps for determining the representative tool orientations are as follows:

- Step1: specify initial tool orientation for representative positions. Blade surface are highly sculptured surface, it's smooth enough that representative positions can be selected uniformly in each milling circle. At the top edge of the blade, broad space means that fewer representative positions have to be determined; at the bottom edge of the blade, narrow space means that more representative positions have to be determined. For each representative position, initial tool orientations are specified with the vector sum determined above. Figure 6 shows the representative positions and the initial tool orientations.

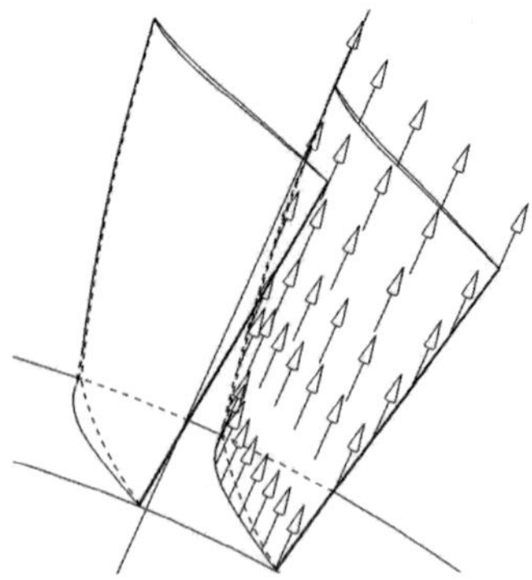

Fig. 6. Representative positions and the initial tool orientations on the blade surface

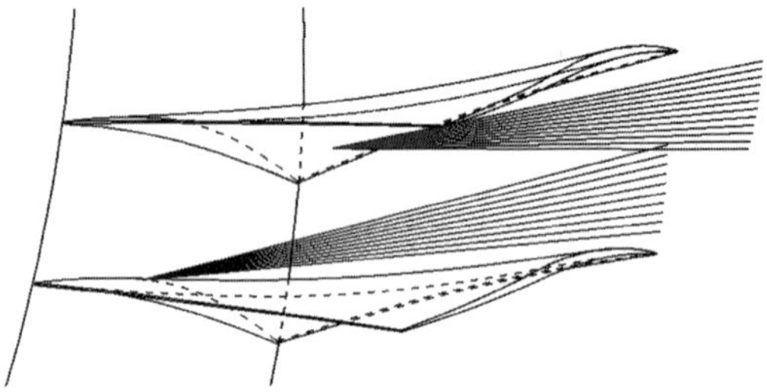

Fig. 7. Tool orientation optimizing process to get collision-free tool orientation

- Step2: interference detection. As for ball-end cutter used in the milling process, check whether collision exists at the current position. Adjust the tool orientation if collision happens. The orientation of the cutter can only be changed by rotating it around the rotary axis of the blade disk with a four-axis machine tool. Figure 7 illustrates the optimizing process.

3.2 Tool Orientation Interpolation and Interference Detection

Optimized representative tool orientations only determine tool orientations for a small portion of the CC points, tool orientations for other CC points will be determined by tool orientation interpolation with representative tool orientations. The common used vector interpolation algorithms are the coordinate interpolation algorithm (CI algorithm), the Euler interpolation algorithm (EI algorithm), and the quaternion interpolation algorithm (QI algorithm). Among the three interpolation algorithms, the rotational velocity between two successive tool orientations interpolated by CI algorithm are not uniform along the toolpath; and for the EI algorithm, there are undesirable quirks in the tool orientations. The QI algorithm can provide smoother tool orientation variation and constant angular velocity, no undesired tool orientations quirks will happen. Therefore, the QI algorithm is employed in this study to interpolate tool orientations for the rest CC points.

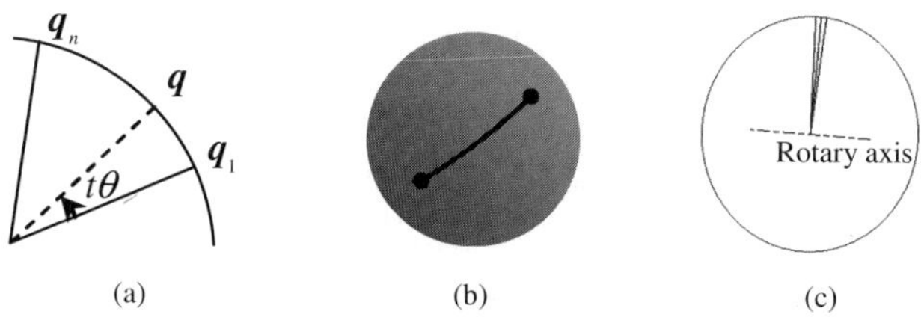

Fig. 8. (a) A step in the interpolation goes from q_1 to q_n across the angle θ. (b) Interpolation curve on the unit sphere. (c) All interpolated tool orientations are on the same arc of the unit sphere.

Given two optimized tool orientations q_1 and q_n, the formula for spherical quaternion interpolation from q_1 to q_n with parameter t can be written as follows[8]:

$$q_i = \frac{\sin(1-t)\theta}{\sin\theta} q_1 + \frac{\sin t\theta}{\sin\theta} q_n, \qquad 0 \le t \le 1, i \in [2, n-1] \tag{1}$$

where

$$t = \frac{i-1}{n-1} \tag{2}$$

$$\theta = \arccos(q_1 \cdot q_n) \tag{3}$$

when q_1 and q_n are close, $\theta \approx 0$, thus the denominator of Equation (1) is closed to 0. In this case, the CI algorithm can be used to avoid division by zeros.

As shown in figure 8(b), tool orientations interpolated by QI algorithm with two representative tool orientations follow the shortest great arc on the unit sphere. In four-axis milling, all optimized representative tool orientations are on one arc on the unit sphere, which means that tool orientations interpolated by QI algorithm also yields the shortest possible interpolation path between the two quaternions on the arc. Therefore, the interpolated tool orientations only rotate about the rotary axis of the blade disk, it's suitable for four-axis milling.

Note that not all tool orientations interpolated by the QI algorithm are collision-free, further collision and interference detection need to be performed as we do to determine the optimized representative tool orientations.

4 Implementation Examples

In order to generate symmetrical spiral milling toolpaths for the blade, toolpaths for suction surface and pressure surface are generated first, then toolpaths on the suctions surface and toolpaths on the pressure surfaces of the blade are connected with each other at the leading edge and trailing edge. Note that toolpaths on the suction surface should have the same number with toolpaths on the pressure surface. Figure 9 demonstrates the connection of toolpaths on both surfaces. In order to avoid gouge at the leading and trailing edge, toolpaths on both surfaces are extended at the leading edge and the trailing edge of the turbine blade. Symmetrical spiral toolpath generated by the proposed algorithm is illustrated in figure 10.

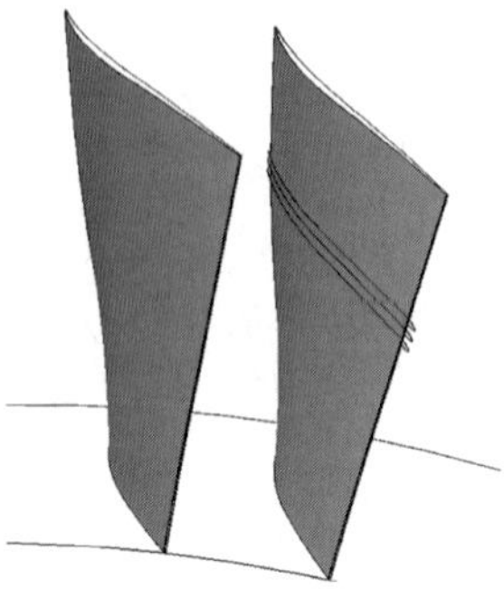

Fig. 9. Connection of toolpaths on the suction surface and toolpaths on the pressure surface at the leading edge and trailing edge

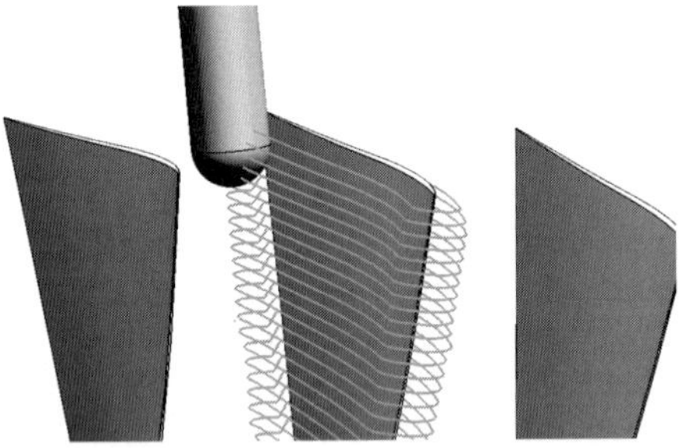

Fig. 10. Symmetrical spiral toolpaths generated by the proposed algorithm

5 Conclusion

This paper introduced a new approach for rough milling of turbine blade disk with four-axis machine tool, it can improve the utilization of different kinds of machine tools. The proposed symmetrical spiral toolpaths generation algorithm consists of two basic steps: cutter-contact curve generation and tool orientation planning. In the first stage, flow line toolpaths were generated for the trimmed blade surface. In the second stage, optimized representative tool orientations were determined and the QI algorithm was employed to generate smooth tool orientations. Finally, computational example was implemented and symmetrical spiral toolpaths was generated for four-axis milling of turbine blade, simulation results show that the proposed algorithm is efficient.

References

1. Madhavulu, G., Sundar, S.A., Ahmed, B.: CAD/CAM solutions for efficient machining of turbo machinery components by Sturz milling method. In: 22nd IEEE International Conference on Industrial Electronics, Control and Instrumentation, pp. 1490–1495. IEEE Press, New York (1996)
2. Ding, S., Yang, D.C., Han, Z.: Boundary-confirmed machining of turbine blades. Proceeding of the Institution of Mechanical Engineers, Part B: J. Engineering Mahufacture 219, 255–263 (2005)
3. Ding, S., Yang, D.C., Han, Z.: Flow line machining of turbine blades. In: Proceeding of the 2004 International Conference on Intelligent Mechatronics and Automation, pp. 140–145. IEEE Press, New York (2005)
4. Monies, F., Redonnet, J.M., Rubio, W., Lagarrigue, P.: Improved positioning of a conical mill for machining ruled surfaces: application to turbine blades. Proceeding of the Institution of Mechanical Engineers, Part B: J. Engineering Mahufacture 214, 625–634 (2000)
5. Young, H.T., Chuang, L.C.: An intefrated machining approach for a centrifugal impeller. Int. J. of Adv. Manuf. Technology 21, 556–563 (2003)
6. Jun, C.S., Cha, K., Lee, Y.S.: Optimizing tool orientation for 5-axis machining by configuration-space search method. Computer-Aided Design 35, 549–566 (2003)
7. Ho, M.C., Hwang, Y.R., Hu, C.H.: Five-axis tool orientation smoothing using quaternion interpolation algorithm. Int. J. Mach. Tools Manuf. 43, 1259–1267 (2003)
8. Dam, E.B., Koch, M., Lillholm, M.: Quaternions, Interpolation and Animation. Deparment of Computer Science, University of Copenhagen (1998)

A Multi-physics Simulation Based Parameters Optimization for Anisotropic Conductive Adhesive Interconnection in Electronic Packaging

ZhengJia Wang, Yuhui Wang, and Zhouping Yin

State Key Laboratory of Digital Manufacturing Equipment and Technology, Huazhong University of Science and Technology, Wuhan, 430074, P. R. China
wangzhengjia@sohu.com, wyh@mail.hust.edu.cn,
yinzhp@mail.hust.edu.cn

Abstract. Flip-chip joining using anisotropic conductive adhesive (ACA) has many advantages. But the reliability of ACA interconnection is still a concern issue. There are many studies about the reliability, but little work was done about the bonding process's effect. It is a coupled field problem which needs multi-physics simulation. In order to improve the reliability of the packaging, a parameters optimization method based on multi-physics simulation was developed. A response surface method was used to reduce the computational cost. A generic model was built as an illustration.

Keyword: Anisotropic conductive adhesive (ACA), reliability, coupled field, multi-physics simulation, optimization.

1 Introduction

Anisotropic conductive adhesive (ACA) Interconnection has many advantages and becomes more and more popular in electronic packaging technology. But the reliability of anisotropic conductive adhesive interconnection is still a concern issue. ACA bonding is a complicated process which involves many physics phenomena such as heat transfer, fluid flow and cure reaction, etc. Over the last few years, many researchers have studied the reliability of ACA joint. Most of those studies are based on experiments. For example, the curing temperature[1], the curing pressure[2-4], the bump height[5-7], and the material properties' effect on the reliability[8] were studied. In those researches, the optimum parameters may be gained by comparing a series of experiments and thus give guides to designers.

Finite element analysis (FEA) has been widely used in analyzing the failures of the electronic packages to explore the directions of design improvement. There are many researches employing FEA to simulate stress/strain development and study the reliability. For example, the reflow process on the reliability of ACA bonding packaging[9], and the moisture induced failure in ACA interconnection were studied[10] respectively. There were studies on both the impact of temperature excursion and moisture absorption through FEA[11]. Though physics phenomena involved in ACA bonding were occurred simultaneously and might couple with each other, those

C. Xiong et al. (Eds.): ICIRA 2008, Part II, LNAI 5315, pp. 896–905, 2008.

researches only studied one physics field at one time[9, 10] or studied several physics fields by employing decomposition method to suppose the different fields bring stains independently[11].

FEA is very useful for engineers' better understanding the reliability behavior during the product design stage. Once the direction of design improvement is found according to FEA, design optimization methodology can be used to find the best path to improve the reliability. Differential evolution(DE) is a powerful optimization method and capable of finding the global optimization even if local minima exist [12]. However, the computational cost is expensive for simulation-based design optimization because FEA is usually very complicated and time-consuming, and a design optimization may need many times of simulations. In order to reduce the computational cost in optimization, a mathematical model was built to approximate the relationship between the system response and the design parameters. Design of experiments(DOE) was used to select a set of input points, and the FEA results at these points was used to generate the response surface of the system.

In this study, a multi-physics finite elements analysis method was used. Parameters optimization was carried out based on the finite element analysis. In order to improve the numerical efficiency of optimization, a response surface method (RSM) was used as metamodel. Furthermore, a differential evolution algorithm is used as the search engine in minimization procedure. This method was demonstrated by a generic model of an electronic package using ACA interconnection.

2 Methods

A typical ACA bonding process was as following: First the ACA was dispensed or placed on substrate, the IC chip was flipped and aligned to the pad on the substrate, and then the ACA was cured by heat and pressure. Under high heat and pressure those conducting particles deformed and contacted with the chip and the substrate. The deformation is maintained by tensile stress in the cured adhesive. After ACA cured, the whole packaging was cooled to room temperature.

There are many factors affecting the reliability of ACA flip chip packaging. Process temperature has great influence on adhesion strength of the ACA interconnection. Cure reaction occurs only at a certain high temperature. Higher temperature enables ACA to cure more quickly, but too high temperature degrades the matrix of ACA and the sharp heating variation may build up serious thermal stress. Pressure is applied to force the conductive particles to contact the chip and substrate, the degree of deformation of the conductive particles can affect the performance of ACF interconnects. If the pressure applied is too great, the metallic layers of the particles maybe cracked, the conductivity of the interconnection will be decreased. Effect of bonding pressure on reliability of joints on flexible and rigid substrates was also studied[3]. There are other factors affect the reliability of ACA interconnection, such as geometry parameters of chip and substrates[5-7]. The properties of ACA such as coefficient of thermal expansion and elastic module also have influences on the reliability [8, 14].

In order to investigate the effects on reliability of different bonding parameters, a parametric finite element model was build. A series of finite elements analyses were carried out on different model parameters. From the results of FEA, a response surface was constructed. In order to select the proper sample points for finite element analysis, a design of experiment method was used. Finally the optimization was implemented to get the optimum values of bonding process parameters and material properties. The whole process was outlined as Fig.1.

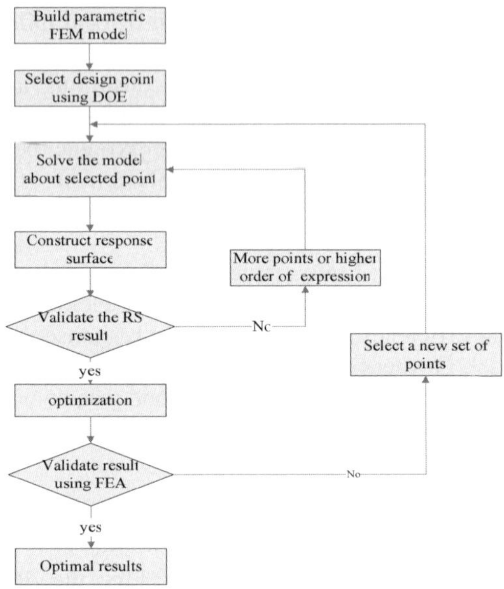

Fig. 1. A flowchart of optimization based on finite element analysis

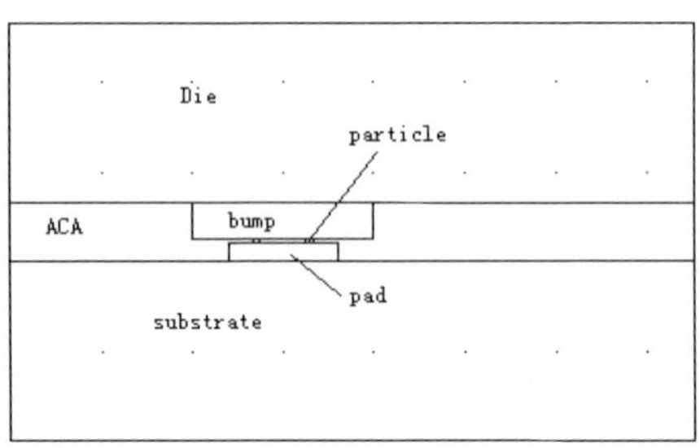

Fig. 2. The structure of a generic ACA interconnection packaging

The generic model used was a RFID packaging with 2 bumps. The structure of the specimen was shown in Fig.2. The chip size was 750x750μm^2 , the bump size was 100x100μm^2, and the pitch was 300μm. The substrate design had a pad size of 60x60μm^2 .The ACA used here had particles with diameter 3.5μm. 2D model was used for simplicity. Due to symmetry, only half the packaging was built.

Table 1. Mechanical and thermal properties of materials(units:SI)

	Density	Modulus	Specific heat	Conductivity	Thermal expansion(ppm)	Poisson's ratio
Silicon	2330	131e9	703	163	4.15	0.27
Nickel	8900	219e9	445	90.7	13.4	0.31
Particle	2200	1.3e9	1100	0.24	70	0.4
ACA	4000	1.450e9-0.482e9	800	150	57(<150℃) 133(>150℃)	0.45 (30℃) 0.49(150℃)
Copper	8700	110e9	385	400	17	0.35
Substrates	1530	2000e6-6000e6	1090	0.12	20	0.3

Table 2. Elastic module of ACA at different temperature

Temperature(℃)	20	40	60	80	100	120	130	180
Modulus(MPa)	1450	1410	1340	1250	1140	899	542	542

Table 3. Design variables and their nominal design value

	Lower bound	Upper bound	Nominal design
T(℃)	160	210	180
F(N)	2	8	5
E(MPa)	2000	6000	4000

Table 1 gives material properties of the packaging[6]. The elastic module of the ACA changes with the temperature, as shown in table 2[6]. Although there were many factors may influence the reliability of the packaging, the bonding force, bonding temperature and the elastic modulus of substrate were selected in this study as illustration. If the stress/strain level is too high, the crack maybe initiate and propagate, the electrical contacts may degraded by cracking in the adhesive joint or by delamination between the adhesive material and the substrate pads or chip bumps. So the minimum of von_Mises was used as optimization objective. Table 3 gives the ranges of design parameters and their nominal design value.

3 Finite Elements Modeling and Analysis

For a multi-physics finite element analysis, the effect in each physics field should be taken into consideration simultaneously. All the govern equation of different physics fields should be solved with a single method. Partial differential equations form the basic laws of science and provide the foundation for modeling a wide range of scientific and engineering phenomena. This kind of equations can be solved by COMSOL, which is a powerful environment for modeling and solving all kinds of problems based on partial differential equations. The model can be built by script programming language. For finite element analysis of ACA bonding, as to the generic model used as illustration, heat transfer and mechanical analysis were carried out and the temperature and displacement of each node were solved simultaneously. The heat transfer was a 2D problem. The mechanic analysis was a plain strain problem.

For a 2D heat transfer problem, the govern equation may be written as

$$\rho C \frac{\partial T}{\partial t} - \frac{\partial}{\partial x}(k_{xx} \frac{\partial T}{\partial x}) - \frac{\partial}{\partial y}(k_{yy} \frac{\partial T}{\partial y}) = Q \quad (1)$$

where T is the temperature, ρ is the density, C is the heat capacity, k is thermal conductivity, k_{xx} is the x component and k_{yy} the y component, Q is a heat source or a heat sink. The hear source Q is zero for the model since there is no heat source inside the packaging during bonding process.

The govern equation of mechanic analysis may be calculated from following equations:

(1) The equilibrium equations:

$$\frac{\partial \sigma_x}{\partial x} + \frac{\partial \tau_{xy}}{\partial y} = -F_x \quad (2)$$

$$\frac{\partial \sigma_y}{\partial y} + \frac{\partial \tau_{xy}}{\partial x} = -F_y \quad (3)$$

where Fx and Fy are the volume forces, σ_x, σ_y the stress in the x, y directory respectively, τ_{xy} is the shear stress.

(2) The strain-stress relation is $\sigma = D\varepsilon$. And the elasticity matrix D is:

$$D = \frac{E(1-\mu)}{(1+\mu)(1-2\mu)} \begin{bmatrix} 1 & \frac{\mu}{1-\mu} & 0 \\ \frac{\mu}{1-\mu} & 1 & 0 \\ 0 & 0 & \frac{1-2\mu}{2(1-\mu)} \end{bmatrix} \quad (4)$$

where E is the elastic module, μ the Poisson's ratio. So the strain-stress relation may be written as:

$$\sigma_x = \frac{E(1-\mu)}{(1+\mu)(1-2\mu)}(\varepsilon_x - \frac{\mu}{1-\mu}\varepsilon_y) \quad (5)$$

$$\sigma_y = \frac{E(1-\mu)}{(1+\mu)(1-2\mu)}(\varepsilon_y - \frac{\mu}{1-\mu}\varepsilon_x) \quad (6)$$

$$\tau_{xy} = \frac{E}{2(1+\mu)}\gamma_{xy} \quad (7)$$

where $\varepsilon_x, \varepsilon_y, \gamma_{xy}$ is normal strain in the x, y direction and shear strain.

(3)The strains may be calculated by:

$$\varepsilon_x = \frac{\partial u}{\partial x} \tag{8}$$

$$\varepsilon_y = \frac{\partial v}{\partial y} \tag{9}$$

$$\gamma_{xy} = \frac{\partial u}{\partial y} + \frac{\partial v}{\partial x} \tag{10}$$

where u , v means displacement in the x , y direction. Substituting the variable in equation (2) and (3) with equations (5)-(10), assuming the thick of the plain as *th*, the governing partial differential equation may be written as following:

$$\rho \cdot th \cdot \frac{\partial^2 u}{\partial t^2} - \frac{\partial}{\partial x}(-\frac{\partial u}{\partial x} \cdot \frac{th \cdot E(1-\mu)}{(1+\mu)(1-2\mu)} - \frac{\partial v}{\partial y} \cdot \frac{th \cdot E\mu}{(1+\mu)(1-2\mu)}) - \frac{\partial}{\partial y}(\frac{E \cdot th}{2(1+\mu)} \cdot (\frac{\partial u}{\partial y} + \frac{\partial v}{\partial x})) = 0 \tag{11}$$

$$\rho \cdot th \cdot \frac{\partial^2 v}{\partial t^2} - \frac{\partial}{\partial y}(-\frac{\partial u}{\partial x} \cdot \frac{th \cdot E\mu}{(1+\mu)(1-2\mu)} - \frac{\partial v}{\partial y} \cdot \frac{th \cdot E(1-\mu)}{(1+\mu)(1-2\mu)}) - \frac{\partial}{\partial x}(\frac{E \cdot th}{2(1+\mu)} \cdot (\frac{\partial u}{\partial y} + \frac{\partial v}{\partial x})) = 0 \tag{12}$$

Considering the physics field involved in the process, the partial differential equations of the domain are composed of (1),(11)and (12). In order to solve the temperature and the strain with a single method and simultaneously, the degrees of freedom of each node include temperature *T*, u and v .

Introducing the virtual temperature *test(T)* and integrate it over all the domain for govern equation of heat transfer (1) leads to the equation:

$$\int_\Omega (\rho C \frac{\partial T}{\partial t} - \frac{\partial}{\partial x}(k_{xx}\frac{\partial T}{\partial x}) - \frac{\partial}{\partial y}(k_{yy}\frac{\partial T}{\partial y}))T' dA = 0 \tag{13}$$

where T' denotes *test(T)*. In following equations, T_t is used to denote $\partial T / \partial t$,T_x is used to denote $\partial T / \partial x$,T_y is used to denote $\partial T / \partial y$ for simplicity.

After applying divergence theorem and rearranging it, the equation will be:

$$\int_\Omega \rho C T_t \cdot T' dA - [-\int_\Omega T'_x k_{xx} T_x dA + \int_{\partial\Omega} T' k_{xx} T_x \cdot n_x dS - \int_\Omega T'_y k_{yy} T_y dA + \int_{\partial\Omega} T' k_{yy} T_y \cdot n_y dS = 0 \tag{14}$$

where n is the normal vector of the boundary.

For a boundary where heat transfer with the surrounding environment by convection, the boundary condition is:

$$n \cdot (k \nabla T) = h(T_{\text{inf}} - T) \tag{15}$$

where h is the heat transfer coefficient and T_{inf} is the ambient bulk temperature. For the right boundary of the model, T_{inf} is the room temperature 25℃ and the heat transfer coefficient is 4.5.

For the boundary with constant temperature, it may be described as:

$$T = T_p \tag{16}$$

where T_p denotes the prescribed temperature. In curing process the top boundary was contacted with the heater, and kept constant by the thermal control system. In curing stage, the top temperature was assigned as T_{top} whose value can be assigned before each time the model was solved. The bottom boundary was T_p =60. In cooling stage, the top and bottom boundaries' heat transfer were by convection

Using the similar method, partial differential equation (11) and (12) can be reformulated and the vale can be specified in the model. The top side was applied load force of T_{top} in curing stage and the load was removed in cooling stage. The left side was the symmetry side and the bottom side was support by the platform. In order to investigate different material's effect, the elastic module of substrate was assumed as E_{sub}. Using those factors a parametric model was built. When the calculating finished, the strain can be gained through equation (8)~(10), and the stress can be gained through equation (5)~(7). If the thermal strain and the initial strain were taken into consideration, the total strain was calculated by equation :

$$\overline{\varepsilon} = \overline{\varepsilon}_{el} + \overline{\varepsilon}_{th} + \overline{\varepsilon}_0 \tag{17}$$

where $\overline{\varepsilon}_{el}$ is the elastic strain, $\overline{\varepsilon}$ is the total strain, $\overline{\varepsilon}_0$ is the initial strain, $\overline{\varepsilon}_{th}$ is the strain caused by thermal can be calculated by equation:

$$\overline{\varepsilon_{th}} = \overline{\alpha}_{vec}(T - T_{ref}) \tag{18}$$

where $\overline{\alpha}_{vec}$ is thermal expansion.

And the total stress was calculated by:

$$\overline{\sigma} = \overline{D\varepsilon_{el}} + \overline{\sigma_0} = D(\overline{\varepsilon} - \overline{\varepsilon}_{th} - \overline{\varepsilon_0}) + \overline{\sigma_0} \tag{19}$$

where $\overline{\sigma}_0$ is the initial stress. In curing stage, the initial stress was zero and the ACA part was not active. In cooling stage, the initial stress was the result from the curing stage and all the parts were active for analysis.

4 Parameters Optimization

According to what described in previous section the optimization problem can be stated as:

min $\sigma = f(F, T, E)$

s.t:

$2 \le F \le 8$ *(N)*

$160 \le T \le 210$ *(℃)*

$2000 \le E \le 6000$ *(MPa)*

In order to find the global minimum value, a differential evolution method is used. To reduce the computational costs, a second order polynomial response surface was used to approximate the objective value. The polynomial expression for the surface approximation[13]:

$$\sigma_i = b_0 + b_1 F_i + b_2 T_i + b_3 E_i + b_4 F_i^2 + b_5 T_i^2 + b_6 E_i^2 + b_7 F_i T_i + b_8 F_i E_i + b_9 E_i T_i + e_i \quad (20)$$

where i is the index of the sample points, $i=1,2,\ldots n$, σ_i is the measured response in design point i, F_i, T_i and E_i the coordinates of design point i; b_j the constants to be determined; e_i the deviation between the fitted curve and the calculated response in design point i and n the number of design points to be evaluated.

To determine the 10 constants b_j in equation (20) at least 10 design points have to be evaluated. Also 3 levels for each design variable are needed to estimate the quadratic terms. A widely used design of experiments for fitting second order response surfaces is the central composite design [13], where 15 design points is used to estimate the second order response surface. Using the sample points defined by central composite design, several FEA were implemented, the result listed in table 4. From the FEM result, the coefficient of the RSM was calculated. The values were: b0=-2.25793e9; b1=9.29765e7; b2=4.0057e7; b3=5611.11; b4=-35.55; b5=3086.42; b6=5.244; b7=166.66; b8=-1902.25; b9=-352.083. To find out if the response surface was a good approximation of the σ_i in the design space, the coefficient of multiple determinations is calculated. If the surface approximation is not acceptable the accuracy of the response surface can be increased by either increase the number of design points or increase the order of the polynomial function (20). The procedure is repeated until acceptable results are attained.

Table 4. The results of selected design variables from FEA

No.	T(℃)	F(N)	E(MPa)	Von_mises(MPa)
1	160	2	2000	12119.1
2	210	8	2000	16578.4
3	160	2	2000	12355.3
4	210	8	2000	16814.7
5	160	2	6000	11089.1
6	210	8	6000	15168
7	160	2	6000	11316.9
8	210	8	6000	15395.8
9	160	5	4000	11702.5
10	210	5	4000	15964.8
11	185	2	4000	13717.1
12	185	8	4000	13950.3
13	185	5	2000	14466.9
14	185	5	6000	13242.4
15	185	5	4000	13833.7

Using the established response surfaces, a DE method optimization was used to find the minimum of the fitted surface with the constraints according to the previous section. The minimum was found at T=160C, F=2N and E=60000MPa and the minimized von-Mises value was 11089.67MPa. The optimum point is at the DOE point, so no more calculation needed. The nominal design is T=180, N=5, E=4000, and the von-Mises value is 13406.9MPa. The optimum result is better than the nominal design. The minimum value is found at lower bound of *T* and *F* and upper bound of *E*. For the lower temperature is closer to the room temperature, so the T-T_{inf} in equation (18) is smaller, and leads to lower stress. The small force leads to slight deformation which results in small strain and small stress. This result is same as the study about the bonding force effect on ACA reliability [15]. The greater elastic module in substrate leads to small stress, which is in accord with the research of [6]. So the final conclusion from this study is that the force and the temperature should be kept as low as possible on condition that the temperature can make the ACA cure enough and the force make the particles deform enough to ensure the mechanical and electronic performance. The elastic module can be keep as high as possible at the same time.

5 Conclusions

A multi-physics finite element analysis simulation was implemented and parametric optimization based on it was developed for electronic package reliability in this paper. It is capable to provide the best direction on how to improve the design within the design space. The central composite design was used in selecting sample points. To reduce the computational cost the RSM was used to fit a second order surface to the simulated stress values. Furthermore, DE optimization algorithm was used to find the global minimum while the local minimum exists. A generic electronic packaging was constructed as an illustration and the curing process was simulated. Using the parametric model, Series of ACA bonding process was performed to find the optimum design. The results showed that the present model of the curing process gives the same trend as the reality.

In this study a simple ACA interconnection packaging was used to state an example of multi-physics finite elements analysis and parametric optimization. The same methodology can also be used to find the optimum designs of electronic packaging reliability. Only two process parameters and the elastic module of substrate were considered in this study, no material properties such as CTE and elastic module of ACA was considered in the optimization process. Considering more factors' effects on the reliability of electronics packaging can be an interesting subject for further studies. Using Failure mechanism and electric performance both as optimization objective function will bring more practical results. Furthermore considering the thermal cycling test and external mechanical loading after the packaging process would bring more accurate results.

Acknowledgements

The work is supported by the Natural Science Fund of China (NSFC) (Project No 50625516), the National Fundamental Research Program (973) (Project No. 2003CB716207) and the 863 program of China under Grant No. 2006AA04A110.

References

1. Chen, X., Zhang, J., Jiao, C.L., Liu, Y.M.: Effects of different bonding parameters on the electrical performance and peeling strengths of ACF interconnection. Microelectronics Reliability 446, 774–785 (2006)
2. Chan, Y.C., Luk, D.Y.: Effects of bonding parameters on the reliability performance of anisotropic conductive adhesive interconnects flip-chip-on-flex packages assembly ii. different bonding pressure. Microelectronics Reliability 42, 1195–1204 (2002)
3. Frisk, L., Seppala, A., Ristolanien, E.: Effect of bonding pressure on reliability of flip chip joints on flexible and rigid substrates. Microelectronics Reliability 44, 1305–1310 (2004)
4. Wu, Y.P., Alam, M.O., Chan, Y.C., Wu, B.Y.: Dynamic strength of anisotropic conductive joints in flip chip on glass and flip chip on flex packages. Microelectronics Reliability 44, 295–302 (2004)
5. Pinardi, K., et.,, al.,: Effect of Bump Height on the Strain Variation During the Thermal Cycling Test of ACA Flip-Chip Joints. IEEE Transactions on Components and Packaging Technologies 23, 447–451 (2000)
6. Wu, C.M.L., Liu, J., Yeung, N.H.: The effects of bump height on the reliability of ACF in flip-chip. Soldering & Surface Mount Technology 13(1), 25–30 (2001)
7. Chiang, W.K., Chan, Y.C.: Reliability of Anisotropic Conductive Film Joints Using Bumpless Chip—Influence of Reflow Soldering and Environmental Testing. Journal of Electronic Packaging 127, 113–119 (2005)
8. Teo, M., et al.: Effects of Anisotropic Conductive Adhesive (ACA) Material Properties on Package Reliability Performance. In: Electronics Packaging Technology Conference, 2003, pp. 718–725 (2003)
9. Yin, C.Y., et al.: Experimental and Modeling Analysis of the Reliability of the Anisotropic Conductive Films. In: 2003 Electronic Components and Technology Conference, pp. 698–702 (2003)
10. Yin, C.Y., et al.: Experimental and Modeling Analysis on Moisture Induced Failures in Flip Chip on Flex Interconnections with Anisotropic Conductive Film. In: 2005 International Conference on Asian Green Electronics, pp. 172–177 (2005)
11. Mercado, L.L., et al.: Failure Mechanism Study of Anisotropic Conductive Film (ACF) Packages. IEEE Transactions on Components and Packaging Technologies 26, 509–516 (2003)
12. Storn, R., Price, K.: Differential evolution – A Simple and Efficient Heuristic for Global Optimization over Continuous Spaces. Journal of Global Optimization 11(4), 341–359 (1997)
13. Box, G.E.P., Wilson, K.B.: On the experimental attainment of optimum conditions. Journal of the Royal Statistical Society, Series B 13, 1–45 (1951)
14. Teo, M., Subodh, G.M., et al.: Correlation of Material Properties to Reliability Performance of Anisotropic Conductive Adhesive Flip Chip Packages. IEEE Transactions on Components and Packaging Technologies 28(1), 157–164 (2005)
15. Yeung, N.H., Chan, Y.C., Tan, C.W.: Effect of Bonding Force on the Conducting Particle With Different Sizes. Journal of Electronic Packaging, Transactions of the ASME 125, 624–629 (2003)

Optimum Path Planning of Robotic Free Abrasive Polishing Process

Guangchao Han[1] and Ming Sun[2]

[1] School of Electronic Information & Mechanics, China University of Geosciences, Hubei Wuhan 430074, China
[2] Faculty of Information Engineering, China University of Geosiences, Hubei Wuhan 430074, China
hgc009@163.com, smw1013@163.com

Abstract. In the rapid spray metal tooling, high efficient polishing process can improve the mold quality and shorten the lead time of the rapid tool. The polishing of the tool is frequently carried out manually, and the introduction of robotic polishing can minimize the production times and enhance the efficiency obviously. Robotic polishing process with free abrasive and soft polishing tool is developed in this paper to fit for the application of commercial industrial robot, which is hard to be controlled online for its close control construction. A partition & flexible mapping method based on CAM is also proposed for the uniform robotic polishing path on the mould curved surface. In order to compensate the elastic deformation and the abrasion of the soft polishing tool, the robotic polishing path should be offset along the direction normal to the surface with the pre-compressed value and the abrasion compensation value to keep a steady normal polishing force. The optimal pre-compressed and abrasion compensation value are verified by the experiments. The blank holder of punch mould produced by rapid spray metal tooling is finally polished to test the robotic polishing system.

Keywords: Polishing, Industrial robot, free abrasive, Path Planning, Rapid spray metal tooling.

1 Introduction

Rapid spray metal tooling (RSMT) has attracted extensive attention in the automobile industries, because it can shorten the period of developing new type automobile [1]. In the RSMT, high efficient polishing process can improve the mould quality and shorten the lead time of the rapid metal tool. But the polishing process is frequently carried out manually, these kinds of operations are iterative, time consuming and require experience. Automation can introduce cost reduction by minimizing production times on such manual finishing operations, which mostly includes the methods of industrial robot and NC machine. The industrial robot has more advantage than NC machine on polishing a large complex metal mould for its flexibility on machining fashion and machining range. This fact has attracted much research to investigate possible methods of designing and implementing robotic polishing systems. A robotic

C. Xiong et al. (Eds.): ICIRA 2008, Part II, LNAI 5315, pp. 906–915, 2008.

die polishing station controlled by a PC and a robot controller, which can exchange the grinding tool automatically so that the operation was completely unmanned [2]. The contact stress for an automated polishing process was modeled and analyzed, which determined the quality of the polished part, not the force exerted on the polishing tool [3]. A high precision polishing robot with a learning-based hybrid position/force controller was developed for polishing PET (Poly Ethylene Terephthalate) bottle molds [4]. An automatic mold polishing system (AMPS) was present, which integrates with mold geometry process kernel, path planner, process planner, and force control robot into a system [5,6]. An automatic planning and programming system was developed based on data from a CAD system for a robotic polishing cell for mold manufacturing [7]. So the path planning and force control has become the research focus of the robotic polishing process.

Most of the industrial robots in the market now, such as Motoman UP20 robots, have a close control system that an user is hardly to intervene or adjust the robotic program when the robot is working except terminating the machining process. (Not including the particular cell that has the open control system especially designed by the robot manufacturer). A Motoman UP20 robot is selected for the RSMT, so a robotic polishing system with free abrasive and soft polishing tool is developed to fit for the selection. And a partition & flexible mapping method basing on CAM module is proposed to make the real even polishing path on the curved mould surface. The control and compensation for the polishing path is also applied to keep the steady polishing force and smooth the robotic polishing process.

2 RSMT and the Robotic Polishing System

DPST is a developing rapid metal tooling technology. The schematic diagram of DPST is shown in Fig.1. Firstly, the ceramic prototype is formed directly from the ceramic roughcast by the robotic milling method before sintering. Secondly, the metal film with excellent wear resistance is spray formed on the ceramic prototype by robotic plasma spraying. Then the sprayed surface layer needs to be supported and the backup materials should usually possess high mechanical property and fine casting character, namely low rate of shrinkage and goodish fluidity.

The sprayed original prototype is no longer necessary after backup and then be broken and separated from the sprayed layer to obtain the metallic mold surface through the mechanical method. Finally, the robotic polishing is used to finish the sprayed surface and the metal mould is gained, which can be applied to industrial production after assembly.

The facilities of the DPST include industrial robot, plasma spaying machine, numerical rotating plate, and high speed electrical polishing & milling spindle. The type of UP20 industrial robot of YASKAWA Company is selected, which has six axes and comes into being 7-axis robot forming system combining with the numerical rotating plate. In the system, different forming functions can be realized by the industrial robot when mounting different executing devices to the robotic end-effector. Consequently, the whole forming process can become concise and flexible. The fund invested on the equipment and the space is also saved at the same time.

RSMT is a developing rapid metal tooling technology [8,9]. The schematic diagram of RSMT is shown in Fig.1. Firstly, the master model is formed by the rapid prototyping method such as SLS or transformed from the part. Secondly, the silicon rubber mould is transformed from the master model and the original sprayed model is also produced from the silicon rubber mould. Then the metal film with excellent wear resistance is formed on the original model by robotic plasma spraying. The original model is no longer necessary after backup and then is broken and separated from the sprayed layer to obtain the metallic mold surface through the mechanical method. Finally, the sprayed surface is finished by robotic polishing and the metal mould is gained, which can be applied to industrial production after assembly.

The robotic polishing process is an important step of the RSMT. The facilities of the robotic polishing system consist of a Motoman UP20 industrial robot, a high speed electrical polishing spindle and a numerical swivel table. Soft polishing tool (made up of unwoven cloth or wool) and free abrasive are also selected for the system, which can weaken the influence caused by the fluctuation of the robotic moving path error. The CAD/CAM system (such as UG NX) is running on a separate workstation.

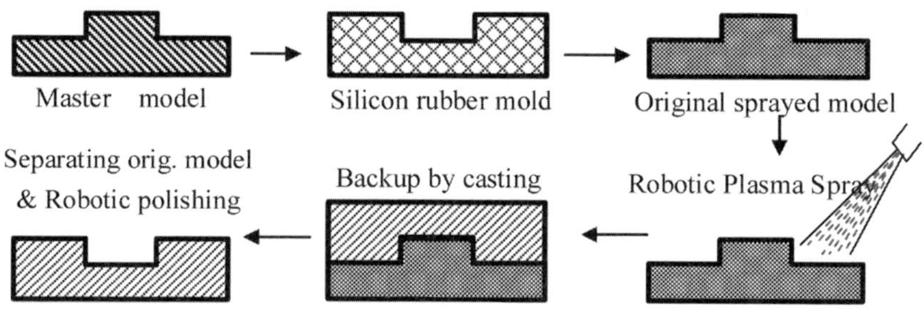

Fig. 1. The schematic diagram of RSMT

3 Path Planning of the Robotic Polishing

Most of the designers usually employ CAD/CAM systems to design workpieces and generate the NC programs for machining process. But the CAD/CAM system can also be used for the robotic path planning because it can edit the multi-axis NC machine programs, which include the information of points on the part's curved surface about surface coordinates and normal vectors. So the robotic machine path can be transformed from the NC machine program and then be adjusted to fit for the different manufacturing processes by offsetting or rotating.

Many engineers usually employ CAD/CAM systems to design workpieces or prepare the NC programs for machining the parts. And the CAD/CAM system can also be used for the path planning of robotic polishing because the information of points on the mould surface about coordinates value and normal vectors can be obtained in the NC programs. So the robotic path planning of RSMT is developed basing on the CAD/CAM system.

In the commercial CAD/CAM software system, such as UG, the multi-axis (max 5 axis) NC milling program can be generated through the CAM module. The axes of the milling tool is usually vertical to the machined surface, so the information of the surface points about coordinates value and the normal vectors can all be included in the NC programs, which can also be fit for the path planning of robotic polishing.

3.1 Path Planning with Partition and Flexible Mapping Method

For the robotic polishing on a complex mould surface, the uniform path interval is important to the final surface quality. The polishing path is usually be achieved by the integral mapping method with fixed driving path intervals, so the actual polishing path intervals projected to the mould curved surface will become uneven with the fluctuation of the surface curvature. The schematic diagram is showed in Fig.2 (a), in which a0a1=a1a2=...=a5a6 are the fixed driving path intervals and b0b1≠b1b2≠...≠b5b6 is the actual polishing path intervals projected on the mould curved surface. So a partition & flexible mapping method is proposed in this paper for generating the actual uniform robotic polishing path on the curved mould surface.

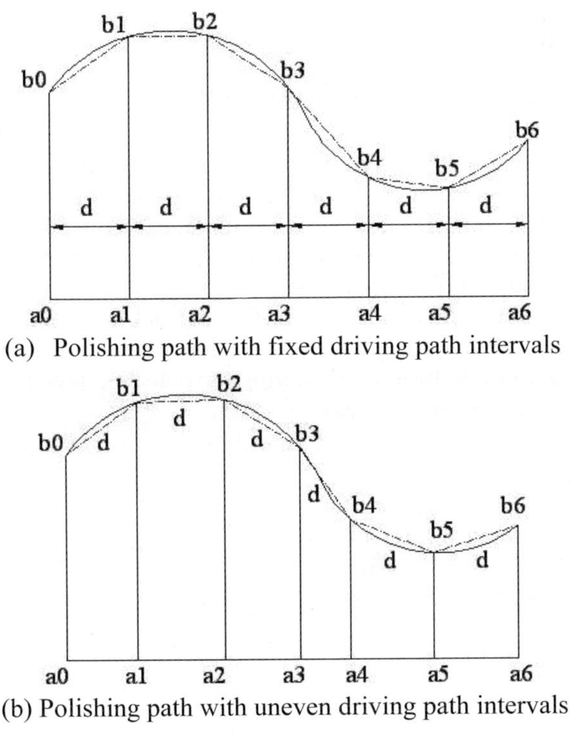

Fig. 2. The schematic diagram of uniform robotic polishing path planning

Firstly, the CAD model of the mould needs to be partitioned into several parts according to the fluctuation of the surface curvature. The partitioned surface fluctuation should be smooth along all the direction except the main fluctuation direction, which can achieve the actual uniform polishing path on the curved mould surface by adjusting the driving path intervals according to the main fluctuation direction. And the uneven driving path intervals will become uniform polishing path after being mapped. The schematic diagram is showed in Fig.2 (b), in which a0a1≠a1a2≠…≠a5a6 are uneven driving path intervals and b0b1=b1b2=…=b5b6 are the uniform NC machining path on the mould curved surface.

Secondly, the track points with uniform distance on each part's contour line can be searched by interpolation arithmetic along the contour line. And the uneven driving path intervals can be obtained after mapping the uniform track points to the underside surface. The UG/Open GRIP programming module is used to compile the programs, which can generate a series of paralleling driving path on the underside surface with the uneven driving path intervals. The uniform multi axis NC machining path can then be generated by mapping the uneven paralleling driving path to the curved surface again.

Thirdly, the multi axis NC machining path of each part should be connected to form an integrated NC path. And the integrated NC path should be transformed into robotic polishing path with the format conversion. Finally, the robotic polishing path needs to be offset for compensating the elastic deformation and the abrasion loss of the soft polishing tool.

4 Control of the Robotic Polishing Path

In the robotic polishing system, online control is hardly applied to the commercial industrial robot for its close control construction. So the soft polishing tool and free abrasive are chosen to compensate some fluctuation caused by the robotic path error. During the robotic polishing process, the angle θ between the tool axis and normal direction of the polished surface should be set between 5° ~ 15° to make the polishing process more smoothly, which is shown in Fig. 3. And the common material of the soft polishing tool is unwoven cloth or wool, so the robotic polishing path control for the elastic deformation and the abrasion during the polishing process of the soft tool is the key to the robotic polishing process.

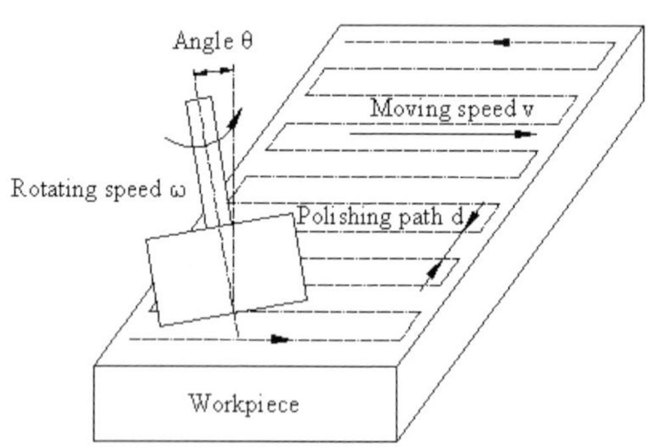

Fig. 3. Sketch of robotic polishing process

4.1 Path Control for the Elastic Deformation

In the robotic polishing process, the polishing force comes into being by the contact press between the soft tool and the polished surface. So the soft tool will make elastic deformation under different polishing force and the effective polishing width will also change. In order to confirm the effective polishing width of the soft tool, the polishing width of the compressed tool is measured with the different pre-compressed value on the 45# steel plate surface. The material of the soft polishing tool with a diameter 30 mm is unwoven cloth, and the scope of the pre-compressed value is from 0.2 to 1.3mm. When the pre-compressed value is over 1.3mm, the shake of the robot is so obvious. The value is not fit for the robotic polishing process. The experimental results are shown in Fig.4, which can be observed that the effective polishing width of the soft tool will come to be steady when the pre-compressed value is greater than 0.8mm. This revealed that the polishing path should offset down about 0.8~1.3mm along the negative normal direction of the polished surface basing on the original polishing position, at which the steady effective polishing width and the initial polishing force can be obtained.

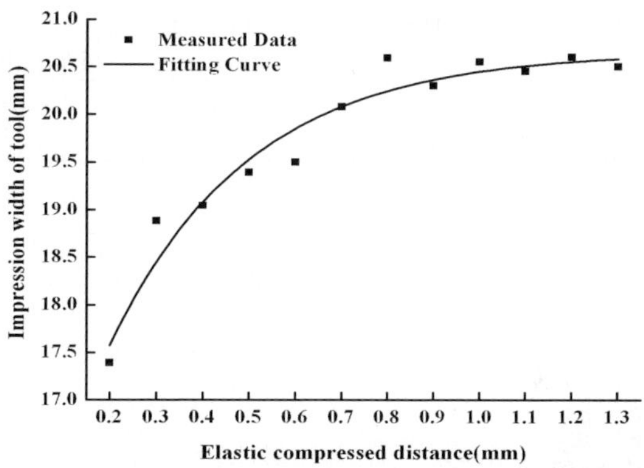

Fig. 4. Relation between the impression width and the compressed distance

4.2 Path Compensation for the Polishing Abrasion

With the path offsetting for the elastic deformation of the soft polishing tool, the wear among the soft polishing tool, free abrasive and the metal mould surface will become more severe. And the polishing force will fluctuate with the abrasion of the soft tool.

The fluctuation character of the polishing force is measured by the experiment, and the experimental parameters are shown in the Table.1. The pre-compressed value can vary from 0.7 to 1.3mm.The polishing path is shown in Fig.5 and the total polishing distance is about 800mm.The polishing force is measured by the 9257A three phase piezoelectricity ergometer and the 5070A-10000 three phase charge amplifier of KISTLER Corp. The experimental situation is shown in Fig.6 and the test result with different pre-compressed value is shown in Fig.7 (a), which appears that the polishing force should be rapid declined at the beginning polishing period, and be fluctuated regularly and declined slowly.

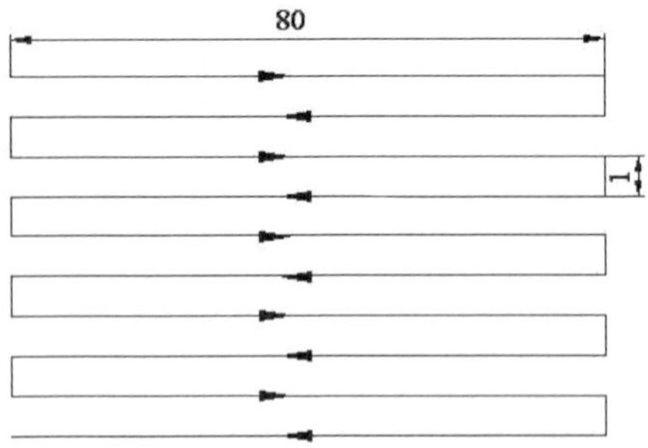

Fig. 5. Polishing path of force measuring

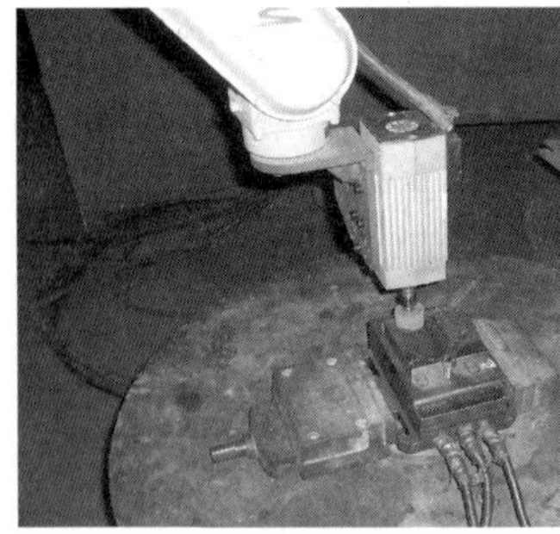

Fig. 6. Situation of the polishing experiment

Table 1. Polishing force fluctuating experimental parameters

Inclination angle(°)	Rotation speed(r/min)	Moving speed(mm/s)	Path interval(mm)
10	3600	10	1
Polished material	Soft tool material	Tool diameter(mm)	Type of free abrasive
45# steel	Unwoven cloth	30	Green SiC

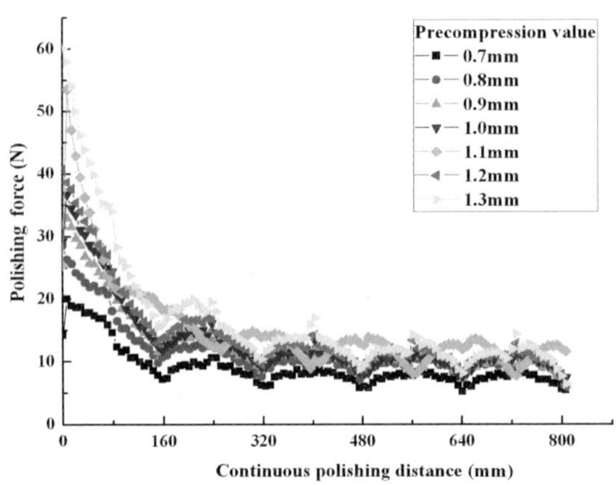

Fig. 7. Polishing force without path compensation

So the robotic polishing path should be adjusted to keep a steady polishing force and polishing process by compensating the abrasion of the polishing tool during the polishing process. The pre-compression value 1.0mm is selected as the control example. The polishing path need to be continuously compensated for the soft tool's continuous abrasion through the polishing process, so the polishing path should be offset every the optimal distance and the offset value for every time is set as 0.1mm according to the

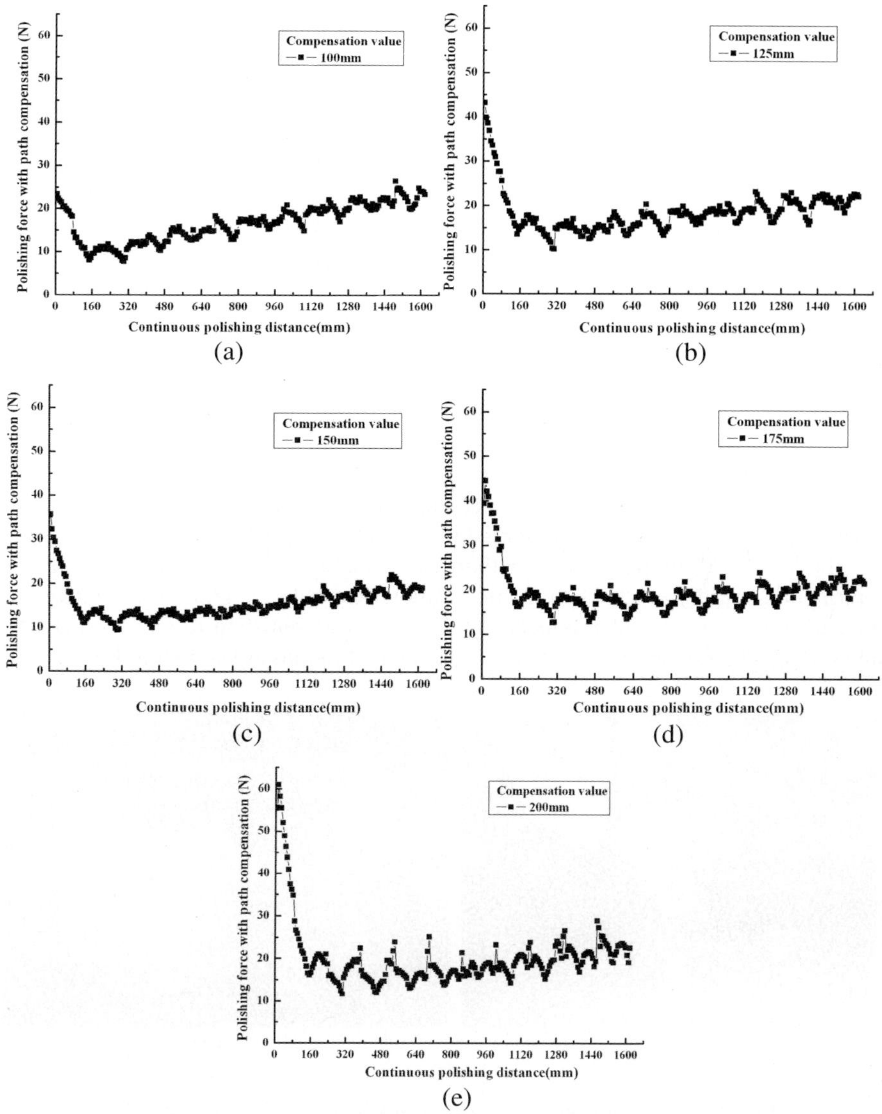

Fig. 8. Polishing force with different path compensating distance

experiment. The optimum distance should be verified by the experiments. The experimental compensation space is set as 100mm, 125mm, 150mm, 175mm and 200mm, respectively, and the total polishing distance is prolonged to about 1600mm. The tested polishing force with different compensation distance is shown in Fig.8 (a) ~ (e).

The deviation of the polishing force in the experiment is calculated in Table.2. From table 2 the optimal polishing path compensation method is probably compensating 0.1mm every 175mm polishing distance, when the pre-compressed value is 1.0mm.

Table 2. Compensation space and deviation of polishing force

Compensation space (mm)	Mean of polishing force (N)	Max deviation with mean force (N)	Sum of deviation square (N2)
100	16.76	9.65	3754.29
125	17.65	7.52	1645.00
150	14.99	7.11	1467.55
175	18.51	6.28	1153.67
200	18.46	10.48	2156.04

5 Summary

In this paper a path planning and control system for robotic polishing process with free abrasive and a soft tool have been developed for the RSMT. A partitioning & flexible mapping method has also been proposed for the robotic polishing path planning. The elastic deformation and the abrasion of the soft polishing tool are controlled and compensated with the robotic polishing path to keep the smooth polishing process. The optimal compensation method is probably compensating 0.1mm every 175mm polishing distance, when the pre-compressed value is 1mm. Finally, the blank holder of the punch mould produced by the RSMT is polished to test the path planning system. The polishing process and the finished mould are shown in Fig.9.

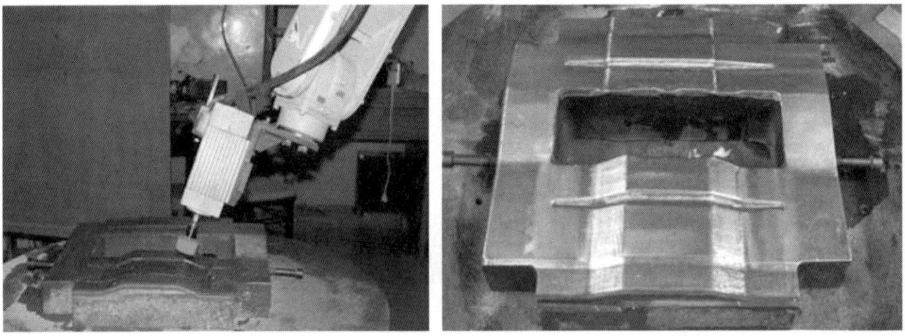

(a) (b)

Fig. 9. Robotic polishing process (a) and the finished blank holder (b)

Acknowledgements

This paper was supported by the Research Foundation for Outstanding Young Teachers, China University of Geosciences (Wuhan) (No:CUGQNL0837), by China Postdoctoral Science Foundation (No. 20070410933) and Project (06-14) Sponsored by Foundation of the State Key Laboratory of Material processing and Die & Mould Technology, China.

References

1. Haiou, Z., Guilan, W., Yunhua, L., et al.: Rapid Hard Tooling by Plasma Spraying for Injection Molding and Sheet Metal Forming. Thin Solid Films 390, 7–15 (2001)
2. Ryuh, B.-S., Park, S.M., Pennock, G.R.: An automatic tool changer and integrated software for a robotic die polishing station. Mechanism and Machine Theory 41, 415–432 (2006)
3. Roswell, A., Xi, F.J., Liu, G.: Modelling and analysis of contact stress for automated polishing. International Journal of Machine Tools & Manufacture 46, 424–435 (2006)
4. Nagata, F., Kusumoto, Y., Watanabe, K., et al.: Polishing robot for PET bottle molds using a learning-based hybrid position/force controller. In: 5th Asian Control Conference, pp. 914–921 (2004)
5. Tsai, M.J., Fang, J.J., Chang, J.L.: Robotic path planning for an automatic mold polishing system. Int. J. Robot. Autom. 19(2), 81–89 (2004)
6. Tsai, M.J., Chang, J.-L., Haung, J.-F.: Development of an Automatic Mold Polishing System. IEEE Transactions on Automation Science and Engineering 2(4), 393–397 (2005)
7. Márquez, J.J., Pérez, J.M., Rios, J., et al.: Process modeling for robotic polishing. Journal of Materials Processing Technology 159, 69–82 (2005)
8. Zhang, H., Han, G., Wang, G.: Development of Direct Prototype Spray Tooling Technology. Die & Mould Technology 19(7), 82–83 (2004)
9. Han, G.-c., Zhang, H.-o., Wang, G.-l.: Robotic milling for Rapid Ceramic Prototyping. Journal of Harbin Institute of Technology(New Series) 12(6), 674–679 (2005)

Circular Sub-window Multi-Step GPI Method in Seam Tracking of Welding Robot Based on 3D Vision

Wenzeng Zhang[1], Zhewei Zheng[2], Xiande Ma[1], Qiang Chen[1], and Dong Du[1]

[1] Key Laboratory for Advanced Materials Processing Technology, Ministry of Education, Dept. of Mechanical Engineering, Tsinghua Univ, Beijing 100084, China
[2] Technology Center, Baotou Beifang Chuangye Dacheng Equipment Manufacturing Co. Ltd., Baotou 014030, China
wenzeng@tsinghua.edu.cn

Abstract. Laser welding requires quite high trajectory accuracy of articulated welding robot. To increase this dynamic trajectory accuracy, a novel 3D seam tracking method is proposed based on stereo visual feedback control, in which a key task is to detect the seam from the vision image. To improve the precision and efficiency of the GPI seam-detecting method, this paper proposed a new method, the multi-step gray projecting integral (MSGPI) method with a circular sub-window. This method applies a circular division in image as the sub-window for detection and the means of GPI values, based on while surpassing the Standard GPI method. It adopts a link table to store edge points gained by Sobel filtering previously to reduce the amount of computation. A threshold method is employed to effectively eliminate noises caused by scratching and rust. The searching range of the line's angle in GPI process is divided into coarse searching and fine searching, which not only ensures detection accuracy but also greatly reduces the amount of computation. The experimental results show that the MSGPI method can achieve rapid and accurate detection for weld seam even if the seam is quite narrow, and can thus greatly improve the trajectory accuracy of industrial robot for laser welding, and the system using this method could meet the demand of high accuracy trajectory tracking.

Keywords: Welding robot; seam tracking; gray projecting integral method; visual servoing.

1 Introduction

Along with the development of manufacturing and processing, some high-speed and high-accuracy jobs, such as laser welding and cutting, require quite high trajectory accuracy. However, nowadays articulated robots only provide customers their positioning accuracy, without offering or guaranteeing their trajectory accuracy, which limits the applications of the welding robots.

As an important sensing method, vision plays an important role in improving the industrial robots' ability in environmental understanding and variance adaptation. In reference [1], a visual servoing system of industrial robots based on position was constructed, and algorithm to estimate the object position and pose with a camera is

C. Xiong et al. (Eds.): ICIRA 2008, Part II, LNAI 5315, pp. 916–926, 2008.

proposed when the distances of several characteristic points were known beforehand. According to this thought, a seam tracking system can be built for laser welding robots to improve the moving trajectory accuracy. In this system, a GPI transform method for seam recognition in trajectory tracking was utilized, and an improved algorithm was proposed to reconstruct the trajectory line and laser focus more precisely [2]. Meanwhile a tool coordinate system was constructed skillfully to facilitate the tool displacement calculation. The modified displacement of the robot is calculated and the robot is finally commanded to move and decrease the trajectory error as soon as possible based on robot kinematics.

A key task and important base of the system above is to detect the seam. It is significant but difficult to extract a weld seam in images when it is extremely narrow. A laser visual sensor with structured light is commonly used for the purpose of avoiding noise caused by welding arc in a welding process. But it also brings some limits in seam detection, because the welding seam is so feeble under structured light that it is easily submerged by noise. Under environmental and arc light, the welded joints exhibit the main characters of a line in the image. Because a curvilinear weld seam has a small curvature, it can be considered as a straight line approximately within a relatively small field.

For line edge detection, the Hough transform method for detecting lines is considered one of the standard techniques, which requires scanning the whole image to obtain line-support regions and then determine the location and properties of the edges [3, 4]. Based on this strategy, various edge detectors and modules have been developed [5, 6]. A gridding Hough transform (GHT) for detecting the straight lines in sports video is fast and uses little memory by using the fact that the interested straight lines in sports video are sparse and long [7]. An inverse problem formulation of finding the location and orientation of straight lines in gray-scale images is in terms of the inverse Radon transform operator, relating the to-be-computed transform to the data, i.e., the observed images [8].

Different from traditional methods based on Hough transform, in order to obtain robust and quick line detection, a new efficient algorithm for robot seam tracking is developed [2], Gray Projecting Integral (GPI), according to the nature of a line projection onto a plane and the gray features of a line in a gray image. In this paper, GPI method and its formula are analyzed, followed by a new method for weld seam detection, multi-step gray projecting integral (MSGPI) method by circular sub-window.

2 Robot Seam Tracking System Base on Vision

The hardware of the established robot visual servoing system is shown in Fig.1. A laser processing tool and two cameras are mounted on the end of articulated robot. The laser focus and trajectory line are imaged in both cameras. The control structure of system is shown in Fig. 2.

The inner and outer parameters of cameras [1], stereo vision coordinates, transform matrix of coordinates between the robot hand and eye [9], and relation matrix between the robot hand and tool are all calibrated beforehand. The laser focus and trajectory line in two images are detected by a threshold segmentation method and GPI transform [2]. Since images in left camera and right camera are matched, the position

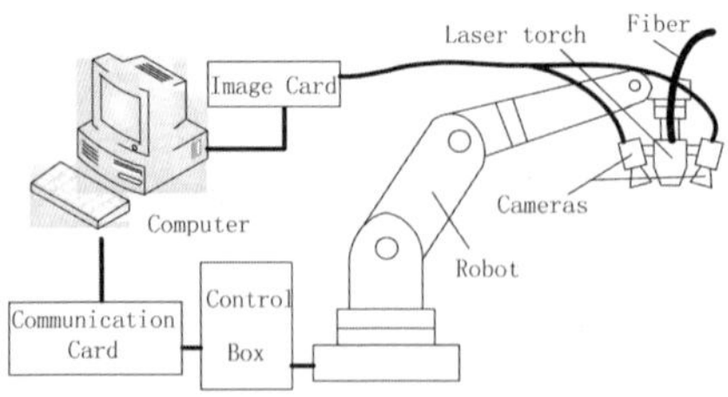

Fig. 1. System hardware components

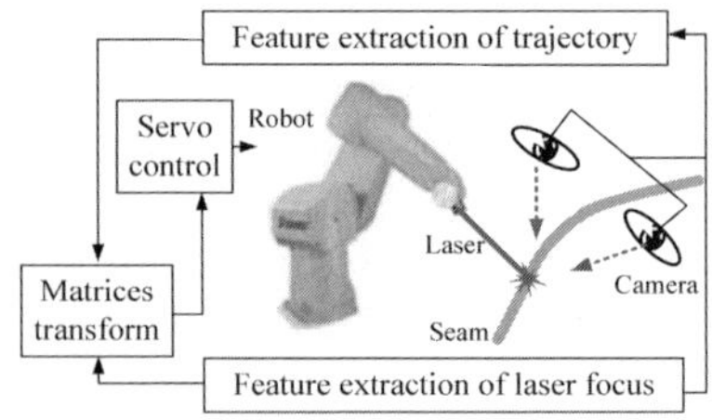

Fig. 2. Principle of the system

of laser focus in the coordinates of left camera can be reconstructed based on the principle of stereo vision reconstruction.

3 GPI Method with Circular Sub-window

3.1 The Principle of GPI Method

In the GPI method, the gray value of pixels are set as coefficients, and pixels in image are mapped onto a curve in projecting parameters space (with the projecting angle of α and projecting position of η) by a projecting operation, as shown in Fig.3a.

Suppose a coordinate system $\{A{:}Oxy\}$ is established and fixed in image with gray distribution function of $f(x, y)$. A sub-window frame is built in the image, shown in Fig. 3b, with the origin $O_s(x_s,y_s)$ in the coordinates $\{A\}$, in which $-b\le u_k\le b$, $-c\le v_k\le c$, and α_k is the angle between u_k-axis and x-axis, called the projecting angle. $[x_i, y_i, 1]$ and $[{}^k u_i, {}^k v_i, 1]$ are the homogeneous coordinates of the same point to deal with in different frames: $\{A\}$ and $\{F_k\}$.

$$\begin{bmatrix} x_i \\ y_i \\ 1 \end{bmatrix} = \begin{bmatrix} \cos\alpha_k & -\sin\alpha_k & x_s \\ \sin\alpha_k & \cos\alpha_k & y_s \\ 0 & 0 & 1 \end{bmatrix} \begin{bmatrix} {}^k u_i \\ {}^k v_i \\ 1 \end{bmatrix}. \tag{1}$$

As for an arbitrary point $P(x, y)$ in sub-window, we have

$$O_s P = l = \sqrt{(x-x_s)^2 + (y-y_s)^2}\,. \tag{2}$$

$$\gamma = \mathrm{atan}[(x_s - x)/(y_s - y)]\cdot \tag{3}$$

The projecting position is

$$\eta = l\cos(\gamma+\alpha)\,. \tag{4}$$

The formula of GPI mapping transform is,

$$G(\eta,\alpha) = \iint_D f(x,y)\sigma[\eta - l\cos(\gamma+\alpha)]\mathrm{d}x\mathrm{d}y\cdot \tag{5}$$

where D is the range of sub-window.

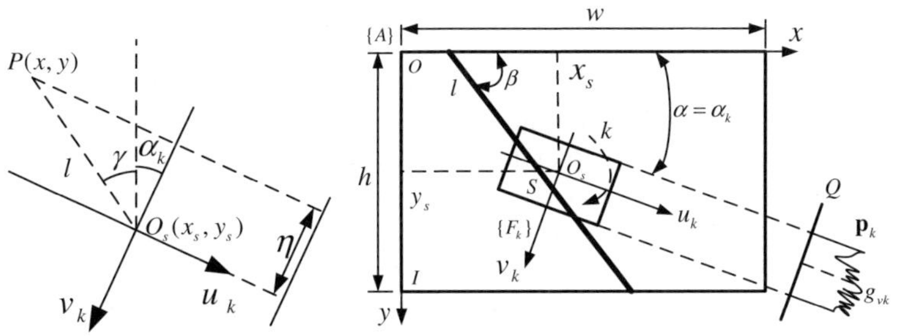

(a) GPI parameters mapping (b) Sub-window and GPI vector

Fig. 3. The principle of GPI method

The straight line in the image space is mapped into a point by the GPI method. Affected by the coefficient of gray values, a white line is corresponding to the points of maximum and a black line the points of minimum. Let

$\alpha_{\min}$ - the original projecting angle; $\alpha_{\max}$ - the final projecting angle; θ - the search step length in angle; $k_{\max}$ - the number of search steps [2] . Then

$$k_{\min}\theta = \alpha_{\max} - \alpha_{\min} \cdot \tag{6}$$

The GPI value related to the projecting position is obtained by the integral along the projecting direction,

$$g_{vk} = \sum_{{}^k u_i=-b}^{b} f(x_i, y_i) \cdot \tag{7}$$

A GPI vector consists of all the GPI values under a projecting angle,

$$\mathbf{p}_k = [g_{1k} \quad g_{2k} \quad \cdots \quad g_{(2c+1)k}]^{\mathrm{T}} \cdot \tag{8}$$

Rotating the sub-window, the GPI vectors under the $k_{\max}$ pieces of projecting angles construct the GPI matrix of the image.

$$\mathbf{G} = [\mathbf{p}_1 \quad \mathbf{p}_2 \quad \cdots \quad \mathbf{p}_k \quad \cdots \quad \mathbf{p}_{k\max}] \cdot \tag{9}$$

Suppose the extremum in G is in row m and column n, then the angle between the straight line and x axis is the projecting direction corresponding to extremum.

$$\beta = \alpha_{\min} + n\theta \cdot \tag{10}$$

The coordinate of the intersecting point of the straight line and v_n -axis is (0, m-c-1) in the frame $\{F_n\}$. By substitute it into the formula (1), the coordinate (x_0, y_0) of this point in $\{A\}$ can be determined. As a result, the equation of the straight line can be obtained according to the formula (11).

$$\begin{cases} y = t\sin\theta + y_0 \\ x = t\cos\theta + x_0 \end{cases} . \tag{11}$$

3.2 Improved GPI Method with Circular Sub-window

According to the analysis of rectangle sub-window of GPI process, there is in fact only a small common part among multiple sub-windows of all rotating angles, which is the inscribed circle of these rectangle sub-windows shown in Fig.4. The content gathered by these sub-windows is different, resulting in that the obtained GPI vectors, strictly speaking, are not comparable. For example, when the straight line lies in the non-common area, i.e. outside the inscribed circle, there will be redundant computation amount of that area without improving the precision. If a square sub-window is adopted, the actual calculating efficiency is only 78.5%.

Thus, an improved GPI method using circular sub-window is proposed, ensuring that the content gathered in rotating sub-window process is the same. To facilitate the calculation, the sub-window can be placed in the center of image. Generally, set the diameter of circular sub-window as 90% of the smaller one of the image height and width, and the sub-window will cover the image area as big as possible.

Since the circular sub-window is adopted, the number of points in the integral column is different, so the extremum in projecting vectors does not always show the place of the straight line, and the GPI values are again not comparable, as shown in Fig.6. The means of GPI values are utilized to solve this problem. The means of GPI values are equal to the results that the GPI values are divided by the number of points in corresponding integral column.

The number of points to integral under some projecting position v_k

$$s = \sqrt{d^2 - 4 \times v_k^2} + 1 \cdot \qquad (12)$$

The means of GPI values are

$$g'_{vk} = \frac{1}{s} \times \sum_{^k u_i = -b}^{b} f(x_i, y_i) \cdot \qquad (13)$$

The feature of the GPI mean matrix obtained is the same as the original GPI matrix, as shown in Fig.7. Fig.8 is obtained when the projecting angle is set as the horizontal axis, and the minima of GPI mean values under this angle, which shows the possible position of straight line, is set as the vertical axis.

It is found that the change of the angles can make great difference to the minima of the GPI mean values, especially near the minimum of the curve in the figure. If a difference is applied to Fig. 6a, the angle difference between the maximum and minimum obtained from Fig.6b is about 9 degrees in this case when the step length is 1 degree. Some angle difference can be defined as the sensitive angle section for projecting. In this case, the sensitive angle section can be found to be 9 degrees from Fig 8b. Fig.9 is obtained by setting the angle corresponding to the minimum point of GPI mean matrix, i.e. the angle of the straight line, as horizontal axis, and the relevant GPI mean value as vertical axis.

It can be said that the change of projecting position makes a great difference to the GPI mean value, especially near the minimum points of GPI mean matrix. Apply a difference operation to Fig. 9a, the angle difference between the maximum and minimum obtained from Fig. 9b is 7 pixels in this case. The width range of this area is

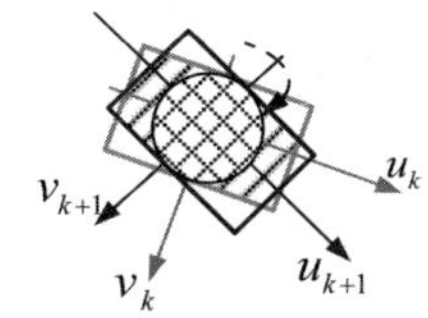

Fig. 4. The same area of rectangle sub-windows

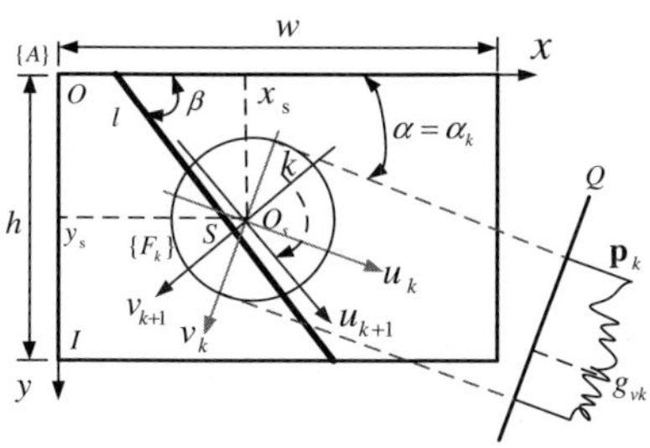

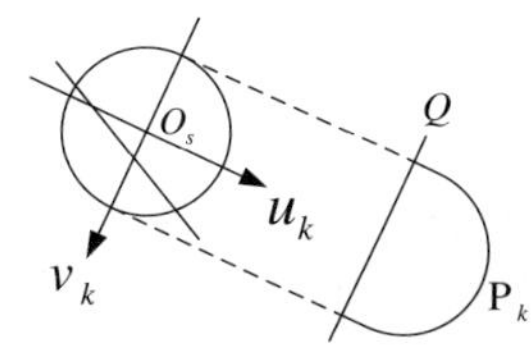

Fig. 5. Improved GPI method **Fig. 6.** GPI vectors with circular sub-window

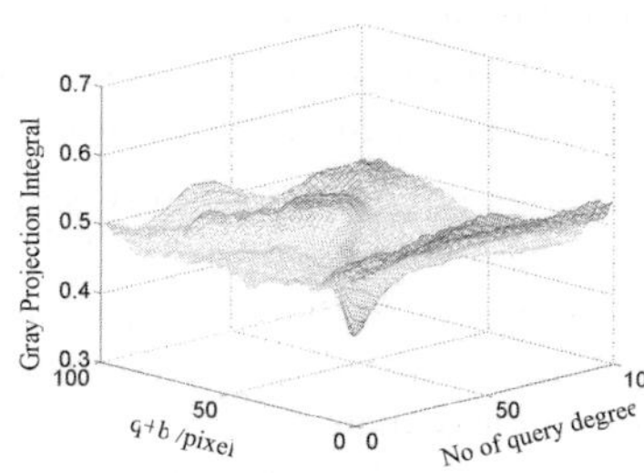

Fig. 7. The GPI mean matrix of welding seam image

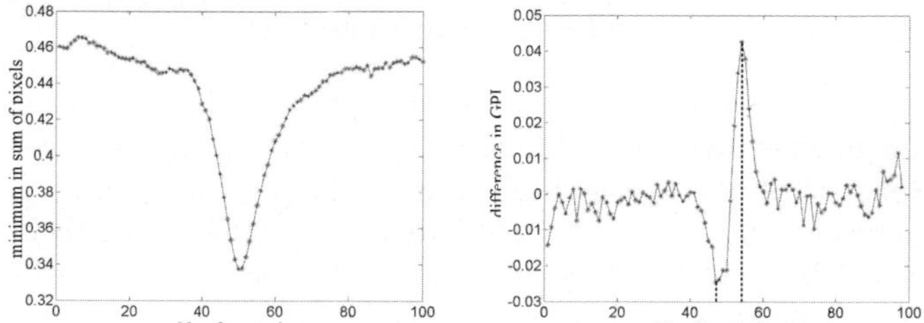

(a) the minimum GPI values under various angles
(b) sensitive angle section obtained by finite difference

Fig. 8. Analysis of sensitive angle section for projecting

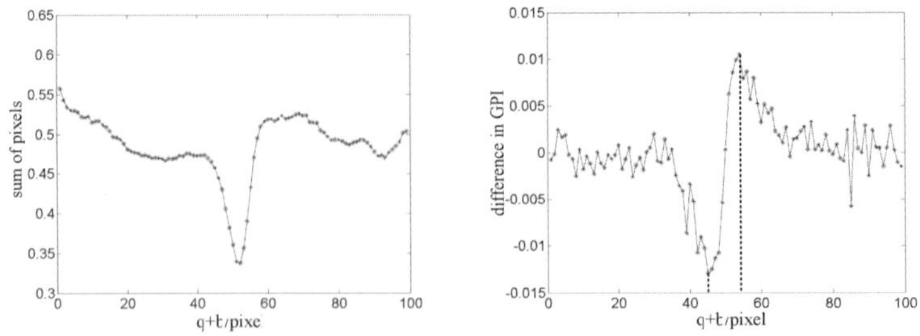

(a) the GPI mean value vector of extremum angle
(b) the projecting width obtained by finite difference

Fig. 9. The analysis of the projecting width of straight line

called the projecting width of straight line. The practical weld seam in the area of sub-window is estimated as 7 pixels, which is close to the analysis result.

4 MSGPI Method

Since the origin searching angle domain is 180 degrees but the sensitive angle section only 9 degrees, large amount of background information brings about a great deal of useless computation. A method to reduce the computation amount is presented below.

1) Extract and save only the edge points, whose gray values are used in consequential GPI transform.

2) Determine the sensitive angle section through previous experiments.

3) Calculate the coarse GPI mean matrix using the sensitive angle section as the searching step angle. Thus the approximate angle range of the weld line can be obtained from the analysis of the coarse GPI mean matrix.

4) Calculate the fine GPI mean matrix using finer searching step angle. Analyse the fine GPI mean matrix and find the accurate angle of the weld line.

4.1 Gray Threshold Method and Edge Detection

Edge detection can be used to extract the edge points along the weld seam. Generally, this is based on gradient image method, which can obtain the intensity and orientation of the edge. Sobel detector is usually used to detect the edge of images.

Scratch and rust are the main noise in weld images. Scratch is usually bright, which can be eliminated by gray threshold method, while rust usually has blurry edges, which can be eliminated by edge intensity threshold.

To self-adapt different weld images, the mean Sobel threshold method is applied.

Gray threshold is:

$$\lim\_g = 1.5 \times \frac{1}{w \times h} \sum f(x, y) \cdot \tag{14}$$

Edge intensity threshold is:

$$\lim\_edge = 2.5 \times \frac{1}{w \times h} \sum S(x, y) \cdot \tag{15}$$

In which the threshold coefficients 1.5 and 2.5 are obtained in experiments.

The experimental results show that this method not only reserves the weld seam information, but also eliminates most noise. In addition, a link table is established to save all the edge points in the circular sub-window, which are obtained by searching the gradient image. In the computing process, the coordinates of the edge points come from this link table, which are used to access the gray value of the original image. This method greatly reduces the amount of computation.

4.2 Multi-Step Searching Using Sensitive Angle Section

From the analysis above, the sensitive angle section of the weld line is 9 degrees, with the coarse searching range of 180 degrees and the searching step angle length of 6 degrees. The fine searching range is 20 degrees, at the range of -10 ~ +10 degrees of the coarse searching results, with the searching step angle length of 1 degree. The total number of searching steps is 50, which is much less than the Standard GPI method. Fig. 10a and 10b are the coarse and fine GPI mean matrix, respectively.

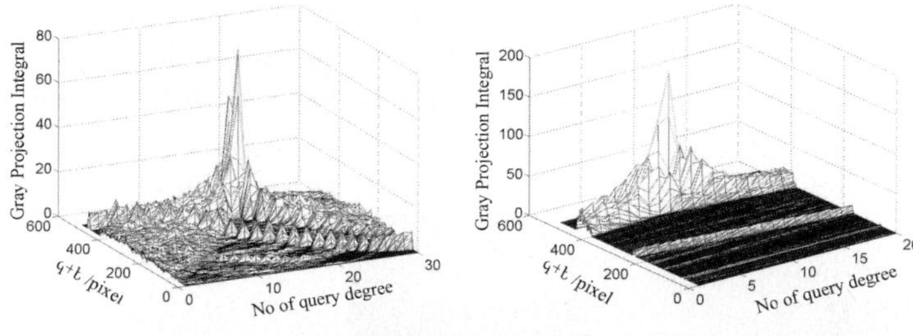

(a) GPI matrix of coarse detection (b) GPI matrix of fine detection

Fig. 10. GPI detection results by coarse and fine steps

5 Experimental Results

The butted gaps of experimental steel sheets which have diverse extent of rust and scratching are in the range of 0.1~0.5 mm. Then 100 weld images in diverse intensity and direction of illumination are captured. The hardware condition: a computer with Pentium 2.4 GHz and 256M memory, and an operation system of Windows XP Professional. Then the Standard GPI method and the new MSGPI method are both programmed in MATLAB 6.5. The Standard GPI method uses small sub-windows of 61 pixels both in length and in width, with each image consuming 33.467 seconds on average. While the MSGPI method uses big circular sub-windows of 259 pixels in radius, with each consuming 4.844 s on average. Compared to the Standard one, the new MSGPI method greatly reduces the time consumption and is thus more favorable for a real-time image processing system of robot welding.

The MSGPI method is then realized by Visual Basic.NET. 100% of the detections have been successful in the finished experiments. The maximum error of the seam location is 2 pixels, while the minimum is less than a pixel. On average, the error of the seam location is sub-pixel. The time consumption of running the program for detection is 0.912s on average. Fig.11a shows the detecting result in one experiment.

By applying MSGPI in the seam robot tracking system, the experimental results show that the trajectory detecting and control system of welding robot based on stereo vision can do quite well in trajectory recognizing, detecting and automatic tracking. The error of tracking is less than 0.5 mm in real-time.

In the experiments, two steel sheets are butted closely, and the tracking speed of robot end is 20 mm/s, with the position and orientation of weld seam (trajectory line) unknown beforehand. Fig.11b shows the image captured before tracking, in which two short parallel white lines are the edges of the adopted sub-window, the long white line is the trajectory line detected by GPI transform method, the large white point is laser focus, and the smaller black point is the anticipated position of the laser focus figured out by stereo vision algorithm, which should be on the seam. Fig.11c shows the image of tracking result, where the laser focus has already bean moved to the anticipated position and goes along with the welding seam.

Experimental results show that the errors in *X, Y, Z* are all less than 0.3 mm, while the spatial distance error is less than 0.4 mm. The spatial distance error of tracking is shown in Fig. 11d. The system can not only recognize the welding seam automatically, but also meet the welding requirement in real-time trajectory tracking.

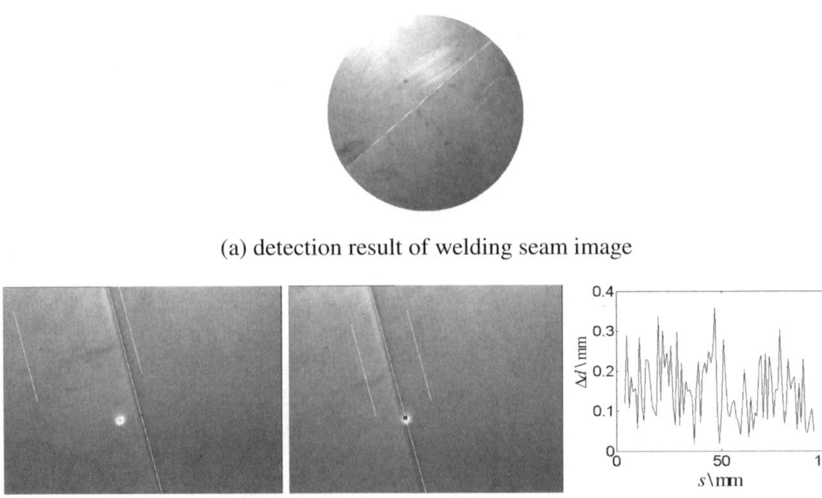

(a) detection result of welding seam image

(b) image before tracking (c) image after tracking (d) tracking distance error

Fig. 11. Detection and tracking results

6 Conclusions

In this paper, a 3D seam tracking method of articulated robot for laser welding based on stereo visual feedback control is proposed, in which a new method for weld seam detection is presented, namely the multi-step gray projecting integral (MSGPI) method with a circular sub-window. This method applies a circular division in image as the sub-window for detection and the means of GPI values, based on while surpassing the Standard GPI method. It also adopts a link table to store edge points gained by Sobel filtering previously to reduce the amount of computation. A threshold method is employed to effectively eliminate noises caused by scratching and rust. The searching range of the line's angle in GPI process is divided into coarse searching and fine searching, which not only ensures detection accuracy but also greatly reduces the amount of computation. The experimental results show that the MSGPI method can achieve rapid and accurate detection for weld seam even if the seam is quite narrow, and can thus greatly improve the trajectory accuracy of industrial robot for laser welding, and the system using this method could meet the demand of high accuracy trajectory tracking.

Acknowledgements

This research was funded by "Tsinghua Basic Research Foundation" (No. JC2007009), Key Laboratory for Advanced Manufacturing by Materials Processing Technology, Ministry of Education, "Hi-Tech Research and Development Program of China" (No. 2007AA04Z258), "The Research Foundation for the Doctoral Program of Higher Education" (No. 20060003069) and "The Seeds Foundation on Student Extracurricular Science and Technology Innovation of Tsinghua University".

References

1. Mana, S., Marcelo, H.: 3D Vision-based Control on an Industrial Robot. In: Proceedings of IASTED International Conference on Robotics and Applications, Florida, pp. 152–157 (2001)
2. Chen, Q., Zhang, W.Z., Du, D., et al.: A new straight line detection method in images for robot seam tracking. China Welding 15(2), 1–5 (2006)
3. Burns, J.B., Hanson, A.R., Reseman, E.M.: Extracting straight lines. IEEE Transaction on Pattern Analysis and Machine Intelligence 8(7), 425–455 (1986)
4. Kahn, P., Kitchen, L., Riseman, E.M.: A fast line finder for vision-guided robot navigation. IEEE Transaction on Pattern Analysis and Machine Intelligence 12(11), 1098–1102 (1990)
5. Venkateswar, V.: Extraction of straight lines in aerial irnages. IEEE Transaction on Pattern Analysis and Machine Intelligence 14(11), 1111–1114 (1992)
6. Nelson, R.C.: Finding line segments by stick growing. IEEE Transaction on Pattern Analysis and Machine Intelligence 16(5), 519–523 (1994)
7. Yu, X.G., Lai, H.C., Liu, S.X.F., et al.: A gridding Hough transform for detecting the straight lines in sports video. In: ICME 2005, p. 4 (2005)

8. Aggarwal, N., Karl, W.C.: Line detection in images through regularized Hough transform. IEEE Transactions on Image Processing 15(3), 582–591 (2006)
9. Shiu, Y.C., Ahmad, S.: Calibration of Wrist-mounted Robotic Sensors by Solving Homogeneous Transform Equations of the Form AX=XB. IEEE Trans. of Robotics and Automation 5(1), 16–27 (1989)
10. Mezouar, Y., Chaumette, F.: Path Planning for Robust Image-based Control. IEEE Trans. on Robotics and Automation 18(4), 534–549 (2002)
11. Huang, N., Abbott, M.G., Beattie, R.J.: Approaches to low level image processing for vision guided seam tracking systems. In: 9th nternational Conference on Pattern Recognition, pp. 601–603 (1988)

Intelligent Assembly for Aero Engine Components

Fritz Klocke, Dražen Veselovac, Thomas Auerbach, and Robert Seidner

Laboratory for Machine Tools and Production Engineering, RWTH Aachen,
Steinbachstraße 19, 52074 Aachen, Germany
T.Auerbach@wzl.rwth-aachen.de

Abstract. In this paper, an intelligent assembly system for a welding process of aero engine components is presented. In contrast to present approaches, the proposed assembly unit is able to automatically align and clamp different rotary components. Furthermore, an optimised orientation of the parts for the adjacent welding process is realised, taking the geometric information of each part into consideration. An optical measurement system is used to orientate the individual components to each other. The controller of the alignment system is implemented by using LabVIEW as a graphical software solution.

Keywords: Assembly, rotary components, align fixture.

1 Introduction

For the assembly of aero engine components such as compressor stages, a precise alignment and clamping device of rotation-symmetric parts is required. In an adjacent welding process the separate parts are centrical welded. As due to the high safety requirements in the aviation sector, the functionality of aero engine components has to be guaranteed. Narrow assembly tolerances are demanded. According to the manufacturer's information the permissible tolerances for concentricity are less than 0.05 mm. The part alignment is currently manually accomplished, so that the assembling process is very time-consuming and causes high production costs.

The positioning of parts can be implemented by the usage of piezoelectric actuators [1, 2]. Thereby the actuator moves the part towards the stimulated direction. Piezoelectric actuators are applied mainly for positioning micro parts as their full length of actuation is about 100 μm [2]. In [3], the alignment of rotation-symmetric components is described. Work pieces are freely movable and outside of the rotation centre positioned on a rotary table. The concentricity deviation of the part is measured during a rotary table's revolution. As a result of the measurement, a series of controlled impacts moves the part directly to the centre of the rotary table within a 2.5 μm tolerance [3].

In the manufacturing area a flexible assembly system is able to align different stage types in a random order. Due to the fact that each aero engine type consists of different parts, an identification of every part is necessary. Currently used assembly systems have a regular clamping fixture selected in dependence on the parts geometry and the identification of the parts is done manually.

C. Xiong et al. (Eds.): ICIRA 2008, Part II, LNAI 5315, pp. 927–935, 2008.

Overall part identification can be done in different ways, as there are mechanical and optical inspection technologies for measuring component properties. In particular optical technologies such as laser triangulation or laser scanning provide the opportunity for non-contact measurements. Due to the high costs of high-resolution optical measurement systems, other measurement systems have to be applied for high-precision alignment processes. Mechanical inspection technologies such as touch probes are more suitable for measurements of narrow tolerance as their resolutions are sufficiently high.

The present paper describes a method to automated align rotation-symmetric aero engine components as a pre-stage for the welding assembly. Based on the procedure described in [3] an application is developed to arrange discs axial-symmetrical to each other. Furthermore the automated part identification, the inspection of the part's geometry and orientation as well as the process documentation is explained, so that the basis concept for an automated and flexible assembly system is presented.

2 Intelligent Assembly Station

In aero engine manufacture processes are applied on a high product variety and within small batch productions. Each compressor needs a specific clamping device for the welding process therefore a modification of the assembly station is very time-consuming. As the welding process is irreversible, the positioning, the orientation and the alignment of the single discs is a critical production stage. Any mistakes of the operator result in a costly post processing or loss of the part.

The presented concept of an intelligent assembly station provides an automated and interacting aligning system. This system assists the operator's activities during the assembly process. Here, the following requirements are fulfilled by the support system:

- Automated part identification and reconfiguration of the clamping device,
- acquisition of the part's geometry and orientation,
- measurement of the part's concentricity,
- automated alignment of the parts,
- and documentation of the assembly process.

Figure 1 shows a principle sketch of the assembly station. On a rigid rack a rotary table is mounted to enable a control of a part's geometry and orientation as well as part's concentricity to each other. Additionally two more linear axes – a horizontal and vertical axis – are implemented to position the sensoring and actuating devices at the dedicated position. The horizontal axis is mounted on the vertical axis, so that part alignment is possible at individual heights of the single components within a drum. The measuring and aligning equipment (1, 4, 5 cp. Figure 1) is positioned at the end of the horizontal axis. As after the alignment process each disc has to be secured in its position, an inner and outer clamping system is implemented into the system. The clamping device itself is not described in this paper.

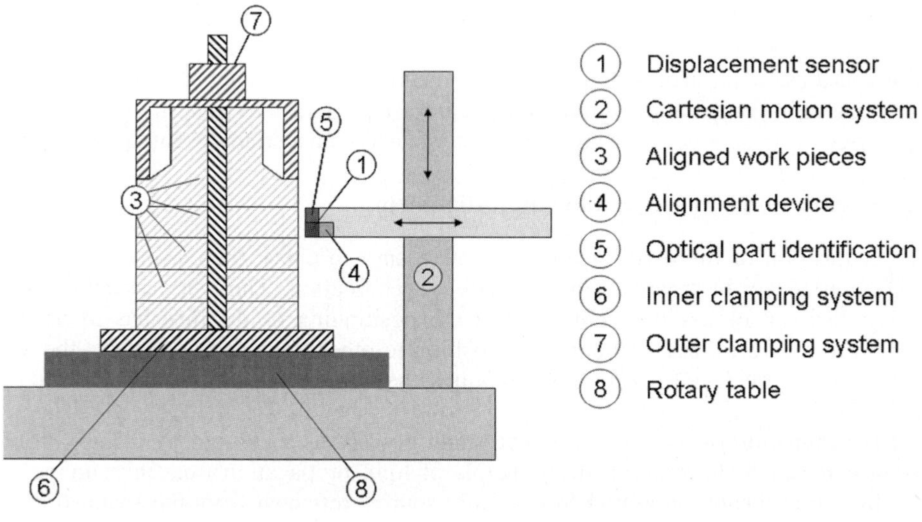

Fig. 1. Concept of the Assembly Station

2.1 Automated Part Identification

The discs are identified by a barcode reader system when arriving at the assembly station. Each disc is tagged by its own specific barcode that is stored in a database. By reading the disc's barcode the part's properties as well as the assembly instructions are downloaded from a database. As additional information of all possible assembly configurations is stored in this database, the software system selects the specified assembly configuration and uploads the required alignment parameters into the clamping system. Following, the operator prepares the assembly device and verifies the workflow for the adjacent assembly process.

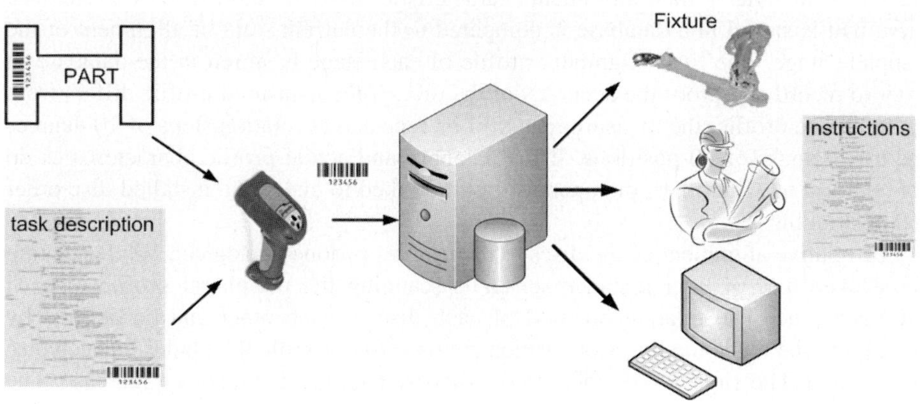

Fig. 2. Part Identification

Compared to other optical scanning systems the barcode devices are chosen because of their ease of use and system integration. The biggest advantage of a barcode based database is the fact that each barcode includes an individual identification (ID) part number in combination with additional information such as measurement reports or configuration parameters, which can be stored and managed in the database.

2.2 Part's Geometry Acquisition and Alignment

The acquisition of the part's geometry is necessary to check the current assembled disc's conformity in regard to the database's specification. Thus, the assembly of a wrong disc can be avoided. Furthermore the positioning of the disc has to be inspected in regard to its circumferential position to other stage components as the assembly of the blades at a later stage requires the correct orientation of the discs to each other.

The acquisition of the part's geometry and position is measured by using a laser distance sensor that works on the principle of light propagation time measurement. Hereby a laser beam is emitted from a light source, reflected from the scanned disc and absorbed by a light sensor. The calculated distance l between beam source and the disc results from the elapsed time t and the speed of light c considering the following physical relationship.

$$l = \frac{t}{2} \cdot c \,. \tag{1}$$

Equation (1) enables the distance calculation of selected positions on the disc. As the concentricity control of the part requires at least three individual positions of measurement, disc or measurement sensor motion has to be integrated into the alignment system. The design of such a system is described in the following chapter.

The elevation profile of each disc type is stored in the database of the support system. Subsequent to the current disc's position, the position among themselves is inspected by measuring their alignment characteristics to each other. Hereby a reference curve that is stored in a database is compared to the current state of alignment of the complete stage. The final alignment profile of each stage is stored in the database in order to record and proof the accuracy of the disc. If the measured profile differs from the reference profile, the measurement will be repeated at rotation steps of 10 degrees and a maximum of 10 positions. If the database and actual profile characteristics do not conform to each other, the operator will be asked to check the installed disc order and positioning.

The relative alignment of the discs to themselves is done analogical. While rotating the stacked disc, a laser distance sensor is scanning the peripheral profile of each individual one. The relative position of each disc to each other can be defined by identifying the blade loading slots, which are used to assemble the blades on each disc of the stage. The slots can be identified easily by measuring a distance increase. The alignment system detects the position of the loading slot and calculates the angular offset related to the required slot position. The offset correction will be done manually by the operator.

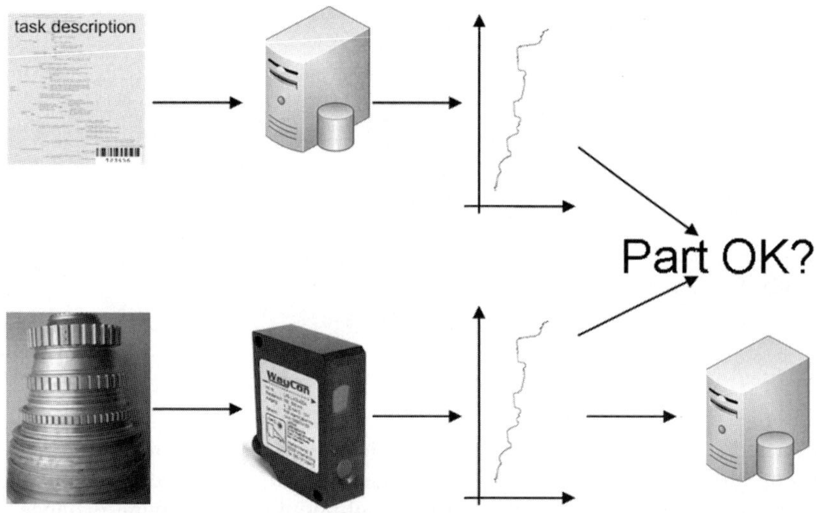

Fig. 3. Optical Part Recognition

2.3 Measurement and Alignment System

An automated measurement and alignment system is integrated in the assembly process to realise the narrow tolerance requirements (Figure 2). Decision criterion for the quality of the assembly process is each disc's concentricity. The measurement system acquires the concentricity of the components and an automated alignment system aligns actively the out-of-position discs by the calculated offset.

The used displacement transducer of the type MT2571 (company Heidenhain) is able to cover a large measurement range and guarantees an accuracy of 2 µm. Based on an incremental material measure the displacement of the probe is photoelectric scanned. Thereby photo sensors are stimulated by incidence of light through a structured scan plate which generates a sinusoidal signal. The periodicity of the signal is a measure for the sensor's displacement. Additionally the measurement probe has an integrated digitization and interpolation unit (10 times interpolation) to increase its resolution.

The measurement probe is mounted on a linear gantry of high precision and mechanical rigidity. The out-of-centre positioned discs are pushed by a sleeve that surrounds the probe. Both parts are attached to the linear gantry of a multi-axis handling system. A pre-condition for the alignment system is that the discs surface finish should not be affected by the procedure in order to meet the claimed quality requirements of the product. Therefore the sleeve has to fulfil certain specifications like higher material deformability. As rubber materials can not be used due to their abrasion behaviour the sleeve is made out of aluminium, a material that enables a non-destructive alignment of the titanium alloy based discs. Abrasive rubber would interfere the following in vacuum executed welding process.

The relative position between sensor and sleeve is important to realise an automated measurement and alignment process procedure. The probe which is springy seated and extended to its limit in the unloaded state is positioned on a disc in a

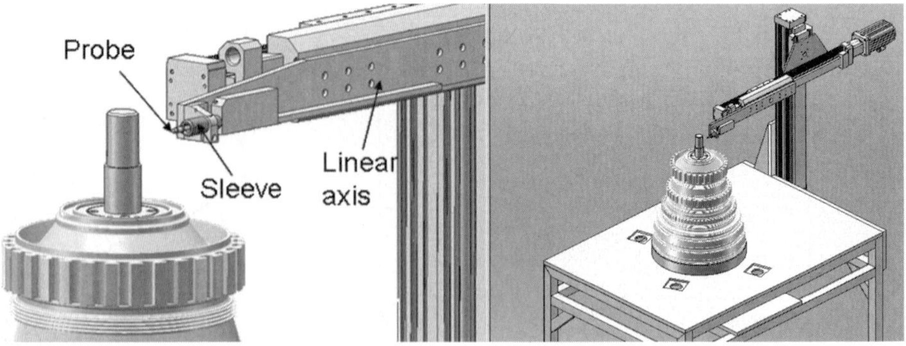

Fig. 4. Measurement and Alignment System

half-retracted state, so that double sided distance measurements are enabled. For the positioning process the carriage is moved towards the disc until the sleeve touches the disc. As at the same time the probe retracts continuously, the moving distance of the sleeve is limited to the probes remaining range of measurement. Therefore the sensor is mounted on the linear gantry keeping a 2 mm security distance to its end position.

To measure the concentricity of the work pieces the rotary assembly system is started after the probe's tip is positioned on one disc's surface. The measurement of one complete revolution shows an oscillation, in which the wave's amplitude is a measure for the part's concentricity. Based on this the needed adjustment of the disc is calculated. As a defined force is needed to realise the part's correction of position and as the applicable force is depending on the friction behaviour of the contact zones, the friction coefficients of the individual and possible friction combinations have to be taken into consideration. Minimum and maximum forces are contemplated to define the force value that enables a first movement and overcomes the static friction. An upper limit is necessary to avoid a deformation of the disc as a result of the load transmission.

After the first alignment step a further measurement of the disc's concentricity is done to check the tolerance requirements. Hereby different outcomes are possible. With the measured value meeting the demanded tolerance of concentricity the alignment process is fulfilled and the disc is clamped to secure its position. Otherwise the software calculates an adjustment force to move the part into position. The procedure is repeated as long as necessary to achieve the demanded tolerances.

2.4 Software Implementation

The demonstrator's software is implemented by using the development environment LabVIEW of the company National Instruments. Next to the graphical language "G" LabView offers numerous methods for controlling external systems as well as extensive functions for data analysis and processing. Programming in NI LabView is done according to the data flow model. As NI LabVIEW supports a number of communication protocols and connection methods, it is qualified for applications in the area of

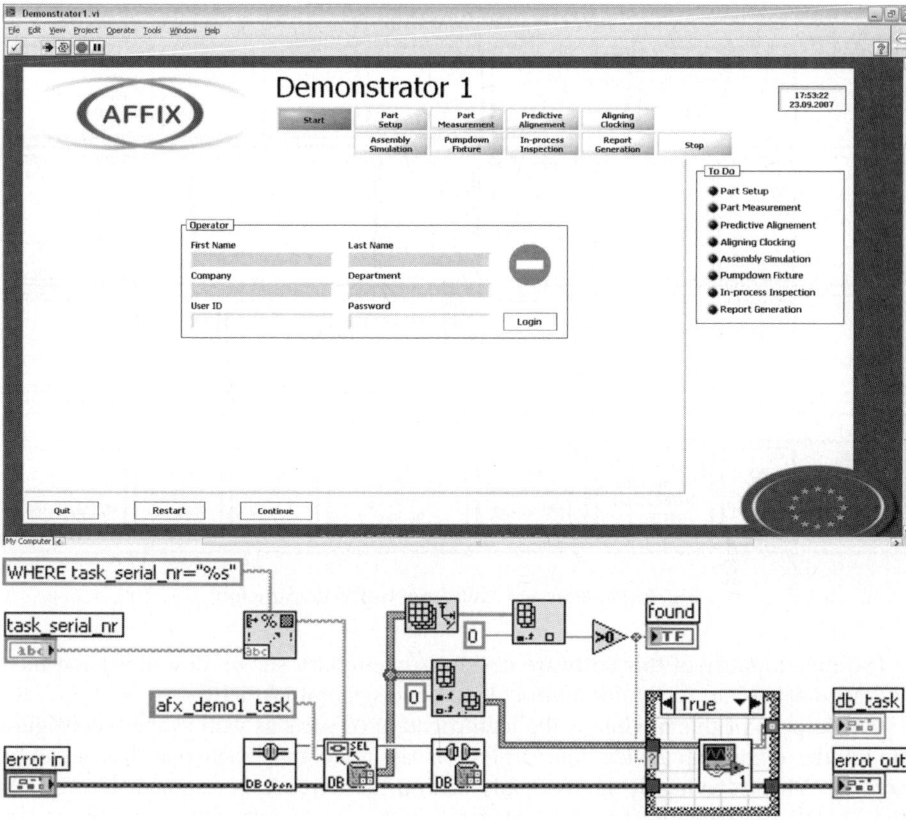

Fig. 5. Example of the Graphical User Interface and Programming Code

measuring, testing and controlling. Figure 3 shows the graphical user interface and programming code of the alignment system.

The integrated software of the test rig has a modular and multilayered structure, which is shown in Figure 4. Due to its modular structure new elements can be easily integrated into the software, exchanged on the application level or adapted to new requirements. The cross-layer communication occurs by defined interfaces whereas modules of high-level layers use the methods and modules of low-level layers to implement the respective tasks.

Virtual instruments are used to access the hardware components of the demonstrator which are controlled by the presentation layer. Due to this fact it is not necessary that each module of the application contains implemented information of the specific hardware's functionality. Thus, a new hardware as an actuator or sensor can be integrated without adapting the new technologies to the modules of the application layer. Hardware components are controlled by the physical layer. Each component of this physical layer has a correspondent element in the presentation layer. For the data exchange respectively the hardware access, modules of the presentation layer use fundamental functions which are defined in the data link layer.

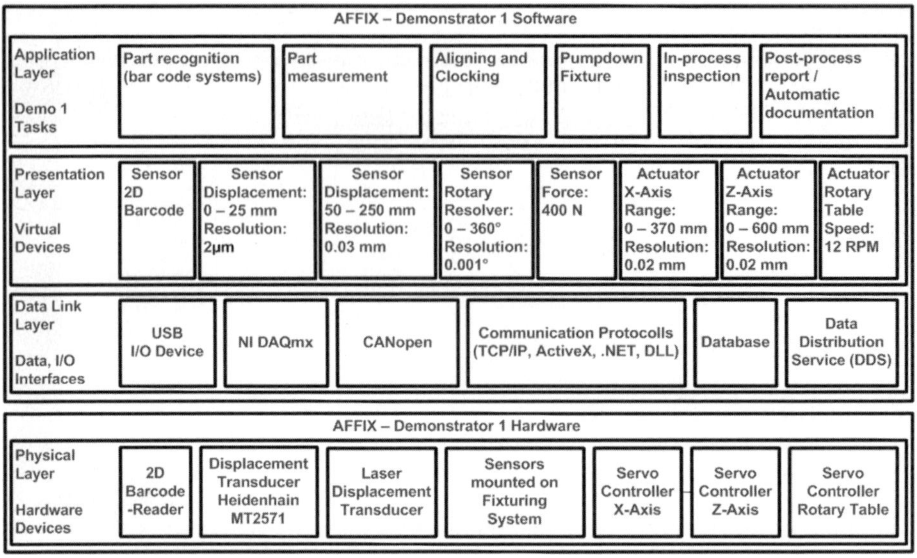

Fig. 6. Modular and Multilayer Software Structure

The functionality of this software design is exemplary shown describing the module "Automated part recognition through barcode systems (APRBC)".

The purpose of this module is the identification of parts as well as the reconfiguration of the clamping device (cp. 2.1). It is assumed that each part has a unique barcode. When arriving at the assembly station the barcode is scanned. Hereby, the module APRBC has not to read or interpret the barcode itself. The actual processing of the barcode information is done by the virtual device "2D Barcode scanner" which provides an ID number or character string to the APRBC module. The APRBC module replicates the acquired information with the reference database to ensure the accurate positioning of the selected part. Obtaining a successful match, the part's information is provided to all modules in order to process the alignment procedure. Due to the modular and multilayer structure other part identification methods such as RFID solutions can be integrated easily into the software module as a replacement for the current identification module. Furthermore, system properties can easily be changed by adapting the virtual element as the functionality of the module APRBC is not affected exchanging an interface between the application and presentation.

3 Summary

The concept of an intelligent assembly station that enables the centric alignment of rotation-symmetric aero engine components has been presented. As this new concept allows the automated alignment of discs within a demanded tolerance range, the assembly task is processed more efficient and less time-consuming compared to current manual processed alignment steps. To fulfil the high safety requirements in the aviation sector several components are integrated into the assembly station to monitor the complete process step. A barcode system indentifies the components and provides information about the assembly procedure to the operator. With a laser distance sensor the part's geometry and orientation is measured and compared to the required position of the part. After orienting each component to each other hand operated the concentricity alignment step is automatically carried out by the system itself. The measurement of the part's concentricity is used to calculate the force needed to correct a part's position. All steps within the assembly process are controlled by a modular and multilayer software which also enables a complete documentation of the process.

Acknowledgement

The reported research is conducted as part of the ongoing European Commission FP6 funded integrated project (FP6-2004-NMP-NI-4) - AFFIX "Aligning, Holding and Fixing Flexible and Difficult to Handle Components". The financial support of the EU and the contributions by the project consortium members are gratefully acknowledged.

References

1. Higuchi, T., Yamagata, Y.: A Micropositioning Device for Precision Automatic Assembly using Impact Force of Piezoelectric Elements. In: IEEE International Conference on Robotics and Automation (1995)
2. Fearing, R.S., Zesch, W.: Alignment of Microparts Using Force Controlled Pushing. In: SPIE Conference on Microrobotics and Micromanipulation (1998)
3. Mears, M.L.: Geometry Estimation and Adaptive Actuation for Centering Preprocessing and Precision Measurement, dissertation, Georgia Institute of Technology (2006)

The Scheduling for Press Shop Based on Operation Constraints Parallel Machine Model

Daoyuan Yu[1], Zhengfeng Li[1], Shunian Yang[1], and Zhili Yao[2]

[1] School of Mechanical Science and Technology, Huazhong University of Science and Technology, 430074 Wuhan, China
[2] DongFeng Automoblie Co., Ltd, 441004 Xiangfan, China
d.y.yu@163.com, zhengfengli@yeah.net, syang1229@yahoo.com.cn

Abstract. This paper presents the new scheduling solution for press shop and the new scheduling model based on operation constraints parallel machine for bidirectional press lines. In this new model, the jobs will be processed from the both terminals of the press line and in the order of machines, and the parallel processed jobs are under the constraints of operation number. In this paper, the constraints relative between operation and time are formulated. Then, the hybrid genetic algorithm with heuristic rules has been devised to solve the problem. In the end, an example is given in which the minimum makespan and load balance among press lines are used as the optimized objects to validate this model, and the scheduling results is obtained which possessed practical application value.

Keywords: scheduling, press shop, parallel machine, hybrid genetic algorithm, operation constraints.

1 Introduction

Taking the most complicated automobile press shop scheduling for example, various kinds of optimum objects for press shop have been studies based on the due date, makespan, inventory and multi-objects, etc, in which many technologies and methods have been investigated such as bound and branch, genetic algorithm, simulation and virtual manufacturing, etc. In paper [1], the optimization model of the storage ration has been presented, and the inventory cost has been optimized considering setup time of production, constraint of the certain supply capacity for downstream production line and the average occupancy fund of inventory. In paper [2], the lot sizing problem has been studied considering individual machine processing ability. In paper [3], an integration job shop production planning and scheduling with setup time and batches has been addressed. And in paper [4], an integrated optimization of production planning and scheduling for multi-stage manufacturing system has been investigated, which consists of press shop, weld-assembly shop and painting shop. Meanwhile, other new technologies such as simulation and virtual manufacturing have also been adopted on scheduling in press shop. In paper [5], the flexsim software has been used in scheduling optimum as the tool for simulation of the bidirectional press line. In

C. Xiong et al. (Eds.): ICIRA 2008, Part II, LNAI 5315, pp. 936–945, 2008.

paper [6, 7], the dynamic scheduling of press shop has been studied in the virtual manufacturing environment.

In the most scheduling research on the press shop, the press shop model is simply assumed as a single shop model, like job shop. In these research based, the press shop scheduling is usually assumed a class typical job shop problem and the research contents are the different optimization objects such as maximum completion time, due date and storage cost under different conditions of processing time, setup time, waiting time, due time, priority of job and so on. But in production activity, the press shop possesses the mixed characteristics of job shop and flow shop, which results that the above-mentioned scheduling fails to be well applied to practice production.

The four major limitations of these investigations are described as follows. (1) The press shop model is assumed a single model like job shop, which is disaccord with the real model. (2) The number of operation of jobs is assumed to be the same without considering affection on process characteristics resulted from the different operation number. (3) The cost is not taken into account of the transferring time, the apparatus cost to place the semi-finished products, management cost and so on, resulted from transportations among different lines or/and workstations. (4) The processing route of the same job varies in every scheduling. The cost of job transferring among lines and workstations varies with the scheduling and is hard to compute. So many scheduling results of press shop are not well adapted to apply in the practice production.

In this paper, the new model of press line is advanced to solve the disaccord with the foundational model and to overcome the above limitations, and a hybrid genetic algorithm was devised to solve the optimization of scheduling.

The remainder of this paper is organized as follows. Section 2.1 gives the description of bidirectional press line. Section 2.2 presents the bidirectional press line model based operation constraints parallel machine. Section 2.3 describes the model of press shop. Section 3 describes how to devise the hybrid genetic algorithm to solve the optimization model. Section 4 gives an example to validate the new model and algorithm. Section 5 gives some conclusion remarks and directions for future work.

2 Press Shop Model Based on Operation Constraints Parallel Machine

2.1 The Description of Press Shop

In the automobile press shop, the real production activities mixes the feature of the job shop and flow shop. The jobs assignment has the characteristics of the job shop, but once when the job begins being processed, operations of the job will be machined in the way of flow mode.

The press jobs are diversity and jobs is consisted of different operations. Commonly, the maximum number of operations among jobs is equal the number of the machines on a press line. For example, if jobs in press shop are consisted 1~5 operations, then, the machines for a line are 5 machines at least.

It is batch production in press shop. Considering the setup time of mould is almost half an hour while the processing time of a job is about several seconds, the batch size is the important factor to obtain more efficiency. In this paper, as the lot sizing plan is not the main issue, for the simple reason, the economic lot size is adopted.

For bidirectional press line, the jobs can be parallel machined on a press production line and the processing starts only from the two terminals of line.

Specially, in real production activity, the process procedure of a job would not be interrupted until the operations of the job are machined completely on the ordinal machines. This means that the job will not be transferred among press lines.So, the scheduling for press shop can be divided into two issues: (a) the scheduling of jobs for one press line and (b) the scheduling for among several press lines.

2.2 The Bidirectional Press Line Model Based on Operation Constraints Parallel Machine

Taken above various factors into consideration as a whole, the new model of bidirectional press line based on the operation constraints parallel machine is put forward in which the jobs have different operation number, and relative process route of the same kind of jobs is determined. The new model is described as follows.

The n kinds of jobs will be machined on one bidirectional line composed of m machines.

(1) One operation is processed on one machine.

(2) The processing procedure of jobs in the same batch is continuous, i.e. the completion time of certain kind job is the start-time of the next.

(3) There are enough number machines to complete all operations of jobs, i.e. the number of machines on one press line is equal to the maximum operation number of jobs.

$m = max\{q_i, i = 1,2\ldots n\}$

Where m is the number of machines on one line and q_i the number of operations of job i.

(4) The operations of one job are processed in the order of machines on one press line until the job is completed. So the total batch processing time of job i can be deduced.

$$P_i = \sum_{k=1}^{bi}\left(\sum_{j=1}^{qi}(p_{ij} + t_{ij}) + R_i\right) + M_i$$

where P_i is the total batch processing time of job i including setup time, b_i is the lot size of jobs, q_i is the operation number, p_{ij} is the processing time of operation j of the job i, t_{ij} is the transferring time of job i from workstation j-1 to workstation j, R_i is the preparing time of every job i which usually is zero, and M_i is the setup time for jobs i.

(5) The processing of jobs starts from the both terminal of the press line, i.e. it is parallel model in which the one terminal is logically represented as parallel machine A and the other as parallel machine B. The logical machine A or B maybe include one or several machines, and the number of machines in the logical machine A or B depends on the operations of job processed on the press line.

(6) In the parallel machine model, the operations of jobs processed simultaneously on one press line are constrained, i.e. the total operations number of two jobs simultaneously processed is not more than the number of machines on the line.

(7) For jobs on two parallel machines, the processing time related to operation number is constrained. Given the machine A as the benchmark, the job *i* is to process on machine A while the job *j* on machine B. It is presented as follows.

(a) the start-time and completion time of first job processed on machine A are formulated as follows.

$S_{a1} = 0;$

$C_{a1} = P_{a1};$

(b) when $q_{ai} + q_{b(j-1)} =< m$

$S_{ai} = C_{a(i-1)};$

$C_{ai} = S_{ai} + P_{ai};$

(c) when $q_{ai} + q_{b(j-1)} > m,$

$S_{ai} = max\{ C_{a(i-1)}, C_{b(j-1)} \};$

$C_{ai} = S_{ai} + P_{ai};$

(d) when $q_{ai} + q_{bj} =< m$ and $q_{a(i-1)} + q_{bj} =< m$

$S_{bj} = C_{b(j-1)};$

$C_{bj} = S_{bj} + P_{bj};$

(e) when $q_{ai} + q_{bj} =< m$ and $q_{a(i-1)} + q_{bj} > m$

$S_{bj} = max\{ C_{a(i-1)}, C_{b(j-1)} \};$

$C_{aj} = S_{aj} + P_{aj};$

(f) when $q_{ai} + q_{bj} > m$, since machine A is the benchmark, the job *i* will be processed on machine A, while the job *j* will be assigned next turn.

Where S_{ai}, C_{ai}, P_{ai} and q_{ai} stand for the start-time, the completion time, the total batch processing time and the operations number of job *i* on machine A while S_{bj}, C_{bj}, P_{bj} and q_{bj} for job *j* on machine B.

2.3 The Press Shop Model

In the real production activities in the automobile press shop, since the processed job is not transferred among lines, the press lines are mutually independent without the procession relation. On the basis of the press line model based on operation constraints parallel machine, the press shop model is described as follows.

The *n* kinds of jobs will be machine on *k* press lines composed of m_i machines.

(1) All the operations of one job are completely machined on one line.

(2) The operations of one job are processed in the order of machines on one press line until the job is completed.

(3) The model of each line is the operation constraints parallel machine model and the start-time and completion time of jobs simultaneously processed satisfy the constraints of operation number.

(4) The production on each press line is parallel, so the scheduling problem of press shop is the balance problem on the basis of the scheduling of one press line.

3 A Hybrid Genetic Algorithm to the Operation Constraints Parallel Machine Model

In the scheduling of press shop based on the operation constraints parallel machine model, there are five key problems to be solved as follows: (1) the partitions of jobs for several press lines, (2) the partitions of jobs for machine A and machine B of each press line, (3) the sequence of jobs processed on parallel machine, (4) the operation constraints of jobs simultaneously machined on parallel machine, and (5) the start-time constraints of jobs processed on parallel machine. According to these above problems, a hybrid genetic algorithm is devised which includes heuristic rules based on the operation and start-time constraints. Firstly, the genetic algorithm is adopted to distribute jobs to the press lines, to partition jobs to two parallel machines of each press line and to sequence jobs processed on one machine, then the heuristic rules are used to determine the start-time and completion time of jobs according to constraints.

3.1 Representation and Initialization

In the last decades, the several kinds of encoding representation have been proposed [8]. Job-based representation is adopted to represent a gene here. Using the reference paper [9], the chromosome is devised to present jobs partition and sequences. A partitioning symbol is presented the separator of jobs for parallel machine of each press line. Other partitioning symbols are presented the separator of jobs for the press lines. The chromosome consists of the codes of jobs assigned to the press shop, one separator indicating the boundary between the two parallel machines of each press line, and other separators indicating the boundary among the press lines. In the chromosome, the code of job does not allow missing and being repeated, asterisks * are used to represent the separator to designate the partition jobs to machine A and machine B, and to represent the boundary of jobs for each press line. Let us consider an example with 16 jobs on three bidirectional press lines in one press shop. The chromosome maybe represent as follows:

[1 5 3 * 6 9 *2 * 4 7 8 * a b c * d e f g]

From the permutation, every two sub-schedules represent the scheduling for one press line. The above example shows details as follows: the sub-schedule [1 5 3 * 6 9] for the first press line, the sub-schedule [2 * 4 7 8] for the second press line and the sub-schedule [a b c * d e f g] for the third press line. The jobs (1, 5, 3, 6, 9) are distributed to the first press line, and jobs (1, 5, 3) are assigned to machine A for the first press line and the sequence of the list indicates the jobs order processed while the other jobs (6, 9) are assigned to machine B for the first press line and the sequence of the list indicates the jobs order processed. Similarly, the jobs (2, 4, 7, 8) to the second press line, job (2) and jobs (4, 7, 8) to the each parallel machine for the second press line, and the jobs (a, b, c, d, e, f, g) to the third press line, jobs (a, b, c) and jobs (d, e, f ,g) to the each parallel machine for the third press line. Generally, for n jobs and k press lines, the legal chromosome contains n symbols of the job and $2k$-1 partitioning symbol, resulting in the total size of (n+$2k$-1).

Initial population is randomly generated by the above rules.

3.2 Crossover Operator

The sub-schedule preservation special crossover operator is used to maintain the offspring chromosome validation. In the chromosome, the sub-schedule is the partition of jobs for each parallel machine. It works with the following three steps.

(1) Obtain the positions of asterisks * from one parent. The partitioning structure of jobs is determinate.

(2) Obtain randomly one sub-schedule from the same parent.

(3) Obtain the remaining codes of jobs from the other parent from left to right and fill the blank position of the offspring in turn.

Parent 1: [1 5 3 * 6 9 * 2 * **4 7 8** * a b c * d e f g]
Offspring 1: [a 9 e * g b * 1 * **4 7 8** * d 2 c * 3 f 6 5]
Parent 2: [a 7 * 9 e * g b 1 4 * d 2 * c 3 8 * f 6 5]

Through the crossover operator, the job partition and the job order are adjusted simultaneously.

3.3 Mutation Operator

The swapping mutation is used in this algorithm, in which two positions are randomly selected and the two selected genes are swapped. The two genes selected may be either jobs or the asterisks or the pipes. The five types of mutation describe as follows.

Chromosome 1: [1 5 3 * 6 9 * 2 * 4 7 8 * a b c * d e f g]
Mutation 1: [**3** 5 **1** * 6 9 * 2 * 4 7 8 * a b c * d e f g]
Mutation 2: [1 5 **6** * **3** 9 * 2 * 4 7 8 * a b c * d e f g]
Mutation 3: [1 5 **2** * 6 9 * **3** * 4 7 8 * a b c * d e f g]
Mutation 4: [1 5 ***** **3** 6 9 * 2 * 4 7 8 * a b c * d e f g]

(1) If two genes are jobs for the same machine, i.e. the both genes are in the same sub-schedule, the jobs order will be altered while the job partition will not be changed.

(2) If two genes are jobs for different machines for the same press line, the jobs order and the job partition will be altered for the press line while the number of jobs for each machine keeps constant.

(3) If two genes are jobs for different machines on the different press line, the job partition will be changed for each press line, not the job number.

(4) If one gene is one job and the other is the asterisk, there two types swapping as follows. (a) If the both genes are representation for the same press line, the jobs order, the job partition and the number of jobs for each machine on the same press line are changed. (b) If the genes are representation for different press lines, the job partition for different press line are changed, and the job partition, the jobs order and the job number for every press line are changed.

(5) If both genes are asterisks, the mutation operation is trivial.

These first three types of mutation could change the jobs partition, the jobs order and the number of jobs for each machine. The forth type of mutation, especial (b) type operator, change the job partition and job order for every press line. These show that the swapping mutation covers all the possibility of chromosome varying.

3.4 Heuristic Rule

In the press shop model based on operation constraints parallel machine, the scheduling of press shop is consisted of the scheduling of one press line and the scheduling among several press lines.

The heuristic rule is based on the operation constraint of the bidirectional press line model mentioned in section 2.2. The start-time and the completion time of jobs processed could be determined through the following heuristic rules based on constraints.

Step 1: Obtain the partition and the sequence of jobs for each logical machine for one press line through decoding the chromosome.

Step 2: Select one logical machine as the benchmark. The jobs for this machine are prior to that for the other machine. Initialize the start-time and the completion time of the first job for the benchmark machine A.

$S_{a1} = 0$;

$C_{a1} = P_{a1}$;

Step 3: Calculate the start-time and the completion time of jobs based on the operation constraints. The procedure of heuristic rule is given as follows.

```
while ( i =1; i< the max number of jobs for machine A)
    if q_ai + q_b(j-1) =<m, then
        S_ai = C_a(i-1);
        C_ai = S_ai + P_ai;
    endif
    if q_ai + q_b(j-1) >m, then
        S_ai = max{ C_a(i-1), C_b(j-1) };
         C_ai = S_ai + P_ai;
    endif
  i++;
    while(j=0;j<the max number of jobs for machine B)
        if q_ai + q_bj =<m and q_a(i-1)+ q_bj =<m, then
            S_bj = C_b(j-1);
            C_bj = S_bj +P_bj
            j++;
      endif;
      if q_ai + q_bj=<m and q_a(i-1) + q_bj >m, then
            S_bj = max{ C_a(i-1), C_b(j-1) };
            C_aj = S_aj + P_aj
            j++;
      endif
    endwhile
endwhile
while (j < the max number of jobs for machine B)
    S_bj = C_b(j-1); C_bj = S_bj +P_bj
    j++;
endwhile
```

3.5 Evaluation and Select

From the chromosome encoding representation, before computing the fitness function value, the chromosome will be decoded, and a well contrived fitness function is important to optimal object. There are several press lines in the press shop, so the chromosome is decoded into several sub-schedule with press lines, and the each sub-schedule is based on the operation constraints parallel machine model for press line.

In the new bidirectional press line model based operation constrained parallel machine, diversified performance objects can be optimized considering various factors. And the object function value needs to be converted to fitness value. The roulette wheel selection, ranking selection and tournament selection may be used as selection mechanism [10]. In additional, the elitist strategy could be combined to preserve the best chromosome in the offspring, to accelerate the evolution and overcome the stochastic errors.

4 An Example

The following example shows how to optimize the maximum makespan of jobs in press shop, which has three bidirectional press lines, and balance the working time of each press line. Considering the thirteen jobs and the maximum of operations of jobs is five, and each press line has five machines. The parameters about jobs are showed in the following table and the time unit is second.

Table 1. Processing parameters of jobs

J / Para	J_1	J_2	J_3	J_4	J_5	J_6	J_7	J_8	J_9	J_{10}	J_{11}	J_{12}	J_{13}
B_i	500	300	400	1000	400	400	600	800	650	700	500	600	1200
M_i	20*60	15*60	30*60	10*60	25*60	25*60	20*60	15*60	15*60	15*60	30*60	20*60	15*60
q_i	3	2	5	1	3	4	3	2	2	2	4	3	1
t_{i1}	1	2	1.5	1.5	1	1	1	1.5	1	1	4	2	2
p_{i1}	3	10	6	8	6	4	3	9	6	4	3	9	5
t_{i2}	1.5	1.5	2		1.5	1.5	1	1	2	2	2	2	
p_{i2}	5	6	10		9	8	6	4	9	6	9	5	
t_{i3}	1.5		1		1	1	1.5				6	1	
p_{i3}	8		3		4	3	7				5	3	
t_{i4}			1			1					2		
p_{i4}			3			6					2		
t_{i5}			1.5										
p_{i5}			6										
P_i	11200	6750	15800	10100	10500	11700	12900	13300	12600	10000	18300	14400	10700

In the model based on operation constraints parallel machine for press shop, the jobs do not transfer between press lines and would be processed in the sequence of the machines, so the relative processing route of jobs is unchangeable. The transportation time between machines is easy to make certain and calculate, and the extraordinary cost of transport is not brought like apparatus to place the semi-finished products. The transportation time could be considered into the total batch processing time and not be calculated specially. The total batch processing time is used as processing time of job, in which the setup time and the economic lot size are considered. The processing time of one job and the total batch processing time of one kind of job could be calculated according to the formula 2.

The above hybrid genetic algorithm is adopted to solve the problem with the makespan object and balance for each press line. Especially, the fitness function is devised to meet the optimal object which is formulated as total makespans added the deviation among press lines. Fix the maximum generation as 1000, the population size as 200 and the crossover possibility as 0.1 and the mutation possibility as 0.5. The elitist strategy is combined here. The jobs partition and jobs order are conducted through the iterative computing, then the start-time and completion time of jobs are educed through heuristic rules based on operation constraints. The one better scheduling result shows as follows. In the figure 1, the rectangle represents the resource for the processing job including time and machines. The width of the rectangle represents the number of machines and the height for processing time. Specially, the data at the top and the bottom of the rectangle respectively represents the completion time and the start-time of the job. From the figure, it is showed that the balance among three press lines and the total processing time is optimized.

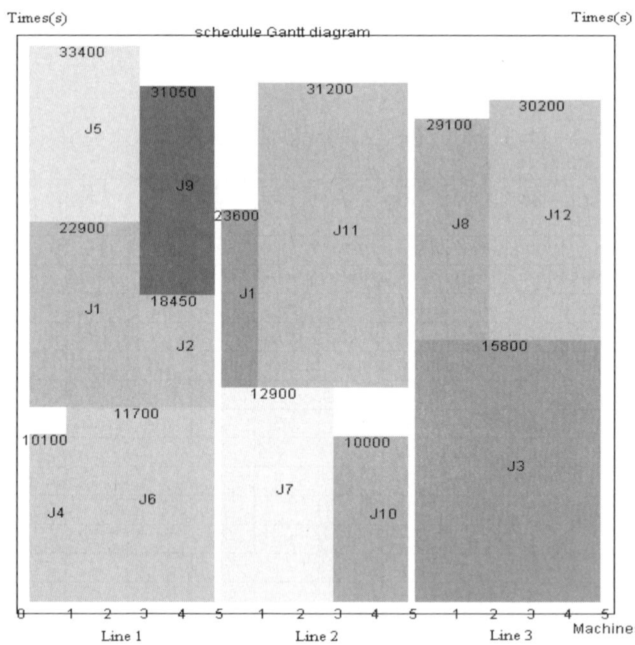

Fig. 1. The scheduling result of the example

5 Conclusion and Prospect

This paper has presented a new scheduling solution for press shop and a new model based on operation constraints parallel machine for bidirectional press line, then the solution combined the genetic algorithm and the heuristic based on operation constraints is given. In this new scheduling method, the main shortcomings of the common-used single job shop model are overcome including the different operations number, the varying transportation time and the cost of extraordinary apparatus and management. And the relative process route is unchangeable, so that the process parameters of jobs are easy to compute and obtain. In the end, the example is demonstrated that the model and the hybrid genetic algorithm are valid and effective.

In the future works, the following three topics will be further investigated: (1) multi-object optimum scheduling for the press shop under many conditions, (2) the better optimum algorithm to solve the model and (3) the scheduling considering the different processing capacity of machines and lines.

Acknowledgement

This work was supported in part by hi-tech research and development program of China: No.2005AA411040.

References

1. Jianfeng, C., Yuexian, Z., Zandong, H.: Optimal Method of Capacitated Lot Sizing Planning in Manufacturing Systems. Journal of Tsinghua University (Science and Technology) 44(5), 605–608 (2004)
2. Weimin, Z., Yan, H.S., Zhao, Z.: Optimization of Inventory Storage Ration in Press Workshops with Set-up Time. Computer Technology and Development 17(4), 5–8 (2007)
3. Zhang, X.D., Yan, H.S.: Integrated Optimization of Production Planning and Scheduling for a Kind of Job-shop. International Journal of Advanced Manufacturing Technology 27(6), 876–886 (2005)
4. Zhang, X.D., Yan, H.S.: Integrated Optimization of Production Planning and Scheduling for Multi-stage Workshop. Chinese Journal of Mechanical Engineering 41(9), 98–105 (2005)
5. Qing, H., Yan, H.S., Lin, C.: Study on Scheduling Simulation of Bi-directional Production Line Based Flexsim. Industrial Control Computer 20(8), 63–64 (2007)
6. Jianfeng, C., Yuexian, Z., Zandong, H.: Research on Scheduling of Automobile Press Shop in Virtual Environment. Journal of Plasticity Engineering 11(6), 84–88 (2004)
7. Jianfeng, C., Yuexian, Z., Zandong, H.: A Virtual Manufacturing System for The Press Production Line of Car Body. Journal of Plasticity Engineering 11(4), 61–66 (2004)
8. Mitsuo, C.R.G., Tsujimura, Y.: A Tutorial Survey of Job-shop Scheduling Problems Using Genetic Algorithms–I. Representation. Computers & Industrial Engineering 30(4), 983–997 (1996)
9. Runwei, C., Mitsuo, G.: Parallel Machine Scheduling Problems Using Memetic Algorithms. Computers & Industrial Engineering 33(3-4), 761–764 (1997)
10. Ling, W.: Shop Scheduling with Genetic Algorithms. Tsinghua University Press, Peking (2003)

Hybrid Intelligent Algorithm for Job-Shop Scheduling under Uncertainty

Guojun Zhang, Chanjuan Li, Jun Zhu, and Haiping Zhu

State Key Laboratory of Digitalization Manufacturing & Equipment, Huazhong University of Science and Technology
chanjuan.li@gmail.com, zgj@mail.hust.edu.cn

Abstract. Production scheduling plays an important role in improving efficiency and reducing cost. One of its core technologies is the establishment of an effective scheduling model and its corresponding optimization algorithms. Nowadays, most researches are concentrated on the optimization algorithms of classical scheduling problems without considering the uncertainties in the real job-shop. Describing the uncertain information in the real job-shops with several stochastic variables, a stochastic multi-objectives and multi-priorities programming model for job-shop scheduling is proposed, in which Time, Cost and Equilibrium serve as the three basic objectives for scheduling. The credibility of the delivery time of different types of work pieces serve as the scheduling constraints. In order to obtain the approximate optimum solution, a hybrid intelligent algorithm which combines Stochastic Simulation, Neural Network with Genetic Algorithm is proposed, and the primary steps are discussed. A case is given to illustrate the feasibility of this model and the method.

Keywords: Job-shop scheduling Stochastic programming Multi-objectives optimization.

1 Introduction

Inchoate research on JSP (Job-shop Scheduling Problem) concentrated on the simple application of integer programming and simulation, which can hardly be used to solve the complex scheduling problem. With the development of related fields and theory of optimization, a great many methods and techniques have been adopted into JSP. Operational research predigests the JSP into a mathematical programming model, using branch-and-bound method and dynamic programming algorithm to realize optimization or approximate optimization. However, OR only suits to simple scheduling problem [1]. Based on theory of control, Gershwin and his fellows expatiate comprehensively the adoption of theory of control in manufacturing system. Limited to the capability of modeling, a lot of predigestion to the environment is a must; the practice to get the optimum solution expands with a exponential characteristic [2]. AI (Artificial Intelligence) is a combination of all the methods for JSP, which aim at enhancing the intelligence of scheduling method. It can smooth the disadvantages of mathematical programming and simulation. Based on the system

C. Xiong et al. (Eds.): ICIRA 2008, Part II, LNAI 5315, pp. 946–956, 2008.

status and deterministic objective of optimization, effective heuristic research and concurrent fuzzy reasoning are conducted to choose the optimum solution and support online decision. Nevertheless, AI is weak in adapting to new environment, and there are 3 main limitations of this method: low speed of operation, insensitive to asynchronisic event in the environment, the system can't be universally adopted [2]. In a job-shop DEDS (Discrete Event Dynamic System), the JSP can be solved by its parsing model and method, such as Petri net. The Petri net can precisely reflect the characteristics of discrete and stochastic etc. in job-shop scheduling [3]. But it's hard to present a model when the principle and methodology are complex. The complexity of manufacturing system makes it hard to express and analyze by a precise analytical model. Simulation can provide an ideal model for quantitative evaluation to guide the scheduling [4]. Whereas, the experimental characteristic make it hard to figure out the general rule, and the value and credibility of the result have much to do with the simulation model, simulation method and the data input. Uncertain theory has also been adopted into the scheduling problem for its stochastic and fuzzy characteristics [5]. Just as AI, it needs a long development cycle time as well as abundant experience etc. Soft computing is also widely adopted into scheduling, such as GA[6] (genetic algorithm), TS[7](Tabu searching), SA[8] (simulated annealing), NN[9](neural network), PSO (particle swarm optimization) etc. Based on the aforementioned methodologies, we can find that each method has its own limit, so researchers start to combine the approximate algorithms to solve scheduling problem. This paper proposed a compounding method which syncretizes simulation and soft computing to solve FJSP (flexible job-shop scheduling problem) under uncertain environment.

As the execution layer between the ERP/MRPII for planning and job-shop layer for operation and control, MES (Manufacturing Execution System) focuses on how to optimize the job-shop scheduling[10]. The essence of scheduling is a decision making constrained by multi-objectives and multi-priorities. The multi-objectives here focuses on the combination of less production time, less total cost and equilibrium of production ability while the multi-constraints focuses on the constraints of process route, machines and delivery time of order in which the priorities differ on different types of work pieces.

Information is the basis of decision making. The scheduling models in previous research are proposed with all the information deterministically given, for example, taking the process time of the work piece on specific machine as deterministic information without considering the priority. Actually, the stochastic information floods the real job-shop, which makes getting the satisfied scheduling a difficult job. In recent years, job-shop scheduling in uncertain environment gradually arouses the attention of researchers, such as study on scheduling problem with fuzzy characteristic. However, in discrete event dynamic system, more parameters are suited to be described by stochastic variable rather than fuzzy variable, such as the process time of work piece, the frequency of machine fault and the interval of order, which can be thought to obey an exponential distribution[11] , so it is of great significance to study scheduling under stochastic constraints.

2 The Stochastic Programming Model with Chance-Constraint

Generally, job-shop problem is depicted by a non-linear programming model. If certain stochastic factors being taken into account, the programming model would differ from the classical model. The concept of chance-constraint and stochastic programming proposed by Liu[12] is depicted as follows:

Assume that X is a decision-making vector; E is a stochastic vector with deterministic distribution. There are r objective functions decided by X and E: $f_i(X,E), 1 \le i \le r$, constrained to p constrained function: $g_j(X,E), 1 \le j \le p$. The objective functions and constrained functions are stochastic, so they can be depicted only by the credibility as follows: $P\{g_j(X,E) \le 0\} \ge \alpha_j, 1 \le j \le p$,P represent the probability of the stochastic event $g_j(X,E) \le 0$, α_j is the credibility. If the objective of programming is to minimize $f_i(X,E), 1 \le i \le r$, choose β_i as the credibility, the objective function would be:

$$\begin{cases} \min \overline{f_i} \\ s.t. \quad P\{f_i(X,E) \le \overline{f_i}\} \ge \beta_i \end{cases}, 1 \le i \le r$$

Above all, the stochastic programming model with multi-chance-constraints and multi objectives is:

$$\begin{cases} \min[\overline{f_1}, \overline{f_2}, ..., \overline{f_r}] \\ s.t. \\ \quad P\{f_i(X,E) \le \overline{f_i}\} \ge \beta_i, 1 \le i \le r \\ \quad P\{g_j(X,E) \le 0\} \ge \alpha_j, 1 \le j \le p \end{cases}$$

$[\overline{f_1}, \overline{f_2}, ..., \overline{f_r}]$ stands for the weighted sum of the *r* variables.

3 Multi-objectives and Multi-priorities Job-Shop Scheduling Strategy

In the job-shop with several pieces of machines, after receiving the production order assigned by the planning section, production process would be arranged and optimized by reasonable scheduling. The scheduling parameter can be depicted by the mathematical format:

There are m pieces of machine available: $\{R_1, R_2, ... R_m\}$

There are n work pieces' task included in the order: $\{T_1, T_2, ... T_m\}$. $T_i (1 \le i \le n)$ is a operation sequence decided by the process route programming, which includes $K_i (1 \le K_i \le m)$ operations and recorded as follows: $T_i = \{OP_{i1}, OP_{i2}, ..., OP_{iK_i}\}$, each operation OP_{ik} can be processed on several machines, and operation on each machine Rj would take you certain time and cost, time function be depicted as $et(OP,R)$, cost function be depicted as $ec(OP,R)$. In the uncertain informative environment, when operation $OP_{ik}(1 \le i \le n, 1 \le k \le K_i)$is being processed on machine $R_j (1 \le j \le m)$,

$et(OP_{ik},R_j)$ and $ec(OP_{ik},R_j)$are two stochastic constants with deterministic distribution, else $et(OP_{ik},R_j)=ec(OP_{ik},R_j)\equiv 0$.

3.1 Work Piece Priority and Chance Constraint

On the premise of following the demand of process route, MES would assign appropriate machine for each operation of each work piece, making sure that the delivery time of order can be met. That is to say, the delivery time is a key constraint in scheduling. As the production order is formed by a consideration of customer order, enterprise planning and operation. The tasks included in the order can be divided into many priorities for many factors such as importance of customer, quantity of order, and the degree of emergency of the requirement. For example, if we divide the work pieces into two group, in one of which the delivery time should be precisely met (called critical work piece) while there can be a flexible space in the other group of work pieces (called ordinary work piece). On this condition, the job-shop resources should satisfy the needs of critical work pieces on first hand to meet the delivery time. The remained resources can then be assigned to the ordinary work pieces. Literature 4 adopted by-directional scheduling strategy, for the critical work piece, reverse order scheduling is adopted, while for the ordinary work piece, sequential scheduling is adopted. However, for uncertain environment in which processing time is stochastic, this strategy for scheduling will bring out many problems. That means the result of the scheduling can hardly meet the delivery time.

In real job-shop, the processing time of work piece on each machine is a stochastic variable obeying certain distribution (exponential distribution in general), that leads to the stochastic characteristic of the production cycle of work piece. We can describe the constraint of delivery time as a chance constraint. The priority of the work pieces can be divided into r subclasses by a high-low order(the element in the same subclass share the same priority): $S_1,S_2,\ldots,S_r$, each subclass has the corresponding credibility of meeting delivery time : $\alpha_1,\alpha_2,\ldots\alpha_r(\alpha_1>\alpha_2>\ldots>\alpha_r)$. The delivery time of each task is deterministic as : $dt_1,dt_2,\ldots,dt_n$, the real production cycle time of each task(including the total processing time and total waiting time) can be calculated and depicted as $pt_1,pt_2,\ldots,pt_n$. The delivery constraint described by chance constraint is

$$\forall T_i \in S_j, P\{pt_i - dt_i \le 0\} \ge \alpha_j, 1 \le i \le n, 1 \le j \le r \qquad (1)$$

There would be a queue waiting when several work pieces are assigned to the same machine, the sequence of processing should be determined by the principle of scheduling. Generally, FIFS (first in first serviced) principle is adopted. Towards different priorities, serving the task with higher priority on first hand is more reasonable to actual demand. At this moment, if there is a queue on a machine waiting for processing while a piece is being processed, after it is processed, the piece in queue with highest priority should be chosen to be processed. The piece of longer waiting time should be processed first within the same priority.

3.2 Proposing a Multi-objectives Function

Shorter production time and lower cost is two basic objectives. For an order to be scheduled, with the complexity of process route of each component differing from others, we can aim at minimize the total production cycle time of the task for all work pieces. η as the credibility, the time objective function can be depicted by chance constraint as follows:

$$\begin{cases} \min \overline{pt} \\ s.t.\ P\{\sum_{i=1}^{n} pt_i \le \overline{pt}\} \ge \eta \end{cases} \tag{2}$$

Meanwhile, we can aim at minimizing the total production cost of the task for all work pieces, taking γ as credibility. The cost objective function can be depicted by chance constraint as follows:

$$\begin{cases} \min \overline{ec} \\ s.t.\ P\{\sum_{i=1}^{n}\sum_{k=1}^{K_i} ec(OP_{ik}, R_j) \le \overline{ec}\} \ge \gamma \end{cases} \tag{3}$$

Another objective of scheduling is the equilibrium of the schedule, which has long been ignored. According to a schedule, if the average load of machine is floating dramatically, we call it an unbalanced scheduling. The disequilibrium of scheduling would cause a loss in coping with the emergency. We introduce the standard deviation in statistics to quantify the equilibrium of scheduling, dividing the whole production cycle time into several isometric time segment, figure out the total working time of the machine in each time segment, than calculate the standard deviation between this total working time and average working time. The smaller the standard deviation, the better the equilibrium of the schedule is.

Assume that the production cycle time is OT, obviously, $OT = \max_{1 \le i \le n} pt_i$, divide OT into N isometric time segments, in each of which the total processing time of all the machines is $\Delta RT_s (1 \le s \le N)$,the standard deviation is $D^2 = \sum_{s=1}^{N} (\Delta RT_s - \frac{1}{N}\sum_{s=1}^{N} \Delta RT_s)^2$, with credibility ν , the objective of equilibrium of schedule is depicted as:

$$\begin{cases} \min \overline{rt} \\ s.t.\ P\{\sum_{s=1}^{N} (\Delta RT_s - \frac{1}{N}\sum_{s=1}^{N} \Delta RT_s)^2 \le \overline{rt}\} \ge \nu \end{cases} \tag{4}$$

3.3 Stochastic Programming Model of Job-Shop Scheduling with Multi-objectives and Multi-priorities

The process route of each work piece and the machines available for each operation are known according to (1) (2) (3) (4), the machines available to operation OP_{ik} is

$AR_{ik} = \{R_{ik}^1, R_{ik}^2, ..., R_{ik}^{H_{ik}}\}$, including H_{ik} elements, the principle for scheduling of task waiting in queue is Higher Priority First Served. The stochastic programming model of job-shop scheduling in uncertain environment is proposed as follows:

$$\begin{cases} \min[\overline{pt}, \overline{ec}, \overline{rt}] \\ s.t.\ \ P\{\sum_{i=1}^{n} pt_i \le \overline{pt}\} \ge \eta \\ P\{\sum_{i=1}^{n}\sum_{k=1}^{K_i} ec(OP_{ik}, R_j) \le \overline{ec}\} \ge \gamma \\ P\{\sum_{s=1}^{N} (\Delta RT_s - \frac{1}{N}\sum_{s=1}^{N} \Delta RT_s)^2 \le \overline{rt}\} \ge \nu \\ P\{pt_i - dt_i \le 0\} \ge \alpha_j, 1 \le i \le n, 1 \le j \le r, T_i \in S_j \end{cases} \quad (5)$$

4 The Design and Implementation of Hybrid Intelligent Algorithm

4.1 Basic Procedures of Hybrid Intelligent Algorithm

Model (5) is too complex to be solved by traditional algorithm, so we adopt the hybrid intelligence which syncretizes stochastic simulation, neural network, genetic algorithm and other critical techniques. The algorithm includes 3 major steps:

Step1: based on the quantity and capability of machine in job-shop, as well as the distribution characteristics of stochastic variables as time and cost etc. Present a simulation model; collect quantities of data samples by simulating.

Step 2: Present the three-layer feed-forward neural networks, use the samples acquired in simulation to weight-train the neural network to approach the stochastic functions in model(5).

Step3: apply the genetic algorithm to solve the optimization problem, including definition of rules for chromosome coding/encoding, initialization and selection of population, the calculation and evaluation of individual fitness, crossover and mutation etc. The calculation of individual fitness will utilize the trained neural network in step2.

4.2 Stochastic Simulations

Stochastic simulations(Monte Carlo simulation) is one of the stochastic system modeling techniques focuses on sample test, the sample of the stochastic variables is based on their probabilistic distribution. There are a lot of complex calculations for probabilities of stochastic variables in model (5), as for the complexity of multi-priorities scheduling, even a schedule sequence is determined, the stochastic variables such as the completion period of each work piece can not be expressed by a explicit. So the stochastic simulation should be integrated with simulation analysis to get the approximate sample data.

According to experience, we can assume the operation time et(OP_{ik},R_j) comply with the exponential distribution with λ_{ikj} as its exponent, depicted as et(OP_{ik},R_j)~exp(λ_{ikj}). The cost of processing is influenced by many uncertain factors, ec(OP_{ik},R_j) can be assumed to comply with normal distribution depicted as ec(OP_{ik},R_j)~ $N(\mu_{ikj},\sigma^2_{ikj})$.

Given a schedule sequence (the concrete machine for each operation) and a group of deterministic sample values for all stochastic variables, which work pieces are being processed is available on theory. Therefore, to present stochastic simulation model on platform of SIMUL8, then run simulation and statistically analyze the critical data acquired, including:

(1) Production time of each work piece pt_i

(2) The processing cost of each work piece $\sum_{k=1}^{K_i} ec(OP_{ik}, R_j)$

(3) The total working time of all devices in each time segment (N segment in all) is ΔRT_s

4.3 Neural Network Approach to the Stochastic Functions

Take the schedule sequence as Vector *Y*, the four constraints in model (5) can be depicted by *Y*'s stochastic function, definition as the following *n+3* functions:

$$\begin{cases} U_1(Y) = \min\{\overline{pt} \mid P\{\sum_{i=1}^{n} pt_i \le \overline{pt}\} \ge \eta\} \\ U_2(Y) = \min\{\overline{ec} \mid P\{\sum_{i=1}^{n}\sum_{k=1}^{K_i} ec(OP_{ik}, R_j) \le \overline{ec}\} \ge \gamma\} \\ U_3(Y) = \min\{\overline{rt} \mid P\{\sum_{s=1}^{N} (\Delta RT_s - \frac{1}{N}\sum_{s=1}^{N} \Delta RT_s)^2 \le \overline{rt}\} \ge \nu\} \\ U_4^{(i)}(Y) = P\{pt_i - dt_i \le 0\}, 1 \le i \le n \end{cases} \tag{6}$$

The stochastic simulation provides abundant data samples, which are used to train a neural network to approach the *n+3* uncertain functions in (6). The neural network is three-layer feed-forward with $\sum_{i=1}^{n} K_i$ input neurons (data input is *Y*), 18 hidden layer neurons and *n+3* output neurons (data output are $U_1(Y)$, $U_2(Y)$, $U_3(Y)$, $U_4^{(i)}(Y)$).

4.4 Genetic Algorithm of Multi-objectives Optimization

Coding, Encoding of Chromosome and Initialization of Population. Besides being simple, the principle for coding of chromosome should also assure any of the chromosomes can get a permissive schedule sequence by encoding. Permissive means meeting the requirements of constraints of process route and process machine. Here designed a coding method for positive integer:

Each bit of the code represents an operation: the first bit represents the first operation of work piece 1, the second bit represents the second operation of work piece 1,…, the K_{1+1} represents the first operation of work piece 2, the rest may be deduced by analogy. If bit j represents operation k of work piece of I, the range of value for bit j is [1,H_{ik}], H_{ik} represents the number of machine available for operation k of work piece i. Looking on the coding principle, once given the collection of machine for each operation and the accurate process time, each chromosome can be precisely mapped into a schedule sequence, meanwhile the process details(when and where) of each operation can be calculated which is solely determined. Also, during the initialization of population, once length bits stochastic positive integers are created with value-range of each bit in $[1,H_{ik}]$, the coding of chromosome is permissive.

The Calculation and Evaluation of Fitness. Individual fitness can be calculated using the trained neural network, if we take $\sum_{i=1}^{n} K_i$ bits coding of random chromosomes as the input of neural network, n+3 output would be acquired. Contraposing data output first prove whether $U_4^{(i)}(Y) \geq \alpha_j, T_i \in S_j$ is right, if not, the delivery time can not be satisfied which means the schedule is not donable. The fitness of chromosome is 0, the corresponding individual being eliminated. Else when $U_4^{(i)}(Y) \geq \alpha_j, T_i \in S_j$ proves to be true, then *U1(Y)*, *U2(Y)* and *U3(Y)*can figure out $\overline{pt}, \overline{ec}, \overline{rt}$, giving the weight of the three objectives(time, cost and equilibrium) w_1, w_2, w_3 on preferential relationship, then calculate $w_1 \overline{pt} + w_2 \overline{ec} + w_3 \overline{rt}$, the smaller the value, the higher the individual fitness is.

Operator of Cross and Mutation. The cross between two parents is operated as follows: exchange the codes presenting the same operation sequence in two chromosomes, and then we will get two sons.

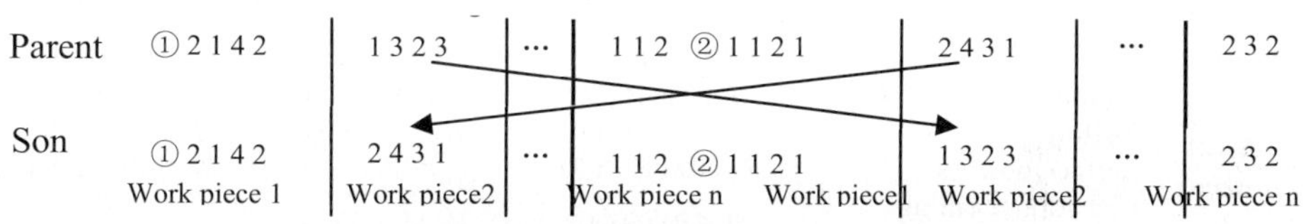

Fig. 1. Process of crossing

The mutation process is as fig.2, bit *j* of parent's chromosome mutates stochastically by certain probability. Notes: if bit j stands for the operation *k* of work piece I, the value range of bit *j* after mutation is $[1,H_{ik}]$.

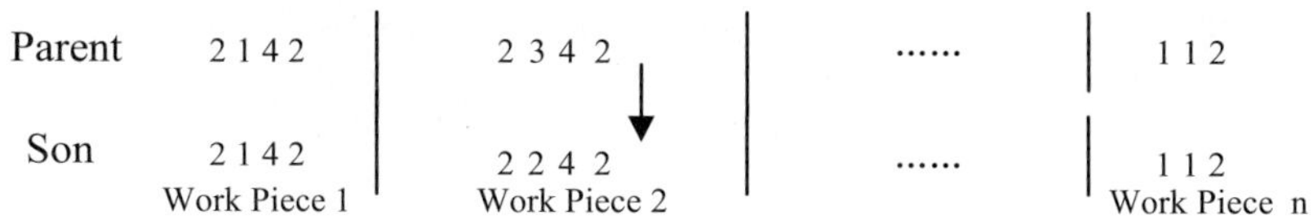

Fig. 2. Process map of mutation

5 Case Study

We apply our study to a car manufacturing enterprise. The mold job-shop accepts the orders for manufacturing of molds, which include orders from both enterprise itself and other company. The manufacturing resources in the job-shop is enough with all necessary machine for mold processing, which include lathe, milling machine, grinding machine, numeral control machine, process center, electric discharge machine etc.(the serial number of machines are $R_1,R_2,\ldots,R_{35}$). Table 1 shows a piece of production order, which includes 3 work pieces waiting for process with delivery time of 270,300,320 respectively. The delivery time of work piece 1 and 2 should be strictly met with credibility99%, while work piece 3 is more flexible with a 50% credibility to meet the delivery time. So, there are two priorities of scheduling. Three work pieces have fixed process route, each operation has many devices available for processing which differ in time and cost. According to experience and historical statistically analysis, the time and cost spent on each machine for one operation are stochastic variables. The time complies with exponential distribution while cost obeys normal distribution, whose parameters are shown in table 1. Take "R_2/20/(18,6)"as an example, it means work piece being processed on machine R_2 with processing time obeying exponential distribution exp(20), cost obeying normal distribution N(18,6). We need to schedule for the order and implement optimum scheduling.

Table 1. Operations and machines available for work pieces

Work piece	Operation	Class of machine available Resource1	Resource2	Resource3
Work piece 1	Lathing	R_2/20/(18,6)	R_3/25/(17,5)	
	Milling	R_7/35/(39,1)	R_8/30/(45,2)	R_{10}/40/(37,1)
	Surface process	R_{30}/100/(125,8)	R_{31}/90/(140,6)	R_{32}/110/(120,8)
	Lineation, Drilling Assembling,Adjustment	R_{20}/40/(50,4)	R_{22}/42/(55,3)	
	Line incision	R_{17}/40/(45,4)	R_{18}/45/(49,3)	
Work piece 2	Lathing	R2/25/(19,2)	R_3/33/(18,2)	R_5/30/(18,1)
	Drilling,Milling	R_8/40/(55,4)	R_{10}/50/(50,3)	
	Surface process	R_{30}/70/(85,8)	R_{31}/67/(90,6)	
	Grinding	R_{25}/50/(60,6)	R_{26}/52/(60,5)	
	Repairing Assembling	R_{20}/100/(110,10)	R_{21}/115/(117,10)	R_{22}/110/(121,9)
Work piece 3	Milling	R_8/60/(102,5)	R_9/70/(85,7)	R_{11}/55/(127,9)
	Surface process	R_{31}/50/(93,6)	R_{32}/60/(55,2)	R_{33}/58/(60,2)
	Electrode NC process	R_{35}/33/(36,4)	R_{30}/30/(42,3)	
	Electric-charge Process	R_{19}/40/(50,4)	R_{16}/39/(60,4)	
	Repairing ,assembling	R_{21}/160/(220,12)	R_{22}/150/(240,10)	

First, present a stochastic programming model, believable probabilities are $\eta=\gamma=\nu=0.8, \alpha_1=0.99, \alpha_2=0.5$. Then use hybrid intelligent algorithm with weights of three objectives being 1/3 respectively to solve the problem. Get 200 groups of data samples through stochastic simulation (each group of data should be acquired by 500 times simulation), train the neural network with these data (15 input units, 18 hidden layer units and 6 output units), and calculate the weight. Finally, using genetic algorithm to find the optimum solution with 15 bits code, cross rate 0.5 and mutation rate 0.01. After 30 generations' evolution, the result of schedule is as follows:

Work piece 1(2,7,30,22,17), work piece 2(5,8,30,25,20), work piece 3(8,32,35,19,22). The numbers in the bracket represent the serial number of machine for each operation. According to experience, this schedule sequence is a approximate optimum solution which has satisfied the requirements of all the chance constraints.

6 Conclusions

After analyzing the stochastic factors as time and cost in production process, we have proposed stochastic programming model based on chance constraints to describe the multi-priorities job-shop scheduling problem aiming at objectives of shorter production time, lower cost and equilibrium of schedule. The advantage of this model is that it reflects the stochastic condition in real job-shop and proposes a hybrid intelligent algorithm which syncretizes many critical techniques such as the stochastic simulation, neural network and genetic algorithm etc., finally, a case study shows that our study can be applied to FJSP to get a approximate optimum solution.

Acknowledgments

The research presented in this paper has been supported by the National Basic Research Program of China (2005CB724107) and the National Natural Science Foundation of China (50575084).

References

1. Philips, T., Revenderen, A., et al.: Theory and Practice of Operational Research, pp. 282–346. China Commercial Press, Beijing (1987)
2. Juanqi, Y.: Synthetically Description and development of FMS Scheduling Research. Journal of Shanghai Jiaotong University 32(5), 124–127 (1998) (in Chinese)
3. Hongsen, Y.: Research and Application of FMS Modeling, Scheduling, Controlling and Simulating. Harbin Institute of Technology (1994) (in Chinese)
4. Law, M.: Simulation series: Part I: Introducing simulation: A tool for analyzing complex systems. Ind. Eng., 46–63 (May 1986)
5. Zhaoqiang, G., Yiren, Z.: Study on Job Shop Fuzzy Scheduling Problem Based on Genetic Algorithm. CIMS 8(8), 616–620 (2002) (in Chinese)
6. Croee, F.D., Tadei, R.: A genetic algorithm for the Job Shop problem. Computer Ops. Res. 22(1), 15–24 (1995)
7. Taillard, E.: Some efficient heuristic methods for the flow shop sequencing problem. Euro. Operation Res. 47(1), 65–74 (1990)
8. Laarhoven, V.: Job shop scheduling by simulated annealing. Operations Research 40, 113–125 (1992)

9. Foo, Y.S., Takefuji, Y.: Integer linear programming neural networks for job-shop scheduling. In: IEEE Int. Conf. on NNS, San Diego, pp. 320–332 (1998)
10. Shuxia, L.: MES certain technologies research under complex information environment. [Doctoral dissertation]. Wuhan (2004) (in Chinese)
11. Peigen, L.: Manufacturing System Performance Analysis Modeling - Theory and Methods. Huazhong University of Science and Technology, Wuhan (1998) (in Chinese)
12. Baoding, L., Ruiqing, Z., Gang, W.: Uncertain programming and application. Tsinghua University Press, Beijing (2003) (in Chinese)

Numerical Study on Viscous Heating of Oil Flow in a Spool Valve

Jian Deng[1], Xueming Shao[1,2], and Xin Fu[2]

[1] School of Aeronautics and Astronautics, Zhejiang University, Hangzhou, 310027, P.R. China
[2] The State Key Lab of Fluid Power Transmission and Control, Zhejiang University, Hangzhou, 310027, P.R. China

Abstract. The temperature distributions around the notches in spool valve were simulated using a finite-volume based CFD code. The temperature increase is due to the viscous heating effect, which is generally significant in high speed oil flow. Two valve spools with different types of notches are investigated, of which spool A is an earlier one, and spool B is an improved one in order to avoid the heat shock. The results show important difference between spool A and spool B, including the local temperature distributions and the maximum temperatures around the notches. As a conclusion, the spool B is evaluated to be safer from heat shock than spool A.

Keywords: Spool valve, CFD, Viscous heating, heat shock.

1 Introduction

Spool valves are widely used in fluid power transmission and control systems. The flow structure inside a spool valve plays an important role on the performance of the valve, thus influencing the property of the whole power system. Therefore, many researchers have focused on their studies on the flow structure inside the valve. Vaughan et al.[1] used the finite difference method to investigate the spool valve flow field and flow force compensation. Wang et al.[2] and Ruan et al. [3] used the PIV method to measure the velocity field in spool chamber. Borghi et al. [4] dealt with the application of a simplified numerical analysis of the flow field inside the compensation port connections of a reference spool valve. Gao [5] investigated the flow structure inside a spool valve with FEM and PIV methods. One can refer to [6–7] for more articles on this topic.

The above mentioned researches focused on the flow behavior in spool valves, treating the working substance inside the valves as an isothermal fluid. However, under particular conditions, the viscous heating effect ought to be taken into account. The engineers from Hitachi (Japan) Ltd found that valve stall was often occurred for some spool valves in cold state. From the appearance of disabled spool valves, they estimated that heat shock occurred at the notch. When the hydraulic oil passes through the notches with very high speed, high shear rate of the fluid leads to a local temperature increase. Local high temperature will induce the deformation of

C. Xiong et al. (Eds.): ICIRA 2008, Part II, LNAI 5315, pp. 957–965, 2008.

the spool. Because the allowable radial clearance between spool and house is generally several micrometers, the deformation of spool will finally cause the valve stalled.

In this paper, as a first sight into this problem, viscous heating in spool valves is numerically investigated. Two valve spools (spool A and spool B) with different notches are studied. First, the numerical method is introduced, followed by an examination of this method by validations on different grid sizes. Second, results are presented and analyzed, including the flow rate predictions under different hydraulic pressure, and the temperature distributions around the notches. In the last section, conclusions are drawn, giving an evaluation to the later improved spool, to predict whether this kind of spool can avoid heat shock or reduce it.

2 Case Description

The spool valves studied in this paper are simplified from that used in a real servo system, in which a spool consists of several groups of notches. The two spools A and B for current investigation each consists of one group of notches are shown in Fig.1. The right side of Fig.1 shows amplificatory view of the notches of spools A and B. Each spool contains three pairs of notches. A1, A2 and A3 are U-shape notches with different sizes. B1, B2, B3 are V-shape notch, K-shape and combined U-shape, respectively. Combination of these different shape notches leads to a specific flow-rate pressure relation. Under a specified pressure (10 Mpa, which is employed as the inlet boundary condition in the simulations), the mass flow rate and the temperature distributions in the spool varies with the valve opening. The opening changes from 1 mm to 6 mm, of which 0 mm and 6 mm refer to closed and fully opened status respectively.

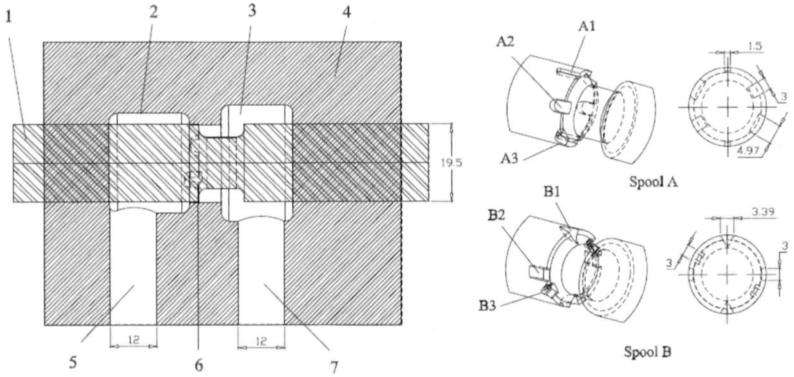

Fig. 1. Configuration of the models, including sectional view of the valve and amplificatory view of the notches: (1) sliding spool, (2) sleeve, (3) chamber, (4) solid block, (5) inlet section, (6) notches, (7) outlet section

3 Numerical Method

For the fluid model, the flow is assumed to be turbulent, Newtonian, and incompressible. A finite volume based code is applied to solve the discretized Navier-Stokes equations. The standard *k-ε* turbulence model is used. The program is based on the pressure-correction method and employee the PISO algorithm. The second order upwind difference scheme (UD) is adopted for the momentum, energy and turbulence equations. Next, the control equations will be introduced.

The continuity equation and momentum conservation equations:

$$\frac{\partial \rho}{\partial t}+\nabla\cdot(\rho\vec{u})=0 \tag{1}$$

$$\frac{\partial}{\partial t}(\rho\vec{u})+\nabla\cdot(\rho\vec{u}\vec{u})=-\nabla p+\nabla\cdot(\vec{\tau}) \tag{2}$$

where p is the static pressure, $\vec{\tau}$ is the stress tensor, given by:

$$\vec{\tau}=\mu\left[\left(\nabla\vec{u}+\nabla\vec{u}^{T}\right)-\frac{2}{3}\nabla\cdot\vec{u}I\right] \tag{3}$$

here, μ is the molecular viscosity, which would be replaced by the effective viscosity ($\mu_{eff}=\mu+\mu_t$, where μ_t is the turbulent viscosity) if taking into account the turbulence.

The *k-ε* turbulence model is used to model turbulent flow. The Reynolds stresses are related to the mean velocity gradients on the basis of the Boussinesq hypothesis. The turbulence kinetic energy, *k*, and its rate of dissipation, *ε*, are obtained from the following transport equations:

$$\frac{\partial}{\partial t}(\rho k)+\frac{\partial}{\partial x_i}(\rho k u_i)=\frac{\partial}{\partial x_j}\left[\left(\mu+\frac{\mu_t}{\sigma_k}\right)\frac{\partial k}{\partial x_j}\right]+\rho G_k-\rho\varepsilon \tag{4}$$

$$\frac{\partial}{\partial t}(\rho\varepsilon)+\frac{\partial}{\partial x_i}(\rho\varepsilon u_i)=\frac{\partial}{\partial x_j}\left[\left(\mu+\frac{\mu_t}{\sigma_\varepsilon}\right)\frac{\partial\varepsilon}{\partial x_j}\right]+C_{1\varepsilon}\frac{\rho\varepsilon}{k}G_k-C_{2\varepsilon}\frac{\rho\varepsilon^2}{k} \tag{5}$$

In these equations, G_k represents the generation of turbulence kinetic energy due to the mean velocity gradients, calculated by:

$$G_k=\frac{\mu_t}{\rho}\frac{\partial u_i}{\partial x_j}\left(\frac{\partial u_i}{\partial x_j}+\frac{\partial u_j}{\partial x_i}\right) \tag{6}$$

The energy equation is in the following form:

$$\frac{\partial}{\partial t}(\rho h)+\nabla\cdot(\vec{u}\rho h)=\nabla\cdot\left(k_{eff}\nabla T+\vec{\tau}_{eff}\cdot\vec{u}\right)+S_h \tag{7}$$

$$h=\int_{T_{eff}}^{T}C_p dT \tag{8}$$

where k_{eff} is the effective conductivity, S_h is the sources of energy. The first two terms on the right-hand side of Eq.(7) represent energy transfer due to conduction, and viscous dissipation respectively. The viscous dissipation term describes the thermal energy created by viscous shear in the flow. The key point of this paper is the activation of this term, which is often negligible under normal conditions. Viscous heating will be important when the Brinkman number, Br, approaches or exceeds unity, where

$$\mathrm{Br} = \frac{\mu U_e^2}{k\Delta T} \tag{9}$$

in which ΔT represents the temperature difference in the system. In current studies, **Br** is in the range of 20~30, greatly exceeding unity. The properties of the fluid (oil) in this study are: ρ = 900kg/m^3, C_p = 1880J/(kg · s), k = 0.12w/(m· k), and μ = 0.036kg/(m· s) (at 25^{0}C).

4 Grid Generation and Its Independence Study

The computational domain includes both the chamber (fluid zone) and the spool (solid zone). Around the notches, tetrahedral cells are generated, which are used for adaptation to the complex geometry shape. In the region far from the notches, such as the inlet and outlet sections of the chamber, prism cells are distributed. Hexahedral or prism cells are preferred, since they provide better accuracy and stability than tetrahedral cells.

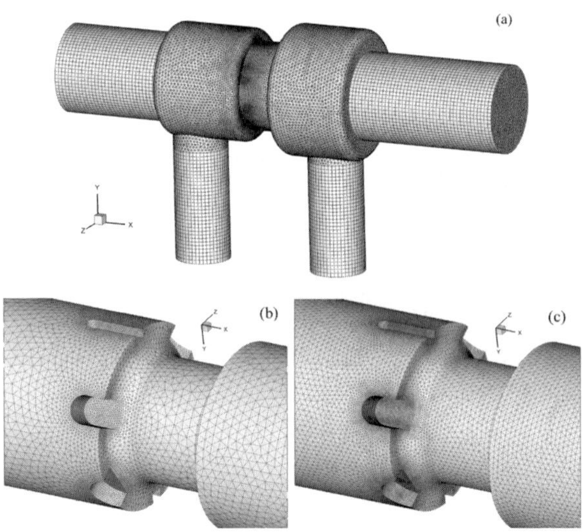

Fig. 2. Computational grid (a) for the whole domain, (b) coarse grid around the notches, (c) fine grid around the notches

The whole computational grid is shown in Fig.2(a): the employed three dimensional grids are hybrid, moreover, the "size function" technique is involved, which allow the refinement of the grid near the notches. In order to obtain a good quality grid and to control the size ratio between two successive cells in space, size function is used for grid generation. The edges of the notches are defined as the sources, where the small features of the model are captured. The cells away from the source are gradually enlarged at a specific ratio of 1.2, till that the cell size reaches the up-limit.

Fig.2(b) and (c) show a coarse and a fine grid respectively. The smallest cell in the coarse grid system is 2mm in length, while that in the fine grid is 1mm. As we have tested, the computations based on both grids can reach converged results, however, which result is more reliable? This requires to be discovered in this section.

As everybody can imagine, different grids could lead to different results. The simulation based on a fine grid is generally more precise than that on a coarse grid. But an extremely fine grid requires a mass of computational resources, which are limited at present condition. In order to establish a grid-independent solution, tests should first be performed. In these tests, length of the grid (the start size) around the notches varies from 0.5mm to 0.05mm, the growth rate of the size function and the up-limit of the size are kept at 1.2 and 1mm respectively. It is found that the solutions converge at the cells number of 1112255, where the maximum temperature is 415K and the flow rate is 1.025kg/s. It is to say that the simulation become grid independent for this size of grid. Therefore, all the following simulations will be carried out on this grid. It takes about 4 hours for a case of calculation on a super-computer with 12 CPUs involved.

5 Flow Structures and Temperature Distributions

In order to study the thermal performance of the valves at different openings, eight cases are studied for each spool (A and B) with the opening varied from 1.0mm to 6.0mm. The results are listed in Table 1, which exhibits the mass flow rate for different openings, the local maximum temperature around each notch, and the global maximum temperature on the spool. The numbering for notches is shown in Fig.1. The local maximum temperature is measured in such a way that we first define a spherical zone, which contains all edges of a certain notch, while not interfering with other notches. The maximum value of temperature in such a spherical zone represents the local maximum temperature for the corresponding notch. However, it should be noticed that the maximum value of these three local maximum temperatures is not always the global maximum temperature, which will be illustrated in the following text.

Fig.3 shows the temperature contours on the spools. We observe that the heat congregates at the bottom of the notches where a strong viscous shear is predicted. The maximum velocity magnitude of the flow through the notches is in the range of 130m/s to 150m/s. As can be visualized from Fig.3, when the valve containing spool A is fully opened, the highest temperature region is located at notch A3, the axial length of which is the smallest. Due to the large flow rate, the heat is greatly transferred downstream. The maximum value of temperature for this case (Case 1) is 492K. When decreasing the valve opening, the heat transmission region downstream the notches is gradually reduced, at the same time the temperature at notch A1 increases, the axial length of which is the largest, while holding the least radial depth and the least circumferential length. With a further decrease of the opening, as shown in Case 5, notch A3 is closed, no flow is allowed to pass by it, so the temperature at this place returns to its original value, about 323K. When the valve opening is decreased to 3.0mm, as shown in Case 6, the high temperature region downstream the notches almost vanishes, in which case the spool has traveled 3mm from the fully opened position. With the more traveling of the spool, to Case 7, notch A2 is shut down, and only notch A1 is available at this time. The highest temperature on spool A under this opening condition is 379K, which is over 100K less than that of the fully opened case. From the temperature distributions, one can predict that stress concentration will occur on the edges of the notches, due to the heat concentration around them, thus inducing the deformation of the spools. When the deformation exceeds the allowable radial clearance, heat shocks occur.

Table 1. Results for different cases

	Case Index	Opening (mm)	Flow rate (kg/s)	Tmax at A1 or B1 (K)	Tmax at A2 or B2 (K)	Tmax at A3 or B3 (K)	Tmax on spool (K)
Spool A	Case1	6.0	2.640	348	430	492	492
	Case2	5.0	1.961	363	426	436	436
	Case3	4.5	1.495	371	414	420	420
	Case4	4.0	1.022	377	419	353	419
	Case5	3.5	0.746	367	428	323	428
	Case6	3.0	0.498	365	408	323	408
	Case7	2.0	0.277	379	323	323	379
	Case8	1.0	0.218	383	323	323	383
Spool B	Case9	6.0	2.411	364	439	460	460
	Case10	5.0	1.852	353	417	433	433
	Case11	4.5	1.592	353	437	441	441
	Case12	4.0	1.363	351	441	443	444
	Case13	3.5	1.104	351	391	394	394
	Case14	3.0	0.871	348	372	330	388
	Case15	2.0	0.588	347	369	329	377
	Case16	1.0	0.296	324	373	324	373

Case9 to Case16 are for spool B. At the fully opened state, as shown in Case 9 of Fig.3, the highest temperature region is located at notch B3, the depth of which is the largest. The maximum value of temperature for this case is 460K. With the decrease of valve opening, notch B3 and notch B1 are shut down one after the other. The highest temperature region is shifted from notch B3 to notch B2 at last. It is noticed that if comparing between spool A and spool B at a same opening, for example case 14 with case 6, one can observe that the high temperature region on spool A has been limited inside the notches, however on spool B, the heat is transferred along the spool surface, even over the other edge of the concavity. This has a positive effect for protecting the valve from heat shock, for the concavity has a small radial depth, the deformation on which could hardly lead to the exceeding over the allowable radial clearance.

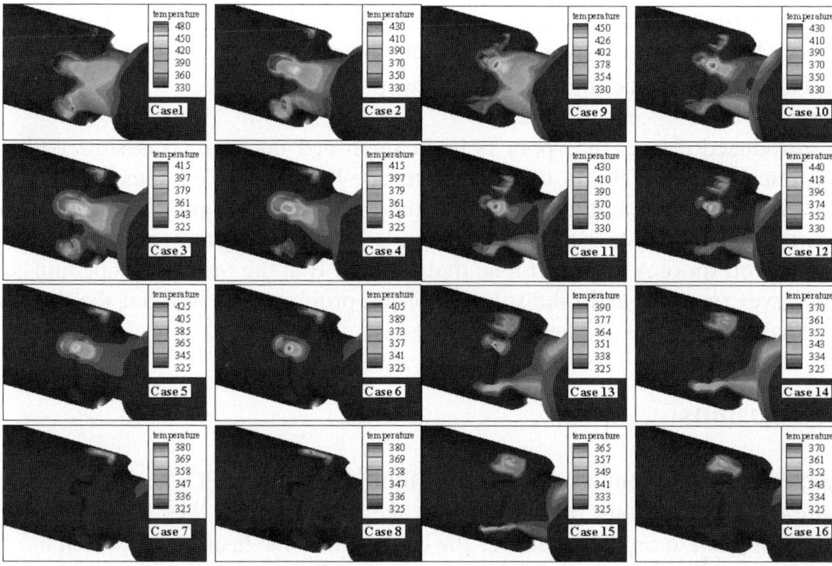

Fig. 3. Temperature distributions around the notches

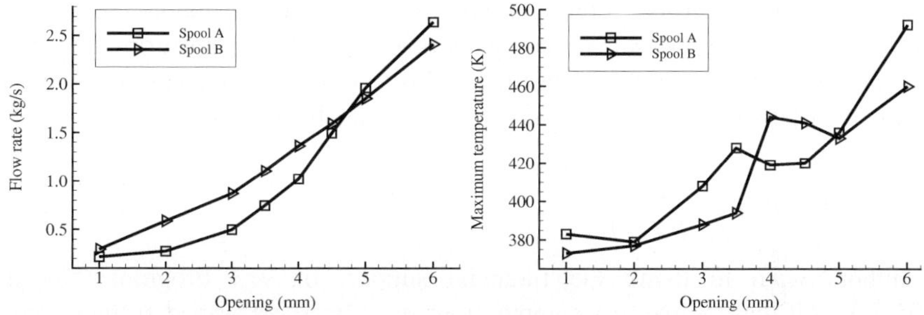

Fig. 4. Flow rates and maximum temperatures at different openings for both spools

Fig.4 shows the flow rate and maximum value of temperature that vary with the opening for both spools. For smaller opening, the flow rate of the valve containing spool B is larger than that of spool A, while beyond the opening of 5mm, the flow rate of valve containing spool B is smaller than that of spool A. This should be avoided to the best of the designers' abilities, for this curve should be kept constant for different spools, in order to obtain the same performance of the valves. The maximum temperatures' variation with the opening is the major focus of this paper. We observe that both curves are not monotone, and keeping a flat level in the range 4mm-5mm opening. In this range, the maximum temperature on spool B is higher than that on spool A, while in other cases of opening, the maximum temperatures on spool B are lower than that on spool A. For the fully opened case, the maximum temperature on spool B is 460K, which is 32K lower than that on spool A, which is

492K. This difference is though very small in general situations, it can be very significant under specific situation, for example the case of which the clearance is very strict. The clearance for the valves we study in current paper is reported to be 6 micrometers.

As introduced above, the spool B is an improved one, which is supposed to be more applicable for its ability to avoid or reduce heat shock. We thus have provided some CFD results, attempting to support the engineers' design. Though it is found that the temperature distributions on the two spools are different, and the maximum temperature on spool A is greater than that of spool B at the maximum opening condition. It serves to guide us in the solution of the problem, but it is not the direct evidence. Therefore, further studies are needed.

6 Conclusions

This paper has carried out a computational fluid dynamics (CFD) analysis of the flow structures and temperature distributions in the spool valves. The numerical studies have been applied in order to discover the causation of the heat shock, which has been supposed to due to the thermal effect. The viscous heating leads to local temperature increase, resulting in deformation of the valve spool. The current studies confirmed these suppositions. Moreover, we investigated two different valve spools. The numerical results predict different thermal behaviors on these two spools. The heat concentration (the high temperature spot) takes place at different positions for spool A compared with spool B. All these results help us to draw a conclusion that spool B is more reliable that spool A, for its ability to avoid heat shock.

Acknowledgment

The authors wish to thank the financial support of 973 Program (No. 2006 CB705400). All these numerical computations have been performed at the Center for Engineering and Scientific Computation (CESC), Zhejiang University. The authors are grateful for this assistance.

References

1. Vaughan, N.D., Jonn, D.N., Burnell, L.R.: The use of computational dynamics in hydraulic valve design. In: Design, Circuit, Component and System Design, pp. 226–244. John Wiley and Sons Inc., New York (1992)
2. Wang, L., Chen, Y., Ruan, X., Lu, Y.: Experimental study on fluid flow in fluid power system. In: The 4th international conference of fluid power transmission and control, Hangzhou, China (1997)
3. Ruan, X.D., Song, X.Q., Yamamoto, F., Wang, L., Shao, X.: PIV experiment of flow field in spool valve chamber. In: The 4th international conference of fluid power transmission and control, Hangzhou, China (1997)

4. Borghi, M., Milani, M., Paoluzzi, R.: Stationary axial flow forces analysis on compensated spool valves. Int. J. Fluid Power 1, 17–25 (2000)
5. Gao, D.R.: Investigations of flow structures inside spool valve with FEM and PIV methods. Int. J. Fluid Power 5, 51–66 (2004)
6. Del, V.G., Lippolis, A.: Three-dimensional analysis of flow forces on directional control valves. Int. J. Fluid Power 4, 15–24 (2003)
7. Amirante, R., Del, V.G., Lippolis, A.A.: Flow forces analysis of an open center hydraulic directional control valve sliding spool. Energy Conversion and Management 47, 114–131 (2006)

Clamping Fixtures for Intelligent Cell Manufacturing

Karol Velíšek, Peter Košťál, and Radovan Zvolenský

Institute of Production Systems and Applied Mechanics, Faculty of Materials Science and Technology, Slovak UniversitY Of Technology, Rázusova 2, 91724 Trnava, Slovak Republic
karol.velisek@stuba.sk, peter.kostal@stuba.sk, radovan.zvolensky@stuba.sk

Abstract. Philosophy of flexible manufacturing cell dedicated for small batch production present production system that manipulates with workpieces and produce from semi products individual parts for concrete final products. Base of the complex automatic production is automation of technological process control, automatic transport, manipulation, feeding, workpiece and tool exchange. Industrial production develops, the new generation production systems – intelligent production systems. Development of new generation production machines and systems demand that they are equipped by adequate fixture devices. These fixture devices are developed with machine together, to don't decrease their production facilities and their time and performance utilizations. Efficiency of fixture device in automatized production systems underlie using efficiency of entire production systems.

Keywords: Intelligent manufacturing, clamping fixture, cell manufacturing, production systems, flexible manufacturing.

1 Introduction

Following to the up rising users individualization trend in field of customer industry, the low series production is also rising. Manufacturers are trying to reach maximal market benefit, by its products, which have to be produced with maximal tact, minimal costs and they also need to be suitable for all individual customer requirements. One way, which can be used for creating of all these requirements is wide using of cell manufacture. Cell manufacture is characterized by wide economical effect which is nearly the same as economical effect of mass or high series production. Cell production also ensures flexible change of manufacturing assortment, which can be changed following to the market requirements.

Modern production cells has in many aspect inbuilt intelligent control system on different level. This intelligent control system ensures better using of such devices. It also ensures manufacturing costs minimalization, as well as manufacturing quality increasing. Such intelligence in these days includes various control algorithms. Such algorithms are able to optimalize manufacturing cell activity following to the various actual external factors. These factors are influencing to the manufacturing process inside of the cell and in connection with manufacturing process, can these factors influence to the whole factory and its parts. Very important parts of intelligent

C. Xiong et al. (Eds.): ICIRA 2008, Part II, LNAI 5315, pp. 966–972, 2008.

manufacturing cells are its peripheral devices, such as for example clamping devices. These devices have to designed, that they are not able to limit abilities of whole manufacturing cell. Better say, whole design process of all peripheral devices have to simple integration of new intelligent functions in to the manufacturing cell and also to the manufacturing process. Such peripheries have to be equipped by proper actuators and sensors to be able effective cooperate with manufacturing cell control system. We are building such manufacturing cell on our department. This cell will ensure manufacturing and assembly operations and we are also developing some peripheral devices such as clamping device with some intelligent functions.

2 Intelligent Flexible Manufacturing and Assembly Cell

Intelligent flexible manufacturing and assembly cell, which is developed at our workplace is created of these main parts:

- industrial robot with Cartesian kinematics, which is equipped by automated tool and grippers changing system
- clamping device, which ensures clamping and fixing of semi products and products during manufacturing and assembly operations
- shelf storage with manipulator, which is used as storage place for semi products and final products
- rotary feeding device, which ensures pallets manipulation between cell workplace and shelf storage.

Whole intelligent, flexible, manufacturing and assembly cell configuration is showed at the figure…

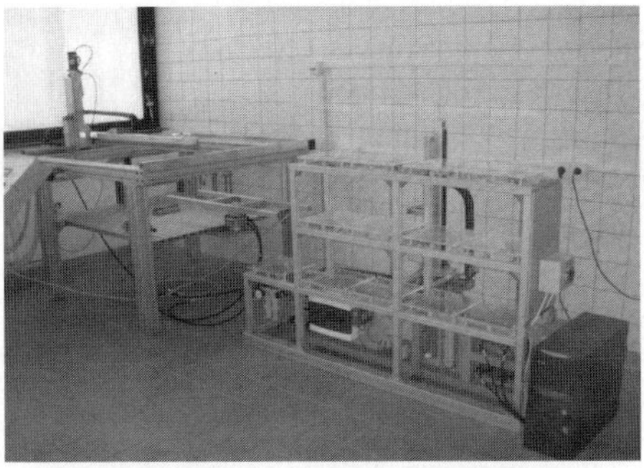

Fig. 1. Intelligent flexible manufacturing and assembly cell

3 Basic Design of Intelligent Clamping Fixture

An robotic work place is realized in laboratories of institute. This work place is equipped by SMC industrial robot with storage system. Both this systems are connected with feeding rotary device. The system is equipped by automated gripper changing system and it is also equipped by pneumatic clamping system, which will contain some basic functions of intelligent clamping system.

Pneumatic driven clamping device will be placed in the working area of industrial robot. This device will be designed by these requirements:

- Clamped dimension to the 70mm – there will be no manipulation with parts, which will overreach this dimension. Robotic arm bearing capacity is 100N.
- Synchronized clamps movement – this requirement is necessary because of rotary parts clamping
- open clamps signalization – to prevent manipulation with clamped part, or to prevent putting the part in the fixture, when there is one part already
- part clamped in fixture device signalization – prevent to the collision of part which are placed in the fixture and which are gripped in robotic arm
- clamped shapes variability – clamping of various shapes – cylinder, square
- Using of changeable clamps – clamps will be changed with help of the gripper
- proper clamps on the fixture signalization – to prevent clamping of oval shaped part with clamps not used for oval shaped parts
- Clamping force regulation ability – it is necessary to use various clamping force for various types of pars.
- All can be realized from own financial sources with minimal costs

According to these requirements was chosen the pneumatic base for proper clamping device. The basic building element of the fixture will be double clamp fixture with marking MHF2. The fixture was produced by firm SMC. The design of the fixture is known as design with synchronized, parallel driven clamps movement. Chosen fixture has maximal clamping dimension 80 mm. More precisely we chose clamping fixture MHF2 20D2 (Fig. 2), which has these basic characteristics:

- clamping precision repeatability ± 0,05mm
- small proportions (174x62x41mm)
- synchronized clamps movement with stroke 2x40mm
- linear bearing with high precision
- double acting

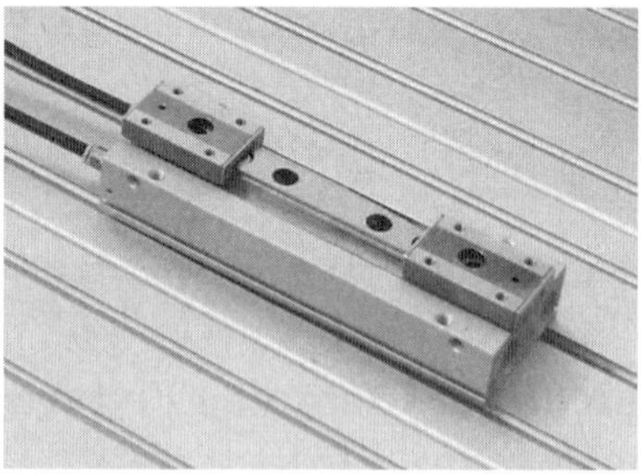

Fig. 2. Clamping device MHF 2

Fixture device is pneumatic driven. Fixture acting is realized by two double acting cylinders. One pressed air input will open the clamps and other one input will close them. Clamps synchronization movement is ensured by geared transfer mechanism. Clamps position can be monitored by one or two sensors. Sensors can be mounted to the fixture with help of grooves. Chosen pneumatic actuator advantages are for example simple design, safeties, reliability, wide clamping dimension, undemanding maintenance, high lifetime small sizes and low costs. Working pressure can be set up from 0,1 to the 0,7 MPa, what means that clamping forces will rise from 30N to the 220N on each clamp. Pressed air can be plugged to the fixture by two ways:

- direct in the piston axis, with help of M5 thread,
- on the flank side of the fixture, with help of M6 thread.

3.1 Clamps Presence Scanning

Also design of monitoring system of claps presence on the fixture body, was created following to some conditions. Most important conditions influenced to the design are sensor sizes, sensor simplicity, its reliability, lifetime, rapid and exact scanning.

For actual needs (it is only important to scant clamps presence, not the type of clamps) is the most proper solution, using of micro switchers. Micro switchers will be placed at clamps holder. Biggest advantage of such scanning is price of micro switchers. Sensors will be placed on the pneumatic fixture body. But we can not do any holes in to the actuator body, that why switchers will be glued. In the future, after design finishing phase, after short fixture running, switchers will be replaced by other more complicated and effective system, which will ensure the clamps presence scanning.

3.2 Work Piece Presence Scanning

There are different ways how to scan presence of work piece in the fixture clamping area. This position can be scanned by various types of sensors such as optical sensor, inductive sensor, camera scanning system and so on. Most effective solution is using of optic sensor, which will be placed in the middle of clamping dimension. Big advantage of optic sensor against to the inductive sensor or against to the capacity sensor is its longer scanning range and there is also a possibility of various material kinds scanning. Camera scanning systems are for this solution vain complicated. For this concrete solution there will be used optical reflex sensor with axial optic, with advantage of optical beam regulation.

Optical reflex sensors are working at principle of optical performance scanning. They are comparing set optical performance value with actual value coming from the environment. Such sensors are able to scan object of various sizes and complexity. Sensor will be placed on the fixture device with help of assembly clip, which will be glued on the side of the fixture device body.

3.3 Clamps Placement Scanning

Proper solution of clamps placement scanning uses standard magnetic sensors. Those sensors can be placed and fixed in grooves which are created and designed on the fixture body, by the fixture producer. Such sensor is scanning increase of magnetic array. Magnetic array increase is made by permanent magnet, which is composed in the piston, placed in the fixture body. The magnetic array will grow with decreasing distance of piston to the sensor. When magnetic array will reach some set up value, the sensor will switch on. Magnetic sensors advantage is its immediate signalization, simple manipulation, immediate and simple placement and on the side of the fixture. These sensors will scan open position of the fixture clamps. This scanning is proper for our design, because we are creating pneumatic driven device and that why there are no other clamps positions such as open and closed.

3.4 Clamping Force Regulation

According to that fact, that we are designing pneumatic driven device, we have to regulate working pressure in ranges from 0,1 to the 0,7 MPa. We will regulate clamping force by very simple principle which will operate with pressure regulation. Pressure change will be realized by electric controlled pressure valve. The input to this valve is 0,8 MPa and on the output we are able to regulate the pressure, thanks to the analogue signal in range of 5 to 15 V.

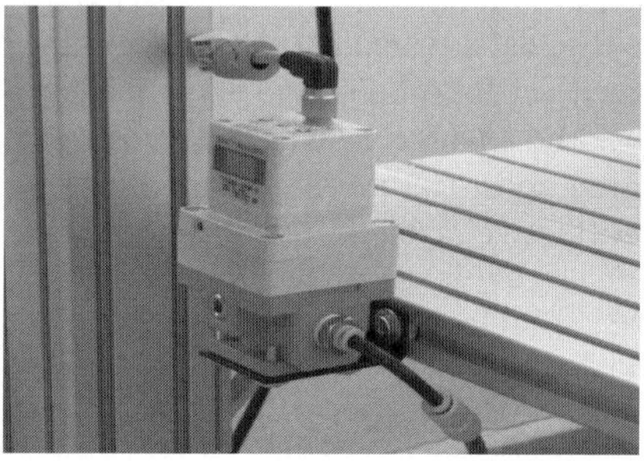

Fig. 3. Pressure valve

Pressure valve is equipped by alphanumerical display, which ensure simple controlling of the device and its also shows the actual pressure value. Except to the switching outputs, there is also other one analogue output for other processing. Advantage of such device is rapid evaluation of clamping force, simple assembly, rigid design and adjustable hysteresis. (Fig. 3)

Whole fixture with all sensors is showed at the Fig. 4. Because this clamping fixture has small dimensions (length is only 174 mm), we must choice the smallest sensors.

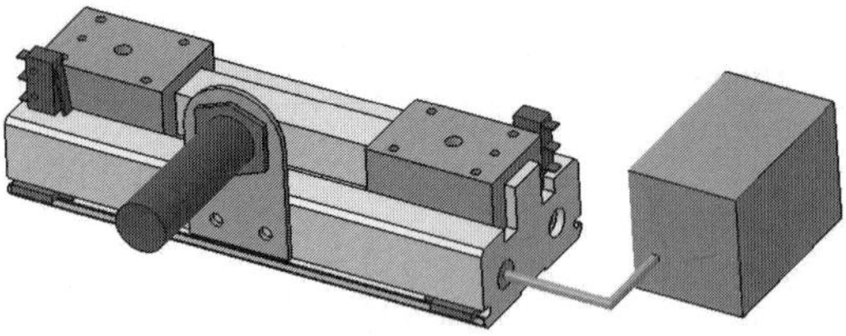

Fig. 4. 3D model of clamping device with sensors

4 Conclusion

For successful position on the market, continue productivity increasing is needed. That why effective using of new technologies in manufacturing process is necessary. Such effective using is also connected with intelligence increasing of single manufacturing and helping devices. Intelligent clamping systems can help to increase reliability of some operations. Automated manufacture can be done more flexible. Such clamping systems are more expensive and complex as classical fixtures, because they have integrated some automated control and measuring units. Intelligent clamping systems are able to prevent to some failures, which are created during the production in automated manufacture and assembly. Designed intelligent pneumatic clamping system will be equipped by sensors. Sensors will scan clamps presence, working product presence, clamps placement and also clamping force regulation. According to the small sizes of pneumatic fixture, we are designing all devices in small sizes, we choose small sizes sensors. Also simple design, simple and reliable assembly and low costs are very important.

By our meaning the best solution for clamping jigs detection are micro switches take to clamping jig holders. They can detect only two states: jig is present – switch is closed, jig is not present – switch is open. This signal will be send to control system.

The best way to workpiece detection is by our meanings to use of an optical sensor. The capacitive or inductive sensors has small range of detection, and detection by camera is very complicated and expensive solution for this case.

The position of clamping jig holder are detected by two magnetic sensors on side of fixture body.

We will reach automated manufacturing process without labour operation by equipping of pneumatic fixtures by sensors. By such solution the productivity and production quality will increase.

Acknowledgment

This paper was created thanks to the national grants:

VEGA 1/3193/06 - **Multifunctional** ***manufacturing and assembly cell.***

VEGA 1/3164/06 - ***Using of intelligent fixtures in manufacturing and assembly processes.***

References

1. Danišová, N., Pastierovič, M., Fidler, B.: Nové generácie upínačov vo výrobnom procese (New generation of clamping fixtures in production). In: Vedecké práce MtF STU v Bratislave so sídlom v Trnave, pp. 21–26 (2006); ISSN 1336-1589. - Č. 21
2. Danišová, N., Zvolenský, R.: Automated flexible manufacturing systems. In: KOD 2006: Zbornik radova / nadát. Simpozijum sa medunarodnim učešcem. 4. Konstruisanje, oblikovanje i dizajn. Palic, 30-31 May 2006, pp. 253–256. Fakultet tehničkih nauka, Novi Sad (2006)

3. DrstvenšEK, I., Pahole, I., KovačIč, M., Balič, J.: Intelligent interface in a flexible production environment. J. mater. process. technol. [Print ed.], May 15, 2005, vol. 164-165, pp. 1309–1316 [COBISS.SI-ID 9462806] (2005), http://dx.doi.org/10.1016/j.jmatprotec.2005.02.074
4. Ficko, M., Drstvenšek, I., Brezočnik, M.: Design of layout of flexible manufacturing system by genetic algorithms. V: MicroCAD, Section J, Production engineering and manufacturing systems, pp. 57–60. University of Miskolc, Innovation and Technology Transfer Centre, Miskolc (2004) [COBISS.SI-ID 8632854]
5. Hrušková, E., Matúšová, M.: Fixture model creation in software Catia V5R15. - 1/3193/06, 1/3164/06. In: RaDMI 2006: Proceedings on CD-ROM / nadát. International Conference, Budva, Montenegro, September 13-17, 2006, pp. 1–4. High Technical Mechanical School of Trstenik, Trstenik (2006)
6. Košál, P., Matúšová, M., Velíšek, K.: Modeling of clamping fixtures. Academic Journal of Manufacturing Engineering 5(2), 65–68 (2007)
7. Matúšová, M., Hrušková, E.: Database of fixture mechanisms. In: RaDMI 2007: Proceedings on CD-ROM of 7th International Conference Research and Development in Mechanical Industy - RaDMI 2007, Belgrade, Serbia, September 16-20, 2007, pp. 613–617. High Technical Mechanical School of Trstenik, Trstenik (2007)
8. Matúšová, M., Javorová, A.: Analyse der Spannvorrichtungen durch Algorithmus. Analýza upínacích prípravkov pomocou algoritmu. In: Materials Science and Technology [online] (2005); ISSN 1335-9053. - Roč. 5, č. 1 [cit. 2005-03-29]
9. Matúšová, M., Katalinic, B., Hrušková, E.: Determination of cutting forces direction and point of acting. In: Annals of DAAAM for 2006 and Proceedings / nadát. International DAAAM Symposium. 17th. Intelligent Manufacturing and Automation: Focus on Mechatronics and Robotics, Viena, Austria, 8-11th November 2006, pp. 241–242. DAAAM International Vienna, Viedeň (2006)
10. Velíšek, K., Danišová, N., Košál, P.: Exploitation of intelligence in roboted assembly. In: Annals of MTeM for 2007 & Proceedings of the 8th International Conference Modern Technologies in Manufacturing, 4th-5th October 2007, pp. 453–456. Technical University of Cluj-Napoca, Cluj-Napoca (2007)
11. Velíšek, K., Javorová, A., Zvolenský, R., Danišová, N., Košt'ál, P.: Multifunctional manufacturing and assembly system. In: Development of Mechanical Engineering as a Tool for Enterprise Logistics Progress: Science Report Project CII-PL-0033-01-0506, pp. 135–158. University of Technology, Poznaň (2006)

Kinematics Constrained Toolpath Planning for Five-Axis Machines

Tao Ye and Cai-Hua Xiong

State Key Lab of Digital Manufacturing Equipment and Technology of China,
School of Mechanical Science and Engineering,
Huazhong University of Science and Technology, Wuhan 430074, P.R. China
taoye@smail.hust.edu.cn, chxiong@mail.hust.edu.cn

Abstract. This paper presents a new general toolpath planning method which considers two important types of constraints: the kinematics constraint and the geometric feature constraints. The contact kinematics theory for rigid bodies is used to incorporate the two types of constraints into our optimization framework. The objective is to maximize the machining efficiency. The proposed method consists of three stages: establishing the mapping between the tool feeding speed with surface curvature, the orientation of the tool and the kinematics of machines; identifying the optimal cutting direction by solving a constrained nonlinear programming problem in the parametric domain; generating streamline-like toolpath and mapping it back to the surface. An example using our toolpath generation method is given to demonstrate its effectiveness.

Keywords: Toolpath, contact kinematics, machining efficiency, streamline, parametric domain.

1 Introduction

Machining of mechanical parts with free-form surfaces usually requires weeks or months which costs large quantity of resources. Therefore, the machining efficiency is critical for industrial practices. Generally speaking, using five-axis machines instead of three-axis machine in free-form surface machining can achieve higher productivity due to the flexibility from the two additional rotational axes. However, machining planning for five-axis machines is much more complicated than for three-axis machines. It is observed that the structural complex aroused from the additional rotational axes induces the anisotropic performance along different cutting directions: 1) the maximum feeding speed which can be achieved is different at different local region and along different feeding directions; 2) the quantity of material removed using different tool orientations and along feeding directions is different. To fully exploit the machining capability of the five-axis machines, the toolpath has to adapt to both the surface geometry and the machine tool kinematics.

There are large quantities of work focusing on optimization of toolpath optimization from geometric perspective. Among them the maximization of local cutting region and minimization of total path length are two mostly involved principles. The

C. Xiong et al. (Eds.): ICIRA 2008, Part II, LNAI 5315, pp. 973–982, 2008.

former are usually realized through local curvature matching or identifying the cutting direction in which the largest cutting width is achieved. Rao et. al. [1] proposed a principle axis method using the projected effective curvature of the cutter to match the local geometry. Through curvature matching, more material can be removed and larger portion of cutter edge would involve in the cutting process. Later, Gray [2,3] developed the rolling ball method in which a variable rolling sphere is constructed at sampled positions on the free-form surface. The difficult iterative checking of gouging and complicated computation in curvature matching methods can thus be avoided. Wang and Tang [4] proposed an orientation optimization for machining using flat-end mill. The silhouette curve of the effective cutting surface is used to match the local geometry. As they separate the generation of cutter location with the determination of cutter orientation, the generated toolpath would not be irregular spaced.

Different from the curvature matching, John and Lee [5] proposed the potential field method which directly identifies the feeding direction along which the maximum cutting width is achieved. The toolpath are then generated tangentially to these directions.

Reducing the total path length is another criterion to increase the machining efficiency[7,8,9,10,11,12]. The total path length can be divided into the productive paths on which the cutter actually cuts the part stock and removes material, and the non-productive paths including the tool lifting and traversing process from one region to another [6]. To achieve high machining efficiency, three major elements need to be optimized: the total length of the productive toolpath, the total length of non-productive toolpath and the total number of tool retractions.

Although toolpath planning methods with the objective to increase the machining efficiency have been studied extensively, we observed that there are not much work concerning about the machine kinematics. Makhanov et al. use a variational grid which adapts to the variation of surface curvature to generate the toolpath. Their method mainly concerns the kinematics error. Kim developed a general framework for finding the optimal sweeping path on 2-manifold. In his method, the motor speed limit is included. But they made assumptions that the tool orientations are pre-assigned during machining.

In this paper, we shall give the relationship between the material removal speed with the kinematical structure of the machines, the cutter geometry, the local surface geometry, and the tool configuration.

The major contributions of our work are:

1) We explicitly give the relationship among the machines' kinematics, the tool feeding speed, and the local surface property.
2) An optimization method which can simultaneously give the tool path geometry and the tool orientation is devised instead of treating the tool orientation data and tool path geometry data separately.

2 Machining Description Using Contact Kinematics

During the machining process, the cutter moves along the part surface. The part surface and the cutter surface contact with each other at the cutter contact point. We shall study the relationship between the motion of this contact point and the feeding speed.

The motion of the cutter contact point in the parametrical space of the surface can be described using the contact kinematics equations for rigid bodies derived by Montana [13,14]

$$\begin{cases} \begin{bmatrix} \dot{u}_w \\ \dot{v}_w \end{bmatrix} = \mathbf{M}_w^{-1}\mathbf{R}_\Psi\left(\mathbf{K}_t+\tilde{\mathbf{K}}_w\right)^{-1}\left(\begin{bmatrix} -\omega_y \\ \omega_x \end{bmatrix}+\tilde{\mathbf{K}}_t\begin{bmatrix} v_x \\ v_y \end{bmatrix}\right) \\ 0 = v_z \end{cases} \quad (1)$$

where $\mathbf{M}$, $\mathbf{K}$, are metric tensor and curvature tensor respectively, $\mathbf{R}_\Psi = \begin{bmatrix} \cos\psi & -\sin\psi \\ -\sin\psi & -\cos\psi \end{bmatrix}$, $\left(v_x \quad v_y \quad v_z \quad \omega_x \quad \omega_y \quad \omega_z\right)^T = V_{l_w l_t}^b$ is the relative body velocity between the contact frames: $L_w(\tau)$ and $L_t(\tau)$, Ψ is the angel between x-axes of the two frames, the subscript t and w represents the tool frame and the workpiece frame respectively. The equations (1) are originally derived assuming that the surfaces are parameterized orthogonally. However, it can be extended to general regular parametrical surfaces and curve-surface contact situation [15]. For simplicity, we shall use equations (1) in our discussion. It can be observed that first equation in (1) establishes the relationship between the motion of the tool and the motion of the cutter contact point in the parametrical space of the part surface. The second equation of (1) imposes a constraint that the feeding direction lies in the tangent space at $(u_w \quad v_w)$.

The part surface is viewed as a 2-manifold with the parametrical description as $S(u,v)$, $S: U \subset \Re^2 \to \Re^3$. A curve on the surface is denoted by $S\left(u(t),v(t)\right)$ or $\gamma(t)$. The length of the curve on the surface can be calculated using the first fundamental form:

$$I = ds^2 = g_{11}\cdot du\cdot du + 2\cdot g_{12}\cdot du\cdot dv + g_{22}\cdot dv\cdot dv \quad (2)$$

where $g_{11} = \frac{\partial S}{\partial u}\cdot\frac{\partial S}{\partial u}$, $g_{12} = \frac{\partial S}{\partial u}\frac{\partial S}{\partial v}$, $g_{22} = \frac{\partial S}{\partial v}\frac{\partial S}{\partial v}$. The surface is said to have a orthogonal parameterization if $g_{12} = 0$.

Now we can give the explicit relationship between the feeding speed and the tool motion using equations (1) and (2):

$$f = ds/dt$$

$$= \sqrt{\begin{bmatrix} \mathbf{e}_1^T\cdot\mathbf{M}_w^{-1}\mathbf{R}_\Psi\left(\mathbf{K}_t+\tilde{\mathbf{K}}_w\right)^{-1}\left(\begin{bmatrix} -\omega_y \\ \omega_x \end{bmatrix}+\tilde{\mathbf{K}}_t\begin{bmatrix} v_x \\ v_y \end{bmatrix}\right) \\ \mathbf{e}_2^T\cdot\mathbf{M}_w^{-1}\mathbf{R}_\Psi\left(\mathbf{K}_t+\tilde{\mathbf{K}}_w\right)^{-1}\left(\begin{bmatrix} -\omega_y \\ \omega_x \end{bmatrix}+\tilde{\mathbf{K}}_t\begin{bmatrix} v_x \\ v_y \end{bmatrix}\right) \end{bmatrix}^T \mathbf{G} \begin{bmatrix} \mathbf{e}_1^T\cdot\mathbf{M}_w^{-1}\mathbf{R}_\Psi\left(\mathbf{K}_t+\tilde{\mathbf{K}}_w\right)^{-1}\left(\begin{bmatrix} -\omega_y \\ \omega_x \end{bmatrix}+\tilde{\mathbf{K}}_t\begin{bmatrix} v_x \\ v_y \end{bmatrix}\right) \\ \mathbf{e}_2^T\cdot\mathbf{M}_w^{-1}\mathbf{R}_\Psi\left(\mathbf{K}_t+\tilde{\mathbf{K}}_w\right)^{-1}\left(\begin{bmatrix} -\omega_y \\ \omega_x \end{bmatrix}+\tilde{\mathbf{K}}_t\begin{bmatrix} v_x \\ v_y \end{bmatrix}\right) \end{bmatrix}} \quad (3)$$

where $\mathbf{G}=\begin{bmatrix} g_{11} & g_{12} \\ g_{12} & g_{22} \end{bmatrix}$, $\mathbf{e}_i$ is the natural basis. It should be noted that equation (3) is true under condition $0=v_z$.

3 Problem Formulation

3.1 Kinematics Relationship between the Motors and the Cutting Process

The maximum feeding speed that the tool could achieve is constrained by the motor speed limits. Here we derive the relationship between the motor speed and the feeding speed. The kinematics relationship is studied based on Lie group theory [16]. Note that an element $\mathbf{g}_{wt} \in SE(3)$ physically represents a configuration of the rigid body in Euclidean space where the subscript w and t represents workpiece frame and tool frame respectively. The twist of the rigid body (or the body velocity of the tool) can be identified using its tangent at the group identity: $\hat{\mathbf{V}}_{wt}^{b}=\mathbf{g}_{wt}^{-1}\cdot\dot{\mathbf{g}}_{wt}\in\Re^{4\times4}$ (The operator $\wedge$ means for $\forall\boldsymbol{\zeta}\in\Re^{3\times1}$, $\boldsymbol{\xi}\in\Re^{3\times1}$, $\hat{\boldsymbol{\zeta}}=\begin{pmatrix}\zeta_x\\ \zeta_y\\ \zeta_z\end{pmatrix}\wedge=\begin{pmatrix}0 & -\zeta_z & \zeta_y\\ \zeta_z & 0 & -\zeta_x\\ -\zeta_y & \zeta_x & 0\end{pmatrix}\in\mathbf{so}(3)$ and if $\boldsymbol{\eta}=\begin{bmatrix}\boldsymbol{\zeta}\\ \boldsymbol{\xi}\end{bmatrix}\in\Re^{6\times1}$ we denote $\hat{\boldsymbol{\eta}}=\begin{bmatrix}\hat{\boldsymbol{\zeta}} & \boldsymbol{\xi}\\ 0 & 1\end{bmatrix}$).

Considering a multi-axis machine, $g_{wt}(\boldsymbol{\theta}(t)): Q\to SE(3)$, $\boldsymbol{\theta}(t)\in Q$, represents the tool configuration of the tool at time t where Q is the joint space of the multi-axis machine. We can further derive the relationship between the joint velocity and the twist of the tool:

$$\mathbf{V}_{wt}^{b}=\mathbf{J}_{wt}^{b}(\boldsymbol{\theta})\cdot\dot{\boldsymbol{\theta}} \tag{4}$$

where $\mathbf{J}_{wt}^{b}(\boldsymbol{\theta})=\left(\left(\mathbf{g}_{wt}^{-1}(\boldsymbol{\theta})\cdot\frac{\partial\mathbf{g}_{wt}}{\partial\theta_1}\right)\vee\cdots\left(\mathbf{g}_{wt}^{-1}(\boldsymbol{\theta})\cdot\frac{\partial\mathbf{g}_{wt}}{\partial\theta_n}\right)\vee\right)\in\Re^{6\times n}$ is called the body Jacobian (where $\forall\boldsymbol{\zeta}\in\Re^{3\times1}$, $\boldsymbol{\xi}\in\Re^{3\times1}$, $\vee:\begin{bmatrix}\hat{\boldsymbol{\zeta}} & \boldsymbol{\xi}\\ 0 & 1\end{bmatrix}\to\begin{bmatrix}\boldsymbol{\zeta}\\ \boldsymbol{\xi}\end{bmatrix}$). We can now explicitly give the relationship between the feeding speed and the joint velocity of the multi-axis machines using equation (3) and (4):

$$\begin{aligned} f &= ds/dt \\ &= \sqrt{\begin{bmatrix}\mathbf{e}_1^T\cdot\mathbf{M}_w^{-1}\mathbf{R}_\Psi\left(\mathbf{K}_t+\tilde{\mathbf{K}}_w\right)^{-1}\boldsymbol{\Lambda}(\boldsymbol{\theta},\dot{\boldsymbol{\theta}})\\ \mathbf{e}_2^T\cdot\mathbf{M}_w^{-1}\mathbf{R}_\Psi\left(\mathbf{K}_t+\tilde{\mathbf{K}}_w\right)^{-1}\boldsymbol{\Lambda}(\boldsymbol{\theta},\dot{\boldsymbol{\theta}})\end{bmatrix}^T \mathbf{G} \begin{bmatrix}\mathbf{e}_1^T\cdot\mathbf{M}_w^{-1}\mathbf{R}_\Psi\left(\mathbf{K}_t+\tilde{\mathbf{K}}_w\right)^{-1}\boldsymbol{\Lambda}(\boldsymbol{\theta},\dot{\boldsymbol{\theta}})\\ \mathbf{e}_2^T\cdot\mathbf{M}_w^{-1}\mathbf{R}_\Psi\left(\mathbf{K}_t+\tilde{\mathbf{K}}_w\right)^{-1}\boldsymbol{\Lambda}(\boldsymbol{\theta},\dot{\boldsymbol{\theta}})\end{bmatrix}} \end{aligned} \tag{5}$$

where $\Lambda(\boldsymbol{\theta},\dot{\boldsymbol{\theta}})=\left(\begin{bmatrix}-\mathbf{e}_5^T\cdot(\mathbf{J}_{wt}^b(\boldsymbol{\theta})\cdot\dot{\boldsymbol{\theta}})\\ \mathbf{e}_4^T\cdot(\mathbf{J}_{wt}^b(\boldsymbol{\theta})\cdot\dot{\boldsymbol{\theta}})\end{bmatrix}+\tilde{\mathbf{K}}_t\begin{bmatrix}\mathbf{e}_1^T\cdot(\mathbf{J}_{wt}^b(\boldsymbol{\theta})\cdot\dot{\boldsymbol{\theta}})\\ \mathbf{e}_2^T\cdot(\mathbf{J}_{wt}^b(\boldsymbol{\theta})\cdot\dot{\boldsymbol{\theta}})\end{bmatrix}\right)$. Also note that the constraint on the tool in the second equation of (1) is expressed as

$$\mathbf{e}_3^T\cdot\left(\mathbf{J}_{wt}^b(\boldsymbol{\theta})\cdot\dot{\boldsymbol{\theta}}\right)=0 \tag{6}$$

3.2 Instantaneous Swept Volume Definition

The objective of our method is to search the toolpath which maximizes the material being removed. The problem is transformed into finding a toolpath on which the maximum instantaneous swept volume is achieved. The instantaneous swept volume is defined as follows:

$$\Im = f\cdot A \tag{7}$$

where f is instantaneous feeding speed, A is the area obtained by projecting the tool surface along the cutting direction which we call the instantaneous swept section. In figure 2, the two curves representing the boundary of the $\boldsymbol{A}$ is obtained through intersecting the actual surface, the ideal surface with a plane defined by surface normal $\boldsymbol{n}$ and $\boldsymbol{n}\times\boldsymbol{t}$ ($\boldsymbol{t}$ is the cutting direction at the CC point).

3.3 Optimal Cutting Stream Field

The general idea of our tool path planning method is to first identify the optimal cutting directions in the parametrical domain of the part surface along which the maximum quantity of material would be removed. Then by properly selecting the streamlines of the generated vector field, the tool path is determined. We shall call the vector field obtained through optimization the optimal cutting stream field. Namely, the optimal cutting stream field is established by solving the following optimization problem:

$$\begin{aligned}&\max_{u_t,v_t,\Psi,\dot{\theta}_t}\ \Im\\ &\textit{subject to}:\ g_i=0\ \ (i=1,2,\ldots k)\\ &\qquad\qquad\quad\ g_j\le 0\ \ (j=k+1,\ldots l)\end{aligned} \tag{8}$$

where $g_i=0$, $g_j\le 0$ are a set of constraints which relates to the kinematics of the machines, the geometric properties of the generated vector field and the configuration of the tool, (u_t,v_t,Ψ) defines the configuration of the tool on the workpiece. We shall introduce the detail form of these constraints in the following section.

At each point in the parametric space of the surface, the optimization problem is solved. Thus the cutting stream field is constructed. The corresponding tool orientation data which is a function of the 3-tuple (u_t, v_t, Ψ) can also be obtained.

3.4 Direction Conforming Constraint

The optimal cutting field should be regular, i.e. the streamline integrated from the vector field should not bifurcate or varies dramatically. Otherwise, the streamline can not be used as the tool path for machining. One way to ensure the vector field to be regular is through confining the identified cutting direction $\dot{\mathbf{u}}_{i,j}$ in the paramedical space within a range. As we are calculating the cutting directions iteratively, this range can thus be controlled by previously obtained directions around it. We incorporate this requirement into our optimization framework using the direction conforming constraint. We define this constraint as

$$\dot{\mathbf{u}}_{i,j} - \sigma \cdot std\left(\dot{\mathbf{u}}_{neighbors}\right) < \dot{\mathbf{u}}_{i,j} < \dot{\mathbf{u}}_{i,j} + \sigma \cdot std\left(\dot{\mathbf{u}}_{neighbors}\right) \tag{9}$$

where $std(\bullet)$ is the standard deviation of $\dot{\mathbf{u}}_{neighbors}$, and σ is a constant. A large value of σ would allow large variation of the streamline while an extremely small value of σ would require the cutting direction almost identical to its neighbors. $\dot{\mathbf{u}}_{neighbors}$ is determined by the sequence we solve our optimization problem. A possible solving sequence and the definition of $\dot{\mathbf{u}}_{neighbors}$ corresponding to this solving sequence is illustrated in figure 1.

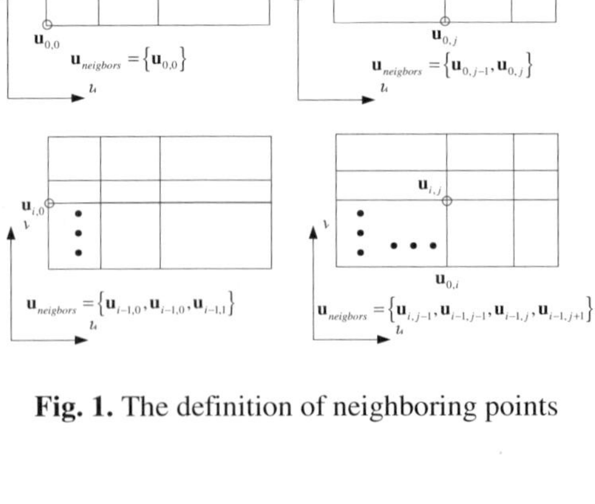

Fig. 1. The definition of neighboring points

3.5 Optimization Problem

Now we present our main optimization problem in details which identifies the cutting stream field:

$$
\begin{aligned}
&\max_{\mathbf{u}_t, v_t, \Psi, \dot{\boldsymbol{\theta}}_t} \ \Im \\
&\mathit{subject\ to}: \ \mathbf{e}_3^T\left(\mathbf{J}_{wt}^b(\boldsymbol{\theta})\cdot\dot{\boldsymbol{\theta}}\right)=0 \\
&\qquad \dot{\mathbf{u}}_{i,j}-\sigma\cdot std\left(\dot{\mathbf{u}}_{neighbors}\right)<\dot{\mathbf{u}}_{i,j}<\dot{\mathbf{u}}_{i,j}+\sigma\cdot std\left(\dot{\mathbf{u}}_{neighbors}\right) \\
&\qquad \dot{\theta}_{i,\min}\le\dot{\theta}\le\dot{\theta}_{i,\max} \quad i=1,2,\cdots n \\
&\qquad g\left(u_t, v_t, \Psi\right)\le 0
\end{aligned}
\tag{10}
$$

The first constraint in (12) ensures the cutting directions lies in the tangent space of the cutter contact point so that the feeding speed can be calculated using (5). The second constraint is the direction conforming constraint as explained in section 3.4. The third constraint requires the feeding speed be constrained by the maximum achievable motor speed. The fourth constraint is interference constraint ensuring no collisions and local interferences happen. In this paper, we shall not go deep to explore the form of the interference constraint. We simply specify a range for the tool to be orientated so that it will nowhere interferes with the workpiece.

4 Numerical Simulation

4.1 Simulation Setup

We test our algorithm on a free form surface as shown in figure 2. The configuration of the machine tool is also shown in figure 4. The five axis machine has two rotation axes and three translation axes. To machine the workpiece, we use a ball-end mill with radius of 5mm. The actual surface is modeled as an offset surface with thickness of 3mm. The scallop height requirement is set to 1.5mm. We assume the rotation axes have speed limits within [-1rad/s, 1rad/s], the translation axes have speed limits within [-200mm/s, 200mm/s].

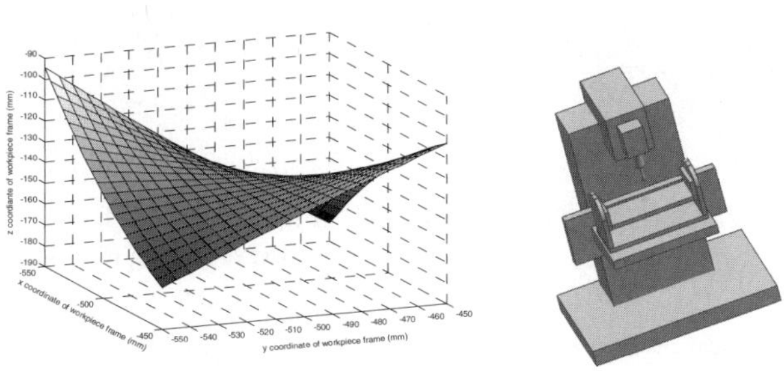

Fig. 2. The test surface and five-axis machine

Figure 3 shows the regularly distributed cutting stream field and streamlines generated by imposing the direction conforming constraint in the optimization process. It can be seen the streamlines are properly spaced.

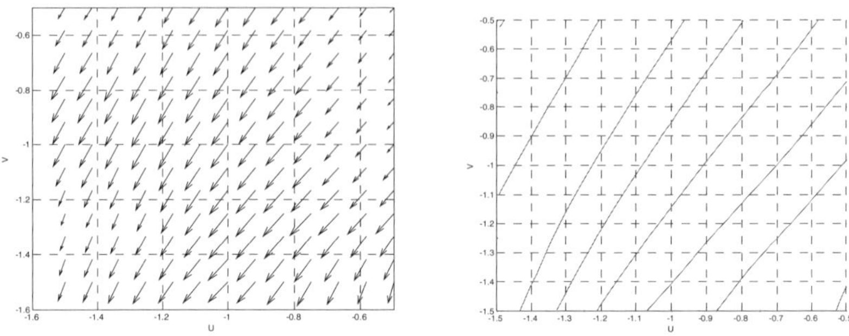

Fig. 3. Cutting stream field generated with direction conforming constraint

4.2 Steamlines Generated Using Scallop Height Constraint

Figure 4 shows the streamlines generated from the cutting streamfield with prescriped scallop height requirement. The streamlines are then mapped to the workpiece frame and the tool orientation data obtained in the optimization can be illustrated. Figure 5 shows one of the toolpath on the workpiece with corresponding tool orientations.

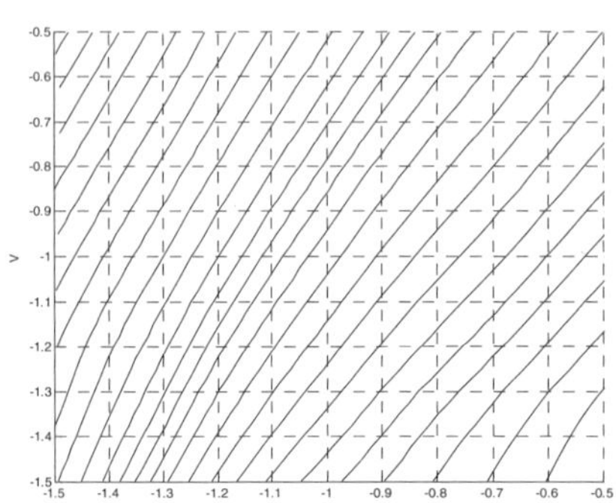

Fig. 4. A set of streamlines used as the toolpath

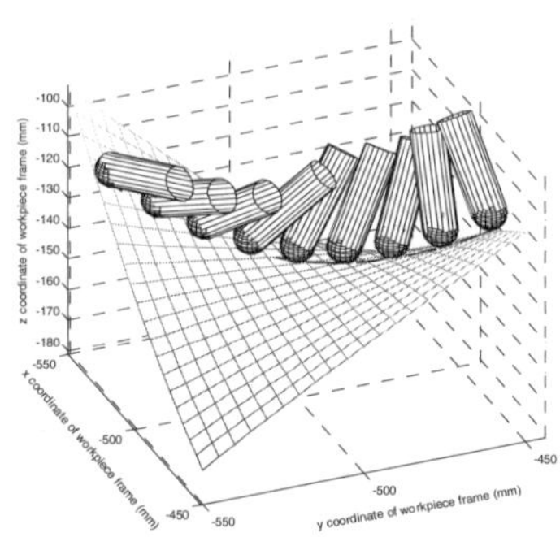

Fig. 5. A toolpath on the workpiece with corresponding tool orientation

It can be seen that, when considering the kinematical effect, the toolpath is quite different from iso-parametric toolpath (the grid lines in figure 7) or the traditional iso-scallop height toolpath which often has an orientation along the boundary of the workpiece. Such choices would not be possible to fully exploit the performance of the machines.

In our method, the scallop height constraint is used to generate a boundary for selecting the adjacent streamline. We mention that redundant paths exist. However, the redundancy can be alleviated by checking the adjacent path and eliminate the redundant part of the path. A strategy has been discussed in [5].

5 Conclusion

We present a new general toolpath planning method for five-axis machining. The method considers the machines' kinematics performance and generates both path geometry and the tool orientation data simultaneously. Compared with traditional iso-parametric and iso-scallop height toolpath generation methods, the toolpath pattern can achieve faster material removal as can be seen from the definition of the objective function of our optimization problem. The toolpath orientation is controlled by the direction conforming constraint. Therefore, the dramatic change and irregular spacing can be avoided which also ensures the realization of better machining performance.

Acknowledgement. This work is supported by the '973' Research Foundation of China (Grant No. 2005CB724100), '863' High-Tech of China (Grant No. 2007AA04Z204) and NSF of China (Grant No. 50775080).

References

1. Rao, N., Ismail, F., Bedi, S.: Tool path planning for five-axis machining using the principal axis method. International Journal of Machine Tools & Manufacture 37(7), 1025–1040 (1997)
2. Gray, P., Bedi, S., Ismail, F.: Rolling ball method for 5-axis surface machining. Computer-Aided Design 35(4), 347–357 (2003)
3. Gray, P.J., Ismail, F., Bedi, S.: Graphics-assisted Rolling Ball Method for 5-axis surface machining. Computer-Aided Design 36(7), 653–663 (2004)
4. Wang, Y., Tang, X.W.: Five-axis NC machining of sculptured surfaces. International Journal of Advanced Manufacturing Technology 15(1), 7–14 (1999)
5. Chiou, C.J., Lee, Y.S.: A machining potential field approach to tool path generation for multi-axis sculptured surface machining. Computer-Aided Design 34(5), 357–371 (2002)
6. Kim, T., Sarma, S.E.: Optimal sweeping paths on a 2-manifold: a new class of optimization problem. IEEE trans. on robotics and automation science 19(4), 613–636 (2003)
7. Arkin, E.M., Held, M., Smith, C.L.: Optimization problems related to zigzag pocket machining. Algorithmica 26(2), 197–236 (2000)
8. Park, S.C., Choi, B.K.: Tool-path planning for direction-parallel area milling. Computer-Aided Design 32(1), 17–25 (2000)
9. Griffiths, J.G.: Toolpath based on Hilbert's curve. Computer Aided Design 26(11), 839–844 (1994)
10. Cox, J.J., Takezaki, Y., Ferguson, H.R.P., et al.: Space-filling curves in tool-path applications. Computer Aided Design 26(3), 215–224 (1994)

11. Makhanov, S.: Optimization and correction of the tool path of the five-axis milling machine - Part 1. Spatial optimization. Mathematics and Computers in Simulation 75(5-6), 210–230 (2007)
12. Anotaipaiboon, W., Makhanov, S.S.: Curvilinear space-filling curves for five-axis machining. 40(3), 350–367 (2008)
13. Montana, D.J.: The Kinematics of Contact and Grasp. The International Journal of Robotics Research 7(3), 17 (1988)
14. Xiong, C.H., Ding, H., Xiong, Y.L.: Fundamentals of Robotic Grasping and Fixturing. World Scientific, Singapore (2007)
15. Nelson, D., Johnson, D., Cohen, E.: Haptic Rendering of Surface-to-Surface Sculpted Model Interaction. In: Proc. 8th Annual Symp. on Haptic Interfaces for Virtual Environment and Teleoperator Systems, Nashville, TN, ASME (1999)
16. Murray, R.M., Li, Z., Sastry, S.S.: A Mathematical Introduction to Robotic Manipulation. CRC Press, Boca Raton (1994)

The Research of Dual NURBS Curves Interpolation Algorithm for High-Speed Five-Axis Machining

Yuyao Li[1], Yuhan Wang[1,2], Jingchun Feng[1], and Jianguo Yang[1]

[1] School of Mechanical Engineering, Shanghai Jiao tong University
[2] State Key Laboratory of Mechanical System and Vibration, Shanghai Jiaotong University, Shanghai 200240,P.R .China

Abstract. To achieve the goal of high-speed and highly accurate machining, this paper proposes a real-time control algorithm based on Taylor's expansion for implementing variable feed rate non-uniform rational B-spline (NURBS) curve. To efficiently compute the NURBS curve and its derivatives in real-time, some effective methods are proposed. In contrast to the existing linear and circular interpolators, the proposed interpolator can maintain small contour errors and feedrate fluctuations. It also can shorten the size of machining code effectively compared with the linear and circular interpolators. At the same time, the NURBS-format milling codes adapting the dual NURBS Curve interpolation algorithm for 5 axis high-speed machining are adopted in this study. Besides, an effective algorithm is adopted to minimize the kinematics error by means of the shortest path scheme.

Keywords: Five-axis machining, NURBS curves, Interpolation, Non-linear error.

1 Introduction

Five-axis machine tools are used for machining complex sculptured surfaces because they have the advantages of reducing the fixture's setup time, improving surface finish with fewer cutter paths and rotating the cutter to the appropriate position and orientation. Traditionally, five-axis machine tools consist of three linear axes and two rotational axes that are orthogonal to the machine coordinate system. Most CNC machines only provide line or arc interpolators and cutter location paths are usually given by a set of lines or arc segments. Such an approach has several inherent disadvantages[1]: (1) the data size becomes quite large and the data transmission load is substantially increased for accurate machining. Considering the machining time and the cost, the conventional five-axis machining is wasteful. (2) The cutting tool must accelerate and decelerate at each line segment, which results in the velocity discontinuities at the linear segment junctions lead to higher accelerations, poor surface finish, lower surface accuracy and longer machining times. These drawbacks suggest that conventional machining methods fail to meet the requirements of high-speed, high accuracy machining in modern industry.

C. Xiong et al. (Eds.): ICIRA 2008, Part II, LNAI 5315, pp. 983–992, 2008.

To overcome the above-mentioned drawbacks, NURBS curve interpolators have been proposed ([2],[3]). It offers a common mathematical form for representing standard analytical shapes. By manipulating the values of control points, weights, and knots, a wide variety of part shapes can be designed using NURBS. And many commercial CAD/CAM systems developed the NURBS function. The major advantages of NURBS can be summarized as following: (1) They offer one common mathematical form for both standard analytical shapes (e.g., conics) and free-form shapes;(2) They provide the flexibility to design a large variety of shapes;(3) They can be evaluated reasonably fast by numerically stable and accurate algorithms;(4) They are invariant under affine as well as perspective transformations;(5) They are generalizations of non-rational B-splines, and non-rational and rational Bezier curves and surfaces.

In this paper, we proposed the Dual NURBS curves interpolation. It develops a orientation spline curve on the basis of the existing 3-axis NURBS codes format. So, there are two spline curves in the interpolation format. And we proposed a variable feed rate interpolation algorithm in this paper to achieve a high machining precision.

2 Choose the Interpolation Scheme

During the design and the machining, there are some questions to solve from the tool-path programming to NC machining. A: Calculating the tool-path expression. B: The inverse kinematics transformation from the workpiece coordinate system to the machine coordinate system.

Considering the sequence of A and B, we have alternative disposing mode, as shown in **Fig. 1.** The post-processor carries out the whole inverse kinematics transformation for the calculation mode 1. The NC unit calculates the tool-path by the ISO data from the CAM system in the machine coordinate system. In this way, the principle interest of NC lies in the interpolation. However, it would cause that the machining velocity and precision is out of control because of the shortage of the machining information.

The calculation mode 2 is the most attractive one, considering that the NC unit carries out the inverse kinematics transformation in real-time. In this way, it defines the tool position and tool orientation in the workpiece coordinate system. Then, the information is imported to the NC unit. The NC unit performs the interpolating and gets a mass of the data points. Then it performs the coordinate transformation in the NC unit. In contrast to the calculation mode 1, the implementation within the NC unit of the transformation calculation at the same level that the position instruction calculation allows ensuring the fidelity between the tool-path really described in the workpiece coordinate system and the programmed tool path ([4]). It improves the follow-up quality of the tool path while respecting the specified federate and minimize the non-linear error theoretically. Here we adopt the calculation mode 2 with a view to the expansibility and the machining quality based on the independent-study open architecture CNC system.

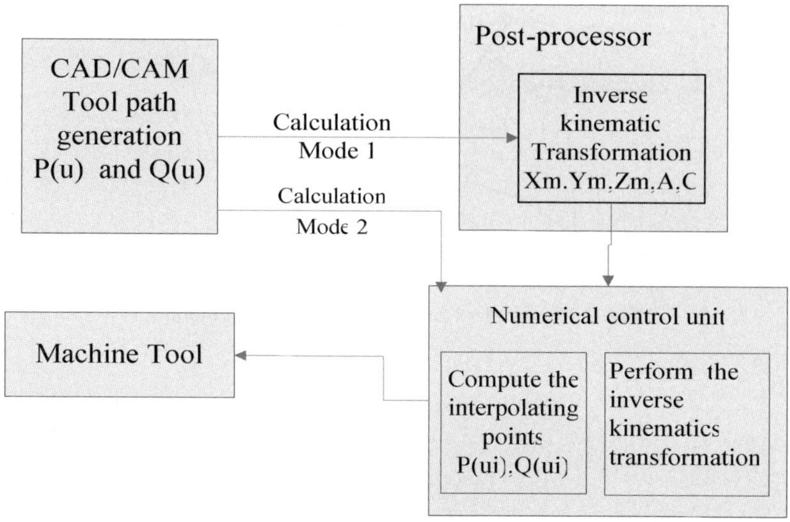

Fig. 1. Date transmission between CAD/CAM system and NC machine tool

3 Dual NURBS Curve Representation

3.1 NURBS Curve Formulation

A NURBS Curve is represented by the following equation [5]:

$$P(u) = \frac{\sum_{i=0}^{n} N_{i,k}(u) w_i C_i}{\sum_{i=0}^{n} N_{i,k}(u) w_i} \tag{1}$$

$P(u)$ is the vector to a point defined at some value of u. C_i represents the control point, w_i is the corresponding weight of C_i. In addition, $N_{i,k}(u)$ is called the blending function of B-spline([6],[9]). u is the interpolation parameter.

3.2 CAM Data Format Description

The dual NURBS interpolation algorithm means the tool position and the tool orientation are respectively determined by the NURBS curves $P(u)$ and $Q(u)$ which defined in the workpiece coordinate system, as shown in **Fig.2**. Curve $P(u)$ expresses the cutter contact (CC) path and $Q(u)$ expresses the path of arbitrary point from the tool axis. The equations are given as follows:

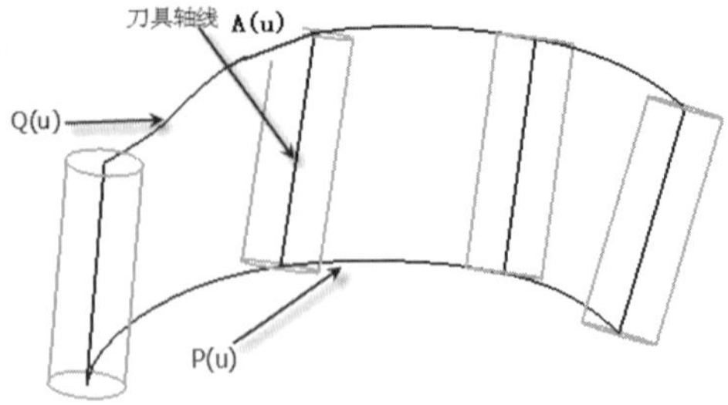

Fig. 2. Tool path of the dual NURBS interpolation

$$P(u) = (Xt(u), Yt(u), Zt(u)) \tag{2}$$

$$Q(u) = (Xh(u), Yh(u), Zh(u)) \tag{3}$$

$$\text{And: } A(u) = (Q(u) - P(u)) / \|Q(u) - P(u)\| \tag{4}$$

where $A(u)$ represents the vector of the tool axes in the workpiece coordinate system. Equation (2) and (4) define the position of the tool-tip point and the vector of the tool axes respectively. So, we propose the dual NURBS-format :

G642

NURBS P_ ;

X_ Y_ Z_ TX_ TY_ TZ_W_ K_ F_ ;

……

NURBSOFF ;

Where G642 is the cutting instruction. P is the order of NURBS, K represents knots, and W represents their associated weights. X_Y_Z_ represents the control points coordinate of the tool-tip spline. TX_ TY_ TZ_ represents the control points coordinate of the orientation spline.

4 Design of NURBS Interpolator

4.1 NURBS Interpolator

Suppose $P(u) = (X_t(u), Y_t(u), Z_t(u)), Q(u) = (X_h(u), Y_h(u), Z_h(u))$ are two NURBS curves to be interpolated, and V is the desired feedrate. We take the curve $P(u)$ for example and curve $Q(u)$ has the same knot vector u. According to differential geometry:

$$\mathrm{V(t)} = \frac{ds}{dt} = \left|\frac{dP(u)}{dt}\right| = \left|\frac{dP(u)}{dt}\right|(\frac{du}{dt}) \tag{5}$$

Or :
$$\frac{du}{dt} = \frac{V(t)}{|dP(u)/du|} \tag{6}$$

where,

$$\left|\frac{dP(u)}{du}\right| = \sqrt{(x'(u))^2 + (y'(u))^2 + (z'(u))^2} \tag{7}$$

$$\frac{du}{dt} = \frac{V(t)}{|dP(u)/du|} = \frac{V(t)}{\sqrt{(x'(u))^2 + (y'(u)^2 + (z'(u)^2}} \tag{8}$$

A computationally efficient solution of Equation (10) is necessary in order to realize a real-time interpolation for this parametric curve. Because the solution of Equation (8) is difficult in the general case, approximation forms are used, based on Taylor's expansion ([7],[8]). As we know, u_{i+1} is a key to minimize the feedrate fluctuation. So, a second-order approximation is used:

$$u_{i+1} = u_i + T\frac{du}{dt}\bigg|_{u=u_i} + \frac{T^2}{2}\frac{d^2u}{dt}\bigg|_{u=u_i} \tag{9}$$

where T is sampling interval, d^2u/dt^2 can be obtained by taking the derivative of Equation (8):

$$\frac{d^2u}{dt^2} = \frac{dV(t)/dt}{dP(u)/du} - \frac{V^2(t)(d^2P(u)/du^2)}{(dP(u)/du)^3} \tag{10}$$

where ,

$$\frac{d^2P(u)}{dt^2} = \frac{x'(u)x''(u) + y'(u)y''(u) + z'(u)z''(u)}{\sqrt{(x'(u))^2 + (y'(u))^2 + (z'(u))^2}} \tag{11}$$

Substituting Equation (8) and (11) into Equation (9) :

$$u_{i+1} = u_i + \frac{VT}{\sqrt{(x'(u))^2 + (y'(u))^2 + (z'(u))^2}}\bigg|_{u=u_i}$$

$$-\frac{(VT)^2\left(x'(u)x''(u) + x'(u)x''(u) + x'(u)x''(u)\right)}{2\left((x'(u))^2 + (y'(u))^2 + (z'(u))^2\right)^2}\bigg|_{u=u_i} \tag{12}$$

where,

$$x = P_x(u), y = P_y(u), z = P_z(u) \tag{13}$$

$$x'(u) = \frac{dP_x(u)}{du}, y'(u) = \frac{dP_y(u)}{du}, z'(u) = \frac{dP_z(u)}{du} \tag{14}$$

$$x''(u) = \frac{d^2P_x(u)}{du^2}, y''(u) = \frac{d^2P_y(u)}{du^2}, z''(u) = \frac{d^2P_z(u)}{du^2} \tag{15}$$

We know the NC unit carries out not only the interpolation process but also the inverse kinematics transformation in the dual NURBS interpolation algorithm from **Fig. 1**. Hence to make sure that all of the computational work can be completed in a sampling period is a key point. However, the computation of a NURBS interpolator is relatively complex and the Clock of the Windows System has a lower accuracy. To overcome the problem and to improve the real-time performance, the RTX (Real-Time Extension) system is added to the Windows System. With the Clock of RTX, the precision can reach 0.1us. Meanwhile, a NURBS curve class in the NURBS++ written in the C++ is introduced to optimize the computation of a NURBS interpolator.

By using this method, the time for the computation of a NURBS interpolator is shown in **Fig 3**. Considering that the sampling interval of servo system is 4 ms, the two methods should be feasible to implement this interpolator. In this study, we use the second-order approximation method considering the radii curvature and the feedrate fluctuation.

Once the new value of u_{i+1} has been obtained, it is substituted into Equation (1) to calculate the next command point $(x_{i+1}, y_{i+1}, z_{i+1})$ along the NURBS curve.

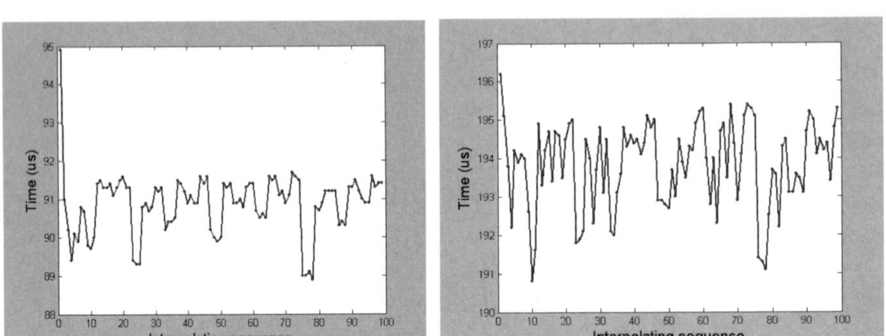

Fig. 3. The CPU time of the NURBS interpolator (a) by using a first-order approximation, and (b) by using a second-order approximation

4.2 Interpolation Error and Feedrate Fluctuation

From the above mentioned interpolation algorithm, we know that the interpolated points of each interpolation cycle lie on the curve. It means that the proposed interpolator doesn't involve inherited errors, but only chord deviation. Chord deviation $\delta(\mu m)$ can be calculated by:

$$\delta = \frac{1000}{k}\left[1-\sqrt{1-\left(\frac{VTk}{2}\right)^2}\right] \tag{16}$$

where $V(mm/s)$ is the desired feedrate, $T(s)$ is sampling interval, and $k(mm/s)$ is curvature. In this study, the sampling interval T is constant. From Equation(16) we can get that Chordal deviation δ, desired federate V and curvature k are correlative. To determine the relation between the chord error and the curve speed, the circular approximation is thus applied. The curvature K_i is:

$$K_i = \frac{\left.\frac{dC_x(u)}{du}\cdot\frac{d^2C_y(u)}{du^2}-\frac{dC_y(u)}{du}\cdot\frac{d^2C_x(u)}{du^2}\right|_{u=u_i}}{\left\|\frac{dC(u)}{du}\right\|^3_{u=u_i}}, \quad \rho_i = \frac{1}{K_i} \tag{17}$$

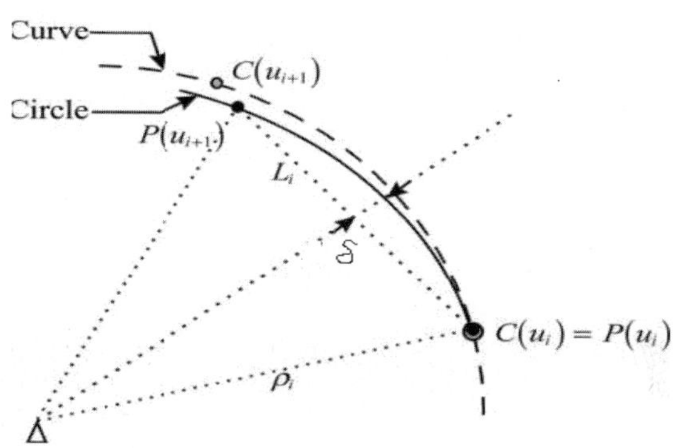

Fig. 4. Estimation of the next interpolated point

From **Fig.4** the chord error δ and the approximated curve speed are derived as:

$$\delta = \rho_i - \sqrt{\rho_i^2 - \left(\frac{L_i}{2}\right)^2}, \quad V(u_i) = \frac{L_i}{T_s} \tag{18}$$

The curve speed $V(u_i)$ corresponding to the chord error δ is then derived as:

$$V(u_i) = \frac{2}{T_s}\sqrt{\rho_i^2 - (\rho_i - ER_i)^2} \tag{19}$$

By setting ER_i as the tolerance value of the chord error, $V(u_i)$ is thus obtained as the acceptable curve speed, and we can get the curve speed is adaptively changed according to the radius of curvature, and the following adaptive-feedrate law is proposed for parametric curves:

$$V(u_i) = \begin{cases} F, & \text{if } \frac{2}{T_s}\sqrt{\rho_i^2 - (\rho_i - ER_i)^2} > F \\ \frac{2}{T_s}\sqrt{\rho_i^2 - (\rho_i - ER_i)^2}, & \text{if } \frac{2}{T_s}\sqrt{\rho_i^2 - (\rho_i - ER_i)^2} \le F \end{cases} \tag{20}$$

Fig. 5 shows the architecture of the interpolator, which mainly includes two function modules: the parameter calculation module, the adaptive feedrate adjustment module. The purpose of the adaptive feedrate adjustment module is to adjust feedrate to reduce chord error into the set tolerance. The parameter calculation module is used to calculate u_{i+1} from u_i and V with second-order approximation. From the parameter calculation module, we can get the u_i at each sampling period. So we can get the series of the knot vector $U = [u_{0T}, u_{1T}, u_{2T}, \cdots]$.

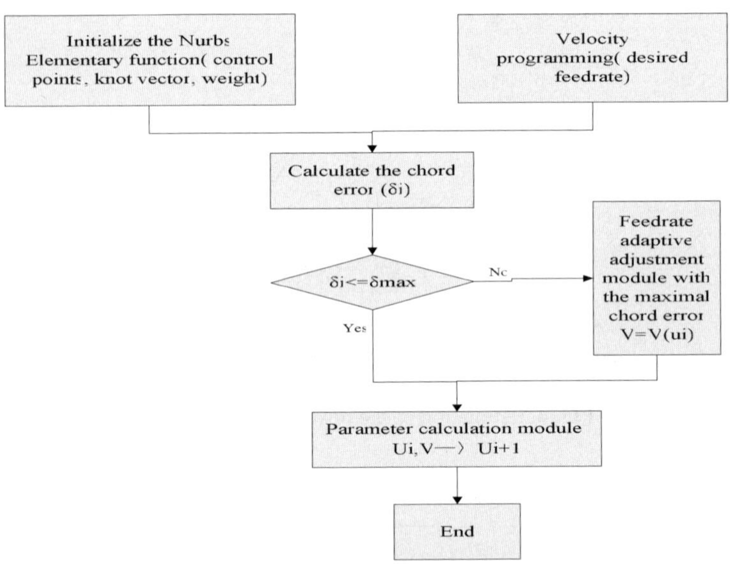

Fig. 5. Architecture of the interpolator

Substituting $U = [u_{0T}, u_{1T}, u_{2T}, \cdots]$ into Equation (2), Equation (3) and Equation (4) respectively. We can get the series of the tool-tip points $[p_{0T}, p_{1T}, p_{2T}, \cdots]$ and the series of the tool-axes orientation $[A_{0T}, A_{1T}, A_{2T}, \cdots]$.

5 Experimental Results

The aim of this experiment is to show how the real-time NURBS machining methods has significant advantages over conventional approaches, such as the size of machining code.

Consider a practical dual NURBS curve as shown in **Fig. 6**. The performance for both the NURBS machining method and the conventional CNC machining are compared in terms of the size of machining codes. It is found that the size of machining code for the conventional approach (fifty segments) is much larger than that for NURBS machining code(fourteen segments). In other words, by using the NURBS machining approach, it can express the more abundant geometrical information for the smaller data. The length of the NC files can be greatly reduced.

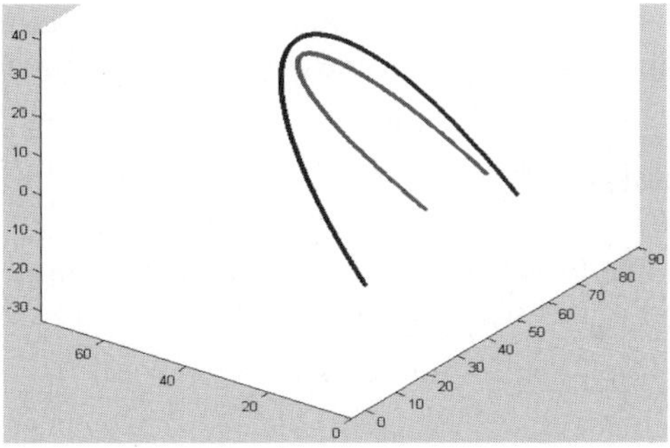

Fig. 6. Dual NURBS tool-path

Fig. 7 (a) and **(b)** show the feedrate command error for the conventional approach with the Look-ahead function and the NURBS machining respectively. In the experiment, the sampling interval T is 4ms, the command feedrate F is 3000mm/min. The resulting feedrate command error shown in Fig. 7 (b) indicates that the NURBS machining approach gave a satisfactory performance. From **Fig. 7(b)**, we see the fluctuation of the feed is kept in 0.006%, namely, the speed is almost equal to the command feed.

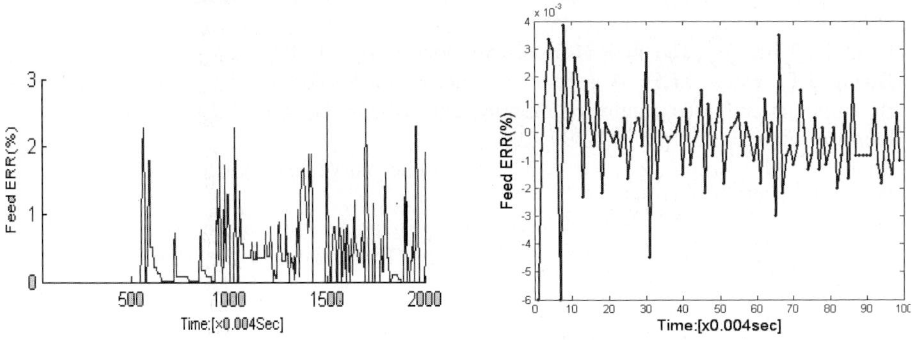

Fig. 7. (a) Feed error of the conventional approach **(b)** Feed error of the dual NURBS approach

6 Conclusions

To overcome the drawbacks in conventional machining, dual NURBS curve interpolators have been proposed. This paper has explored the feasibility of a real-time NURBS command generator. In the dual NURBS machining, NC unit contain not only the interpolating module but also the coordinate transformation module. Therefore, the key issue is to make sure that all of the computational tasks can be competed in a sampling period without sacrificing geometric precision too much in this study. In this paper, we adopt the Taylor's second-order approximation, which converts the NURBS representation into servo control commands. The results of this study suggest that Taylor's second-order approximation is a good choice. In addition, the experimental results also show that the feedrate fluctuation is kept in 0.004%, and the size of machining code for the dual NURBS machining approach is much smaller than for the conventional method. All of these indicate that the dual NURBS machining approach has significant advantages over the conventional approach.

Acknowledgements

The authors would like to acknowledge the National Natural Science Foundation of China for the support of this research (No.50575138).

Reference

1. Cheng, M.Y., Tsai, M.C., Kuo, J.C.: Real-time NURBS command generator for CNC servo controllers. International Journal of Machine Tools & Manufactures 42, 801–813 (2002)
2. Farouki, R.T., Tsai, Y.F.: Exact Taylor series coefficients for variable-feed rate CNC curve interpolators. Compute. Aid. Des. 33, 155–165 (2001)
3. Yeh, S.S., Hsu, P.L.: Adaptive-feed rate interpolation for parametric curves with a confined chord error. Compute. Aid. Des. 34, 229–237 (2002)
4. Affouard, A., Duc, E., Lartigue, C., Langeron, J.M., Bourdet, P.: Avoiding 5-axis singularities using tool path deformation. Int. J. Mach. Tools Manuf. 44(4), 415–425 (2004)
5. Piegl, L.: On NURBS: a surve[J]. IEEE Computer Graphics and Applications 1, 55–71 (1991)
6. Piegl, L., Tiller, W.: The NURBS Book. Springer, Berlin (1995)
7. Huang, J.T., Yang, D.CH.: A generalized interpolator for command generation of parametric curves in computer controlled machines. In: ASME Japan/USA Symposium on FlexibleAutomation, vol. 1, pp. 393–399 (1992)
8. Shpitalni, M., Koren, Y., Lo, C.C.: Real-time curve interpolators. Compute-Aided Des. 26(11), 832–838 (1994)
9. Tsay, D.M., Huey, C.O.: Application of rational B-splines to the synthesis of cam-follower motion programs. Journal of Mechanical Design, Transactions of the ASME 115(3), 621–626 (1993)

Numeric-Symbolic Solutions to Analyses of Forward Position and Singularity Configuration for 3-RPS Parallel Mechanism

Jinge Wang, Qiang Wang, and Qian Yu

College of Mechanical Engineering and Automation, Xihua University,
Chengdu China 610039
wangjg@mail.xhu.edu.cn

Abstract. Based on Groebner base method, numeric-symbolic solutions to forward position analysis for a 3-RPS parallel mechanism and computer symbolic manipulating technique are proposed. A set of nonlinear polynomial equations are transformed into a set of equivalent triangularization equations by using the following operations: ordering of variables, forming all pairs of polynomials, finding S-polynomial, reduction etc. The analytical solutions in the closed form are obtained. The jacobian matrix and the equation in numeric-symbolic form for determining singularity configuration are derived. The maneuverability of the parallel mechanism and singularity configuration are investigated. The numerical examples are given for the illustration.

Keywords: Groebner base, parallel mechanism, forward position analyses, maneuverability, singularity configuration.

1 Introduction

The Groebner base method, proposed by Buchberger in 1965, is a method for forming standarded base of a nonlinear polynomial system. It has been attracted more and more attention by researchers and developed quickly in theory and application. Now the Groebner base method is seem as a basic solution method for a set of nonlinear polynomial equations by many mathematicians of symbolic math and automatic reasoning in Europe and selected as core algorithm for POSSD of EC.

Parallel robot has a wide development prospect as a new kind robot. Lower-Mobility Parallel Robots have attracted the attention of many researchers because of the simple structure and low cost [2-7]. The analysis of forward position for a 3-RPS parallel mechanism is given in this paper and the jacobian matrix for the mechanism is derived. Then the analysis of maneuverability and singularity for the mechanism are given.

2 The Analysis of Forward Position

(1) Constrained equations

A 3-dof parallel mechanism consists of a base platform (A_1 , A_2 , A_3) and an upper platform (B_1 , B_2 , B_3) connected by drive legs (l_1 , l_2 , l_3) with the

C. Xiong et al. (Eds.): ICIRA 2008, Part II, LNAI 5315, pp. 993–1002, 2008.

lengths l_1 , l_2 and l_3 ,as shown in fig1.The upper and base platforms adopted with regular triangle layout and the circumradius are R and r respectively. The spherical joints of drive leg are arranged on the upper platform and the revolute pairs are fixed on the base platform. The three dimensional unit vectors u_1 , u_2 , u_3 represent revolute axes. The angles between revolute axes and X-axis areλ_1 , λ_2 and λ_3 . For the lengths of three drive legs are known, the position and orientation of moving platform can be obtained.

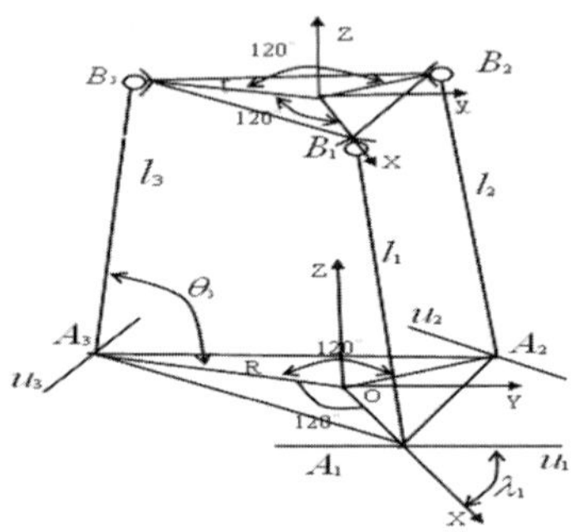

Fig. 1. kinematic architecture of a 3-RPS mechanism

In the fixed coordinate system OXYZ which is fixed on the base platform, the origin O is the centre of figure of triangle and the Z-axis is upward and vertical to base platform, the direction of X-axis is point O to A_1; in the coordinate system CXYZ which is fixed on the upper platform, the origin C is the centre of figure of triangle and the Z-axis is upward and vertical to upper platform, the direction of X-axis is point C to B_1.In terms of the geometric relation between the upper and base platform, the coordinates of three spherical joints in the coordinate system OXYZ can be expressed as follow:

$$\begin{cases} B_{iX} = A_{iX} - l_i \cos\theta_i \sin\lambda_i \\ B_{iY} = A_{iY} + l_i \cos\theta_i \cos\lambda_i \quad \text{(i=1,2,3)} \\ B_{iZ} = l_i \sin\theta_i \end{cases} \tag{1}$$

where θ_i is roll between drive leg and base platform, as shown in figure1.

The three side lengths of triangle platform are expressed as follow:

$$\begin{cases} (B_{1X} - B_{2X})^2 + (B_{1Y} - B_{2Y})^2 + (B_{1Z} - B_{2Z})^2 = |B_1B_2|^2 \\ (B_{2X} - B_{3X})^2 + (B_{2Y} - B_{3Y})^2 + (B_{2Z} - B_{3Z})^2 = |B_2B_3|^2 \\ (B_{1X} - B_{3X})^2 + (B_{1Y} - B_{3Y})^2 + (B_{1Z} - B_{3Z})^2 = |B_1B_3|^2 \end{cases} \tag{2}$$

Substituting the trigonometric formulas $\cos\theta_i = \frac{1-x_i^2}{1+x_i^2}$, $\sin\theta_i = \frac{2x_i}{1+x_i^2}$ (i =1,2,3)

into (2),we have:

$$\begin{cases} f_1 = a_{11}x_1^2x_2^2 + a_{12}x_1^2 + a_{13}x_1x_2 + a_{14}x_2^2 + a_{15} = 0 \\ f_2 = a_{21}x_2^2x_3^2 + a_{22}x_2^2 + a_{23}x_2x_3 + a_{24}x_3^2 + a_{25} = 0 \\ f_3 = a_{31}x_1^2x_3^2 + a_{32}x_1^2 + a_{33}x_1x_3 + a_{34}x_3^2 + a_{35} = 0 \end{cases} \quad (3)$$

where, $a_{ij}\,(i = 1,2,3;\ j = 1,2,3,4,5)$ are given by the structure and input parameters of mechanism.

(2) Elimination of equations

Based on Groebner base method, we can transform the polynomial equations (3) into triangularization standard base by using the following operations: ordering of variables, forming all pairs of polynomials, finding S-polynomial, reduction etc.

$$\begin{cases} g_1(x_3) = 0 \\ g_2(x_2, x_3) = 0 \\ g_3(x_1, x_2, x_3) = 0 \end{cases} \quad (4)$$

$$g_1(x_3) = \sum_{i=0}^{16} e_i x_3^i = 0,\ g_2(x_2, x_3) = x_2 + \sum_{i=0}^{15} s_i x_3^i = 0,\ g_3(x_1, x_3) = \sum_{i=0}^{5} h_i x_1 x_3^i + \sum_{i=0}^{14} k_i x_3^i$$

where $e_i(i = 0,1,\cdots 16)$, $s_i(i = 0,1,\cdots 15)$, $h_i(i = 0,1,\cdots 5)$, $k_i(i = 0,1,\cdots 14)$ are the functions of the structure parameters. We can get the symbolic solutions of x_1, x_2, x_3 by finding equation (4) and get θ_1, θ_2 and θ_3 by back substituting the results into half-angle formulas. Then we can get the coordinate of spherical joints in base coordinate system and the rotation transformation matrix of upper coordinate system by substituting the results into (1).

3 Manipulability and Condition Number

The maneuverability evaluation has two indexes: manipulability and condition number.

(1) manipulability

We can evaluate manipulability based on jacobian matrix. The manipulability proposed by Yoshikawa is also suitable for parallel robot and mechanism which originally aim at series redundant robot. The manipulability is defined as follow:

$$W = |\det([J])|$$

where $[J]$ is jacobian matrix.

Manipulability is a variable which can reflect the ability of robot's output lever to achieve a poison and attitude and an index of judging the flexibility of robot in some poison and attitude. The parallel mechanism is in singular status when W=0 and in nonsingular status when W>0. We should avoid approaching singularity configuration because the flexibility gets minimum when the parallel mechanism is under the singularity configuration.

(2) condition number

Salisbury puts forward to using the condition number of jacobian matrix as index of robot flexibility. In the paper, we adopt Frobenius norm and it defined as the evolution of square sum of each element. The condition number of jacobian matrix is defined as follow:

$$Cond([J]) = \sqrt{tr([J]^T[J])} \cdot \sqrt{tr([J]^{-1T}[J]^{-1})}$$

where tr is the matrix trace. It is a sum of each element which is in diagonal line of matrix.

The condition number reflects the flexibility and maneuverability of parallel mechanism. The parallel mechanism can get best property of motion transmission when $Cond([J]) = 1$ and it is located at singularity configuration when $Cond([J]) = \infty$.The condition number of matrix is an amplification factor of input rate relative deviation. So it is given with less value rate in the operation range.

4 The Analysis of Singularity Configuration

We can use rotation transformation matrix to express the coordinate of pivot point in base coordinates system as follow:

$$\vec{B}'_i = [T]\cdot\vec{b}_i + \vec{C} \quad (i=1,2,3) \tag{5}$$

where $\vec{B}'_i$ is a position vector of pivot point in the fixed coordinates system, $[T]$ is a spin matrix of moving coordinate system CXYZ for fixed coordinate system and : $[T]=\begin{bmatrix} c\beta c\gamma & -c\beta s\gamma & s\beta \\ c\gamma s\alpha s\beta + c\alpha s\gamma & c\alpha c\gamma - s\alpha s\beta s\gamma & -c\beta s\alpha \\ -c\alpha c\gamma s\beta + s\alpha s\gamma & c\gamma s\alpha + c\alpha s\beta s\gamma & c\alpha c\beta \end{bmatrix}$, $\vec{b}_i$ is a position vector of pivot point in the moving coordinates system, $\vec{C}$ is a position vector of origin C in fixed coordinates system. The position vector between point A and B and the length of each drive leg are expressed as follow:

$$\left|\vec{A}_i - \vec{B}'_i\right|^2 = l_i^2 \quad (i=1,2,3) \tag{6}$$

The three branches and revolute pairs of mechanism will limit the motion of three spherical joints on upper platform, when the axes u_1 , u_2 , u_3 present tangent distribution in base level of 3-DOF parallel mechanism. The point B_1 , B_2 , B_3 must move in three vertical planes $y=0$, $y=-\sqrt{3}x$, $y=\sqrt{3}x$,respectively. From the characteristic, the following geometry constraints can be obtained,

$$\begin{cases} Y_c = -rc\beta s\gamma \\ X_c = r(c\beta c\gamma - c\alpha c\gamma + s\alpha s\beta s\gamma)/2 \\ \tan\gamma = -s\alpha s\beta/(c\alpha + c\beta) \end{cases} \tag{7}$$

Substituting the element of rotation matrix and (7) into (5) and (6), we have:

$$\begin{aligned} l_1^2 &= \left(rc\gamma c\beta + r\left(c\beta c\gamma - c\alpha c\gamma + s\alpha s\beta s\gamma\right) - R\right)^2 \\ &\quad + \left(r\left(s\alpha s\gamma - c\alpha s\beta c\gamma\right) + Z_c\right)^2 \\ l_2^2 &= \frac{1}{4}\Big[\left(-\sqrt{3}rc\beta s\gamma - r\left(c\alpha c\gamma - s\alpha s\beta s\gamma\right) + R\right)^2 \\ &\quad + \left(3rc\beta s\gamma + \sqrt{3}r\left(c\alpha c\gamma - s\alpha s\beta s\gamma\right) - \sqrt{3}R\right)^2 \\ &\quad + \left(r\left(c\alpha c\gamma s\beta - s\alpha s\gamma\right) + \sqrt{3}r\left(c\gamma s\alpha + c\alpha s\beta s\gamma\right) + 2Z_c\right)^2\Big] \\ l_3^2 &= \frac{1}{4}\Big[\left(\sqrt{3}rc\beta s\gamma - r\left(c\alpha c\gamma - s\alpha s\beta s\gamma\right) + R\right)^2 \\ &\quad + \left(3rc\beta s\gamma - \sqrt{3}r\left(c\alpha c\gamma - s\alpha s\beta s\gamma\right) + \sqrt{3}R\right)^2 \\ &\quad + \left(r\left(c\alpha c\gamma s\beta - s\alpha s\gamma\right) - \sqrt{3}r\left(c\gamma s\alpha + c\alpha s\beta s\gamma\right) + 2Z_c\right)^2\Big] \end{aligned} \tag{8}$$

Derivativing of Equation (8) with respect to t and write it in the matrix form,

$$[A][\dot{x}] = [B][\dot{L}] \tag{9}$$

where $[\dot{x}] = [\dot{\alpha} \quad \dot{\beta} \quad \dot{Z}_c]^T$, $[\dot{L}] = [\dot{l}_1 \quad \dot{l}_2 \quad \dot{l}_3]^T$, $[A]$、 $[B]$ are 3 by 3 matrices, a_{ij} , b_{ij} (i =1,2,3 , j =1,2,3) are the functions of the structure parameters and input parameters of the mechanism , and

$$\begin{cases} b_{11} = l_1, \quad b_{12} = 0, \quad b_{13} = 0 \\ b_{21} = 0, \quad b_{22} = l_2, \quad b_{23} = 0 \\ b_{31} = 0, \quad b_{32} = 0, \quad b_{33} = l_3 \end{cases}$$

$$a_{23} = Z_c + \frac{r}{2}s\alpha(\sqrt{3}c\gamma - s\gamma) + \frac{r}{2}c\alpha s\beta(c\gamma + \sqrt{3}s\gamma)$$

$$a_{33} = Z_c - \frac{r}{2}s\alpha(\sqrt{3}c\gamma + s\gamma) + \frac{r}{2}c\alpha s\beta(c\gamma - \sqrt{3}s\gamma)$$

$$
\begin{cases}
a_{11} = \dfrac{r}{4(1+c\alpha c\beta)}(\dfrac{r}{2}c\beta(c\gamma)^2 \\
\quad s\alpha\left(-3c(2\alpha)+2c(\alpha-\beta)+c(2(\alpha+\beta))+5c(2\beta)+2c(\alpha+\beta)\right) \\
\quad +c\beta s\gamma(4Z_c c\alpha(c\alpha+c\beta)-6Rs\beta-2R(c\alpha)^2 s\beta \\
\quad +rs\alpha\left(4c\alpha(c\alpha+c\beta)+\left(3+(c\alpha)^2\right)(s\beta)^2\right)s\gamma) \\
\quad +c\gamma(-2Rc\beta s\alpha(c\alpha+c\beta)+Z\, s(2\alpha)s(2\beta) \\
\quad -\dfrac{1}{4}rc(2\beta)s(2\beta)s\gamma\left(11c\alpha+5c(3\alpha)+2c\beta\left(-9+c(2\alpha)c\beta\right)\right)s(2\beta)s\gamma)) \\
a_{12} = \dfrac{r}{32(1+c\alpha c\beta)}(2c\gamma(-16Z_c(c\alpha c\beta(1+c\alpha c\beta+(s\alpha)^2-4Rs\beta\left(-7+c(2\alpha)\right) \\
\quad +4c\alpha(3rc\gamma+c\beta(6R+r(7c\alpha+\left(-7+2c(2\alpha)c\beta\right)c\gamma) \\
\quad +5rc\gamma(s\alpha)^2 s\beta+3rc\gamma s(2\beta)(-7+c(2\alpha))-4(c\beta s\alpha(16R+19rc\alpha c\gamma) \\
\quad -2s(2\alpha)s\beta(-2Z_c+Rs\beta)+2rc\gamma(4(s(3\alpha))^2 \\
\quad +s\alpha(s\beta)^2(3+(s\alpha)^2))s\gamma+24Rr(8c\beta \\
\quad +c\alpha(-9+c(2\beta))(s\alpha s\gamma)^2 s\beta r(2(24(c\beta)^2 \\
\quad +(c\alpha)^2(1-9c(2\beta))s\alpha)+3c(3\beta)s(2\alpha))s(2\gamma)) \\
a_{13} = Z_c - rc\alpha c\gamma s\beta + rs\alpha s\gamma
\end{cases}
$$

We only list the above element of $[A]$ because the length is limited.

From the equation (9), we can get $\det([B]) = l_1 l_2 l_3 \neq 0$ .Let $\det([A])$ be equal 0 and expand :

$$
\begin{aligned}
&a_{11}a_{22}a_{33} + a_{21}a_{32}a_{13} + a_{31}a_{12}a_{23} \\
&-a_{13}a_{22}a_{31} - a_{12}a_{21}a_{33} - a_{11}a_{23}a_{32} = 0
\end{aligned} \tag{10}
$$

Let $x = \tan\dfrac{\alpha}{2}$ and substituting trigonometric identity $\sin\alpha = \dfrac{2x}{1+x^2}$, $\cos\alpha = \dfrac{1-x^2}{1+x^2}$ into (10), we can get a 16 degree polynomial equation of X, viz.

$$
\sum_{i=0}^{16} f_i x^i = 0 \tag{11}
$$

where $f_i (i = 0,1,2...16)$ is function concerning structure parameters and output variant β, Z_c . The equation (11) is a surface equation of α, β, Z_c . As soon as β, Z_c are specified, the cross section curve of the surface equation by finding (11).

5 The Numeric-Symbolic Method of Polynomial Function

Symbolizing Z_c and β and digitizing other structure parameters, we adopt the follow symbol,

$$\begin{cases} U = Z_c \\ V = \sin\beta \\ W = \cos\beta \end{cases} \tag{12}$$

Then the each element of polynomial can be written as follow:

$$T = \sum_{k=1}^{m} t_k (Z_c)^{u_k} (\sin\beta)^{v_k} (\cos\beta)^{w_k} = \sum_{k=1}^{m} t_k (U)^{u_k} V^{v_k} (W)^{w_k} \tag{13}$$

where t_k is constant, u_k 、 v_k 、 w_k are power of integers of Z_c 、 $\sin\beta$ 、 $\cos\beta$, respectively, m is the number of terms.

The power exponent matrix $[M]$ is introduced to do Numeric-symbolic computation for the polynomial T .

$$[M_k] = [u_k, v_k, w_k] \qquad M_k \in R^3 \tag{14}$$

So, we can rewrite (14) as follow:

$$T = \sum_{k=1}^{m} [t_k, M_k] \tag{15}$$

Expression of any polynomial can be expressed by using the above polynomial variable and get the analytic expression of each coefficient element f_i in equation (11) by applying the Numeric-symbolic algorithm.

6 Example

Case 1: The structure parameters of spatial parallel mechanism are listed as follow: $R = 50mm, r = 25mm, l_1 = 240mm, l_2 = 200mm, l_3 = 180mm, \lambda_1 = 90^\circ, \lambda_2 = 210^\circ, \lambda_3 = 330^\circ$.

16 teams solution can be received based on Groebner base method. There are 8 teams real solution and 8 teams complex solution. Substituting the solutions into original equation, we can prove that the solution is right. We list the θ_1, θ_2 and θ_3 which given by the 8 teams real solution in table1.

The real solution of forward position for spatial parallel mechanism

	1	2	3	4	5	6	7	8
θ_1	-74.611	-72.340	-50.265	-49.209	49.265	50.265	72.340	74.611
θ_2	-81.604	-83.863	-69.296	-81.221	81.221	69.296	83.863	81.602
θ_3	-70.581	-62.520	-84.810	-71.365	71.365	84.810	62.520	70.581

Case2: The structure parameters of spatial parallel mechanism are listed as follow: R=30mm、 r=6mm.The analysis of maneuverability as follow:

(1)The analysis of manipulability and condition number of some different positions and attitudes are respectively shown in figure 2 and figure 3. We can get the manipulability and condition number of mechanism when the center of upper platform C is static and the upper platform only rotate around the Y-axis in figure 2 (a) and figure 3 (a) .There are the manipulability and condition number of mechanism when the upper platform keep a fixed attitude and displace along Z-axis in figure 2 (b) and figure 3 (b) .The manipulability and condition number of mechanism when the center of upper platform C is static and the upper platform only rotate around X-axis and Y-axis in figure 2 (c) and figure 3(c).

(2)The relationships between the circumradius of base platform R and manipulability, condition numbers are shown in figure 4 and there are relationships between the circumradius of upper platform r and manipulability, condition number in figure 5.

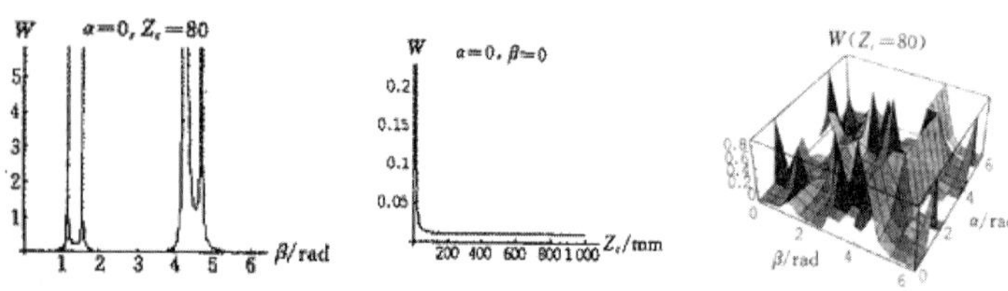

(a) (b) (c)

Fig. 2. The manipulability of position and orientation

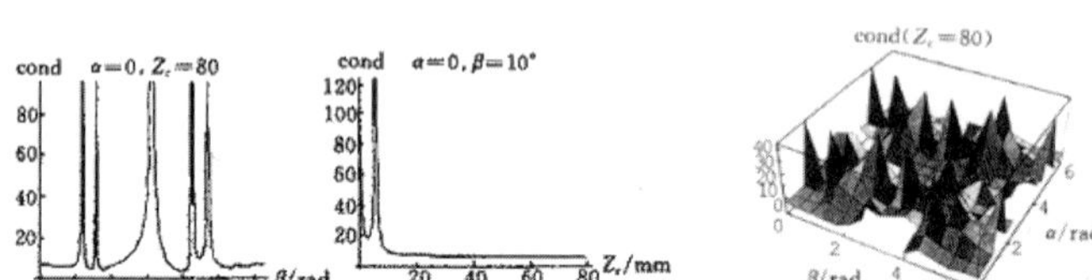

(a) (b) (c)

Fig. 3. The condition number of position and orientation

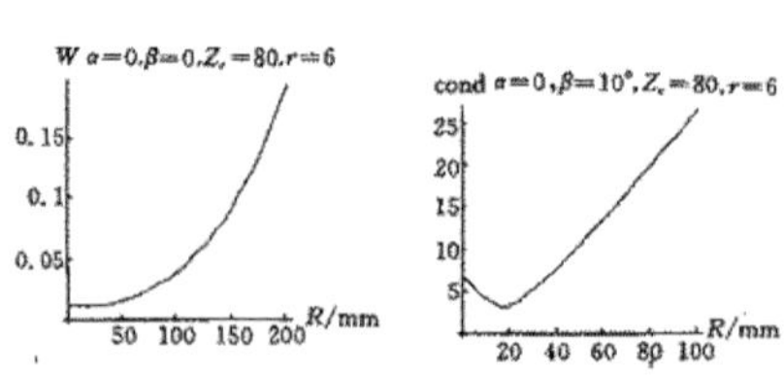

Fig. 4. Relationship between R and manipulability

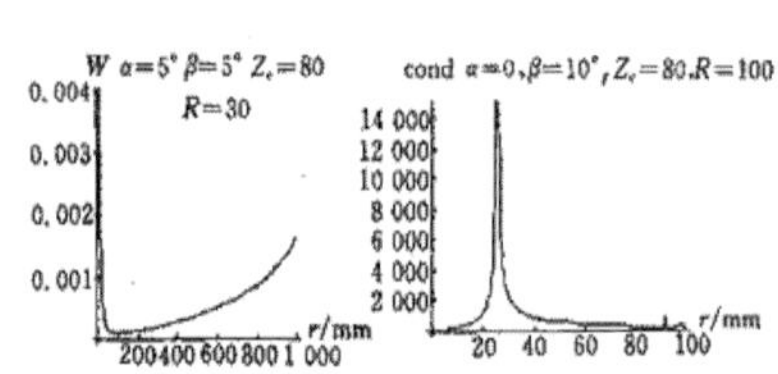

Fig. 5. Relationship between r and condition number

Case3: the structure parameters are the same as case 2. We have the analysis of singularity as follow:

We can figure the singularity graph of parameters space by calculating. There are curves of Z_c=80 , Z_c =60 in figure6 (a) and the cures of β =5° , β=15°are shown in figure6(b).There are singularity curves of R=30 , R=60 and R=90 when r=6、Z_c =100 in figure7.

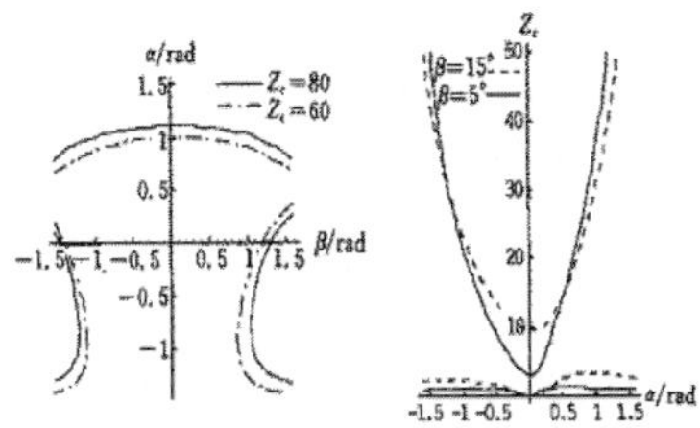

(a)

Fig. 6. The singularity curves in parameters space

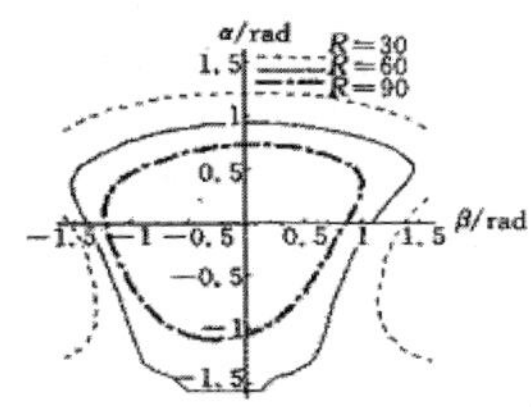

(b)

Fig. 7. The relationship between R and singularity configuration

7 Conclusion

(1)The paper present the forward position analysis for a spatial parallel mechanism based on Groebner base method. A set of nonlinear polynomial equations are transformed into a set of equivalent triangularization equations by using the method and the analytical solutions in the closed form are obtained.

(2)The jacobian matrixes of 3-RPS parallel mechanism are derived and the analysis of manipulability and condition number are given in the paper. The analytical expression about distinguish singularity of the 3-RPS parallel configuration is derived and the singularity cure equation can be obtained. The each element of jacobian matrix and coefficient of singularity discriminant can be expressed as numeric-symbolic polynomial by using numeric-symbolic method. The on-line operation of maneuverability and singularity configuration discrimination become simple and effective because the numeric-symbolic calculates is off-line.

(3)The relationship between parameter changing and maneuverability, singularity configuration can be obtained in the paper. The result obtained from the paper has an important influence in kinematics design of the mechanism.

References

1. Hang, L.-b.: Research on kinematics of the robots' mechanism Southeast university, Doctor Degree dissertation, pp. 21–46 (2001)
2. Lee, K.-M., Shah, D.K.: Kinematic Analysis of a Three Degrees of Freedom In-Parallel Actuated Manipulator. IEEE Journal of Robotics and Automation 4, 3 (1988)
3. Huang, Z., Kong, J.-f., Fang, Y.-f.: Mechanism theory and controlling system of parallel robot. China machine press (1997)

4. Yu, J.-j., Wang, J., Huang, Z.: Workspace analysis of deficient-rank 3-RPS parallel platform mechanism. Machine Design and Research (1998)
5. Rao, Q., Bai, S.-x.: Manipulability analysis and definition of 6-6 Steward Robot. ROBOT 11, 345–349 (1994)
6. Fan, S.-w., Xu, L.-j.: Forward solution of position and analysis of working space for a new typed hybrid virtual axle machine tool. J. Machine Design 8, 27–29 (2002)
7. Fan, S.-w., Xu, L.-j.: Close Form Solution to Singularity Configuration of a New Type Parallel Machine Tool. Journal of University of Electronic Science and Technology of China 4, 369–373 (2002)
8. Xu, L.-j., Fan, S.-w.: A Numeric-Symbolic Approach for Analysis of Singular Position Surfaces and Workspace Boundary Surfaces of Robotic Manipulators. Mechanical Science and Technology 19, 6 (2000)

A Genetic Optimization Approach to Optimize the Multi-head Surface Mount Placement Machine

Wei-Qing Lin and Guang-Yu Zhu

College of Mechanical Engineering and Automation, Fuzhou University, Fuzhou, Fujian Province, P.R. China
zhugy@fzu.edu.cn

Abstract. The genetic algorithm (GA) for multi-head surface mounting machines is studied, and it has two contributions to the multi-head case, one is that the algorithm has a special crossover operation; the other is that its mutation operation is composed of exchange operator and inversion operator. Experimental results show that the proposed approach gives good robot assembly time and less movement of the feeder carrier and PCB table.

Keywords: Genetic algorithm, PCB.

1 Introduction

As the application of the Surface Mounting Technology (SMT), Surface Mount Machine (SMM) has been wildly used to produce a complete Printed Circuit Board (PCB), and have been looked as most important device in the process of printing PCB. Generally, the path optimization of placement is a combinatorial optimization problem and is known to be NP-hard [1] and discrete type [2]. The scheduling problem of SMM is consisted of two related ones, reel assignment problem (RAP) and pick-and-placing problem (PAPSP). The second problem is generally regarded as Traveling Salesman Problem (TSP) [3] to single-head surface mounting machines, for solving this problem, traditional Genetic Algorithm (GA)[4~6] has been used successfully, but along with the development of SMM Technology the machine structure become more complex, nowadays the number of Head is often eight or more, so these algorithms can not be used efficiently without any improvement. In this paper, a GA algorithm is proposed to solve PAPSP when the positions of feeder racks are given in a four-head surface mounting machine. The proposed GA algorithm has a_randomly selected crossover operator and a mutation operation composed of exchange operator and inversion operator. Experimental results show the proposed GA algorithm is effective and good results for printing three types of PCB are achieved.

2 Problem Statement and Mathematic Model

Varieties of PCB assembly machines have been developed to improve the production rate. The multi-head surface mounting machine is popular used because of its

C. Xiong et al. (Eds.): ICIRA 2008, Part II, LNAI 5315, pp. 1003–1012, 2008.

characters of high mounting speed with relatively low cost. Just this type of machine is studied in this paper. Figure 1 shows a schematic diagram of a multi-head surface mounting machine.

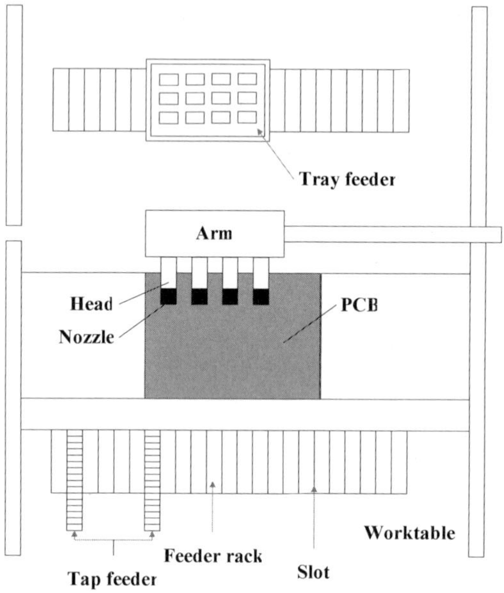

Fig. 1. Schematic diagram of a multi-head surface mounting machine

In the target multi-head mounting machine, components are supplied to the machine by reels. Each reel contains only one type of components. Two feeder racks are located on both sides of conveyor and each feeder rack has a number of slots for reels. The actual pick-and-place unit is the arm, which has multiple heads. The arm always moves from one location to another along a straight line at a constant speed. The heads pick up components from feeders and place them on the board. Since the distance between adjacent heads is equal to integer times the distance between two adjacent slots, the arm can pick multiple components simultaneously by one pickup operation, which is called simultaneous pickup. Each head has a nozzle that grips and holds a component until it is placed on the board. Nozzles of different diameters are used depending on the size of the component to be retrieved. The nozzle is automatically changed at the automatic nozzle changer (ANC) when it can not grip the required component. The assumptions made in solving the PAPSP for four-head mounting machine are as follows:

1. The number of heads is not limited.
2. The order in which the heads operate in placing the components is predetermined as follows: the first head places its component at first, the second head places its component secondly, and so on.

3. The number of reels required to complete the job is, at most, equal to the capacity of the feeder racks.

While mounting a PCB, a cycle consists of the pick-and-place movements. During the first phase of a cycle, the heads pick up components from reels sequentially or simultaneously. During the next phase of a cycle, the arm moves to the board and places the components sequentially. The nozzle at each head may be changed while the arm moves from the last mounting position in a cycle to the first pickup position in the next cycle. The cycle can't be stop until all components are mounted in PCB, finally the PCB is carried away and a new PCB replays it by conveyor.

The mathematic model made is as follows: $T_1(i)$ represents the pickup time in the ith cycle, the time is spent while the heads moving along slot and picking all of components in *i*th cycle. $T_2(i)$ represents the placing time in the *i*th cycle, the time is spent while the heads leaving from slot to mounting position and placing all of components in *i*th cycle. D_{ij} represents the moving time of heads from the final placing position in *i*th cycle to the first pickup position in *j*th cycle. x_{ij} is binary system variable which is used to judge if *i*th cycle is adjacent to *j*th cycle. The parameter p represents the cycle sum. The objective function of the optimization problem is as follow:

$$\min \sum_{i=1}^{p} T_1(i) + \sum_{i=1}^{p} T_2(i) + \sum_{\substack{i,j=1 \\ i \neq j}}^{p} D_{ij} x_{ij} \tag{1}$$

Constraint conditions:

$$x_{ij} \in \{0,1\}, i, j = 1, 2, \cdots, p, i \neq j \ . \tag{2}$$

$$\sum_{i=1}^{p} x_{ij} = 1, i = 1, 2, \cdots, p \tag{3}$$

$$\sum_{j=1}^{p} x_{ij} = 1, j = 1, 2, \cdots, p \tag{4}$$

$$\sum_{i=1}^{p} \sum_{j=1}^{p} x_{ij} = p - 1 \tag{5}$$

And, the terms in (2)~(5) ensure each cycle should be done once.

3 Genetic Algorithm

3.1 Chromosome Coding

GAs work by creating a population of individuals and each individual represents a possible solution to a given problem. The property of each individual is described by using a chromosome. In the GA the sequence of mounting components is represented by the chromosome, and *i*th node in chromosome is represented the component to be mounted on the PCB in the *i*th order. A chromosome used to four-head surface mounting machine case is showed in the figure 2. From figure 2, we can know there are eight components to be mounted, components 1,2,3,5 would be mounted in cycle 1; components 4,6,7,8 would be mounted in cycle 2. In cycle 1 the first node indicates that the machine mounts the component 1 firstly, the component 3 will be mounted 7 is mounted and the sixth node indicates the component 8 is mounted, and so on.

Fig. 2. Chromosome

3.2 Genetic Operations

3.2.1 Evaluation and Selection of Chromosome

The fitness of chromosome is defined as the total assembly time which is calculated by equation (1). If assembly time is less, then the fitness of chromosome will be larger. The individual with the largest fitness in population will be selected and kept to next generation.

3.2.2 Crossover Operation

Crossover operator is a key to the genetic algorithm's power is achieved by the cross of links. Parameter crossover rate pc is given in range [0,1] and random variable r will be generated in range [0,1]. If the value of pc is larger than r, the crossover would be done, otherwise skipped. The process of crossover operation is showed as follows:

Step 1. Two parents are selected randomly (showed in the figure 3).

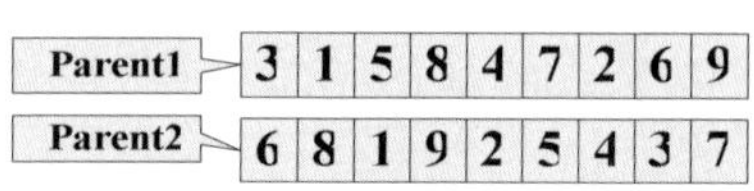

Fig. 3. Crossover operator

Step 2. Generate a initial node, the nodes which locate on its left side are moved to the end of right side. Then first node of offspring can be decided. For example, if node "1" is generated randomly as the initial node, in parent1 node "3" should be moved to the end of right; in parent2 node "6","8" should be moved to the end of right in order(showed in the figure 4). The first node of offspring is "1".

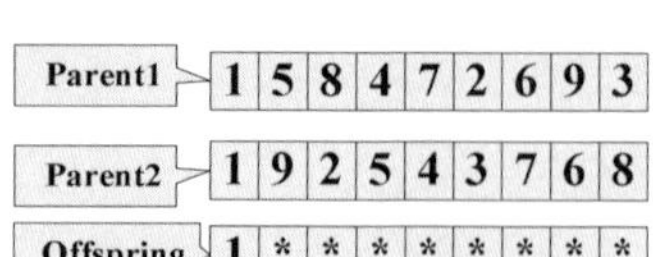

Fig. 4. Crossover operator

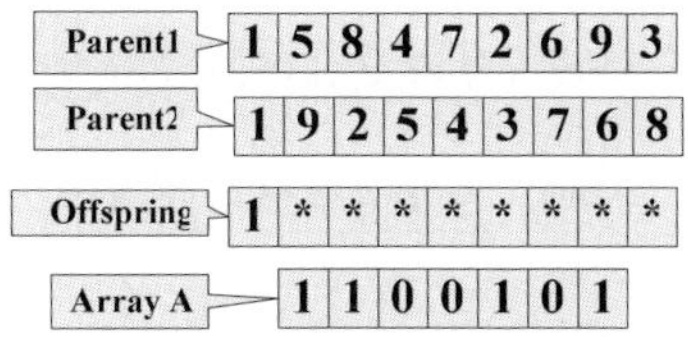

Fig. 5. Crossover operator

Step 3. Generate a binary array A randomly(showed in the figure 5)

Step 4. The next node is selected according to corresponding position's value in binary array A. For example, if A(1) =1, the second node is decided by Parent 1. As the second node is "5" in Parent 1, the "5" is selected as second node of offspring, then the nodes before "5" in paraent 2 are moved to the right end side in order. The parent 1, parent 2 and offspring in Fig 5. is shifted and showed in Fig 6. If A(1)=0, the second node is decided by Parent 2. the "9" is selected, at same time, the parent 1 is shifted.

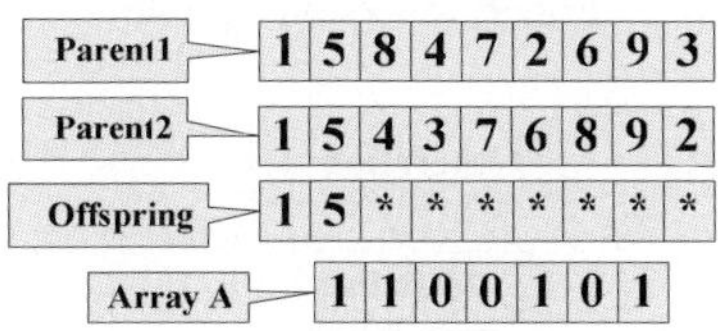

Fig. 6. Crossover operator

Step 5. Repeat the step 4 until all nodes of Offspring are achieved (showed in figur7).

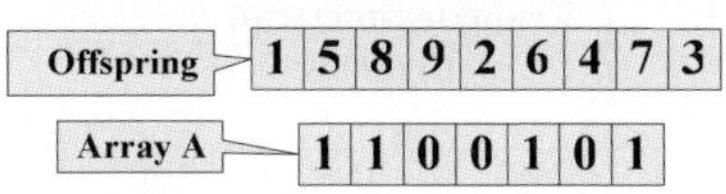

Fig. 7. Crossover operator

3.2.3 Mutation Operation

Mutation has the effect of local search an increasing the diversity of a population. This operator is a secondary guarantee that the genetic search can access the whole search region. It ensures useful schemata will not lose and the searching will not converge to local points prematurely. We use the exchange operator and inversion operator as a mutation operator. Parameter mutation rate *pmjh* and parameter inversion rate *pmfz* are given in the range [0, 1] and variable *r1* and *r2* are generated randomly in range [0, 1]. When the value of *r1* is smaller than *pmjh*, mutation operation is done, otherwise skipped; and if the values of *r1* and *r2* are smaller than *pmjh* and *pmfz* respectively, both operations are done; if the value of *r1* is smaller than *pmjh* and the value of *r2* is not smaller than *pmfz*, only exchange operation is

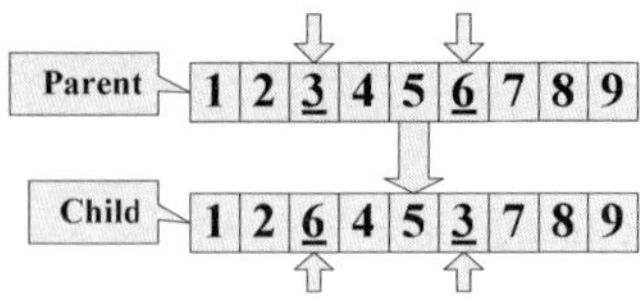

Fig. 8. Exchange operator

done. Exchange operator exchanges two genes in a link. Figure 8 shows the exchange operator.

The inversion operator means a segment is taken from a parent link and is inversed to form a new link. Figure 9 shows the inversion operator.

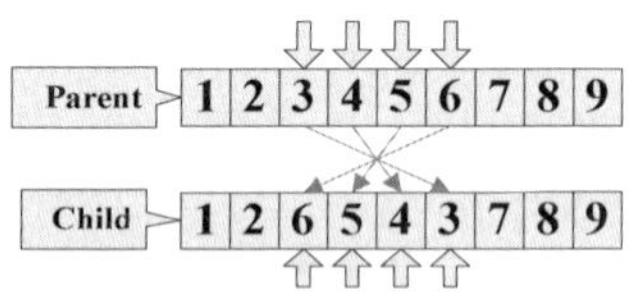

Fig. 9. Inversion operator

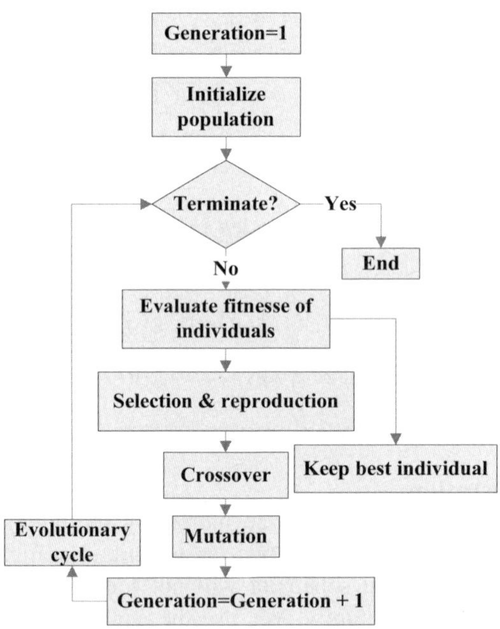

Fig. 10. Flowchart of GA

3.3 The Flowchart of GA

First of all, initial links composed of many feasible mounting orders are generated, those links are assembled as a parent chromosome population, i.e. initialization of chromosome; then individuals' fitness in parent population should be evaluated by equation (1), the individual which fitness is largest in the population is selected and kept to next generation. Crossover and mutation operations are done to generate next new population, then the new population is used as parent population, and the evolution steps mentioned above are repeated until the times of cycle come to the number given. The best individual with the largest fitness in the whole process of searching as the optimization order will be finally got by using GA. The flowchart of the GA is showed in figure 10.

4 Simulation Results

We consider a real dual-gantry multi-head tool that has four heads and 52 slots at each feeder rack. Tap feeder width is 17 mm and the distance between each feed is 8.5 mm. There are three PCB tested.

Their figure dimension is 200mm×300mm. Three simulation results are showed in table 1. The population size *pop_size*=10, the crossover rate *Pc*=0.9, the mutation exchange rate *Pmj*=0.01, the mutation inversion rate *Pmfz*=0.9.

Table 1. Simulation Result

Questions	1	2	3
Number of components	20	40	80
Component style	4	8	16
Nozzle style	2	4	8
Number of heads	4	4	4
GA(sec)	3.0033	5.8378	11.4292
Figure of evolution process	Figure 13	Figure 14	Figure 15

The optimization sequence which comes from PCB 1 composed by 20 components is showed in figure 11 and evolution process is graphically shown in figure 12. Pick-up and placement route is showed in figure 13. Component style and the optimization sequence which comes from PCB 1 can be gotten as follow:

{1,2,3,4,5} ={a1,a2,a3,a4,a5} ∈ component **a**
{6,7,8,9,10} ={b1,b2,b3,b4,b5} ∈ component **b**
{11,12,13,14,15} ={c1,c2,c3,c4,c5} ∈ component **c**
{16,17,18,19,20} ={d1,d2,d3,d4,d5} ∈ component **d**

Optimization sequence:

5	7	4	20	17	19	3	15	12	11	16	13	18	8	9	2	1	6	10	14
a5	*b2*	*a4*	*d5*	*d2*	*d4*	*a3*	*c5*	*c2*	*c1*	*d1*	*c3*	*d3*	*b3*	*b4*	*a2*	*a1*	*b1*	*b5*	*b4*
Cycle1				*Cycle2*				*Cycle3*				*Cycle4*				*Cycle5*			

Fig. 11. Optimization sequence for 20 components

So the optimization sequence can be showed in figure 11. In cycle 1, the first pickup components are a5 and b2, because the distance between their positions in slot is equal to the distance between head 1 and 2, so they can be picked up simultaneity. And second component is a4, the third component is d5. Then heads move from slot to PCB, the first component which is needed to place is a5, and next are b2, a4, d5 in order. And so on. the whole process of pick-and-place sequence can be showed in figure 12.

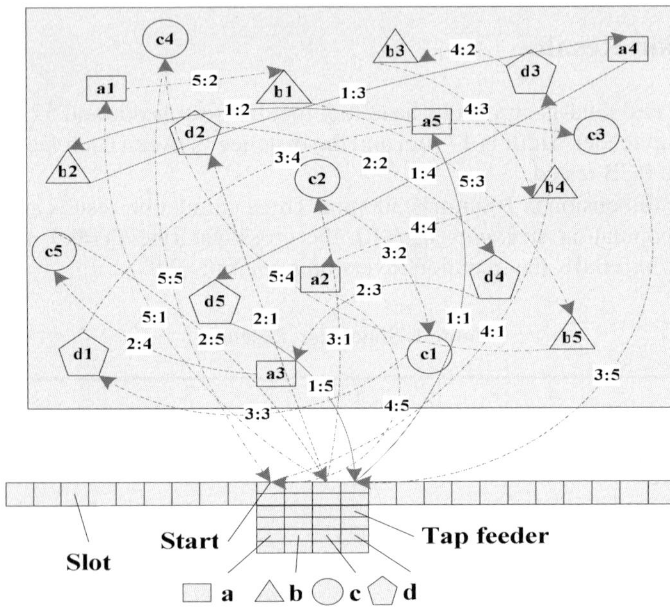

Fig. 12. Pick-up and placement route for 20 components

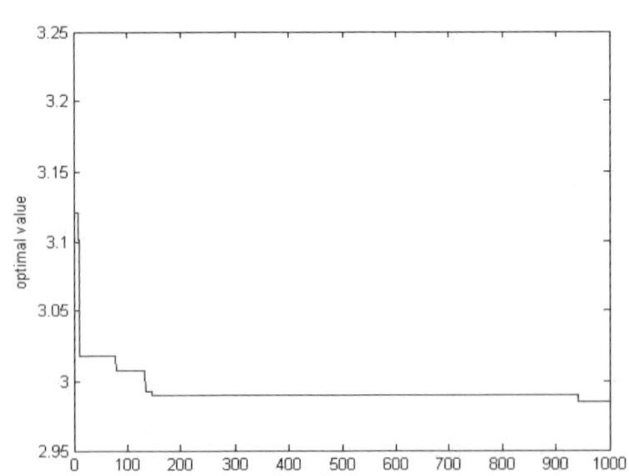

Fig. 13. Evolution process to mount PCB 1

The evolution process for PCB 2 and PCB 3 is showed in figure 14 and figure 15.

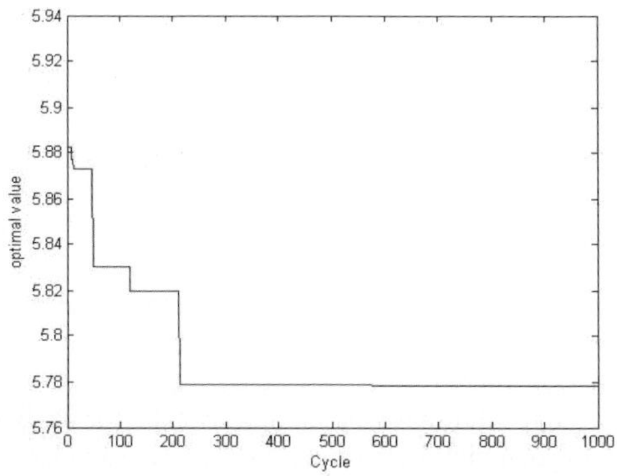

Fig. 14. Evolution process to mount PCB 2

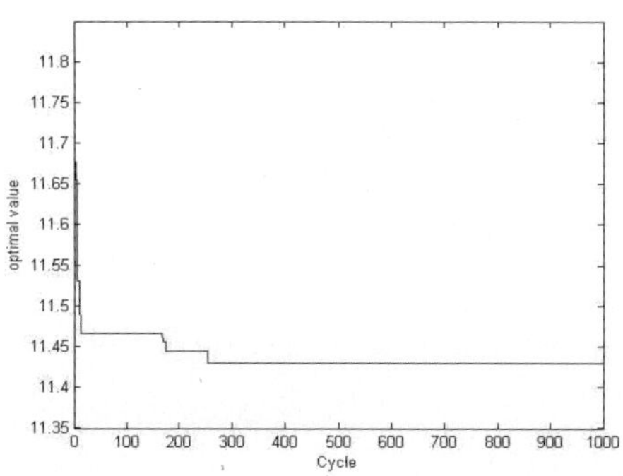

Fig. 15. Evolution process to mount PCB 3

5 Conclusions

In this paper, a GA algorithm is developed to solve the problem of minimizing the PCB assembly time for multi-head surface mounting machines. At same time, some experiments have been done. Experimental results show the proposed GA algorithm is effective and good results for printing three types of PCB are achieved.

Acknowledgments

This work is supported by the Young Talent Fund of Fujian Province(2006F3074) and the project of Office of Education of Fujian Province (JB06054).

References

1. Burkeek, Cowlingpi, Ralfk: New models and heuristics for component placement in printed circuit board assembly. In: Proceedings of the 1999 IEEE International Conference on Information, Intelligence and Systems(ICIIS 1999), pp. 133–140. IEEE Press, Los Alamitos (1999)
2. Laarhoven, P.V., Zijm, W.: preparation and numerical control in PCB assembly. International Journal Flexible Manufacture System 3, 187–207 (1993)
3. Leipulut, N.: Optimization of the movements of a component placement machine. European Journal of Operation Research 38(2), 167–177 (1989)
4. Leumc, Wongh, J.: Planning of component placement/insertion sequence and feeder setup in PCB assembly using genetic algorithms. Journal of Electronic Packaging, Transactions of the ASME 115(4), 424–432 (1993)
5. Khoolp, N.: A genetic algorithm-based planning system for PCB component placement. International Journal of Production Economics 54(3), 321–332 (1998)
6. Loh, T.S., Satich, T.S., Bukkapatnam, D., Kwon, H.: A genetic algorithm for sequential. part assignment for PCB assembly. Computer & Industrial Engineering 40(4), 293–307 (2001)

A Method of General Stiffness Modeling for Multi-axis Machine Tool

Rong Yan, Fangyu Peng, and Bin Li

National NC System Engineering Research Center,
Huazhong University of Science and Technology, Wuhan 430074
zwm8917@263.net

Abstract. In this paper, a new method for computing general stiffness model at tool tip for multi-axis machine tool is presented. The formula of general stiffness model at tool tip is derived from virtual-work principle and point transformation matrix method. Point transformation matrix method indicates the transformation relationship of elastic displacement on both ends of flexible axes as well as the transformation relationship of force. By multiplying the point transformation matrix, the final stiffness matrix at tool tip will be obtained efficiently. In this modeling method, the final stiffness matrix is composed of local compliance matrixes according to their contribution to the final stiffness matrix.

Keywords: Multi-axis Stiffness Point transformation matrix.

1 Introduction

Compared with traditional three axis machining, multi-axis machining offers more flexibility for machining complex surface, but at the same time it comes up with the problem that the rigidity of the machine tool is unsatisfying [1]. Obviously, the rigidity characteristic of multi-axis machine tools has a direct effect on machining performances. Therefore, during machining planning process of multi-axis machine tools, we should not only focus on the geometry characteristic of workpiece surface and motion capacity of the machine tool, but also take into account the rigidity characteristic of multi-axis machine tool.

Generally, when discussing the rigidity characteristic of the multi-axis machine tool system, the stiffness model is appropriately simplified due to the complex machine structure. For instance, the deflection of the tool-tool holder is only considered (Philippe et al [2], 2006 ; G.M. Kim et al [3], 2003). This simplified model is reasonable under the assumption that the rigidity of the machine base and other parts is infinite compared with tool and tool holder. However, it will be not feasible to obtain precise mechanics model by this way if any of the following conditions exists. The first one is that machine axes are spindly so that the deflection of machine axes affects the deflection of the tool tip greatly. The second is that the rigidity of machine joints is unsatisfying so we can't ignore the effect on the deflection of the tool tip resulted from their deformation. Salgado [4] discovered by the experiment of machine rigidity characteristic that the deflection of machine joints could reach 50－60% of the total

C. Xiong et al. (Eds.): ICIRA 2008, Part II, LNAI 5315, pp. 1013–1021, 2008.

deflection at tool tip, which means the influence on the deflection at tool tip caused by the deflection of machine joints can't be neglected. The rigidity characteristic of multi-axis machine tools is affected by many factors such as machine axes, machine joints and tool-spindle. So when analyzing the rigidity characteristic, we should synthetically concern all these factors in order to get accurate stiffness model of machine tool.

2 General Stiffness Model of Multi-axis Machine Tools

During machining process, once force F acts on the tool tip, small deflection will take place at the tool tip due to the elastic deflection of the machine joints [5], the flexible machine axes and tool-spindle. With the assumption of small deflections, the deflection at the tool tip can be expressed as:

$$\delta v = \delta v_1 + \delta v_2 \ . \tag{1}$$

where δv_1 is the deflection at the tool tip caused by the deflection of the machine joints, δv_2 is the deflection at the tool tip caused by the deflection of the flexible machine axes and tool-spindle.

According to the principle of virtual-work and the formula (**1**):

$$\delta w = F^T \delta v = F^T \delta v_1 + F^T \delta v_2 = \delta w_1 + \delta w_2 \ . \tag{2}$$

The total virtual-work δw of multi-axis machine tool system is the sum of the virtual-work δw_1 on the condition of the deformation of machine joints and the virtual-work δw_2 on the condition of the deformation of machine axes and the tool-spindle.

2.1 General Compliance Matrix Model for Multi-axis Machine Tools Only Concerning about the Deformation of Machine Joints

If only the deformation of machine joints is taken into account, the formula is obtained: $\delta w_1 = F^T \delta v_1$ based on the principle of virtual-work, where δv_1 is the deformation of machine joints caused together by gravity and force F. Therefore a relationship between force and displacement at tool tip is:

$$\delta v_1 - \delta v_{1,gravity} = S_{t1} F \ . \tag{3}$$

where $\delta v_{1,gravity}$ is the displacement at tool tip due to the deflection of the machine joints affected by the gravity. S_{t1} is the general compliance matrix at the tool tip in the machine coordinate system (*CSo*) expressed as [6]:

$$S_{t1} = J_j^{(o)} K_j^{-1} \left(J_j^{(o)} \right)^T \ . \tag{4}$$

where K_j is an n×n order diagonal matrix which consists of the stiffness of the machine joints. n is the number of machine joints of multi-axis NC machine tools.

$J_j^{(o)}$ is a Jacobi matrix which presents the relationship between differential displacement in the machine coordinate system (*CSo*) and that in joint space [7]. It is derived from kinematics model for multi-axis NC machine tools [8].

2.2 General Compliance Matrix Model for Multi-axis Machine Tools only Concerning about the Deflection of Machine Axes and Tool-Spindle

If only the deflection of the machine axes and tool-spindle is taken into account, the formula is obtained: $\delta w_2 = F^T \delta v_2$ based on the principle of virtual-work, where δv_1 is the deformation of the machine axes and tool-spindle caused together by gravity and force *F*. Therefore a relationship between force and displacement at the tool tip is:

$$\delta v_2 - \delta v_{2,gravity} = S_{t2} F \quad . \tag{5}$$

where $\delta v_{2,gravity}$ is the displacement at the tool tip due to the deflection of the machine axes and tool-spindle affected by the gravity. S_{t2} is the general compliance matrix at the tool tip in the machine coordinate system (*CSo*).

From the relationship of force and displacement in the formula (**5**), the compliance matrix S_{t2} at the tool tip can be established without considering the affection of the gravity. Furthermore, the point transformation matrix will be used to establish S_{t2} in the following.

(1) Establish the point transformation matrix between frame A and frame B

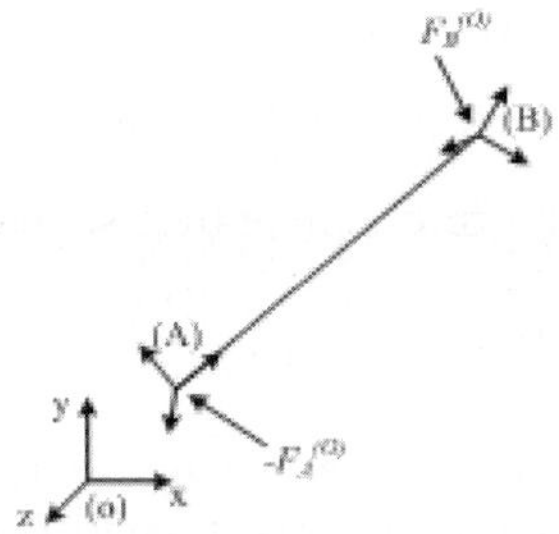

Fig. 1. Force Model of AB linkage

Consider a link with frame A and frame B rigidly attached at either end, and another frame O which will serve as the reference frame, as shown in Fig. 1. The relationship of force at the point A and the point B is expressed as follows:

$$F_A^{(o)} = \begin{pmatrix} I & 0 \\ \left(R_A^{(o)} P_B^{(A)}\right)\times & I \end{pmatrix} F_B^{(o)} = J_{B,force}^{A(o)} F_B^{(o)} \quad . \tag{6}$$

where $J_{B,force}^{A(o)}$ is the point transformation matrix which transforms force vector from point B to point A with respect to the reference frame O. We use the notation $P\times$ to represent the linear transformation of a cross product with a vector $p \in R^3$.

In the reference frame O, there is a relationship of velocity between A and B:

$$\begin{cases} v_A^{(o)} = v_B^{(o)} + w_B^{(o)} \times \left(R_B^{(o)} \times P_A^{(B)} \right) \\ w_A^{(o)} = w_B^{(o)} \end{cases}$$

From the relationship of velocity the relationship of differential displacement between A and B is obtained as:

$$\delta v_A^{(o)} = \begin{pmatrix} I & -\left(R_B^{(o)} P_A^{(B)} \right) \times \\ 0 & I \end{pmatrix} \delta v_B^{(o)} = J_{B,disp}^{A(o)} \delta v_B^{(o)} \quad (7)$$

where $J_{B,disp}^{A(o)}$ is the point transformation matrix expressing the relationship of differential displacement between B and A with respect to the reference frame O.

(2) Establish the transformation relationship of compliance matrix between any frame i and the reference frame O

Assuming matrix $R_i^{(o)}$ the coordinate transformation matrix between frame i and the reference frame O, and assigning $J_i^{(o)} = \begin{pmatrix} R_i^{(o)} & 0 \\ 0 & R_i^{(o)} \end{pmatrix}$, the transformation relationship of force and displacement from frame i to frame O is:

$$F^{(o)} = J_i^{(o)} F^{(i)} \ , \ \ \delta v^{(o)} = J_i^{(o)} \delta v^{(i)} \ . \quad (8)$$

As $\delta v^{(i)} = S^{(i)} F^{(i)}$, with the expression (**8**), thus:

$$\delta v^{(o)} = J_i^{(o)} \delta v^{(i)} = J_i^{(o)} S^{(i)} F^{(i)} = J_i^{(o)} S^{(i)} \left(J_i^{(o)} \right)^T F^{(o)} .$$

As $\delta v^{(o)} = S^{(o)} F^{(o)}$, with the expression above, we have:

$$S^{(o)} = J_i^{(o)} S^{(i)} \left(J_i^{(o)} \right)^T \ . \quad (9)$$

Formula (**9**) is the transformation relationship between the compliance matrix *S* in frame i and that in frame O. Similarly, the transformation relationship between the stiffness matrix *K* in frame i and that in frame O:

$$K^{(o)} = J_i^{(o)} K^{(i)} \left(J_i^{(o)} \right)^T \ . \quad (10)$$

(3) Establish the general compliance (stiffness) matrix of two linkages

Assuming two linkages AB and BC connect in series, as shown in Figure 2. Three joints A, B, C are rigid, therefore we only concern about the deformation of linkage AB and BC. A and B represent the origins of the two machine axes respectively. It's already known that $K_{AB}^{(A)}$ is the stiffness matrix of linkage AB in frame A, and $K_{BC}^{(B)}$ is that of BC in frame B. We would like to obtain the general stiffness matrix $K_C^{(o)}$.

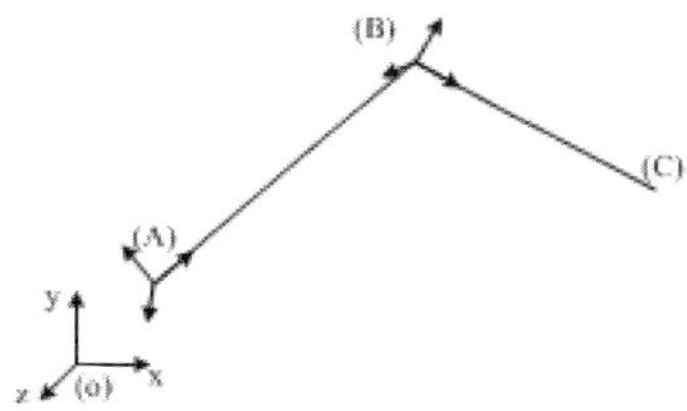

Fig. 2. Model of two linkages

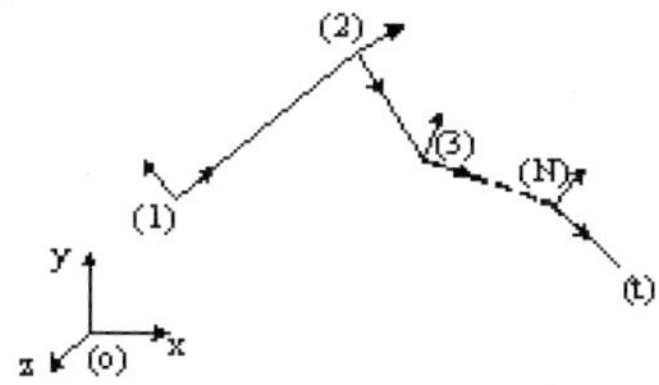

Fig. 3. Model of *N* series of linkages

Step 1: calculate the displacement $\delta v_B^{(o)}$ caused by link AB flexibility
If there is force $F_C^{(o)}$ acting on C, we can compute the force $F_B^{(o)}$ transformed to B, then the displacement $\delta v_B^{(o)}$ caused by the compliance of flexible link AB when the force $F_B^{(o)}$ acts on B using (**9**):

$$\delta v_B^{(o)} = S_{AB}^{(o)} F_B^{(o)} = J_A^{(o)} S_{AB}^{(A)} \left(J_A^{(o)}\right)^T F_B^{(o)} \quad . \tag{11}$$

where $S_{AB}^{(o)}$ is the compliance matrix of linkage AB with respect to frame o.

Step2: calculate the displacement $\delta v_{C,1}^{(o)}$ caused by $\delta v_B^{(o)}$
The displacement on C is calculated using (11), together with (**6**) and (**7**):

$$\begin{aligned}\delta v_{C,1}^{(o)} &= J_{B,disp}^{C(o)} \delta v_B^{(o)} = J_{B,disp}^{C(o)} S_{AB}^{(o)} F_B^{(o)} = J_{B,disp}^{C(o)} J_A^{(o)} S_{AB}^{(A)} \left(J_A^{(o)}\right)^T F_B^{(o)} \\ &= J_{B,disp}^{C(o)} J_A^{(o)} S_{AB}^{(A)} \left(J_A^{(o)}\right)^T J_{C,force}^{B(o)} F_C^{(o)}\end{aligned} \quad .$$

Step 3: calculate the displacement $\delta v_{C,2}^{(o)}$ caused by link BC flexibility
From local compliance matrix of link BC, $S_{BC}^{(B)}$, we compute the displacement $\delta v_{C,2}^{(o)}$ caused by $F_C^{(o)}$ due to the flexibility of link BC only. By Formula (**10**), the displacement $\delta v_{C,2}^{(o)}$ is obtained as:

$$\delta v_{C,2}^{(o)} = S_{BC}^{(o)} F_C^{(o)} = J_B^{(o)} S_{BC}^{(B)} \left(J_B^{(o)}\right)^T F_C^{(o)} \quad .$$

where $S_{BC}^{(o)}$ is the compliance matrix of link BC in frame O.

Step4: Compose the overall compliance matrix
The total displacement of C due to the flexibility of links AB and BC is the sum of the individual displacements expressed in the reference frame O:

$$\delta v_C^{(o)} = \delta v_{C,1}^{(o)} + \delta v_{C,2}^{(o)} = \left[J_{B,disp}^{C(o)} J_A^{(o)} S_{AB}^{(o)} \left(J_A^{(o)}\right)^T J_{C,force}^{B(o)} + J_B^{(o)} S_{BC}^{(B)} \left(J_B^{(o)}\right)^T \right] F_C^{(o)} = S_C^{(o)} F_C^{(o)} \quad .$$

where $S_C^{(o)}$ is the overall compliance matrix of the two linkages on point C:

(4) Establish the compliance matrix of N series of linkages
Above method can be used to compute the stiffness matrix of N serially-connected flexible linkage at the end-effector *t*, as shown in Figure 3.

The contribution of flexibility of link *Nt* to the compliance matrix $S_{t2}^{(o)}$ is:

$$S_{t2}^{(o)} = J_N^{(o)} S_{Nt}^{(N)} \left(J_N^{(o)}\right)^T$$

The contribution of flexibility of Link $N-1, N$ to the compliance matrix $S_{t2}^{(o)}$ is:

$$S_{t2}^{(o)} = J_{N,disp}^{t(o)} J_{N-1}^{(o)} S_{N-1,N}^{(N-1)} \left(J_{N-1}^{(o)}\right)^T J_{t,force}^{N(o)}$$

The contribution of flexibility of Link $i, i+1$ to the compliance matrix $S_{t2}^{(o)}$ is:

$$S_{t2}^{(o)} = J_{i+1,disp}^{t(o)} J_i^{(o)} S_{i,i+1}^{(i)} \left(J_i^{(o)}\right)^T J_{t,force}^{i+1(o)}$$

......

The contribution of flexibility of Link 12 to the compliance matrix $S_{t2}^{(o)}$ is:

$$S_{t2}^{(o)} = J_{2,disp}^{t(o)} J_1^{(o)} S_{1,2}^{(o)} \left(J_1^{(o)}\right)^T J_{t,force}^{2(o)}$$

If no statement of the mark at top right corner of matrix is specified, compliance matrix and stiffness matrix both mean matrixes with respected to the base frame O. So $S_{t2}^{(o)}$ can be simplified as S_{t2} .Based on the analysis above, we compose the contribution of all flexibility of all the linkage to the compliance matrix S_{t2} at the end *t*:

$$S_{t2} = \sum_{i=1}^{N-1} J_{i+1,disp}^{t(o)} J_i^{(o)} S_{i\,i+1}^{(i)} \left(J_i^{(o)}\right)^T J_{t,force}^{i+1(o)} + J_N^{(o)} S_{N\,t}^{(N)} \left(J_N^{(o)}\right)^T . \quad (12)$$

If at the same time the deflection of the machine joints is taken into account, the general compliance matrix at the end *t* is obtained using (**1**), (**3**), (**4**), (**5**) and (**12**):

$$S_t = S_{t1} + S_{t2} = J_j^{(o)} \left(K_j\right)^{-1} \left(J_j^{(o)}\right)^T + J_N^{(o)} S_{N\,t}^{(N)} \left(J_N^{(o)}\right)^T + \sum_{i=1}^{N-1} J_{i+1,disp}^{t(o)} J_i^{(o)} S_{i\,i+1}^{(i)} \left(J_i^{(o)}\right)^T J_{t,force}^{i+1(o)} \cdot \quad (13)$$

and the general stiffness matrix is then: $K_t = S_t^{-1}$

3 Example of Stiffness Analysis of a Five-Axis Machine Tool

This kind of machine tool consists of 5 machine axes: two translational axes and three rotational axes as shown in Figure 4(a). If translational axes X and Z are located at 1m and 0.5m and rotational axes C1, B2, A2 turn to 45º,-30º, 30º respectively, the general stiffness matrix at tool tip of this machine tool is calculated in this case.

In order to establish local stiffness matrix of A2 axis, two local coordinate systems, called CS6 and CS7, are established in Fig.4.b.Taking into account all the deflection of machine joints, flexible axis A2 and tool-spindle, the formula of general stiffness matrix of this kind of 5-axis machine tool with special milling tool is derived from expression (**13**):

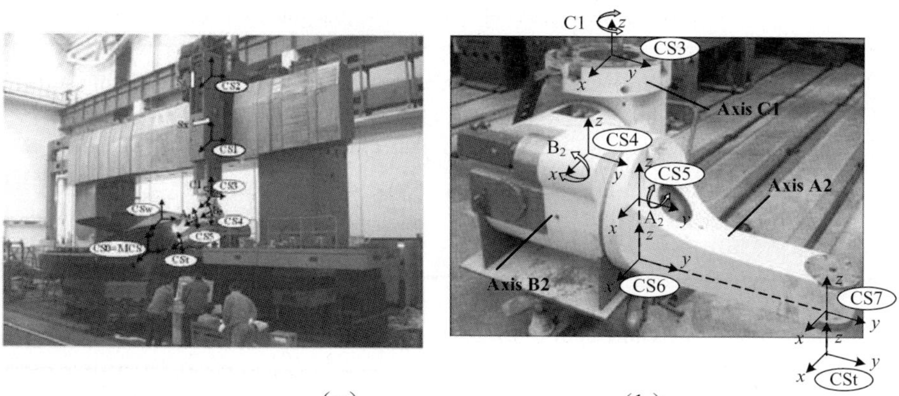

Fig. 4. Kinematical schematic and reference frame of a five-axis machine tool

$$K_t = S_t^{-1} = \left[J_j^{(o)} \left(K_j\right)^{-1} \left(J_j^{(o)}\right)^T + J_{7,disp}^{t(o)} J_6^{(o)} S_{67}^{(6)} \left(J_6^{(o)}\right)^T J_{t,force}^{7(o)} + J_7^{(o)} S_{7t}^{(7)} \left(J_7^{(o)}\right)^T \right]^{-1} . \quad (14)$$

In the expression (**14**), both of the point transformation matrix, namely $J_{7,disp}^{t(o)}$ and $J_{t,force}^{7(o)}$, and Jacobi matrix, namely $J_j^{(o)}$ and $J_7^{(o)}$, can be obtained directly from the kinematics model of this machine tool in VC platform. The stiffness of the machine joints, flexible axis A2 and tool-spindle is shown in Table 1, Table 2 and Table 3, respectively, which is measured by experiment.

Table 1. Stiffness coefficient of machine joints

stiffness coefficient of machine joints	k_X (MN/m)	k_Z (MN/m)	k_{C_1} (MN·m/rad)	k_{B_2} (MN·m/rad)	k_{A_2} (MN·m/rad)
	120.00	140.00	2.02	3.29	0.87

In the expression(**14**), stiffness matrix K_j is a 5×5 order diagonal matrix consist of the stiffness coefficient of each machine joint (listed in Table 1) expressed as:

$$K_j = \begin{bmatrix} k_X & 0 & 0 & 0 & 0 \\ 0 & k_Z & 0 & 0 & 0 \\ 0 & 0 & k_{C_1} & 0 & 0 \\ 0 & 0 & 0 & k_{B_2} & 0 \\ 0 & 0 & 0 & 0 & k_{A_2} \end{bmatrix} = \begin{bmatrix} 120.00 & 0 & 0 & 0 & 0 \\ 0 & 140.00 & 0 & 0 & 0 \\ 0 & 0 & 2.02 & 0 & 0 \\ 0 & 0 & 0 & 3.29 & 0 \\ 0 & 0 & 0 & 0 & 0.87 \end{bmatrix}$$

In the expression(**14**), $S_{67}^{(6)}$ is local compliance matrix of the flexible A2, of which the contrary matrix is the stiffness matrix $K_{67}^{(6)}$ expressed as:

Table 2. Stiffness coefficient of the machine axis A2

axial stiffness (MN/m)	radial stiffness (MN/m)		bending stiffness (MN.m/rad)			coupling stiffness (MN)	
K_{xx,A_2}	K_{yy,A_2}	K_{zz,A_2}	$K_{\theta_x m_x,A_2}$	$K_{\theta_y m_y,A_2}$	$K_{\theta_z m_z,A_2}$	K_{ym_z,A_2}	K_{zm_y,A_2}
791.97	1.01	0.91	1.94	10.95	12.16	3.04	2.74

Table 3. Stiffness coefficient of tool-spindle

axial stiffness (MN/m)	radial stiffness (MN/m)		bending stiffness (MN.m/rad)			coupling stiffness (MN)	
$K_{zz,t}$	$K_{xx,t}$	$K_{yy,t}$	$K_{\theta_x m_x,t}$	$K_{\theta_y m_y,t}$	$K_{\theta_z m_z,t}$	$K_{xm_y,t}$	$K_{ym_x,t}$
32.40	18.40	18.40	0.50	0.50	0.12	1.67	1.67

$$S_{67}^{(6)} = \left(K_{67}^{(6)}\right)^{-1} = \begin{bmatrix} K_{xx,A_2} & 0 & 0 & 0 & 0 & 0 \\ 0 & K_{yy,A_2} & 0 & 0 & 0 & K_{ym_z,A_2} \\ 0 & 0 & K_{zz,A_2} & 0 & -K_{zm_y,A_2} & 0 \\ 0 & 0 & 0 & K_{\theta_x m_x,A_2} & 0 & 0 \\ 0 & 0 & -K_{zm_y,A_2} & 0 & K_{\theta_y m_y,A_2} & 0 \\ 0 & K_{ym_z,A_2} & 0 & 0 & 0 & K_{\theta_z m_z,A_2} \end{bmatrix}^{-1} = \begin{bmatrix} 0.001 & 0 & 0 & 0 & 0 & 0 \\ 0 & 3.95 & 0 & 0 & 0 & -0.99 \\ 0 & 0 & 4.38 & 0 & 1.10 & 0 \\ 0 & 0 & 0 & 0.52 & 0 & 0 \\ 0 & 0 & 1.10 & 0 & 0.37 & 0 \\ 0 & -0.99 & 0 & 0 & 0 & 0.33 \end{bmatrix}$$

In the expression(**14**), $S_{7t}^{(7)}$ is local compliance matrix of tool-spindle, of which the contrary matrix is the stiffness matrix $K_{7t}^{(7)}$ expressed as:

$$S_{7t}^{(7)} = \left(K_{7t}^{(7)}\right)^{-1} = \begin{bmatrix} K_{xx,t} & 0 & 0 & 0 & K_{xm_y,t} & 0 \\ 0 & K_{yy,t} & 0 & -K_{ym_x,t} & 0 & 0 \\ 0 & 0 & K_{zz,t} & 0 & 0 & 0 \\ 0 & -K_{ym_x,t} & 0 & K_{\theta_x m_x,t} & 0 & 0 \\ K_{xm_y,t} & 0 & 0 & 0 & K_{\theta_y m_y,t} & 0 \\ 0 & 0 & 0 & 0 & 0 & K_{\theta_z m_z,t} \end{bmatrix}^{-1} = \begin{bmatrix} 0.08 & 0 & 0 & 0 & -0.26 & 0 \\ 0 & 0.08 & 0 & 0.26 & 0 & 0 \\ 0 & 0 & 0.03 & 0 & 0 & 0 \\ 0 & 0.02 & 0 & 2.87 & 0 & 0 \\ -0.02 & 0 & 0 & 0 & 2.87 & 0 \\ 0 & 0 & 0 & 0 & 0 & 8.33 \end{bmatrix}$$

Substitute matrix K_j, $S_{67}^{(6)}$ and $S_{7t}^{(7)}$ into the formula (**14**) to get the final result:

$$K_t = \begin{bmatrix} 2.48 & 1.85 & 2.04 & -0.29 & 0.27 & 0.28 \\ 1.85 & 1.75 & 1.69 & -0.31 & 0.20 & 0.27 \\ 2.04 & 1.69 & 2.09 & -0.24 & 0.16 & 0.22 \\ -0.29 & -0.31 & -0.24 & 0.33 & -0.06 & -0.08 \\ 0.27 & 0.20 & 0.16 & -0.06 & 0.23 & 0.10 \\ 0.28 & 0.27 & 0.22 & -0.08 & 0.10 & 0.21 \end{bmatrix}$$

4 Conclusion

This paper put forward a method of general stiffness modeling for multi-axis machine tool. Taking account the deflection of the machine joints, the flexible axes and tool-spindle, a general stiffness model for multi-axis machine tool is established by principle of virtual-work and point transformation matrix. This kind of method can be commonly used to establish general stiffness model for different kinds of multi-axis machine tools without fussy dynamics expressions. At present this method has been used for stiffness modeling of both standard milling tool and special milling tool of 5-axis machine tools. Furthermore it's helpful to set relevant indexes for stiffness performance evaluation and guide machining process in available working space [9].

Acknowledgements

The authors would like to thank the anonymous referees for their valuable comments and helpful suggestions. This work was supported by Major State Basic Research Development Programme of China (2005CB724101) during all the period of this research.

References

1. Tsutsumi, M., Saito, A.: Identification and compensation of systematic deviations particular to 5-axis machining centers. International Journal of Machine Tools and Manufacture 43(8), 771–780 (2003)
2. Depince, P., Hascoet, J.-Y.: Active integration of tool deflection effects in end milling. Part 1. Prediction of milled surfaces. International Journal of Machine Tools & manufacture 46, 937–944 (2006)
3. Kim, G.M., Kim, B.H., Chu, C.N.: Estimation of cutter deflection and form error in ball-end milling processes. International Journal of Machine Tools & Manufacture 43, 917–924 (2003)
4. Salgado, M.A.a., de Lacalle, L., Lamikiz, L.N.a., MuÃÃoa, A.a., SÃÃnchez, J.A.a.: Evaluation of the stiffness chain on the deflection of end-mills under cutting forces. International Journal of Machine Tools and Manufacture 45(6), 727–739 (2005)
5. Uriarte, L., Herrero, A., et al.: Error budget and stiffness chain assessment in a micromilling machine equipped with tools less than 0.3mm in diameter. Precision Engineering 31, 1–12 (2007)
6. Tsai, L.W.: Robot analysis: the mechanics of serial and parallel manipulators, pp. 260–297. John Wiley & Sons, New York (1999)
7. Youlun, X.: Robotics. Mechanics Engineering Press, Beijing (1993)
8. Yaoxiong, H., Qihuo, X., Yanhong, Z.: Kinematics Model and its Solution for NC Machines of Arbitray Configuration. Chinese Journal of Mechanical Engineering 38(10), 31–36 (2002)
9. Rong, Y., Fangyu, P., Bin, L.: General stiffness analysis for multi-axis machine tool. Global Design and Manufacture to Gain a Competitive Edge, ICADAM (2008)

Symbolic Solutions for Direct Displacement and Manipulability Analyses of 3-DOF Parallel Machine Tools Using Groebner Base Method

Qiang Wang, Kang Luo, and Jin-ge Wang

College of Mechanical Engineering and Automation, Xihua University,
Chengdu China, 610039
wq_py123@163.com

Abstract. Based on Groebner base method and computer symbolic manipulating technique, symbolic solutions for direct displacement analysis of a three-DOF spatial parallel machine tool are proposed in this paper. A set of nonlinear polynomial equations are transformed into a set of equivalent triangularization equations by using the following operations: ordering of variables, forming all pairs of polynomials, finding S-polynomial, and reduction etc. The analytical solutions in the closed form are obtained. The Jacobian matrix is derived and symbolic technique is introduced into the procedure of derivation of Jacobian matrix. The manipulability of the parallel machine tool is investigated. Two numerical examples are given for illustration.

Keywords: Parallel machine tool direct displacement analysis Groebner base Manipulability Computer symbolic manipulating technique.

1 Introduction

Parallel machine tool, developed in the middle of 1990s, is a new type machine tool with high rigidity, response speed, machining accuracy, strong environment adaptability and high added value of technology. As the result of synthesizing machine tools with robot technology, parallel machine tool is called virtual axis machine tool. Recently many researchers studied with the solution for direct displacement of parallel machine.

The Groebner base method, proposed by Buchberger in 1965, is a method for forming standard base of nonlinear polynomial system. It has been attracted more and more attention by researchers and developed quickly in theory and application. Now the Groebner base method is seem as basic solution method for a set of nonlinear polynomial equations by many mathematicians of symbolic math and automatic reasoning in Europe and selected as core algorithm for POSSD of EC.

Manipulability is an important index for evaluation of parallel machine tool. Yoshikawa put forward the concept of manipulability in 1983 and Salisbury presented the index for evaluation of condition number of jacobian matrix [1-7]. Based on Groebner base method, the forward position solution for parallel machine tool can be obtained and the jacobian matrix can be derived in this paper.

C. Xiong et al. (Eds.): ICIRA 2008, Part II, LNAI 5315, pp. 1022–1029, 2008.

2 Groebner Base Method

(1) To list the variables by sorting on dictionary in each polynomial, as

$x_1 \prec_T x_2 \prec_T x_3 \prec_T \cdots \prec_T x_n$;

(2) To give set G, the polynomials compose the polynomial system F after ordering.

(3) To form the set B about all pairs of polynomials in G: $B = \{(f_i, f_j) \mid f_i, f_j \in G, i \neq j\}$

(4) To computes S-polynomial of the element $h = SP(f_i, f_j)$ and removes it from B. The (f_i, f_j) is a pair of polynomials in B, then $B = B - \{(f_i, f_j)\}$

(5) To standardize the S-polynomial (by one times or many times reduction) : $h' = NF(F,h)$, it is brought into G if $h' \neq 0$.Update B: $B = B \cup \{\{g,h'\} \mid g \in G\}$, the (4)and (5) is under procedure in new B. To calculate until the B is empty $G = \{f_1, f_2, f_3, \cdots f_n\}$ is obtained.

(6)To simplify G to the simplest Groebner standard base, the equivalent triangularization equations of polynomial equations is obtained.

$$\begin{cases} g_1(x_1) = 0 \\ g_2(x_1, x_2) = 0 \\ \vdots \\ g_n(x_1, x_2, \cdots, x_n) = 0 \end{cases}$$

3 Solution for Direct Displacement of Parallel Machine Tools

A 3-dof parallel mechanism consists of a base platform （B_1, B_2, B_3） and an upper platform （M1, M2, M3） connected by drive legs, as shown in fig1.There are two drive legs (l_1, l_2) connected base platform by hook joint (B_2, B_3) and connected upper platform by spheric hinge (M_2, M_3).The other drive leg (l_1) fixed on base platform by moving pair and connected upper platform by hook joint (M_1).The mechanism can displacement along Z-axis and rotate around X-axis and Y-axis. We invert the mechanism on worktable and fix the base platform on the framework of machine tool. The worktable accomplishes feed motion in X, Y direction by servo-actuator drive. As long as the degree of freedom of NC Machine tool is given, the two sports combine for operation. The layout of parallel machine tool is shown in figure2 [8~10].

The coordinate is designed as follow: the origin of fixed coordinate system R_0 is the point B_1 in base platform, the direction of Z_0-axis is point $B_1$to M_1, The direction of X_0-axis is B_1O; the origin of moving coordinate system R_1 is the point M_1 in upper platform, the direction of X_1-axis is point X_1 to O_1, the Z-axis is vertical to platform.

The coordinates of spherical joints M_i in the fixed coordinate system R_0 can be expressed as follow:

$$\begin{bmatrix} \vec{M}_i \\ 1 \end{bmatrix} = \begin{bmatrix} M_{ix} \\ M_{iy} \\ M_{iz} \\ 1 \end{bmatrix} = \begin{bmatrix} & [T] & & \vec{M}_1 \\ 0 & 0 & 0 & 1 \end{bmatrix} \begin{bmatrix} a_i \\ b_i \\ c_i \\ 1 \end{bmatrix} \quad (i = 2,3)$$

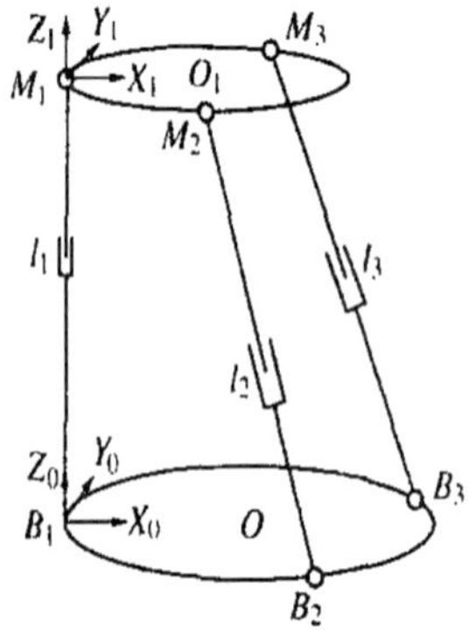

Fig. 1. 3-dof parallel mechanism

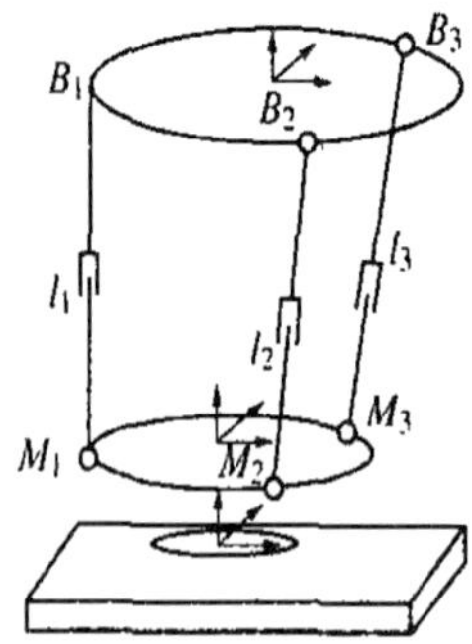

Fig. 2. The layout of parallel machine tool

Where a_i ,b_i ,c_i (i=2,3)is the coordinates of spherical joints M_i in the moving coordinate system R_1,$[T] = R(Y,\alpha) \bullet R(X,\beta)$, .Expand the above equation ,we have:

$$\vec{M}_i = \begin{bmatrix} a_i \cos\alpha + b_i \sin\alpha \sin\beta + c_i \sin\alpha \cos\beta \\ b_i \cos\beta - c_i \sin\beta \\ -a_i \sin\alpha + b_i \cos\alpha \sin\beta + c_i \cos\alpha \cos\beta + l_1 \end{bmatrix} \quad (i = 2,3) \tag{1}$$

The constraint equation of the mechanism can be expressed:

$$(M_{ix} - B_{ix})^2 + (M_{iy} - B_{iy})^2 + (M_{iz} - B_{iz})^2 = l_i^2 \qquad (i = 2,3) \tag{2}$$

We can rewrite (2) as follow:

$$\begin{cases} C_1 \cos\alpha \cos\beta + C_2 \sin\alpha \cos\beta + C_3 \cos\alpha \sin\beta + C_4 \sin\alpha \sin\beta \\ +C_5 \cos\alpha + C_6 \sin\alpha + C_7 \cos\beta + C_8 \sin\beta + C_9 = 0 \\ D_1 \cos\alpha \cos\beta + D_2 \sin\alpha \cos\beta + D_3 \cos\alpha \sin\beta + D_4 \sin\alpha \sin\beta \\ +D_5 \cos\alpha + D_6 \sin\alpha + D_7 \cos\beta + D_8 \sin\beta + D_9 = 0 \end{cases} \tag{3}$$

Thereinto, C_i, D_i (i=1~9) are functions concerning the structure parameters and input variables.

Substituting the half-angle formulas $x = \tan(\alpha/2)$, $y = \tan(\beta/2)$ and trigonometric $\sin\alpha = 2x/(1+x^2)$, $\cos\alpha = (1-x^2)/(1+x^2)$, $\sin\beta = 2y/(1+y^2)$, $\cos\beta = (1-y^2)/(1+y^2)$ into(3), we have:

$$\begin{cases} f_1 = m_1x^2y^2 + m_2xy^2 + m_3y^2 + m_4x^2y \\ \quad + m_5xy + m_6y + m_7x^2 + m_8x + m_9 = 0 \\ f_2 = n_1x^2y^2 + n_2xy^2 + n_3y^2 + n_4x^2y \\ \quad + n_5xy + n_6y + n_7x^2 + n_8x + n_9 = 0 \end{cases} \tag{4}$$

Where m_i, n_i (i=1~9) are functions concerning the structure parameters and input variables. Based on Groebner base method, we can transform the polynomial equations (4) into triangularization standard base as follow:

$$\begin{cases} g_1(x)=0 \\ g_2(x\ ,y)=0 \end{cases} \tag{5}$$

$$g_1(x)=\sum_{i=0}^{8} s_i x^i=0,\quad g_2(x,y)=y+\sum_{i=0}^{7} t_i x^i=0$$

where, $s_i(i=0,1,\cdots,8)$, $t_i(i=0,1,\cdots,7)$ are functions concerning the structure parameters. We can get the symbolic solution of x, y by finding equation (5) and get α, β by back substituting the result into half-angle formulas. Then we can get the coordinate of point M_2, M_3 in fixed coordinate system by substituting the result into (1).

4 Manipulability Analyses

4.1 Jacobian Matrix

$\vec{\omega}$ is absolute angular velocity of upper platform, $\dot{l}_i(i=1,2,3)$ are driving velocity of the three telescopic links, $\vec{\omega}_i$ is angular velocity of driving link, $\vec{r}_i$ is a vector of point o_1 to hinges center M_1 and $\vec{e}_i=(\vec{M}_i-\vec{B}_i)/l_i$, $\vec{e}_x$, $\vec{e}_y$, $\vec{e}_z$ are unit vectors which along coordinate axis.

Because velocity of each hinges center Mi are equal, we can get:

$$\dot{l}_1\vec{e}_z+\vec{\omega}\times\vec{r}_i=l_i\vec{\omega}_i\times\vec{e}_i+\dot{l}_i\vec{e}_i \quad (i=2,3) \tag{6}$$

The dot product of $\vec{e}_i$ and (6) is as follow:

$$\vec{e}_i\cdot(\dot{l}_1\vec{e}_z+\vec{\omega}\times\vec{r}_i)=\dot{l}_i \quad (i=2,3) \tag{7}$$

And

$$\vec{\omega}=\omega_x\vec{e}_x+\omega_y\vec{e}_y \tag{8}$$

Substituting (8) into (7) and rewrite, we have:

$$[A][\theta]=[B][\varphi] \tag{9}$$

Where $[\theta]=[\dot{l}_1,\omega_y,\omega_x]^T$, $[\varphi]=[\dot{l}_1,\dot{l}_2,\dot{l}_3]^T$, $[A]=(a_{ij})\in R^{3\times3}$, $[B]=(b_{ij})\in R^{3\times3}$

a_{ij}, b_{ij} are functions concerning the structure and orientation parameters.

$$[\theta]=[A]^{-1}[B][\varphi]=[J][\varphi] \tag{10}$$

Let $\left[A\right]=\left[\vec{u}_1,\vec{u}_2,\vec{u}_3\right]$, if it have inverse matrix $\left[A\right]^{-1}$and it can be expressed as $\left[A\right]^{-1}=\left[\vec{u}_1^{\prime},\vec{u}_2^{\prime},\vec{u}_3^{\prime}\right]$, we have:

$$\vec{u}_1^{\prime}=\frac{\vec{u}_j\times\vec{u}_k}{\left(\vec{u}_j\times\vec{u}_k\right)\cdot\vec{u}_i} \tag{11}$$

Where, We can get the jacobian matrix $[J]=[A]^{-1}[B]$ by giving 1, 2, 3 to i , j, k in turn.

4.2 Evaluation of Manipulability

① Manipulability
We can evaluate manipulability based on jacobian matrix. The manipulability proposed by Yoshikawa is also suitable for parallel robot and mechanism which originally aim at series redundant robot. The manipulability is defined as follow:

$$W=\left|\det([J])\right|$$

Manipulability is a variable which can reflect the ability of parallel machine tool to achieve a poison and attitude and an index of judging the flexibility of machine tool in some poison and attitude. The parallel mechanism is in singular status when W=0 and in nonsingular status when W>0. We should avoid approaching singularity configuration because the flexibility gets minimum when the parallel mechanism is under the singularity configuration.

②Condition number
Salisbury puts forward to using the condition number of jacobian matrix as index of robot flexibility .In the paper, we adopt Frobenius norm and it defined as the evolution of square sum of each element. The condition number of jacobian matrix is defined as follow:

$$Cond([J])=\sqrt{tr([J]^{T}[J])}\cdot\sqrt{tr([J]^{-1T}[J]^{-1})}$$

Where tr is the matrix trace. It is a sum of each element which in diagonal line of matrix.

The condition number reflects the flexibility and maneuverability of parallel mechanism. The parallel mechanism can get best property of motion transmission when $Cond([J])=1$ and it is located at singularity configuration when $Cond([J])=\infty$.The condition number of matrix is an amplification factor of input rate relative deviation. So it is given with less value rate in the operation range.

5 Example

Case 1: The structure parameters of spatial parallel mechanism are listed as follow:
R =500mm, r =400mm, l_1 =500mm, l_2 =500mm, l_3=350mm,

Table 1. The real solution of forward position for spatial parallel mechanism

i	1	2	3	4
α	70.1513910	52.21973787	37.71268292	19.9180160
β	7.54440603	29.28271667	-30.51932061	-9.27315999

$\vec{M}_2' =$ (400mm,-400mm,-10mm), $\vec{M}_3' =$ (400mm, 400mm, 10mm),

$\vec{B}_2 =$ (500mm,-500,-10mm), $\vec{B}_3 =$ (500mm, 500mm, 10mm).

8 teams solution can be received based on Groebner base method. There are 4 teams real solution and 4 teams complex solution. Substituting the solutions into original equation, we can prove that the solution is right. We list the real solution in table 1.

Case2. The structure parameters of spatial parallel mechanism are listed as follow: l_1 =350mm, l_2 =350mm, l_3 =400mm and the other structure parameters are the same as case 2. The analysis of maneuverability as follow:

(1)The relationship between the circumradius of base platform R and manipulability when $\alpha = 27.06311722$, $\beta = 40.25357409$, l_1 =300mm are shown in figure 3.The relationship between R and manipulability are shown in figure 3(a) and there are relationships between R and condition number in figure3(b).
(2)The analysis of manipulability and condition number of some different positions and orientations are respectively shown in figure4 and figure 5. We can get the manipulability and condition number of mechanism when the center of upper platform M_1 is static and the upper platform only rotate around the X-axis in figure4 (a) and figure5 (a) .There are the manipulability and condition number of mechanism when the upper platform keep a fixed orientation and displace along Z-axis in figure4 (b) and figure5 (b) .The manipulability and condition number of mechanism when the center of upper platform M_1 is static and the upper platform only rotate around X-axis and Y-axis in figure4 (c) and figure 5(c).

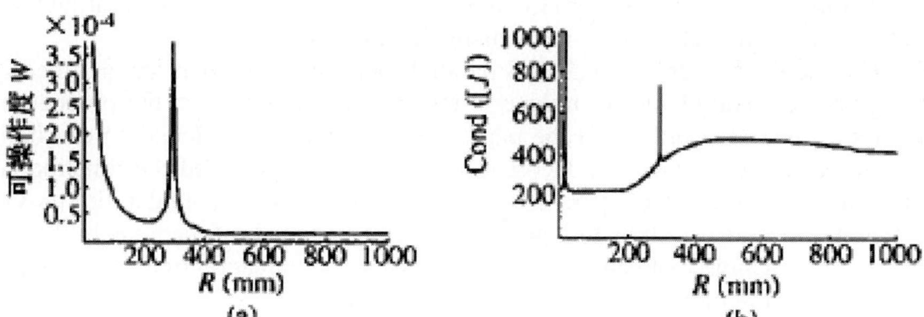

Fig. 3. The relationship between R and manipulability

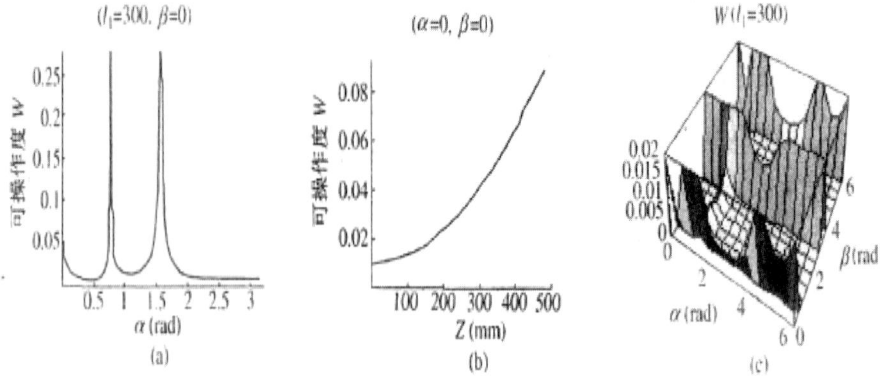

Fig. 4. The manipulability of position and orientation

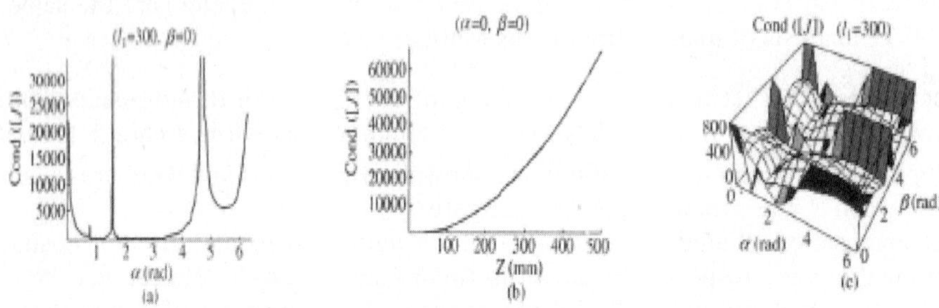

Fig. 5. Te condition number of position and orientation

6 Conclusions

(1) In this paper a set of origin equations are transformed into a set of equivalent triangularization equations by using Groebner base method and 8 terms solution to forward position for spatial parallel mechanism are obtained.

(2) The Jacobian matrixes of 3-RPS parallel mechanism are derived and the computer symbolic manipulating technique is introduced for transform the procedure of derivation to matrix operation in the paper. The efficiency of calculation can be improved because the elements of Jacobian matrix can be expressed the function concerning structure parameter. Effect of changing parameter on manipulability provides conveniently to study machine tool performance. The analysis of manipulability for 3-DOF parallel machine tool can be obtained by use two evaluation indexes (manipulability and condition number) base on Jacobian matrix.

(3) The relationship between circumradius and maneuverability can be obtained in the paper. The result obtained from the paper prove the machine tool have perfect manipulability, when circumradius change in some range.

References

1. Huang, L.B.: Research on kinematics of the robots' mechanism-including discussion of solving method for nonlinear algebra equations. Southeast university (2001)
2. Li, L., Chen, G.: Symbolic Approach for the Problems of Mechanism Based on Groebner Base Method. Mechanical Science and Technology for Aerospace Engineering 17, 5–7 (1998)
3. Liu, M.L.: Theory and Application of Groebner Basis. Science press (2000)
4. Yoshikawa, T.: Manipulability of robotic mechanisms. International Journal of Robotics Research 4(2), 3–9 (1987)
5. Salisburg, J.K., Craig, J.: Articulated hands kinematic and force control issues. International Journal of Robotics Research 1(2), 12–15 (1982)
6. Rao, Q., Bai, S.X.: Manipulability analysis and definition of 6_6 Steward Robot. Robot 16, 345–349 (1994)
7. Huang, Z., Kong, J.F., Fang, Y.F.: Mechanism theory and controlling system of parallel robot. China machine press (1997)
8. Fan, S.W., Xu, L.J.: Forward solution of position and analysis of working space for a new typed hybrid virtual axle machine tool. Machine Design 8, 27–29 (2002)
9. Fan, S.W., Xu, L.J.: Close Form Solution to Singularity Configuration of a New Type Parallel Machine Tool. Journal of University of Electronic Science and Technology of China 4, 369–373 (2002)
10. Xu, L.J., Fan, S.W., Xu, X.M.: A New Type of Hybird Five Degrees of Freedom Vitual Axis Machine Tool. China Patent ZL.01107247.4 (2003-08-6)

Application of High Speed Machining in Impeller Process

Mingjun Feng, Xuehui Wang, Can Zhao, and Guangbin Bu

College of Mechanical Engineering, Heilongjiang Institute of Science and Technology, Harbin, China, 150027
mingjunfeng.ky@163.com

Abstract. For improving previous compressor impeller's machining efficiency, the new process routine and tool parameters were adjusted by using high speed machining(HSM), which can decrease machining time and the types of tools. The high efficient machining process was proved by tests, and it had been shown that the time of machining was shorter. Improvement measures were taken to deal with the problems of vibration ripples which occurs in the improvement process.

Keywords: Impellor, HSM, Machining Process.

1 Introduction

Some compressor impeller used to adopt conventional processing methods machining,which can meet the yield requirements of not much order quantities.But with the increasing of order quantities and the decreasing cost, conventional processing should not meet the needs of market.How to improve the efficiency of impeller machining,reduce cost have made production decision maker puzzled a lot.

Making impeller machining process high speed has become a weapon to settle the above contradiction. But, whether it is simply to improve the speed can attain the object or not,whether it is the increase of machining speed can affect the quality of product,especially the decrease of fatigue life of high speed rotating impeller,which is the problem difficult to solve for each enterprise.Thus improving product machining efficiency considers not only the machining speed but also the whole process.

Our center adopts synthetical means which can improve machining efficiency 100% and reduce cost 30%.Consequently other enterprise also improve the process of high efficiency machining and achieve great economic benefits and social benefits.

2 Product Analyses

The working characteristics of impeller is high speed rotating,which has high requirements about dynamic balance,dimension precision,form and position precise for the parts.As shown on Fig.1.High requirements have been brought forward to machining :

C. Xiong et al. (Eds.): ICIRA 2008, Part II, LNAI 5315, pp. 1030–1037, 2008.

1)The contour of the impeller blade is obtained by rigor calculation,whose form and position precision should be ensured during the machining.Such complicated three dimension curved surface should only adopt multi-axis NC machining.

2)The impeller is mounted inside a small space of engine, which has high form precise request, such as the maximum external diameter flop less than 0.03mm, impeller face run out less than 0.01mm.

3)For the consideration of pneumatic efficiency, the requirement of impeller surface is high.

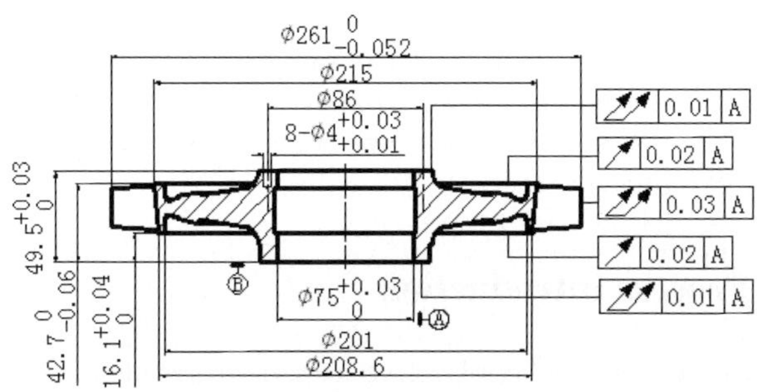

Fig. 1. Product process requirement diagram

The material of the impeller is 2A70 aluminum alloy which has better processability,but is easier to scratch and bump, whose rigidity is poor and is easier to appear vibration ripples.These all require us consider the arrangement of process carefully, improve product efficiency by the premise of assuring the quality.

3 Previous Process Introduction

The impeller has finalized many years,which is always processed with the conventional NC machining methods.The main process routine is shown as Fig.2.

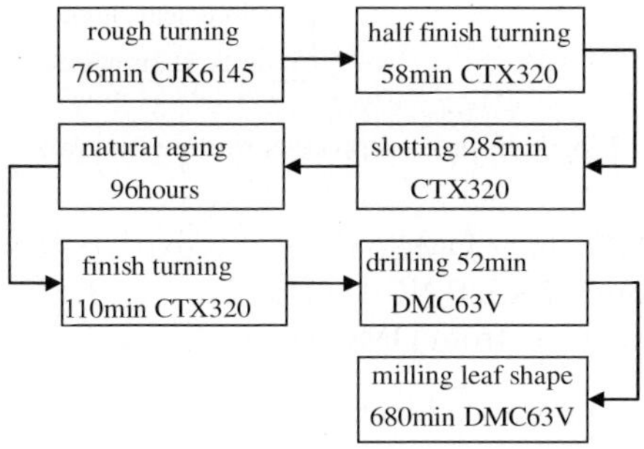

Fig. 2. Previous process routine diagram

The characteristics of the process are as follows:

1)Finishing three procedures on CTX320 NC lathe,which is easier to ensure the requirements of coaxiality radial run out and face run out.

2)Times of clamping are few,which reduce the conveying times of workpiece and avoid the possibility of scratch and bump by this means;

3)DMC63V is processed with drilling and milling leaf shape to ensure precise requirement;

4)The spaces of CTX320 is small,whose power axle output power is insufficient when slotting,which causes tool breaks many times due to the problem of chip removal and power,the time of slotting is longer;

5)Milling leaf shape adopts conventional four-axis NC machining center whose maximum speed is 10000rpm,machining efficiency is lower.

The above can be seen that the key to the process improving lies on slotting and milling leaf shape two procedures.

4 Improved Process Introduction

After the introduces of Mikron 600U (five-axis high speed machining center), the high speed process exploration has been developed.After trial and error,we adjust the process routine to achieve the improving efficiency by the premise of not changing procedure.

The improved process routine is shown as Fig.3, which has follow adjustments:

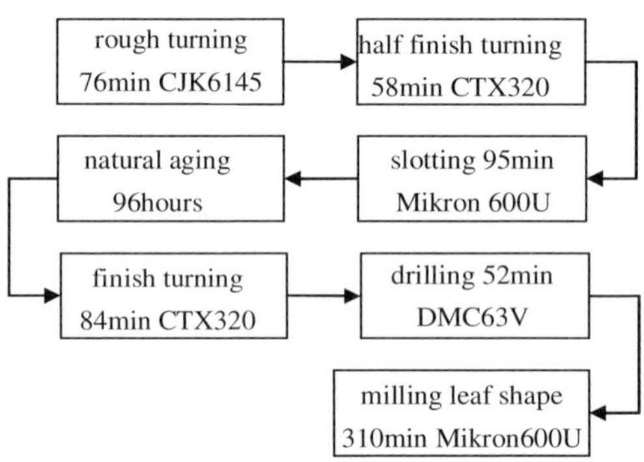

Fig. 3. Improved process routine diagram

1)Change four-axis NC center DMC63V to five-axis HSM Mikron600U.

2)Change slotting from CTX320 NC lathe to five-axis HSM Mikron600U.

3)Change milling leaf shape from DMC63V to five-axis HSM Mikron600U.

These adjustments have follow advantages:

1) Less machining time behaves two aspects:one is the greatly shorten of slotting time,from 285min reduce to 95min;the other is milling leaf shape time,because the increasing of spindle speed from 6500rpm to 10500rpm~16000rpm ,the feed speed

rises from 1300mm/min to 2100~3200mm/min,thus brings the greatly increasing of machining efficiency,the machining time reduces from 680min to 310min.

2) Less types of tools. It behaves two aspects: one is the reducing of special tool on CTX320 for slotting; the other is the cost reducing by reusing of dull tool which is used for milling leaf shape on CTX320 when slotting.

3) Less finishing time after the improved frock.

5 High Speed Process Implementation Theory Foundation

The real machining must have form process as the guidance,but the finalized product, the implement of new and high efficiency machining process must satisfy acceptance conditions or change better ,which need the support of theory and test.

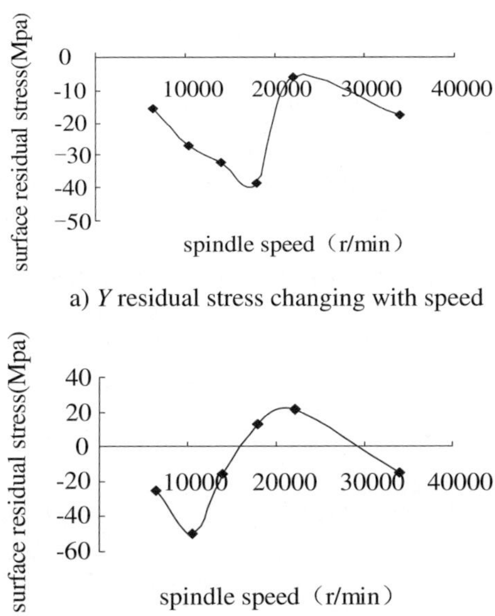

a) *Y* residual stress changing with speed

b)*X* residual stress changing with speed

Fig. 4. Surface residual stress change with spindle speed

The index of the machined surface quality is expressed as the characteristics and size of surface roughness[1], surface residual stress, surface work hardening and so on. Therefore ,before we set up the process ,we proceed and tests a lot.

The conclusion of test is as follows:

With the increasing of spindle speed, surface residual stress has made great changes (Fig.4). It occurs surface residual tensile stress when the speed rises to 18000r/min,which is not what we hope so.So we fix the speed under 18000r/min.

Figure 5 shows that the surface microstructure has not changed and the size of crystal grain is almost identical with the changing of machining speed. We also find

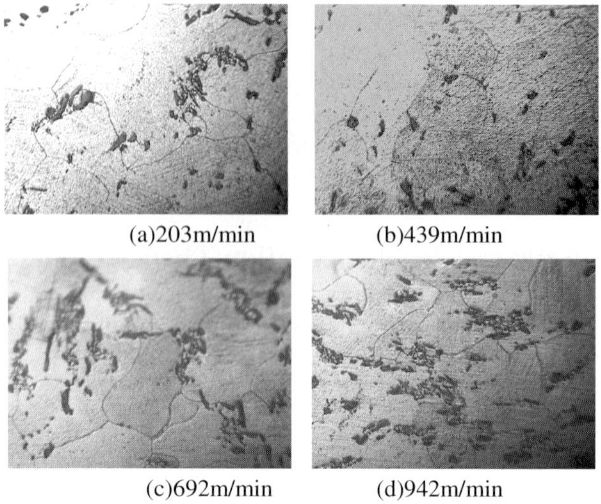

Fig. 5. Surface microstructure at each speed

that the leaf surface does not appear surface layer microcrack though fluorescent inspection.From these two aspects we can make a conclusion that the changing of machining speed has few influence on the fatigue property of product.

The surface roughness has the trend of decrease with the increase of machining speed,but it will be in a stable state when the machining speed rises to definite extents(> 400m/s)[2].This shows that the increase machining speed avails to the improvement of product quality from the aspects of surface roughness,which is of great advantage to the improvement of process.

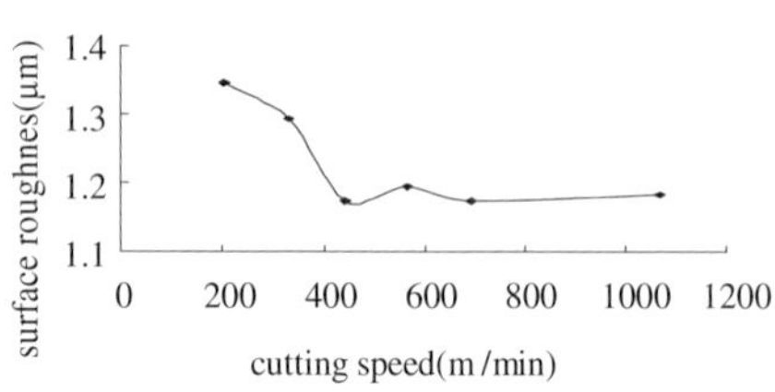

Fig. 6. Changes of surface roughness

Surface hardness is increasing with the improved machining speed, which appears maximum hardness about 420m/min. And followed the phenomenon of the decrease of hardness, appears minimum hardness at almost 570m/min.According to the principle of similarity compared with previous product,we select the machining hardness above previous field as machining field(dashed as Fig.7)

It can be found by the tests that above items are close or better than previous process product,which establish an important basis for high speed process and also can carry out new process for the product machining.

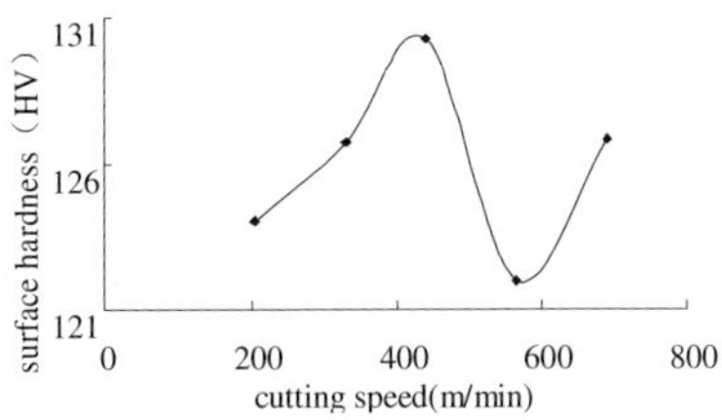

Fig. 7. Changes of surface hardness

6 Specific Improvement Measures

6.1 Slotting

According to the deficiency of output power of power axles about original process, UG software reprogram has been adopted to change slotting procedure to proceed on MikronHSM600U.The main work includes as follows:

1)Using UG software program realize four-axis machining.

2)Using HSM strategy of small cutting depth and deep-feed make cutting force and heat less,distortion less.

3)Using integrated horniness alloy end mill slotting at the upper of slot leads to less machining resist force and higher efficiency;adopting finish dull ball mill at the root of slot machining not only meet the requirement of leaf foot fillet but also realize the reuse of tool ,reduce product cost.

4)Making full advantage of high speed spindle of the equipment improves machining efficiency.

5)Utilizing the frock of leaf machining decreases the number of design and manufacture of frock, reduces cost.

6.2 Milling Leaf Shape

The efficiency of original milling leaf shape procedure is limited by spindle speed and each axle response speed.With the introduction of new equipment,the study of high speed leaf shape milling process has been brought into effect.Beacuse the programming of five-axis consumes lots of times and need do more tests,we decide to proceed high speed based on present four-axis program.This has follow advantages:

1)Utilizing the high speed properties of equipment increases machining speed and feed speed,improves product efficiency effectively.

2)Improving bases on previous program which optimize parameters of speed , feed and so on,the work is less.As the contents of program has no changes,so does the tool path and the shape of leaf,the quality of product has good guarantee.

This method also has shortage, that is it does not change the machining method,inherit the limitation of original conventional machining,can not adjust tool path to the change of high speed machining.

In order to overcome these shortages we must adopt five-axis NC programming. At present, we are in the study of NC programming and make great progress[3].If it succeeds,which must go to a new step for efficiency and quality.

6.3 Problem Occurred in Improvement of Process and Disposal Measurement

With the increasing of machining speed, the quality problem also occurs .All kinds of process means have been taken according to these problems.

The root of leaf occurs linear ripples as Fig.8.Improvement instruments is to adopt four blades ball milling tool machining, increase the pressure flux of cooling fluid, change the direction of spraying, make cooling fluid spray to the top of tool and avoid the shelter of adjacent leaf. Thus the root leaf ripples does not appear.

The machining of top leaf edge is easier to appear vibration ripples as Fig.9. Three aspects can be started with [4]:firstly, the proper selecting of tool which will be narrated on the followings; secondly, the decreasing of input excited energy through matching parameters of machining reasonably so that avoid the appearances of ripples; thirdly,dividing leaf into upper and lower two sections,the upper 5mm field adopts 10500r/min machining, the lower adopts 15000r/min.Therefore the differences between two speed are small ,the link field has no evident difference.

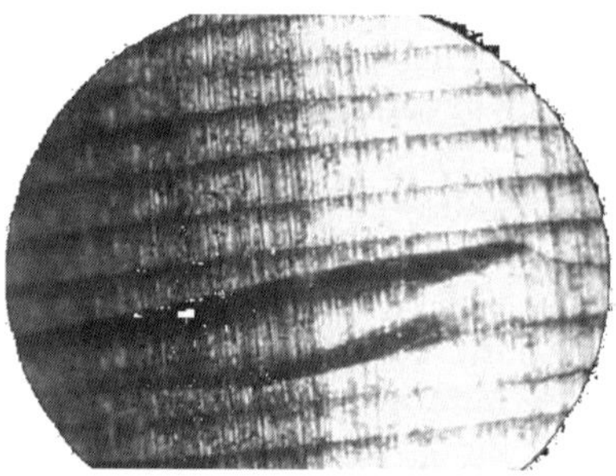

Fig. 8. Root leaf ripple micrograph

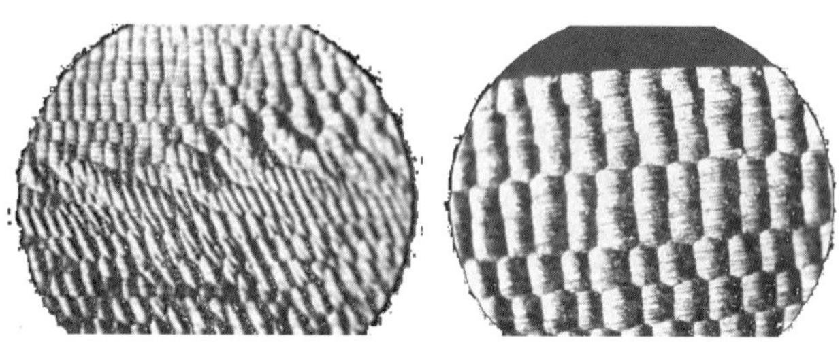

a) vibration texture b) normal machining texture

Fig. 9. Top leaf surface texture

The two face run out of hub oversize. Improvement measure is to design special frock and use special tool and clamp only once.

$8-\phi 4^{+0.03}_{+0.01}$ Aperture oversize,surface scratches. Improvement measure is to select special combination drilling and reaming integration tool.

6.4 Tool Selection

In order to solve the vibration problem brought by the changing of HSM process, many tool parameters has been tested to select most suitable one.

Two kinds of horniness alloy tool materials are tested about several tool angles:one is Lanzhi 10F,the other is Zigong YG6X.The tool is selected from which does not ripples on leaf surface.The result of test is shown as table 1.

It is found that there is no evident difference between the two kinds of materials by means of test.Consider the cost, we finally select Zigong tool material.

Table 1. Parameters and results of tool test

Diameter (mm)	No.	rake angle (°)	relief angle (°)	helical angle (°)	slot deep (mm)	edge (mm)	machining condition
φ10	1	8	10	45	2.6	0.8	ripples
	2	8	12	45	2.3	0.5	ripples
	3	8	12	40	2.3	0.3	ripples
	4	12	14	40	2.0	0.5	no ripples

7 Conclusion

The common methods of impeller high speed machining has been studied,which grope one way of improvement for impeller high speed machining process.

It is necessary to fully master the product before improving the process to ensure the final property of product invariability.So the test is very essential.The process improvement is based on that and advance step by steps should be obeyed during the improvement.For example,the increasing of speed is based on the original program and changes little, based on which explore five-axis machining.

It is necessary to find the source of problems carefully and propose improvement opinions when the process problems occur. Doing some process tests to find the key to questions is very essential.

References

1. Wang, X.: Mechanical Manufacture Technology. China Machine Press, Beijing (1995) (in Chinese)
2. Zhang, S., Liu, S., Bu, G.: Experimental Research on Surface Roughness of Aluminum Alloy Blade in HSM. J. Tool Engineering 41, 21–24 (2007) (in Chinese)
3. Jiang, R.: Integral Impeller Machining Tool-path Planning and NC Program Automatic Generation. Harbin Institute of Technology, Harbin (2007) (in Chinese)
4. Jia, X.: Method of Elimination Thin Workpiece Ripples. Machinist Metal Cutting 23, 3 (1984)

The Influence of Material Removal on the Modal Change of Blade

Guangbin Bu[1], Can Zhao[2], Dunwen Zuo[1], and Min Wang[1]

[1] College of Mechanical & Electrical Engineering, Nanjing University of Aeronautics & Astronautics, Nanjing, China, 210016
buguangbin@sina.com

[2] College of Mechanical Engineering, Heilongjiang Institute of Science and Technology, Harbin, China, 150027
canzhao@sohu.com

Abstract. The influence of material removal on the modal change of blade was investigated by FEM simulation and experiment. It was found that the modal of blade was complex. Natural frequency of blade distributed nonuniform: it was denseness in some areas and sparseness in others. Frequency was changed with the material removal: modal frequency decreased with the material removal in whole manufacture process; decreased slope appeared at the process beginning and it was became decreased slowly at the middle and end of process. The machined surface was defaced because cutting force frequency was near some state's modal frequency and resonance was arisen. Base one this research, the spindle speed was changed with the manufacture proceed. The rate of blade finished products was improved by this way.

Keywords: impeller blades, modal, HSM.

1 Instruction

Blade type part was a curve surface thin wall cantilever. The stiffness of it was weak and was easy to vibrate. The vibration of blade was arisen under the drive of periodic cutting force and friction force between cutter and workpiece in the milling process, so the final surface was defaced. In order to solve the problem, a lot of method was used in manufacture practice, such as: appropriate tool chosen, cutting parameters chosen, cutting fluid chosen, and so on. Those methods had blindness in a way, because it had not been investigated that the change of blade vibrates with the material removal. It often got half the result with twice the effort.

The cutting parameters were chosen base on the designed modal frequency in traditional blade manufacture process. But, the designed modal frequency was according to the final state of manufacture, the influence of roughcast was not taken into consideration. This caused the limitation of cutting parameters, and arose cutting vibration in somewhere on the cutting surface. The method of trial and error was often used to solve this problem in machining practice, a series of experiments were done, and a set of relative reasonable parameters was chosen. So the parameters always were conservative with low cutting efficiency.

C. Xiong et al. (Eds.): ICIRA 2008, Part II, LNAI 5315, pp. 1038–1046, 2008.

2 FEM Modal Simulation

Analysis of structure natural vibration is also called modal analysis. This analysis was used to recognize the mode shape and frequency of structure. Any structure or part all has natural frequency and corresponding mode shape. These belong to the natural characters of the structure or part. The fact of modal analysis is calculation of eigenvalues and the eigenvectors of vibration characteristic equation [1].

Typical non-damping free vibration equation is

$$[M]\left\{\ddot{X}\right\}+[K]\{X\}=0 \tag{1}$$

Where $[M]$ is mass matrix, $[K]$ is rigidity matrix, $\left\{\ddot{X}\right\}$ is accelerate vector, $\{X\}$ is displacement vector.

If $\{X\}=\{\phi\}\sin(\omega t+\varphi)$, then $\left\{\ddot{X}\right\}=-\omega^2\{\phi\}\sin(\omega t+\varphi)$, they are substituted into equation (1), we obtain equation (2).

$$([K]-\omega^2\{M\})\{\phi\}=0 \tag{2}$$

Equation (2) is called vibration characteristic equation. Modal analysis wants to solve this equation and obtain egenvalues ω_i and the eigenvectors $\{\phi_i\}$ of it.

Through a series formula derivations, the result has obtained as (3) shown.

$$\omega_i^2=\frac{\{\varphi\}_i^T[K]\{\varphi\}_i}{\{\varphi\}_i^T[M]\{\varphi\}_i}=\frac{k_i}{m_i} \tag{3}$$

Where k_i is modal stiffness, m_i is modal mass.

From equation (3) we can see, natural frequency is decided by modal stiffness and modal mass. And those two is decided by rigidity matrix, mass matrix and modal eigenvectors. In the manufacture process, rigidity matrix and mass matrix change with material removal, also the modal eigenvectors changes. There is some internal relationship between them. While one changes, others also change. It is too complex to give out an analytic relationship with an equation. So we used FEM to do some qualitative analysis about modal change with material removal.

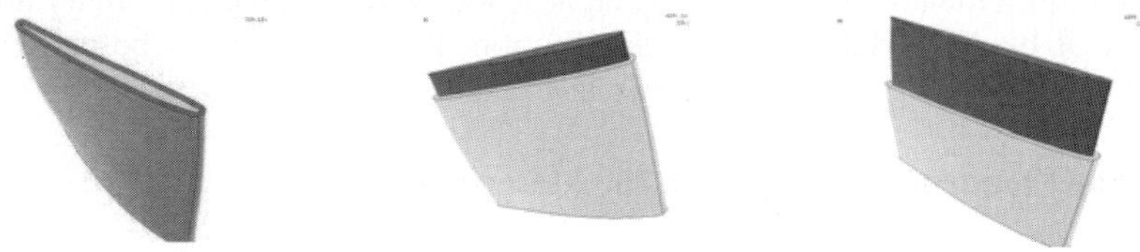

(a) Uncut model (b) Cut 5mm model (c) Cut 15mm model

Fig. 1. Blade model of simulation

Modal simulation is use FEM to solve equation (2). ANSYS was used as FEM tool to obtain modal result in this research.

Roughcast model was built to simulate the material removal process. As Fig.1 (a) shown, the model inside was the design model of blade, out it was the roughcast. Cutting process is continuous roughcast removal process, as Fig1 (b) & (c) shown.

2.1 Decides the Section of Modal Frequency

The max spindle speed of milling center was 42000rmp, and four teeth mill was used. So the max frequency of cutting force was: $42000/60\times4=2800$ Hz. According to this result, the section of frequency in FEM simulation set as 0Hz~3000Hz.

After model built, meshed and solved, following results were obtained.

2.2 Modal Frequency Distribution

There were 25 ranks of modal in the set frequency section in uncut model's FEM simulation. If the difference value of two ranks modal frequency was less than 30Hz, we defined them were close section. There were two close sections in Fig.2 as the squares shown. If the difference value of two ranks modal frequency was less than 50Hz, we consider them were secondary–close section. There were four secondary-close sections in Fig.2 as the triangles shown.

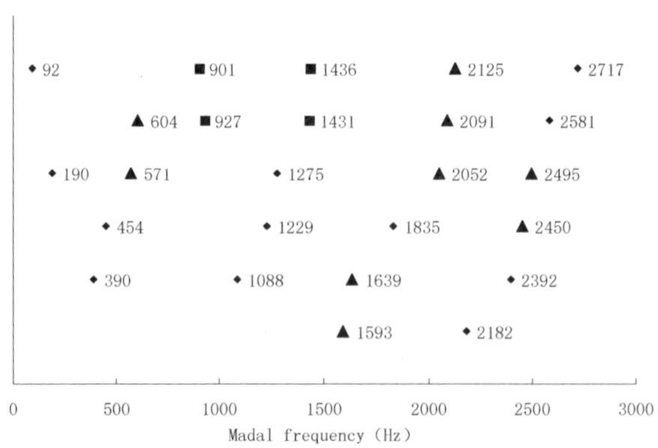

Fig. 2. Modal frequency distribution of uncut model

The requirement of spindle speed chosen was arisen by the catholicity and heterogeneity of blade modal frequency distribution. It was avoided to be chosen that the frequency close range and secondary close range.

2.3 The Frequency Change with the Material Removal

As equation (3) shown, the frequency was decided by modal mass and modal stiffness. Those two factors were changed with material removal, so the frequency changed. While the decrease of modal mass was superiority, modal frequency was inclined to go up; otherwise modal frequency was inclined to go down.

The curve of modal frequency change with the material removal was obtained by FEM simulation, as Fig.3 shown.

Following conclusion could be made from Fig.3:

① Modal stiffness was inclined to drop and dropped faster than modal mass with material removal in whole manufacture process. So every rank modal frequency presented a dropped incline in whole process. The main drop was happened at the beginning of cutting process (cutting height less than 10mm). In this stage, several ranks of frequency dropped sharply. This illustrated that modal stiffness dropped sharply. Out this range, frequency dropped smoothly, and the modal stiffness dropped relative slowly.

② Modal mass was also dropped with material removal. It was in a secondary condition compared with modal stiffness. But in the area frequency line was horizontal, modal mass and modal stiffness dropped at same rate. In the area frequency line went up, modal mass dropped fast than modal stiffness.

③ Frequency interval of two interfacing rank became closer with material removal.

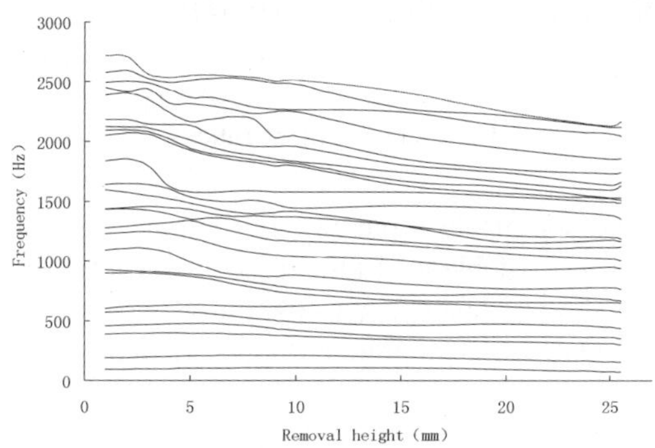

Fig. 3. Change of modal frequency with material removal

3 Experiment Research

3.1 Experiment System

The whole measure system was built up with impact sinker, MTI KD300 Fotonic sensor, USB data collection system, uTek modal analysis software, computer and assistant clamp and so on [2], as Fig.4 shown.

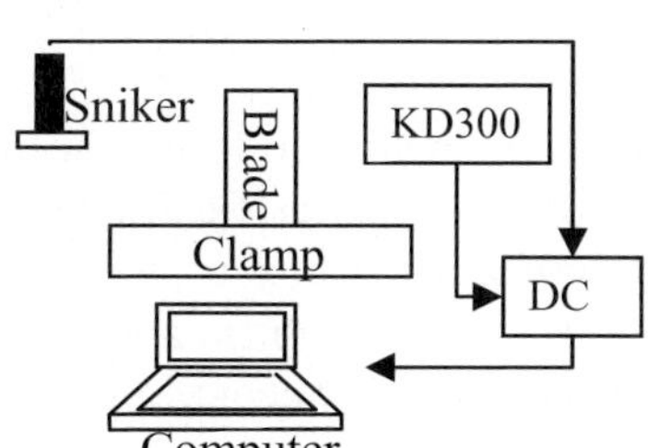

Fig. 4. Experiment system

3.2 Experiment Process

Six blades with different state were cut with WEDM, as fig.5 shown. Their states respectively were: rough (1#), cut 1 circle (2#), cut 3 circles (3#), cut 6 circles (4#), cut 25 circles (5#), finished (6#). There was a section of wheel at the end of each blade, as holder for clamp. The integer weight of blade and holder is less than 50 gram. It was clamped in a table vice. Optical fiber was maintained in a milscale adhere on the table vice by the magnet. It was 1mm that the distance between the end of fibre and surface of blade by adjust the milscale. After connected the equipment as fig.4 shown, the test of modal could begin.

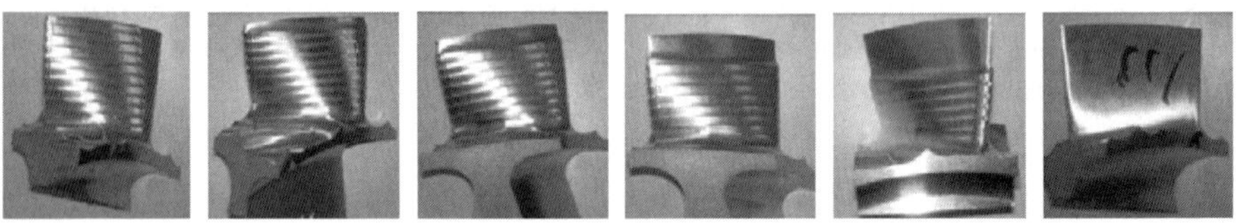

(a) 1# (b) 2# (c) 3# (d) 4# (e) 5# (f) 6#

Fig. 5. Experiment Blades

The method of MISO (Multiple Input Single Output) was used to earn the mode shape and modal frequency of blade. Eight input positions were equispaced on the back of blade, as Fig.6 shown. The out put position was on the middle of blade front. The weight of impact sinker was 100 gram equipped with an aluminum alloy head.

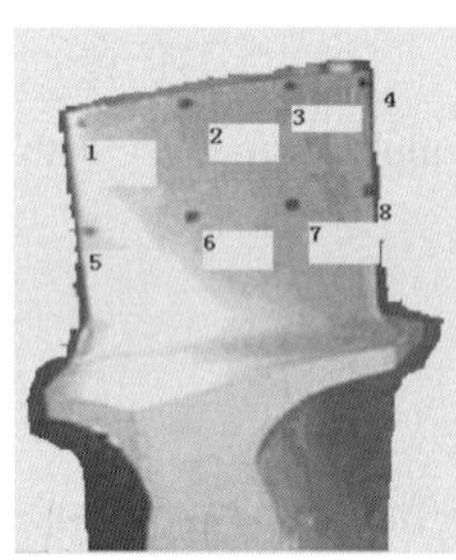

Fig. 6. Input position

3.3 Experiment Result

This type blade has a lot of levels modal, 10 levels modal were detected in this experiment. The frequency distribution was as fig.7 shown. The distribution was not symmetrical, the section of 400Hz~1200Hz was sparse, there were only two levels; while the section of 1200Hz~1600Hz was thick, and there were three levels. Thickness or sparseness limited the spindle speed choice, more sparse more choice.

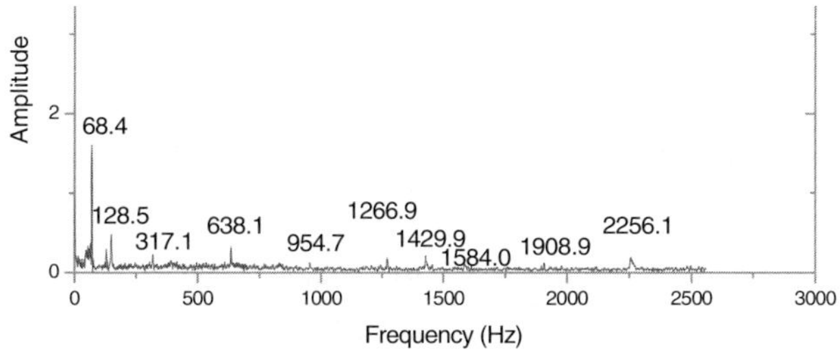

Fig. 7. The frequency distribution of 1#

The experiment demonstrated that every level frequency decreased with the material removed. We focused on the frequency near the cutting force frequency (about 1200Hz) which was frequency of rank 5, 6, and 7.

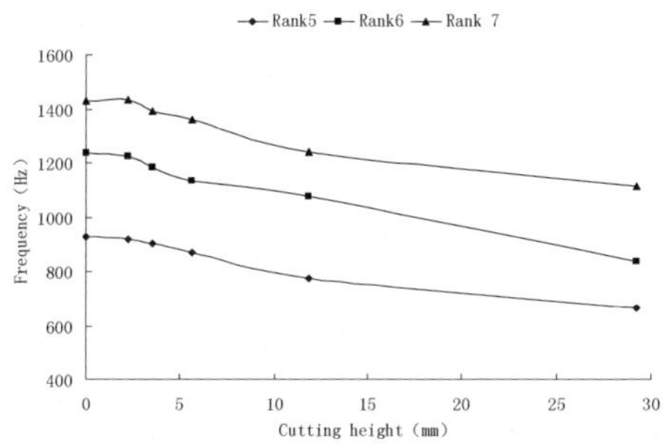

Fig. 8. Frequency change of with material removal

3.4 Compare with FEM Simulation

Frequency could be detect in experiment was compared with the simulation's in Table.1. We found that, the error between them was small; the maximal error is 79Hz; the minimum error is 5Hz; mean error is 32Hz. So the FEM simulation was reliable.

Errors were produced by these two reasons. First, material in ANSYS modal simulation is an elastic body without any damp, but the aluminum alloy is a damp alloy. Second, there was some inaccuracy between model of simulation and actual blade.

N/A in Table.1 refers to the modal frequency was not detected by experiment. Because the experiment was a MISO test, there were many ranks of undetected frequency. If want to avoid this, the method MIMO (Multi Input Multi Output) must be used.

Table 1. Modal frequency compare

Unit:Hz

Rank	1	2	3	4	5	6	7	8	9	10	11
Test	68	128	317	N/A	N/A	N/A	638	N/A	954	N/A	1266
FEM	73	156	302	355	436	570	648	762	940	1163	1185
Error	5	28	15	N/A	N/A	N/A	10	N/A	14	N/A	79

Table 1. *(continue)*

Rank	12	13	14	15	16	17	18	19	10	21
Test	N/A	1429	N/A	N/A	1584	N/A	N/A	1903	N/A	2256
FEM	1355	1487	1509	1533	1630	1661	1739	1858	2045	2279
Error	N/A	58	N/A	N/A	46	N/A	N/A	45	N/A	23

In whole material removal process, the FEM result coincided to the experiment result, as FIg.9 shown.

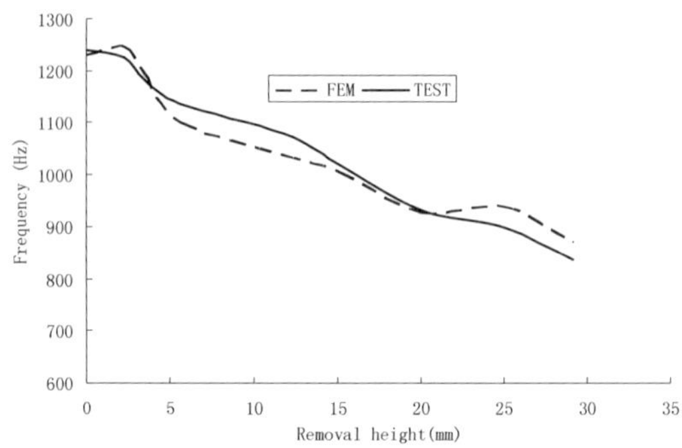

Fig. 9. Test and FEM frequency compare of rank 11

4 Thc Influence of Blade Modal

There are two types of cutting vibration. One is chatter, the other is resonance. The typical character of resonance is that outside force's frequency is near some rank of natural frequency of the system. Resonance destroyed surface of the blade [3,4]. If the resonance was avoided the rate of blade finished products would be improved. Base on this theory, our research can be used to determine the spindle speed of blade manufacture.

To choose the spindle speed, following experiment was done. First the frequency was changed modal frequency to spindle speed, Fig.10 was obtained. Some unused line was deleted to make the figure clear. 16krmp and 30krmp were chosen as the spindle speed, as dash line in Fig.10. While the blade was machined, we predicted that the vibration would happen at 3.8mm according to 16kmp, and 3.8mm~5.2mm according to 30kmp.

After machining, the blade was observed and measured under a microscope to find the vibration position. As Fig.11 shown, the vibration section of 16krpm is from 2.8mm to 3.7mm, the middle position is 3.3mm; the section of 30krmp is form 4.2mm to 5.8mm, the middle position is 5.0mm. The position error was 0.5mm to 16kmp, and 0.4 to 30krmp. Consider the average modal error between FEM and test (32Hz, according to spindle speed is 480rmp), less than 1mm is an acceptable error [5]. So we could say our prediction was successful.

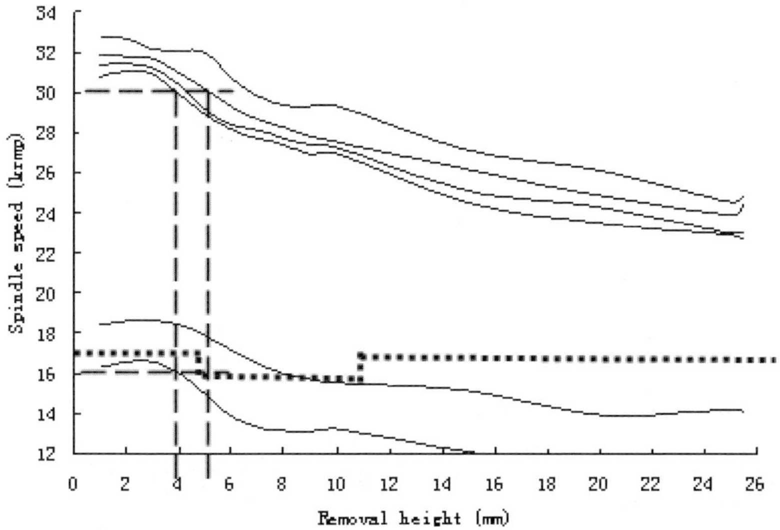

Fig. 10. Vibrate spindle speed change with material removal

As dot line show, the spindle speed in blade manufacture practice was changed to avoid the vibration. After machined over 10mm, the speed can be increase more because the stiffness increased at the cutter contacting position. But if the deferent value of two spindle speed is more than 2000rmp, there is an obvious unacceptable line on the surface of blade. So the speed was chosen as dot line. The rate of blade finished products was improved form 60% to 99% by this way.

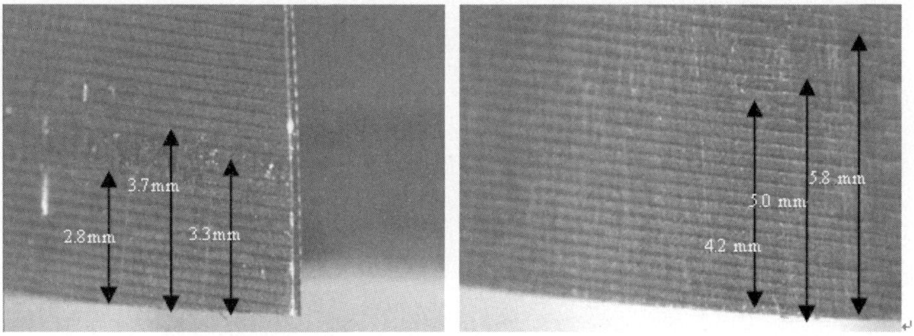

(a) Machined with 16kmp (b) Machined with 30kmp

Fig. 11. The vibration position of machining

5 Conclusions

It is not neglectable that the influence of material removal on the modal change of blade while machining it. Modal changed very complex can not be expressed by a formula. FEM is a good method to analysis the modal change, and it has a reliable accuracy. Base on the result of FEM, the vibration can be predicted and the manufacture spindle speed can be recommended.

References

1. Zhang, J., Liu, X.: Principle and Numerical Methods of modal analysis to Turbomachinase. National Defence Industry Press, Beijing (2001) (in chinese)
2. Heylen, W., Larmnaese, S., Sas, P.: Modal Analysis Theory and Testing. Beijing Insistute of Technology Press, Bejing (2001) (in chinese)
3. Li, L., Zha, W.-w.: Influence of Chatter on High-speed Milling of the Thin-wall Components. Journal of Yancheng Institute of Technology (Natural Science Edition) 19(2), 9–13 (2006) (in chinese)
4. Wang, T., He, N., Li, L.: Vibration In High-speed Milling of Thin-wall compments. Transactions of Nanjing University of Aeronautics & Astronautics 24(2), 112–117 (2007)
5. Song, Q., Ai, X., Yu, S.: Research on Stability and Surface Finish In High-speed Milling Process. Manufacturing Technology & Machine Tool 4, 40–43 (2008) (in chinese)

Research on Cutting Parameters Optimization of High-Speed Milling Based on Orthogonal Experiment

Yubo Liu, Can Zhao, Jinping Hu, and Mingjun Feng

Mechanical Engineering Department, Heilongjiang Institute of Science and Technology, Harbin 150027, China
{Yubo Liu,Can Zhao,Jinping Hu,Mingjun Feng}ysclx@126.com

Abstract. This article takes aluminum alloy(2A70)impeller as a high speed cutting test, chooses the cemented carbide cutters, the influences of different cutting on the roughness of blade finished surface was analyzed and investigated. First using orthogonal array for multi-factor analyses the effect of each factor in high-speed milling, then adopting the range analytical method to analyze the trial results, and point out the primary and secondary influence order of each factor to the surface roughness, and determine the most superior cutting condition. The experimental results show that best surface roughness can be obtained by selecting the appropriate cutting parameters for the aluminum alloy impeller vane. The experimental results also show that there is a definite significance to guide how to choose milling parameters for curved face's high speeding machining.

Keywords: high-speed milling; aluminum alloy; surface roughness; cutting parameters.

1 Introduction

High-speed cutting technology is one of processing technology whose main characteristics are high cutting speed, high feed speed and high processing accuracy, the development is more rapid nearly 20 years and it's the direction of advanced manufacturing technology development. With the development of high-speed machining technology, the cutting surface quality analysis and control of advanced manufacturing technology is that one of the issues to be resolved. In high-speed milling, machine cutting parameters optimization related to product quality, processing efficiency and processing economy, has been the focus of high-speed cutting research over the years. From the viewpoint of kinetics, high-speed cutting system is a complex dynamic system [1].With the improvement of cutting speed, dynamic characteristics in high-speed cutting and the general rate cutting is quite different. People encountered insurmountable obstacles in raising cutting speed is that the machine will be in a strong vibration when cutting speed is much lower than the maximum speed, that is cutting instability, in addition to the rapid tool wear and damage, the existence of this phenomenon will leave vibration ripples on the surface, affects surface processing precision and surface roughness, even damage to themselves or tools, machine equipment, the cutting can not continue, therefore, measures must be taken to curb vibration in surface processing, so that the advantages of high efficiency,

C. Xiong et al. (Eds.): ICIRA 2008, Part II, LNAI 5315, pp. 1047–1055, 2008.

high-precision processing and low-cost of high-speed cutting application are in full play, thus enable high-speed machining technology further promoting use in production [2]. At present, high-speed cutting parameters can not be selected like ordinary cutting through cutting manual, high-speed processing has no integral process parameters table and high-speed cutting database. In actual production, according to processing materials, processes features and others, determine the best cutting speed and feed rate through testing [3].Cutting parameters optimization is from the high-speed cutting process in-depth and systematic study.

From the viewpoint of dialectical materialism and cutting research development, various cutting elements have inevitable link, and they are interaction and mutual influence, to profoundly understand and grasp these links, a great deal of arduous research and testing are needed, CNC machine tools in cutting process, to reduce the vibration technology system to ensure that cutting stability and improve the processing parts surface quality, we must optimize the cutting parameters.

Parts surface rough is an important indicator to measure parts quality and machining performance, and the current high-speed cutting surface roughness formation mechanism is not perfect. So through cutting experiment, study the impact factors of high-speed cutting surface roughness, find the best machine cutting parameters.

2 Orthogonal Experiment

Orthogonal experiment has been used widely in engineering analysis to optimize performance characteristics by means of settings of design parameters. Orthogonal experiment is also strong tool for the design of high quality systems. Optimize designs are for quality, performance, and cost. Orthogonal experiment presents a systematic approach that is simple and effective. Orthogonal experiment was developed by Taguchi. It involves the stages of system design, parameters design, and tolerance design. System design involves the application of scientific and engineering knowledge required in manufacturing a product; parameter design is employed to find optimal process values for improving the quality characteristics; and tolerance design consists of determining and analyzing tolerances in the optimal settings recommended by parameter design. In this study, parameter design is adopted to achieve the optimal levels of process parameters that lead to low surface roughness [4].

By applying orthogonal experiment based on orthogonal arrays, the time and cost of experiments can be reduced. Here, Orthogonal experiment methods a special design of orthogonal arrays to learn the whole parameter space with only a small number of experiments. Taguchi recommends the use of the S/N ratio for the determination of the quality characteristics implemented in engineering design problems. The S/N ratio for the determination of the quality characteristics implemented in engineering design problems. The S/N ratio characteristics can be divided into three stages: smaller the better, nominal the best and larger the better, signed-target type. Since the purpose of this study is to minimize surface roughness within the optimal levels of process parameters, the smaller the better quality characteristic is selected.

In addition to the S/N ratio, a statistical analysis of variance can be employed to indicate the impact of process parameters on surface roughness. In this way, the optimal levels of process parameters can be estimated. The results of the aforementioned subjects are given in the following sections.

3 Experiment Scheme Design

3.1 Experimental Conditions

The experiment is done in HSM600 CNC 5-axis high-speed machining centre made in Switzerland Mikron, CNC system is Heidenhain ITNC530. Parts for processing are impeller blades, spindle up to 42000r/min, feed rate 40m/min, positioning accuracy 0.008mm, repeat positioning accuracy 0.005mm.

Experiment material is aluminum alloy (2A70), cutting tools used of ball-cutter ground by carbide alloy rods 30F, blade length 13 mm, cutter length 32 mm, the number of teeth 4, radius 5 mm, total length 114.6 mm. Choose tool material strength and toughness, strong thermal shock resistance and dynamic balance experiments have been done, can be used for high-speed cutting. SJ-201P surface roughness detector made in Japan MITUTOYO is used for detection installations, digital filtering can be satisfied with the results, high-precision surface roughness testing can be completed, measurement range -200 to +150.

3.2 Experimental Environment

Working conduction: shop temperature23℃,relative humidity 52℃ ~ 55℃, machine idling, vibration sensor vibration acceleration 0.3G, fixture revolving round beating ≤ 0.002mm, cutting tool surface integrity after cutting and no wear, experiment using fuel-air cooling.

3.3 Experimental Method

In high-speed machining, there are many impact factors for machined surface roughness such as processing, work piece materials, cutting tool materials cutting parameters and so on plays an important role. Judging from the current situation, the biggest affecting factor for high-speed milling parts surface quality is cutting parameters, the correct choice of cutting parameters can effectively increase productivity and ensure the necessary processing quality and economy.

This test has been used in parts processing procedures, machines blade surface by changing cutting parameters cutting surface, according to actual production situation and manufacturers recommend, select the testing cutting speed from 2100 mm/min to5400mm/min, cutting step 0.2mm ~ 0.4mm, each tooth feed rate 0.02mm / tooth ~ 0.08mm/tooth. Experiment factors and level as shown in table 1.

Table 1. Experiment factors level

Level	*A* Feed rate (mm/min)	*B* Feed per tooth (mm/tooth)	*C* Depth of cut (mm)
1	2100	0.02	0.2
2	3600	0.05	0.3
3	5400	0.08	0.4

It's an experiment design of 3 factors and 3 levels, so 3 levels orthogonal table is choose. Only 3 factors, otherwise there are four columns in $L_9(3^4)$ orthogonal table, it's entirely arranged. Test data, surface roughness values and S/N recorded in table 2.

Table 2. Experiment design using of $L_9(3^4)$ orthogonal array

Level	*A* Feed rate (mm/min)	*B* Feed per tooth (mm/tooth)	*C* Depth of cut (mm)	Empty series	R_a values (μm)	S/N ratio (dB)
1	1(2100)	1(0.02)	1(0.2)	1	1.39	- 2.86
2	1(2100)	2(0.05)	2(0.3)	2	1.27	- 2.08
3	1(2100)	3(0.08)	3(0.4)	3	1.31	- 2.34
4	2(3600)	1(0.02)	2(0.3)	3	1.11	- 0.91
5	2(3600)	2(0.05)	3(0.4)	1	1.51	- 3.58
6	2(3600)	3(0.08)	1(0.1)	2	1.21	- 1.66
7	3(5400)	1(0.02)	3(0.4)	2	1.19	- 1.51
8	3(5400)	2(0.05)	1(0.2)	3	1.16	- 1.29
9	3(5400)	3(0.08)	2(0.3)	1	1.47	- 3.35

4 Data Analysis of Orthogonal Experiment

Arrange test by using orthogonal table is representative, more fully reflect various factors and level's impact for indicators, and so experiment with orthogonal arrangement can reduce the number of tests. Then signal to noise ratio (S/N) as a indicator to measure product quality sounds, through statistical analysis of various test method to identify strong anti-interference capability and good adjustment, stable performance best parameters combination for improving product quality.

4.1 Data Calculation

In the analysis of signal and interference ratio, performance characteristics can be divided into smaller-the-better characteristic, smaller-the-better characteristic and definite purposed characteristic. The value of S/N shows products are interfere lever with noise factor in the production process, therefore, greater S/N value, the products less noise factor interference to produce better products [5]. The smallest surface roughness is achieved in this test through optimizing cutting parameters; therefore, quality characteristic is used for smaller-the-better characteristic in this article. Smaller-the-better characteristic calculation formula:

$$\eta = 10\lg\frac{1}{\frac{1}{n}\sum_{i=1}^{n} Y_i^2} = -10\lg\left(\frac{1}{n}\sum_{i=1}^{n} Y_i^2\right) \tag{1}$$

Where n is the number of tests; Y_i is the value of surface roughness for the i th test.

The R_a values measured from the experiments and the S / N ratio values are listed in Table 2, for determining factors effects on response. Below analyzes the primary and secondary order impact on the indicators from various factors and the optimal combination factors with level by extremum difference analysis.

The R_a response table for each level of the process parameters was created in an integrated manner, the R_a response results are given in Table 3. On the other hand, the same procedure for the S/N response table was applied; the S/N response results are listed in Table 4.

In Table 3, k_{ij} expressed the sum of test indicators data of corresponding level i in j column of the of the, i = 1, 2, 3, for example, A column, $k_{11}=1.39+1.27+1.31=3.97$; B column, $k_{12}=1.39+1.11+1.19=3.69$; C column, $k_{12}=1.39+1.21+1.16=3.76$; $\bar{k}_{ij}=\frac{k_{ij}}{3}$, $i=1,2,3$.

Table 3. R_a Response for Surface Roughness

Level	A Feed rate (mm/min)	B Feed per tooth (mm/tooth)	C Depth of cut (mm)
k_{1j}	3.97	3.69	3.76
k_{2j}	3.83	3.94	3.85
k_{3j}	3.82	3.99	4.01
$\bar{k}_{1j}$	1.323	1.23	1.253
$\bar{k}_{2j}$	1.277	1.313	1.283
$\bar{k}_{3j}$	1.273	1.33	1.337
R_j	0.05	0.1	0.084

R_j :The difference between maximum-minimum R_a response values.

4.2 Analysis of the S/N Ratio

Determine factors importance. The same column in Table 3, the difference of maximum subtract minimum among $\bar{k}_{1j}$, $\bar{k}_{2j}$ and $\bar{k}_{3j}$ called extremum denoted by R_j . Generally speaking, different extremum in different column shows different impact on test indicators with changing factors level. The larger extremum shows that larger impact on test indicators with changing factors level, column with the largest extremum, larger impact on test indicators when the level of that factor changed, that is we have to consider major factors. From the table that extremum of *B* factor R_B =0.1 is the largest, showed that *B* factor has the biggest impact on parts' surface roughness; the extremum of A factor R_A =0.05 is the smallest showed that A factor has smaller impact on parts' surface roughness.

Table 4. S/N response table for surface roughness

Level	*A* Feed rate (mm/min)	*B* Feed per tooth (mm/tooth)	*C* Depth of cut (mm)
k_{1j}	- 7.28	- 5.28	- 5.81
k_{2j}	- 6.51	- 6.59	- 6.34
k_{3j}	- 6.15	- 7.35	- 7.43
$\bar{k}_{1j}$	- 2.43	- 1.76	- 1.94
$\bar{k}_{2j}$	- 2.05	- 2.32	- 2.11
$\bar{k}_{3j}$	- 2.05	- 2.45	- 2.48
R_j	0.38	0.69	0.54

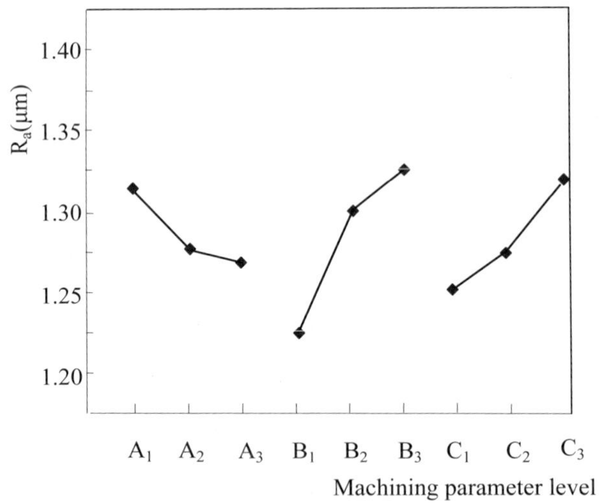

Fig. 1. Effect on *Ra* from each factor

4.3 Drawing Trend Graph

Further trend graph can draw shows A, B, C three factors affecting the high-speed milling aluminum alloy (2A70) surface roughness. We can see the index change with various factors changing in Fig.1and Fig.2.

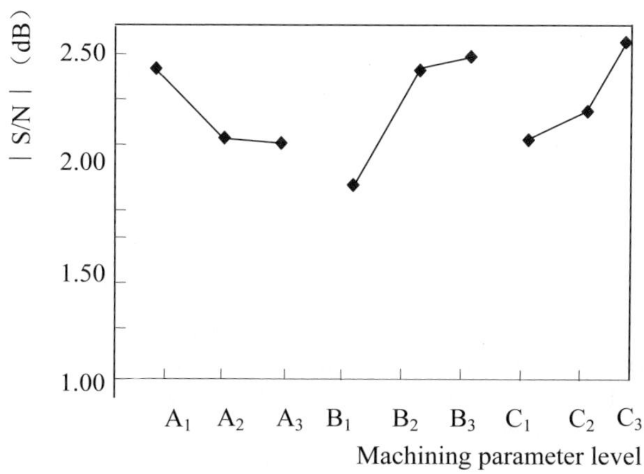

Fig. 2. Effect on S/N from each factor

For each factor, index (expressed by the average roughness $\bar{k}_{1j}$, $\bar{k}_{2j}$ and $\bar{k}_{3j}$ of each factor used in every level) as longitudinal coordinates, factors level as abscissa for factors - index graph. From Fig.1 we can see, if getting better surface processing quality so that minimum surface roughness value, corresponding to the best cutting parameters combination is $B_1C_1A_3$, that is

B_1 : feed per tooth, the first lever, 0.02

C_1 : Depth of cut, the first lever, 0.2

A_3 : feed rate, the third lever, 5400

According to the above signals and interference ratio analysis, the best level of cutting parameters is the level when signal and interference ratio is greater[6].The different effects on S/N for various factors , B factor (feed per tooth) is the greatest impact, and S/N rise significantly with feed per tooth increasing, that shows components surface roughness increasing with feed per tooth to increase variable, this conclusion can be obviously drawn through the observation of feed per tooth different parts' morphology (Fig.3).This followed by C factor (Depth of cut), the last is A factor (feed rate).

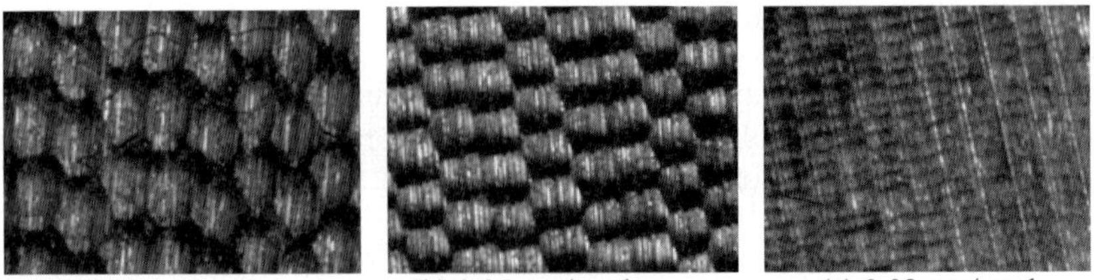

(a) 0.08mm/tooth (b) 0.05mm/tooth (c) 0.02mm/tooth

Fig. 3. Surface profile according to the feed per tooth

According to calculation results and above analysis, a set of conclusions can be drawn.

1. Primary and secondary of various factors effects on index (roughness)

According to the data in the line of extremum R_j indicates that the second and third column is larger, the first is minimum. This reflects when B and C factors level changed, fluctuations in indicators are the largest, when A factors level changed, fluctuations in indicators are the least. According to the order of extremum from the primary and secondary factors:

primary——————————————→secondary

feed per tooth, feed rate, Depth of cut

Comprehensive test results can be seen feed per tooth (B factor) is the most important, followed by the Depth of cut (C factor); finally, feed rate (A factor). Therefore, in order to be processed at the lower blade surface roughness, you can choose smaller feed per tooth.

2. Better production conductions

From the meaning of k_{1j} , k_{2j} and k_{3j} we can see that various factors difference which are in columns k_{1j} , k_{2j} and k_{3j} . in fact, only reflects the factors fluctuations in indicators due to level changed, and keep other factors level from the effects, so combined simply good level of all factors will be better production conditions. However, in fact, should distinguish between the primary and secondary factors, for the main factor, according to certain requirements select the best level, for secondary factors which can be based on savings, convenience, and other aspects consider to choose a level. From Table 3 and 4 that better production conditions is $B_1C_1A_3$, feed per tooth (B factor) 0.02 mm / tooth, Depth of cut (C factor) 0.2 mm, feed rate (A factor) 5400 mm / min, given the smallest surface roughness value, surface quality is optimal.

5 Conclusions

In order to study deeply impact laws on spindle speed, feed rate and feed per tooth for surface roughness orthogonal experiment is designed, through extremum analysis and factors effect on R_a 、 S / N , detailed analyze test results and draw the following conclusions:

1. The experiment studies various factors impact on high-speed milling surface roughness, gets the primary and secondary influence order of each factor to the surface roughness and optimal processing method. The parts' surface structure under different feed per tooth was observed in scanning electron microscope; supply a test basis for the optimization of high-speed milling system.

2. To reduce surface roughness, spindle speed should be appropriately increased; the feed rate and feed per tooth should be reduced. But the choice of parameters should also meet technological requirements to consider the premise of milling efficiency.

3. In various factors, the effect of feed per tooth is the most. During the test, for aluminum alloy(2A70) impeller leaves free curved surface, a number of tests were done for leaves on 5-axis high-speed machining center, preliminary draw the following conclusions: feed speed around 5400 mm / min, Depth of cut about 0.2 mm feed per tooth 0.02 mm / tooth, optimal surface quality obtained.

References

1. King, P.I., Vaughn, R.L.: A Synaptic view of High-Speed Machining from Salmon to the Present. In: Komanduri, S.K., et al. (eds.) M. High Speed Machining, pp. 1–13. ASME, U.S.A (1984)
2. Ko, T.J., Kim, H.S., Park, S.H.: Machineability in NURBS Interpolator Considering Constant Material Removal Rate. J. International Journal of Machine Tools Manufacture 45, 665–671 (2005)
3. Wang, S., Zhao, J., Ai, X., Lu, Z.: Theoretical Research of Surface Roughness for HSM. Mechanical Engineer 10, 3–5 (2004)
4. Yang, W.H., Tang, Y.S.: Disign optimization of cutting parameters for turning operations-baded on the Taguchi mothod. Mater Process Tecthol. 84, 122–129 (1998)
5. Zhang, C., Zhang, Y., Li, Z., Liu, Y.: Research and application of cutting parameters of high-speed machining based on Taguchi method. J. Modern Manufacturing Engineering 8, 78–80 (2006)
6. Fang, Y., Li, F., He, Q., Chen, X.: Selection of optimum process parameters of surface roughness in high-speed cutting. Journal of Tianjin Polytechnic University 25, 58–60 (2006)

Dynamical Research Based on a New Type of Reconfigurable Robot

Yanhui Wei[1], Dexin Xu[1], Yanbin Gao[1], Jie Zhao[2], and Hegao Cai[2]

Coll of Automation of HEU, 2.Robotics Institutes of HIT, Harbin, Harbin, Heilongjiang Province, China
wyhhit@163.com

Abstract. Currently, the reconfigurable robot has become a hot topic for its diverse configurations. In this thesis, a new type of reconfigurable robot system is proposed, whose main modules are cylinders, which makes its structure quite compact and dexterous. Taking this kind of robot as an example, some new methods for robot module modeling and reconfiguration modeling are figured out, according to which a reconfigurable robot of any configuration can set up a dynamical model for itself automatically. By analyzing the velocities, forces and torques of each module, the dynamical functions of the robot are established, using the Newton-Euler method. Finally the six degree of freedom PUMA robot is used to carry out the experimental simulation to test the reliability and applicability of this method proposed in this thesis.

Keywords: Reconfigurable robots, Modular robots, Dynamical.

1 Introduction

As time goes on, people's life pace is speeding up more quickly, more and more intelligent and diverse tools are needed to improve our life quality and life pace. Reconfigurable robot modules can build up many robot work configurations quickly according to the demand of actual environments and tasks, which makes the idea of 'one set of modules create multiple robot work configurations' a reality. And according to the requirement of diversity and small batch for flexibly manufacturing, this becomes an effective method to shorten the developing period and cut costs, which promises a wide vision applied to social development[1].

Many researches on the reconfigurable robot have been done at home and abroad. Chen and Yang et al. from Nanyang Technology University in Singapore used the robot modules produced by ATMEC to study the configuration design, kinematics, and dynamics[2-3]. CHAPELLE[4] developed the closed form approximate symbolic solutions using the genetic algorithm. Li and Zhang from Northeast University discussed module structure of reconfigurable robot. The reconfigurable unit of robot proposed by Zheng and et, al can be classified into three basic types, i.e. vacillate, rotate and auxiliary units. feature of combined assemble of robot was also analysed. A five-legged walking robot was assembled by using these types of basic units. A reconfigurable tracked robot was developed by Wang from Beihang University. In a word, researches on reconfigurable robots focus on the configuration design, kinematics and dynamics.

C. Xiong et al. (Eds.): ICIRA 2008, Part II, LNAI 5315, pp. 1056–1065, 2008.

Generally, a 4*4 homogeneous transformation matrix is used to build the dynamical model and determine the joint position relationships. On the basis of mechanics theory, dynamical robot models are established. However, the configurations of reconfigurable robots can be quite different, that is, they will change as actual work situations, and their dynamical models are not easy to build. This thesis aims to find a method that enables the robots to set up dynamical models and dynamical functions automatically.

2 Reconfigurable Robot System

The reconfigurable modular robot system is quickly assembled from functional modules according to the requirement of work conditions and tasks, and therefore the modules themselves must possess these features below: a) each module must can finish a certain function individually; b) each module should have its own drive system, which has a small mass and moment of inertia so as to obtain the optimal motion and action performance; c) all modules must have good assembling and communication capacities d) all modules should have sort of data processing capacity, that is, on one hand, the control software should meet the robot reconfiguration ability; on the other hand, it should have some information fault tolerance capacity.

These modules are driven by DC servo motor. Besides the characteristics of ordinary reconfigurable robots, these modules are smaller, more dexterous, and faster compared with the RMMS (Developed by Carnegie Mellon University); the configurations are different from those of PowerCube series modules produced by AMTEC Co. Ltd (Germany), and their configurations are more compact and practical. The elementary modules are shown in Fig.1, and some built up models are shown in Fig.2.

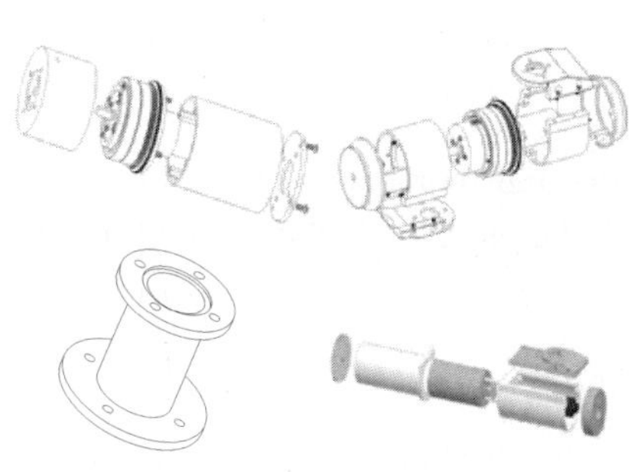

Fig. 1. The machine structure of modular

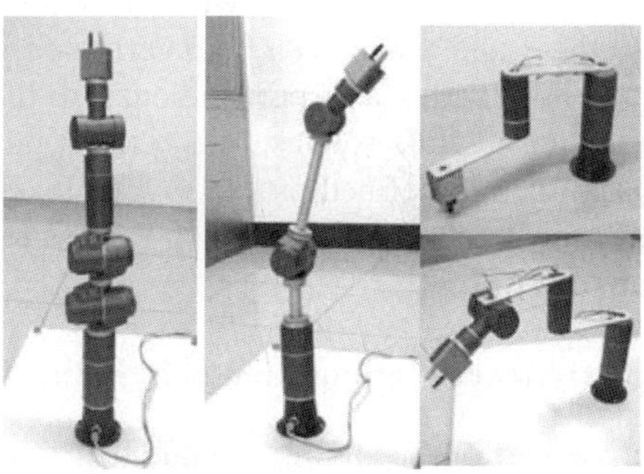

Fig. 2. Configuration of reconfigurable modular robot

3 Dynamical Modeling of the Modules of the Reconfigurable Robot

3.1 Dynamical Simulation of Rotary Module

These two components of one rotation module that rotate relative to each other are modeled separately, and suppose the component that fixes the motor to be Link 1; the component that rotates to be Link 2. The initial joint frame of rotary component are fixed at the bottom of Link 1 (point A.), with z axis perpendicular to the joint face inward, and x and y axes can be determined using the right hand rule; position C is where the module tip frame lies, where z axis is perpendicular to the joint face, and this frame changes as the rotary module rotates. When the rotation angles are all zeros, all their orientations are defined as shown in Fig.3. The mass centers and moments of inertia of Link 1 and Link 2 relative to their own frames respectively can be calculated using the software of Pro/E.

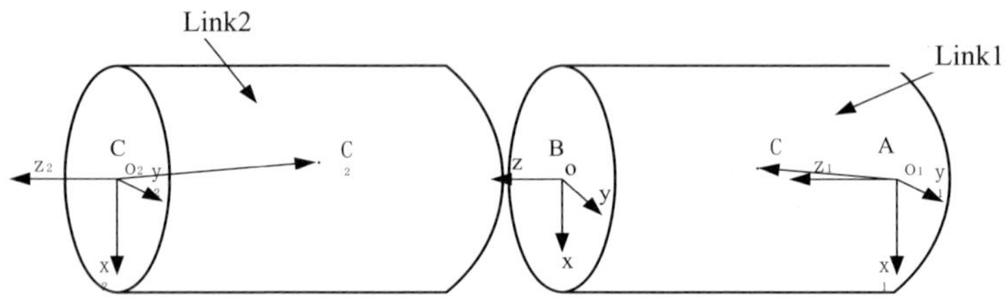

Fig. 3. The dynamical model of a rotary module

3.2 Dynamical Simulation of a Rotary Module

Let the component fixing the motor be Link 3, and the rotation part Link 4. In order to make the reconfiguration between modules as convenient as possible, the origin of swing module is built in the location (D) where this module connects with last module. The z axis is perpendicular to the joint surface inward; position E is where the joint frame is established, with the z axis identical with the joint rotation axis, and also the x and y axes can be determined via right hand rule; the module tip frame is set up at F, with z axis perpendicular to the joint surface, and this frame transforms as the swing module rotates. When the rotation angles are all zeros, the orientations of this frame are defined as Fig.4. The mass centers and moments of inertia of Link 3 and Link 4 relative to their own frames respectively can be calculated using the software of Pro/E.

3.3 Dynamical Simulation of a Sliding Module

Let the part of the sliding module that fixes the motor be Link 5, and the sliding component be Link 6. Similarly, set the origin of the translation component frame at the center of the joint surface where Link 5 connects with last module; build the joint Frame 6 at the center of the other joint surface of Link 5; since the fixed and sliding parts of the translation module superpose with each other, and as the sliding part moves, the overlay area varies, we have to set frame 7 at the center point J inside the sliding part, with the same orientation with frame 6; make the origin of Frame 8 at the center point K outside the translation part. All the coordinate systems are shown in Fig.5. Finally, the mass centers and moments of inertia of Link 5 and Link 6 relative to Frame 5 and Frame 8 respectively can be computed with the help of Pro/E.

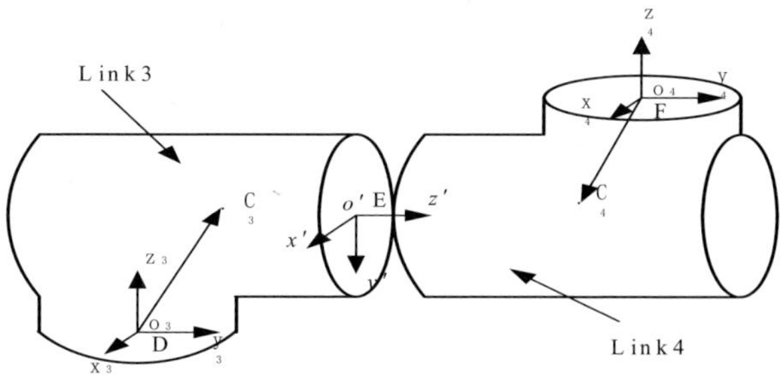

Fig. 4. Dynamical model of a swing module

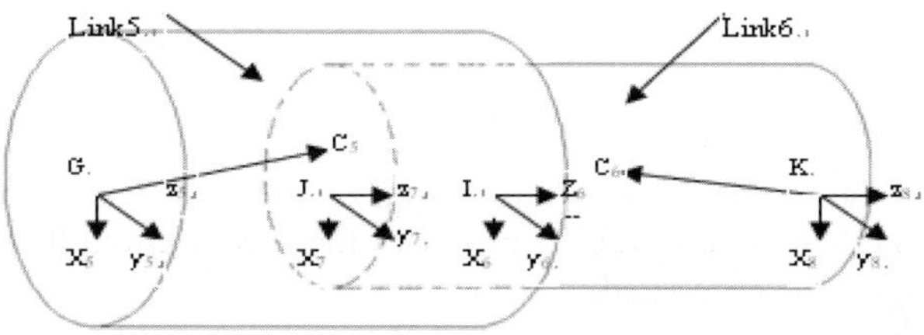

Fig. 5. Dynamical model of a sliding module

3.4 Modeling the Reconfiguration between Modules

After connecting the rotary module with the swing module, Link 2 of the rotary module and Link 3 of the swing module become one, and we should treat them as a whole in dynamical computation, and therefore we must know the mass center and moment of inertia of the whole body. The masses, mass centers, and moments of inertia of Link 2 and Link 3 relative to Frame 2 and Frame 3 respectively are already known, and when connecting these two parts together, let Frame 2 and 3 coincident to make a new coordinate system – Frame 5. The reconfigured model is shown in Fig.6. The positions of these two links relative to the new mass center don't change, so that we can find the new mass center using the moment balance principle. Via coordinate transformation, the mass center can be transformed into the joint coordinate system.

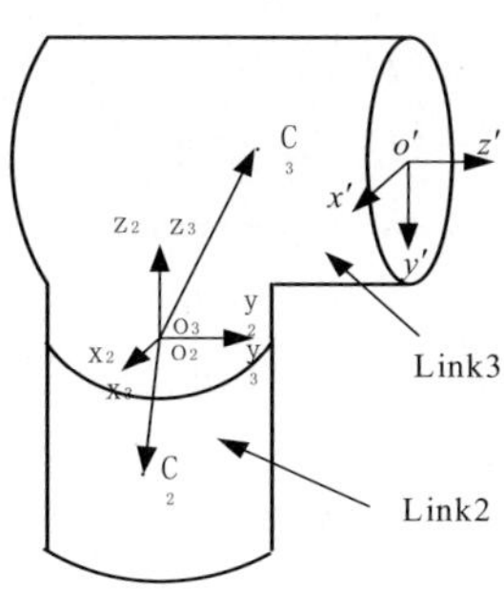

Fig. 6. Dynamical model of the reconfiguration

Suppose the coordinates of the mass center of Link 2 relative to Frame 5 is (x_2, y_2, z_2), and similarly, that of Link 3 is (x_3, y_3, z_3). The mass of Link 2 is m_2, and that of Link 3 is m_3. Then the mass center coordinates are

$$\begin{cases} x = x_2 + \dfrac{m_3}{m_2 + m_3}(x_3 - x_2) \\ y = y_2 + \dfrac{m_3}{m_2 + m_3}(y_3 - y_2) \\ z = z_2 + \dfrac{m_3}{m_2 + m_3}(z_3 - z_2) \end{cases} \tag{1}$$

The coordinates of the mass center relative to the swing joint frame are

$$(x_c, y_c, z_c)^T = (x, y, z,)^T \left(T_D^E\right)^{-1} \tag{2}$$

We already know the moments of inertia of Link 2 and Link 3 in Frame 2 and Frame 3 respectively, and then the moment of inertia of the reconfigured links relative to the new Frame 5 can also be computed.

$$I_c = I_{c2} + I_{c3} \tag{3}$$

Through coordinate transformation, we can also obtain the moment of inertia in the mass center coordinate system. If we know the moment of inertia relative to frame *T'* and are required to compute that relative to another frame, the parallel theorem and similarity transformation can be employed. Suppose that frame T_c' has the same origin, that is, $o_c x' y' z'$, and R is the rotation matrix from T_c to T_c'. Then the moment of inertia relative to T_c' is

$$I_c' = R^c I_c R^T \tag{4}$$

When these two frames have translations relative to each other, then the moments of inertia are

$$\begin{cases} {}^oI_{x'} = {}^cI_{x'} + m(r_2^{\,2} + r_3^{\,2}) \\ {}^oI_{y'} = {}^cI_{y'} + m(r_1^{\,2} + r_3^{\,2}) \\ {}^oI_{z'} = {}^cI_{z'} + m(r_1^{\,2} + r_2^{\,2}) \\ {}^oI_{x'y'} = {}^cI_{x'y'} + mr_1r_2 \\ {}^oI_{y'z'} = {}^cI_{y'z'} + mr_2r_3 \\ {}^oI_{x'z'} = {}^cI_{x'z'} + mr_1r_3 \end{cases} \tag{5}$$

Where $r = [r_1 \quad r_2 \quad r_3]^T$ is the radius vector mapping from origin o of Frame T' to origin o_c of Frame T_c.

In this way, we can compute the mass center position relative to the joint frame and the moment of inertia relative to the mass center frame, and consequently the dynamical model for the configurations of each reconfigurable robot can automatically be built up.

4 Fstablish the Dynamics Functions

4.1 The Velocity Analysis for Each Module

In order to describe the motion states of each Link, we employ the symbols below: c_i is the center of mass of Link i; ${}^iv_{ci}$ is the centroid velocity vector of Link i; ${}^i\dot{v}_{ci}$ the centroid acceleration vector of Link i; ${}^iv_i$ and ${}^i\dot{v}_i$ are the velocity vector and acceleration vector of the origin o_i of Frame i respectively; ${}^i\omega_i$ and ${}^i\dot{\omega}_i$ the angular velocity vector and angular acceleration vector of Link i respectively. ${}^il_i$ is the radius vector from o_{i-1} to o_i, ${}^i\rho_i$ from o_{i+1} to c_i, and ${}^ih_i$ from o_{i-1} to c_i, where ${}^ih_i = {}^il_i + {}^i\rho_i$. Then the angular velocity, angular acceleration, velocity, and acceleration can be expressed in the iterative formulas below.

$$ {}^{i+1}\omega_{i+1} = R_{i+1,\ i}\left({}^i\omega_i + \dot{q}_{i+1}\,{}^ie_i\right) \tag{6}$$

$$ {}^{i+1}\dot{\omega}_{i+1} = R_{i+1,\ i}\left({}^i\dot{\omega}_i + \ddot{q}_{i+1}\,{}^ie_i + \dot{q}_{i+1}\,{}^i\omega_i \times {}^ie_i\right) \tag{7}$$

$$ {}^{i+1}\dot{v}_{i+1} = R_{i+1,\ i}\,{}^i\dot{v}_i + {}^{i+1}\dot{\omega}_{i+1}\times{}^{i+1}l_{i+1} + {}^{i+1}\omega_{i+1}\times\left({}^{i+1}\omega_{i+1}\times{}^{i+1}l_{i+1}\right) \tag{8}$$

$$ {}^iv_{ci} = {}^iv_i + {}^i\omega_i \times {}^i\rho_i \tag{9}$$

$$ {}^i\dot{v}_{ci} = {}^i\dot{v}_i + {}^i\dot{\omega}_i \times {}^i\rho_i + {}^i\omega_i \times\left({}^i\omega_i \times {}^i\rho_i\right) \tag{10}$$

Where $R_{i+1,i}$ is the rotation matrix from Frame $i+1$ to frame i, and these transformation can be expressed using this 3*3 matrix

$$ R_{i-1,\ i} = \begin{bmatrix} \cos\theta_i & -\sin\theta_i\cos\alpha_i & \sin\theta_i\sin\alpha_i \\ \sin\theta_i & \cos\theta_i\cos\alpha_i & -\cos\theta_i\sin\alpha_i \\ 0 & \sin\alpha_i & \cos\alpha_i \end{bmatrix} \tag{11}$$

Since this is an orthonormal matrix, it can be rewritten like this

$$ R_{i-1,\ i} = R^{-1}_{i,\ i-1} = R^{T}_{i,\ i-1} \tag{12}$$

Then we obtain:

$$R_{i,\,i\text{-}1}=\begin{bmatrix}\cos\theta_i & \sin\theta_i & 0\\ -\sin\theta_i\cos\alpha_i & \cos\theta_i\cos\alpha_i & \sin\alpha_i\\ \sin\theta_i\sin\alpha_i & -\cos\theta_i\sin\alpha_i & \cos\alpha_i\end{bmatrix} \tag{13}$$

4.2 The Mechanics Analysis for Each Module

The joint forces imposed on Link i are ${}^iF_J$ – the force that Link *i-1* exerts on module i in joint J_i and M_J – the moment that Link *i-1* exerts on module i in joint J_i. These two items contain the forces and moments that result in by the constraints forces, drive forces, frictions and so on.

The external forces exerted on Link i are ${}^iM_i$– the external force that is exerted on Link i and simplified into a resultant force at the center of mass c_i, that is, the principle vector of external forces, and ${}^iM_e$ – the external force that is exerted on Link i and simplified into a resultant torque at the center of mass c_i, that is, the principle torque of external forces.

After simplifying all the external forces into a resultant force ${}^iF_i$ at the mass center c_i and a resultant torque ${}^iM_i$, using the Newton-Euler function, we can obtain.

$${}^iF_i = m_i\,{}^i\dot{v}_{ci} \tag{14}$$

$${}^iM_i = {}^cI_i\,{}^i\dot{\omega}_i + {}^i\omega_i \times ({}^cI_i\,{}^i\omega_i) \tag{15}$$

The relationship between the resultant forces and torques and joint forces and torques are like this.

$${}^iF_{J_i} = R_{i,\,i+1}\,{}^{i+1}F_{J_{i+1}} + {}^iF_i + m_i g \tag{16}$$

$${}^iM_{J_i} = {}^iM_i + R_{i,\,i+1}\,{}^{i+1}M_{J_{i+1}} + {}^ih_i \times ({}^iF_i - m_i g) + {}^il_i \times R_{i,\,i+1}\,{}^{i+1}F_{J_{i+1}} \tag{17}$$

4.3 The Dynamical Model of Reconfigurable Robot

The whole algorithm for the reconfigurable robot dynamical problems using Newton-Euler function, that is, given the motion parameters of all the links, q_i, $\dot{q}_i$, $\ddot{q}_i$, i=1,2,…,n, compute all the drive forces and torques Q_i, i=1, …, n, can be realized through two iteration. The first iteration is to compute the velocities and accelerations of all the links from Link *1* to Link n, and apply Newton-Euler function to each link, which is the forward kinematics iteration. The initial condition is that the base does not move. And if it does, ${}^0\omega_0$=0, ${}^0\dot{\omega}_0$=0. The second iteration involves the computation of drive forces and the counterforces from Link n to Link *1*, which is the inverse dynamics iteration. The initial conditions are $M_{J_{n+1}} = M_{end}$, $F_{J_{n+1}} = F_{end}$. If the end manipulator is free in space, M_{end}, F_{end} are equal to zeros.

1. The forward iteration is used to compute the velocities, accelerations, i=0,1,…,n-1.

$$^{i+1}\omega_{i+1} = R_{i+1,\ i}\left({}^{i}\omega_i + \dot{q}_{i+1}\,{}^{i}e_i\right) \tag{18}$$

$$^{i+1}\dot{\omega}_{i+1} = R_{i+1,\ i}\left({}^{i}\dot{\omega}_i + \ddot{q}_{i+1}\,{}^{i}e_i + \dot{q}_{i+1}\,{}^{i}\omega_i \times {}^{i}e_i\right) \tag{19}$$

$$^{i+1}\dot{v}_{i+1} = R_{i+1,\ i}\,{}^{i}\dot{v}_i + {}^{i+1}\dot{\omega}_{i+1} \times {}^{i+1}l_{i+1} + {}^{i+1}\omega_{i+1} \times \left({}^{i+1}\omega_{i+1} \times {}^{i+1}l_{i+1}\right) \tag{20}$$

$$^{i}v_{ci} = {}^{i}v_i + {}^{i}\omega_i \times {}^{i}\rho_i \tag{21}$$

$$^{i}\dot{v}_{ci} = {}^{i}\dot{v}_i + {}^{i}\dot{\omega}_i \times {}^{i}\rho_i + {}^{i}\omega_i \times \left({}^{i}\omega_i \times {}^{i}\rho_i\right) \tag{22}$$

$$^{i+1}F_{i+1} = m_{i+1}\,{}^{i}\dot{v}_{ci} \tag{23}$$

$$^{i+1}M_{i+1} = {}^{c}I_{i+1}\,{}^{i+1}\dot{\omega}_{i+1} + {}^{i+1}\omega_{i+1} \times ({}^{c}I_{i+1}\,{}^{i+1}\omega_{i+1}) \tag{24}$$

2. The inverse iteration returns the forces and torques, $i = n$, n -1, … , 1

$$^{i}F_{J_i} = R_{i,\ i+1}\,{}^{i+1}F_{J_{i+1}} + {}^{i}F_i \tag{25}$$

$$^{i}M_{J_i} = {}^{i}M_i + R_{i,\ i+1}\,{}^{i+1}M_{J_{i+1}} + {}^{i}h_i \times {}^{i}F_i + {}^{i}l_i \times R_{i,\ i+1}\,{}^{i+1}F_{J_{i+1}} \tag{26}$$

$$Q^{M}{}_{i} = R_{i-1,i}\,{}^{i}M_{J_i} \cdot {}^{i-1}e_{i-1} \tag{27}$$

When considering the weight of links themselves, let $^{0}\dot{v}_0 = g$, that is, the support effect exerted on the robot base is equivalent to the gravity acceleration g upward. Then we can treat all the modules including the base in the same way.

5 Examples

The dynamical simulation of a reconfigurable robot needs the help of ADAMS as the simulation experimental platform. Since the modeling capacity of ADAMS is not very strong, instead we take Pro/E to simulate the whole reconfigurable robot, and define the involving parameters. Then import the model into ADAMS, determine the motion joints and constraints, add regulation functions, gravity, loads and other parameters, and finally start the simulation.

Build a six degree of freedom PUMA robot using the reconfigurable modules, and compute all the dynamical parameters through the reconfiguration modeling method. The built dynamical model is shown in Fig.7. The dynamical emulation results are displayed in Fig.8 and Fig.9.

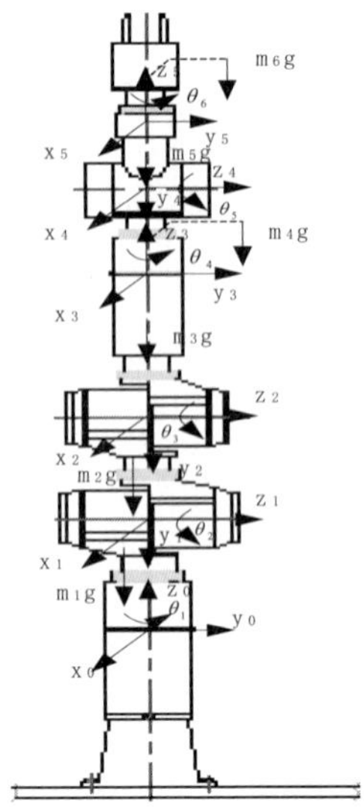

Fig. 7. Dynamical diagram of PUMA robot with six degrees of freedom

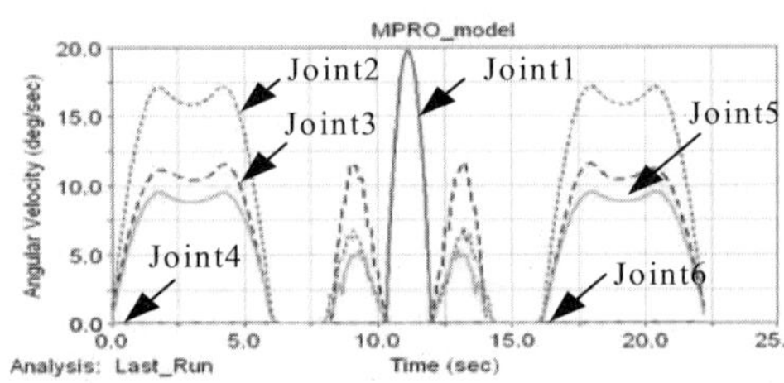

Fig. 8. Joint velocity curves

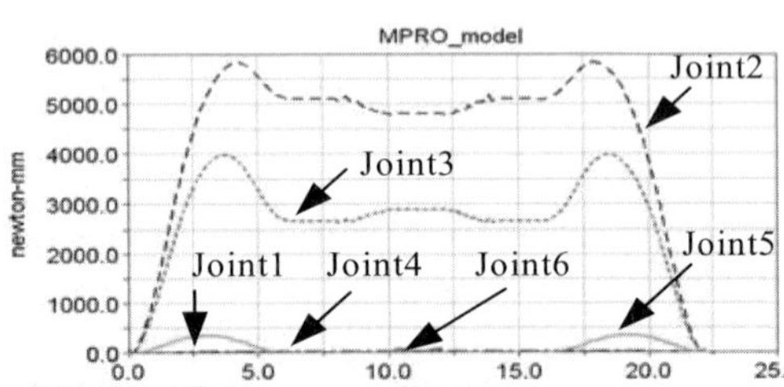

Fig. 9. Joint force curves

6 Conclusions

In this thesis, a new type of reconfigurable modular robot system is proposed. These modules are independent with each other from the angle of functions, dynamics, and kinematics. Through dynamical simulations with this system, we can reach the conclusions below:

1. The dynamical model of the reconfigurable robot can be built automatically from each single dynamical model of each module and the reconfiguration simulation.
2. Via Newton-Euler forward and inverse iteration method, the dynamical functions for robot of any configuration can be set up automatically.
3. The dynamical simulation of the reconfigurable robot with six degrees of freedom suggests that this method can analyze the joint velocities acceleration and torques of the robots with all kinds of configurations.

Acknowledgement

This project is supported by Heilongjiang postdoctoral Foundation of China（LRB-KY 02029）, and partially supported by Program for Changjiang Scholars and Innovative Research Team in University（PCSIRT）(IRT0423) and The National High Technology Research and Development Program of China(2006AA04Z220).

References

1. Liu, S.N., Chen, Y., Zhang, W.J.: Modular Robots and Computer-aided Design. Robot 1, 16–22 (1999)
2. Chen, I.M.: Rapid response manufacturing through a rapidly reconfigurable robotic workcell. Robotics and Computer Intergrated Manufacturing 17, 199–213 (2001)
3. Yang, G.l., Chen, I.M.: Task-based optimization of modular robot configurations: minimized degree-of-freedom approach. Mechanism and Machine Theory 35, 517–540 (2000)
4. Chapelle, F., Bidaup, P., Philippe, B.: Closed form solutions for inverse kinematics approximation of general 6R manipulators. Mechanism and machine theory 39, 323–338 (2004)
5. Li, S.J., Zhang, Y.L., Zhao, M.Y.: Modules and configuration design of reconfigurable modular robots. Journal of northeastern university (Natural science) 25, 78–81 (2004)
6. Zheng, H.J., Wang, J.S., Li, T.M.: Reconfigurable robot unit structure design and assembly character analyses. Chinese Journal of mechanical engineering 39, 34–37 (2003)
7. Wang, T.M., Zou, D., Chen, D.S.: Mechanism design and control method of reconfigurable tracked robot. Journal of Beijing university of aeronautics and astronautics 31, 705–708 (2005)

The Modeling and Simulation of Dynamic Error on Turn-Milling Centre

Lida Zhu[1], Gang Li[1], Ertao Chen[2], Cong Su[1], and Wanshan Wang[1]

[1] School of Mechanical Engineering and Automation, Northeastern University, Shenyang 110004, China
[2] Shenyang Ligong University, Shenyang, 110168, China
zld1999@gmail.com

Abstract. The complex surface with high precision can be obtained on turn-milling centre, but its dynamic error is very complicate and difficult compensation, which affect directly machining accuracy of tool path. According to motion characteristics of turn-milling centre, the coordinate transformations of each kinematical pair among coordinate system are built by the homogeneous coordinate transformation, and the error mathematical models are derived to get five compensation quantities of kinematic pair's location and orientation. Then the dynamic error that comes from flexible body in motion process is simulated by virtual prototype technology. Therefore, the method provides theoretical basis of error compensation for modern machine tool and has application value.

Keywords: turn-milling centre; dynamic error; coordinate transformation; modeling; simulation.

1 Introduction

With the rapid development of scientific technology, numerical control machine of turn-milling function is suitable for machining the complicated and high-efficient products. The turn-milling centre enables completely machining of work pieces with different shape elements without changing the set-up and the complex surface of high precision to satisfy the military project. But its dynamic error is very complicate and difficult compensation, which directly affect machining accuracy of tool path [1][2].

Dynamic error mainly includes machine tool structural characteristics, deflection of components joint and components bending deformation in motion process. When machining speed is low, the error may be neglected; when machining speed is high, the error is also big. Parts are processed in motion process, so dynamic error is very important to machining accuracy. Many people researched error components on machine tool. Okafor[3] researched Derivation of machine tool error models and error compensation procedure for three axes vertical machining centre using rigid body kinematics. Jun [4] researched CNC machine accuracy enhancement through real-time error compensation. Dynamic error on turn-milling centre is rarely researched. Dynamic error that comes from flexible body in motion process is researched in this paper.

C. Xiong et al. (Eds.): ICIRA 2008, Part II, LNAI 5315, pp. 1066–1075, 2008.

2 The Homogeneous Coordinate Transformation of Kinematics Pairs among Coordinate System

2.1 Turn-Milling Centre Characteristics

The turn-milling centre is a newly emerging machining process, which tends to make use of the advantages of both turning and milling. The productivity could be much greater in comparison to the conventional processes like turning or milling. The turn-milling centre can realize five-axis linkages which include the movement of X, Y, Z direction and the rotation of C axis and B axis in machining process. A very important advantage is also that it enables completely machining of work pieces with different shape elements without changing the set-up. The turn-milling centre offers the possibility of product, besides flat and cylindrical shapes, more complicated ones, for example, ellipses, screw-threads etc. It has been shown that surface quality obtained by turn-milling process is better than that of conventional milling process [1][5].Figure.1 shows turn-milling centre.

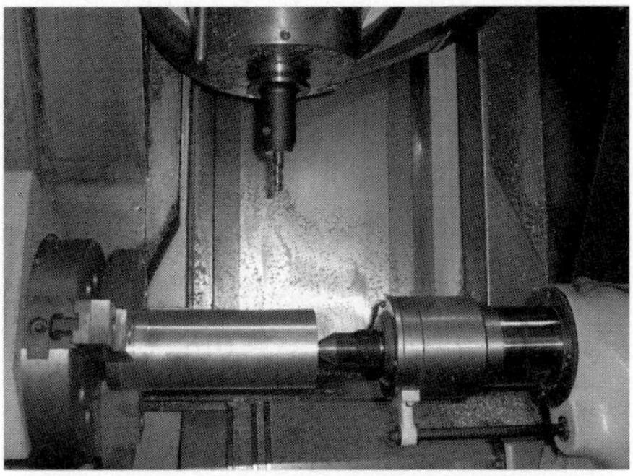

Fig. 1. Turn-milling centre

2.2 The Homogeneous Coordinate Transformation

The turn-milling centre is a five-axis machine tool with type of 3T2R (three motion axes and two rational axes). Figure.2 shows five axes motion and rational direction of turn-milling centre. *W* coordinate system is regarded as based coordinate system. *Z* axis is movement of slide on bed. *X* axis is movement of cross slide on slide. *Y* axis is movement of tool carrier on cross slide in $45°$ direction.

According to robot kinematics principle, the homogeneous coordinate transformation of kinematics pairs among coordinate system is expressed [6]:

$$T_{V,U} = \begin{bmatrix} n_x & o_x & k_x & p_x \\ n_y & o_y & k_y & p_y \\ n_z & o_z & k_z & p_z \\ 0 & 0 & 0 & 1 \end{bmatrix} = \begin{bmatrix} n & o & k & p \\ 0 & 0 & 0 & 1 \end{bmatrix} \tag{1}$$

where, *n, o, k* is respective cosine vectors of three directions, *p* is displacement vectors.

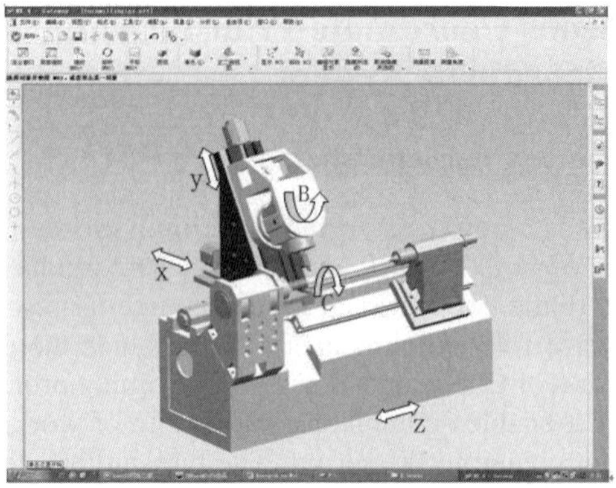

Fig. 2. The 3D assembling model of turn-milling centre

$(T_{V,U})^{-1} = T_{U,V}$

$$(T_{V,U})^{-1} = \begin{bmatrix} n_x & n_y & n_z & -p \cdot n \\ o_x & o_y & o_z & -p \cdot o \\ k_x & k_y & k_z & -p \cdot k \\ 0 & 0 & 0 & 1 \end{bmatrix} \tag{2}$$

In without error condition, displacement pair has a translational degree of freedom and rational pair has a rational degree of freedom.

(1) When the moving distance is z in *Z* axis direction, $T_{W,Z}$ expresses *Z* coordinate system relative to W coordinate system. When the moving distance is x in *X* axis direction, $T_{Z,X}$ expresses *X* coordinate system relative to *Z* coordinate system. When the moving distance is y in *Y* axis direction, $T_{X,Y}$ expresses *Y* coordinate system relative to *X* coordinate system.

$$T_{W,Z} = \begin{bmatrix} 1 & 0 & 0 & 0 \\ 0 & 1 & 0 & 0 \\ 0 & 0 & 1 & z \\ 0 & 0 & 0 & 1 \end{bmatrix} \tag{3}$$

$$T_{Z,X} = \begin{bmatrix} 1 & 0 & 0 & x \\ 0 & 1 & 0 & 0 \\ 0 & 0 & 1 & 0 \\ 0 & 0 & 0 & 1 \end{bmatrix} \tag{4}$$

$$T_{X,Y} = \begin{bmatrix} 1 & 0 & 0 & y \\ 0 & 1 & 0 & y \\ 0 & 0 & 1 & 0 \\ 0 & 0 & 0 & 1 \end{bmatrix} \tag{5}$$

(2) When the moving distance is β in B axis direction, $T_{Y,B}$ can express B coordinate system relative to Y coordinate system. $T_{B,P}$ can express P (workpiece)coordinate system relative to B coordinate system.

$$T_{Y,B} = \begin{bmatrix} 1 & 0 & 0 & -d_1 \\ 0 & \cos\beta & -\sin\beta & -d_1 \\ 0 & \sin\beta & \cos\beta & 0 \\ 0 & 0 & 0 & 1 \end{bmatrix} \begin{bmatrix} \cos 45° & -\sin 45° & 0 & 0 \\ \sin 45° & \cos 45° & 0 & 0 \\ 0 & 0 & 1 & 0 \\ 0 & 0 & 0 & 1 \end{bmatrix} \tag{6}$$

$$T_{B,P} = \begin{bmatrix} 1 & 0 & 0 & -L\sin 45° \\ 0 & 1 & 0 & -L\cos 45° \\ 0 & 0 & 1 & 0 \\ 0 & 0 & 0 & 1 \end{bmatrix} \tag{7}$$

where, L is length from tool point to B axis. d_1 is height from B axis to across slide.

(3) When the moving distance is α in C axis direction, $T_{W,C}$ can expresses C coordinate system relative to W coordinate system. $T_{C,S}$ can expresses S (spindle) coordinate system relative to C coordinate system. $T_{S,Q}$ can expresses Q (tool point)coordinate system relative to S coordinate system.

$$T_{W,C} = \begin{bmatrix} \cos\alpha & -\sin\alpha & 0 & 0 \\ \sin\alpha & \cos\alpha & 0 & 0 \\ 0 & 0 & 1 & 0 \\ 0 & 0 & 0 & 1 \end{bmatrix} \tag{8}$$

$$T_{C,S} = \begin{bmatrix} 1 & 0 & 0 & 0 \\ 0 & 1 & 0 & 0 \\ 0 & 0 & 1 & d_2 \\ 0 & 0 & 0 & 1 \end{bmatrix} \tag{9}$$

$$T_{S,Q} = \begin{bmatrix} 1 & 0 & 0 & 0 \\ 0 & 1 & 0 & 0 \\ 0 & 0 & 1 & L_0 \\ 0 & 0 & 0 & 1 \end{bmatrix} \tag{10}$$

where, L_0 is length of workpiece. d_2 is height from spindle tail to chuck.

(4) In without error condition, Q (tool point) coordinate system and P (workpiece) coordinate system are coincident in space, so $T_{S,Q} = T_{W,P}$.

$$T_{W,C} \cdot T_{C,S} \cdot T_{S,Q} = T_{W,Z} \cdot T_{Z,X} \cdot T_{X,Y} \cdot T_{Y,B} \cdot T_{B,P} \tag{11}$$

$$T_{P,Q} = T_{P,W} \cdot T_{W,Q} = I \tag{12}$$

where, I is unit matrix. Figure.3 shows attachment chain of coordinate system in turn-milling centre.

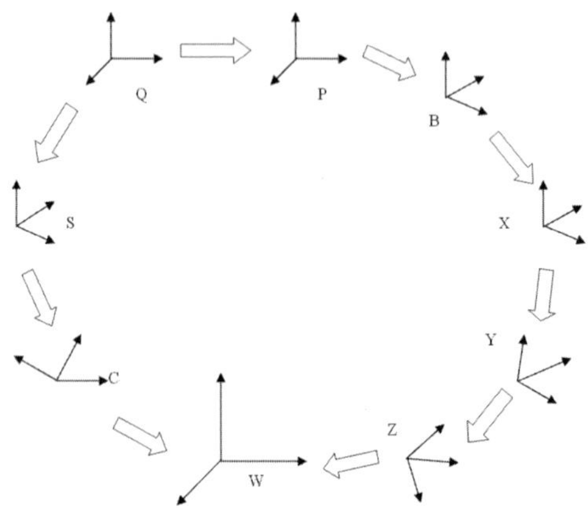

Fig. 3. The attachment chain of coordinate system in turn-milling centre

2.3 The Error Compensation

In error condition, Q (tool point) coordinate system and P (workpiece) coordinate system are separated in space, ${}^{e}T_{P,Q} = {}^{e}T_{P,W} \cdot {}^{e}T_{W,Q} \neq I$. According to robot kinematics differential transform principle, in order to meet ${}^{e}T_{P,Q} = {}^{e}T_{P,W} \cdot {}^{e}T_{W,Q} = I$, error compensation quantity of position and orientation will be got.

$$dT_{P,Q} = \frac{\partial T_{P,Q}}{\partial z}\Delta z + \frac{\partial T_{P,Q}}{\partial x}\Delta x + \frac{\partial T_{P,Q}}{\partial y}\Delta y + \frac{\partial T_{P,Q}}{\partial \alpha}\Delta \alpha + \frac{\partial T_{P,Q}}{\partial \beta}\Delta \beta \tag{13}$$

Where, Δz , Δx , Δy , $\Delta \alpha$, $\Delta \beta$ are respective error compensations of z, x, y, C, B.

$$\frac{dT_{W,Z}}{dx} = \begin{bmatrix} 0 & 0 & 0 & 0 \\ 0 & 0 & 0 & 0 \\ 0 & 0 & 0 & 1 \\ 0 & 0 & 0 & 0 \end{bmatrix} \tag{14}$$

$$\frac{dT_{Z,X}}{dx} = \begin{bmatrix} 0 & 0 & 0 & 1 \\ 0 & 0 & 0 & 0 \\ 0 & 0 & 0 & 0 \\ 0 & 0 & 0 & 0 \end{bmatrix} \tag{15}$$

$$\frac{dT_{X,Y}}{dx} = \begin{bmatrix} 0 & 0 & 0 & 1 \\ 0 & 0 & 0 & 1 \\ 0 & 0 & 0 & 0 \\ 0 & 0 & 0 & 0 \end{bmatrix} \tag{16}$$

$$\frac{dT_{Y,B}}{dx} = \begin{bmatrix} 0 & 0 & 0 & 0 \\ 0 & \sin\beta & -\cos\beta & 0 \\ 0 & \cos\beta & \sin\beta & 1 \\ 0 & 0 & 0 & 0 \end{bmatrix} \tag{17}$$

$$\frac{dT_{W,C}}{dx} = \begin{bmatrix} \sin\alpha & -\cos\alpha & 0 & 0 \\ \cos\alpha & \sin\alpha & 0 & 0 \\ 0 & 0 & 1 & 0 \\ 0 & 0 & 0 & 1 \end{bmatrix} \tag{18}$$

3 Simulation of Dynamic Error

In order to get the dynamic error that comes from flexible body in motion process, virtual prototype technology provides modern advanced method for turn-milling

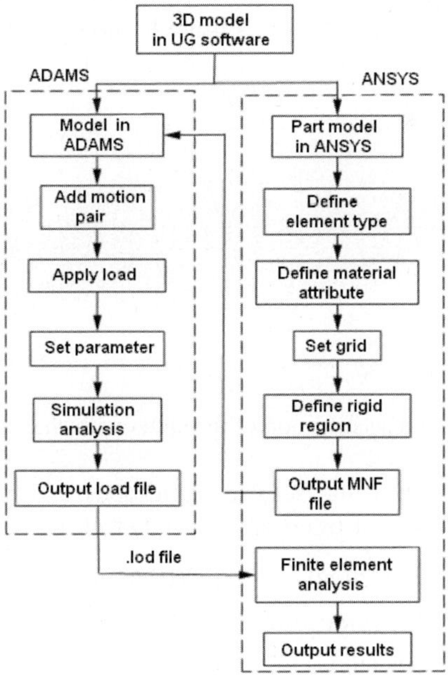

Fig. 4. The flowchart of co-simulation of rigid-flexible coupling system

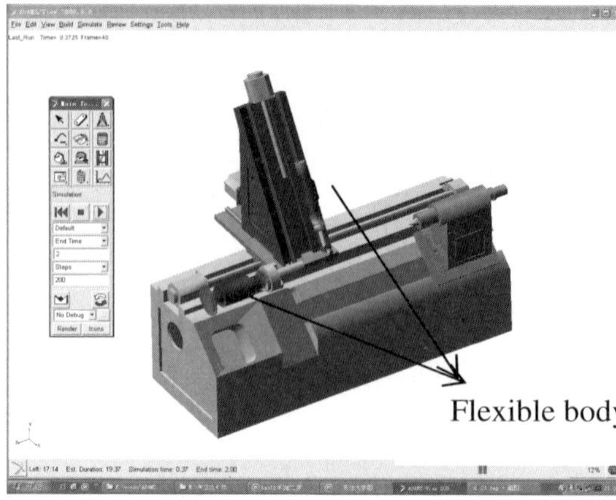

Fig. 5. The model of rigid-flexible coupling system of turn-milling centre

centre design. The method that the machining centre important components are regarded as flexible bodies and the other parts are rigid bodies to form the rigid-flexible coupling system in the simulation process is close to actual conditions. Therefore, co-simulation of rigid-flexible coupling system for turn-milling centre is significant and has application value. Figure.4 describes the flowchart of co-simulation of rigid-flexible coupling system. Figure.5 shows rigid-flexible coupling system of turn-milling centre.

Initial condition (empty load): the maximum cutting velocity of turn-milling centre is $0.5\,m/s$ and acceleration is $9.8\,m/s^2$ .Figure.6 shows velocity and acceleration of the cutter with sine and cosine curves.

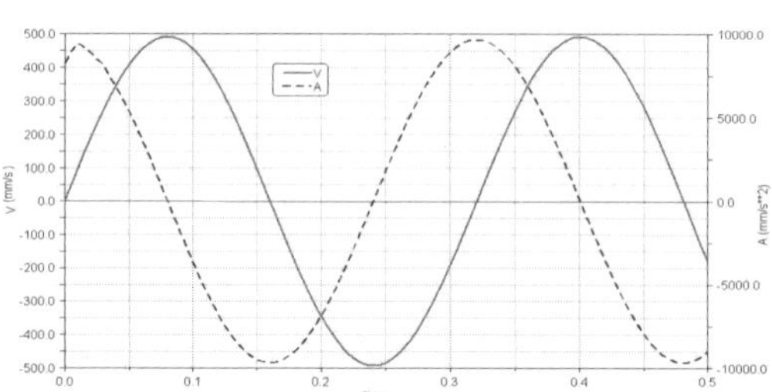

Fig. 6. Velocity and acceleration of the cutter with sine and cosine curves

The simulation difference value between rigid body and flexible body is to get dynamic error. The five degrees of freedom are set as follows:

$$\begin{cases} X: disp(time) = 25 * \cos(19.6 * time) \\ Y: disp(time) = 25 * \cos(19.6 * time) \\ Z: disp(time) = 25 * \sin(19.6 * time) \\ \quad B: velo(time) = 45d * time \\ \quad C: velo(time) = 100 * time \end{cases} \tag{19}$$

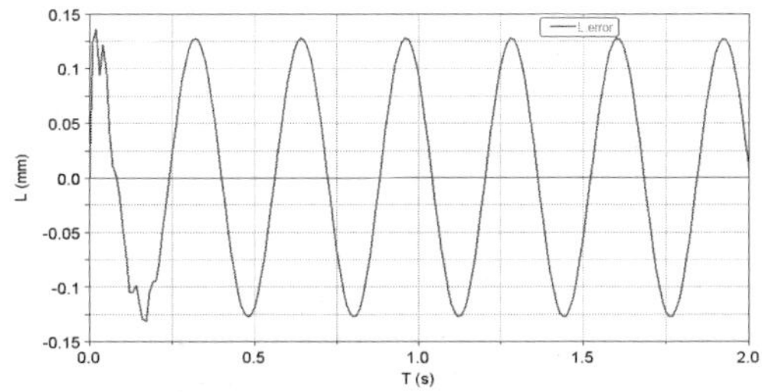

Fig. 7. Dynamic error in Z direction

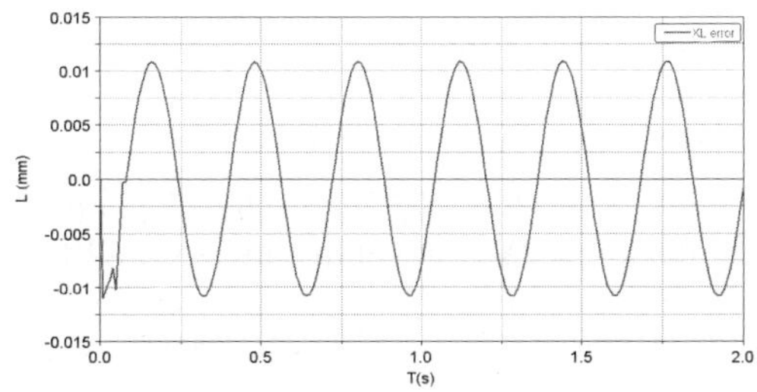

Fig. 8. Dynamic error in X direction

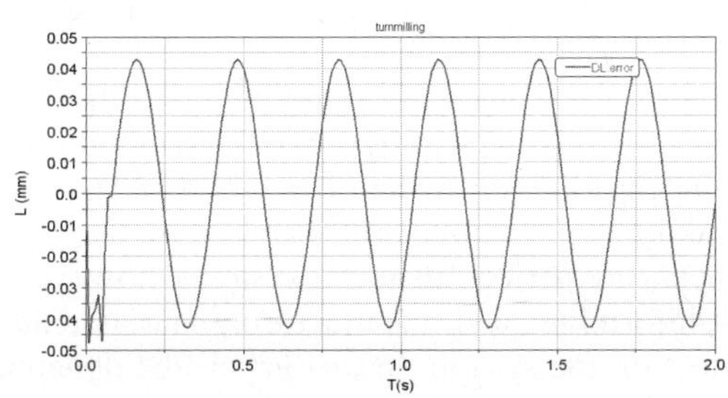

Fig. 9. Dynamic error in Y direction

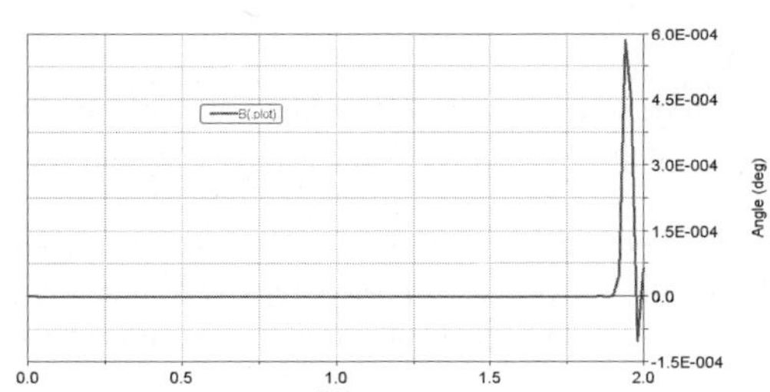

Fig. 10. Dynamic error in B rotation angle

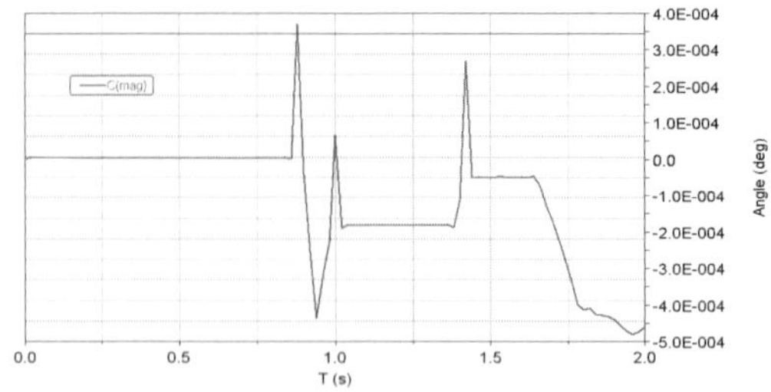

Fig. 11. Dynamic error in C rotation angle

We can see simulation results from the above figures. Figure.7 shows dynamic error in Z direction and maximum displacement is 0.15mm. Figure.8 shows dynamic error in X direction and maximum displacement is 0.011mm. Figure.9 shows dynamic error in Y direction and maximum displacement is 0.043mm. Figure.10 shows dynamic error in B rotation angle and maximum angle is 6×10^{-4}. Figure.11 shows dynamic error in C rotation angle and maximum angle is 5×10^{-4}.

4 Conclusions

1) According to motion characteristics of turn-milling centre, the error mathematical models are derived to get five compensation quantities of kinematical pair's location and orientation.
2) The dynamic error that comes from flexible body in motion process is simulated by virtual prototype technology. So, the method provides theoretical basis of error compensation for modern machine tool and has application value.
3) Generally speaking, the dynamic error is based on the assumption that the system's components are perfect. In actual systems, however, clearances, friction, material non-uniformities and manufacturing and assembly errors can have a significant effect on the system. In this paper, the dynamic error for the turn-milling centre and a co-simulation method are developed.

References

1. Savas, V., Ozay, C.: Anaysis of the surface roughness of tangential turn-milling for machining with end milling cutter. Journal of Materials Processing Technology 186, 279–283 (2007)
2. Zverev, I.A., In, U.E., Yong, K.H.: An elastic deformation model of high-speed spindle units. International Journal of Precision Engineering and Manufacturing 7(3), 39–46 (2006)
3. Ni, J.: CNC machine accuracy enhancement through real-time error compensation. International Journal of Manufacture Science and Engineering 119, 717–725 (1997)
4. Okafor, A.C., Ertekin, Y.M.: Derivation of machine tool error models and error compensation procedure for three axes vertical machining center using rigid body kinematics. International Journal of Machine tools&Manufacture 40, 1199–1213 (2000)

5. Cao, Y.Z., Altintas, Y.: A general method for the modeling of spindle-bearing systems, Transactions of the ASME. Journal of Mechanical Design 126(8), 1089–1094 (2004)
6. Ren, Y.Q., Yang, J.G.: Study on decoupling of synthesis error compensation for a 5-axis CNC machine tool. Chinese journal of mechanical engineering 40(2), 56–59 (2004)
7. Zaeh, A., Siedl, D.: A New Method for Simulation of Machining Performance by Integrating Finite Element and Multi-body Simulation for Machine Tools. Annals of the CIRP 56(1), 383–386 (2007)
8. Wu, N.X., Sun, Q.H.: Development of Kinematics Simulation System for CK1416 High Speed/Precision NC Lathe. Journal of Southwest Jiaotong University 38(5), 544–546 (2003)
9. Mujber, T.S., Szecsi, T., Hashmi, M.S.: Virtual reality applications in manufacturing process simulation. Journal of Materials Processing Technology 156(11), 1834–1838 (2004)

Predictive Force Model Based Variable Feedrate Scheduling for High-Efficiency NC Machining

Yuwen Sun, Daidi Li, Fei Ren, and Dongming Guo

School of Mechanical Engineering, Dalian University of Technology,
Dalian, 116024, China
{Yuwen.Sun,Daidi.Li,Fei.Ren,Dongming.Guo}, xiands@dlut.edu.cn

Abstract. For improving machining efficiency, variable feedrate optimization instead of constant feedrate becomes very important under constraints of surface roughness and dynamic milling force. In this paper, a predictive force model is established for ball-end milling with considerations of cutter deflection and change of feedrate direction. The corresponding cutting force coefficients are regressed from the experimental data. Then the cutting force model is used for scheduling variable feedrate along the given toolpaths, and formulas of iterative optimization of feedrate are further given. The proposed feedrate scheduling strategy is tested under various machining conditions. Experimental results show that the proposed method can effectively reduce machining time while ensuring machining quality.

Keywords: Cutting forces; Ball-end mill; Feedrate scheduling; NC machining.

1 Introduction

Ball-end milling is used extensively in the machining of sculptured surfaces such as propellers and turbine blades in automobile, aerospace, die/mold industries. During the cutting process, instantaneous cutting force has to be controlled within a specified value since it is related to reducing tool deflection and avoiding tool breakage, chipping or excess tool wear. The cutting force has become one of the most considerable process parameters in milling. In this case, it is very important to adopt predictive force model based feedrate scheduling strategy for high-efficiency ball-end milling especially under situations of frequent changes of machining allowances. Thus, dynamic milling force can be controlled at an acceptable level while trying to increase feedrate.

Although commercial CAM software packages are helpful to select suitable tool type, tool paths and machining allowances, research on feedrate scheduling is still a challenge task. Li [1] established a solid model-based milling process simulation and optimization system integrated with CAD/CAM for 3-axis end milling. After chip parameters necessary for predicting milling force was extracted, milling force was predicted using an empirical model. Then feedrate was optimized to satisfy machining requirements such as productivity and quality. Yun [2] developed a mechanistic cutting force model and machined surface errors for steady cuts under fixed cutting conditions were predicted. Then the cutting force model and surface error prediction

C. Xiong et al. (Eds.): ICIRA 2008, Part II, LNAI 5315, pp. 1076–1085, 2008.

method were extended to transient situations using the moving edge-node Z-map model to calculate the varying cutting configurations efficiently. Also, off-line feedrate scheduling was shown to be more accurate by applying instantaneous cutting coefficients. Guzel [3] proposed a strategy of increasing productivity in sculpture surface machining via off-line piecewise variable feedrate scheduling based on the force system model. A mathematical model was developed for the prediction of cutting force system in ball end milling of sculpture surfaces. This physical force model was used for selecting varying and 'appropriate' feed values along the tool path in order to decrease the cycle time in sculpture surface machining. In addition, Erdim [4] introduced a feedrate scheduling approach based on the mechanics of the process. Both the proposed feedrate scheduling strategy and the previous strategy were compared theoretically and experimentally for 3D ball-end milling of free-form surfaces. It was shown that the machining time could be decreased significantly along the tool path using force based feedrate-scheduling strategy.

This paper proposes a cutting force based feedrate scheduling strategy to achieve high productivity while maintaining high quality of parts for ball-end milling. The cutter is not assumed as a rigid object and both the tool deflection and change of feed direction are incorporated into the proposed model. Then based on the prediction model of cutting force, the feedrate is scheduled and further optimized.

2 Establish of Cutting Force Model

2.1 Cutting Force Model

The used cutting force model is based on the previous studies of Lee [5]. Here, the model is enhanced in such a way that cutter deflection as well as different ways of obtaining cutting coefficients is considered in the model to improve the prediction accuracy. Theoretically, the ball-end mill can be viewed as a set of disk elements with infinitesimal thickness along the axial position.

Let $\mathrm{d}F_t$, $\mathrm{d}F_r$ and $\mathrm{d}F_a$ be the differential cutting forces in tangential, radial, and axial directions acting on an infinitesimal cutting edge element, and these forces can be calculated with the following expressions [5]

$$\begin{pmatrix} \mathrm{d}Ft(i,\theta,z) \\ \mathrm{d}Fr(i,\theta,z) \\ \mathrm{d}Fa(i,\theta,z) \end{pmatrix} = \begin{pmatrix} Kte \\ Kre \\ Kae \end{pmatrix} \mathrm{d}S + \begin{pmatrix} Ktc \\ Krc \\ Kac \end{pmatrix} tn(\psi_{ij},\theta,k)\mathrm{d}b \tag{1}$$

where i represents the number of the cutting edge on the ith axial disk element. θ is the cutter rotational angle. ϕ_i is the angle between the ith cutting edge and the z axis. ψ_{ij} is the rotational angle of the jth element of the ith cutting edge. $\mathrm{d}b$ is differential cutting edge length in the direction perpendicular to the cutting velocity. $\mathrm{d}s$ is differential length in axial direction. k is the angle in a vertical plane between a point on the flute and the z-axis. $t_n(i,\psi_{ij},k)$ is normal undeformed chip thickness. Fig.1 shows the cutter geometry of a ball-end mill, and the above parameters can be seen in

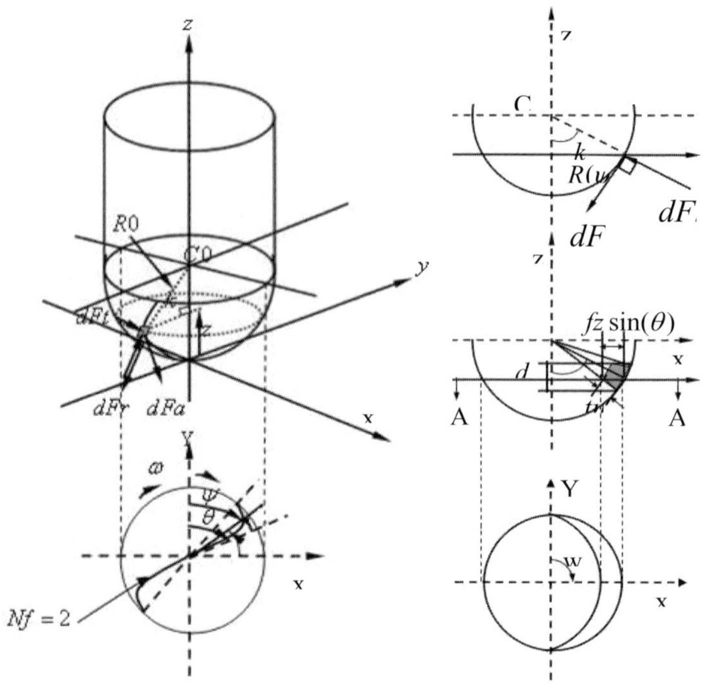

Fig. 1. Geometry of ball-end mill

Fig.1. *Kte* , *Kre* and *Kae* (N/mm) are tangential, radial, and axial edge force coefficients respectively. *Ktc* , *Krc* and *Kac* (N/mm^2) are tangential, radial and axial cutting force coefficients respectively.

dF_t , dF_r and dF_a in $X-Y-Z$ global coordinate system are expressed as follows

$$\begin{pmatrix} dFx(i,\theta,z) \\ dFy(i,\theta,z) \\ dFz(i,\theta,z) \end{pmatrix} = \begin{pmatrix} -\cos\psi & -\sin k\sin\psi & \cos k\sin\psi \\ \sin\psi & -\sin k\cos\psi & \cos k\cos\psi \\ 0 & \cos k & \sin k \end{pmatrix} \begin{pmatrix} dFt(i,\theta,z) \\ dFr(i,\theta,z) \\ dFa(i,\theta,z) \end{pmatrix} \tag{2}$$

The cutting force components at an arbitrary cutter rotation angle θ can be calculated by the following expressions

$$\begin{pmatrix} Fx(\theta) \\ Fy(\theta) \\ Fz(\theta) \end{pmatrix} = \begin{pmatrix} \sum_{j=1}^{Nf}\sum_{i=1}^{Ni}\sum_{Zi=Z\min}^{Zi=Z\max} dFx(i,\theta,zi) \\ \sum_{j=1}^{Nf}\sum_{i=1}^{Ni}\sum_{Zi=Z\min}^{Zi=Z\max} dFy(i,\theta,zi) \\ \sum_{j=1}^{Nf}\sum_{i=1}^{Ni}\sum_{Zi=Z\min}^{Zi=Z\max} dFz(i,\theta,zi) \end{pmatrix} \tag{3}$$

where *Nf* is the number of cutting edges, *Ni* is the number of the elements engaged in cutting on the *ith* cutting edge of the milling cutter.

As mentioned above, the machining direction has to be considered in the process of calculating the undeformed chip thickness. The relationship between $tn(i,\psi_{ij},\beta)$ and the tool path direction is expressed by Eq. (4). And this calculation method has been generalized for complex surfaces machining.

$$tn(i,\psi_{ij},\beta) = fz\times\sin(\psi_{ij}+\beta)\times\sin(\theta) \tag{4}$$

where β is defined according to the work piece geometry and the tool path direction. Both point $P(x,y,z)$ and point $Q(x1,y1,z1)$ are points lying in the tool trajectory, and point $Q(x1,y1,z1)$ is next to point $P(x,y,z)$. Vector $\overrightarrow{PQ}$ expresses the feed direction of the tool. β is the angle between $\overrightarrow{PQ}$ and the xoy plane and it can be calculated when the tool path is given.

When the cutter is under the action of the cutting force F_x, F_y and F_z, spring deflection occurs [6]. However, the spring deflection of the cutter along Z axial is much less than that of along X and Y axial, so the cutter spring deflection along Z axial can be neglected. Theoretically, since the tool shank can be supposed as a cantilever, the spring deflection produced by F_x and F_y can be calculated based on the cantilever theory. $\delta x(\theta,z)$ and $\delta y(\theta,z)$, which are displacements along X and Y axial directions caused by F_x and F_y can be obtained by Eq. (5).

$$\begin{aligned}\delta x(\theta,z) &= \frac{Fx}{2.0ER0^4}[<Ctx(\theta)-z>^3 - (L-z)^3 + 3.0(L-z)^2(L-Ctx(\theta))]\\ \delta y(\theta,z) &= \frac{Fy}{2.0ER0^4}[<Cty(\theta)-z>^3 - (L-z)^3 + 3.0(L-z)^2(L-Cty(\theta))]\end{aligned} \tag{5}$$

where function <x> is defined as <x>=x if x>0. otherwise, <x> =0. $Cx(\theta)$ and $Cy(\theta)$ are instantaneous centers of cutting forces along X and Y axial directions at a cutter rotation angle θ, and Eq.(6) is their expressions. dMx and dMy are moments of the cutting elements engaged in cutting.

$$Ctx(\theta) = L - \left(\sum_{j=1}^{Nf}\sum_{i=1}^{Ni} dMx \Big/ Fx\right), Cty(\theta) = L - \left(\sum_{j=1}^{Nf}\sum_{i=1}^{Ni} dMy \Big/ Fy\right) \tag{6}$$

In this case, the new instantaneous chip thickness can be written as following

$$\begin{aligned}&tn'(i,\psi_{ij},\beta) = tn(i,\psi_{ij},\beta) - tt\\ &= tn(i,\psi_{ij},\beta) - \sqrt{\delta x^2(\theta,z) + \delta y^2(\theta,z) - [\delta x(\theta,z)/\tan\psi_{ij} - \delta y(\theta,}\end{aligned} \tag{7}$$

2.2 Cutter/Work Piece Intersection Model

In this paper, Z-Map model is used to determine which part of the cutter is engaged with the work piece at any instant of machining time. It is very important to find the cutter-work piece engagement domain due to its direct influence on the accuracy of cutting force calculation. The tool reference system $o-xyz$ and the part reference system $O-XYZ$ are first defined, as it is shown in Fig.2. Using Z-Map model, the

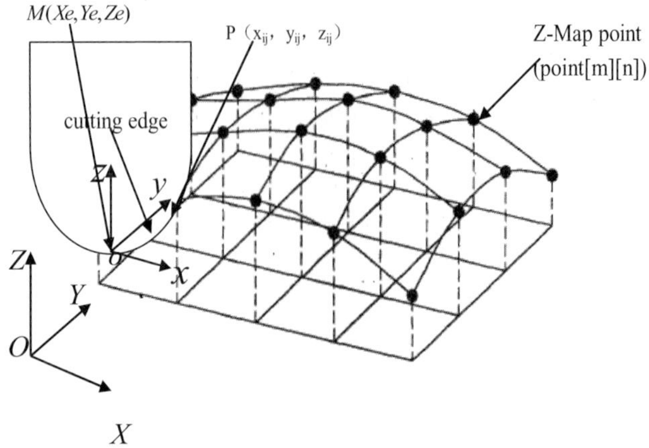

Fig. 2. The Z-Map model and the relationship between tool and work part reference frames

cutter and work piece are meshed into small elements whose projection into the XOY plane is square. Size selection of mesh elements depends on desired level of accuracy in the simulation, etc. The smaller the mesh size is divided, the better the accuracy of the cutting force prediction is and at the same time the longer the calculation time is. Therefore, the size of the mesh elements is selected according to the required machining accuracy of the work piece. As shown in fig.2, the heights of the nodal points of the mesh elements in the work piece surface in $O-XYZ$ global coordinate system are denoted by a 2D array point[m][n].

Given the cutter tip location $M(Xe, Ye, Ze)$ and the cutter rotational angle, all the locations of discrete points on the cutting edges are calculated in terms of $O-XYZ$ global coordinates. Therefore, the instantaneous work piece heights at each of the $X-Y$ coordinates of discrete points on the cutting edges are also determined by comparing the cutting edges with work piece heights at these points. At the same mesh grid node, point[m][n] is the height of work piece surface and P (x_{ij}, y_{ij}, z_{ij}) is a point on the cutting edge in $X-Y-Z$ global coordinates. If and only if{ point[m][n]> z_{ij} }, P (x_{ij}, y_{ij}, z_{ij}) is in cutting and the height of work piece surface point[m][n] equals to z_{ij} , or else P (x_{ij}, y_{ij}, z_{ij}) is not engaged in cutting. In the next increment, the cutter tip travels one grid again. Repeating the process, the lengths of cutting edges and the work piece surface topography can be obtained and the instant force can be calculated in the simulation.

2.3 Cutting Coefficient Calculation

As mentioned in the above section, the resulting cutting forces are determined by summing up the cutting forces of each discrete element. They can be calculated by using Eq. (1) and for doing so the cutting coefficients and edge coefficients must be known first. Usually, these coefficients, Kte , Kre , Kae , Ktc , Krc and Kac , are regressed with Eq.(1) and Eq.(8)

$$\begin{pmatrix} Ktc \\ Krc \\ Kac \\ Kte \\ Kre \\ Kae \end{pmatrix} = \begin{pmatrix} a_{00} & a_{01} & a_{02} & a_{03} & 0 & 0 \\ a_{10} & a_{11} & a_{12} & a_{13} & 0 & 0 \\ a_{20} & a_{21} & a_{22} & a_{23} & 0 & 0 \\ 0 & 0 & 0 & 0 & a_{34} & 0 \\ 0 & 0 & 0 & 0 & 0 & a_{45} \\ 0 & 0 & 0 & 0 & 0 & a_{56} \end{pmatrix} \times \begin{pmatrix} 1 \\ z_{ij} \\ z_{ij} \times z_{ij} \\ z_{ij} \times z_{ij} \times z_{ij} \\ 1 \\ 1 \\ 1 \end{pmatrix} \tag{8}$$

where Ktc, Krc and Kac vary with z_{ij}, and Kte, Kre, Kae are invariable when the tool and the work piece are given.

3 Feedrate Scheduling Strategies

3.1 Initial Feedrate Optimization

Feedrate optimization plays a key role in free-form surface machining for improving machining efficiency. Keeping constant force in milling is very important for obtaining better stability of the cutting process and improving the machined surface topography. Hence, in sculptured surface machining it is expected that piecewise feedrate is scheduled so as to keep a constant milling force.

In this paper, maximum force method is introduced to optimize the feedrate. Firstly, required data of force modeling module such as tool and work piece data and constant feedrate v_0 are given in advance. Secondly, based on the cutting force model, maximum forces are predicted for each cutter step, and these data are saved into a file from which the maximum force $F_{\max}$ in the cutting progress is selected. After setting reasonable constant cutting force value F of cutting process, corresponding feedrate v_n for each cutter step can be obtained by Eq. (9).

$$v_n = v_0 \frac{F}{F_{\max}} \tag{9}$$

However, v_n gained by Eq. (9) can not always satisfy the machining requirement very well and sometimes it needs to be further optimized. Based on the feed value v_n, new federate v_{n1} at each cutter step can be gained according to the following formula.

$$v_{n1} = v_n + \frac{(F - F_{\max 1})(v_n - v_0)}{F_{\max 1} - F_{\max}} \tag{10}$$

where $F_{\max 1}$ is the maximum force using v_n in the cutting process. After further optimization, the purpose of keeping constant force in milling can be achieved better.

3.2 Iterative Optimization of Feedrate

Although v_{n1} for each cutter step obtained according to the above formula (10) usually satisfy engineering requirements very well, in some special cases frequent change of feedrate could shorten the cutter life significantly. Meanwhile, the machining precision of the work piece is also influenced more or less due to the machine tool's response lag caused by the frequent change of feedrate. To some extent these disadvantages mentioned above can be remedied remarkably by adjusting the change frequency of the feedrate. For this goal the following introduces a method to further optimize feedrate iteratively.

Generally, the cutting force changes linearly with the cutting depth. Based on this premise, some segments are divided between maximum depth and minimum depth in order to obtain piecewise feedrate scheduling along the given tool path. In each segment, average cutting depth is derived and then average feedrate of this segment is calculated. Consequently, the whole feedrate curve is consisted of some piecewise feedrate segments. Thus, the abrupt change of feedrate can be avoided or alleviated effectively. In the process of feedrate optimization, when the feedrate varies from v_1 to v_2 what should be noted is that the displacement S must satisfy Eq.(11)

$$S = \frac{(v_1 - v_2)(v_1 - v_2)}{720000a} \leq S_1 \tag{11}$$

where a is the feed acceleration of the cutter.

4 Experiments Validation

Before implementing feedrate optimization in free-form surface machining, the coefficients in the cutting force prediction model must be determined and the veracity of the cutting force model must also be validated. In this section, two experiments are introduced and they are experiments for calibrating force coefficients and feedrate scheduling validation. Both experiments are based on 45 steel which is usually used for automobile prototype production dies. And the same tool, a 10 mm diameter, 30° helix angle, 2 flutes, tungsten carbide ball-end mill, is used in the two tests. The first experiment concerns obtaining the cutting force data used for regressing cutting coefficients. The following compares the results of the simulated cutting force with measured cutting force in a certain cutting condition and tool geometry. And then the reasons that cause the deviations between the measured and simulated forces are analyzed. Based on the force model, the feedrate scheduling approach is validated by real sculptured surface machining in the second experiment.

Table 1. Work piece material and cutting parameter

Part material	45# steel				R_0		10mm			Helical angle		30°		Nf	2
Feedrate (mm/min)	20					50					100				
ap (mm)	1	2	3	3.5	4	1	2	3	3.5	4	1	2	3	3.5	4

4.1 Experimental Calibration of Force Coefficients

To obtain empirical force coefficients, 15 sets of slot cutting tests were performed on a vertical machining center. The spindle speed was set to 1000 rpm. Cutting parameters, fz and ap, are shown in Table 1. Instantaneous cutting forces in the X, Y and Z directions were measured using a three component piezoelectric force dynamometer. The coefficients, Kte, Kre, Kae, Ktc, Krc and Kac, are determined from above cutting tests using the measured cutting forces as input data.

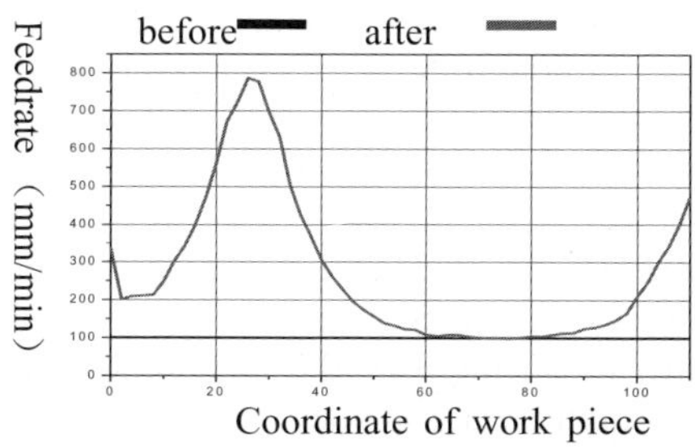

Fig. 3. Feedrates in constant and adaptive machining

From the experiment, it can be seen that the simulated and measured cutting force results. From this it can be seen that the established cutting force prediction model is validated. Among the three cutting forces along the x axis, y axis and z axis directions, the prediction accuracy of the cutting force along the Z axis direction is best. Deviations of the other two cutting forces are also under control within an allowable value and they are mainly caused by the tool runout.

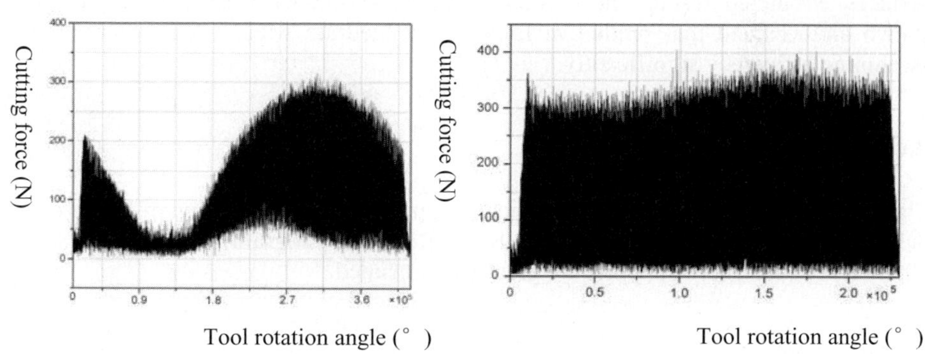

Fig. 4. Measured forces in constant and adaptive feedrate machining

4.2 Feedrate Scheduling Validation

The feedrate scheduling approach is performed not only for the plane in which the feed is horizontal direction but also for complex free-form surface in which the feed is in non-horizontal direction. In federate scheduling validation, the CL (cutter location)

path is a sinusoidal curve with small amplitude along the cutting-depth direction. The spindle speed was set to 1000 rpm and the constant feedrate was 100 mm/min. The interval value d between two adjacent tool paths is given according to Eq. 12. The machining error h is set as 0.04mm.

$$d = 2.0\times\sqrt{h(2.0\times R_0 - h)} \tag{12}$$

Where R_0 represents the radius of the cutter. The machining experiments of constant feedrate and adaptive feedrate machining are performed. Fig.3 shows the feedrate scheduling curves in two experiments. The measured force results in both experiments are shown in Fig.4. Although the feedrate in constant machining is only set as 100mm/min, there still exists dramatic change of cutting forces from about 50 N to 300N. In force based machining the feedrate is scheduled piecewisely, so it is normal that the cutting force changes within a small range. It is not necessary to try to keep constant cutting force using iteration strategy in case the feedrate changes dramatically. From the machining experiments it can be seen that the predictive force based feedrate scheduling strategy can improve the machining efficiency over 40% compared with the constant feedrate strategy.

5 Conclusions

In this paper, a predictive force model is established for ball-end milling with considerations of cutter deflection and change of feedrate direction. And based on the 45 steel and the tungsten carbide ball-end mill, tests are performed to calibrate the cutting coefficients. Then the validation of force model is proved by the experiment. Both constant feedrate and force-based feedrate scheduling strategies in machining are compared theoretically and experimentally for 3D ball-end milling of free-form surfaces. Predicted results show good agreements with Measurement results. It is shown and verified that predictive force based feedrate strategy can improves the machining efficiency significantly.

Acknowledgments

This research is supported by the National Natural Science Foundation of China under the grant no. 50775023 and Chinese Basic Research Program under the grant no. 2005CB724100. These supports are greatly appreciated.

References

1. Li, Z.Z., Zheng, M., Zheng, L., Wu, Z.J., Liu, D.C.: A solid model-based milling process simulation and optimization system integrated with CAD/CAM. Mater. Process. Technol. 138, 513–517 (2003)
2. Yun, W.S., Ko, J.H., Lee, H.U.: Development of a virtual machining system, Part 3: cutting process simulation in transient cuts. Int. Mach. Tools Manuf. 42, 1617–1626 (2002)

3. Guzel, B.U., Lazoglu, I.: Increasing productivity in sculptured surface machining via off-line piecewise variable feedrate scheduling based on the force system model. Int. J. Mach. Tools Manuf. 44, 21–28 (2004)
4. Erdim, H., Lazoglu, I., Ozturk, B.: Feedrate scheduling strategies for free-form surfaces. Int. J. Mach. Tools Manuf. 46, 747–757 (2006)
5. Lee, P., Altintas, Y.: Prediction of ball-end milling forces from orthogonal cutting data. Int. J. Mach. Tools Manuf. 36, 1059–1072 (1996)
6. Ni, Q.M., Li, C.X., Wu, G.L., Ruan, X.Y.: Modeling and simulation of Milling forces for flexible ball-end milling cutters. Chin. J. Mech. Eng. 38, 108–112 (2002) (in Chinese)

Design of Redundant Robot for Automated Painting of Large and Complex Surface

Shiqi Li[1], Yang Liu[1], and Ming Xie[2]

[1] School of Mechanical Science & Engineering, Huazhong University of Science & Technology, Wuhan, China
[2] School of Mechanical& Aerospace Engineering, Nanyang Technological University, Singapore
sqli@mail.hust.edu.cn, liuyang-hust@163.com, mmxie@ntu.edu.sg

Abstract. This paper presents a spray-painting robot which has eight DOFs and can be used to automate the painting of a very large and complex surface. The robot is named as XN-600-2 with eight revolute joints which are independently driven by a single mechanical-power supplier (i.e. a motor). The developed robot is more compacter in structure than TX90 made by Staubli. We first present our robot prototype. There are four modular units in it, each of which has two independent joints which can move bi-directionally. Then, we discuss the strength and vibration of the robot, and show some simulation results when robot is in different working states. Finally, we discuss the harmonious response of the robot driven by the motor mounted in the basement.

Keywords: redundant robot, spray painting, uni-drive concept.

1 Introduction

Spray painting is an important process for the manufacture of many durable products, such as automobiles, furniture and appliances. The uniformity of paint thickness on a product can strongly influence the quality of the product. Paint gun trajectory planning is critical to achieve the uniformity of paint thickness. Numerous works related to trajectory planning were published. Some confront the challenge of automatic generation of a 3D paint path[1][2], and some build a geometry library for CAD-guided robotic system[3][4][5]. Also, some try to equip the robot with laser range sensors to obtain an accurate scan of the part or mounting some camera in order to develop a vision-guided robotic system[6]. These works are all based on the existing robots, in which the DOFs and structure impose some limitations.

In a robotic painting station, the spray gun is mounted on the wrist of a six degree of freedom industrial robot such as Staubli or ABB at a workshop of automobile. Such a scenario remains until now. Although these robots move fast and efficient and get a good precision painted in some parts like door of automobile, it's not enough when the surface to be painted is complex or very large. If a spray-painting robot has many degrees of freedom, it will have a superior ability to flex, reach, and approach a large volume in its workspace with infinite number of configurations. It also can be used in soldering and assembling when the tool mounted is changed. And since the

C. Xiong et al. (Eds.): ICIRA 2008, Part II, LNAI 5315, pp. 1086–1095, 2008.

tool for painting is lighter, the hyper redundant robot can be used to support the tool. There are many ways to achieve "light weight, multiple DOFs" properties, such as, new structure material application, modularization, compact joint design and light body design, and so on. The last two ways are widely used.

Joint mechanism design has been a bottle neck for constructing compact, strong and maneuverable robot. There are many joint designs for robot, like universal joint or active joint, etc. Until now, the most compact and dexterous joint is the angular swivel joint [7][8], which is built by Professor Choset at Carnegie Mellon University in USA. The most difference between the design and the others is all rotation axes of the revolute joints are not parallel or perpendicular to each other, but angular, which save much joint space. Choset designed an elephant-trunk mobile robot with 14 DOFs using the angular swivel joint mounted a camera to search in remains.

Since the actuator often contributes a significant portion of the module weight, this is reduced in the proposed design by replacing the actuator with a pair of clutches. There are some researchers who design robots with one motor driven. For instance, a snake robot with twenty DOFs driven by single motor was designed and implemented in 1998[9][10]. The snake robot has some one-to-many coupling device which connect main shaft to several joints. That can be done with eight parallel splitter of motion and serial splitter of motion. Every joint will be controlled by a clutch and a brake. However, for uni-drive concept the biggest challenge is the clutches control. Dr. Karbasi who is at university of Waterloo in Canada developed a 2-axis gantry robot based on the modular uni-drive concept[11][12] in 2003 and did some experimental for the position and velocity of the modules regulated by controlling the engagement time of the clutches using the pulses width modulation technique. The PWM technique may be a way for precision control for the uni-drive robot.

The spray painting robot for complex and large surface needs multiple modular units. A fully modular re-configurable robot consisting of a set of standardized modules can be configured to different structures for different painting task. Using uni-drive concept with modularity and compact joint design may be a solution to achieve a spray painting mechanisms which provide flexibility, ease of maintenance, and fit for huge complicated surface. In the following sections, we introduce the snake robot which was designed in our lab. We will show its mechanical structure (section 2), kinematic analysis (section 3), strength analysis (section 4), vibration analysis (section 5).

2 Mechanical Structure of The Robot

Some concept of single-motor-driven(SMD) can be seen in[10][11]. The SMD provides a new way to design robot arms compared to conventional design philosophy which simply advocates the one-to-one coupling between actuators and joints. The robot named as XN-600-2 is shown in Fig.1. XN-600-2 is look like a big snake, of which length is 1400mm and the radius is nearly 100mm and the weight is nearly 60kg. If the robot is mounted a painting tool as TX90XL made by Staubli, then the robot can be used in spray-painting. Compared to TX90XL, the load capacity of XN-600-2 is 1kg which is less than TX90XL, but XN-600-2 has two more DOFs as their nearly length. And the more DOFs will make the robot more fit for painting the surface of cavity in automobile workshop.

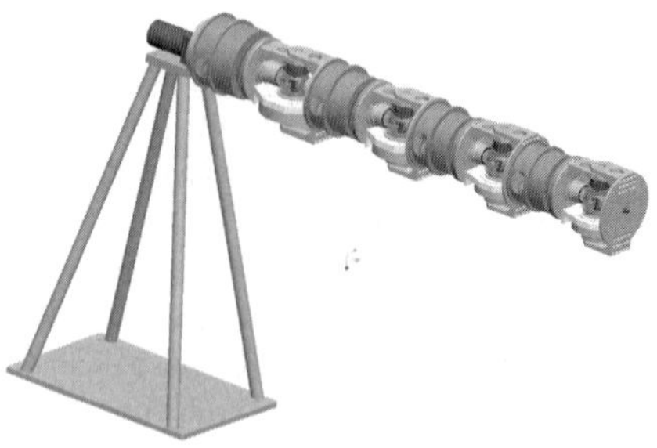

Fig. 1. 3D model of XN-600-2

There are eight independent revolute joints in it. The motor mounted in the basement supplies energy to robot through the main shaft of joint one by one. There are two motions in every joint, one is main motion, and the other is joint motion. When the motor is running, main motion is transferred to every joint of the robot by main shaft and gear box. And when the joint clutch is on or off, the joint can get or refuse energy from the main motion. That is joint motion. The clutch box is the coupling device which couple mechanic and electric. Since the clutch is the most important device in the robot, the frequency and the ratio of the clutch can be great influence for the precision of the joint.

The eight joints can be divided into four same modular units shown in Fig.2, each of which is made up by twisting and pivoting joint mounted together. The main shaft of the modular unit closed to the basement can be driven by DC motor, and transfer motion from joint to joint through the twisting and pivoting joints. The joint will be driven by the harmonic driver which is mounted in the joint when the clutches are on. There are two clutches and one brake in one joint, which can control the robot turning around or reverse. And there is a gear reducer in the DC motor. The speed coming out from motor is 375 rpm, which is fit for harmonic drive working in the state of high efficiency.

The main motion through joint will meet the twisting joint firstly. As shown in Fig.3, the twisting joint gets the main motion from the main shaft by the gears which are connected clutches. We designed a central hole for the main shaft to mount in twisting joint that would make the joint very compact. When the clutch is on, the speed reducer will get motion from main shaft directly and the house of twisting joint will be driven at the same time.

From Fig.3, it is shown that main motion which is going out from twisting joint is same to that going into, so the pivoting joint can get same main motion with twisting joint. The clutches of pivoting joint with their bevel gears are set up perpendicularly, as shown in Fig.4.

Each of clutches or brake in pivoting joint is mounted with two bevel gears. One of the gears which are connected clutch is used to transfer main motion of joint, and the other is used to drive the speed reducer. When the brake is on and clutch is off, the three bevel gears in the center of joint will transfer main motion through pivoting joint. And if either of the clutches is on and the brake is off, the speed reducer will get the motion by the two bevel gears which are mounted on the input shaft of speed reducer and that is the joint motion of pivoting joint. The control diagram is seen in Fig.5.

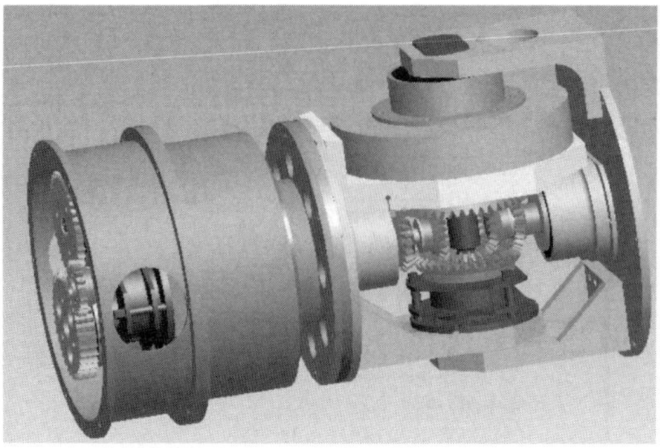

Fig. 2. 3D model of modular unit

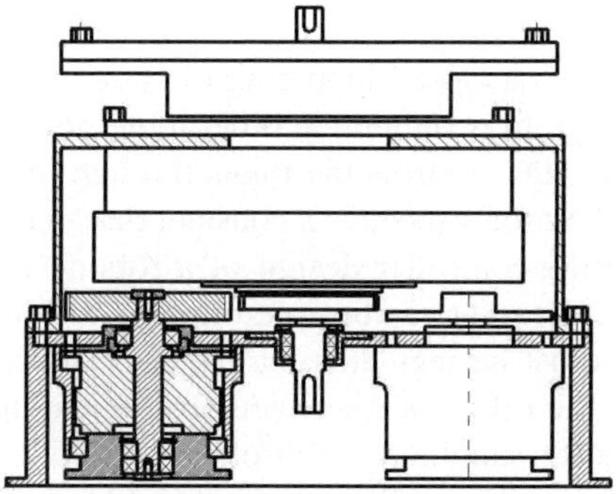

Fig. 3. Design of twisting joint

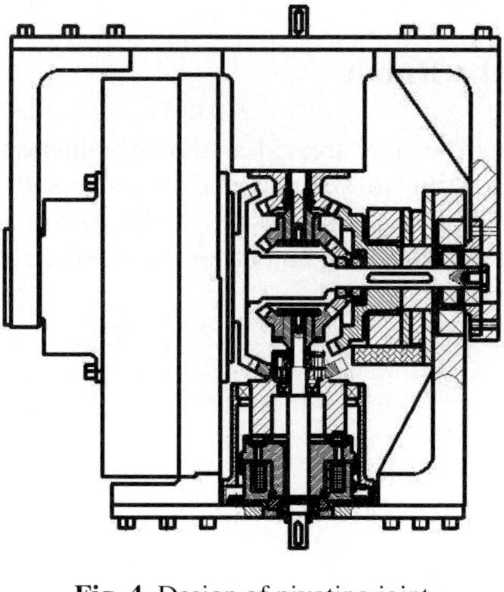

Fig. 4. Design of pivoting joint

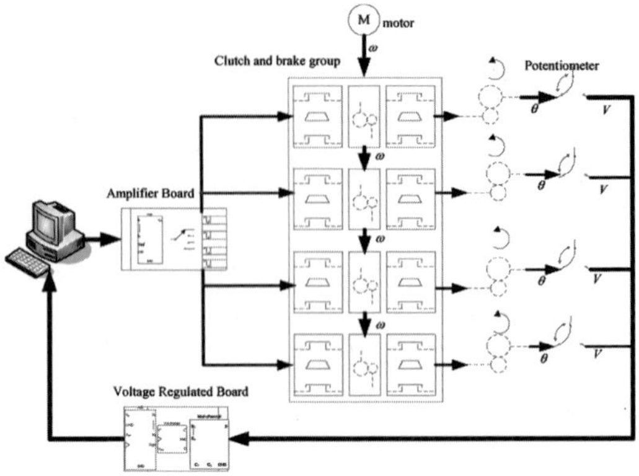

Fig. 5. Control diagram for XN-600-2

From Fig.5, we know it is a closed-loop control system for XN-600-2. The central PC in which a control program is running in order to get joint angles by some potentiometers mounted in joints. PC controls the joints through the clutch and brake working together. And the DC motor's speed is a constant that make thing easy.

The discontinuous PWM controller design of a robotic manipulator has been reported [13]. The angle of the joint can be controlled by the engagement of clutch, but the velocity of the joint must be regulated by the ratio and frequency of the engagement of clutch, which is the difference between position control and velocity control. The discontinuous (on–off) stabilizing controller is used in XN-600-2 which was determined from a continuous controller designed for the nonlinear average model of the PWM controlled system. Linear clutch mounted in the joint will be good for the velocity control, but it's not easy to be manufactured.

3 Kinematics for the Robot

Since a robot's mechanism can be treated as the combination of a set of open kinematics-chains, it is interesting to simulate theoretical results for the modeling and analysis of an open kinematic-chain. Based on the design of XN-600-2 shown in Fig.1, we can establish the frame assignment for the robot, as shown in Figure 6.

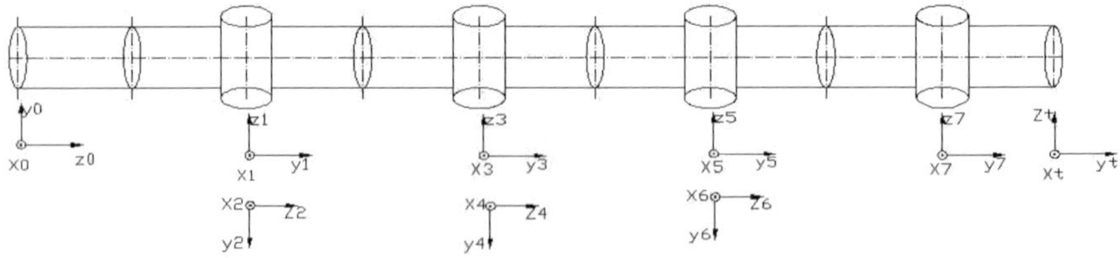

Fig. 6. Reference frame of XN-600-2

Based on the frame assignment, the DH parameters of XN-600-2 can be obtained. The results are shown in Table 1.

Table 1. D-H parameter table

link number	α	a	θ	d
1	-90^0	0	0^0	350
2	90^0	0	0^0	0
3	-90^0	0	0^0	350
4	90^0	0	0^0	0
5	-90^0	0	0^0	350
6	90^0	0	0^0	0
7	-90^0	0	0^0	350
8	90^0	0	0^0	0
T	0	100	0^0	0

Fig.7 shows 3D view of XN-600-2 with eight degrees of freedom based on the DH parameters in Table 1.

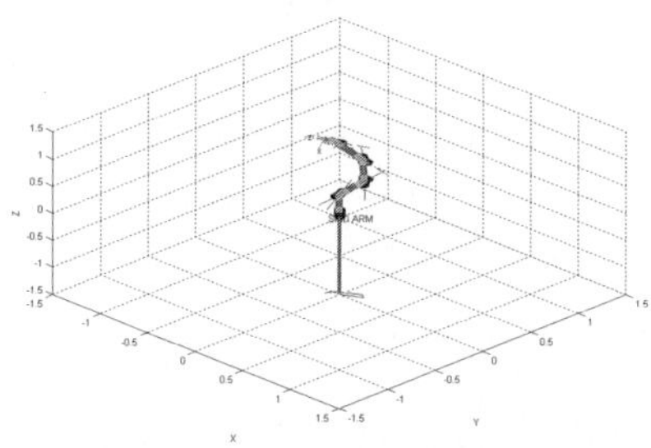

Fig. 7. Kinematic simulation for XN-600-2

For the first modular unit, we can get the two transform matrices, one is twisting joint's coordinate frame with respect to the basement's coordinate system, and the other is the pivoting joint's coordinate frame with respect to twisting joint's coordinate system.

$$ {}_1^0T = \begin{bmatrix} c_1 & -s_1 & 0 & 0 \\ 0 & 0 & 1 & l_1+l_2 \\ -s_1 & -c_1 & 0 & 0 \\ 0 & 0 & 0 & 1 \end{bmatrix}, \quad {}_2^1T = \begin{bmatrix} c_2 & -s_2 & 0 & 0 \\ 0 & 0 & -1 & 0 \\ s_2 & -c_2 & 0 & 0 \\ 0 & 0 & 0 & 1 \end{bmatrix}, $$

Transformation matrices of the other modular units are same like above one. At last, we can get the coordinate frame transform matrix of nozzle with respect to the basement, ${}_8^0T = {}_1^0T\,{}_2^1T\,{}_3^2T\,{}_4^3T\,{}_5^4T\,{}_6^5T\,{}_7^6T\,{}_8^7T$. Since it is perpendicular between the axes of twisting joint and pivoting joint, ${}_8^0T$ owns some zero what make the forward kinematic solution quickly.

4 Strength of the Robot

Since the ratio of length and radius is very large and the weight is not small, the strength of the robot is very important when it is mounted a nozzle for a painting task. We build a FEM model of XN-600-2 for the structure analysis, as shown in Fig.8.

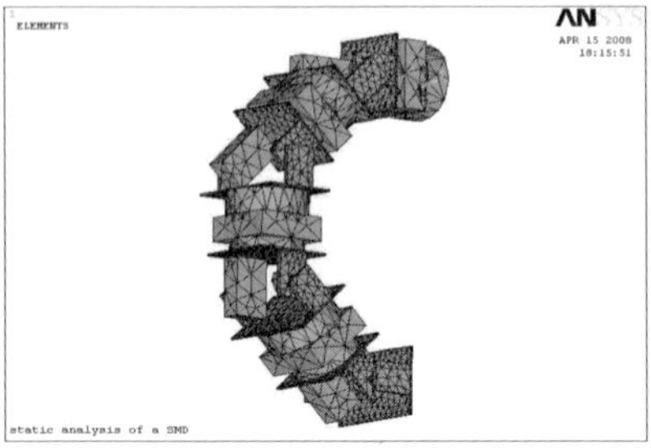

Fig. 8. The FEM model of XN-600-2

When the robot is working obey the rule, e.g.: $\theta_t = 50t + 50$, $\theta_p \in [0, 60]$, the displacement and the maximum stress of robot are changed as shown in Fig.9.

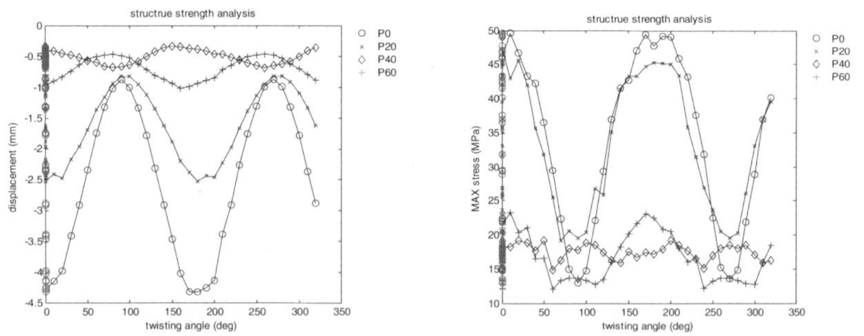

Fig. 9. Strength analysis for XN-600-2.P0 represent pivoting angle is zero ; P20 represent pivoting angle is 20deg; P40 represent pivoting angle is 40deg; P60 represent pivoting angle is 60deg

From the Fig.9, we can see when the pivoting angle is zero that means the robot in horizontally, the distortion of robot is the biggest. Since the robot posture is changed, the maximum error of nozzle is 3.5mm. We are sure that the distortion is not over the limitation of material and will be changed when the robot is working. The errors need a new way to be compensated. When the robot is used in painting task, the pivoting and twisting joints will not obey the rule of joint angle changed shown in the Fig.8. But the most dangerous of structure has been covered and the strength of the robot is enough for a painting tool.

5 Vibration of the Robot

Since the robot is driven by a DC motor, every joint in the robot will get same main motion, that is to say, the oscillation of joints are all coming from the main motion. Fig.10 shows the modes of structure as different postures.

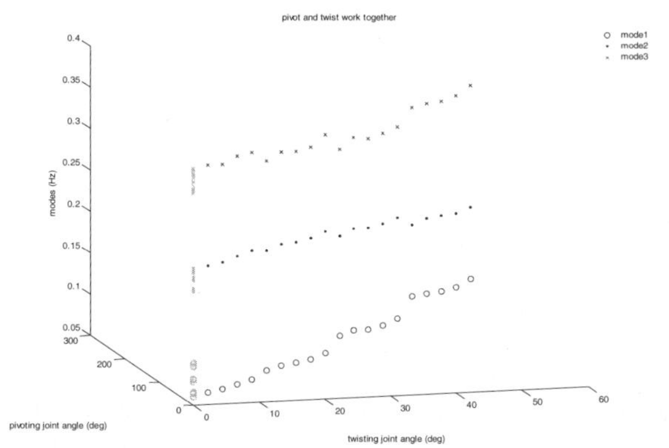

Fig. 10. The modular analysis of XN-600-2 as different postures

From Fig.10, the modes of structure have no any big changes when the angle of twisting joint is changed from 0 to330 degrees and the pivoting joint is changed from 0 to 60 degrees. In fact, the twisting joint has no big impact to the modes changed and the modes of structure changed with the angle of pivoting joint are nearly same to the pivoting and twisting joint work together.

The DC motor can be regulated from 0 to 375rpm, which is equal to an exciter exciting the robot from 0 to 6.25Hz. The following is the harmonious response of the robot, as shown in Fig.11.

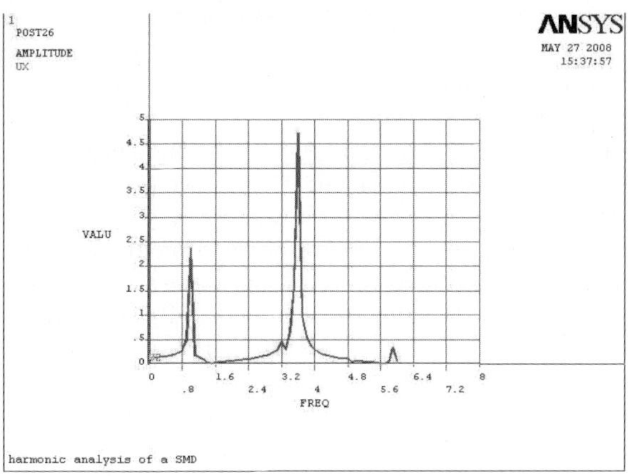

Fig. 11. XN-600-2 harmonic response

From the Fig.11, we can see the points of sympathetic vibration are 1Hz and 3.5Hz. It is required that the motor speed can not nearly 60rpm and 210rpm, otherwise, it will make XN-600-2 vibrate uncontrollable. Fortunately, the modes of structure seen in Fig.10 are not a big part of frequency scope at the time of motor speed regulating, which may be a good thing for robot control.

6 Conclusion

In this paper, we present a design of an eight DOFs robot for painting task. This design obeys the concept of single-motor-driven with strong strength and large running scope and compact structure. This robot can be used to assemble or solder if the tool mounted in the end of robot is changed.

With compact joint design and using one motor to drive many independent joints, we may build a robot owned many advantages such as cost reduction, weight reduction and space reduction. In addition, if get off some speed reducers from the robot for some multi-support task such as rescuing in remains, it'll miniaturize the body of the robot than present one, while maintaining the same power of the motor in the base. This may open a new avenue toward the investigation of mini and dexterous robot for search and rescue into places not accessible or dangerous for mankind.

Acknowledgements

The research works are generously funded by CAST foundation of China. Contributions from J.Guo and Z.W.Su have been greatly appreciated by the authors.

References

1. Chen, H.P.: Automated Robot Trajectory Planning for Spray Painting of Free-Form Surfaces in Automotive Manufacturing. In: Proceedings of the 2002 IEEE International Conference on Robotics & Automation, pp. 450–455 (2002)
2. Suh, S.H., Woo, I.K., Noh, S.K.: Development of an automatic trajectory planning system (atps) for spray painting robots. In: IEEE International Conference on Robotics and Automation on 1991, pp. 1948–1955 (1991)
3. Kwok, K.S., Louks, C.S., Driessen, B.J.: Rapid 3-D Digitizing and Tool Path Generation for Complex Shapes. In: IEEE international Conference on Robotics and Automation, pp. 2789–2794 (1998)
4. Tse, W.C., Chen, Y.H.: A robotic system for rapid protoryping. In: IEEE International Conference on Robotics and Automion, vol. 3, pp. 1815–1820 (1997)
5. Vincze, M., Biegelbauer, G.: Painting Parts Automatically at Lot Size One, Robot Sensing, 2004. In: ROSE 2004. International Workshop on 2004, pp. 35–40 (2004)
6. Zaki, A., Eskander, M.: Spray Painting of a General Three-Dimensional Surface. In: Proceedings of the 2000 IEEE/RSJ International Conference on Intelligent Robots and Systems, pp. 2172–2177 (2000)
7. Shammas, E.A., Choset, H.: Orientation Preserving Angular Swivel Joint,US Patent Number 6,871,563 (2005)

8. Shammas, E.A., Wolf, A., Brown, H., Choset, H.: New Joint Design for Three-dimensional Hyper Redundant Robots. In: Proceedings of the 2003 IEEE/RSJ International Conference on Intelligent Robots and Systems, pp. 3594–3599 (2003)
9. Zhu, H.H., Xie, M., Lim, M.K.: Modular Robot Manipulator Apparatus, PCT/SG00/0002 (2000)
10. Xie, M.: Fundamentals of Robotics: Linking Perception to Action, 1st edn. World Scientific, Singapore (2003)
11. Karbasi, H., Huissoon, J.P., Khajepour, A.: Uni-drive modular robots:theory, design,and experiments. In: Mechanism and machine. Theory, vol. 39, pp. 183–200 (2004)
12. Karbasi, H.: Uni-drive modular robots. PhD Thesis, Department of Mechanical Engineering, University of Waterloo, Waterloo, Canada (2003)
13. Ramirez, H.S., Zribi, M., Ahmad, S.: Pulse width modulated control of robotic manipulators. In: Proceeding of the 29th IEEE Conference on Decision and Control, vol. 1, pp. 366–367 (1990)

Intellectualized Structural Synthesis and Classification of the 3-DOF Space Parallel Robot Mechanisms

Fanghua Liu[1,2], Hongtao Wu[2], and Lüzhong Ma[3]

[1] School of Mechanical& Electrical Engineering, Nanjing University of Aeronautics& Astronautics, NanJing 210016
[2] School of Mechanical& Power Engineering, Jiangsu University of science and technology Jiangsu, 2120003
[3] College of Mechanical Engineering, Jiangsu University Jiangsu, 2120013
cylfhua@163.com, mehtwu@163.com, mlz@ujs.edu.cn

Abstract. Based on the theory of structural synthesis and classification of degenerate-rank parallel robot mechanisms, which uses the units of single open chain limb. An intelligent, systematic and effective new method is put forward, which utilizes intelligent structural synthesis and classification of the parallel robot mechanisms with VB. The method produces a series of models according to the output movement characteristics of activated platform and degrees of freedom, and provides the foundation for a series of work such as kinematics and dynamics analysis. The new method makes the structural synthesis of 3-DOF space parallel robot mechanisms automated. It is of universal significance and can be applied to mechanisms with other kinematics output types. Previous methods were repetitious, tedious inefficient and prone to mistakes The new method overcomes these problems and paves a new for synthesis research development and has good application prospect.

Keywords: Parallel robot mechanisms, Single open chain limb.

1 Introduction

Some scholars have done much research about structural synthesis and classification of the mechanisms. HUNT[1] presented the way based on the screw theory[2], It has good guiding meaning for the problem of the structural synthesis and classification of the parallel mechanisms. HARA, et al[3], studied the structural synthesis and classification of the micro-motion manipulator according to the characteristic of the Jacobin matrix. HERVE[4] researched the structural synthesis and classification of the 3DOF translational parallel mechanisms using the group theory of mathematics. A new way was put forward by Yang, et al[5], based on the theory of structural synthesis and classification of degenerate-rank parallel robot mechanisms which uses the units of single open chain limb. These ways can be used to explain the mechanisms, which have been found, and to synthesis many new mechanisms, but these ways put forward mainly depended on the experience, knowledge, wisdom and association or inference of the designer, and the course of the structural and classification is very complex, repetitive and inefficient. With the rapid development of the computer and calculation

C. Xiong et al. (Eds.): ICIRA 2008, Part II, LNAI 5315, pp. 1096–1104, 2008.

technology, it posed an arduous task for the scholar of the mechanisms, that is, to set about exploiting the thought function of the computer and making the structural synthesis and classification automated. This paper implements the thorough study on the research of documentation[6] ,exploiting a set of intellectualized structural synthesis and classification Software with VB based on the units of single open chain limb and utilizing the intellectualized structural synthesis and classification of the three-degree of space parallel robot mechanisms. It can get a series of different 3-DOF space parallel mechanisms. Applying this program provides the convenience for research about structural synthesis and classification of the mechanisms. The intellectualized method is very important for the enlarging the scope of the selective preference and innovation design of the mechanisms.

2 Theoretical Foundation of Parallel Mechanisms Structural Synthesis

The procedure based on the theory of structural synthesis and classification of degenerate-rank parallel robot mechanisms which uses the units of single open chain limb according to Ref.[6]is presented below :

(1) List the output matrix, U^p, of the parallel robot mechanisms which should be synthesized. Write the expression of U^p according to the demand of the design.

(2) Select structural type of single open chain (SOC) limb. Select the satisfactory structural type from all the known SOC limbs, the output of which should contain all the output of U^p.

(3) Determine the minimum limbs, $n_{\min}$, of the parallel mechanisms. If the output matrix of SOC limb is in complete correspondence with the output matrix of the parallel robot mechanisms which should be synthesized, the $n_{\min}$ is two according to the minimum limbs of the parallel mechanisms which at least is two. If the output of SOC limb exceed the expected output of the parallel mechanisms, and require all the limbs are the same. Take the 3-DOF translational parallel mechanisms for example, $\hat{\xi}^p$ is the rotational numbers of expected output of the parallel mechanisms, $\hat{\xi}^o$ is the rotational numbers of expected output of the single open chain limb , we have $n_{\min} = \hat{\xi}^o - \hat{\xi}^p = 1$.

(4) Determine the rank, ξ_j^l, of the fundamental loop. We obtain the rank of the fundamental loop

$$\sum_{j=1}^{n-1} \xi_j^l = \sum_{i=1}^{m} f_i - M \tag{1}$$

where f_i is the degree of freedom of the ith kinematics pair, and M is the mobility of the mechanisms. Apparently, there are many allocation plans which satisfy Eq. (1) , the numeric of ξ_j^l of different fundamental loop may be the same or different.

(5) Determine the distributed mode of SOC limb between the moving platform and static platform. If the rank of SOC limb, ξ=6, it can be allocated in any place, or allocation will be determined by the intersection of Eq. (2) and the rank of fundamental loop.

$$U^{p} = \bigcap_{i=1}^{n} U_i^{o} \tag{2}$$

where U^{p} is the output matrix of the moving platform? U_i^{o} is the output matrix of the ith SOC limb, it relates to the type of the SOC limb and the distributed mode of SOC limb between the moving platform and static platform.

(6) Get the parallel mechanism. We can get the relation of kinematics pair in the SOC limb of the parallel mechanism and the relation of allocation between different SOC limbs.

(7) The synthesis of the parallel mechanisms with all the active joints located on the static platform. We get the parallel mechanism, which only consist of $n_{\min}$ limbs from step (6), if all the active joints located on the static platform, that is $n = M$, we must add ($M - n_{\min}$) SOC limbs. The limbs which are added may be the same as original SOC limbs or different, but the aim is meeting the requirements of U^{P} and eq.(1).

(8) Delete the passive joint. Following the decision rule for the passive joint, we can delete the mechanism, which consists of the passive joint during the course of the synthesis.

(9) Select the active joint. We select the active joint following the selected rule for the active joint to make sure of realizing the expected output of motion.

(10) Investigate the coupling degree, k, of the mechanisms. We can get coupling degree of the mechanisms from Eq. (3) and Eq. (4), and we can know the complexity of the mechanisms.

$$\Delta_j = \sum_{i=1}^{m_j} f_i - I_j - \xi_j =$$

$$\begin{cases} \Delta_j^{-} = -5, -4, -3, -2, -1, \textit{ soc applied restrain to the mechanism, it makes mobility red} \\ \Delta_j^{0} = 0, \textit{ soc is noneffective to mobility of the mechanism} \\ \Delta_j^{+} = +1, +2, +3, \ldots\textit{ soc adds mobility of the mechanism } \Delta_j^{+} \end{cases} \tag{3}$$

where f_i is the degrees of freedom of the ith kinematical pair, I_j is the number of active input of jth SOC limb, ξ_j is the minimum of the ranks in all the loops which are composed of the jth SOC limb (as for the first loop of SOC limb, because can not be composed of loop, so ξ_j =0). Δ_j is the restriction degree which jth SOC limb applied to the mechanism.

(11) Displacement of the generalized kinematical pair. In order to make the P pair motive rapidly and improve efficiency, we can use parallelogram 4R mechanism to displace some or all the P pairs, but we should make sure of the output matrix does not change.

3 The Research on Intellectualized Structural Synthesis and Classification of 3-DOF Space Parallel Mechanism

3.1 The Flow Chart of Programming of Intellectualized Structural Synthesis and Classification

Accordance with the process based on the theory of structural synthesis and classification of degenerate-rank parallel robot mechanisms which uses the units of single open chain limb, software of intellectualized synthesis, following the flow chart of programming (Figure 1)

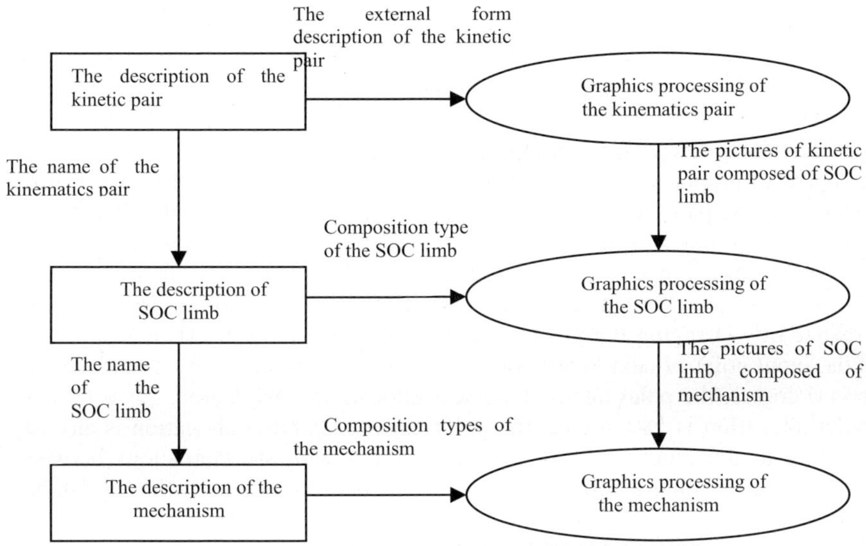

Fig. 1. The flow chart of programming

3.2 The Realization of Intellectualized Structural Synthesis and Classification

3.2.1 Generation of the Kinetic Pairs

Any mechanisms are made of the *SOC* limbs, the *SOC* limbs are made of the kinetic pairs, so if we want to realize the output of the mechanisms, we must utilize the output P, R, S, C pairs with VB programming. first, the external form description of the kinetic pair is expressed by polar coordinates method□that is we can get a point relative to the base point in the polar coordinate system by use of (α, l), Line segment can be expressed by use of changing the angle and the length of line in the polar coordinate system $L = (\alpha, l_1) - (\beta, l_2)$. Arc can be expressed by use of setting radius of arc, the start angle and the end angle of arc. We can get the kinetic pair through linking the line segment into graphics and linking the arc into graphics. The output of the kinetic pair as shown in Fig.2.

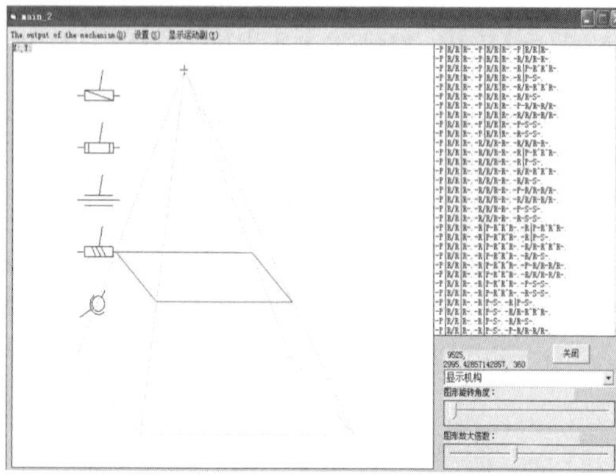

Fig. 2. The output of the kinetic pair

3.2.2 The Generation of the Single Open Chain Limb

The output of graphics of the single open chain limb is based on the output of graphics of the kinetic pair. We can define the input and output point of the SOC limb form the output of graphics of the kinetic pair, and then link different kinetic pairs according to the types of SOC limbs. The patterns of links between kinetic pairs and the SOC limbs are: parallel, coincidence, stigmatic, coplanar, random, vertical, They can be realized by changing the polar angle between the output point of kinematics pair and the input point of next kinetic pair, such as the polar angle of coincidence allocation is 0 degree, the polar angle of vertical allocation is 90 degree, the polar angle of parallel allocation is 180 degree, the polar angle of parallel allocation is any degree. According to the kinetic pair in fig.2 combining with six allocations between the kinetic pair generating a series of single open chain, thus establishing a database of

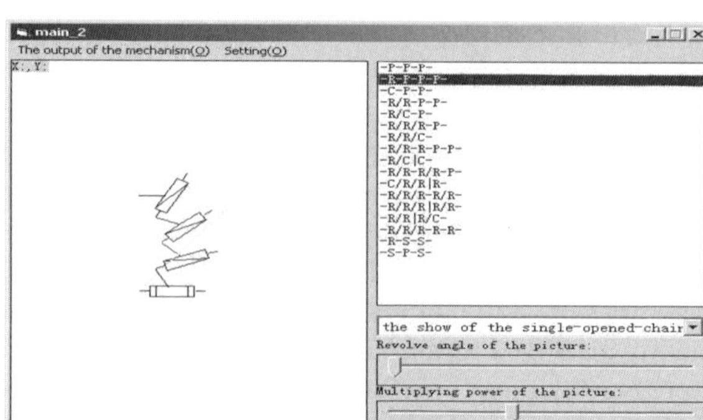

Fig. 3. The output of the *SOC* limb

single chain. The single open chain database includes single open chain information such as the specific composition of the kinetic pair, connectivity, in addition to that, preservation of the functional parameters set of some specific operating procedures. A single chain is the role of the database program can access the database, called models of graphics output, which must be completed space-integrated parallel mechanism for a single chain database. The role of the single open chain database is to make program access and call the database, achieve graphics output of mechanism models. Take the SOC limb -R-P-P-P-for example, the output of the SOC limb as shown in Fig.3.

3.2.3 The Output of Three-Degree of Space Parallel Mechanism

We can realize some functions as follows according to the output of the SOC limbs, associating to the numbers of limbs and the allocation pattern of SOC limbs between the moving platform and the static platform which can be determined by the characters of the parallel mechanisms, ① we can select the mechanisms with different limbs, as there are two types of three-degree of space parallel mechanisms, which have two limbs and three limbs respectively. ② we can calculate the numbers of the different types of mechanisms□by setting program to index, record and summate the numbers of mechanisms. ③we can know the structure of the different types of the mechanisms, which is the display of the mechanisms, can be realized by use of access, calling program to different databases. ④we can enlarge the picture of mechanism, change revolve angle of the limb of the mechanism and so on, that is we can amend the parameter of the program such as default the length of link, amplification factor, staggered angle between different kinetic pairs and revolve angle to realize the changes.

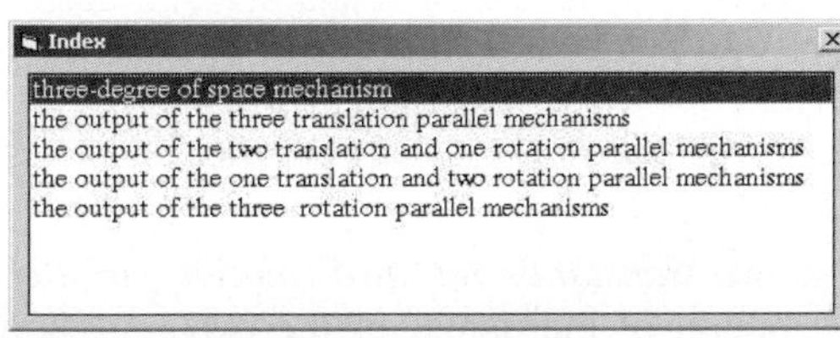

Fig. 4. The interface of the output

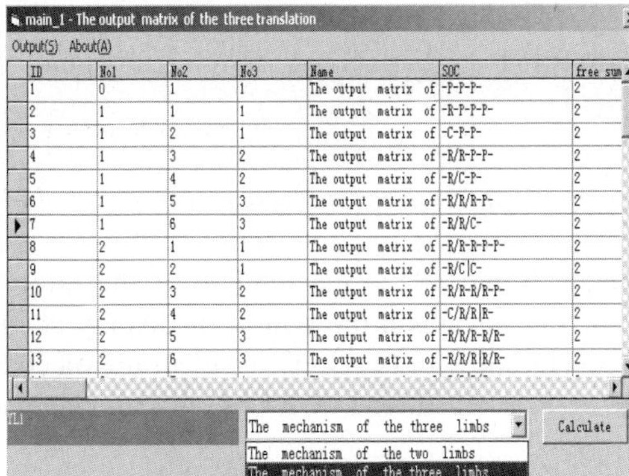

ID	No1	No2	No3	Name	SOC	free sum
1	0	1	1	The output matrix of	-P-P-P-	2
2	1	1	1	The output matrix of	-R-P-P-P-	2
3	1	2	1	The output matrix of	-C-P-P-	2
4	1	3	2	The output matrix of	-R/R-P-P-	2
5	1	4	2	The output matrix of	-R/C-P-	2
6	1	5	3	The output matrix of	-R/R/R-P-	2
7	1	6	3	The output matrix of	-R/R/C-	2
8	2	1	1	The output matrix of	-R/R-R-P-P-	2
9	2	2	1	The output matrix of	-R/C|C-	2
10	2	3	2	The output matrix of	-R/R-R/R-P-	2
11	2	4	2	The output matrix of	-C/R/R|R-	2
12	2	5	3	The output matrix of	-R/R/R-R/R-	2
13	2	6	3	The output matrix of	-R/R/R|R/R-	2

Fig. 5. The interface of the output

The interface of the output of three-degree of space parallel mechanisms is shown in Fig.4, when we touch the button of three translation parallel mechanism, it will display the frame of limb selection, button of the numbers calculation of the mechanisms and button of the output of the mechanisms as shown in Fig.5. If we touch the button of the output of the mechanisms, we can get all the output of the three translation parallel mechanisms.

3.2.3.1 The output of three translation parallel mechanisms. If we touch the button of the output of the three translation parallel mechanisms in Fig.4, and select frame of the mechanism of the three limbs, calculate the numbers of the mechanisms and touch the button of display in Fig.5, we will get the output of the mechanisms as show in Fig.6, if we select the mechanism which is made up of -P-P-P-, -R-P-P-P-, -C//R//R⊥R limbs , this mechanism will appear as in Fig.6.

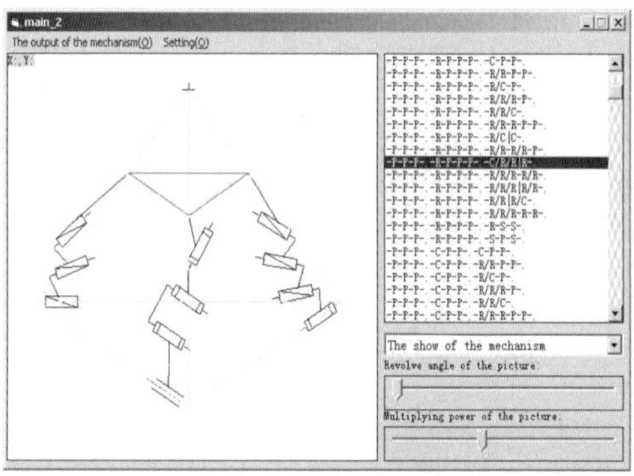

Fig. 6. The button of display

3.2.3.2 The output of two translation and two rotation parallel mechanisms. Similarly, if we touch the button of the output of the two translation and one rotation parallel mechanisms in Fig.4, and select frame of the mechanism of the three limbs, calculate the numbers of the mechanisms and touch the button of display in Fig.7, we will get the output of the mechanisms as show in Fig.7, if we select the mechanism which is made up of-R-P-P-P-, -R//R//R-P-, -R//C⊥C limbs, this mechanism will appear as in Fig.7.

3.2.3.3 The output of one translation and two rotation parallel mechanisms. If we touch the button of the output of the one translation and two rotation parallel mechanisms in Fig.4, and select frame of the mechanism of the three limbs, calculate the numbers of the mechanisms and touch the button of display in Fig.8, we will get the output of the mechanisms as show in Fig.8, if we select the mechanism which is made up of-R-P-P-P-, -R//R//R-P-, -C//R//R⊥R limbs, this mechanism will appear as in Fig.8.

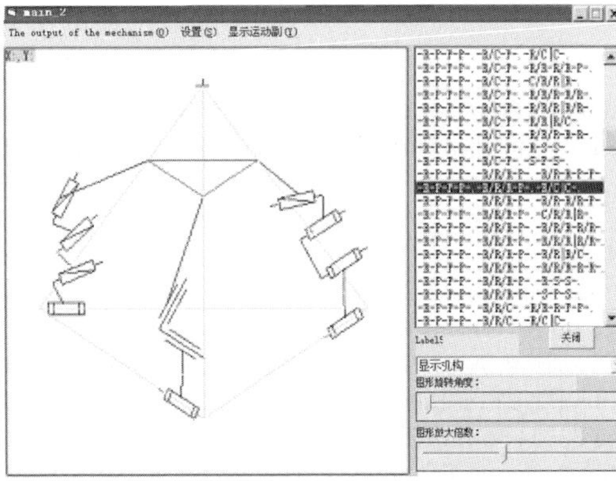

Fig. 7. The output of two translation and two rotation parallel mechanisms

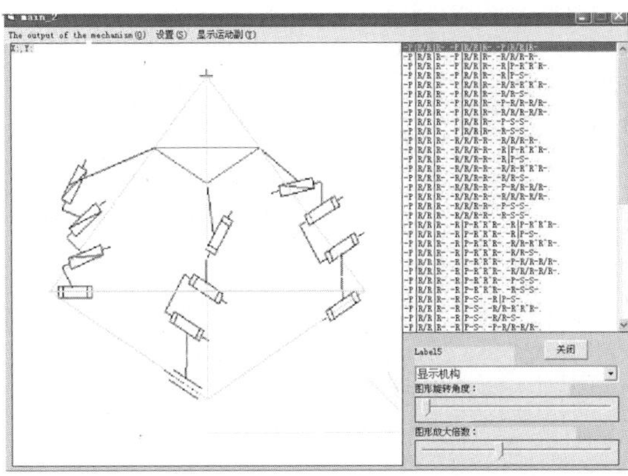

Fig. 8. The output of the one translation and two rotation parallel mechanisms

4 Conclusion

(1) A new method with VB programming which utilizes the intelligence structural synthesis and classification of the parallel robot mechanisms is put forward, based on the units of single-opened chain limb and according to the relations between the output matrix of the mechanism and the output matrix of the SOC limb, and with this new method for structural synthesis of 3-DOF space parallel robot mechanisms.

(2) This intellectualized method provides a theoretical basis for designing the mechanisms of the multi-degree of freedom vibration absorption that the author is studying.

(3) We can get the mechanisms of the parallel robot mechanisms rapidly in the course of the synthesis, saving time and labors, by making the structural synthesis automation.

(4) The intelligent, systematic, general and effective method is of universal significance and is used for the structural synthesis of degenerate-rank parallel robot mechanisms with other kinematics output types.

References

1. Hunt, K.H.: Kinematic geometry of mechanisms. Clarendon Press, Oxford (1978)
2. Ball, R.S.A.: A Treatise on the Theory of Screws. Cambridge University Press, London (1900)
3. Hara, A., Gosselin, C.M.: Synthesis of parallel micromanipulators. ASME J. of Mechanisms 111, 34–46 (1989)
4. Herve, J.M.: Structural synthesis of 'parallel' robots generating spatial translation. In: 5th IEEE Int. Conference on Advanced Robotics, pp. 808–813. IEEE Press, Pisa (1991)
5. Yang, T.L., et al.: Structural Synthesis and Classification of the 3DOF Transnational Parallel Robot Mechanisms Based on the Units of Single opened Chain. Chinese Journal of Mechanical Engineering 8, 31–36 (2002)
6. Yang, T.L.: Robot Mechanisms Topological Theory, pp. 55–80 (2005)

The New Design of Digital Servo Robot Controller

P.S. Pa and C.M. Wu

Graduate School of Toy and Game Design, National Taipei University of Education,
No.134, Sec. 2, Heping E. Rd., Taipei City 106, Taiwan
myhow@seed.net.tw

Abstract. Servos have been widely used in robots in various fields and a plurality of toys. To keep functioning, servos are controlled by PWM signals constantly sent from a servo controller, but the controller often has its limitations in performance. A servo interface device comprising a CPLD is designed that not only provides simultaneous control over more servomotors, but can also compute and generate the PWM signals needed by the servos. In addition, the servo interface device can be directly integrated with another single chip to achieve division of control, in which the single chip takes care of sensing, communication, connection and other interactive functions while the CPLD provides multiple-axis servo control. More importantly, when the single chip is communicating with a computer or performing other external communication tasks, the normal operation of the servos will not be affected by brief pauses of the MCU resulting from the communication tasks.

Keywords: Robot, Toy, Servo, CPLD, PWM, Single Chip.

1 Introduction

The motion of a walking robot comprising a plurality of servos can be generally characterized by two, three, four, six or more legs. The plurality of servos provides the walking robot with a higher degree of freedom and allows easier adaptation to the environment, as opposed to a wheeled robot. Now that the existing environment has not developed completely into an environment suitable for wheeled robots to move around, it is the walking robots that will have more effective use in human society in the long run. Moreover, while the wheeled robots move forward without any anticipatory actions, the walking robots are designed to imitate the actions of living creatures while walking, so that we can anticipate their actions according to human experience and are less likely to feel threatened by the robots. Nowadays, several research institutions are dedicated to the development of walking robots, and it is believed that significant advances will some day be achieved that allow walking robots to work not only for but with humans. The research of the biped robot combines different disciplines such as mechanism, mechanics of machinery, electronic engineering, control engineering, biological engineering, and robotics. The major research content includes: the design of the leg mechanism, gait planning, walking track, and balance & control theories. In 1977, Gollidary & Hemani adopted Langrangian's dynamics theory to deduce and linearize the mathematic model of the kneeless biped robot to

C. Xiong et al. (Eds.): ICIRA 2008, Part II, LNAI 5315, pp. 1105–1114, 2008.

analyze its stability, manipulability, and observability. In 1980, Miyazaki & Arimoto applied the Singular Perturbation method to categorize the dynamic behaviors of the biped robot into the fast mode and slow mode, and designed the controller based on the method. In 1986, Railbert published his book 「The Balance of the Robot with feet」, which is regarded as the most pioneering and contributive research for all oil-pressure-driven robot with one, two, or four feet [1-2]. Grishin et al. (1994) designed a biped robot with 2 degrees of freedom (DOF) of full load. The robot is composed of a pelvis and two stretched feet. Its mechanic system has 4 DOF, 2 spinning and 2 moving, and minus 2 restraints. The total length of the two feet is a constant. The pelvisis kept at the center between two feet. To prevent from toppling over, the leg of the robothas been installed a feet vertical to the ground. From the side view, it liked a 3 linkage movement. Therefore, the biped robot is able to walk straight on the floor. The first generation of the Japanese Honda robot was developed by Honda R & D Center (Hirai, 1997) [3]. The robot has no body but with a high pelvis that connects the arms. It is a biped robot with "loaded" 12 DOF, including: 3 DOF in the hip, 1 DOF in the knee, and 2 DOF in the ankle. There are 5 linkages with 4 DOF from the front view, and 7 linkages with 6 DOF from the side view. The weight of two feet is only around 5 ~ 10% of the total weight. If the load of the arms has little impact on the balance, and the proportion of the weight of the two arms to the total weight is small, the robot will be able to up and down the stairs, walk on a slope with less than 10% degree, turn, and step back [4].

A walking track for robots to follow is necessary before successfully driving the robot to walk or move something from one place to another place. There are several ways to generate the walking track. One is through observing the qait of real human [5] another by instant calculation. In 1970, Vukobratovic et al. adopted the numerical methods to calculate the dynamic walking track of the biped robot [6]. Kato applied the same method to generate the dynamic walking track for his biped robot, WL-10RD [7]. However, it takes a long time to calculate the reference track when the robot is walking, and it is hard to adjust to different surface. Unless the CPU can calculate faster or the algorithm is simplized, the numerical method still has the problem of slow calculation. Other methods to generate the walking track include: inputting the least power [8], using actuator of the neural network and using the genetic algorithm [9]. The DOF of the robot's arm depends on the type of robot and flexibility like human arms can be achieved. There are 6 DOF in human arm-and-wrist mition. The upper arm around the shoulder juncture has two DOF for rotating and swinging. The elbow juncture has the 3rd DOF. The 4th DOF is for spinning the wrist. The 5th DOF is for the up and down movement of the wrist. The right and left movement of the wrist is the 6th DOF. Operations of the fingers and thumb are other additional DOF. The robot arm kinematics is about the movement operation of the robot arm during a period of time relative to a fixed coordinate system. In traditional analysis, the robot's base is regarded as a reference point, and other movements must be based on such reference point. When we know about all positions of junctures and linkage on the robot's arm, then we can calculate the exact position of the arm's terminal in the space. This is a question about the direct kinematics. The reversed question is to decide the target position of the juncture and the linkage to enable the robot's arm to move to the specific positions and directions in the space. The reversed question is more difficult and may have more than one answer [10]. Modern commercial robots equip with the hybrid spin and slip junctures, connected by the arm linkage or the wrist parts of the robot's arm. The spin juncture controls the movement of two linkages in a specific degree, and the slip juncture controls only the line movement between the two linkages. Theoretically, other juncture relationship is possible. However, in reality, only the two junctures are adopted. The serial combination of the juncture and the linkage is called a chain. The chain is open or closed. Every linkage end of the chain only connects to a juncture point. Open chain refers to a chain that does not connect to linkages that are closer to the base. A chain that connects a linkage to the prior juncture point is called the closed chain. The main type in modern industrial robots is the open chain [11]. The analysis and control of the robot's arm requires the development of the analysis and control method. An arm with multiple juncture points is impacted by many force interactions and external environment, and it requires a more complex analysis. Researches of Paul about the homogenous transformation matrix method and the coordinate transformation in the analysis of the robot's kinematics are useful references [12-13].

A walking robot is a compact embodiment of modern science and technology, encompassing such fields as electronics, electrical engineering, information technology, control engineering, mechanics and robotic kinematics. In the past few decades, considerable progress has been made in the study of robots, propelling the conditions for further development to mature. However, a walking robot requires highly non-linear walking control and is not supported by a stationary base, making it far more difficult to control the motion of the walking robot than a fixed robotic arm in a factory. In order to achieve higher stability, a more complicated control system is called for to accurately control a walking robot's walking speed, acceleration, moving angle and applied torque. In addition, kinematic theories such as the zero moment point (ZMP) theory must also be applied to maintain the robot's overall balance while walking. Robots have had plenty of applications in our daily life and show vast potential in the future. More particularly, the walking robots can be integrated with different external devices as needed so as to serve different purposes such as exploration, transportation, substitution for manpower and perform dangerous tasks for man. The multiple-axis servo interface device of this study can reduce the tasks of a main control chip to communication or sensing. For example, while the device of this study carries out servo control, it thereby provides effective division of control over the robot. This lowers not only the threshold for relevant research and development, but also the R&D cost of the robot.

2 Experimental Setup

The chip used in this study is EPM1270T144C5ES from the MAX II series of ALTERA. The chip has 1270 logic elements (LEs), 116 general I/Os, an 8 K bit user Flash memory and an operating voltage of 3.3V. The chip's internal structure is shown in Figure 1, wherein the I/O states and pin locations corresponding to the desired control functions can be planned by the user. The multiple I/Os on the chip also allow the expansion of servo control. Moreover, the chip has an extremely short pin-to-pin delay time (about 5 ns) that enables continuous generation of several sets of PWM signals needed by the servos, without delay. The chip delivers higher performance as the number of servos it controls increases. Quartus II 7.2, a development platform from ALTERA, was used in the experiments and research of this study.

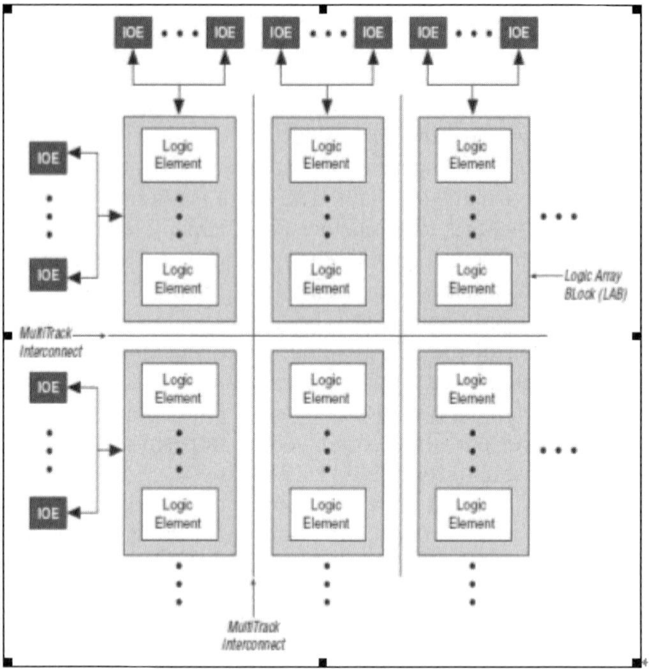

Fig. 1. Internal structure of ALTERA MAX II

3 Results and Discussion

Servo control is conducted through pulse-width modulation to rotate and maintain the angle of motion, as shown in Figure 2, which illustrates, by way of example, the control mechanism of an S03T servo manufactured by Grand Wing Servo-Tech in Taiwan. In Figure 2, the pulse width ranges from 0.5 ms to 2.3 ms and the angle of rotation ranges from 0° to 180°. The relation between the angle of rotation and the pulse width is given by the following equation:

$$Y = 0.5 + 0.01X \tag{1}$$

wherein Y is the pulse width to be generated, expressed in the unit of ms, and X is the angle to be rotated by the servo, expressed in degrees.

In addition to being controlled by the pulse width, servos require a fixed period to deliver maximum performance. Figure 3 schematically shows the period at which the S03T servo of Grand Wing Servo-Tech is controlled by PWM signals. If it is desired to control the servo, PWM signals having a corresponding pulse width must be sent thereto continuously at a fixed period, so as to maintain the servo's angle. Therefore, a controller has to generate the PWM signals incessantly to keep the servo working.

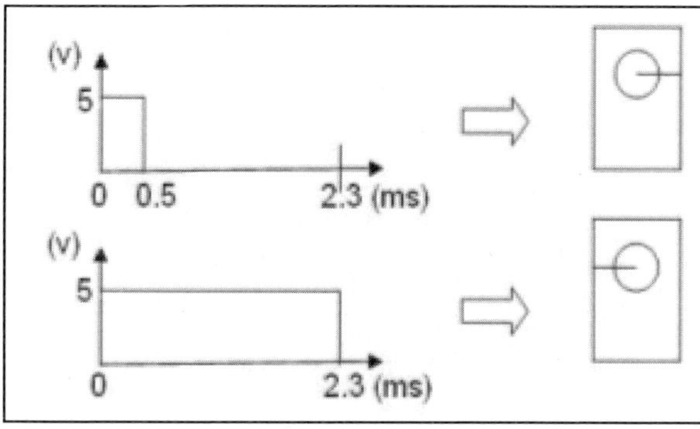

Fig. 2. Schematic drawing of servo control through pulse-width modulation

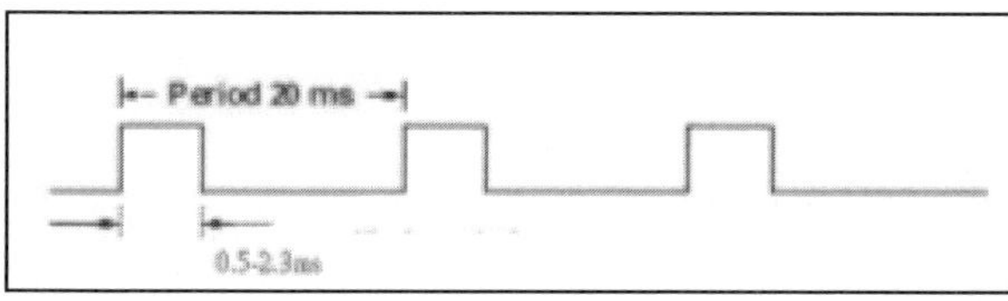

Fig. 3. Schematic drawing showing the period at which the servo controlled by PWM signals

However, the servo controllers available on the market usually generate PWM signals in a sequential manner. In other words, a PWM signal is generated only after the previous one is generated, which are the pulse analysis diagrams of a commercially available 24-axis servo controller, respectively. The controller controls 24 servos, each requiring a time ranging from 0.5 ms to 2.3 ms. Assuming each motor is intended to provide an angular motion of 90°, the above-given equation for calculating angle and pulse width yields a pulse width of 1.4 ms. Thus, the total time it takes to send 24 PWM signals having a pulse width of 1.4 ms sequentially is 1.4 ms $\times$ 24 (axes) = 33.6 ms, which is longer than the predetermined period. Therefore, when the number of servos controlled by a controller increases to a certain extent, the period at which the servos are supposed to be controlled may be violated. In this study, the waveforms of PWM signals from each control panel were captured by a 32-channel logic analyzer recently developed by Zeroplus, as shown in Figure 4, so that the pulse widths of the PWM signals were observed along with the period of successive pulses.

The device designed in this study not only generates plural sets of PWM signals accurately, but more importantly, allows easy integration with control chips of other types. Therefore, in this study, a simple communication interface was designed into the system structure of the device, as shown in Figure 5, whereby a user only has to provide the device with such binary-code information as the servos to be controlled and the corresponding angles, to engage the device in servo control, while the MCU carries on other communication tasks and other external tasks.

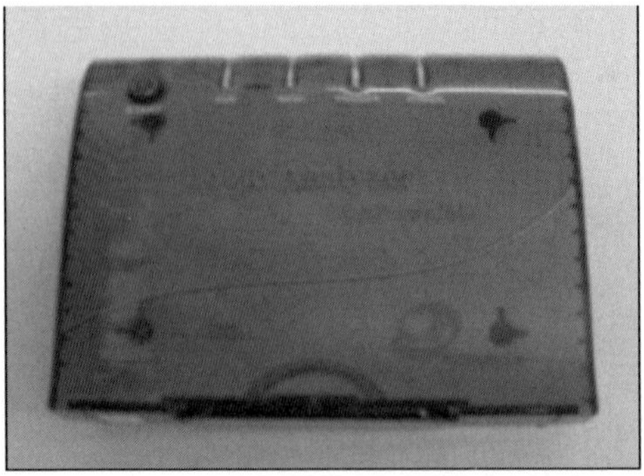

Fig. 4. Logic analyzer

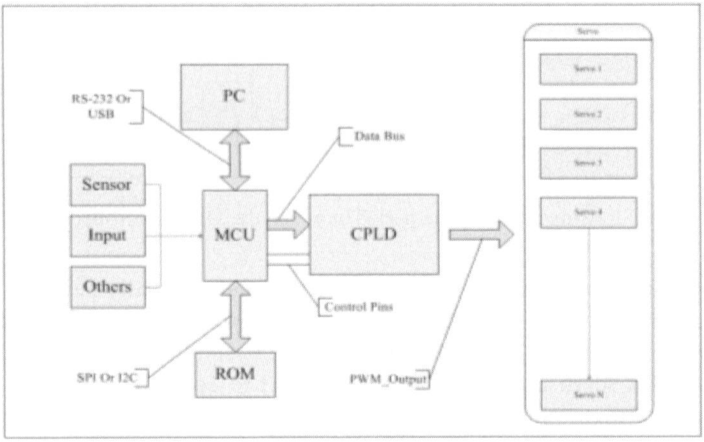

Fig. 5. System structure of the controller of this study

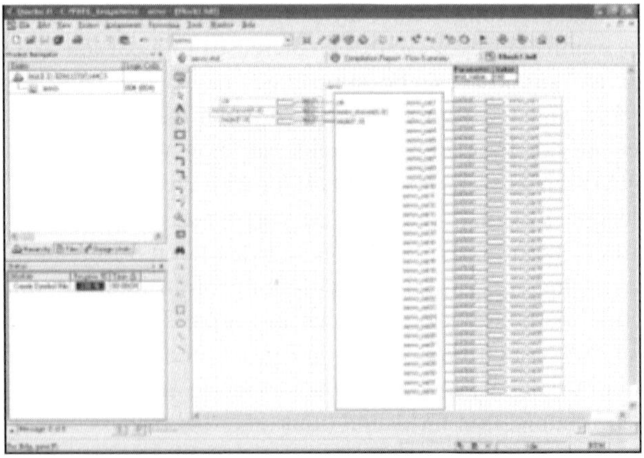

Fig. 6. Input and output structure of the servo controller

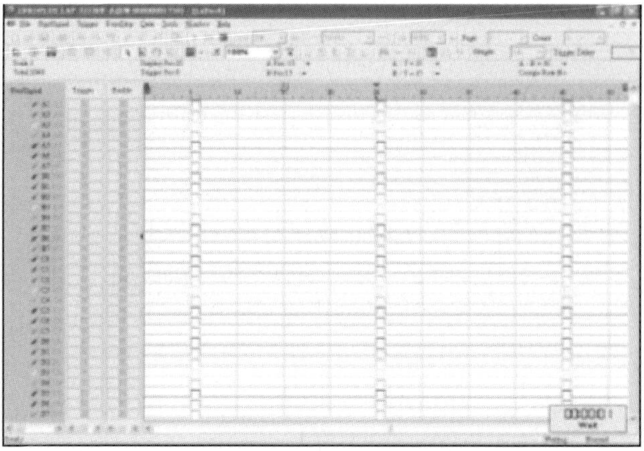

Fig. 7. Pulse analysis diagram of the servo controller of this study

The servo interface device of this study was designed with very high speed integrated circuit hardware description language (VHDL) and has an input and output structure shown in Figure 6. It is shown in Figure 8 that the required input signals are Clock_in (1 bit), angle (8 bits) and Motor_select (5 bits) while the output signals are 32 PWM output pins and an angle-restricting parameter of 180. Through a combination of these input and output signals, simultaneous control of 32 servos can be achieved.

The servo control device of this study was intended to control 32 servos. Since simultaneous serial and parallel control was conducted directly by hardware after the circuit was planned and completed, the delay time in PWM signal generation was almost negligible (about 5 ns). Figure 9 is a 32-channel PWM pulse analysis diagram of the circuit designed in this study. It is found in Figure 7 that all the pulses were

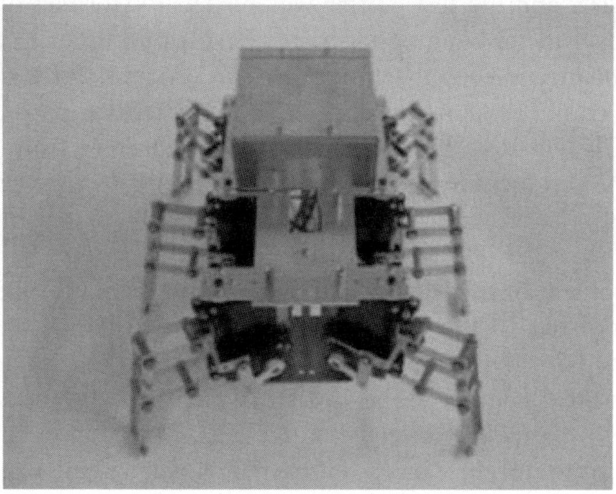

Fig. 8. Test carrier of this study

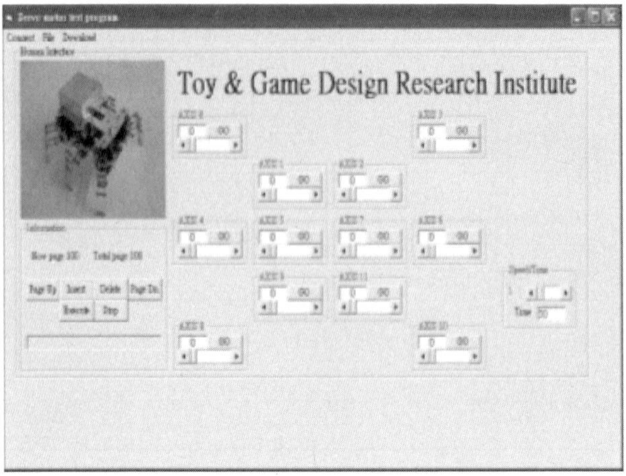

Fig. 9. Man-machine interface program for testing purposes of this study

generated at substantially the same time and all the periods between successive pulses were approximately 20 ms. Consequently, not only were the PWM signals needed by each axis generated accurately, but the accuracy of the periods were also effectively controlled. With this design, the same effects can be realized even if there are more than a hundred servos to be controlled. All it needs is a minor alteration of the description of the circuit and a CPLD chip with a higher capacity, if necessary. Moreover, through division of control, the servos will keep operating stably even if the MCU pauses to perform other tasks.

In order to verify the performance and reliability of the server controller of this study, a six-legged robot comprising 12 servos was designed and manufactured as a test carrier, as shown in Figure 8. The mechanism design of the test carrier was done with Pro-E software, and the test carrier was physically formed of aluminum plates processed by a sheet metal bending machine. Besides, in order to edit the actions of the robot, a computer-end man-machine interface program for testing purposes was written in Visual Basic, as shown in Figure 9. The interface program can communicate with the MCU via RS-232 and send servo parameters from the man-machine interface end to the servo controller of this study through a single chip. After integrating the aforementioned components, practical research on servo control was conducted.

Further development of this study shall involve integration of the RS-232 communication circuit into the CPLD chip, allowing a user to connect a computer to the CPLD through no more than a voltage-converting IC, so that control signals can be sent directly from the computer to the CPLD, or alternatively, the MCU can communicate directly with the CPLD through the RS-232. In that case, a single chip needs only one I/O to control all the servos. Figure 10 shows a design structure for further development of this study.

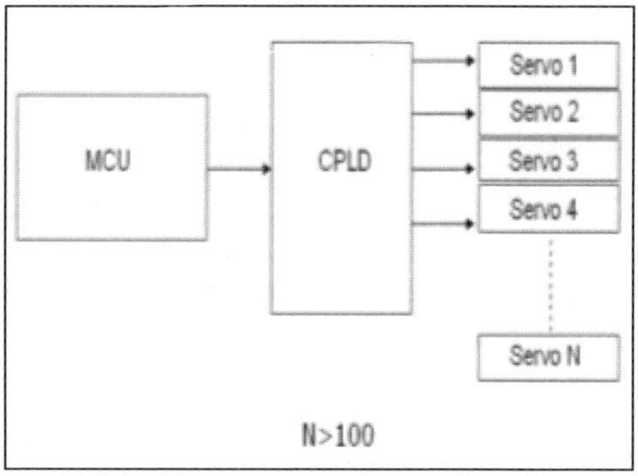

Fig. 10. System structure for further development of this study

4 Conclusions

In this study, a servo motor control interface device comprising a CPLD was designed and produced along with a computer-end man-machine interface program. By actually controlling a six-legged robot as a test carrier of this study, the performance of the device was verified. It is found that the device can be directly integrated with a variety of single chips and generate the required PWM signal pulse width more accurately, so as to control servomotors. Furthermore, operations of the servomotors will not be affected even though the main single chip is communicating with a computer or performing other tasks. Nowadays, most of the commercially available servo controllers can only control 24 axes each. However, demands for higher degrees of freedom and movable joints are bound to increase significantly, and it is very probable that the palm alone of a future robot will include more than a dozen servos. Therefore, if each of the servos is still controlled by sequentially generated signals, not only will the performance of the MCU be compromised, but the problem of unsynchronized control will also occur, hindering subsequent introduction of motion equations and gait planning. With the control method of this study, the efficiency of the MCU can be greatly enhanced while synchronism among servos is improved, which also facilitates follow-up studies and relevant verifications.

References

1. Golliday, C.L., Hemami, H.: An Approach Analyzing Biped Locomotion Dynamics and Designing Robot Locomotion Control. IEEE Transactions on Automation Control 22(6), 963–972 (1997)
2. Miyazaki, F., Arimoto, S.A.: Control Theoretic Study on Dynamical Biped Locomotion. ASME Journal of Dynamic Systems Measurement and Control 102, 233–239 (1980)
3. Hira, K.: Current and Future Perspective of Honda Humanoid Robot. In: Proceedings of 1997 IEEE/RSJ International Conference on Intelligent Robots and Systems, pp. 500–508 (1997)

4. Sadain, P., Rostami, M., Thomas, E., Bessonnet, G.: Biped Robots: Correlations between Technological Design and Dynamic Behavior. Control Engineering Practice 7, 401–411 (1999)
5. Ambarish, G.: Postural Stability of Biped Robots and the Foot-Rotation Indicator (FRI) Point. The International Journal of Robotics Research 18, 523–533 (1999)
6. Frank, A.A.: An Approach to the Dynamic Analysis and Synthesis of Biped Locomotion Machines. Med. Biol. Eng. 8, 465–476 (1970)
7. McGeer, T.: Passive Walking with Knees. In: IEEE Intgernational Conference on Robotics and Automation, vol. 3, pp. 1640–1645 (1998)
8. Shih, G.L., Zhu, Y., Gruver, W.A.: Optimization of the biped robot trajectory. In: Proceedings of IEEE International Conference on Decision Aiding for Complex Systems, vol. 2, pp. 899–903 (1991)
9. Meifen, C., Kawamura, A.: An Evolutionary Design Scheme of Neural Oscillatory Network for Generation of Biped Walking Patterns. In: 5th International Workshop on Advanced Motion Control, pp. 666–671 (1998)
10. Denavit, J., Hartenberg, R.S., Kinematic, A.: Notation for Lower-Pair Mechanisms Based on Matrices. ASME Journal of Applied Mechanics, 215–221 (1995)
11. Shih, C.L., Chi, C.T., Lee, Y.W.: Walking Experiment of a Biped Robot with Individual DC Motor Current and Position Control. In: The Fourth International Power Electronics Conference, Tokyo, Japan, pp. 1249–1254 (2000)
12. Tai, J.C., Liao, H.T., Chen, C.T.: Electric and Mechanical Integration, p. 307. Kao Lee Books, Taipei (2003)
13. Jones, B.A., Walker, I.D.: Practical Kinematics for Real-Time Implementation of Continuum Robots. IEEE Transactions on Robotics 22(6), 1087–1099 (2006)

Computer Vision Based Autonomous Navigation for Pin-Point Landing Robotic Spacecraft on Asteroids

Shuang Li

College of Astronautics, Nanjing University of Aeronautics and Astronautics, Nanjing 210016, China
lishuang@nuaa.edu.cn

Abstract. Computer vision based autonomous navigation scheme for pin-point landing of robotic spacecraft on asteroids is considered. Due to the long communication delay and complicated dynamic environment close to asteroids, traditional spacecraft navigation and control using the deep space network (DSN) is not suitable for the precise and safe landing of robotic spacecraft on asteroids. It is necessary to develop new generation autonomous navigation algorithms for future asteroid landing missions. To meet this requirement, this paper presents computer vision based autonomous relative navigation (VARN) algorithm. Firstly, architecture and function of VARN is introduced; secondly, feature detection and tracking algorithm is given out; then, VARN basing on Levenberg-Marquardt (LM) iteration is defined in detail. Finally, the validity of the proposed navigation scheme is confirmed by computer simulation.

Keywords: pinpoint landing, autonomous navigation, computer vision.

1 Introduction

Recent years have witnessed a considerable resurgence of interest in small bodies' exploration missions. It is believed that the elemental composition of these bodies may offer scientists insight into the formation and evolution of the solar system. National Aeronautics and Space Administration (NASA), European Space Agency (ESA) and Japan Aerospace Exploration Agency (JAXA) have already implemented small body landing mission or sample return missions. On February 12, 2001, NASA's NEAR-Shoemaker spacecraft made the first landing of a robotic spacecraft on an asteroid by use of five pre-planned maneuvers [1, 2]. JAXA's MUSES-C robotic spacecraft has succeeded in touching down to the surface of asteroid Itokawa by use of optical navigation sensors and implemented an asteroid sampling attempt on November 26, 2005 [3, 4]. ESA's ROSETTA robotic spacecraft is voyaging to rendezvous with comet 67P/Churyumov-Gerasimenko, and after entering orbit around the comet in 2014, a small lander named Philae will be released onto the icy nucleus and perform scientific investigation [5].

Issues of landing robotic spacecraft on small bodies have already been studied since the 1970's. Meissinger proposed a soft landing scheme, which used a feedback control with a radar altimeter and a three-beam Doppler radar system to achieve landing at Eros' north polar region with a low-impact velocity [6]. Simulation environment and

C. Xiong et al. (Eds.): ICIRA 2008, Part II, LNAI 5315, pp. 1115–1126, 2008.

autonomous control algorithms for landing on comets are investigated in Refs.7 and 8. Gaskell investigated autonomous landmark detection for spacecraft navigation and developed a simulation environment for asteroid approach and landing navigation [9, 10]. Cheng discussed autonomous landmark tracking orbit determination strategy for planetary landing mission [11]. Misu developed image/optical guidance schemes for the MUSES-C sample and return mission [3].

Because of the long communication delay induced by the large distances between the target asteroid and base stations on the earth, the traditional mode of navigating spacecraft with open loop control is not suitable for Pin-Point Landing (PPL) of robotic spacecraft on asteroids, so, asteroid landing operations must be performed autonomously by use of on-board sensors. Optical tracking of craters was first used operationally for navigation by the Near Earth Asteroid Rendezvous (NEAR) mission to asteroid Eros [12, 13], then by the MUSES-C mission to asteroid Itokawa [3]. It has proven to be a powerful data type for determining spacecraft orbits above the target for low altitude orbiting and landing. Tracking individual landmarks, which are small craters, enables orbit determination accuracies on the order of several meters [13]. Few published researches, however, have addressed the topic of a landmark tracking based asteroid landing navigation algorithm, which is a core program of the six freedom degree relative navigation required after image processing is complete. In this paper, Vision based Autonomous Relative Navigation (VARN) algorithm is proposed for pinpoint landing robotic spacecraft on asteroids basing on optical navigation camera measurement.

This paper is structured as follows. Section 2 describes the architecture and function of the VARN. The image processing technology used in the VARN is introduced in section 3. The autonomous navigation algorithm basing on Levenberg-Marquardt (LM) iteration is formulated in Section 4. In Section 5, preliminary simulations and results are discussed. Finally, Section 6 contains the conclusions.

2 Architecture and Function of VARN

Compared with the traditional planetary landers, the new generation smart robotic lander should have the capability of autonomous precise relative navigation. The sketch of the VARN for precise asteroid landing is depicted in fig.1. The full structure of the autonomous navigation scheme proposed in this paper can be divided into two blocks according to their functions: image processing (part I) and navigation algorithm (part II). The former part includes feature points/landmarks detection and tracking; the latter part comprises navigation measurement construction and LM iterative navigation algorithm.

The navigation procedure is performed as follow: First, gray images of the target asteroid surface are acquired by use of an optical navigation camera, and then onboard software autonomously performs natural landmark/feature identification and tracking. Next, the line-of-sight vector from the spacecraft to the center of each landmark can be constructed from the image coordinates in the navigation camera focal plane. Finally, the six-freedom degree relative position and attitude can be estimated by use of LM iterative algorithm.

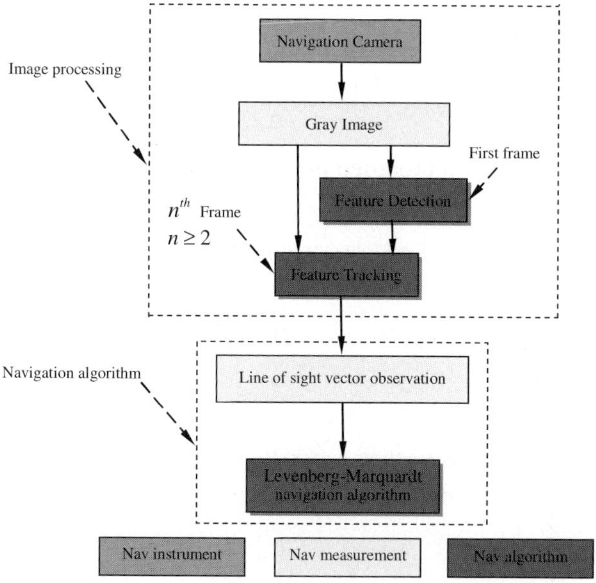

Fig. 1. Sketch of VARN for precise asteroid landing

3 Image Processing in VARN

Feature points, feature windows and features are not strictly distinguished here. Surfaces of asteroids generally appear highly textured, so good features to detect and track are expected to be plentiful. Gray images of around the prescribed landing site are acquired by optical navigation camera, and then on-board software autonomously performs natural landmark/feature detection and tracking. The coordinates of the point at the center of the landmark can be computed by use of center finding technology [9, 13].

Features detection and tracking are the groundwork of autonomous navigation proposed in this paper. Because of the emphasis of the paper is autonomous navigation algorithm, so we elected to implement the proven feature detection and tracking algorithms instead of redesigned our own.

3.1 Feature Detection

Let $I(p,q)$ be function defining image intensity for an image. We would like to determine if an image window containing M pixels centered on pixel $P=(p,q)$ is distinctive enough to be considered as a feature. First, G matrix is computed by the partial derivatives of image intensity

$$G = \begin{bmatrix} \sum_{k=1}^{M} \left(I_p^k\right)^2 & \sum_{k=1}^{M} I_p^k I_q^k \\ \sum_{k=1}^{M} I_p^k I_q^k & \sum_{k=1}^{M} \left(I_q^k\right)^2 \end{bmatrix} = \begin{bmatrix} a & b \\ b & c \end{bmatrix} \tag{1}$$

$$I_p(p,q)=\frac{I(p+1,q)-I(p-1,q)}{2}$$
$$I_q(p,q)=\frac{I(p,q+1)-I(p,q-1)}{2} \tag{2}$$

According to the criterion proposed in [14~16], the image window is considered as a feature if the two eigenvalue λ_1 and λ_2 of G are greater than a threshold λ_t (i.e, $\lambda_2 > \lambda_1 > \lambda_t$). In order to avoid solving eigenvalue problem, this criterion can be modified as follows

$$(a-\lambda_t)(c-\lambda_t)>0 \quad a>\lambda_t \tag{3}$$

3.2 Feature Tracking

Shi-Tomasi-Kanade feature tracker seeks to minimize the intensity differences ε between two successive image frame I and J

$$\varepsilon = \sum_{k=1}^{M}\left(J^k - I^k\right)^2 \tag{4}$$

Generally speaking, ε is not equal to zero because of existence of image distortion and noise contamination in the course of imaging. When ε reaches its minimum value, feature tracking can be considered as accomplishment.

$$\left(\varepsilon = \sum_{k=1}^{M}\left(J^k - I^k\right)^2\right) \Rightarrow \min \tag{5}$$

4 VARN Algorithm

After the image processing (IP) is completed, the line-of-sight vector from the spacecraft to the landmarks can be reconstructed, and then the spacecraft states can be estimated using LM iterative algorithm.

4.1 Navigation Camera Model

Here, a perspective projection model, usually known as pin-hole camera model, is adopted to simulate navigation camera measurement process. A perspective projection model represents an idealization of any optical sensor and allows position in a 2D camera image to be inferred from the 3D position.

The camera model projects an object point $\left(x^c, y^c, z^c\right)$ to a pixel point (u,v) on the image plane according to the following relations

$$u = f\frac{x^c}{z^c}$$
$$v = f\frac{y^c}{z^c} \tag{6}$$

where, f is the focal length of the navigation camera.

4.2 Geometry Relationship and Co-linearity Equations

The line-of-sight vector $\mathbf{b}_i^c$ defined by the line from the ith image point to the navigation camera exposure center in the camera-fixed coordinate system ($o_l x_l y_l z_l$) can be reconstructed by

$$\mathbf{b}_i^c = \frac{1}{\sqrt{(\overline{x}_i^c)^2 + (\overline{y}_i^c)^2 + f^2}} \begin{bmatrix} -\overline{x}_i^c \\ -\overline{y}_i^c \\ -f \end{bmatrix} \tag{7}$$

Where, $\overline{x}_i^c = x_i^c - x_0^c$ and $\overline{y}_i^c = y_i^c - y_0^c$ are the displacements of image coordinates along the x_c and y_c axis from the optical projection center $c(x_0^c, y_0^c)$, f is the focal length of navigation camera, the superscript c denotes the camera coordinate Σ^c.

For simplification, it is assumed that the coordinates of spacecraft are equal to those of the navigation camera perspective center. The coordinates of the perspective center in the landing coordinate system Σ^l is $o(x^l, y^l, z^l)$ and the coordinates of the ith landmark/feature in Σ^l is $F_i(x_i^l, y_i^l, z_i^l)$. So, the line-of-sight vector $\mathbf{l}_i^l$ defined by the line from the camera exposure position o to the ith landmark/feature location is represented in the landing site-fixed coordinate system by

$$\mathbf{l}_i^l = \frac{1}{\sqrt{(x_i^l - x^l)^2 + (y_i^l - y^l)^2 + (z_i^l - z^l)^2}} \begin{bmatrix} x_i^l - x^l \\ y_i^l - y^l \\ z_i^l - z^l \end{bmatrix} \tag{8}$$

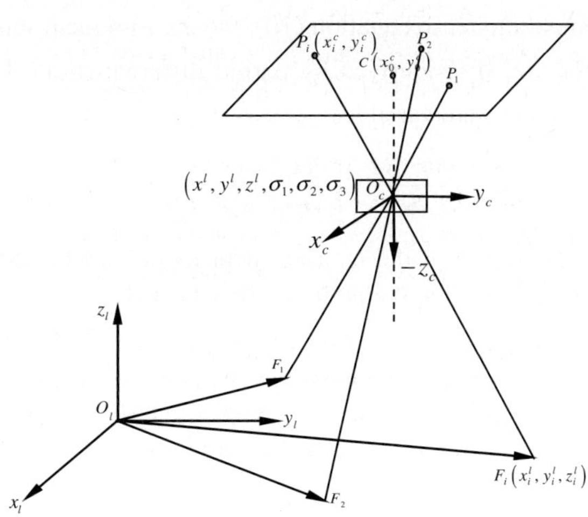

Fig. 2. Relative geometrical relationship between the spacecraft and landmarks

Obviously, the line-of-sight vector $\mathbf{b}_i^c$ and $\mathbf{l}_i^l$ are co-linear for the ideal pin-hole navigation camera. Thereby, the following geometry relationship, called the co-linearity equation, can be derived

$$\mathbf{b}_i^c = \mathbf{A}\mathbf{l}_i^l \tag{9}$$

Where, $\mathbf{A}(\boldsymbol{\sigma}) = \mathbf{I}_{3\times 3} + \dfrac{8[\boldsymbol{\sigma}\times]^2 - 4(1-\boldsymbol{\sigma}^T\boldsymbol{\sigma})[\boldsymbol{\sigma}\times]}{(1+\boldsymbol{\sigma}^T\boldsymbol{\sigma})^2}$ is the coordinate transformation matrix from the landing site-fixed coordinate system to the camera-fixed coordinate system. $\boldsymbol{\sigma}$ are the Modified Rodrigues Parameters (MRPs).

4.3 Navigation Measurement Model

The inherent navigation camera properties produce some measurement noise. When measurement noise is considered, the navigation measurement can be modeled as

$$\tilde{\mathbf{b}}_i^c = \mathbf{m}_i(\mathbf{x}) + \boldsymbol{\upsilon}_i \tag{10}$$

Where, $\tilde{\mathbf{b}}_i^c$ denotes the line-of-sight measurement from the ith landmark/feature; $\mathbf{m}_i(\mathbf{x}) = \mathbf{A}(\boldsymbol{\sigma}_i)\mathbf{l}_i^l(\mathbf{p})$ is the ideal imaging model of the perspective projection, which has been defined in equation (9); $\mathbf{x} \triangleq \left[\mathbf{p}^T, \boldsymbol{\sigma}^T\right]^T$ is the spacecraft state variables for six degree-of-freedom navigation. The navigation camera noise $\boldsymbol{\upsilon}_i$ is modeled as a zero mean white Gaussian process with covariance matrix of measurement errors R_i.

4.4 Measurement Sensitivity Matrix

From the measurement model in equation (10), the measurement sensitivity matrix for the ith landmark/feature, $\mathbf{h}_i$ is derived by partial differentiation of the measurement model with respect to the state variables

$$\mathbf{h}_i = \frac{\partial \mathbf{m}_i(\mathbf{x})}{\partial \mathbf{x}} = \begin{bmatrix} \dfrac{\partial \mathbf{m}_i}{\partial \mathbf{p}} & \dfrac{\partial \mathbf{m}_i}{\partial \boldsymbol{\sigma}} \end{bmatrix}_{3\times 6} \tag{11}$$

Where, the partial derivative of the measurement model with respect to the position vector $\mathbf{p}$ and attitude parameter $\boldsymbol{\sigma}$ can be written as [17]

$$\frac{\partial \mathbf{m}_i}{\partial \mathbf{p}} = \mathbf{A}_i(\boldsymbol{\sigma})\frac{\partial \mathbf{l}_i^l(\mathbf{p})}{\partial \mathbf{p}} = -\frac{\mathbf{A}_i(\boldsymbol{\sigma})\left(\mathbf{I}_{3\times 3} - \mathbf{l}_i^l\mathbf{l}_i^{lT}\right)}{\sqrt{\left(x_i^l - x^l\right)^2 + \left(y_i^l - y^l\right)^2 + \left(z_i^l - z^l\right)^2}} \tag{12}$$

$$\frac{\partial \mathbf{m}_i}{\partial \boldsymbol{\sigma}} = \frac{4}{\left(1+\boldsymbol{\sigma}^T\boldsymbol{\sigma}\right)^2}\left[\mathbf{A}_i\mathbf{l}_i^l\times\right]\left[\left(1-\boldsymbol{\sigma}^T\boldsymbol{\sigma}\right)\mathbf{I}_{3\times 3} - 2[\boldsymbol{\sigma}\times] + 2\boldsymbol{\sigma}\boldsymbol{\sigma}^T\right] \tag{13}$$

4.5 LM Navigation Algorithm

The autonomous vision based relative navigation scheme using the LM algorithm is formulated in the following sections.

First, define the navigation measurement set and measurement prediction set

$$\tilde{\mathbf{Y}} = \begin{bmatrix} \tilde{\mathbf{b}}_1^c \\ \tilde{\mathbf{b}}_2^c \\ \vdots \\ \tilde{\mathbf{b}}_N^c \end{bmatrix}, \hat{\mathbf{Y}}_k = \begin{bmatrix} \mathbf{m}_1(\hat{\mathbf{x}}_k) \\ \mathbf{m}_2(\hat{\mathbf{x}}_k) \\ \vdots \\ \mathbf{m}_N(\hat{\mathbf{x}}_k) \end{bmatrix} \tag{14}$$

Where, $\tilde{\mathbf{b}}_i^c$ denotes the line-of-sight measurement from the ith landmark/feature, $\mathbf{m}_i(\hat{\mathbf{x}}_k)$ stands for measurement prediction of the ith landmark/feature and N is the available line-of-sight vector measurement.

Then, the measurement residual set and sensitivity matrix are given by

$$\Delta\mathbf{Y}_k = \tilde{\mathbf{Y}} - \hat{\mathbf{Y}}_k = \begin{bmatrix} \tilde{\mathbf{b}}_1 - \mathbf{m}_1(\hat{\mathbf{x}}_k) \\ \tilde{\mathbf{b}}_2 - \mathbf{m}_2(\hat{\mathbf{x}}_k) \\ \vdots \\ \tilde{\mathbf{b}}_N - \mathbf{m}_N(\hat{\mathbf{x}}_k) \end{bmatrix} \tag{15}$$

$$\mathbf{H}_k = \left[\mathbf{h}_{1,k}, \mathbf{h}_{2,k}, \cdots, \mathbf{h}_{N,k}\right]^T \tag{16}$$

Where, $\mathbf{h}_{i,k} \triangleq \mathbf{h}_i(\hat{\mathbf{x}}_k)$

The essential function of the relative navigation is to compute an optimal state estimate $\hat{\mathbf{x}}$ for $\mathbf{x}$ by use of nonlinear least squares technique, which minimizes a weighted sum of the measurement residual set.

The LM algorithm provides an iterative solution as follows [17]

$$\Delta\mathbf{x}_k = \mathbf{P}_k \mathbf{H}_k^T \mathbf{W} \Delta\mathbf{Y}_k \tag{17}$$

$$\mathbf{P}_k = \left(\mathbf{H}_k^T \mathbf{W} \mathbf{H}_k + \eta \mathbf{\Gamma}_k\right)^{-1} \tag{18}$$

$$\hat{\mathbf{x}}_{k+1} = \hat{\mathbf{x}}_k + \Delta\mathbf{x}_k \tag{19}$$

Where, η is the weight coefficient, $\mathbf{\Gamma}_k = diag\left(\mathbf{H}_k^T \mathbf{W} \mathbf{H}_k\right)$. The weight matrix $\mathbf{W}$ is the inverse of the measured covariance matrix in the minimum variance estimation sense.

In order to implement the LM navigation algorithm, an initial state variable $\hat{\mathbf{x}}_0$ is required to begin the algorithm and the stopping condition of iteration with an accuracy dependent tolerance is given by

$$\delta J = \frac{\left|J_k - J_{k-1}\right|}{J_k} \leq \lambda \tag{20}$$

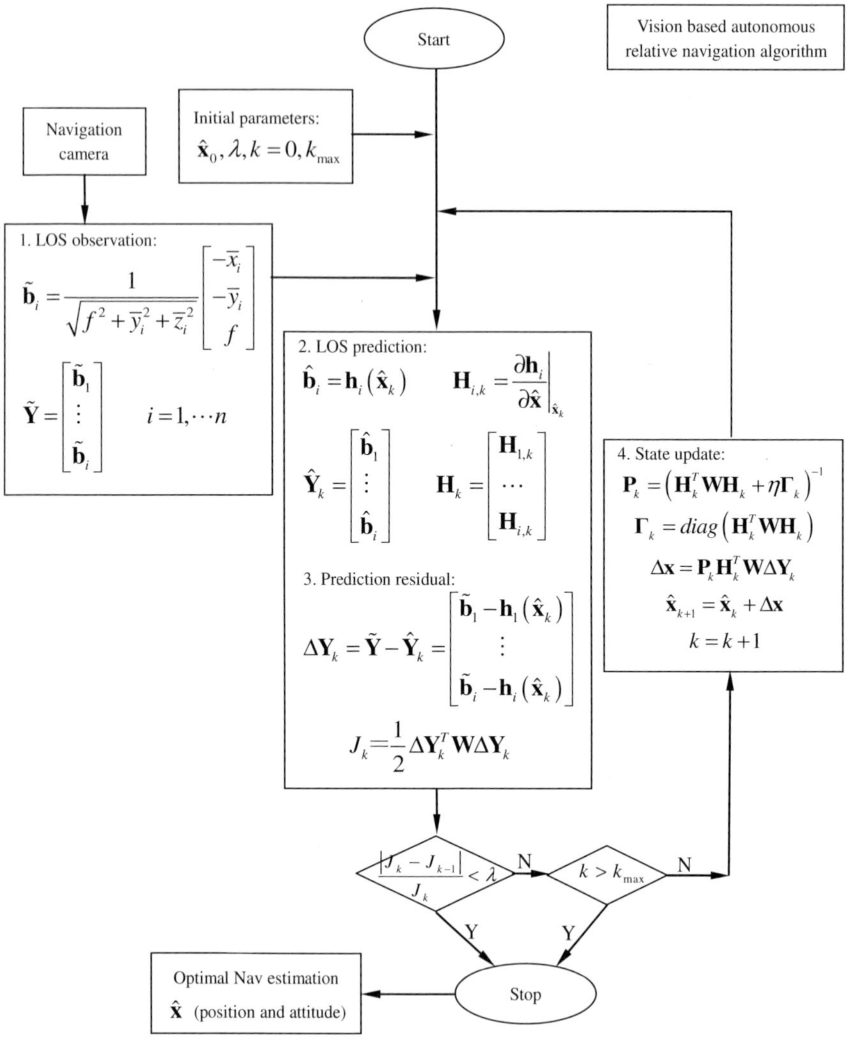

Fig. 3. Flowchart of vision based autonomous relative navigation

where, λ is the prescribed threshold quantity. If equation (20) is not satisfied, then the update procedure is iterated with the new estimate as the current estimate until the process converges, or the maximum allowed number of iterations ($k_{\max}$) is exceeded.

5 Simulations and Results

In order to confirm the validity of autonomous navigation algorithm proposed in this paper, preliminary computer simulations in MATLAB/Simulink environment have been performed with the assumption that Eros is the target asteroid.

The feasibility of feature detection and tracking algorithm is validated by compute simulation. The images used in the simulation are from the surface images of the asteroid 433 Eros taken in the NEAR Shoemaker's mission [18]. Suppose the size of original image taken by navigation camera is 256×256 in pixels and the size of search window is 48×48, simulation results are showed in fig.4 and fig.5. The simulation results show the feature window can be detected and tracked properly.

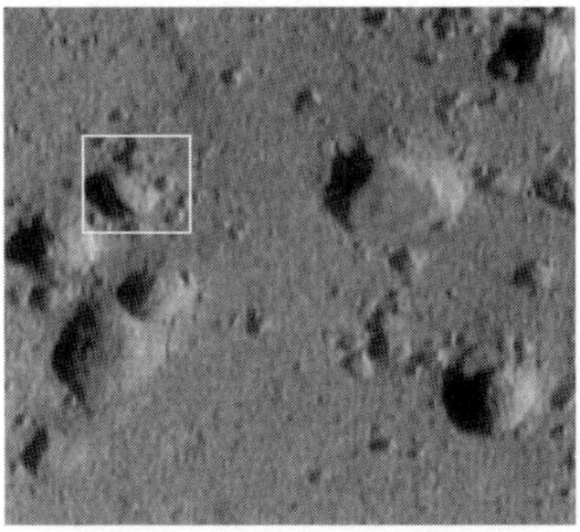

Fig. 4. Features detection in first frame

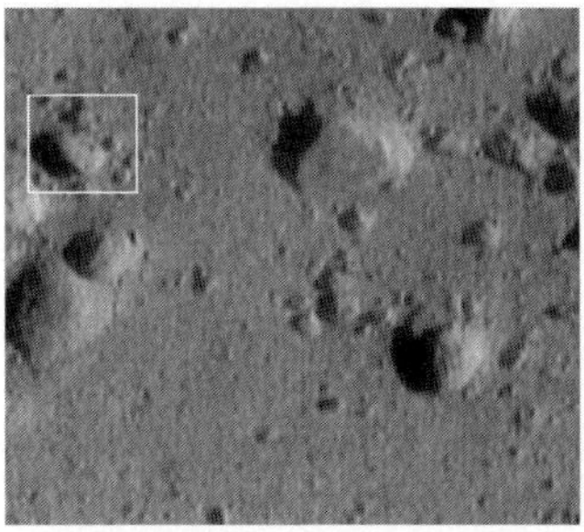

Fig. 5. Features tracking in subsequent frame

Suppose the planned landing time spans $\tau = 430s$, optical navigation camera focal length $f = 0.05m$. CCD navigation camera provides measurement outputs at a 2 second sample period, with the measurement error covariance $\sigma_{pixel} = 1.0\times10^{-6} m^2$. The LM iterative parameters are set to $k_{\max} = 10$ and $\lambda = 0.1$. Spacecraft initial states are given out in table 1.

Table 1. Spacecraft initial state parameters

Initial simulation parameters						
x_0	y_0	z_0	–50	50	500	(m)
v_{x0}	v_{y0}	v_{z0}	0.01	–0.075	–0.2	(m/s)
σ_{10}	σ_{20}	σ_{30}	0.09	–0.04	0.03	$(\cdot)$
ω_{x0}	ω_{y0}	ω_{z0}	0.1	0.1	0.1	$(\deg/s)$

Fig.6 and fig.7 give the navigation position and attitude output errors. The difference between the referenced position of spacecraft and the estimated position, that is navigation position error, is plotted in fig.6. The difference between the referenced attitude of spacecraft and the estimated attitude, that is navigation attitude error, is depicted in fig.7. The simulation results show that the computer vision based autonomous navigation algorithm proposed in this paper can assure the navigation output errors converging to zero. In the final landing phase, the navigation position errors and the navigation attitude errors are less than 1m and 0.1deg respectively; this navigation accuracy can satisfy the requirement of soft landing on asteroids.

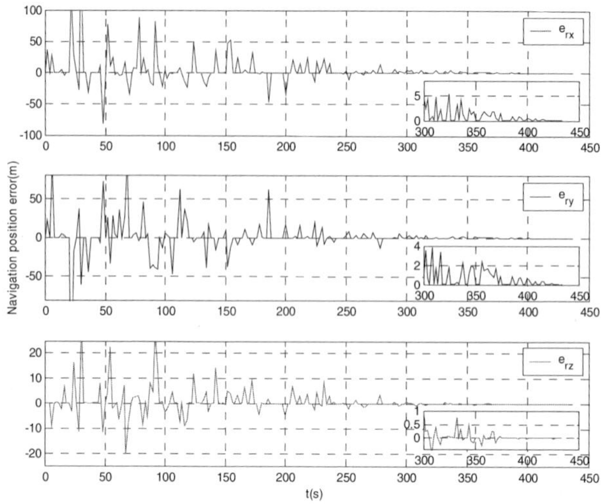

Fig. 6. VARN navigation position error

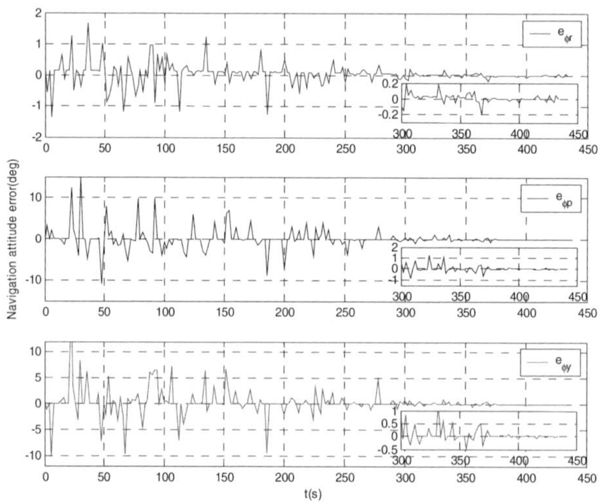

Fig. 7. VARN navigation attitude error

Though the navigation outputs produce relatively larger navigation errors at the beginning phase, the magnitude of navigation errors are gradually decreased and converge toward zero with the navigation successive progress. In the first instance, the observed line-of-sight vectors of the landmarks are too close in an angular sense, which leads to poor geometric placement and convergence difficulty arises. With the spacecraft approaching the target asteroid, the observed line-of-sight vectors become dispersed while the geometric relations are becoming better and better, so the navigation output errors are becoming smaller and smaller.

6 Conclusion

This paper has considered the issues of computer vision based autonomous navigation algorithm for future robotic asteroid landing or sample return mission. Traditional deep space network (DSN) navigation mode is not practical for landing robotic spacecraft on asteroid. Autonomous navigation schemes based on landmark tracking for landing robotic spacecraft on asteroids are proposed. The simulation results show that the proposed scheme's navigation accuracy satisfies the requirement of soft landing asteroid and the navigation scheme is feasible. Further studies on navigation image processing, especially landmark detection and tracking techniques, will be performed in our future work.

Acknowledgement

Project supported by the Natural Scientific Research Innovation Foundation in Nanjing University of Aeronautics and Astronautics (Grant No. Y0813-HT).

References

1. Veverka, J., et al.: The landing of the NEAR Shoemaker spacecraft on asteroid 433 Eros. Nature 413(6854), 390–393 (2001)
2. Dunham, D.W., et al.: Implementation of the first asteroid landing. Icarus 159(2), 433–438 (2002)
3. Misu, T., Hashimoto, T., Ninomiya, K.: Optical Guidance for Autonomous Landing of Spacecraft. IEEE Transactions on Aerospace and Electronic Systems 35(2), 459–473 (1999)
4. Kubota, T., et al.: An autonomous navigation and guidance system for MUSES-C asteroid landing. Acta Astronautica 52(2-6), 125–131 (2003)
5. Ferri, P.: Mission operations for the new Rosetta. Acta Astronautica 58(2), 105–111 (2006)
6. Meissinger, H.F., Greenstadt, E.W.: Design and Science Instrumentation of an Unmanned Vehicle for Sample Return from the Asteroid Eros, NASA SP-267, 1971, pp.543-560 (1971)
7. de Lafontaine, J.: Autonomous spacecraft navigation and control for comet landing. Journal of Guidance, Control, and Dynamics 15(3), 567–576 (1992)
8. Dawson, S., et al.: Autonomous controlled landing on cometary bodies. Advances in the Astronautical Sciences 99(2), 1175–1193 (1998)
9. Gaskell, R.W.: Landmark navigation and target characterization in a simulated Itokawa encounter. In: AAS/AIAA Astrodynamics Specialists Conference, Lake Tahoe, CA, August 7-11 (2005)
10. Gaskell, R.W.: Small body simulations for navigation approach and landing. In: AIAA Space Conference and Exposition, vol. 3, pp. 1613–1620 (2005)
11. Cheng, Y., Miller, J.K.: Autonomous landmark based spacecraft navigation system. Advances in the Astronautical Sciences 114(suppl.), 1751–1765 (2003)
12. Antreasian, P.G., et al.: The design and navigation of the near Shoemaker landing on Eros. Advances in the Astronautical Sciences 109(II), 989–1015 (2002)

13. Owen, J., et al.: NEAR Optical Navigation at Eros. Advances in the Astronautical Sciences 109(II), 1075–1087 (2002)
14. Benedetti, A., Perona, P.: Real-time 2-D feature detection on a reconfigurable computer. In: 1998 IEEE Computer Society Conference on Computer Vision and Pattern Recognition, pp. 586–593 (1998)
15. Jianbo, S., Carlo, T.: Good features to track. In: 1994 IEEE Computer Society Conference on Computer Vision and Pattern Recognition, pp. 593–600 (1994)
16. Tommasini, T., et al.: Making Good Features Track Better. In: 1998 IEEE Computer Society Conference on Computer Vision and Pattern Recognition, pp. 178–183 (1998)
17. Schaub, H., Junkins, J.L.: Analytical Mechanics of Space Systems. AIAA Education Series, pp. 11–12, 107–112 . AIAA, Reston (2003)
18. http://near.jhuapl.edu

Research on the Application of a Marsupial Robot for Coal Mine Rescue

Jie Zhao, Gang Liu, Yubin Liu, and Yanhe Zhu

State Key Laboratory of Robotics and System, Harbin Institute of Technology, Harbin, 150001, China
jzhao@hit.edu.cn, liuxing338@163.com, liuyubin@hit.edu.cn, yhzhu@hit.edu.cn

Abstract. A marsupial robot with strong practicability for coal mine rescue is presented with the discussion and analysis to the complicated environment in the mine disaster and the existing robots for coal mine rescue. The marsupial robot mainly consists of a mother robot and a baby robot. The mother robot carrying the baby robot comes into the mine well under the tele-operation of the command center. When meeting impassable obstacles or is trapped, the mother robot releases the baby robot. Then, the baby robot will go further into the mine well by itself to rescue the survivors. The marsupial robot not only enlarges the scale of rescue, but also increases the probability of successfully rescuing the trapped miners. Consequently the rescue task can be completed perfectly. The marsupial robot has a good potential of development and perspective of application.

Keywords: marsupial robot, mother robot, baby robot, coal mine rescue.

1 Introduction

In recent years, the ratio of coal mine accidents has greatly descended in the developed countries such as America, while it still has been high in China [1], [2] and [3]. With the development of economy in China, the requirement for energy increases constantly, which urges many coal companies to excessively exploit coals, meanwhile these companies undercapitalize to the safety in production, so that coal mine accidents such as fire damp explosion, ceiling board collapse, water disaster and traffic accidents happen frequently. However, the fire damp explosion is the most serious one and the scale of death toll caused by it is maximal. After an explosion accident such as gas or grime happens, the scene under the mine well becomes very abominable, abnormally complicated and awfully unstructured (shown in Fig. 1). It is difficult for rescuers to go into the mine well at the first time, so it delays precious rescue time. The accident experts and decision-makers can not give estimation and make decisions without required information and the trapped miners resultantly lost their life.

A marsupial robot for coal mine rescue which is similar to a kangaroo is presented here. This marsupial robot can carry all kinds of testing and measuring equipments such as sensors and necessary rescue goods such as food and medicines to go into the mine well before rescuers, reach the depth of the mine well with its ability to climb

C. Xiong et al. (Eds.): ICIRA 2008, Part II, LNAI 5315, pp. 1127–1136, 2008.

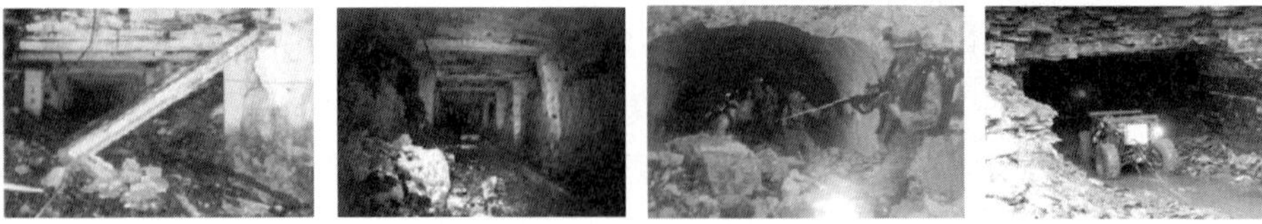

(a) (b) (c) (d)

Fig. 1. The scenes after coal mine disaster happened

over obstacles, explore the damage of accidents, surroundings and the trapped miners, and feed back these information by form of sound, image and data to the control center by wireless and wire communication. The marsupial robot can make up for many deficiencies of a single robot in walking, climbing over obstacles, functions, power, energy and communication, so it has important significance to improve the ability of meeting an emergency and rescuing, reduce casualties and make decisions. Meanwhile it establishes the base for the study, application and popularization of robotics.

2 Status Quo of Research and Application for Coal Mine Rescue Robot

America has been studying coal mine rescue robot for many years. At present, there are many universities, research organizations and companies developing coal mine rescue robot aiming at different usage. American DiscoverMiner Corporation has been devoted to developing relevant technology for abandoned mines rescue robot [1] and [4]. MinBot-XA shown in Fig. 2(a) is the prototype of rescue robot made by this company. But MinBot-XA is not capable of negotiating the structure of hard rock mines with wheels and tractors in deep explorations. Simply turning over on a side or sliding down shallow holes will render them inoperable. As wireless operation through hundreds of feet of rock is impossible because of signal disruption, wire management of such robots does make the long-range control problem considerable but short range solution possible. To improve an ability of adapting to terrain, this company has developed a robot called MOLE (Mine Observational Locomotion Experimenter), as shown in Fig. 2(b). MOLE's wheel is a cylinder. Its former and back section connected by vertical shaft and its above and underside section is symmetry, So it can not overturn and has a better adaptation to the terrain than MinBot-XA.

Fig. 3(a) shows an Andros V-2 robot developed by America Mine Safety and Health Administration [5] and [6]. It can travel through an underground mine in conditions that might be unsafe for miners to pass through. The 50-inch tall, 1200-pound machine that is equipped with navigation and surveillance cameras, lighting and a manipulator arm can travel up to 5000 feet and monitor and sample air. Fig. 3(b) shows a robot developed by Carnegie Mellon University's Robotics Institute called Groundhog [7], [8] and [9]. It looks like a golf cart on steroids. It uses lasers to "see" in dark tunnels and map abandoned mines — some of the most dangerous work in the business. Sandia's Intelligent Systems and Robotics Center (ISRC) has developed a robot called RATLER, as shown in Fig. 3(c) [10]. It has the closest configuration to that would ultimately provide the optimum robotic capabilities.

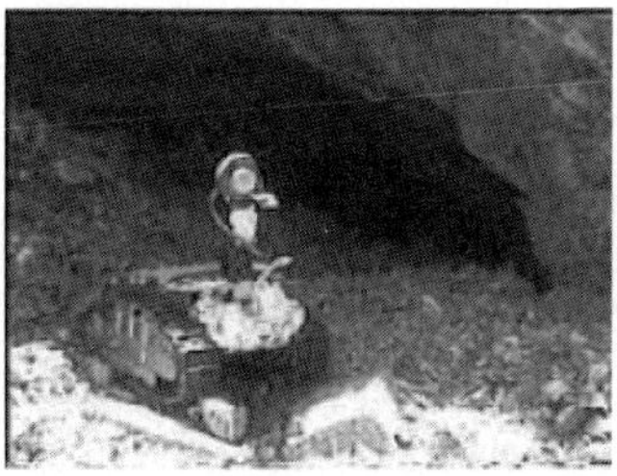

(a) MiniBot robot

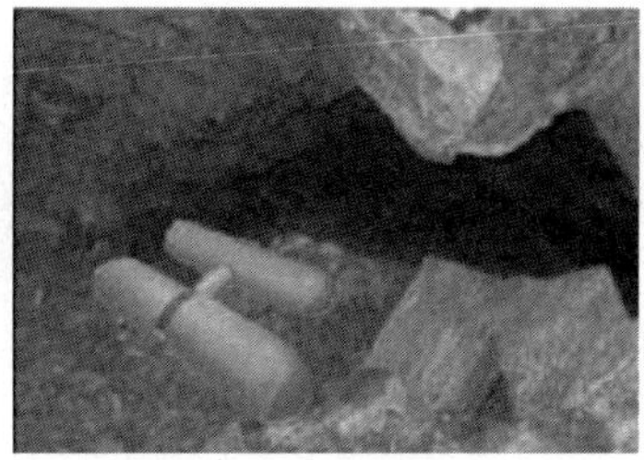

(b) MOLE robot

Fig. 2. The rescue robots developed by American DiscoverMiner Corporation

The snake-like robots which are developed by Tokyo Institute of Technology, called SOURYU-I, SOURYU-II and SOURYU-III [11] and [12]. SOURYU-III are connected as crawler vehicles composed of three crawler bodies connected with active joints capable of posture change, as shown in Fig. 3(d). The front and rear bodies can swing symmetrically, with the center body between them, in vertical and lateral directions by coupled drive of two stable axes at the joints. The front and rear screw axes for this motion are driven concurrently by two motors mounted on the center body. Furthermore, the crawlers of all three bodies are driven concurrently by one motor via the power transmission axis. So, the vehicle has high mobility, though it has only 3 degrees of freedom.

SGI and the University of Electro-Communication of Japan jointly have developed a snake-like rescue robot, as shown in Fig. 3(e) [13] and [14]. KOHGA is constructed using multiple small vehicle units, which are connected by four 2-DOF active joints and three 3-DOF passive joints. KOHGA consists of eight units, and each unit has its own function and travel driving crawlers. The units of KOHGA are connected in series and resultantly KOHGA has a long and thin structure so that it can enter narrow openings. The first units from both ends are respectively equipped with a CCD camera, but no crawlers are attached in order to make it light. The second units have the right and left crawlers which are driven co-accessibly. The other units also have the right and left crawlers which are driven independently.

China University of Mining and Technology made a principle prototype of coal mine search and rescue robot in 2006 [2], as shown in Fig. 3(f). CUMT-1 is expected to go into mine well to search the site and send information and images back, which can provide important field information to the rescue commander. Meanwhile it can carry emergency pharmacy, food, water and self-rescue tools to help the trapped survivors to save themselves and flee. CUMT-1 can be tele-operated to walk 300 meters with wireless communication. Now the walking test outdoors has been finished.

At present, the application instances of robot for coal mine rescue have been seldom reported because of the existing technology problem. On November 24, 1998, the Willow Creek Coal Mine (just north of Helper, Utah) suffered a serious fire. In December, Sandia's personnel went to the site to conduct a preliminary investigation of the robot's suitability accompanied with the RATLER [10]. The robot was tele-operated into the mine and it showed good capability of mobility, even on the steep

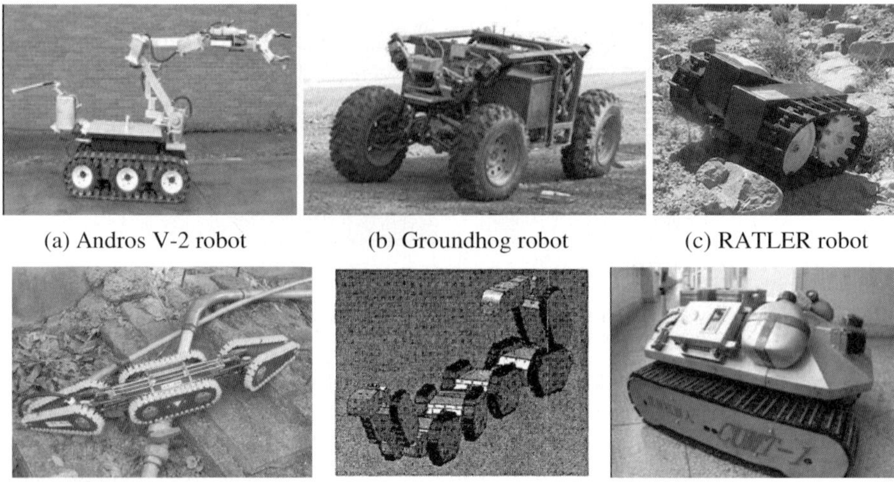

(a) Andros V-2 robot (b) Groundhog robot (c) RATLER robot

(d) SOURYU-III robot (e) KOHGA robot (f) CUMT-1 robot

Fig. 3. The rescue robots developed by other research organizations or universities

slopes of the mine. Exceptionally good vision was available to the operator when a FLIR (Forward-Looking Infrared) video camera was used. With current power levels and frequencies, the range for positive radio frequency (RF) control was approximately 250 feet in a straight, steeply dipping drift. In January 2006, a coal mine disaster happened in American West Virginia, American MSHA accompanied the V-2 to the site to conduct the rescue task, which carried three cameras and gas sensor, had the ability of night vision, used wire communication and had 1500 meters working distance. When V-2 was used to identify the location of 13 trapped miners and find way to enter into, it plunged into silt and failed to rescue [15].

3 The System Structure of the Marsupial Rescue Robot

When a mine disaster happens, the site under the mine well will become greatly abominable, abnormally complicated and awfully unstructured. So from getting into mine well to fulfilling rescue task, a robot will experience all kind of obstacles, walk for a far distance and spend much more time. During this course, a bulky robot will not get through confined gap and rove further after going into mine well deeply. And not only is a small robot limited by the integration of volume, weight, communication and performance and so on, but also the energy stored in cells will be exhausted before reaching target district. Consequently the small robot fails to realize the rescue task. But the marsupial robot can make up for many deficiencies of a single robot in walking, climbing over obstacles, functions, power, energy and communication. Here, the marsupial robot for coal mine rescue adopts a sharing control operation mode based on that the tele-operation is primary and the local independence is secondary. It mainly consists of a mother robot, a baby robot, a remote control center, a remote communication and power system, a sensor system and a lighting system. Its schematic diagram is shown in Fig. 4.

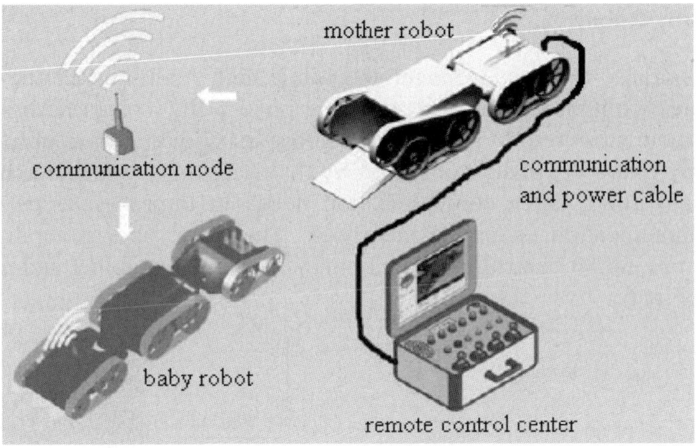

Fig. 4. The schematic diagram of the marsupial robot

3.1 The Mother Robot

The mother robot is an independent and whole unit, with the ability of walking, climbing over obstacles, detecting and measuring. And it can carry food and pharmacy to supply necessary rescue to the wounded. There will be a lot of falling coal blocks after explosion. And according to the analysis of coal quality in China, a coal block doesn't exceed 500 mm. So to adapt to the utmost unstructured environment composed of all kinds of bodies damaged by accidents, the mother robot must be able to climb over the obstacles of 500 mm, walk on all kinds of roads and debris with different sizes, span over the entrenchments under 600 mm consisting of debris, and pass the alleyway over 600 mm long. A tracked structure with double units is adopted for the mother robot to increase the adhesion to ground. Also it supplies a "pocket" used in carrying the baby robot which can enter and get out of the mother robot through the "pocket". Because the mother robot communicates with and gets power from the remote control center via a cable, the mother robot has a mechanism of dragging and releasing the cable. Moreover, it carries various detecting sensors. The schematic diagram of the mother robot is shown in Fig. 5.

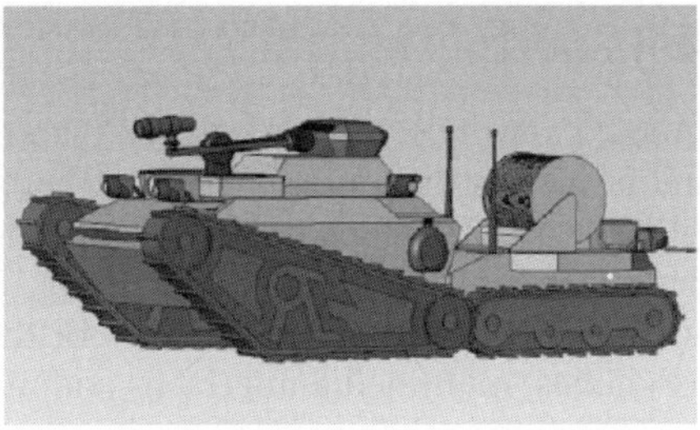

Fig. 5. The schematic diagram of the mother robot

3.2 The Baby Robot

The baby robot also is an independent and whole unit. As discussed above, the robot will experience complicated terrain under the mine well, so it is necessary to bring forth much more strict requirements for its ability of climbing over obstacles. Therefore, the baby robot is serially connected by multiple joints just like a snake. Otherwise, the baby robot takes communication nodes to improve the performance of wireless communication under the mine well. The baby robot generally includes a head unit, a tail unit, a control unit, a communication node cabinet and a power unit, as shown in Fig. 6.

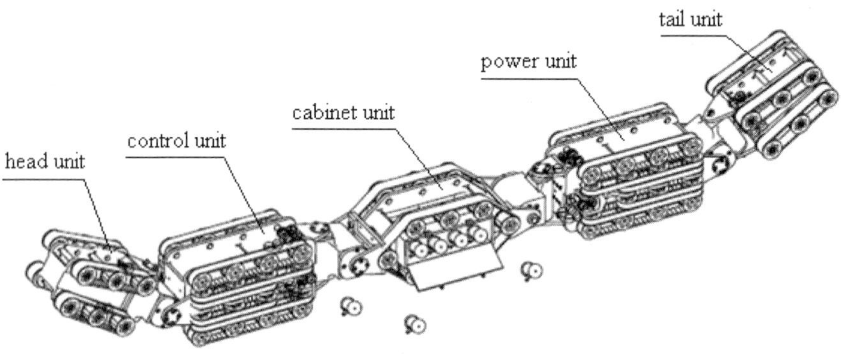

Fig. 6. The schematic diagram of the baby robot

Each unit is connected by active and passive joints and this may enhance the ability of adaptation to the complicated terrain. Each of unit is equipped with motors, retarders and drivers and so on. The cameras are installed in the head unit and the tail unit, thus the image of forth and back of the baby robot can be transmitted back to the remote control center and it is propitious to the commander to make an accurate judgment. The control unit mainly controls the motion of baby robot, deals with the information of sensors and communicates with the mother robot. The cabinet unit has a door that may be opened or closed and in which there are many communication nodes. The power unit takes a biggish lithium polymer cell and supplies power for each unit.

3.3 The Remote Control Center

The main function of remote control center is to realize man-machine mutual control, receiving information and broadcasting communication. Therefore, the remote control center adopts a suitcase-like structure, which not only has a friendly interface, but also can be expediently carried to the rescue site, as shown in Fig. 7. There are a LCD with touching screen, a control system and outside devices in the suitcase. The control panel includes handles, switches, multimedia interfaces and indicator lights and so on. The remote control center can be connected to more far decision-making center through internet and let experts or decision-makers in different places give evaluation and make accurate decisions without attendance using remote conference system so that the ability of the whole emergency reaction is improved.

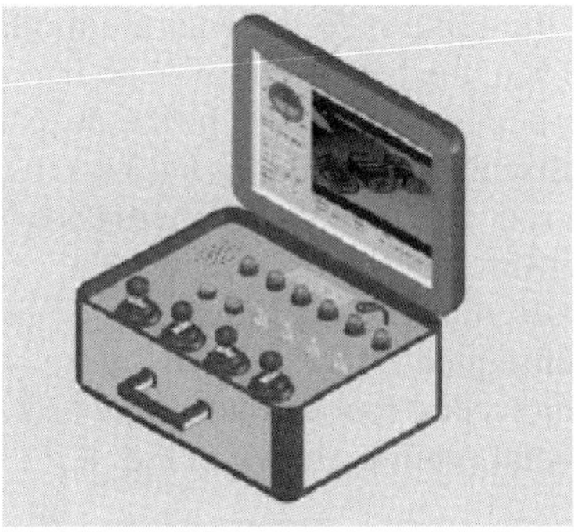

Fig. 7. The remote control center

3.4 The Remote Communication and Power System

The mother robot doesn't carry an energy source. It obtains the power from and communicates with the control center through a cable which can be dragged and released. The baby robot has its own cell module and can independently work. It communicates with the mother robot through wireless net and microwave. Based on the mother robot, the baby robot communicates to the remote control center through the multiple communication nodes released.

3.5 The Sensor System

To acquire the situation under the mine well, The mother robot and baby robot both carry vision sensors, gas sensors, sound sensors and environment detecting sensors to search and rescue survivors and feed back these information by form of sound, image and data to the remote control center to assist the experts to make judgments and decisions. To reduce the volume and integrate expediently, the sensors adopt MEMS techniques and uniform RS232 interface such as C_2H_4 sensor, C_2H_6 sensor, C_2H_2 sensor, CH_4 sensor, CO sensor, O_2 sensor, H_2 sensor, temperature sensor, moisture sensor and wind speed sensor.

3.6 The Lighting System

Because the lighting in the site is not favorable after mine disaster happens, the mother robot and baby robot carry lighting devices which is propitious to collect images of the site and make accurate judgments for the decision-maker.

4 The Rescue Process of the Marsupial Robot

When an accident happens and it is time to work for the marsupial robot, the mother robot carries the baby robot and drags the communication and power supply cable to go into the mine well under the control of the control center. If the dragging force is much bigger or the cable is trapped by some obstacles, the mother robot will release the cable and keep roving. When meeting an impassable obstacle such as that the gap of alleyway is confined or the cable is to the end, the mother robot releases the baby robot and keeps working. Then, the baby robot will go into the mine well by itself and release the communication nodes on the way. In the deep well, the baby robot sends the image, sound and other sensor information back to the mother robot through the communication nodes released, and then the mother robot feeds this information back to the remote control center through the cable. After the control center gets the information, it sends the control command to the mother robot and baby robot via the communication system. Consequently, the control center can acquire the information of the site and control the marsupial robot to fulfill the task of rescuing survivors. The rescue process of the marsupial robot is shown in Fig. 8.

5 The Key Problems for Research on the Marsupial Robot

The marsupial robot will face unpredictable, complicated and unstructured surroundings after mine disaster happens. For examples, the entrance is narrow, the void is limited, there is water on the ground, there is explosive eroding gas, there are debris and unstable structures all round, it is lack of illumination and the communication is difficult. Hence, the research on the marsupial robot must solve the following key problems. (1) The mother robot and baby robot must be able to flexibly climb over obstacles under a complicated and unstructured surrounding. Otherwise, they must have the capability of anti-explosion, water-proof, dust-proof and anti-shock to meet the requirement of mine environment. (2) For the mother robot needs to release the baby robot at the proper time and callback it after completing rescue task, an appropriate releasing and recovery structure and a control method must be studied. (3) It must be studied that the least cables is used to realize much more far distance and stable multi-signal and multi-channel net transmission under the condition of having

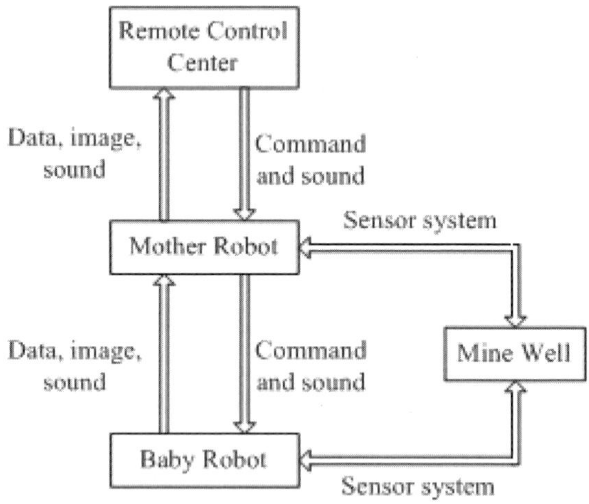

Fig. 8. The rescue process of a marsupial robot

rock dispersion and more obstacles. (4) The remote control station carried easily with integrated man-machine mutual interface must also be studied. It can control the mother robot and baby robot, receive the information of image, sound and sensor data from the marsupial robot and has an ability of multimedia and remote net communication. (5) It is necessary to study high-powered MEMS gas and environment detecting sensors and solve the problem of general interface. The sensors must have a small volume, high reliability and the capability of anti-explosion and interface integration.

6 Conclusion

This paper discusses and analyzes the existing robots for coal mine rescue, and presents a marsupial robot with strong practicability for coal mine rescue. Also, the system structure, a working flow and the key problems for studying on the marsupial robot are discussed in detail. When this cooperative marsupial robot composed of a mother robot and a baby robot is applied to the rescue of survivors in the disaster of coal mine, it not only enlarges the scale of the rescue, but also increases the probability of successfully rescuing the trapped miners, so the rescue task can be completed perfectly. Thus, the marsupial robot has a good potential of development and foreground of application and establishes a stiff base for the research, development and application of robotics.

Acknowledgments. This work was supported by a grant from the National High Technology Research and Development Program of China (863 Program) (No. 2007AA041501).

References

1. United States Mine Rescue Association, http://www.usmra.com
2. Yong, W., Hua, Z., Yong-sheng, W., Gang, C., Yun-wang, L.: Current Status and Technical Problems in Research of Coal Mine Rescue Robot. J. Coal Mine Machinery 28(4), 107–109 (2007)
3. Hua, Z.: Current Status and Technical Problems in the Research of Coal Mine Rescue Robot. J. Journal of Xuzhou Institute of Technology 22(6), 5–8 (2007)
4. American DiscoverMiner Company, http://www.discoveryminer.com
5. Remotec, http://www.remotec-andros.com
6. Mine Safety and Health Administration, http: http://www.msha.gov
7. Nuchter, A., Surmann, H., Lingemann, K., Hertzberg, J., Thrun, S.: 6D SLAM with an application in autonomous mine mapping. In: 2004 IEEE International Conference on Robotics and Automation, April 26–May 1, vol. 2, pp. 1998–2003 (2004)
8. Baker, C., Morris, A., Ferguson, D., Thayer, S., Whittaker, C., et al.: A Campaign in Autonomous Mine Mapping. In: IEEE International Conference on Robotics and Automation, 2004, April 26–May 1, vol. 2, pp. 2004–2009 (2004)
9. Thrun, S., Thayer, S., Whittaker, W., Baker, C., Burgard, W., et al.: Autonomous exploration and mapping of abandoned mines. J. Robotics & Automation Magazine 11(4), 79–91 (2004)
10. Sandia's Intelligent Systems and Robotics Center (ISRC), http://www.sandia.gov

11. Takayama, T., Hirose, S.: Development of Souryu-I Connected Crawler Vehicle for Inspection of Narrow and Winding Space. In: 26th Annual Conference of the IEEE, Japan, October, vol. 1, pp. 143–148 (2000)
12. Masayuki, A., Takayama, T., Hirose, S.: Development of "Souryu-III": Connected Crawler Vehicle for Inspection inside Narrow and Winding Spaces. In: Proceedings of 2004 IEEE/RSJ International Conference on Intelligent Robots and Systems, September 28–October 2, vol. 1, pp. 52–57 (2004)
13. Kamegawa, T., Yamasaki, T., Igarashi, H., Matsuno, F.: Development of The Snake-like Rescue Robot "KOHGA". In: Proceedings of the 2004 IEEE International Conference on Robotics & Automation, Japan, April 26–May 1, vol. 5, pp. 5081–5086 (2004)
14. Miyanaka, H., Wada, N., Kamegawa, T., Sato, N., Tsukui, S., et al.: Development of an unit type robot "KOHGA2" with stuck avoidance ability. In: 2007 IEEE International Conference on Robotics and Automation, Tokyo, April, pp. 3877–3882 (2007)
15. Securities Information, http://www.secinfo.com

Crucial Technology Research on Pipeline Jet Cleaning Robot

Ding Feng, Chaobin Huang, Kui Zhou, Peng Wang, Jin Liu, and Shouyong Li

School of Mechanical Engineering, Yangtze University, Jingzhou, Hubei, 434023, China
fengd@yangtzeu.edu.cn, fengd0861@yahoo.com

Abstract. The pipeline cleaning is an important method to improve the use efficiency of the pipeline. The traditional cleaning methods, such as manual cleaning, chemical cleaning and mechanical cleaning, can not meet the need of cleaning the pipe well. Due to the advantages such as high cleaning efficiency and low cleaning cost and easy to realize mechanization and convenient operation and safe and reliable, etc. The high pressure jet cleaning was used widely in recent years. However, it is a challenge for workers to work in the high pressure environment. In view of this, the method of combining the high pressure water jet cleaning technology with the robot technology is presented in the paper. In addition, the research on the crucial method of the robot which has important significance in the further research and development of the pipeline cleaning robot has been studied in the paper.

Keywords: pipeline; cleaning; robot; crucial technology.

1 Introduction

The traditional pipeline cleaning technologies which include manual cleaning, chemical cleaning, mechanical cleaning, pig cleaning and vapor cleaning etc have made great contributions to the pipeline cleaning [1]. Pipe scaling is a universal phenomenon in industry. Carbonate scale, sulfate scale and silicate deposition can be absorbed strongly by the pipe which makes effective pipe diameter reduced, affect the safety and benefit of the equipment operation. The traditional cleaning methods can not meet the need of cleaning the pipeline. Comparing with mechanical cleaning and chemical cleaning method [2, 3], high pressure water jet cleaning has many advantages such as high cleaning efficiency, low cleaning cost, easy to realize mechanization, convenient operation, safe and reliable and so on. But if we clean the hard-scale only by high pressure jet, the pressure should reach more than 70 MPa, sometimes even reach more than 150Mpa. It is a great challenge for workers to work in so high pressure environment. If we clean the pipeline by the way that high pressure combining with the robot technology, we not only can solve the problems of cleaning the pipe, but also can solve the pollution problems and the safety problems of workers. So, scientists are embarking on the study of the robot which can move and clean in the pipeline intelligently.

C. Xiong et al. (Eds.): ICIRA 2008, Part II, LNAI 5315, pp. 1137–1144, 2008.

2 Status of Pipeline Cleaning Robot

The research on pipeline cleaning robots concentrates primarily in the robots for cleaning the ventilating duct of Central Air Condition. The research on the aspect of

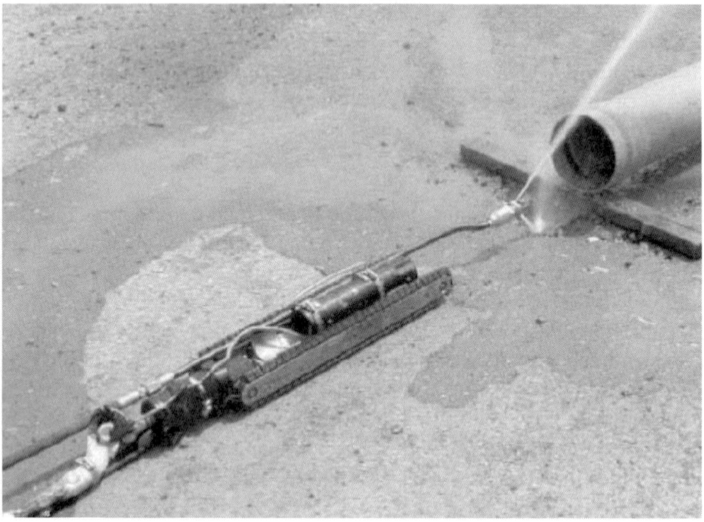

Fig. 1. Pipeline Jet Cleaning Robot of Stone-age Company

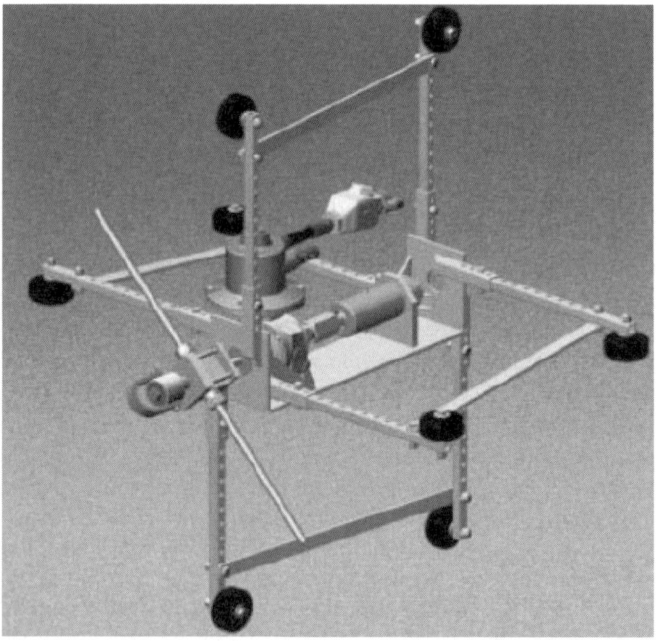

Fig. 2. Bracket with no Power for Pipeline Cleaning

pipeline cleaning robots is relatively less, only the Stone-age Company has done many researches about it whose pipeline cleaning robot is driven by track(figure 1), but the robot can not suit the pipe diameters well, and lateral alignment is bad and the cleaning effect is not excellent. The pipeline jet cleaning robot of Stone-age Company is shown in Figure 1. In order to clean the medium-small pipeline, the research on intelligent cleaning equipment which has small and weight moving carrier and high-efficiency and multi-functional walking mechanism is the trend [4].

The research on the robot inside the pipeline is very backward in China. The experimental prototype of the robot inside the pipeline has been researched in Harbin Institute of Technology. Tsinghua University, Donghua University and Shanghai University and Tianjin University have done many researches on the pipeline robot which mainly aim at the cleaning of the ventilating duct and the pipeline detection, etc. The pipeline cleaning robots combining with high pressure jet have not been researched at present and the cleaning of pipeline mostly adopts the cleaning method without dynamic towline. The bracket with no power for pipeline cleaning is shown in Figure 2.

3 The Study on the System of the Pipe Jet Cleaning Robot

The Pipeline Jet Cleaning Robot mainly is constituted by six parts which is shown in the Figure 3. The matching of each parameter of the system and the interface of each part must be suit one another, namely, each part should suit each other. The match between the pump and the nozzle can generate anticipant working condition; meanwhile, they can suit the running speed of the robot. The movement of the robot can be controlled and coordinated remotely, and be coordinated with the deploying and retracting of the high pressure hose and the cable wire to avoid the high pressure hose and the cable wire bearing larger force. The dynamic of the robot should overcome various resistances. And the robot can adjust running speed according to the condition inside the pipeline to achieve high cleaning efficiency.

3.1 Monitoring System

The monitoring system is composed of a waterproof camera carried by robot body, extra-pipe monitor and extra-pipe controlling box. The internal condition of the pipe is photographed by the waterproof camera installed in the proper position of the pipe body when the robot is moving inside the pipe, and the relative video signal is transferred to the extra-pipe monitor by the signal cable carried by the robot. The operators identify the cleaning and the fouling distribution inside the pipe and control walking speed of the robot, such as reducing the speed in the place where the scaling is severe, to clean the pipe inner surface with highest efficiency and best effect. The waterproof camera can be rotated with 360 degree [5].

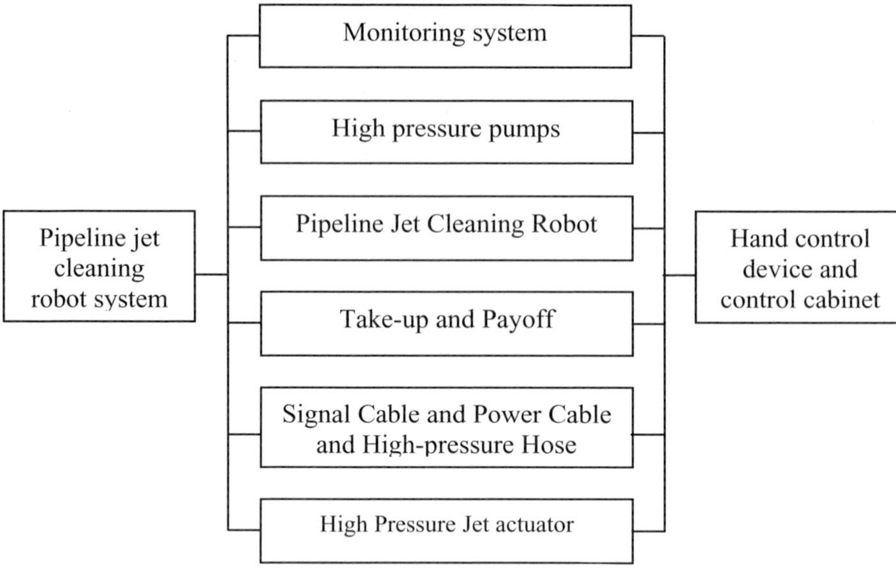

Fig. 3. Component of Pipeline Water Jet Cleaning System

3.2 High Pressure Pumps

High pressure pumps are composed by power plant, high pressure pump, pneumatic pressure-regulated valve, safety valve, booster pump, filtering system and control cabinet, etc. The structure of pump groups is shown in the Figure 4.

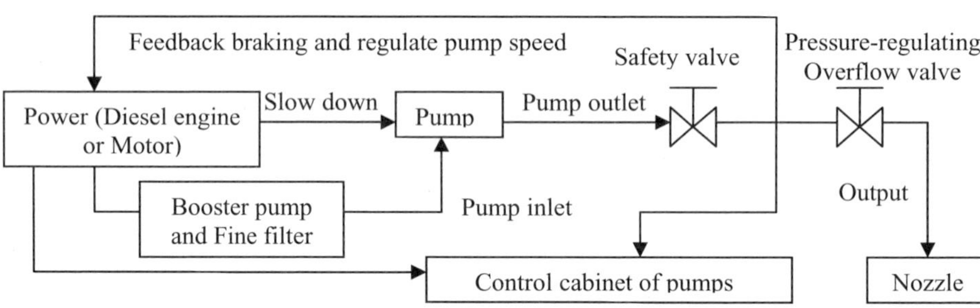

Fig. 4. Structure of Pump Groups

3.3 Pipeline Jet Cleaning Robot

The pipeline jet cleaning robot is not only the actuator of the pipeline cleaning system but also the intelligent equipment which connects another three parts to show the whole function. It plays the role as a relay station, and the function of the pipeline jet cleaning robot is shown in Figure 5.

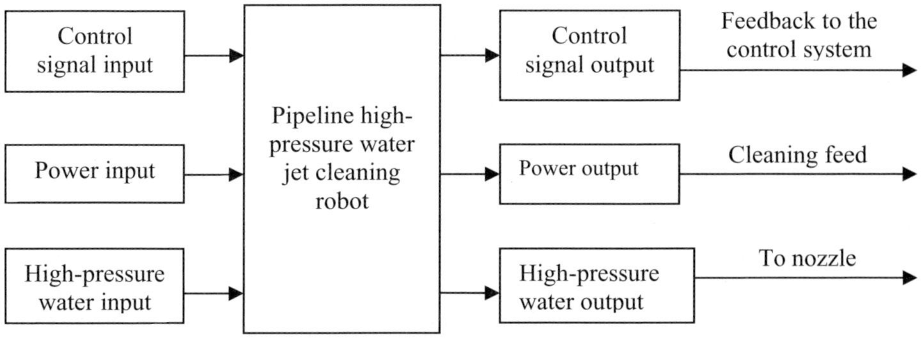

Fig. 5. Function of the Pipeline Jet Cleaning Robot

3.4 Take-Up and Payoff

The robot need tow the signal cable, the power cable and the pressure hose when it is working inside the pipeline. In order to avoid the cable and pipeline being stretched breaking accidentally and the cable being winded, the robot need the take-up and pay-off to take-up and pay-off synchronously.

3.5 Signal Cable and Power Cable and High-Pressure Hose

The signal cable is a coaxial video-signal cable which is the bridge connecting the information between the internal pipe cleaning monitoring system unit and extra-pipe monitoring system unit, at the meantime, it is responsible for transmitting the video signal of the airborne camera to the monitor outside the pipe. The power cable transfer the external alternating current to the servo motor installed in the robot body. The signal cable and the power cable can be packaged together and be installed in the high strength wire rope with the fixture to increase the tensile strength of the cable. The high-pressure hose is composed by a high-pressure hose which is about 250 meters long and a high-pressure steel pipe installed in the body, which is responsible for transferring the water pressurized by the high-pressure pumps to high-pressure rotating cleaning nozzle to clean the pipeline.

3.6 High Pressure Jet Actuator

The pressure jet actuator plays the role of rapidly shunting and jetting the high-pressure water pressurized by the high-pressure pumps according to a certain jet stream and angle to the surface of the pipeline, and the main component of the actuator is the high-pressure cleaning sprinkler. The sprinkler is connected with the body by the high pressure rotating sealing joint and drive the nozzle to rotate with the rotary moment generated by it to perform the cleaning of the surface of the pipe. The cleaning standoff distance can be adjusted by the pressure jet actuator according to different pipe diameter.

The 2D high-pressure rotating sprinkler is used as the pressure jet actuator according to the characteristics of cleaning the internal pipeline surface which is composed by the nozzle, the spray boom and rotary joint. The structure and the connection form of the sprinkler have decided the eccentricity of the nozzle and the jet angle, the speed of the sprinkler can be adjusted through adjusting the eccentricity of the nozzle and the jet angle. The offset nozzle generated the moment enough to rotate the sprinkler because the rotating dynamical of the high-pressure rotating sprinkler comes from water jet itself.

The nozzle is a key component of the high-pressure rotating sprinkler and the affect of which is significant in the property and the efficiency of high pressure jet cleaning. In view of the jet beam states and the effect to the working surface, the nozzle is mainly divided into cylindrical nozzle and fan efficiency nozzle. The research shows that the cylindrical nozzle is better than the fan efficiency nozzle in high pressure jetting. The cylindrical nozzle is better than the fan efficiency nozzle with the better effect and high permeability when the cylindrical nozzle has the same nozzle diameter, pressure and distance from the nozzle to the working surface and working time as the fan efficiency nozzle. The efficiency of the fan efficiency nozzle is lower is because that most jet energy is losing in the nozzle when the jet is being diffused.

4 Analyses on Operation of the Robot Structure

4.1 Walking Mechanism

The main forms of the mobile robot structure of the pipe robot are as followings: track type, outrigger, wheel, snake traveling, creep-walking and amoeboid locomotion and so on [6]. The snake traveling robot, the creep-walking robot and the amoeboid locomotion robot are suitable to work in the smooth pipeline wall or on the ground and under water. The track mobile robot is suitable for working on the uneven road surface well and can touch the surface well. While, the track mobile robot cannot turn easily because of its large volume, and it need keep the track tense, what's more, the structure is complex. The outrigger robot is proper for the rough surface and the loading capacity is high. But both of the control system and the mechanical structure are complicated and the moving speed is slow. The wheeled robot can move quickly and turn easily and has good concentricity. The radial wheeled robot can keep its central axis consistent with the central axis of the pipeline. But the area touched with the surface is smaller and cannot keep the attachment pulling force easily.

In order to improve the quality of cleaning, the central line of the high-pressure rotating sprinkler must keep the same center with the central line of the pipeline, which can ensure the distance between the high-pressure water jet from each sprinkler and the pipe wall can meet the need of the best target distance. So we should consider the concentricity problem of the high-pressure rotating sprinkler when we design the robot. At the same time, the structure of the radial wheel form can be preferentially considered and the width of each wheel can be enlarged appropriately to increase the cable dragging force when the robot is working in the pipeline.

4.2 Driving Mode

There are mainly two ways when the robot is moving and cleaning inside the pipeline: external cable power supply and storage battery power supply. Considering the robot need the force towing cable to tow the high-pressure hose and the signal cable and other equipments and the distance of pipeline is shorter in single-cleaning, the pipeline jet cleaning robot adopts the way of external cable power supply. So, the pipeline jet cleaning robot can also be called cable pipeline jet cleaning robot.

There are three ways of driving the robot commonly: hydraulic driving, pneumatic driving and electric driving. The electric driving mainly includes stepping motor, dc servo motor and ac servo motor. The requirement of environment is strengthened when the robot is driven by hydraulic driving and pneumatic driving and it is complex to be operated. Comparing with the hydraulic driving and pneumatic driving, the structure of electric driving is simpler and it is easy to seal and control the speed. So, ac servo motor is commonly used to drive the robot and the planet-gear decelerator is used as the reducer of the robot.

4.3 Transmission Mode

How to transfer the driving force to the driving gear after the force from the servo motor is reduced by the reducer on the basis of satisfying adaptability of the pipe is the current important technical task in the course of choosing the robot transmission mode. In the designing process, it can be achieved by the device of force transform and the mechanism of synchronous belt transmission.

4.4 Scheme of Variable Diameter Pipe Adaptability

The bracing arm will be shrunk because of the resistance and the robot will pass the deformation place under the driving force, when the robot touch the dust and the deformation place which are caused by the manufacturing error and the deformation caused by the local scaling and bigger local pressure in the working. The bracing arm can be opened as an umbrella under the effect of the spring and the robot can restore the original steady state when it go back to the normal section of the pipeline again. The whole process is the course of variable diameter pipe adaptability. The robot can go through the deformation and achieve the goal of cleaning the pipe effectively with the adaptability.

5 Conclusions

Firstly, high pressure jet combined with the pipeline robot not only can solve the difficult problems of cleaning the pipe but also can solve the environment pollution problems and the safety problems of the operator. Secondly, the analysis and research on the crucial technologies of the pipeline cleaning robot, such as the system design and the body structure design, can guide the design of the pipeline cleaning robot.

References

1. Jianxun, S., Yiqiang, C., Yun, Z.: The technology of High-Pressure Water Jet Cleaning. J. Pipeline Technology & Equipment 4, 40–44 (2001)
2. Guozhi, Q., Zhiming, T.: Application of High Pressure Water Jet Cleaning Technique. J. Pipeline Technology & Equipment 1, 38–40 (2001)

3. Kulekci, M.K.: Processes and Apparatus Developments in Industrial Water Jet Applications. J. Machine Tools & Manufacture 42, 1297–1306 (2002)
4. Xinhua, F.: Simulation Research on Pipeline Jet Cleaning Robot. D. Daqing Petroleum Institute (2007)
5. Gua, J.S., de Silva, C.W.: Development and Implementation of a Real-time Open-architecture Control System for Industrial Robot Systems. J. Engineering Applications of Artificial Intelligence 17, 469–483 (2004)
6. Song, J., Limin, M., Yuqing, G., Shen, L.: Research of Control System of the Ventilating Duct Cleaning Robot. J. Electrical Drive 36, 26–29 (2006)

A Novel Self-navigated Inspection Robot along High-Voltage Power Transmission Line and Its Application

Gongping Wu[1], Xianjin Xu[1], Hua Xiao[1], Jinchun Dai[1], Xiaohui Xiao[1], Zhenglie Huang[2], and Liping Ruan[2]

[1] College of Power and Mechanical Engineering, 430072, Wuhan University, China
[2] Ningbo Bull Electric Company Limited
gpwu@whu.edu.cn

Abstract. In order to reduce maintenance cost, increase reliability of line detection and speed up industrialization, a novel self-navigating inspection robot along 220kv overhang power transmission live line is proposed in this paper. The key technologies are discussed and both software and hardware structure are introduced systematically. There are three main features as follows: (1) Robot with only six freedom degrees is designed into double anti-symmetrical arms, interactive sliding and suspending structure, which enables rolling or crawling along the overhead transmission line and striding the obstacles autonomously. (2)Several key technologies such as GPS-GIS, machine vision, multi-electromagnetic sensors technology are adopted to fulfill global environments detection, rough recognition and the exact location and attitude recognition respectively. (3) Non-contact supply technology is utilized in electrical energy supply in line. Operating pictures and inspection results are also shown, which demonstrate that the robot has the ability of self-inspection without collision and has great application prospects for engineering application.

Keywords: High-voltage transmission lines; Self-determination inspection robot; Mobile robot mechanism; Environment detection and identification; Non-contact power supply unit.

1 Introduction

High-voltage power line inspection plays an important role in the power grid maintenance, which aiming at electrical/ mechanical malfunction diagnosis and the first hand field information collection for condition based maintenance. At present, the general way of power transmission line inspection adopted is manual work and helicopter power line inspection sometimes. As known to all, robot inspection features advantages such as higher inspection precision than the manual inspection, lower cost than the helicopter inspection and inspection blind-area-free, which make the inspection robot more competitive in the field of high-voltage power line maintenance especially when there are difficult places of access such as primitive forest, large rivers and so on. And hence the study of the inspection robot for high-voltage transmission line (hereinafter referred to as inspection robot) has become a hot topic in both application and research field.

C. Xiong et al. (Eds.): ICIRA 2008, Part II, LNAI 5315, pp. 1145–1154, 2008.

In the past two decades, some mobile robots for flexible cable structure have being developed, including a type of cable-climbing mechanism for Cable-stayed bridge [1], an arbitrary gradient cable robot [2], a type of climbing mechanisms of Cable-I Robot [3] and an Inspection Robot for power transmission lines [4], but all of them can only move along those flexible cables without obstacles.

In [5], a double-arm mobile robot prototype was developed by the Robot Research Institute in Wuhan University, China. Based on their former achievements in [6], a new manipulator with wheel-claw hybrid mechanism is proposed which is capable of moving along those flexible cables with obstacles and conducting on-line inspection autonomously.

The robot which introduced systematically here has passed experiment and field tests. The paper is organized as follows: In the following section the structure of the transmission line is introduced and the systematic configuration of the inspection robot presented. In section 3 several key technologies adopted in the prototype are introduced with the mobile mechanism configuration, environment detection, obstacle identification with hybrid multi-sensors system and non-contact power supply technologies detailed respectively. In the forth section the prototype and its field test information are given and conclusion and acknowledgement are made in the fifth and last section.

2 Systematical Mechanism Configuration

As shown in Fig. 1, the inspection tasks are performed by the robot carrying detection instruments while rolling/crawling along the overhead transmission line. A typical structure of the working environment consists of conductors, suspension and tensile clamps, insulator chains, and dampers [6], etc. And the working condition of the inspection robot features characteristics such as strong electromagnetic environment for taking the live line as working path and semi-structure for the unknown local environment, which make it tougher to perform on-line inspection or testing.

Generally there are two principle kinds of inspection tasks: One is autonomous motion including the obstacle identification, motion planning, obstacle overcoming without collision etc. The other is autonomous inspection for locating the attached structures such as insulator chains, clamps, dampers and so on. To achieve above

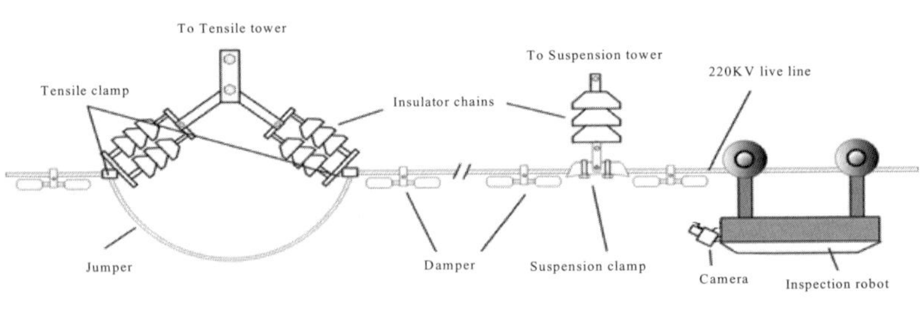

Fig. 1. Inspection environment along moving path-overhead transmission line

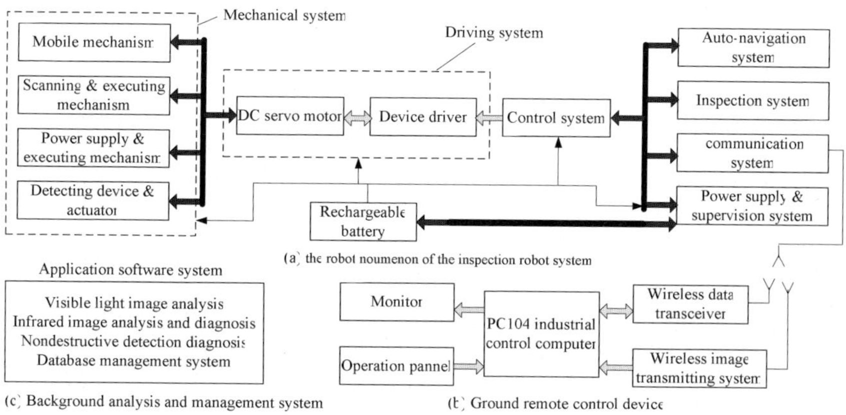

Fig. 2. The schematic structure of the inspection robot system

functions, the author and teammates have developed a dual control function system—remote control or autonomous control. System schematic structure is shown in Fig.2, from which we get the whole system is composed of mechanical noumenon, ground remote control device, background analysis and management software. The critical technologies will be introduced in section 3.

3 Critical Technologies

The critical technologies applied in the proposed inspection robot are detailed in turn mainly concerned with three aspects such as motion mechanism, environment identification and non-contact power supply.

3.1 Motion Mechanism

In consideration of the transmission-line structure and the requirement of inspection tasks, the robot here is designed into anti-symmetrical double-arm and suspending structure [6], [7], which is shown in Fig. 3. Each robot arm has two rotation degrees of freedom (DOF) to realize rotation of robot arms on two axes. There are one driving wheel and a pair of clamp on the end of arm, enabling the robot to roll along non-obstacle section and to loose/grasp the line while overcoming obstacles respectively. Between the two arms, there is also an interactive translation DOF available for their interactive sliding and transposition along the guide rail.

As shown in Fig. 3 (a) and (b), the robot has six joints totally, where Joint 1 is imaginary joint, Joint 8 is horizontal translation joint, and the other four are rotating joints. The axis of Joint 2 and Joint 6 and axis of translation Joint 8,are horizontal, intersecting perpendicularly with that of Joint 3 and Joint 5 respectively. As shown in the Fig. 3.(c), the gripper mechanism is composed of the clamping bar(1-1), rotary pair(1-2), constraint rotary pair(1-3) and gripper jaw(1-4) which are arranged symmetrically in the transverse direction of the cable. The equipotential mechanism is a profiling mechanism which is made up of translational prismatic pair omitted in

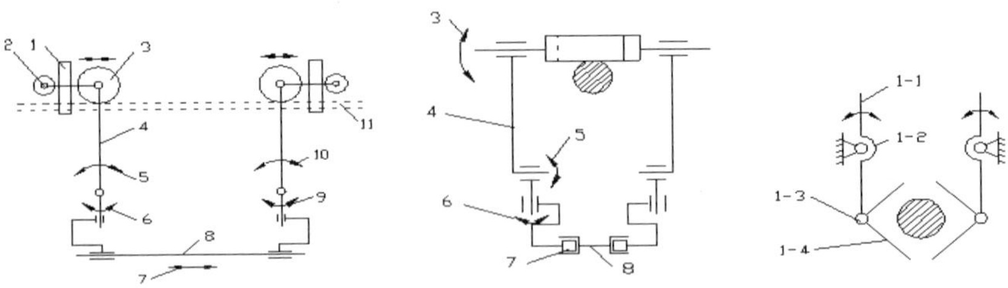

(a) Mechanism schematic (b) Anti-symmetrical arrangement (c) Gripper mechanism

Fig. 3. Inspection robot mechanism schematic: 1—Gripper mechanism; 2—Driven wheel; 3—Driving wheel(Joint 1); 4—Short arm; 5—Rotating joint around horizontal axis (Joint 2); 6—Rotating joint around perpendicular axis (Joint 3); 7—Translation joint (Joint 4); 8—Changeable long arm; 9—Joint 5; 10—Joint 6; 11—live line; 1-1—Clamping bar; 1-2—Rotary pair; 1-3—Constraint rotary pair; 1-4—Gripper jaw.

Fig. 3. Through programming of three basic actions such as translation along Joint 1, tow arms interactive translation along Joint 8, rotation of Joint 2/Joint 6, and rotation of Joint 3/Joint 5, the robot can overcome all kinds of obstacles along the transmission line.

The kinematical simulation and physical experiments have testified the effectiveness of the above mechanism and in Fig.4., the simulated postures of the robot when striding the insulator chains both in collision and without collision situation are given.

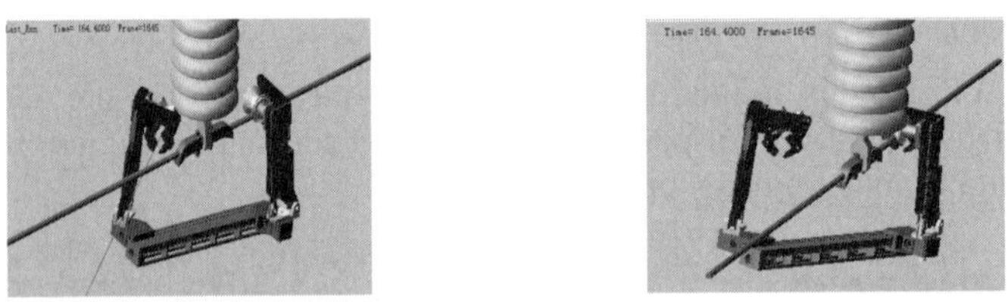

(a) collision posture (b) collision avoiding posture

Fig. 4. The simulation poses under collision and non-collision circumstances

From the discussion above we can draw a conclusion that the proposed robot has several following advantages. First, the simpler structure design compared with the three-arm or multi-arm robots cuts down the weight and size effectively and makes it easier to control. Secondly, the gripper mechanism lies between the driving and driven wheels ensuring at least two grasping points at any conditions. Moreover, the motion of a clamp pair is realized utilizing a steel wire and fixed pulley, thus self-adaptive and balance keeping ability of the clamp is ensured and control task can be concerned on control of the clamp force other than position.

The methods of modeling the mobile mechanism and finding the kinematics inverse solution are shown in [8].

3.2 Environment Identification

3.2.1 Global Environment Identification

The global environment is composed of the inspection environment and the moving space needed for motions along the live line. The former environment includes the mechanism parameters of live line and ground line between adjacent towers, the assembled structures attached to the line, and the location parameters, first two of which are utilized for the scanning platform control, and the rest is used to nominate the related documents. Moreover, the moving space is detailed in the Fig. 5. Supposing there are n towers and thus $n-1$ spans. Taking T_k as the k th tower, D_k the range of the k th span, d_j the estimated real-time distance, and the o_{k+1} the designed distance to the T_{k+1} tower, we can establish the transmission line database(TLDB) for a given transmission line and fulfil the estimation of the d_k through global position system module, and then get the cable structure parameters to decide motion direction utilizing k and hence accomplish the rough recognition of the global environment.

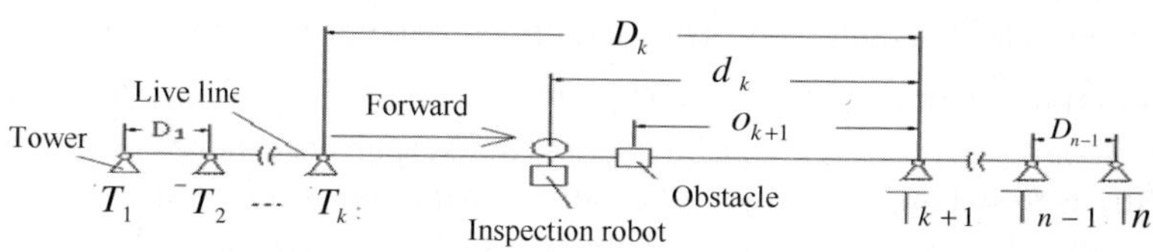

Fig. 5. Motion space of robot

From the GPS module, the robot longitude/latitude and height coordination in the T_{i-1} tower can be obtained and written as (B_0, L_0, H_0) at the kth tower and its location in the k th span as (B_1, L_1, H_1). The receipted longitude/latitude coordination in the WGS-84 system can be transformed to Beijing 54 Coordinate Systems and be coded as X, Y, Z which follows (1).

$$\begin{cases} X = (N+H)\cos B \cos L \\ Y = (N+H)\cos B \sin L \\ Z = [N(1-e^2)+H]\sin B \end{cases} \tag{1}$$

where $N = a/\sqrt{1^2 - e^2\sin^2 B}$, stands for the curvature in prime vertical and $e^2 = (a^2-b^2)/a^2$, a and b denote the semi major axis of ellipsoid and eccentricity of ellipsoid in Geodetic Coordinate Systems respectively.

And then, the approximate distance robot away from the T_i tower can be calculated according to (2) ,where the deflection of the cable is neglected :

$$d_j = D_j - \left(\sqrt{x_1^2+y_1^2+z_1^2} - \sqrt{x_0^2+y_0^2+z_0^2}\right) \tag{2}$$

3.2.2 Local Environment Detection

As shown in Fig. 6, the local environment includes the assembled obstacles such as the damper and the insulator chains and so on. According to the integrated mobile mechanism and its working conditions the striding motion plan can be programmed into four steps. In the first step the effective working space is deduced by the electromagnetic sensors' outputs analysis. In the further step the arms end manipulator (clamp and wheel) loose the cable to avoid the collision directed by electromagnetic sensors. The following step is striding during which the robot transposes from one side of the obstacle to the other side. In the fourth step the attitude of the arm relative to the live line is recognized enabling clamp and wheel grasping the line precisely. Whereas structural limitation of the clamp and wheel, the accumulative errors of kinematic pair clearance, wind loads, the centroidal changes and flexibility introduced may lead to the uncertainty of the relative position and attitude between arm end and inspection path. Among all four stages, only the second one fulfills offline motion plan based on given environment adopting amplified geometric model to offset the accumulative errors mentioned above. During the rest stages local motion plan based on the multi-electromagnetic sensor system in unknown environment is accomplished. So the distribution of multi-electromagnetic is of great importance. In Fig. 6(a), the obstacle detecting sensors is illustrated, where the sensor D_1、D_3 are arranged in driving-wheel shaft for damper detection and D_2、D_4 mounted in internal sides of the arm detecting the tensile clamps and suspension clamps. Fig. 6(b) shows the multi-electromagnetic sensors schematic distribution of one arm, with which the attitude estimation is made and the sensors groups are named as A, B, C group respectively. The group A and B are mounted symmetrically and group C in the clamp bracket of robot's arm featuring the following three characters: (1) Each of the three group has their common axis l_A、l_B and l_C. (2) Group A and B is symmetric to each other and their common axis l_A、l_B are parallel to x direction of the cable and the axis l_C is perpendicular to it with equal distance to l_A、l_B. (3) The group mumbers are placed equidistantly with each other. The arm attitude estimation is decided utilizing the information fusion of the sensor groups' outputs. For example, group A *and* B give out whether the current plane of the arm is parallel or perpendicular to the cable and the group C decides the relative position in y direction. This kind of relative detecting method has been testified in the experiments and field tests and the results show that arm attitude estimation is robust to load current disturbance, θ angle between the normal line of the cable transversal surface and coaxial magnetic field.

According to the inspection direction in Fig.6(a), we can take arm II as the detecting arm and arm I as referenced one. During the obstacle detection, the sudden change of the sensors outputs suggests there be a certain kind of obstacle corresponding to a certain value. An example is also shown in Fig. 7, where the vertical coordinates values mean the four detecting sensors outputs $v_i (i = 1,2,3,4)$, and horizon coordinate stands for time t under load current of 80A.

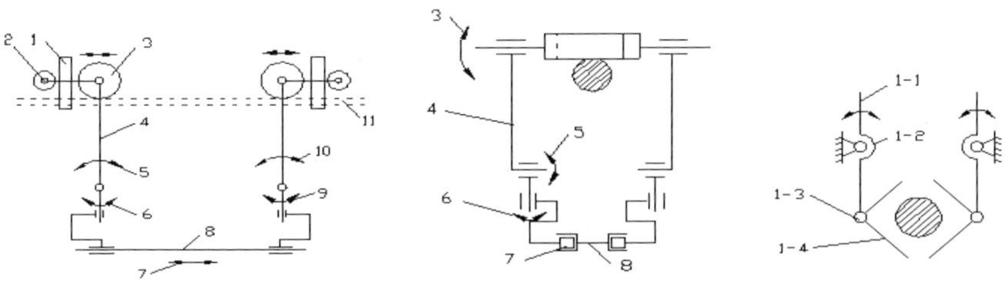

(a) Mechanism schematic (b) Anti-symmetrical arrangement (c) Gripper mechanism

Fig. 6. Distribution plan of the sensor arrays

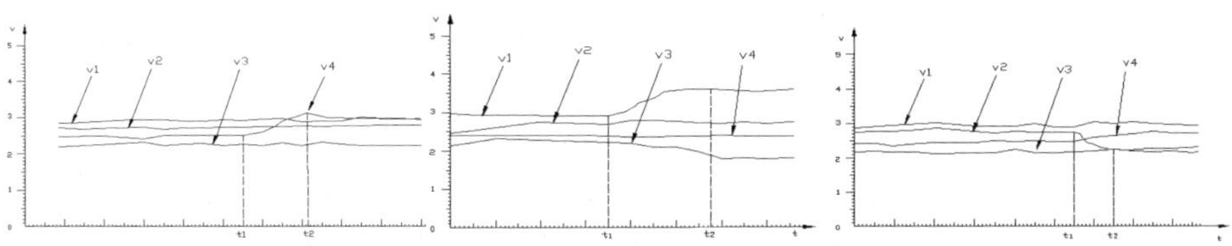

(a) Damper signal (b) Suspension clamp (c) Tensile clamps

Fig. 7. Responding signal of three kinds of obstacles

During the process of grasping / loosing the cable, it is necessary to adjust the arm pose relative to the cable continuously. And hence the cable can be mapped by the attitude sensor arrays. As shown in Fig. 6(b), there are $2m-3$ observe points a_{12}、a_2、a_{23}、a_3、……、$a_{(m-1)m}$ decided by sensors in group A and thus l_A can be divided into $2m-2$ sub working spaces named as A_{12}、A_{21}、A_{23}、A_{32}、……、$A_{m(m-1)}$, where m is the number of sensors in group A. And the sensor numbers of group B and C are m, n respectively. In the Fig.8, m, n equal to 8 and 4 respectively. It's clear that at time t_1 the outputs of sensor A_1 and A_2 have the same value which is maximum among outputs of all six other sensors indicating that the cable is equidistant to A_1 and A_2. Moreover, these two sensors are the nearest to the cable and thus the cable can be mapped to a_{12} in the central axis l_A. Then we can find the corresponding location of the manipulator end relative to the path at various times and the relationships can be noted as $\{A_{p,q}, B_{rs}, C_{wx}\}$,where $p = 2,3.\cdots,8$, $q = 1,2,\cdots,7, and \quad p \neq q$, $r = 2,3.\cdots,8, s = 1,2,\cdots 7, and \quad r \neq s, and \quad w = 2,3.\cdots,8, x = 1,2,\cdots 7, and \quad w \neq x$. From analysis above we can draw a conclusion that arm attitude relative to the cable is uniquely defined by a three-array-sensor system.

3.2.3 Local Environment Recognition Based on Machine Vision

The camera is mounted in the front side of the robot noumenon with an angle of 30 degrees between optical central axis and the inspection direction. Under such

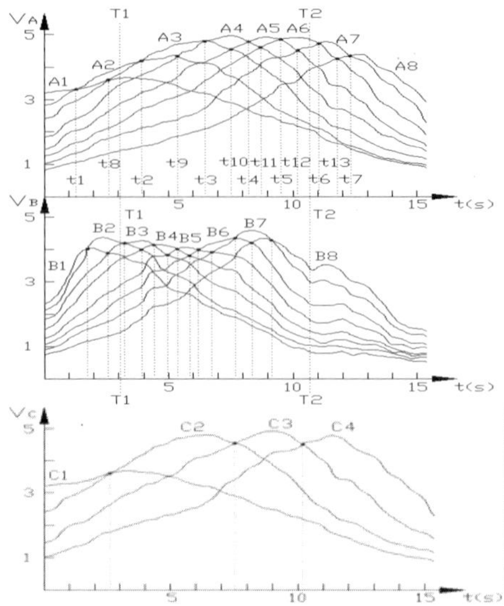

Fig. 8. The attitude signals in field test

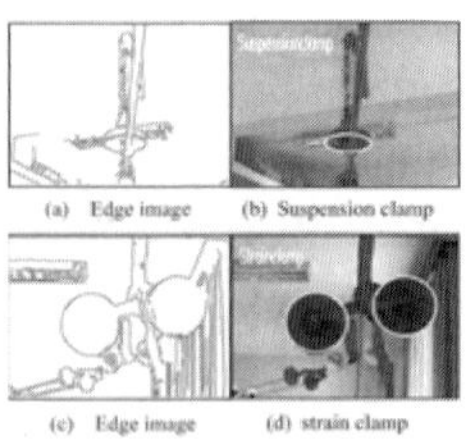

Fig. 9. Identification in lab

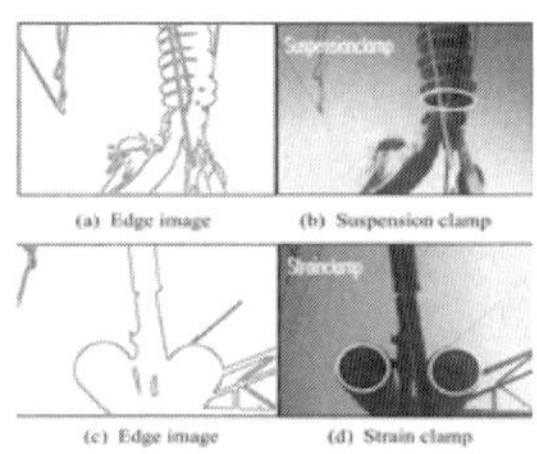

Fig. 10. Identification in field test

condition, the side of damper, the bottom of insulator chains and clamps are injected on camera imaging plane as linear, circular or elliptical geometric figures under constraints respectively. It is these figures that are chosen as the detection result of different obstacles. Considering of the structural characteristics of 220KV overhang high voltage transmission line discussed above, an obstacle recognition strategy is put forward through constraints conditions, circle/ellipse detection method based on existence probability map, and multi-objective and layered decision-making. The obstacle tracing verification strategy based on the Kalman-predictor are also introduced with recognition quality and reliability enhanced greatly. In Fig. 9 and Fig. 10 the identification results of different obstacles both in the experiment and field test are given out.

3.3 Non-contact Power Supply

As shown in Fig. 11, the power supply system is composed of electromagnetic transformer, switch regulator, rechargeable battery, supervisory circuit and DC-DC modules. In our design, the ferromagnetic coil is designed into split structure, whose opening and closing executed by mechanism mounted in the arm end (omitted). Moreover, the ferromagnetic coil must be under proper control to lower magnetic resistance of the executive mechanisms if battery is full or opening/closing motion undergoes. Through theoretical analysis and orthogonal tests the related parameters such as ferromagnetic material , structural size, the number of coils, the current and battery loads can be obtained and optimized.

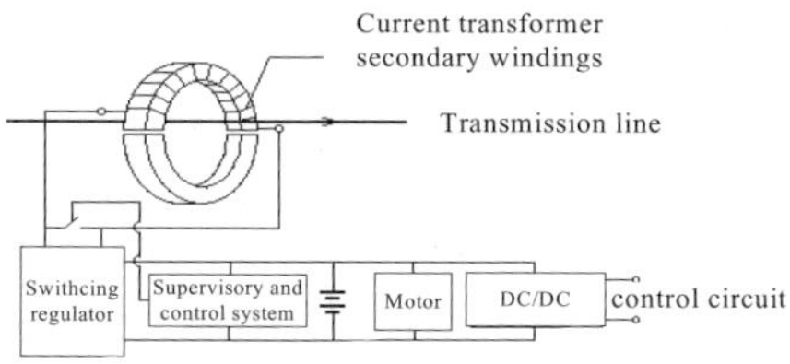

Fig. 11. Engery supply structure

4 Inspection Robot Prototype and Applications

In this paper, the transmission line type is LGJ-185/30, diameter of which is 18.88 mm, density is 3.473×103 kg/m3 and elastic modulo 7,600MPa. The tensile force of cable is 500 N. The robot noumenou of prototype is about 30Kg weights. Total external size is about 760*300*670mm(L*W*H). The power supply is about 40W, the electromagnetic compatibility satisfies 500KV transmission line. The maximum control distance and image transmission distance are about 5Km with rate of 22f/s. The robot has been used in field live line inspection many times and relative pictures of the field operation are shown in Fig. 12(a). Visible light images and infrared image given by the robot are also shown in Fig. 12(b).

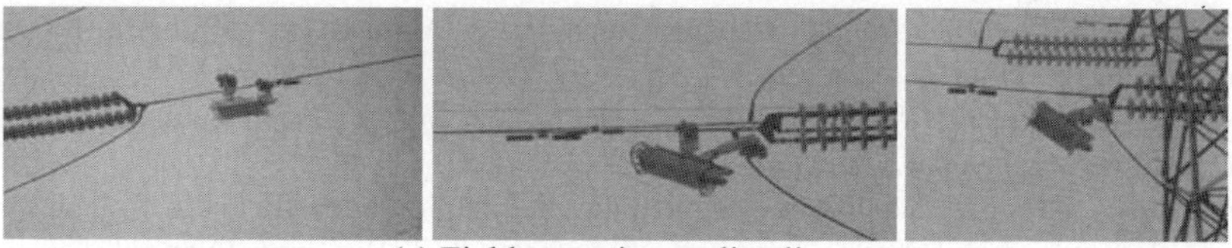

(a) Field operation on live line

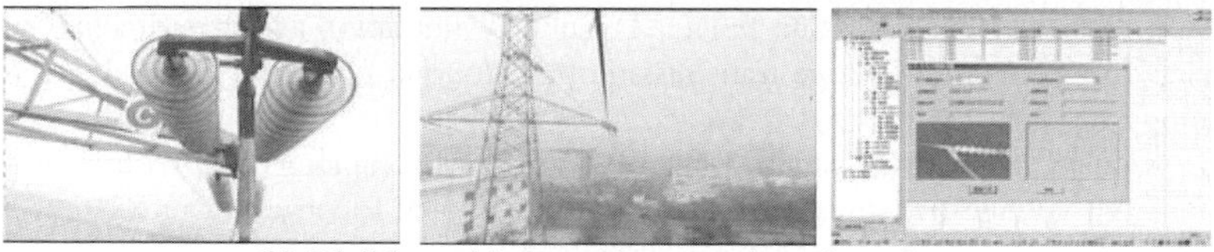

(b) Visible and infrared images given by robot

Fig. 12. Field live line inspection operation

5 Conclusions

In this paper a novel self-navigation inspection robot system are introduced systemically and briefly for the limited length. In the following papers, researches of each part of the system will be discussed in detail respectively. The improved self-navigated inspection robot along high-voltage power transmission line has been applied in the 220KV single conductor transmission line in electric power supply company in Hubei Province and Guangxi province and highly appraised by customers. Further improvement of robot research will be focused on the machine vision servo system and the information fusion of vision section with the multi-electromagnetic sensors to speed up inspection and enhance reliability. The design of inspection robot can also provide a reference for further research in special robots and be introduced into inspection robot for other purposes such as ice-breaking.

Acknowledgement

This paper is supported by the National High Technology Research and Development Program of China under Grant NO: 2002AA420110, 2005AA420010, 2006AA04Z202, National Natural Science Foundation of China under Grant NO:50575165. Thanks for the cooperation and support from Ningbo Bull Electric Company Limited , Wuhan electric power supply company, Hubei province, Guangxi electric power supply company, Nanyang electric power supply company and Institute of Automation Chinese Academy of Science.

References

1. Zhang, J.L., Lu, T.S., Wang, J.G.: Study on cable-climbing mechanism for cable-stayed bridge. J. China Mechanical Engineering 12, 1348–1451 (2001)
2. Fengyu, F.Y.Z., Aiguo, W., Yibin, L., et al.: Development of a mobile robot for inspection of high voltage overhead power transmission lines. J. Automation of Electric Power Systems, 89–91 (2004)
3. Luo, J., Zhao, B., Lu, T.S.: Periments and analysis of climbing mechanisms of Cable-I Robot. J. China Mechanical Engineering 12, 121–122 (2001)
4. Xiong, Y.L., Xiong, C.H.: Review of grasping and manipulation for multi-fingered robotic hands. Journal of Huazhong University of Science & Technology (Natural Science and Technology Edition) 32, 5–10 (2004)
5. Xiao, X.H., Wu, G.P., Du, E., Shi, E.T.L.: Dynamics simulation and experimental study of inspection robot for high-voltage transmission-line. Journal of Center South University of Technology 12, 726–731 (2005)
6. Wu, G., Xiao, X., Xiao, H., Dai, J., Bao, W., Hu, J.: Development of a mobile inspection robot for high voltage transmission lines. J. Automation of Electric Power System 30, 91–93, 107 (2006)
7. Gongping, W., Xiaohui, X., Sanping, L.: Kinematics Simulation of Inspection Robot for Power Transmission Line Based on Pro/e and Adams. J. Wseas Transaction on Power System 1(3), 674–679 (2006)
8. Wu, G., Xiao, X., Xiao, H., Dai, J.: Development of a Mobile Inspection Robot for High Voltage Power Transmission Line. Automation of Electrie Power Systems 30(13), 90–94 (2006)

Coriolis Moments in Manipulators: Demonstrative Experiment and Mathematical Analysis

Kang Luo, Cheng-zhong Deng, Jin-ge Wang, and Qiang Wang

School of Mechanical Engineering and Automation, Xihua University, Chengdu, P.R. of China
luoscit@163.com

Abstract. This paper deals with the problem of how to demonstrate the Coriolis moments in manipulators by an experimental way. This paper brings together the whole solution to the demonstrative experiment plan—from the choice of the device, to the operation of the experiment. Through the use of a differential, a simplest two-DOF spatial mechanism is presented as a manipulator where the Coriolis moments can be analyzed in a systematic way. The phenomenon of the experiment clearly demonstrates the existence of Coriolis moments, and furthermore, the quantity relationship between the moment and the corresponding factors is also obtained.

Keywords: Coriolis moment, Manipulator, Differential, Experiment, Mathematical Analysis.

1 Introduction

In general, a dynamic equation for a serial manipulator could be written symbolically in the form

$$\vec{\tau} = M(\vec{\Theta})\ddot{\vec{\Theta}} + V(\vec{\Theta},\dot{\vec{\Theta}}) + G(\vec{\Theta})$$

where $\vec{\Theta}$ and $\vec{\tau}$ are the vectors of joint coordinates and the corresponding joint torques respectively, $M(\vec{\Theta})$ is the mass matrix of the manipulator, $V(\vec{\Theta},\dot{\vec{\Theta}})$ is a vector of centrifugal and Coriolis terms, and $G(\vec{\Theta})$ is a vector of gravity terms.[1][2]

Centrifugal terms are easy to understand while Coriolis ones difficult to imagine. So it is significant to design an experiment to make people well understand Coriolis force/moment in two aspects: first, a directly demonstration of the existence of Coriolis forces/moments, and second, an obviously reflection of the factors that greatly affect Coriolis forces/moments.

As shown in Fig.1(a), a differential is one of the most typical mechanisms with such engineering applications as motion composition or decomposition. This two-DOF mechanism can be thought of a spatial mechanism and can even be classified as the simplest manipulator, with the planetary gear 2 as the end link and its holder 4 as the first link(refer to Fig.1(b)). This device could be designed to a smaller and lighter one because of its parallel structure featuring such an advantage that the two heavy

C. Xiong et al. (Eds.): ICIRA 2008, Part II, LNAI 5315, pp. 1155–1162, 2008.

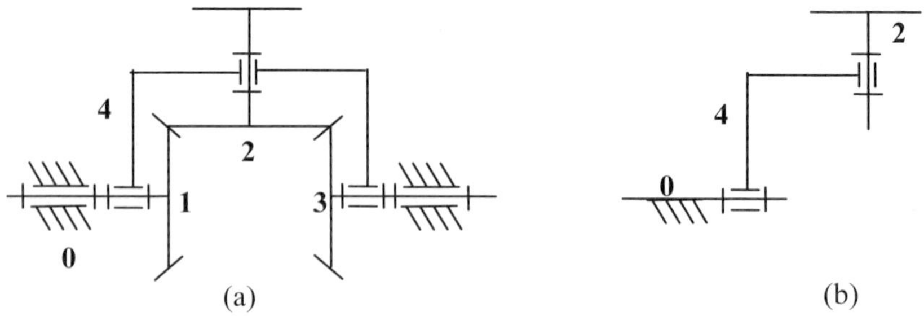

Fig. 1. A differential in (a) is equivalent to a two-DOF spatial manipulator in (b) plus a parallel structure such that both motors could be placed on the fixed frame, rather than on the moving arm

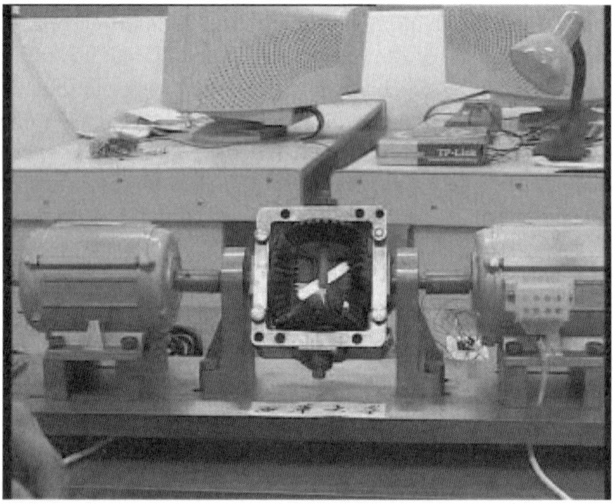

Fig. 2. A differential can be used as an experimental device for observing Coriolis moments

motors can be placed on the fixed frame 0, driving two central gears 1 and 3 rather than two links directly(refer to Fig.2).

2 Mathematical Analysis

2.1 Acceleration of a Point E on the Planetary Gear

A differential is of two-DOF such that when ω_1 and ω_3 are given as constant inputs, ω_4 and ω_2 can be easily obtained as constant outputs,

It is significant to recognize that ω_2 means the relative angular velocity of the planetary gear 2 with respect to the holder 4. So, the actual angular velocity of gear 2 should be the sum of two vectors: $\vec{\omega}_2$ and $\vec{\omega}_4$, demonstrating a composition of two spatial constant rotations in perpendicular.

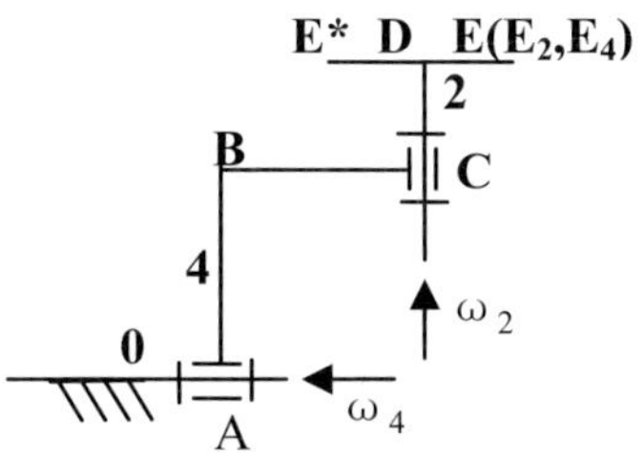

Fig. 3. Analysis on the Coriolis moment of the point couple E and E* is conducted

As shown in Fig.3, the very basic equation on position relationship can be established as follows

$$\vec{r}_{AE} = \vec{r}_{AC} + \vec{r}_{CE}. \tag{1}$$

By differentiating (1), we get

$$\dot{\vec{r}}_{AE} = \dot{\vec{r}}_{AC} + \dot{\vec{r}}_{CE}. \tag{2}$$

Expanding (2) yields

$$\dot{\vec{r}}_{AE} = \vec{\omega}_4 \times \vec{r}_{AC} + (\vec{\omega}_4 + \vec{\omega}_2) \times \vec{r}_{CE} = \vec{\omega}_4 \times (\vec{r}_{AC} + \vec{r}_{CE}) + \vec{\omega}_2 \times \vec{r}_{CE}.$$

Briefly we obtain

$$\dot{\vec{r}}_{AE} = \vec{\omega}_4 \times \vec{r}_{AE} + \vec{\omega}_2 \times \vec{r}_{CE}. \tag{3}$$

Conducting the time-derivation operation on both sides of (3) results in

$$\ddot{\vec{r}}_{AE} = \vec{\omega}_4 \times \dot{\vec{r}}_{AE} + \dot{\vec{\omega}}_2 \times \vec{r}_{CE} + \vec{\omega}_2 \times \dot{\vec{r}}_{CE}. \tag{4}$$

It is important to point out again that although $\vec{\omega}_4$ can be thought of a constant vector, $\vec{\omega}_2$ is a variable vector due to its changing direction.

Expanding (4) by referring to (3) produces

$$\ddot{\vec{r}}_{AE} = \vec{\omega}_4 \times (\vec{\omega}_4 \times \vec{r}_{AE} + \vec{\omega}_2 \times \vec{r}_{CE}) + (\vec{\omega}_4 \times \vec{\omega}_2) \times \vec{r}_{CE} + \vec{\omega}_2 \times [(\vec{\omega}_4 + \vec{\omega}_2) \times \vec{r}_{CE}]$$
$$= \vec{\omega}_4 \times (\vec{\omega}_4 \times \vec{r}_{AE}) + \vec{\omega}_4 \times (\vec{\omega}_2 \times \vec{r}_{CE}) + (\vec{\omega}_4 \times \vec{\omega}_2) \times \vec{r}_{CE} + \vec{\omega}_2 \times (\vec{\omega}_4 \times \vec{r}_{CE}) +$$
$$\vec{\omega}_2 \times (\vec{\omega}_2 \times \vec{r}_{CE})$$

where

(a) the first item $\vec{\omega}_4 \times (\vec{\omega}_4 \times \vec{r}_{AE})$ can be defined as "convected acceleration", denoted as $\vec{a}_{E4}$,

(b) the last item $\vec{\omega}_2 \times (\vec{\omega}_2 \times \vec{r}_{CE})$ can be defined as "relative acceleration", denoted as $\vec{a}^{\,r}_{E2E4}$,

(c) and the other items altogether can be defined as "Coriolis acceleration", denoted as $\vec{a}^{\,k}_{E2E4}$ which can be transformed to a simplified expression as follows

$$\begin{aligned}
&\vec{a}^{\,k}_{E2E4} \\
&= \vec{\omega}_4 \times (\vec{\omega}_2 \times \vec{r}_{CE}) + (\vec{\omega}_4 \times \vec{\omega}_2) \times \vec{r}_{CE} + \vec{\omega}_2 \times (\vec{\omega}_4 \times \vec{r}_{CE}) \\
&= \vec{\omega}_2 (\vec{\omega}_4 \cdot \vec{r}_{CE}) - \vec{r}_{CE} (\vec{\omega}_4 \cdot \vec{\omega}_2) + \vec{\omega}_2 (\vec{\omega}_4 \cdot \vec{r}_{CE}) - \vec{\omega}_4 (\vec{\omega}_2 \cdot \vec{r}_{CE}) + \\
&\vec{\omega}_4 (\vec{\omega}_2 \cdot \vec{r}_{CE}) - \vec{r}_{CE} (\vec{\omega}_2 \cdot \vec{\omega}_4) \\
&= 2[\vec{\omega}_2 (\vec{\omega}_4 \cdot \vec{r}_{CE}) - \vec{r}_{CE} (\vec{\omega}_4 \cdot \vec{\omega}_2)] \\
&= 2\vec{\omega}_4 \times (\vec{\omega}_2 \times \vec{r}_{CE}).
\end{aligned}$$

The differential has such a structure that $\vec{\omega}_4 \perp \vec{\omega}_2$, which means $\vec{\omega}_4 \cdot \vec{\omega}_2 \equiv 0$ and which results in

$$\vec{a}^{\,k}_{E2E4} = 2\vec{\omega}_2 (\vec{\omega}_4 \cdot \vec{r}_{CE}) . \tag{5}$$

Finally we have

$$\vec{a}_E = \vec{a}_{E4} + \vec{a}^{\,r}_{E2E4} + \vec{a}^{\,k}_{E2E4} . \tag{6}$$

2.2 Inertial Moment of a Point Couple E and E*

On the planetary gear shown in Fig.3, chose a point couple E and E*—symmetrical with each other to point D—under the assumption of each point possessing a unit mass.

First we obtain the inertial force of point E and E* respectively, as follows

$$\vec{F}^i_E = -m_E \vec{a}_E = -\vec{a}_E ,$$

and

$$\vec{F}^i_{E*} = -m_{E*} \vec{a}_{E*} = -\vec{a}_{E*} .$$

Compared with the inertial force, we are now more interested in the inertial moment about point D caused by $\vec{F}^{\,i}_E$ and $\vec{F}^{\,i}_{E*}$. Taking into account of $\vec{r}_{DE*} = -\vec{r}_{DE}$, we have the sum of the mentioned moments as follows

$$\vec{M}^i_D(\vec{F}^i_E) + \vec{M}^i_D(\vec{F}^i_{E*}) = \vec{r}_{DE} \times \vec{F}^i_E + \vec{r}_{DE*} \times \vec{F}^i_{E*} = -\vec{r}_{DE} \times (\vec{a}_E - \vec{a}_{E*}) . \tag{7}$$

Subscribing (6) into (7) and regrouping the items yield

$$\vec{M}^i_D(\vec{F}^i_E) + \vec{M}^i_D(\vec{F}^i_{E*}) = -\vec{r}_{DE} \times [(\vec{a}_{E4} - \vec{a}_{E4*}) + (\vec{a}^{\,r}_{E2E4} - \vec{a}^{\,r}_{E2*E4*}) + (\vec{a}^{\,k}_{E2E4} - \vec{a}^{\,k}_{E2*E4*})] .$$

According to the aforementioned definition of "convected acceleration", "relative acceleration" and "Coriolis acceleration", we can compute above expression item by item.

(a) For the first item, we have

$$\begin{aligned}
\vec{M}_{convected} &= -\vec{r}_{DE}\times(\vec{a}_{E4}-\vec{a}_{E4*})\\
&= -\vec{r}_{DE}\times[\vec{\omega}_4\times(\vec{\omega}_4\times\vec{r}_{AE})-\vec{\omega}_4\times(\vec{\omega}_4\times\vec{r}_{AE*})]\\
&= -\vec{r}_{DE}\times\{\vec{\omega}_4\times[\vec{\omega}_4\times(\vec{r}_{AE}-\vec{r}_{AE*})]\}\\
&= -2\vec{r}_{DE}\times[\vec{\omega}_4\times(\vec{\omega}_4\times\vec{r}_{DE})]\\
&= -2\vec{r}_{DE}\times[\vec{\omega}_4(\vec{\omega}_4\cdot\vec{r}_{DE})-\vec{r}_{DE}(\vec{\omega}_4\cdot\vec{\omega}_4)]\\
&= -2\vec{r}_{DE}\times\vec{\omega}_4(\vec{\omega}_4\cdot\vec{r}_{DE})+2\vec{r}_{DE}\times\vec{r}_{DE}\omega_4^2\\
&= 2\vec{\omega}_4\times\vec{r}_{DE}(\vec{\omega}_4\cdot\vec{r}_{DE}).
\end{aligned}$$

This moment is generally nonzero, taking the fact into consideration that $\vec{\omega}_4$ is a constant vector whereas $\vec{r}_{DE}$ rotates by both $\vec{\omega}_2$ and $\vec{\omega}_4$, shown in Fig.4 as follows. Obviously $\vec{M}_{convected}$ is always along the rotating axis of gear 2.

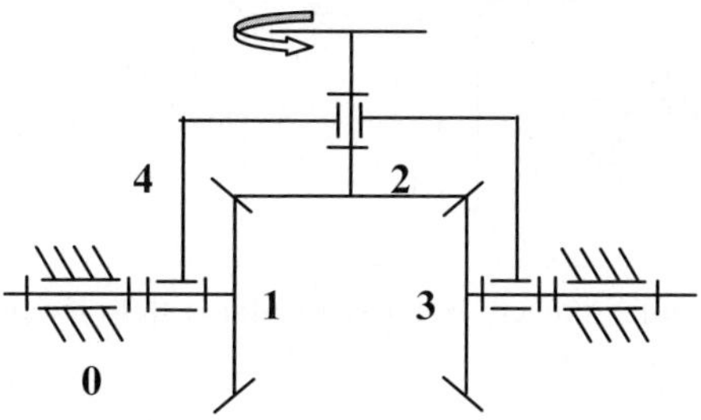

Fig. 4. The axis of the moment concerning the first item is parallel to the axis of planetary gear.

(b) It is followed with respect to the second item that

$$\begin{aligned}
\vec{M}_{relative} &= -\vec{r}_{DE}\times(\vec{a}^{\,r}_{E2E4}-\vec{a}^{\,r}_{E2*E4*})\\
&= -\vec{r}_{DE}\times[\vec{\omega}_2\times(\vec{\omega}_2\times\vec{r}_{CE})-\vec{\omega}_2\times(\vec{\omega}_2\times\vec{r}_{CE*})]\\
&= -2\vec{r}_{DE}\times[\vec{\omega}_2\times(\vec{\omega}_2\times\vec{r}_{DE})]\\
&= -2\vec{r}_{DE}\times[\vec{\omega}_2(\vec{\omega}_2\cdot\vec{r}_{DE})-\vec{r}_{DE}(\vec{\omega}_2\cdot\vec{\omega}_2)]\\
&= 0.
\end{aligned}$$

Note that we have taken into account of such a structure of the differential that

$$\vec{\omega}_2\cdot\vec{r}_{DE}=0$$

(c) Finally, the last item can be treated by replacing it with (5):

$$\begin{aligned}
\vec{M}_{Coriolis} &= -\vec{r}_{DE}\times(\vec{a}^{\,k}_{E2E4}-\vec{a}^{\,k}_{E2*E4*})\\
&= -\vec{r}_{DE}\times[2\vec{\omega}_2(\vec{\omega}_4\cdot\vec{r}_{CE})-2\vec{\omega}_2(\vec{\omega}_4\cdot\vec{r}_{CE*})]\\
&= 2\vec{r}_{DE}\times\vec{\omega}_2(\vec{\omega}_4\cdot\vec{r}_{EE*}).
\end{aligned}$$

This moment is generally nonzero, taking the fact into consideration that $\vec{r}_{DE} \perp \vec{\omega}_2$ and $\vec{r}_{E*E}$ rotates by both $\vec{\omega}_2$ and $\vec{\omega}_4$.

In fact this moment is referred to as Coriolis moment whose axis is perpendicular both to line DE and to the axis of the planetary gear, shown in Fig 5. And obviously $\vec{M}_{Coriolis}$ is always perpendicular to $\vec{M}_{convected}$, so it is possible and reasonable to treat them independently.

In addition, the magnitude of the Coriolis moment is a cosine variable with φ, an angle between EE* and the fixed axis of ω_4. It follows that

$$M_{Coriolis} = 2\omega_2\omega_4 r_{DE} r_{EE*} \cos\varphi \tag{8}$$

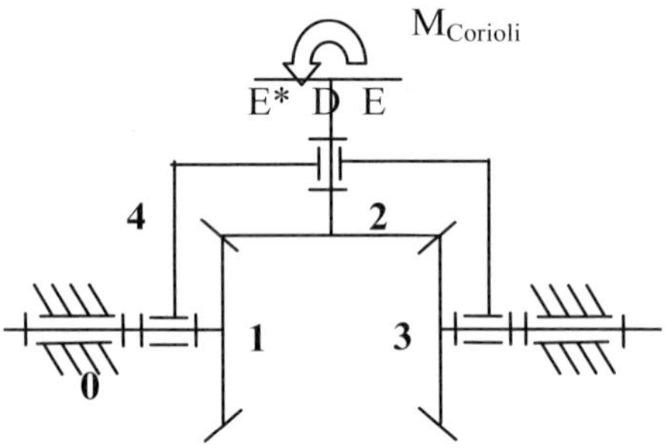

Fig. 5. The axis of the Coriolis moment is perpendicular both to the line EE* and to the axis of the planetary gear

3 Coriolis Moment and the Related Experiment

Now we focus on the Coriolis moment in a differential. In order to manifest the Coriolis effects, we connect a bar on the planetary gear via a revolute pair shown in Fig.6. By this way, such a device can be presented that an experiment on the Coriolis moment can be done as follows.

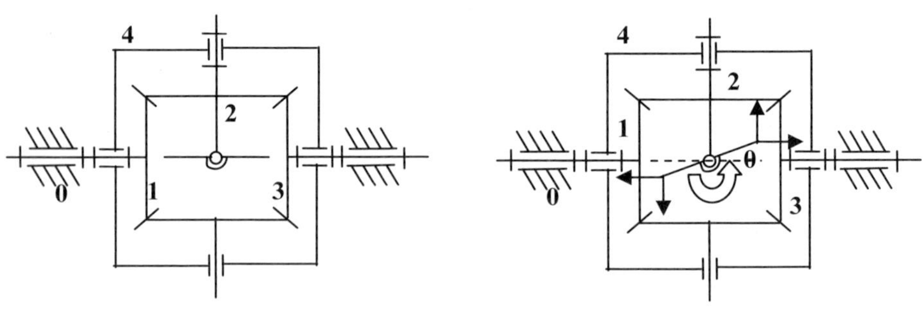

(a) in case that $\omega_2 \neq 0$ and $\omega_4 = 0$ (b) in case that $\omega_2 \neq 0$ and $\omega_4 \neq 0$

Fig. 6. (a) The bar keeps horizontal. (b) The bar tilts to a balanced position by θ.

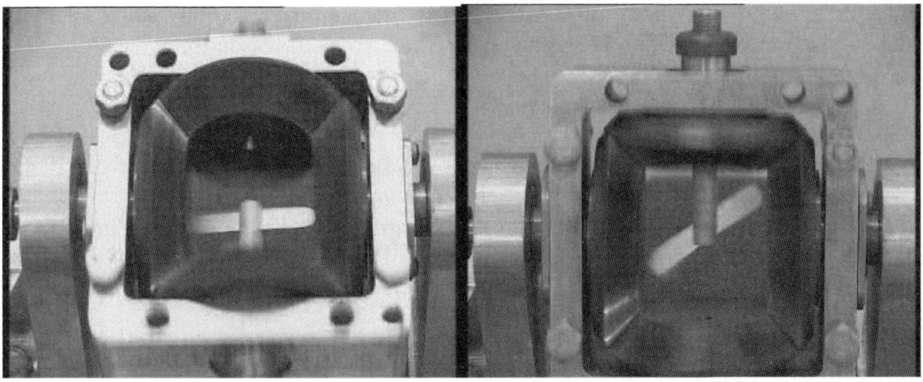

(a) in case that $\omega_2 \neq 0$ and $\omega_4 = 0$ (b) in case that $\omega_2 \neq 0$ and $\omega_4 \neq 0$

Fig. 7. (a) The bar keeps horizontal. (b) The bar tilts to a balanced position by θ.

In the first case that $\omega_2 \neq 0$ and $\omega_4 = 0$, there are only balanced centrifugal forces, leaving the connected bar to keep horizontal. In the second case that neither ω_2 nor ω_4 is zero, Coriolis moment appears and the bar tilts to a balanced position.

A basic conclusion can be drawn that it is Coriolis moment that makes the rod EE^* lose its balance and begin to tilt. And the Coriolis phenomenon can be illustrated by this unique simple way.

Here we have the photo pictures of the experiments in our laboratory shown in Fig.7.The phenomena of the experiment demonstrate the rationality of all the analysis above on Coriolis moments.

One of the important tasks in the future research deals with how to measure such parameters as the Coriolis moment and the tilting angle θ. We couldn't achieve this goal without integrating intelligent analysis techniques. Taking θ as an example, although there are sensors to obtain the information on tilting angle precisely, the compound spatial rotations prevent such devices from being mounted on the rod EE^* because the rotations tend to lead the cables to be twisted with each other. Identification by machine vision techniques seems to be a good choice, but we have to face challenges such as how to rotate the camera in a spatial way to keep it always in perpendicular with the plane formed by both rod EE^* and the axis of planetary gear 2. Now the wireless techniques could provide another solution to this application. Since some IC devices, e.g. cc2510 with RF transceiver, are highly suited for systems where size limitations and low power consumption are required, all the cables, including power cables and data cables, can be mounted totally on the rod EE* itself by means of tinny batteries and wireless communication techniques. So, by this way, the complicated spatial rotations could no longer be a big barrier to such measurement systems.

4 Conclusions

a). A differential is actually a two-DOF spatial manipulator and can be used to study on the Coriolis phenomena theoretically and experimentally.

b). A differential is actually of a parallel structure featuring the advantage of being able to place the heavy motors on the fixed frame so as to lessen the measurement of the experimental device.
c). A systematic mathematical analysis is carried out on the Coriolis moment on the arms of a manipulator.
d). In a differential, Coriolis moments are always perpendicular to convected moments, which makes it possible to research them independently.
e). A very perceivable phenomena is obtained through experiment in the lab and the result is coincident with the theoretical analysis.

References

1. Craig, J.J.: Introduction to Robotics. Addison-Wesley Publishing Company, Menlo Park (1986)
2. Spong, M.W., Vidyasagar, M.: Robot Dynamics and Control. Wiley, New York (1989)
3. Agrawal, S.K., Ryu, J.-C.: Design of Dissipative and Stable Assist Robots. Journal of Mechanical Design 129, 1251–1255 (2007)

Applications of the Fuzzy Immune PID Control and the Genetic Algorithm in the Automated Pharmacy System

Xuefeng Zhao, Chao Yun, Yuanyuan Wang, and Wei Wang

School of Mechanical Engineering and Automation,
Beihang University, 100083 Beijing, P.R. China
zxf801112@163.com

Abstract. In order to solve the existing problems such as inefficiency prescription-processing and high errors in hospitals, the automated pharmacy system is developed, which actualizes the automation of medicines-filling, medicines-storage and medicines-dispensing. Medicines are dispensed by the lifter system, which possess the characteristics of nonlinear, time-varying and complex. A fuzzy adaptive PID control method is presented based on the immune feedback regulating law and the adaptive ability of fuzzy logic ratiocination. The academic analysis and simulation results indicate the validity of the controller. The storage and retrieval efficiency is crucial factor in estimating the performance of the automated pharmacy. The scheduling policy, a multi-objective optimization, is proposed and solved by the genetic algorithm. Experiment results and computer simulations have proved the feasibility and effectiveness of the strategy in dynamic allocating the storage-positions and ensure the smoothness of filling and dispensing. So the good performance and high efficiency of the automated pharmacy system are achieved.

Keywords: Automated pharmacy system; Fuzzy immune PID control; Dynamic model; Genetic algorithm; Storage allocation.

1 Introduction

Some matured automated pharmacy systems have already appeared in overseas markets, which mainly include manipulator, robopharma and separating machines. The manipulator delivers the packages and realizes the automatic input and output of medicines. But manipulator can just dispose one package once and separate filling and dispensing process that finally causes the system to work inefficiently. The robopharma, a sloping cabinet, is composed of canals storing medicines. Although dispensing components issue the packages in output port automatically, manual filling of medicines in input port causes huge workload and high cost. The automatic separating machines are used to seal plastic bottles for the bulked medicines [1-3].

Automated pharmacy system is still on primary stage in our country. The intelligent pharmacy is developed by the Shenzhen 999 Company directing to solve the capsule and imbibe pieces. The vertical carousel of Shenyang Airplane Corporation possesses high adaptability to different packages, but it is semi-automatic.

C. Xiong et al. (Eds.): ICIRA 2008, Part II, LNAI 5315, pp. 1163–1172, 2008.

Since the hospitals of China mostly depend on box-packaged medicines, they have the particularity of the huge variety and amount of medicines. The pharmacy mentioned above can not meet all the demands. Therefore, the automated pharmacy system, which is suitable to the domestic hospital, is developed to fulfill the demands of dispensing and filling automatically. The significant criteria for evaluating the performance of an automated pharmacy system are throughput, accuracy and speed in dispensing and filling, and retrieval and storage efficiency.

The lifter system, dispensing system, must ensure speed under the condition of accuracy. Since it starts and stops frequently and violently in accord with the electronic prescription, so it possesses the characteristics of complex, non-linear and time-varying. In order to attain good dynamic performance, the fuzzy PID control method that based on the immune feedback mechanism is proposed. The simulation results indicate that fuzzy immune PID controller has superior ability than conventional PID controller [4-5].

The storage and retrieval efficiency depends largely on the dynamic scheduling, which is a multi-objective and multi-constraint optimization problem. After analyzing the constraints and objectives, an optimization model is put forward and the genetic algorithm is proposed to solve the problem. Experimental results show that the algorithm is capable of allocating storage-position efficiently and dynamically [6].

2 Introduction System Functions and Implements

2.1 Mechanical System

The automated pharmacy system can manage and store certain medicines to assure the supplying of medicines, dispensing medicines accurately and rapidly based on the hospital electronic prescription in real-time and put the packages at accurate position automatically or semi-automatically. It includes filling system, dedicated storage system, dispensing system, sorting system, control and management system and interface system with HIS (Hospital Information System). The entire system is shown in the Fig.1.

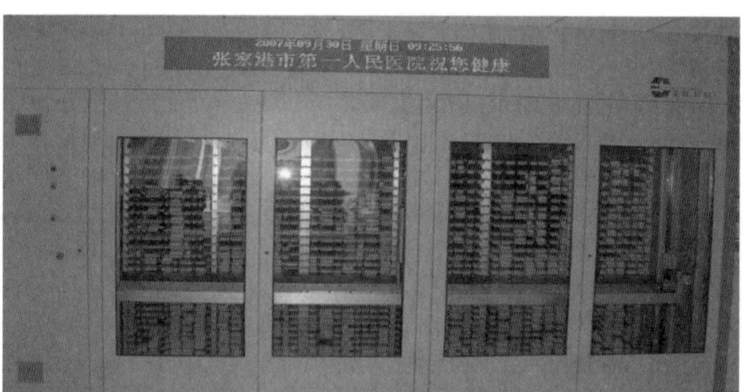

Fig. 1. Automatic pharmacy system

The storage cabinet, composed of matrix arranged slopping canals, achieves the dedicated storage. The manipulator fills the packages in the input port. After filling phase, the packages slide down in the direction of output port due to the force of gravity. All packages are stopped by flaps of the output port. Meanwhile, the next package will slide to the stop plate after the first package delivered by lifter and packages-output devices.

The filling devices mainly include vertical guide-rail, horizontal guide-rail and manipulator installed on the vertical guide-rail. When some packages need to be filled, they are sent to the manipulator by conveyor belt. After that, the slider installed on the horizontal-guide moves in the horizontal direction and drives the vertical guide-rail to move synchronously. Meanwhile, the manipulator moves along the vertical guide-rail. The parallel actions realize the column and row orientations. After the position storing the packages is attained, the manipulator automatically sends out the packages to the specific canal.

The dispensing components are consisted of the lifter installed on two vertical guide-rails and the electromagnet mounted on the lifter. If the packages in certain position need to be picked out, the lifter moves instantly to the certain row location. Then the electromagnet corresponding column will drive the flaps to act to send out the packages out of the canals to the lifter. At the same time, the sensors fixed on the lifter monitor the amounts of the packages to match with the real amounts. Finally, the lifter delivers the packages to the sort window for patients.

2.2 Control and Management System

The hierarchical control and management system is divided into four layers: management-layer, monitoring-layer, controlling-layer and executing-layer. The system is a comprehensive application of automatic control technology, information technology and computer communication network technology. The flow diagram is shown in Fig.2. The server computer receives the prescription information from HIS or requests from filling terminal. After that, the server computer orders the filling or dispensing assignments, based on the optimal scheduling strategy, to the monitoring-layer. Then, the monitoring system control the executing devices to operate via the control units, it also monitors the status and detects the protection state at the same time. The server decides the next assignments according to the feedback information from the monitoring-layer [7].

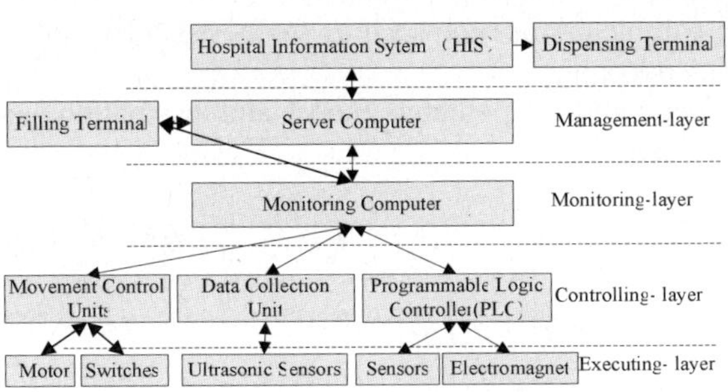

Fig. 2. Diagram flow of the control and management system

3 Introduction System Functions and Implements

3.1 Dynamic Model

The lifter system is driven by two servo transmission devices, and it is mainly consisted of two vertical guide-rails, sliders installed on two vertical guide-rails, lifter fixed to sliders and its attachment as electromagnet, counterweights and pulleys. The motors drive lifter moving in the vertical direction. Meanwhile, the counterweights move in keep with the lifter through the ropes and pulley block. Two motors must turn synchronously; otherwise the lifter will slope in certain angle. The sloping cannot ensure the correspondence between electromagnets and flaps of canals, and it leads to unsmooth sliding of packages. Since the acceleration and jerk should always be in the range of acceptable limits and the vibration levels are kept in a minimum, the dynamic characteristics of lifter should be studied in-depth to accomplish good performance [8-9]. The simplified dynamic model of the lifter system is shown in Fig.3.

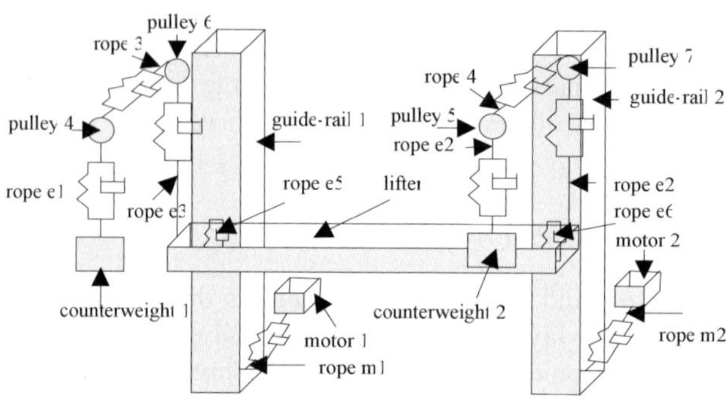

Fig. 3. Simplified schematic of the lifter system

As the lifter moves, more speedy vibration may also be stemmed from distortion of the guide-rail, In this case, the guide-rail is assumed as a spring. The stiffness of the guide-rail varies against the lifter vertical position which in turn may cause parametric vibration. In order to obtain a better control system for lifter vibration reduction, a new method which incorporates the parameter variation dynamic is required. In this control system, some time-varying parameters should be calculated or measured continuously. The parameters of rope such as stiffness coefficient and damping coefficient are taken into account.

The system's kinetic energy, potential energy and dissipation energy are shown as (1), (2), (3) respectively.

$$T = \frac{1}{2}m\dot{x}^2 + \frac{1}{2}m_1\dot{x}_1^{\,2} + \frac{1}{2}m_2\dot{x}_2^{\,2} + \frac{1}{2}J_4\dot{\theta}_4^{\,2} + \frac{1}{2}J_5\dot{\theta}_5^{\,2} + \frac{1}{2}J_6\dot{\theta}_6^{\,2} + \frac{1}{2}J_7\dot{\theta}_7^{\,2} + \frac{1}{2}J_1\dot{\theta}_1^{\,2} + \frac{1}{2}J_2\dot{\theta}_1^{\,2} \,. \tag{1}$$

$$\begin{aligned}V &= \frac{1}{2}k_{m1}(\theta_1-\theta_{10})^2+\frac{1}{2}k_{m2}(\theta_2-\theta_{20})^2+\frac{1}{2}k_{e3}(x-\theta_6 r)^2+\frac{1}{2}k_{e4}(x-\theta_7 r)^2\\ &+\frac{1}{2}k_3(\theta_4-\theta_6)^2+\frac{1}{2}k_4(\theta_5-\theta_7)^2+\frac{1}{2}k_{e1}(\theta_4 r-x_1)^2\\ &+\frac{1}{2}k_{e2}(\theta_5 r-x_2)^2+\frac{1}{2}k_{e5}(x-x_1')^2+\frac{1}{2}k_{e6}(x-x_2')^2\ .\end{aligned} \tag{2}$$

$$\begin{aligned}D &= \frac{1}{2}c_{m1}(\dot\theta_1-\dot\theta_{10})^2+\frac{1}{2}c_{m}(\dot\theta_2-\dot\theta_{20})^2+\frac{1}{2}c_{e3}(\dot x-\dot\theta_6 r)^2+\frac{1}{2}c_{e4}(\dot x-\dot\theta_7 r)^2\\ &+\frac{1}{2}c_3(\theta_4-\theta_6)^2+\frac{1}{2}c_4(\dot\theta_5-\dot\theta_7)^2+\frac{1}{2}c_{e1}(\dot x-\dot\theta_4 r)^2+\frac{1}{2}c_{e2}(\dot x-\dot\theta_5 r)^2\\ &+\frac{1}{2}c_{e5}(\dot x-\dot x_1')^2+\frac{1}{2}c_{e6}(\dot x-\dot x_2')^2\ .\end{aligned} \tag{3}$$

Where, the meaning of the main parameters is defined concretely. *m* denotes mass of object; *J* denotes inertia; *k* and *c* denote the spring and damping coefficient; *x* denotes displacement; θ denotes angle; the differential coefficient of *x* denotes the velocity; the differential coefficient of θ denotes the angular velocity; *r* denotes the radius of pulley. The lower tags represent the parts according to the Fig.3. Take the parameter k_{m1} for example, *k* denotes the spring as mentioned above, *m1* is equivalent to the rope *m1* between the motor 1 and the guide-rail 1, so the parameter k_{m1} denotes the spring coefficient between the motor 1 and the guide-rail 1. θ_{10}, θ_{20} are turning angle of the motor shaft respectively; *x'1, x'2* are the displacement of slider in theory, when the motor turns over the angle θ_1, θ_2 respectively.

Based on the above equations and the second class Lagrange (4), the system dynamics are modeled by the nonlinear differential (5).

$$\frac{d}{dt}\left(\frac{\partial T}{\partial \dot x_i}\right)-\frac{\partial T}{\partial x_i}+\frac{\partial V}{\partial x_i}+\frac{\partial D}{\partial \dot x_i}=Q\ . \tag{4}$$

$$[M]\{\ddot X\}+[C]\{\dot X\}+[K]\{X\}=\{Q\}\ . \tag{5}$$

Where *[M]* denotes mass matrix, and it includes mass of lifter, counterweights and inertia of motors and pulley block. *X* denotes state matrix, the extended vector is $X=[x\ x1\ x2\ \theta1\ \theta2\ \theta4\ \theta5\ \theta6\ \theta7]^T$. *[K], [C]* denotes spring matrix and damping matrix, which is time-varying and consistent. The two matrixes vary according to the variables of *X*. *Q* denotes generalized inspire force, which is relative to the torque of motors.

3.2 Fuzzy Immune PID Controller

Immune is a characteristic physiological reaction of biological body. Immune system of biology could produce relative antibody to resist invading anti-source from extraneous. After antibody combines with anti-source, a serial reaction will be brought to destroy antibody by swallowing effect or producing special enzyme. The most important part of biological immune system is lymph cell, it concludes *T* cell generated by thymus (including assistant cell T_H and suppressive cell T_S) and *B* cell generated by marrow. When antibody invades the body and is absorbed by surrounding cell, it transmits the message to *T* cell, that is, transmits to T_H cell and T_S cell, and then stimulates *B* cell. *B* cell generates antibody to remove anti-source. When there is much anti-source, T_H cell is more and T_S cell is little in the body, thus more *B* cells will be produced. As the decrease of anti-source, T_S cell increases, which restrains the creation of T_H cell, then *B* cell decreases accordingly. After some time-interval, immune feedback system trends to a balance, the cooperation between restrain principle and main feedback principle is done by the fast reaction of immune feedback principle to anti-source and steady immune system.

Regular raising PID controller algorithm is as follows:

$$U_{PID}(k) = U_{PID}(k-1) + k_p((e(k) - e(k-1)) + \frac{k_i}{k_p} e(k) + \frac{k_d}{k_p}(e(k) - 2e(k-1) + e(k-2)) . \tag{6}$$

Where, K_P, K_I, K_D is coefficient of proportion, integral and derivative, so immune PID controller algorithm is:

$$\begin{aligned} \Delta u(k) &= k_{p1}((e(k) - e(k-1)) + \frac{k_i}{k_p}(e(k) + \frac{k_d}{k_p}(e(k) - 2e(k-1) + e(k-2)) \\ &= k_{p1}((e(k) - e(k-1) + k_i^{'} e(k) + k_d^{'}(e(k) - 2e(k-1) + e(k-2)) . \end{aligned} \tag{7}$$

$$k_{p1} = K(1 - \eta f(u(k), \Delta u(k))) . \tag{8}$$

Immune PID controller is designed by learning from immune principle of biology system. Its nonlinear is realized mainly by $f(u(k), \Delta u(k))$. Fuzzy control bases at simulating human thinking way, which solves well the controlled object problem such as nonlinear, large delay, large inertia, fluctuant parameter, without accurate description of controlled model, so it is widely used in all kinds of controlled system. Fuzzy controller could approach to any linear or nonlinear functions. Meanwhile, it is also an effective way to construct nonlinear function. The fuzzy controller in this paper adopts the same structure as in [10-11]. It has two input variable and one output variable. The two input variables are the output of immune controller $u(k)$ and its variation $\Delta u(k)$ apart, output variable is the suppressing-quantity of TS cell f $(u(k),\Delta u(k))$.

3.3 Simulation Based on the Fuzzy Immune PID Controller

To demonstrate the effectiveness of the designed controller, the simulations are done in the Matlab statements. According to the above dynamic model and real condition applied in Zhang Jiagang Hospital, the actual velocity is about 1.0 *m/s*. The initial parameters of PID control are $K_P=1000$, $K_I=0$, $K_D=60$. The simulation curves are shown in Fig.4, Fig.5, Fig.6.

Fig.4 shows the output and error of lifter system with routine PID controller and fuzzy immune PID control method respectively. The fuzzy immune PID method has faster response rate and better tracking performance and it basically realizes the no error control of system, while the routine PID control has the defects of lower response rate, longer delay time and regulating time and larger overshoot.

According to the Fig.5 and Fig.6, when there is disturbance because of the reasons of external world, the fuzzy immune PID control system can suppress the disturbance quickly and the lifter fluctuation is smaller and restoring time is relatively short. So the fuzzy immune PID controller has robustness against the parameters vibrations.

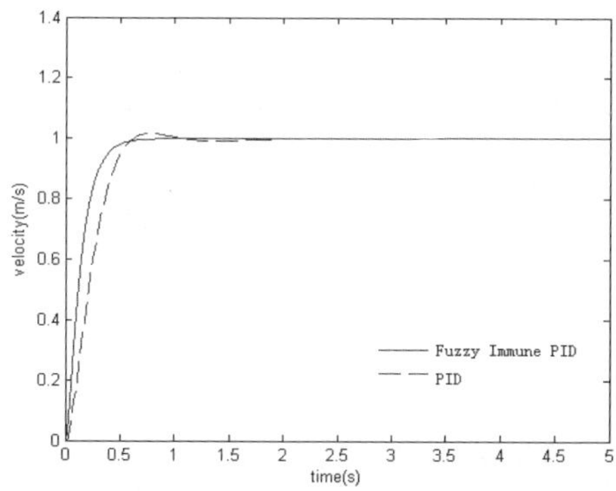

Fig. 4. Response results for classical PID controller and fuzzy immune PID controller

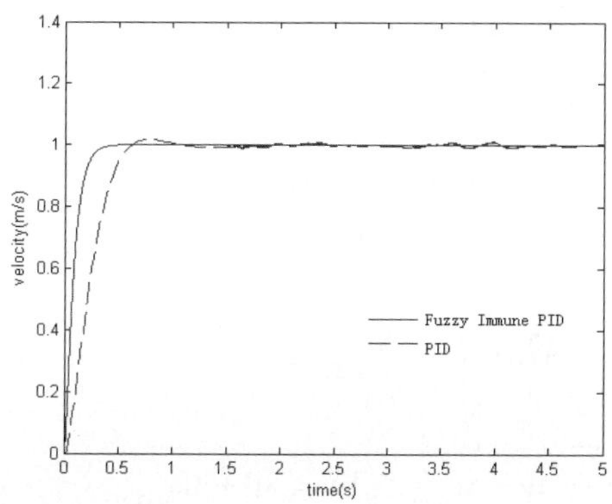

Fig. 5. Comparison of the response curve under random disturbance

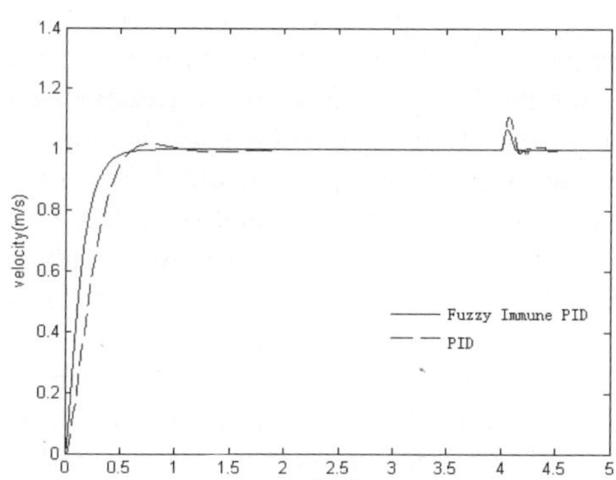

Fig. 6. Comparison of the response curve under the disturbance of 4s

4 Storage-Location Optimization

4.1 Problem Description

The scheduling optimization must take the following factors into account such as the particularity of medicines storage, the irregularity of packages size, the diversity of canals and the parallel operations in dispensing and filling.

To ensure the smooth input and output of packages, it is significant to confine the distance between the packages and the canals in a certain extent, or it will cause a series of problems, such as less sliding force, overlaps and jam of packages and other problems affecting the normal operation of implementation. It is of importance to enhance the efficiency of inputting and outputting drugs, cutting costs, and improving space utilization to optimize the canal specifications, the layout of canals and the layout of drugs as well. The optimization problem is described as the following:

$$MinE = \sum_{i=1}^{p}\sum_{R=1}^{q} I_i \bullet R \ . \tag{9}$$

$$MinS = \sum_{j=1}^{n} W_j \ . \tag{10}$$

$$MinT = \sum_{i=1}^{m} H_i \ . \tag{11}$$

$$MinM = \sum_{i=1}^{l}\sum_{j=1}^{k_i} F_{ij} S_{ij} \ . \tag{12}$$

$$s.t. \qquad w + w_{\min} \le W < w + w_{\max} \ . \tag{13}$$

$$h + h_{\min} \le H < h + h_{\max} \ . \tag{14}$$

where, I_i reflects the frequency of dispensing, which is smaller while the frequency is greater; R denotes the area number; p denotes the varieties of packages; q denotes the area sum; n and m denote the amount of width specification and height specification respectively; F_{ij} denotes the using frequency of the drugs in position *(i, j)*; S_{ij} denotes the distance between drug-outputting mouth and canal *(i, j)*; l is the layers' amount; k_i denotes the amount of columns in layer k; w and h is the width and height of packages respectively; W and H are the width and height of canals; w_{min}, h_{min}, w_{max} and h_{max} denote the min-distance and max-distance between the canal and drug width and height.

The objective (9) ensures the optimization of canals distribution. Equation (10) and (11) ensure the minimum specifications of width and height of canals respectively. Equation (12) ensures that packages in higher retrieve and storage frequency are located in nearer canals relative to the output mouth. Equation (13) and (14) represent the restrictive conditions in space [12].

4.2 Simulation Based on the Genetic Algorithm

The GA based decision methods on scheduling rules start from an initial population, i.e. a chromosome set. The size of this set is fixed and every chromosome represents a group of combining rules which can be used to describe concrete scheduling projects. After populations of each generation produce, the weights of rules are calculated relative to individual performance index. These rules are represented respectively by every gene of every chromosome in this generation. And these values will be used as the basic data in fitness values calculation. Populations of every generation produce going through three genetic manipulation processes: i.e. selection, crossover and mutation. The chromosomes with the best fitness value are exported as the combination of the best rules after the whole process implements pre-established times.

The genetic algorithm is adopted in the system to allocate the storage-position effectively. The system develops the fitness of chromosomes based on the objectives and constrains. The system rationally designs gene codes, fitness function, initial population and genetic manipulation in order to achieve optimal allocation results. The real code technology is adopted, which includes much information as the storage location, the width and the height of the canals and the layout of the canals. For example, gene code 12110354704559 denotes packing 1 and 2 are stored in this layer, and package 1 occupies three canals in width of 35 *mm* and height of 45 *mm*, and package 2 occupies one canal in width of 47 *mm* and height of 59 *mm*. The canals layout of this layer is in the width order of 35 *mm*, 45 *mm*, 35 *mm*, 45 *mm*.

The experiments are carried out according to the real packages information. By experiments, it is found that population size 70 and generation number 500 make a relatively stabilized objective value. Meanwhile, crossing probability is 0.8, and mutation rate is 0.1. The fitness curve of 10 kinds of packing and 70 canals is shown in Fig.7. The GA gains optimizing results in convergence and improves greatly the dispensing frequency. The genetic algorithm elevates greatly the retrieval and storage efficiency. The layouts of the packages reduce time in fetching and filling.

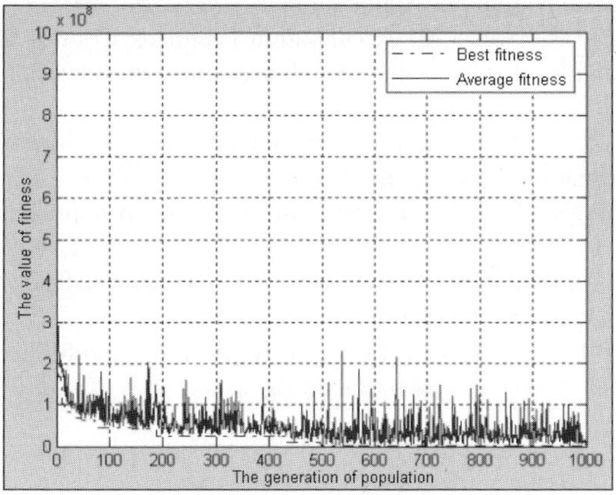

Fig. 7. Fitness variety curve

5 Conclusion

In the paper, the automatic pharmacy system is developed to actualize the automation of filling, storage and dispensing medicines. It has been applied in the hospital of Zhang Jiagang, actualizing the speed of 10 second/prescription in dispensing-prescription. In order to attain good performance of the automated pharmacy system, a fuzzy adaptive PID control method is proposed based on the dynamic characteristic of lifter system, and a scheduling optimization model is presented and the genetic algorithm is applied to solve the optimization problem, The simulation results indicate that the controller has effectively reduced the vibration of the lifter, elevated the precision of positioning and the speed of dispensing prescription. The algorithm has effectively elevates the restore and retrieve efficiency. So the good performance of the automated pharmacy system is obtained.

Reference

1. Bridget, C.: Hospital Pharmacy Staff Attitudes towards Automated Dispensing before and after Implementation. Hospital Pharmacy 11, 248 (2001)
2. Mathew, P.: Medication Errors. Clinical Pediatrics 4, 287 (2003)
3. Chritopher, J.: A Real Life Look at Automated Pharmacy Workflow Systems. National Association of Chain Drug Stores 1, 29 (2005)
4. Liu, J.K.: Advanced PID Control and Matlab Simulink. Publishing House of Electronics Industry, Beijing (2004)
5. Wang, Y.: Fuzzy Immune PID Type Controller Design and Simulation. Computer Simulation 19, 67–69 (2002)
6. Zhang, P., Tain, G.H.: New Hybrid Genetic Algorithm Solving the Order-picking Optimization Problem of a Multi-carousel System. Chinese Journal of Mechanical Engineering 40, 34–38 (2004)
7. Cai, S., Chen, L., Wang, H.C.: The Research and Implement of College Affair Integration Management System. Computer Applications 27, 327–329 (2007)
8. Lee, Y.M., Kang, J.K., Sul, S.K.: Acceleration Feedback Control Strategy for Improving Riding Quality of Elevator System. IEEE Transaction on industrial electronics 40, 1375–1379 (1999)
9. Ai, Y.T., Wang, Z., Li, L.X.: Study on the Active Vibration Control of High-speed Traction-elevator. Journal of vibration and shock 26, 56–59 (2007)
10. Ying, H., Siler, W., Buckley, J.J.: Fuzzy Control Theory: A nonlinear case. Automatica 26, 513–520 (1990)
11. Ding, Y.S., Ren, L.H.: A New Fuzzy Self-tuning Immune Feedback Control System. Control and Decision 15, 443–446 (2000)
12. Wang, L., Zheng, D.Z.: A Modified Genetic Algorithm for Job Shop Scheduling. The International Journal of advanced Manufacturing Technology 20, 72–78 (2002)

A Needle-Holding Robot for Ultrasound Guided Percutaneous Hepatic Microwave Ablation and Initial Experiments

Shuangcheng Deng[1], Lipei Jiang[1], Yingyu Cao[1], Ping Liang[2], He Ren[2], Tong Lu[2], and Yang Wang[2]

[1] Opto-Mechatronic Equipment Technology Beijing Area Major Laboratory, Beijing Institute of Petrochemical Technology, Beijing 102617, China

[2] Department of Ultrasound, General Hospital of PLA, Beijing 100853, China

{dengshuangcheng,lipei,caoyingyu}@bipt.edu.cn, liangping301@hotmail.com

Abstract. A needle-holding robot for percutaneous hepatic microwave ablation is developed. The overall architecture of the robot is introduced first with the explanation of the mechanism of 3D motion tracking. Two experiments were conducted, one to quantify the force required for motion tracking, the other to assess the performance of motion tracking. The result of force-measuring experiment shows that the force required for rotation and radial translation motion tracking are less than 15 grams, which indicates the high sensitivity of the holding robot. The result of in-vivo animal trial performed on a swine shows that the holding robot is accurate enough in tracking the 3D motion of the ablation needle, which allows for stable and precise holding of the needle compared to that of freehand holding.

Keywords: medical robot, microwave ablation, motion tracking, robotic hand.

1 Introduction

Hepatocellular carcinoma presents over 1 million cases per year worldwide [1-3]. In recent years, an increasing interest has been focused on interstitial ablative approaches for the treatment of unresectable liver tumors[4-5]. Local tissue ablation is performed with lower morbidity than conventional resection therapy, and it is very suitable for percutaneous and other minimally invasive approaches.

Local microwave ablation is one of the percutaneous hepatic tumor ablation means. In clinical practice, it's intra-operative procedure is typically performed in three steps. First, the target tumors are localized by means of intrao-perative ultrasonography (IOUS). Second, the microwave ablation needle is inserted into the target tumor center by the surgeon under the guidance of IOUS. Last, the surgeon holds the ablation needle and its accessory cables manually and real tumor ablation begins.

The second step requires simultaneous manual handling of the IOUS probe and the ablator needle, which is a challenging task prone to significant errors even in the hands of the most experienced physicians. Meanwhile, the two-dimensional nature of IOUS

C. Xiong et al. (Eds.): ICIRA 2008, Part II, LNAI 5315, pp. 1173–1182, 2008.

imaging leads to significant variations in results among users. Respiratory motion and liver surface deformation are two of the most significant sources of error. Therefore, there has been a recent interest in robots for US-guided hepatic tumor ablation therapy by several groups (e.g., [6-8]). An hepatic ablation robot system would provide significant benefit by providing consistent reliable guidance to interventions, enabling automatic needle placement, and avoiding fatigue and occasional musculoskeletal injury of the sonographer [9].

However, more attention is paid to the needle placement step than the needle holding step. Actually, the latter plays an as important role as the former in efficient tumor destruction. The needle holding step typically consumes 5-10 minutes, which is 1/3-2/3 of the whole ablation procedure's 15-20 minutes duration. It is in this step that the real ablation of the tumors begins. During the holding process, respiratory motion of the patient in deep anaesthesia will make the needle swing horizontally and periodically. Meanwhile, liver surface deformation may slowly push the ablator needle outward or pull it downward. These two factors will introduce displacement to the needle location and may affect the ablation effect.

So the surgeon must be totally absorbed in the needle holding task and try to follow the patient's respiratory motion and keep the needle in a dynamic balance. However, needle holding is a tedious and time-consuming work and there often are too many cases to be handled in a day. In our clinic practice in General Hospital of PLA in China, a physician has to do 6-13 ablation cases per day. Handling so many cases restlessly is very easy to make the physician exhausted and absent-minded. Absent-minded needle holding is error-prone, and may lead to errors or even the failure of the surgery.

So we try to develop an needle-holding robot system in which robotic hand manipulate the microwave ablation needle and hold it instead of the hands of the physician, keep it in a stable position in the surgical context of liver cancer ablation.

Literature has shown that hepatic respiratory motion are complex, with cranio-caudal(axial), lateral, and anterior-posterior(elevation) motion, in addition to movement due to deformation of tissues[10-12]. The needle's motion during procedures arises from the hepatic motion and is also a 3D motion. So the holding robot must be able to track all these motions in 3D space.

The overall architecture of our holding robot is introduced first with the explanation of the mechanism of 3D motion tracking. Two experiments were conducted, one to quantify the force required for motion tracking of the robot, the other to assess the sensitivity and accuracy of motion tracking. Experiment results show that the force required for rotation and radial translation tracking are less than 15g, which indicates the high sensitivity of the holding robot. Experiment results also show that the holding robot is accurate in tracking the motion of the ablation needle, which allows for stable and precise holding of the needle compared to that of freehand holding. Robotic needle holding can free the two hands of the surgeon, so that more effort can be concentrated on monitoring the ablation procedure, which in turn guarantees good ablation effect.

2 The Needle-Holding Robot

2.1 System Overview

Fig. 1(a), 1(b) shows the overall architecture of our ablation needle holding robot. Major system components include:

• Robot arm : The robot arm has 3 DOFs and consists of one horizontal rotation arm, one elevation adjusting arm, one bend and one grip. The horizontal rotation arm can rotate horizontally around the robot body, and the elevation adjusting arm is used to position the holding hand in appropriate elevation. The grip can rotate horizontally around the bend to adjust the azimuth of the holding hand. The robot arm can be manually positioned at arbitrary point in the 3D space and it can automatically lock itself at that position.

• Robotic holding hand (See Fig. 1(c)): The robotic holding hand has 3 DOFs and is the major component for 3D motion tracking. It consists of one clamp, one rotation & translation motion sensing system, one rotation tracking motor & component, one radial-translation tracking motor & component and one dual-spring elevation tracking component. It has three functions: to clamp one or two microwave ablation needles, to sense the 3D motion of the needle, and to perform 3D motion tracking task.

• Robot controller: The controller provides overall application control for the robot. Its main task is to collect the motion direction signals from the holding hand, and to drive the motors to implement the 3D motion tracking.

When a microwave ablation procedure begins, the surgeon can drag-and-drop the robot arm to its position in the 3D space. The arm can automatically lock itself at that position when the surgeon releases the grip. The needle is clamped and the controller powered on. The robot is ready for tracking after resetting. If the needle moves due to the patient's respiration and soft tissue deformation, the robotic holding hand will sense this motion and send the motion direction signal to the controller. The controller then commands the motors to track the needle's 3D motion synchronously.

2.2 Mechanism of 3D Motion Tracking

2.2.1 Cranio-caudal(Axial) and Lateral Motion Tracking

The mechanism of cranio-caudal (axial) motion and lateral motion tracking for holding robot is illustrated in Fig. 2(a). The combination of axial and lateral motion will cause the needle to move toward one direction in the horizontal plane. The needle's motion consequently may result in two types of motion of the robotic holding hand: rotation around the rotation axis, and radial-translation.

When the clamp is propelled to rotate around the rotation axis by the force applied on the needle, light baffle 1 will rotate synchronously. If light baffle 1 does not block any of the left and right photo-couplers, no signal is sent to the controller and the rotation tracking motor doesn't work. If it blocks the left or right photo-coupler, the block signal that indicates the motion direction of the needle will be sent to the controller, and the rotation tracking motor starts to work which leads to the holding robot's rightward or leftward rotation tracking of the needle's motion.

When the clamp is propelled to translate radially by the force applied on the needle, light baffle 2 will translate synchronously. If it blocks the front or back photocoupler, the block signal will be sent to the control box, and the radial-translation tracking motor starts to work which leads to the holding robot's centrifugal or centripetal translation tracking of the needle's motion.

The combination of rotation and radial-translation tracking makes it feasible to track arbitrary trajectory of the needle's horizontal motion(see Fig. 2(b)).

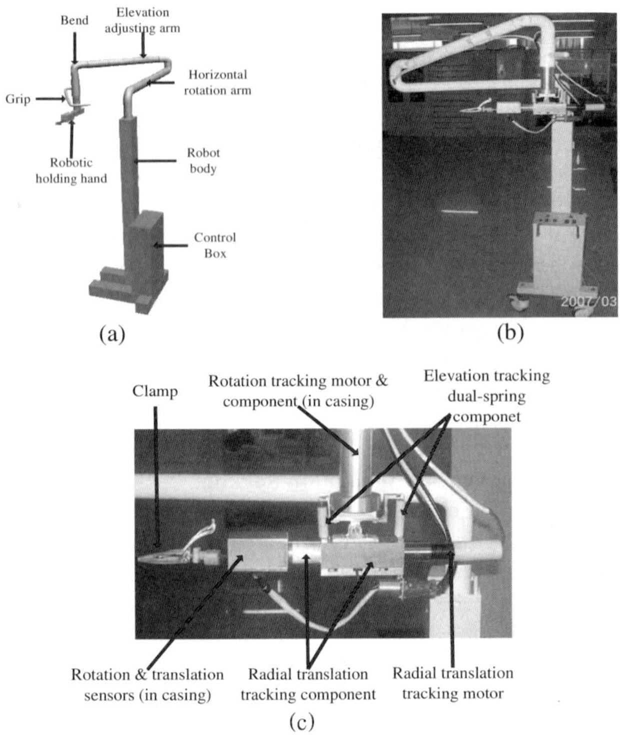

Fig. 1. Overall system architecture

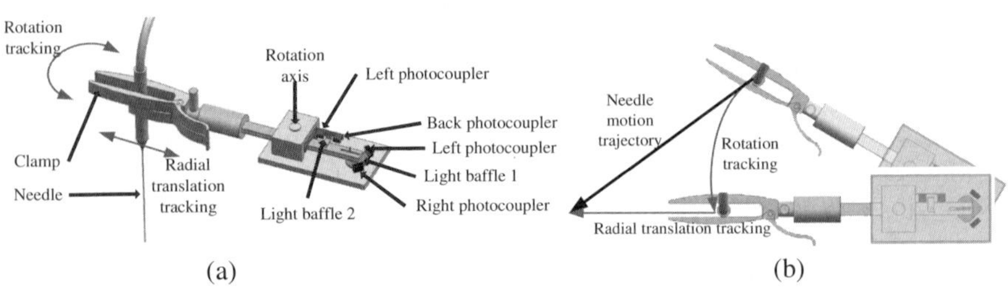

Fig. 2. Mechanism of axial and lateral motion tracking

2.2.2 Anterior-posterior (Elevation) Motion Tracking

Literature and clinical practice both indicate that the elevation motion magnitude is small, sometimes it can even be neglected. So we just utilize a simple dual-spring component to implement passive tracking of the needle's elevation motion (see Fig. 3).

The front spring and back spring combine to maintain the dynamic balance of the holding hand when not tracking. If the needle is pushed-up or pulled-down by the liver motion or tissue deformation, one spring will be compressed while the other tensioned, thus a torque is formed which will elevate or depress the holding hand according to the needle's motion in the elevation direction.

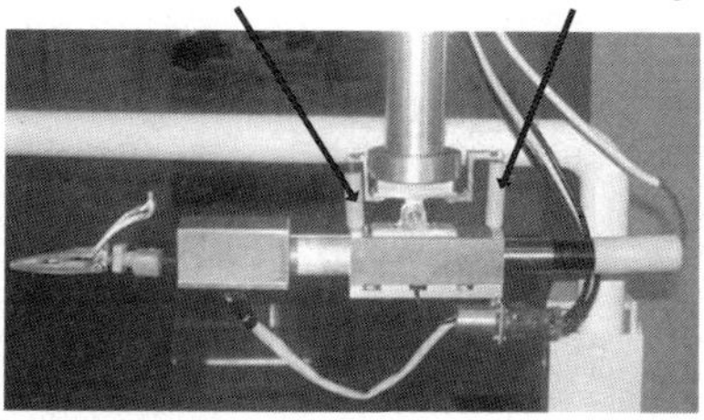

Fig. 3. Mechanism of elevation tracking

The sensitivity of the elevation tracking can be easily adjusted by replacing the two springs.

3 Experiments and Discussion

3.1 Force Measuring Experiment

We devised a simple force measuring device and conducted an experiment to determine how much force should be applied to the needle shaft in order for the holding robot to track its motion.

Fig. 4(a) shows all the devices used in this experiment. One FSS1500 (Honeywell Inc.) force sensor was used to measure the force. It was soldered on a finger-like electronic board to form a simple force-measuring device(see Fig. 4(b)).

Fig. 4(c) shows the configuration of the experiment. In initial state the needle was motionless. When the holding robot began to work, the needle was fiddled toward one direction with the force-measuring device. Force applied on the needle shaft propelled the robotic holding hand to move and to start tracking the motion of the needle. The maximum output voltage of the force sensor in this process was recorded and converted to its corresponding force value, which is the force required for the robot to track motion in this direction.

Several cases were covered in the experiment. For rotation tracking, the forces required for leftward and rightward rotation tracking were measured respectively. For radial-translation tracking, the forces required for centrifugal and centripetal translation tracking were measured respectively. Elevation tracking is subdivided into two groups, one is push-up tracking, the other is pull-down tracking. For both push-up and pull-down tracking, the forces are measured respectively when the robotic hand was at the innermost, halfway and outermost position. (see Fig. 4 (d))

20 data were recorded for each case. The results are shown in Table 1.

Table 1 indicates that the average force required for the robotic hand to track leftward is 8.43g with the range of 6.96-9.50g. For rightward tracking, the range is 6.06-10.25g, and the mean value is 8.02g. Both the forces required for leftward and rightward tracking are very small, which means the force required for rotation tracking is very small.

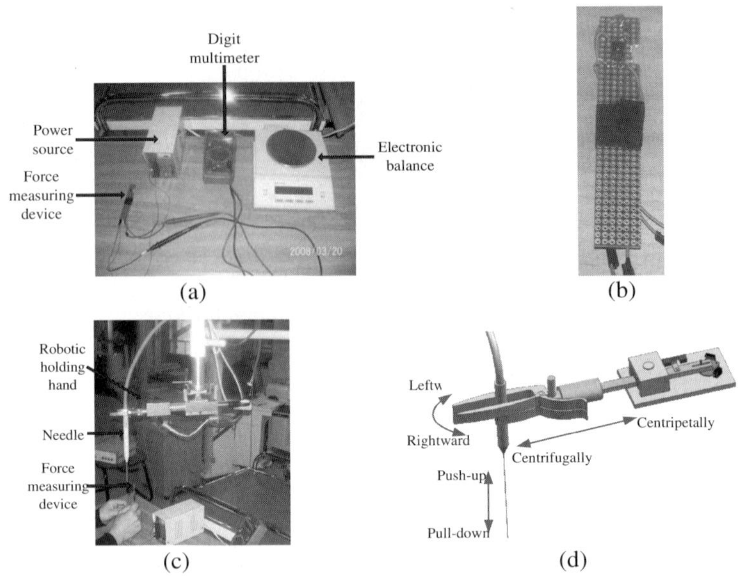

Fig. 4. Force measuring experiment

Table 1. Maximum force required for different cases

Cases		Mean(g)	Min(g)	**Max(g)**
rotation tracking	Leftward	8.43	6.96	9.50
	Rightward	8.02	6.06	10.25
radial translation tracking	Centrifugally	12.06	10.25	14.00
	Centripetally	12.38	10.10	14.30
push-up tracking	Innermost	182.60	174.45	199.62
	Halfway	167.47	160.66	175.65
	Outermost	137.57	125.46	149.73
pull-down tracking	Innermost	150.04	140.29	161.41
	Halfway	122.99	112.72	134.00
	Outermost	111.50	101.64	119.77

The force for centrifugal tracking varies from 10.25 to 14.00g, the mean value is 12.06g. For centripetal tracking the range is 10.10-14.30g and the mean value is 12.38g. From this we can learn that the force for radial-translation tracking is 4g bigger than that for rotation tracking. This conforms to the discussion of the motion tracking mechanism.

For innermost push-up tracking, the mean force is 182.60g，the range is 174.45-199.62g。 When the hand is at halfway the mean force is 167.47g，the range is 160.66-175.65g. For outermost push-up tracking, the mean force is 137.57g, the range is 125.46-149.73g. The force required for innermost push-up tracking is the biggest, and that for outermost is the smallest. The force required for push-up tracking lies between 120-200g.

For innermost pull-down tracking, the mean force required is 150.04g with the fluctuation of 140.29-161.41g. For halfway pull-down tracking, the mean value is 123.00g, the range is 112.72-134.00g. For outermost pull-down tracking, the mean value is 111.50g, the range is 101.64-119.77g. The force required for pull-down tracking lies between 100-160g, and it is 20-40g smaller than that for push-up tracking.

In conclusion, the force required for rotation and radial translation tracking are less than 15g. This enables the holding robot to sensitively and swiftly track the 3D motion of the needle. The force for elevation tracking varies from 100-200g, and it can be adjusted while required.

3.2 In Vivo Animal Trial

We conducted an animal trial on a swine to assess the accuracy and sensitivity of the holding robot. The configuration of the animal test is shown in Fig. 5(a). The experiment was performed as follows: First one microwave ablation needle was inserted into the swine's liver under the guidance of IOUS, but no real ablation was executed. The needle and its accessory cable were then held by our holding robot while its motion tracked by the electromagnetic measurement system and motion data recorded and analyzed on the personal computer.

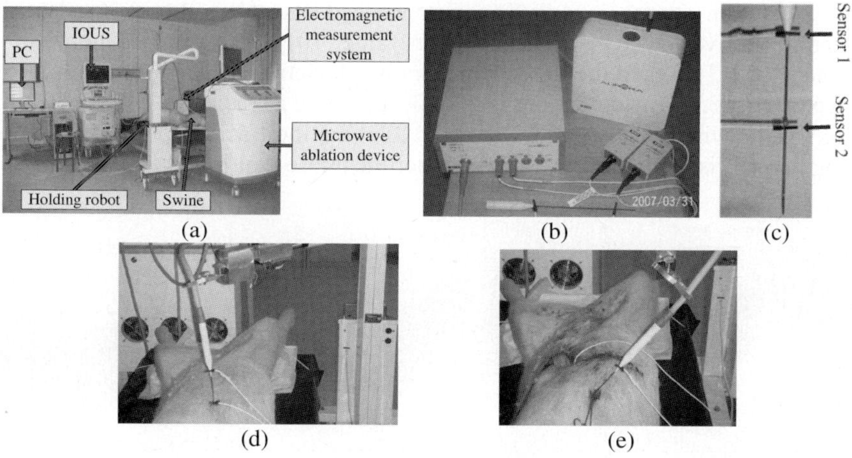

Fig. 5. In vivo animal trial

Aurora (Fig. 5(b), Northern Digital Inc.) was used as the electromagnetic measurement system to track the motion of the ablation needle during the experiment. Two 6D sensors, which can estimate all pose parameters of the needle, facilitated motion tracking and data analysis. Sensor 1 was fastened to the upper part of the needle shaft at a fixed position through the experiment and was motionless to the needle. But sensor 2 was not fastened, it was just sleeved around the lower part of the needle shaft and could slide axially or laterally and rotate.(see Fig. 5(c))

Two cases were covered in the experiment. In case 1, the swine was not opened and sensor 2 was fastened to the swine skin at the needle entry point(Fig. 5(d)). In case 2, the swine was opened, and sensor 2 was fastened to the liver surface at the needle entry point(Fig. 5(e)).

During the experiment in both cases, sensor 2 could float with the swine's skin or liver respectively. If the holding robot was so sensitive and accurate in motion tracking that sensor 1 could follow the motion of sensor 2 synchronously, the distance between sensor 1 and 2 would not change through the experiment. Otherwise it would increase while the needle was pushed outward and would decrease while the needle pulled inward. So we could resort to the distance of the two sensors to evaluate the performance of the holding robot.

The results of the animal test are illustrated both in Fig. 6 and Table 2.

688 data was collected in case 1. In the experiment, x axis means lateral, y axis means cranio-caudal(axial), z axis means anterior-posterior(elevation). Fig. 6(a), 6(b) and 6(c) are the results of case 1. 6(a), 6(b) is the 3D trajectory of sensor 1 and 2 respectively, and 6(c) is the fluctuation of the distance between sensor 1 & 2. From 6(c) we can learn that the distance had kept almost constant with slight deviations. The maximum positive deviation from the mean value (77.45mm) is 1.38 mm with the percentage of 1.78%, and the maximum negative deviation is -1.14 mm with the percentage of 1.47%.

682 data were covered in case 2(Fig. 6(d), 6(e) and 6(f)). Fig. 6(d), 6(e) show the 3D trajectory of sensor 1 & 2 respectively, and 6(f) denotes the fluctuation of the distance between sensor 1 & 2. The distance had also kept almost constant. The maximum positive deviation from the mean value (101.85mm) is 1.33 mm with the percentage of 1.31%, and the maximum negative deviation is -1.17 mm with the percentage of 1.15%. These deviations are almost the same as in case 1.

The small deviations in both cases imply good motion-tracking performance of the holding robot. Visual monitoring during experiment also confirmed this conclusion.

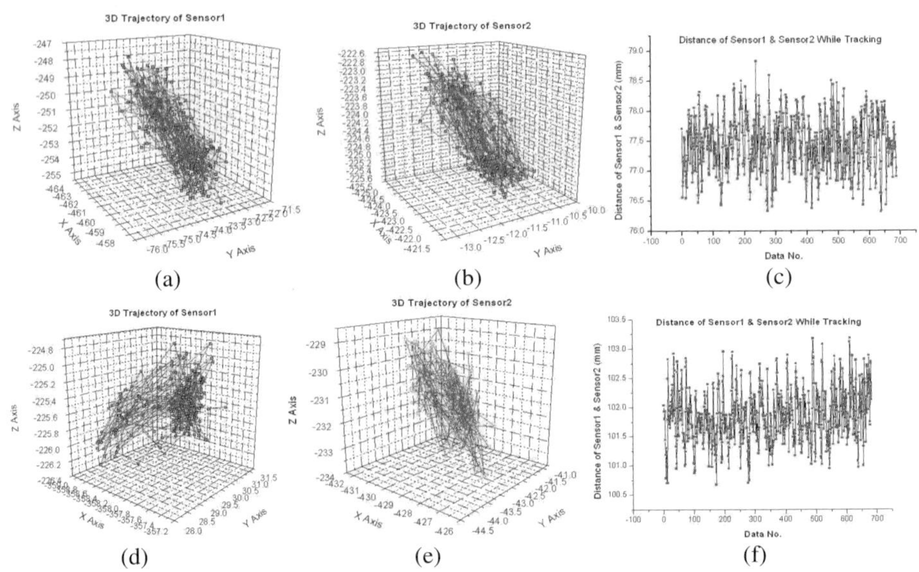

Fig. 6. Results of animal trial

Table 2. Variation of the distance between sensor 1 & 2

	Mean (mm)	Min(mm)	Max(mm)	Range(mm)
Case 1	77.45	76.31	78.83	2.52
Case 2	101.85	100.68	103.18	2.51

4 Conclusion

A needle-holding robot has been developed for ultrasound guided percutaneous hepatic microwave ablation. It can accurately sense and track 3D motion of the ablation needle secondary to respiration and tissue deformation during clinical ablation procedures and allows for stable and precise holding of the ablation needle compared to that of manual holding by the surgeon.

A force-measuring experiment was conducted to quantify the force required for motion tracking of the robot. Experiment results show that the force required for rotation and radial translation tracking are less than 15g. This enables the holding robot to sensitively and swiftly track the 3D motion of the needle. The force for elevation tracking varies from 100-200g, and it can be adjusted while required.

We also conducted an in vivo animal trial with a swine. In this experiment, we resort to the variation of the distance between two electromagnetic sensors to evaluate the performance of the holding robot. Both two cases covered in this experiment have shown satisfactory results. The distance had kept almost constant with slight deviations. The maximum positive and negative deviation from the mean value is less than 2mm with the percentage less than 2%. The small deviations imply good motion-tracking performance of the holding robot. Visual monitoring during experiment also confirmed this conclusion.

Acknowledgment

The work was supported by the Science & Technology Plan sponsored by Beijing Municipal Science & Technology Commission under the Key Project grant H060720050330, and supported by the Science & Technology Plan sponsored by Beijing Municipal Commission of Education under grant 08010921003, and supported by Funding Project for Academic Human Resources Development in Institutions of Higher Learning Under the Jurisdiction of Beijing Municipality.

References

1. Nakakura, E., Choti, M.: Hepatocellular Carcinoma: Current Management Recommendations. Advances on Onc. 16, 12–18 (2000)
2. Nakakura, E.K., Choti, M.A.: Management of hepatocellular carcinoma. Oncology 14, 1085–1098 (2000)
3. Choti, M.A., et al.: Management of hepatic metastases. Transpl. Surg. 5, 65–80 (1999)
4. Bleicher, R.J., et al.: Radiofrequency ablation in 447 complex unresectable liver tumors: lessons learned. Ann. Surg. Oncol. 10, 52–58 (2003)

5. Scott, D.J., et al.: Accuracy and effectiveness of laparoscopic vs open hepatic radiofrequency ablation. Surg. Endosc. 15, 135–140 (2001)
6. Gobbi, D.G., Peters, T.M.: Interactive intraoperative 3D ultrasound reconstruction and visualization. In: Dohi, T., Kikinis, R. (eds.) MICCAI 2002. LNCS, vol. 2488, pp. 156–163. Springer, Heidelberg (2002)
7. Hong, J.S., et al.: A Motion Adaptable Needle Placement Instrument Based on Tumor Specific Ultrasonic Image Segmentation. In: Dohi, T., Kikinis, R. (eds.) MICCAI 2002. LNCS, vol. 2488, pp. 9–16. Springer, Heidelberg (2002)
8. Salcudean, S.E., et al.: Robot Assisted Diagnostic Ultrasound – Design and Feasibility Experiments. In: Taylor, C., Colchester, A. (eds.) MICCAI 1999. LNCS, vol. 1679, pp. 1062–1071. Springer, Heidelberg (1999)
9. Vanderpool, H.E., et al.: Prevalence of carpal tunnel syndrome and other work-related musculoskeletal problems in cardiac sonographers. Journal of Occupational Medicine 35, 604–610 (1993)
10. Davies, S.C., Hill, A.L., Holmes, R.B., Halliwell, M., Jackson, P.C.: Ultrasound quantitation of respiratory organ motion in the upper abdomen. Br. J. Radiol. 67, 1096–1102 (1994)
11. Korin, H.W., Ehman, R.L., Riederer, S.J., Felmlee, J.P., Grimm, R.C.: Respiratory kinematics of the upper abdominal organs: A quantitative study. Magn. Reson. Med. 23, 172–178 (1992)
12. Shimizu, S., Shirato, H., Xo, B., Kagei, K., Nishioka, T., Hashimoto, S., Tsuchiya, K., Aoyama, H., Miyasaka, K.: Three-dimensional movement of a liver tumor detected by high-speed magnetic resonance imaging. Radiother. Oncol. 50, 367–370 (1999)

An Application of Psychoacoustic Metrics to Improve Sound Quality of Fission Air-Conditioning Unit

Jixuan Yuan, Qibai Huang, Zhanxin Liu, Li Hu, and Ruiqiang Wang

School of Mechanical of Science and Engineering, Huazhong University of Science and Technology, Wuhan Hubei Province 430074, China
yuanjixuan@gmail.com, qbhuang@mail.hust.edu.cn, hustliuzx@gmail.com, hunklin@163.com, wrq406@gmail.com

Abstract. The application of using sound quality metrics evaluation to improve the noise radiated by fission air-conditioning unit is studied in this paper. Compared to A-weighted Sound Pressure Level (SPL) ——a traditional measurement to sound, sound quality metrics are better, because they are unanimous with the subjective feeling of human being. The noise caused by compressor vibration is the major noise source of the fission air-conditioning unit through the analysis of the loudness spectrum. Some improvements are carried out to reduce the noise radiated from the compressor vibration, and the result is satisfactory.

Keywords: Psychoacoustics, Sound Quality, Fission Air-conditioning Unit.

1 Introduction

The complexity of sounds gives them a multidimensional character from both acoustics and human perception points of view. [1] It is necessary in sound quality research to address the relationship between sound and human cognition. Sound quality can be defined as following:" Sound quality is the perceptual reaction to the sound of a product that reflects the listener's reaction to the acceptability of that sound for that product; the more acceptable, the greater the sound quality. [2]" Sound quality evaluation has emerged as a very active research area. It deals with the human's subjective response to sounds (mainly noise), and aims to achieve better sound design. Applied psychoacoustics is usually the starting point of any sound quality evaluation. In particular, many sound quality evaluations to air-conditioning unit have been recently carried out. Psychoacoustic parameters are measurable and objective characteristics of sound. They provide a way to measure several aspects of the subjective sensation that sounds can produce on human listeners.

There are many kinds of air-conditioning units' noise: compressor noise, air acoustic noise, structure noise, electronic motor noise, and others. Each possesses particular features. Therefore, it is very difficult to address all the features at the same time. And sound quality studies often focus on comfortable feelings.

It is reported that in indoor machine of the fission air-conditioning unit, 50% ~ 60% of total sound energy is caused by air acoustic noise, mainly by air system, and other noise is radiated by vibration and electronic motor. In outdoor machine of the fission air-conditioning unit, 60% ~ 70% of total sound energy is caused by air acoustic

C. Xiong et al. (Eds.): ICIRA 2008, Part II, LNAI 5315, pp. 1183–1191, 2008.

noise, and other noise is caused by the compressor vibration, the electronic motor and total machine shell vibration. Although the noise radiated by vibration is not the major noise in indoor machine, it is emphasized that the structure noise would annoy human being much more than air acoustic noise. If we want to decrease the noise of fission air-conditioning unit, the structure noise is the main target.

2 Sound Quality Metrics

The air-conditioning units' noise is taken more seriously by the production plant at present. However, sometimes the products are complained about their noise while it is not a high value measured in A-weighted SPL. On the contrary, sometimes the products' noise is acceptable but its A-weighted SPL measurement value is very high. Such results lead the fact that it is uncertain of the practicability of the traditional A-weighted SPL measurement. Because of the simulating auditory system of human being, there are a group of A-weighted filters mainly attenuate low frequency. That is to say, if the main composition of the noise is low frequency, it is suitable to use sound quality metrics, not A-weighted SPL measurement, to evaluate the effect of the noise to the auditory system of human being.

Sound quality metrics have been developed in order to predict how the average person will receive particular characteristics of sounds. Many of these metrics have been standardized and are widely accepted, however, others are still under being defined. Most metrics have been developed to model either the perception of intensity, spectral balance, modulations, etc. Some of the most important metrics are introduced in the following:

2.1 Loudness

There are two major methods of computing loudness, one due to Stevens and the other to Zwicker. The basic difference between them is the way they deal with the phenomenon of masking, the reduction of sensitivity by noise in a stronger frequency band to noise in other band. We shall discuss the latter.

"Loudness is defined as that attribute of auditory sensation in terms of which sounds can be ordered on a scale extending from quite to loud."(Moore, 1997) The loudness that measures one's subject perception in the Sound Pressure Level (SPL) was described in ANSI S1.8 (1989) and ANSI S1.13 (1995), the formula is shown below:

$$SPL = 10\log_{10}\left(P_{rms}^2 / P_{ref}^2 \right) dB \ . \tag{1}$$

where SPL is the sound pressure level, P_{rms} is the root mean squared pressure (rms) of the measured acoustic signal, and P_{ref} is a reference pressure equal to the rms pressure of the quietest sounds that are just audible. Typically in air $P_{ref} = 20\mu Pa$.

In order to approximate the perception of loudness better, several psychoacoustically based models have been proposed. A model based on Zwicker's work has become standardized in ISO 532B (ISO, 1975) and is used as an intermediate calculation for several other metrics.

Because critical bandwidth plays an important role in loudness, the loudness on the slopes of the frequency selectivity characteristic of the human being's auditory system may also play an important role. The excitation level versus critical-band rate pattern represents the pattern that describes not only the influence of critical bandwidth, but also that of the slopes. Therefore, it seems reasonable to use the excitation level versus critical-band rate pattern as a basis from which the loudness of the complex may be constructed. Because it can be seen that the two tones influence each other in the creation of the total loudness, even though they are spectrally separated, it may be useful to treat total loudness as an integral of value that we have to find, but which can be drawn as a function of critical-band rate. If such an integral leads to the loudness that is given in sone, the value we require has to have the unit of sone/Bark. In this case, total loudness, given as the integral of this value over critical-band rate, will lead to the unit of sone.

As usual, it is called the value that required "specific loudness" with the symbol N'. Loudness, N, is then the integral of specific loudness in mathematical expression:

$$N = \int_0^{24\,Bark} N'dz \ . \tag{2}$$

where the integral is taken over all critical-band rates.

Stevens' law says sensation belonging to the category of intensity sensations grows with physical intensity according to a power law. In consequence of that law, we have to assume that a relative change in loudness is proportional to a relative change in intensity. Specific loudness is developed by using this power law. Instead of using the total loudness as the value in question, specific loudness is used. Additionally, instead of intensity excitation has to be used. With a constant of proportionality k, relating the specific loudness N' and its corresponding increment $\Delta N'$ to the excitation E and its corresponding increment ΔE, we can formulate the power law as an equation using differences:

$$\frac{\Delta N'}{N'} = k\frac{\Delta E}{E}, \text{ or } \frac{\Delta N'}{N'+N'_{gr}} = k\frac{\Delta E}{E+E_{gr}} \ . \tag{3}$$

If values N'_{gr} and E_{gr} corresponding to the internal noise floors at very low values of N' and E, respectively, are added. Threshold in quiet is assumed to be produced by such internal noise. Using the threshold factor, which is helpful in describing the relationship between masking sound and masked threshold produced by that sound, we are able to calculate the excitation E_{gr} producing threshold in quiet by the test-tone excitation E_{TQ}, using the equation:

$$E_{gr} = {}^{E_{TQ}}\!/_{s} \ . \tag{4}$$

where *s* is the ratio between the intensity of the just-audible test tone and the intensity of the internal noise appearing within the critical band at the test tone's frequency. This ratio was effectively used for calculating masked threshold produced by external sounds. Here it is used to estimate the internal noise using the knowledge of threshold in quiet.

Treating this equation of differences as a differential equation, it can be solved by using the reasonable boundary condition that excitation equal to zero leads to specific loudness equal to zero, i.e. $E=0$ leads to $N'=0$. The relation is found here:

$$N' = N'_{gr}\left[\left(1+\frac{sE}{E_{TQ}}\right)^{k} - 1\right]. \tag{5}$$

This can be transformed into the final expression using a reference specific loudness

$$N' = N'_{0}\left(\frac{E_{TQ}}{sE_{0}}\right)^{k}\left[\left(1+\frac{sE}{E_{TQ}}\right)^{k} - 1\right]. \tag{6}$$

The most important value in this equation is the exponent *k*. It can be approximated quite simply by using the dependence of the loudness of uniform-exciting noise as a function of its level, as mentioned in the preceding section. Because (6) can be approximated for large values of *E*, for which the influence of threshold in quiet is negligible, as

$$N' \sim \left(\frac{E}{E_{0}}\right)^{k}. \tag{7}$$

The exponent of 0.23 is the value of *k*. for frequencies in the neighborhood of 1 kHz, for which the threshold factor is *s*=0.5, and with the additional boundary condition that a 1-kHz tone with a level of 40 dB has to produce exactly 1 sone as total loudness, the equation

$$N' = 0.08\left(\frac{E_{TQ}}{E_{0}}\right)^{0.23}\left[\left(0.5+0.5\frac{E}{E_{TQ}}\right)^{0.23} - 1\right] sone/Bark . \tag{8}$$

This is the final equation from which specific loudness can be calculated quantitatively. In this equation, E_{TQ} is the excitation at threshold in quiet and E_0 is the excitation that corresponds to the reference intensity $I_0 = 10^{-12}\, W/m^2$. The value "1" in the parenthesis of (6) has been exchanged by the value (1-*s*), i.e. 0.5, with the consequence that the specific loudness reaches asymptotically the value $N'=0$ for small values of *E*.

2.2 Sharpness

Because of the auditory system construction of human being, the shape of the spectrum is an important characteristic of the sound. If there is too much high frequency content in the signal, it feels sharp. If there is too much low frequency content in the signal, it feels dull. The spectral envelope can produce a smoother spectrum shape which can be plotted on a logarithmic frequency scale, and the perception of sharpness tightly relates to the shape of the spectral envelope.

Although a universally accepted standard for Sharpness does not yet exist, a model that originated with von Bismark and has been modified by Zwicker is given by:

$$S = c \times \frac{\int_0^{24} N'(z)\, g(z)\, z dz}{N} acum \ . \tag{9}$$

Where N' is the Specific Loudness, z is the critical band rate in Bark, N is the total Loudness in sones, and $g(z)$ is a weighting factor that emphasizes sound at higher critical band rates. This weighting factor can be defined by:

$$g(z) = \begin{Bmatrix} 1 & for\ z \le 16 \\ 0.066e^{0.172z} & for\ z > 16 \end{Bmatrix} . \tag{10}$$

With c=0.11. Aures has suggested replacing the total loudness in the denominator of Equation(2) with $\ln(0.05N+1)$. This version of the Sharpness metrics then becomes:

$$S = c \times \frac{\int_0^{24} N'(z)\, g(z)\, z dz}{\ln(0.05N+1)} acum \ . \tag{11}$$

Aures' Sharpness is a good model of the perception of sharpness.

3 Description of the Experiment

3.1 Instruments and Environment of the Experiment

Firstly, the study of noise produced by the fission air-conditioning units requires recording different existing noises under variable working process: cooling, heating, dehumidifying, etc. The DAT recording contains a B&K 4188 microphone connecting to a B&K 7701 data recorder. B&K 7701 data recorder supplies a data recorder instrument that allows time history data to be recorded directly to disk for subsequent play back and analysis. In all cases, a 10.5s sample was recorded and the sampling rate was 44100Hz. In order to avoid the influence of air acoustic noise, a windshield was used to wrap the microphone. When signals were recorded and exported as wave data format (.wav), a B&K Sound Quality Analyzer 7698 was used to analyze these signals and play them back.

Using the same recording equipment, a 1 kHz, 94dB SPL reference signal was recorded with a B&K 4231 calibrator. This signal was used subsequently to calibrate the sound levels for the room experiments. The temperature in the experiment room is 22□ and the background noise is 30 dB during the experiment. The target temperature is 20□ in cooling process, while 30℃ in heating process.

The laying drawing of microphone is shown as Fig. 1, where the Cartesian coordinates of the microphone is (45.5, 13.5, 60).

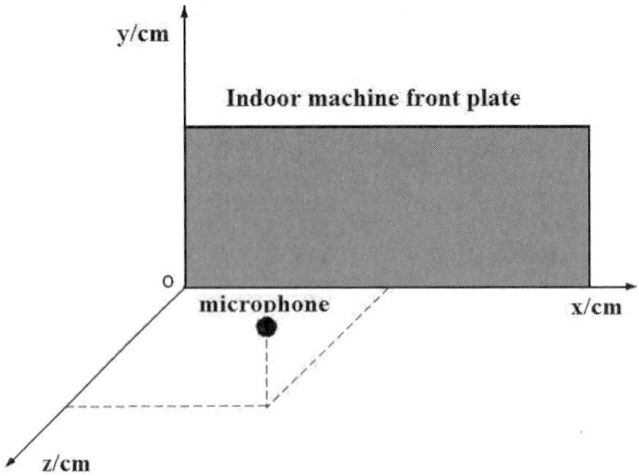

Fig. 1. Layout drawing of microphone

3.2 Result Analysis

During the experiment, it could be heard that the compressor in the outdoor machine is always working under either cooling or heating process when the target temperature is not arrived. Meanwhile, people in the experiment room heard some noise and felt uncomfortable when it ran. This result indicates that there must be some relationships between compressor running and uncomfortable feeling. A lot of researches show the uncomfortable feeling was caused by the noise of outdoor machine compressor shell vibration. Fig 2 shows the SPL in acoustic A-weighted SPL under different cross-flow fan speed, while Fig 3 shows the Loudness under different conditions.

Clearly, SPL increases with the rising of the air speed. And so does Loudness. The figure shows that the higher the air speed is, the less the SPL gaps between different processes are. However, a tiny difference between Fig 2 and Fig 3 can be observed at the fast air speed.

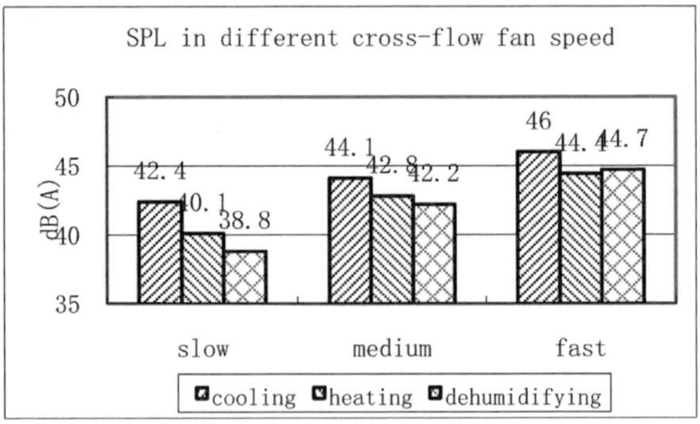

Fig. 2. SPL in different working process

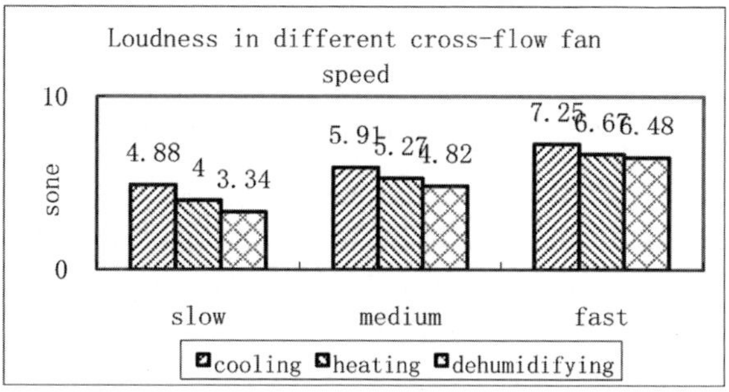

Fig. 3. Loudness in different working process

Research shows that with the increasing value of A-weighted SPL, the noise loudness curve caused by structure noise changes more rapidly than the one by the air acoustic noise. Even if the two noises are at the same SPL, the loudness value of the structure noise is louder than the air acoustic noise. That means although the main noise energy of the outdoor machine is caused by air acoustic energy, the measures to reduce the compressor noise should be firstly carried out, if our main target is to improve the sound quality of the fission air-conditioning unit.

Research [7, 8] also shows that even at the same SPL, sharpness caused by structure noise is higher than the noise caused by electronic fan, because air acoustic noise is a wideband noise but the noise radiated from compressor shell contains the components of medium and high frequency with its discrete spectrum.

4 Compare Before and After Improvement

In order to improve the sound quality of noise radiated from air-conditioning unit, we should place the reducing noise radiated by compressor in priority. Fig 4 shows the loudness spectrum before some improvements are carried out on the fission air-conditioning units. The noise is very boresome with its high loudness. In this figure the area surrounded by the loudness curve between 7 Bark to 10 Bark can be observed very large, that is to say, if we want to reduce the loudness, we must reduce the noise in this area firstly.

After series of researches including time domain analysis, frequency domain analysis, and correlation analysis of noise and vibration applied to the shell of the compressor and the front plate upon indoor machine, the result indicates that the noise curve from 7 Bark to 10 Bark correlates to the vibration caused by both the fins through which the finned tube drilled and the front plate upon indoor machine. Consequently, in order to reduce the stimulation on the fins and front plate in indoor machine, the finned tube of the compressor is rearranged, the refrigerant in the tube is cycled more smoothly, damping material and sound absorption material is stuck to the front plate. With all the steps being carried out, significant decrease in loudness spectrum was shown in Fig 5 while sharpness-time diagram was plotted in Fig 6.

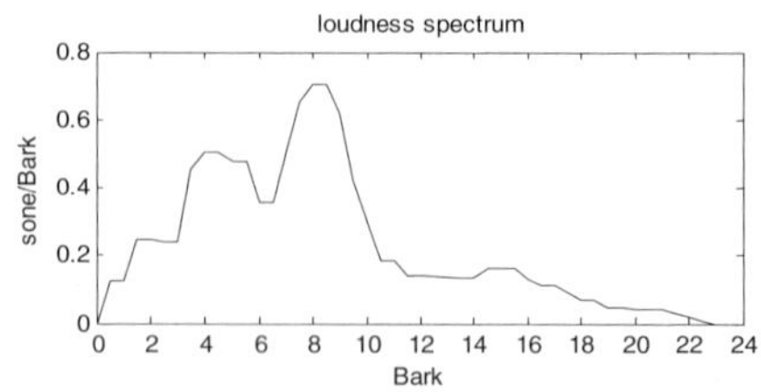

Fig. 4. Loudness spectrum before improvement

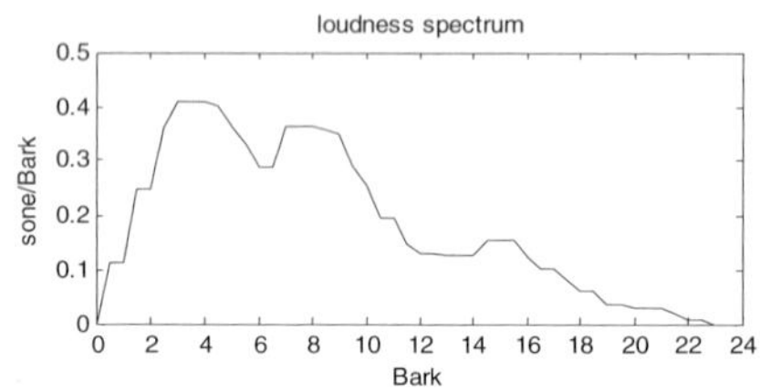

Fig. 5. Loudness spectrum after improvement

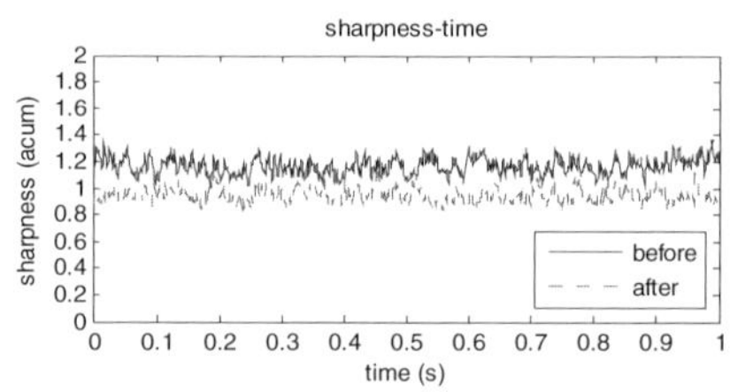

Fig. 6. Sharpness-time compare between before and after improvement

After improvement, total loudness value is decreased from 4.88 sone to 4.07 sone; sharpness value is decreased from 1.17 acum to 0.96 acum. And the sound of indoor machine is felt more comfortable than before.

5 Conclusions

In this article, sound quality has a significant effect on improving the subjective feeling of the fission air-conditioning unit. Psychoacoustic metrics values of certain fission air-conditioning unit are calculated before and after improvement, the following conclusions are drawn:

1) A-weighted SPL is not as good as the sound quality metrics to simulate subjective feelings of human being.

2) The experimental result shows that loudness and sharpness are both decreased which are unanimous with the comfortable feeling of human being.

3) It is the first step to improve the compressor sound quality because structure noise due to compressor vibration is the major noise origin source of fission air-conditioning unit.

References

1. Zwicker, E., Fastl, H.: Psychoacoustics: Facts and Models, 2nd edn. Springer, Berlin (1999)
2. Lyon, R.H.: Designing for Product Sound Quality. Marcel Dekker, Inc., New York (2000)
3. Hastings, A.: Sound Quality of Diesel Engines. PHD thesis, Purdue University (2004)
4. Gonzalez, A., Ferrer, M., de Diego, M., Piñero, G., Garcia-Bonito, J.J.: Sound quality of low-frequency and car engine noises after active noise control. Journal of Sound and Vibration 265(3), 663–679 (2003)
5. Susini, P., McAdams, S., Winsberg, S., Perry, I., Vieillard, S., Rodet, X.: Characterizing the sound quality of air-conditioning noise. In: Applied Acoustics, vol. 65(8), pp. 763–790 (2004)
6. Kuwano, S., Namba, S., Okamoto, T.: Psychological evaluation of sound environment in a compartment of a high-speed train. Journal of Sound and Vibration 277(3), 491–500 (2004)
7. Kuwano, S., Namba, S.: Air-conditioner noise and noise quality. The Journal of the Acoustical Society of America 87(s1), 134 (1990)
8. Ingham, R., Otto, N., McCollum, T.: Sound quality metric for diesel engines. In: SAE 1999-01-1819 (1999)

Modeling, Analysis and Control for a Robotic Roadheader

Junli Li, Yuanzong Li, and Zisheng Lian

College of Mechanical Engineering, Taiyuan University of Technology,
No.79 West Yingze Street, Taiyuan, Shanxi, China, 030024
ljltyut@163.com

Abstract. The problems of parameters uncertainty, disturbances, system vibration and asymmetric dynamic performance existed in asymmetric cylinder controlled by symmetric proportion valve system. To solve these problems, the models of the forward and inverse kinematics and the electro-hydraulic proportion system for a robotic roadheader were established. In combination with the equilibrium point steady theory and the output error equation polynomial, a model reference adaptive controller was designed. The simulation results show that the designed model reference adaptive controller can effectively achieve accurate velocity control of the roadheader's cutter.

Keywords: roadheader; kinematics; electro-hydraulic proportion; model reference adaptive control.

1 Introduction

The boom-type roadheader, one of the partial-size tunneling machines, consists of upper framework, traveling mechanism and working mechanism (Fig.1). The working mechanism of the boom-type roadheader, simplified into a robotic model as shown in Fig.2, has four primary links termed as gyration platform, boom, telescope mechanism and cutter, and connected by rotation joints at O_1 and O_2 and by translational joint at O_3. Their motions are actuated by extension and retraction of three pairs of gyration platform cylinder(ab), boom cylinder(cd) and telescope mechanism cylinder(ef), respectively. The length d of the telescope mechanism is constant during swing motion of the boom.

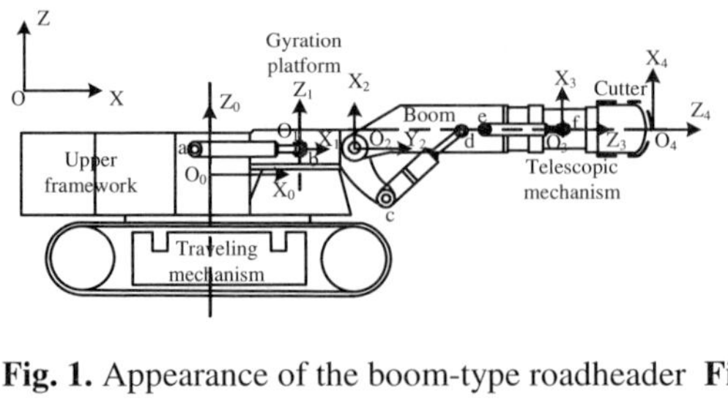

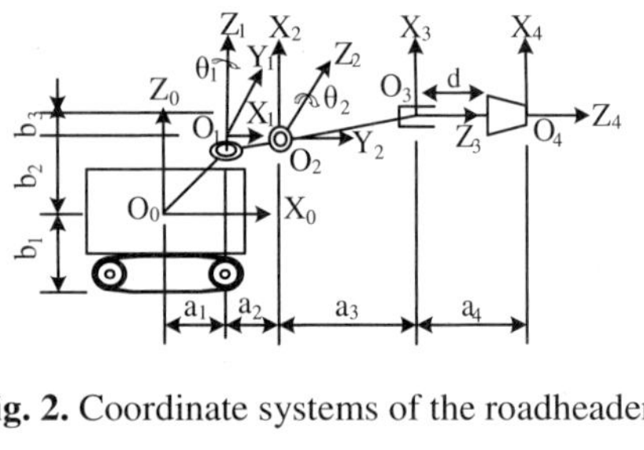

Fig. 1. Appearance of the boom-type roadheader **Fig. 2.** Coordinate systems of the roadheader

C. Xiong et al. (Eds.): ICIRA 2008, Part II, LNAI 5315, pp. 1192–1200, 2008.

In the past decades, the boom-type roadheader were operated manually, which resulted in position and orientation errors of the cutter. The goal of this project is to develop an automatic product that no longer relies on the operator's skill and endurance to maximize roadheader's performance. Therefore, this paper focuses on the controller design of the roadheader's cutter swing velocity based on the model of the robotic roadheader kinematics and the hydraulic system.

2 Kinematics Model of the Roadheader

The coordinate systems are established by the Denavit-Hartenberg representation[1]. As shown in Fig.2, $O_0X_0Y_0Z_0$ is the body coordinate system; $O_iX_iY_iZ_i$ (i=0,1,2,3) is the joint coordinate system; $O_4X_4Y_4Z_4$ is the cutter coordinate system. The joint variables are angles θ_1, θ_2 and displacement d. Table 1 presents D-H link para- meters of the robotic roadheader.

Table 1. Denavit-Hartenberg link parameters

Link	a_{i-1}	α_{i-1}	d_i	θ_i	Joint variable
1	a_1	0°	b_2	θ_1 (0°)	θ_1
2	a_2	-90°	0	θ_2 (-90°)	θ_2
3	b_3	-90°	a_3+d	0	d
4	0	0	a_4		

2.1 Forward Kinematics

Based on the D-H rules, the homogeneous coordinate transformation matrix of the cutter relative to the body coordinate system is presented by

$$ {}^0_4T={}^0_1T\,{}^1_2T\,{}^2_3T\,{}^3_4T=\begin{bmatrix} \cos\theta_1\cos\theta_2 & \sin\theta_1 & -\cos\theta_1\sin\theta_2 & b_3\cos\theta_1\cos\theta_2-(a_3+a_4+d)\cos\theta_1\sin\theta_2+a_2\cos\theta_1+a_1 \\ \sin\theta_1\cos\theta_2 & -\cos\theta_1 & -\sin\theta_1\sin\theta_2 & b_3\sin\theta_1\cos\theta_2-(a_3+a_4+d)\sin\theta_1\sin\theta_2+a_2\sin\theta_1 \\ -\sin\theta_2 & 0 & -\cos\theta_2 & -b_3\sin\theta_2-(a_3+a_4+d)\cos\theta_2+b_2 \\ 0 & 0 & 0 & 1 \end{bmatrix} \tag{1} $$

The point O_4 can be determined in the body coordinate system $O_0X_0Y_0Z_0$ by the vector ${}^0P$

$$ {}^0P={}^0_4T*{}^4P_{O4}=\begin{bmatrix}{}^0x & {}^0y & {}^0z & 1\end{bmatrix}^T \tag{2} $$

where

$$ \begin{aligned} {}^0x&=b_3\cos\theta_1\cos\theta_2-(a_3+a_4+d)\cos\theta_1\sin\theta_2+a_2\cos\theta_1+a_1 \\ {}^0y&=b_3\sin\theta_1\cos\theta_2-(a_3+a_4+d)\sin\theta_1\sin\theta_2+a_2\sin\theta_1 \\ {}^0z&=-b_3\sin\theta_2-(a_3+a_4+d)\cos\theta_2+b_2 \end{aligned} \tag{3} $$

From Eq.(3), joint angles and velocities can be got as follows:

$$ \theta_2=2\arctan\frac{b_3-\sqrt{b_3^2+(a_3+a_4+d)^2-({}^0z-b_2)^2}}{a_3+a_4+d-{}^0z+b_2} \tag{4} $$

$$ \dot{\theta}_2=\frac{1}{(a_3+a_4+d)\sin\theta_2-b_3\cos\theta_2}v_z \tag{5} $$

$$\theta_1 = \arcsin\frac{{}^0y}{b_3\cos\theta_2 - (a_3+a_4+d)\sin\theta_2 + a_2} \tag{6}$$

$$\dot{\theta}_1 = \frac{v_y + [b_3\sin\theta_1\sin\theta_2 + (a_3+a_4+d)\sin\theta_1\cos\theta_2]\dot{\theta}_2}{b_3\cos\theta_1\cos\theta_2 + a_2\cos\theta_1 - (a_3+a_4+d)\cos\theta_1\sin\theta_2} \tag{7}$$

where v_y and v_z are the horizontal and the vertical swing velocity of the cutter, respectively.

2.2 Inverse Kinematics

Inverse kinematics is computation of the joint displacement, angle and velocity from the end-effector position and velocity. From Fig.3 and Fig.4, angle θ'_2 is

$$\theta'_2 = \arcsin\frac{h-h_j}{O_2O_4} + \arcsin\frac{m_0}{O_2d} \qquad (h_j<h\le h_{max}) \tag{8}$$

$$\theta'_2 = \arcsin\frac{h-h_j}{O_2O_4} - \arcsin\frac{m_0}{O_2d} \qquad (-h_w\le h\le h_j) \tag{9}$$

Length l_1 of cylinder cd is

$$l_1 = \sqrt{O_2c^2 + O_2d^2 - 2\times O_2c\times O_2d\times\cos(\gamma_0+\theta'_2)} \tag{10}$$

$$\gamma_0 = \angle cO_2d = \arctan\frac{m_2}{m_3} + \arcsin\frac{m_0}{O_2d} \tag{11}$$

The first-order derivatives of Eqs.(8), (9) and (10) are as follows:

$$\dot{\theta}'_2 = \frac{1}{\sqrt{O_2O_4{}^2 - (h-h_j)^2}}\dot{h} \tag{12}$$

$$\dot{l}_1 = \frac{O_2c\times O_2d\times\sin(\gamma_0+\theta'_2)}{l_1\sqrt{O_2O_4{}^2-(h-h_j)^2}}\dot{h} \tag{13}$$

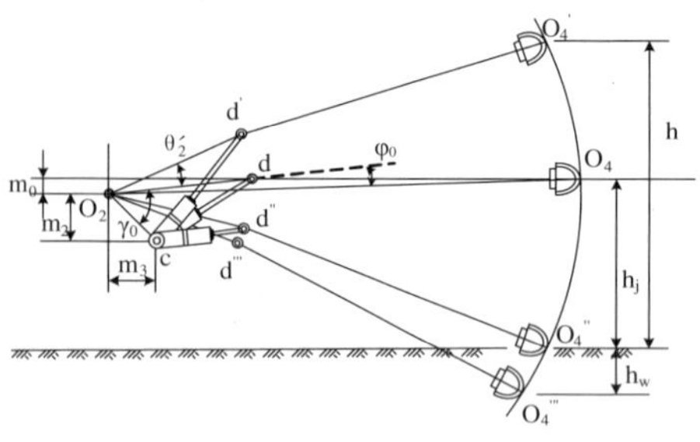

Fig. 3. Link geometry of the vertical swing

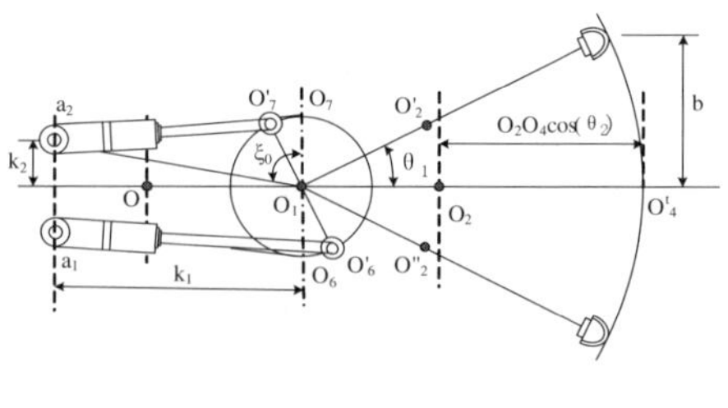

Fig. 4. Link geometry of the horizontal swing

Since $h={}^0z+b_1$, $h_j=b_1+b_2+b_3$, $\theta_2=-90^o-\theta'_2$, $m_0<<O_2d$, we can get $\dot{h}={}^0\dot{z}=v_z$, $\dot{\theta}_2=-\dot{\theta}'_2$. Omitting $\varphi_0=arcsin(m_0/O_2d)$, Eqs.(8), (9), (12) and (13) can be got by

$$\theta_2' = \arcsin\frac{{}^0z - b_2 - b_3}{O_2O_4} \qquad (-b_1-h_w \le {}^0z \le z_{max}+b_1) \tag{14}$$

$$\dot{\theta}_2 = \frac{-1}{\sqrt{O_2O_4^{\,2} - (h - h_j)^2}}\dot{h} \tag{15}$$

$$\dot{l}_1 = \frac{O_2c \times O_2d \times \sin(\gamma_0 + \theta_2')}{l_1\sqrt{O_2O_4^{\,2} - ({}^0z - b_2 - b_3)^2}} v_z \tag{16}$$

From Fig.4, we can got

$$\xi_0 = \angle a_2O_1O_7 = 90^\circ - \arctan\frac{k_2}{k_1} \tag{17}$$

$$\theta_1 = \arcsin\frac{b}{O_1O_2 + O_2O_4 \cdot \cos(\theta_2)} = \arcsin\frac{b}{L} \tag{18}$$

where $L=O_1O_2+O_2O_4\cos(\theta_2)$.

Respectively, the length l_{2ret} and l_{2ext} of the retraction and extension cylinder are as follows:

$$l_{2ret} = \sqrt{a_2O_1^{\,2} + O_1O_7^{\,2} - 2\times a_2O_1 \times O_1O_7 \times \cos(\xi_0 - \theta_1)} \tag{19}$$

$$l_{2ext} = \sqrt{a_2O_1^{\,2} + O_1O_7^{\,2} - 2\times a_2O_1 \times O_1O_7 \times \cos(\xi_0 + \theta_1)} \tag{20}$$

Since $b={}^0y$, thus $\dot{b}={}^0\dot{y}=v_y$. The first-order derivatives of Eqs.(18),(19) and (20) are

$$\dot{\theta}_1 = \frac{1}{\sqrt{(O_1O_2 + O_2O_4\cos(\theta_2))^2 - {}^0y^2}}\left(v_y + \frac{O_2O_4\sin(\theta_2)\,{}^0y}{O_1O_2 + O_2O_4\cos(\theta_2)}\dot{\theta}_2\right) \tag{21}$$

$$\dot{l}_{2ret} = v_{2ret} = -\frac{a_2O_1 \times O_1O_7 \times \sin(\xi_0 - \theta_1)}{l_{2ret}}\dot{\theta}_1 \tag{22}$$

$$\dot{l}_{2ext} = v_{2ext} = \frac{a_2O_1 \times O_1O_7 \times \sin(\xi_0 + \theta_1)}{l_{2ret}}\dot{\theta}_1 \tag{23}$$

3 Hydraulic System Modeling

The robotic roadheader uses an open center hydraulic system consisting of a variable pump with pressure and load-sensing com- pensator, an electro-hydraulic proportional directional valve and three pairs of asym- metric hydraulic cylinders. The pressure compensator adjusts the pump displacement according to the actual need of the sys-tem flow rate in order to keep the pressure constant. By keeping the pressure drop stream resistor constant, the load-sensing compensator represents a output flow rate control for the pump[2].

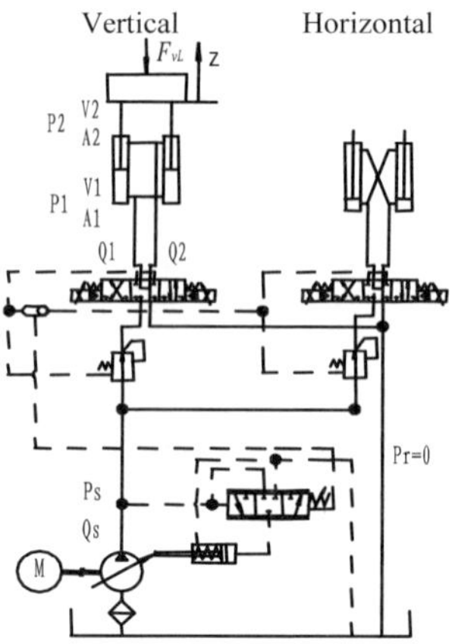

Fig. 5. Electro-hydraulic system

As shown in Fig.5, the electro-hydraulic proportional directional valve is simplified into a directional valve and a fixed differential reducing valve[3]. The steady state flow rate equations of the valve are given by

$$Q_1 = C_d w k_v u_v \sqrt{\frac{2}{\rho}\Delta P_1} = \begin{cases} C_d w k_v u_v \sqrt{\frac{2}{\rho}\Delta P} & u_v \geq 0 \\ C_d w k_v u_v \sqrt{\frac{2}{\rho} P_1} & u_v < 0 \end{cases}$$
$$Q_2 = C_d w k_v u_v \sqrt{\frac{2}{\rho}\Delta P_2} = \begin{cases} C_d w k_v u_v \sqrt{\frac{2}{\rho} P_2} & u_v \geq 0 \\ C_d w k_v u_v \sqrt{\frac{2}{\rho}\Delta P} & u_v < 0 \end{cases} \quad (24)$$

where Q_1 and Q_2 is the flow rate of non-rod and with-rod cavity, respectively; P_1, P_2 and P_r are the pressure of non-rod cavity, with-rod cavity and return oil, respectively; c_d is the orifice flow discharge coefficient; w is the orifice gradient of valve; ΔP is the spring setting pressure of load-sensing valve; ρ is the hydraulic fluid density; k_v is the electromagnetic proportional coefficient; u_v is the input voltage to drive the spool of the proportional valve.

3.1 Vertical Swing Cylinder Modeling

The flow rate continuity equations of the non-rod cavity and with-rod cavity in the vertical swing cylinder can be expressed as follows[4]:

$$Q_1 = A_1 \frac{dz}{dt} + \frac{V_1}{\beta}\frac{dP_1}{dt} \quad (25)$$

$$Q_2 = A_2 \frac{dz}{dt} - \frac{V_2}{\beta}\frac{dP_2}{dt} \quad (26)$$

where A_1 and A_2 are the effective area of the non-rod cavity and with-rod cavity, respectively; z is the displacement of the cylinder piston; V_1 and V_2 are the volume of the non-rod cavity and with-rod cavity, respectively; P_1 and P_2 are the pressure of the non-rod and with-rod cavity, respectively; β is the bulk modulus of hydraulic oil.

The flow rate relation between the non-rod cavity and the with-rod cavity can be expressed approximately as follows:

$$\frac{Q_1}{Q_2} = \frac{A_1}{A_2} \tag{27}$$

So combining Eqs.(24), (27) into (25), (26), the flow rate continuity equations are

$$C_d w k_v \sqrt{\frac{2}{\rho}\Delta P} u_v(t) = A_1 \dot{z} + \frac{V_1}{\beta}\dot{P}_1 \tag{28}$$

$$\frac{A_2}{A_1} C_d w k_v \sqrt{\frac{2}{\rho}\Delta P} u_v(t) = A_2 \dot{z} - \frac{V_2}{\beta}\dot{P}_2 \tag{29}$$

Given that the load is rigid, the force balance equation at the vertical swing hydraulic cylinder is

$$F = P_1 A_1 - P_2 A_2 = m\ddot{z} + c\dot{z} + F_{vL} \tag{30}$$

where F is the hydraulic drive force; m is the total mass of the piston and the load; c is the viscous damp coefficient; F_{vL} is the external load force in vertical direction.

Merging the Laplace transformation of Eqs.(28), (29) and (30), the piston displacement and the velocity equation are obtained by

$$z(s) = \frac{b_u U(s) + b_f s F_{vL}(s)}{(a_2 s^2 + a_1 s + a_0)s} \tag{31}$$

$$v_z(s) = \frac{b_u U(s) + b_f s F_{vL}(s)}{a_2 s^2 + a_1 s + a_0} \tag{32}$$

where $a_1=c$; $a_2=m$; $b_f=-1$; $a_0 = \frac{\beta}{V_1}A_1^2 + \frac{\beta}{V_2}A_2^2$; $b_u = \frac{A_1}{V_1}\beta K + \frac{A_2^2}{A_1 V_2}\beta K$; $K = C_d w k_v \sqrt{\frac{2}{\rho}\Delta P}$.

3.2 Horizontal Swing Cylinder Modeling

The modeling of horizontal swing cylinder is similar to that of vertical swing cylinder. Thus the piston displacement and velocity of the horizontal swing cylinder are

$$y(s) = \frac{d_u U(s) + d_f s F_{hL}(s)}{(e_2 s^2 + e_1 s + e_0)s} \tag{33}$$

$$v_y(s) = \frac{d_u U(s) + d_f s F_{hL}(s)}{e_2 s^2 + e_1 s + e_0} \tag{34}$$

where y is the displacement of the horizontal swing cylinder piston; F_{hL} is the external load force in horizontal direction; V_{h1} is the total volume of the inlet cavity; V_{h2} is the total volume of the outlet cavity; A is the total effective area of non-rod and with-rod cavity; R is the radius of the gyration platform; J is the inertia of the boom system; $d_f = -L$; $d_u = (\frac{1}{V_{h1}} + \frac{1}{V_{h2}})\beta ARK$; $e_0 = (\frac{1}{V_{h1}} + \frac{1}{V_{h2}})\beta A^2 R$; $e_1 = \frac{c}{R\sin\theta_1}$; $e_2 = \frac{J}{R\sin\theta_1}$.

4 Design of the Adaptive Controller

In the models shown above, the strong dynamic nonlinearity and system parameters uncertainty are the main problems in controlling the swing velocity of the robotic roadheader's cutter[5]. Hence the adaptive control is designed as a solution.

Generally, the controlled system can be expressed as follows[6][7]:

$$A(p)v(t) = B(p)u(t) \tag{35}$$

where $v(t)$ is the velocity output; $u(t)$ is the voltage input; p is the differential operator d/dt; $A(p) = p^n + \sum_{i=0}^{n-1} a_i p^i$; $B(p) = \sum_{j=0}^{m} b_j p^j$.

Then, the referential model is

$$A_M(p)v_M(t) = B_M(p)u_M(t) \tag{36}$$

where $A_M(p) = p^n + \sum_{i=0}^{n-1} a_i^M p^i$; $B_M(p) = \sum_{j=0}^{m} b_j^M p^j$; $a_0^M, \cdots a_{n-1}^M, b_0^M, \cdots b_m^M$ are unknown parameters.

When the perfect input $u_M(t)$ is given, the task of the adaptive controller is to find the system input that can make the system output $v(t)$ follow the output $v_M(t)$of the reference model asymptotically. The velocity reference model of the horizontal and vertical swing cylinders can be got as $m=0, n=2$ according to Eqs.(32) and (34).

The steady equations $H(p)=p^2+0.75p+0.125$ and $D(p)=1$ are chosen to make $H(p)D(p)/A_M(p)$ strictly steady according to the theory of the adaptive control[8].

Thus, the output error is

$$e_d(t) = D(p)e(t) = e(t) = v - v_M \tag{37}$$

The state variable filter and adjustable law of the adaptive controller are

$$\xi_i = \left[\frac{1}{H(p)}u(t) \quad \frac{p}{H(p)}u(t) \quad \frac{1}{H(p)}v(t) \quad \frac{p}{H(p)}v(t) \quad v(t) \quad \frac{B_m(p)}{H(p)}u_m(t) \right] \tag{38}$$

$$K_i = -\int_0^\infty \gamma_i \xi_i e_d(t)dt \qquad i = 1,2,3,4,5,6 \qquad \gamma_i > 0 \tag{39}$$

The input of the controlled system is

$$u(t) = \sum_{i=1}^{6} K_i \xi_i \tag{40}$$

Based on the steady theory, the model reference adaptive controller, which can be applied to the roadheader hydraulic and boom system control, is gained in Fig.6.

5 Simulation and Result

In order to illustrate the approach of the model reference adaptive controller, step voltage is used as input, and given F_{hL}=2.5kN, F_{vL}=1.17kN, U=6V. The velocity error, the reference model output and the control model output, three parameters of system velocity responses with the adaptive controller are shown in. Fig.7 and Fig.8.

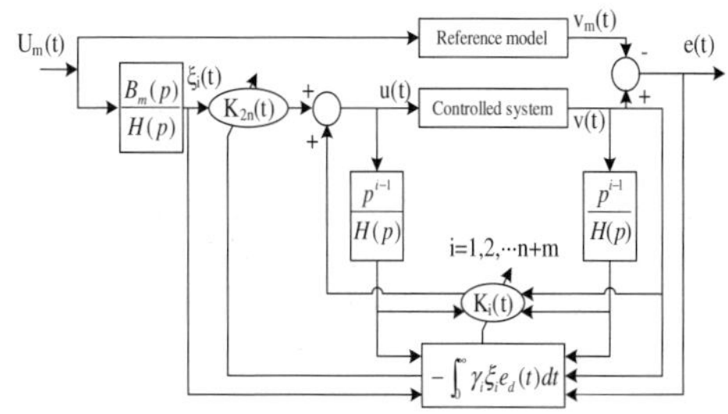

Fig. 6. Diagram of the model reference adaptive controller

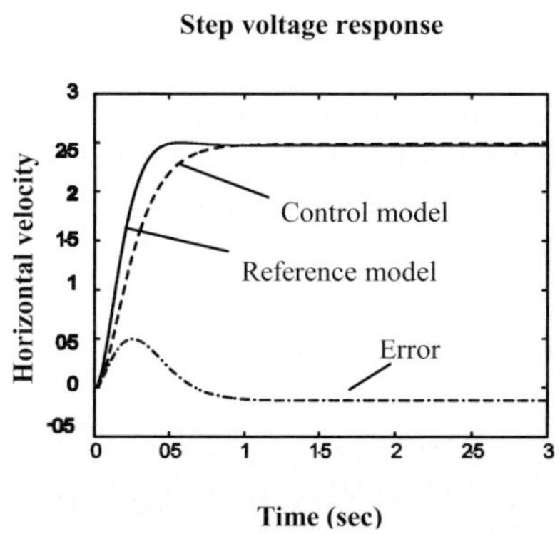

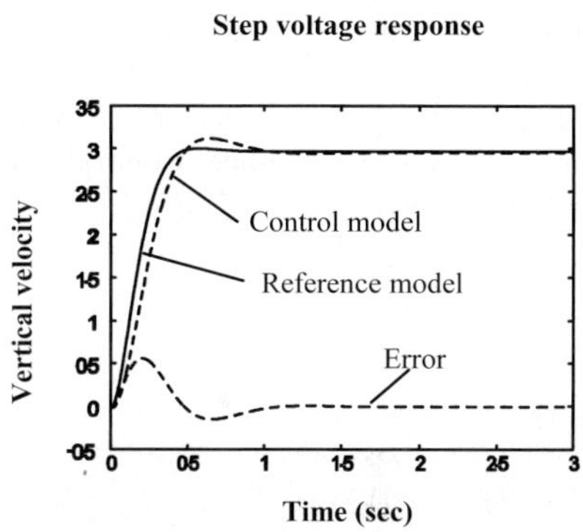

Fig. 7. The horizontal swing velocity response **Fig. 8.** The vertical swing velocity response

Fig.7 shows the horizontal swing velocity response of the cutter. Fig.8 shows the vertical swing velocity response of the cutter. The simulation studies clearly confirm that the model reference adaptive controller can be effectively applied to the velocity control of the robotic roadheader's cutter.

6 Conclusion

The boom-type roadheader is simplified into a robot, and its forward and inverse kinematics model and the hydraulic system model are established. As a solution to problems such as strong nonlinear of the kinematics model, parameters uncertainty, disturbance and asymmetric dynamic performance of the electro-hydraulic proportional system, a model reference adaptive controller using equilibrium point steady theory has been proposed to improve the swing velocity control of the roadheader's cutter. Simulation studies demonstrate the effectiveness of the proposed controller. The cutter position controller and the authentic control system design will be carried out to further the research in this field.

References

1. Xiong, Y.L.: Robotics. China Mechanical Press, Beijing (1993)
2. Xu, Y.M.: Analysis and Design for Electro-Hydraulic Proportional Control System. China Mechanical Press, Beijing (2005)
3. Chen, Q.G., Ji, Y.F., Wu, W.R.: Load Independent Flow Distribution Control Sytem. J. Hydraulic and Pneumatic 10, 10–11 (2003)
4. Zhang, W.H.: The Research of Non-symmetry Oil Cylinder System Controlled by Symmetry Valve and Characteristic. Changchun Photo Electronic and Mechanical College, Changchun University of Science and Technology (2002)
5. Zhang, D.Q., He, Q.H., Hao, P.: Trajectory Tracking Control of Hydraulic Excavator. Journal of Jilin University: Engineering and Technology 5, 490–494 (2005)
6. He, Q.H., Zhang, D.Q., Huang, Z.X., Zhang, X.H.: Adaptive Control of Hydraulic Excavator Manipulator. Journal of Tongji University 9, 1259–1263 (2007)
7. Chen, X.H., Li, Y.J., Zhou, J.: Adaptive control. Northwestern Protechnical University Press, Xi'an (2003)
8. Wu, Z.X., Zhang, L.C., Zhao, C.L.: Adaptive Controller and Its Application in Force System of Asymmetric Cylinder Controlled by Symmetric Valve. Chinese Journal of Mechanical Engineering 6, 50–53 (2007)

Automatic Excavation Planning of Hydraulic Excavator

Hui Shao, Hiroshi Yamamoto, Yuki Sakaida, Takashi Yamaguchi, Yuji Yanagisawa, and Akira Nozue

Incorporated Administrative Agency Public Works Research Institute, Construction Technology Research Department, Advanced Technology Research Team. 1-6, Minamihara, Tsukuba-shi, Ibaraki 305-8516 Japan
shao77@pwri.go.jp

Abstract. This paper describes an efficient trajectory planning method for hydraulic excavator tasks including a complete excavation/loading work cycle. Also provided is an effective method for analyzing geometric trajectories satisfying mechanical-geometric constraints. Additionally, a continuous excavation and shaping method is introduced for trench digging. In order to improve excavation efficiency, we reduced the work cycle for rough excavation but increased the work cycle for finishing excavation (shaping) using similar digging trajectories. Experimental continuous excavation and shaping was conducted and the results were evaluated. The key quantifiable benefits of this automatic technology include the liberation of human workers from many of the work processes, potential increase in work productivity, and significant labor savings.

Keywords: Trajectory Planning, Hydraulic Excavator, Automatic Excavation, Backhoe.

1 Introduction

Some research on the development of robotic excavators has produced a number of successful results, such as the Automatic Excavator [1], [2], [3], [4]. However, most of the research on terrestrial excavation is focused on simple earthmoving or partial work, rather than on automatic operation of the full excavation process including trench shaping, and the majority of reports do not discuss excavation accuracy. There are also many studies on the development of tele-operated excavators, controlled by means of levers on a remote control panel or by the operator controlling a "master", a scaled-down replica of the excavator, to operate the slave excavator [5], [6]. Although tele-operation technology frees workers from exposure to harsh environments, high-performance operation cannot be assured compared with on-board operation, due to the time delay effect of the remote controller or Man-Machine (MMI) Interface display.

The objective of our study was to dig a trench with the designed shape, including dumping the soil, using only automatic operations. The excavator was equipped with a GPS, laser scanner, and camera [8], as well as sensors that provided 3D topographic information.

C. Xiong et al. (Eds.): ICIRA 2008, Part II, LNAI 5315, pp. 1201–1211, 2008.

This paper first describes an effective analysis method for trajectory restrictions due to robot mechanical structure constraints. Then, a trapezoid trajectory as the base shape of the design is introduced. In the full excavation work process the balance between efficiency and accuracy is considered by regulating the work circle of the rough digging and the shaping excavation. The bucket tip is designed to follow the predetermined excavation trajectory, and the continuous excavation experiment is executed in the test yard using Kanto loam that does not contain any large or hard obstacles such as big stones or steel pipes. The operation efficiency for completing one cross section of the trench by automatic excavator is compared with the operator's operation. Lastly, in order to evaluate the bucket performance in following the trajectory, the experimental results of the shaping action in the air space measurements from the sensors and TS (Total Station) are presented and compared.

2 System Statement and Overview

2.1 Control System Statement

The system has the following characteristics:

- This is a tele-operating computer-assisted system. A digital signal generated by the remote controller is introduced to the planning component as a switching signal for Remote and Automatic modes.
- The machine is a free unit not connected to any external systems. (Small Specified Low-Power Radio Wireless and Wireless LAN are set.)
- The proposed system can be used at construction sites, such as for trenching, for example, to improve productivity by means other than human effort.

2.2 Machine System Overview

The excavator is a classic backhoe system, as shown in Fig. 1, with 4 degrees of freedom. The geometrical specifications are listed in Table 1. Potentiometers are installed on the swing, boom, arm and bucket joints as angle sensors. The excavator is equipped with three operation modes: on-board operation, remote operation, and automatic operation. In this study, the operation scenario was such that the excavator

Table 1. Backhoe geometrical specifications

Backhoe parameter	Value
Boom length	4600 mm
Arm length	2519 mm
Bucket length	1230 mm
Swing joint range	–180° to 180°
Boom joint range	–71° to 44°
Arm joint range	31° to 152°
Bucket joint range	–33° to 144°
Bucket bottom angle	49°
Bucket volume	0.5 m^3
Joint position sensors	4 potentiometers

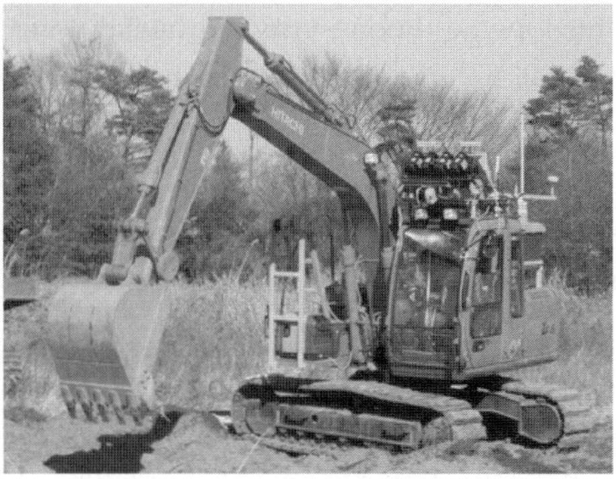

Fig. 1. Photograph of backhoe excavator

and dump truck traveled under remote control operation. After reaching their destination (confirmed by MMI PC), the operation mode was switched to automatic mode, and autonomous excavation and loading planning began. As the first planning step, using topographic information, automatic continuous digging and dumping for trench excavation assuming flat ground was designed and tested.

2.3 Control System Overview

As shown in Fig. 2, the control system for automatic excavation and dumping operation consists of a planning component and a control component. The planning component, a main feature of this study, was constructed in the xPC Target environment of Matlab Simulink, and comprises a Master PC and Slave PC with wireless LAN connection. The FF-PID (FeedForward-Proportion Integration Deviation) controllers are designed in the control component.

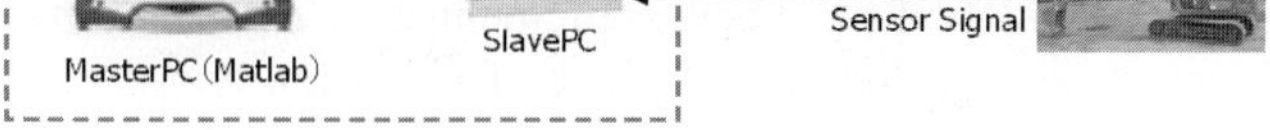

Fig. 2. Control system overview

3 Coordinate System

Coordinate system assignment is shown in Fig. 3. The origin is placed at the rotational center of the excavator body using the height of the boom foot pin. The ground level (GL) from the crawler is about -1.5 m in the coordinate.

$\theta_1, \theta_2, \theta_3, \theta_4$ are defined swing, boom, arm and bucket joint angle, separately. The orientation of the bucket can be specified by the value of the joint variable θ_4 relative to the x3 axis, or by the angle θ_{bucket} (also expressed as the bucket) relative to the x0 axis, where $\theta_{bucket} = \theta_2 + \theta_3 + \theta_4$. In our case, the orientation angle θ_{bucket} of the bucket based on the x0-y0 plane of the origin coordinate is used to specify the orientation of the bucket, as shown in Fig. 4.

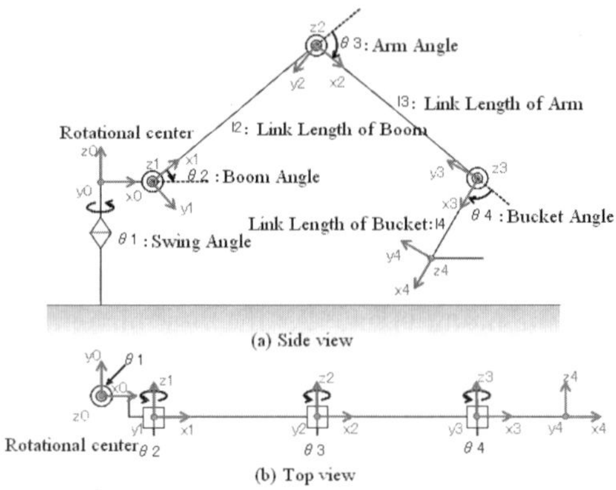

Fig. 3. Coordinate system of excavator

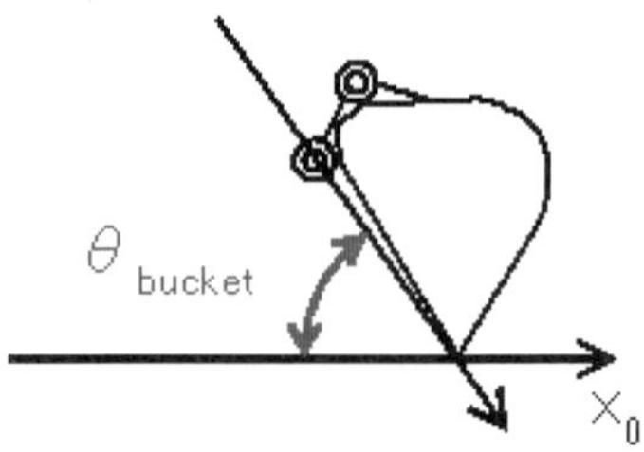

Fig. 4. Orientation angle of bucket

4 Trajectory Analysis (Geometric Analysis)

For automated operation, it is necessary to determine whether or not the end-effect position is reachable. This computation is frequently used for calculating the reachability constraint [2]. Singh uses digging height z and orientation angle, to determine digging distance x from the coordinate origin which differs from our method. In our case, however, the reachability orientation angle constraint contour figure has been complemented, as shown in Fig. 5(a), (b). The color changing from blue (downward) to red (top) shown in the right vertical axis displays the angle range from about -73° to 341° . In Fig.5 the vertical reachable range of the bucket end-effect are also displayed.

A fast lookup table method has been implemented to determine the bucket reachability orientation angle θ_{bucket} in the x-z plane. The method works as follows: The x and z dimensions are divided into discrete intervals (2 cm and 10 cm, respectively). For each (x, z) pair mapped to a (row, column) of the table, a maximum and a minimum orientation angle θ_{bucket} will automatically be found from the table file. So, if a candidate digging point is determined, a reachable orientation angle can be found that satisfies the following formula:

$$\theta_{bucket\_min} <= \theta_{bucket} <= \theta_{bucket\_max} \tag{1}$$

In this process, due to (x, z) pair mapping errors, the determined reachable orientation angles θ_{bucket_min} and θ_{bucket_max} will contain errors to some extent.

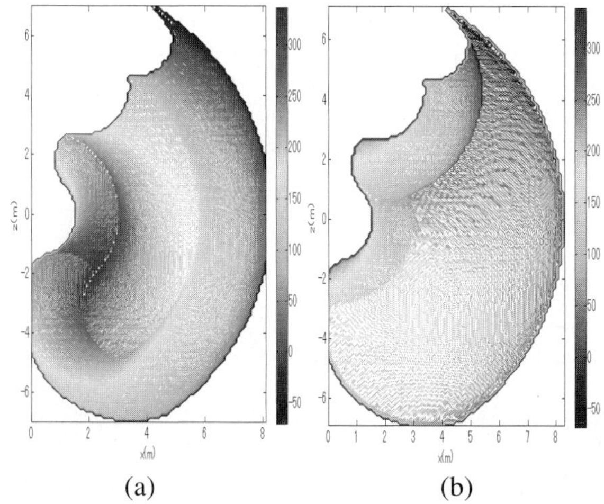

Fig. 5. Maximum and minimum reachable angle at each location on the x-z plane

1) Initial location

Initial location is selected as the point where it is easiest to move to the excavation start location with the excavator in the proper position.

2) Moving to the excavation start location

The designed move to the excavation start location takes into consideration the starting acceleration and stopping deceleration of the boom, arm and bucket joint's motions, and the rotation action considers the stopping deceleration. The digging start location is selected as the point where it is easiest to produce sufficiently large force required for excavation based on the operator's skills. For continuous digging operation, the first digging start location is decided, and then the other digging start location is calculated by decreasing the deviation of the coordinate value of the first digging start location. The deviation is calculated based on the number of digging times, trench depth and inclination. The number of finishing digging times can be set freely.

3) Trapezoid digging trajectory

As our task was to complete a trapezoid trench, skilled operators' operating trajectories for completing one cross section of a trapezoid trench were measured. The requirements for the trench were 1:1 slope, 1 m depth, 2 m bottom length, and one-side shaping with dumping at ground level (GL). The digging radius of our backhoe is about 8 m, and the operator selected an appropriate digging start point at about far 7 m from boom foot-pin. One example of the digging pattern of a skilled operator with shallower and longer dragging is given. Fig. 6 shows a side view of the vertical cross section of trench digging. The digging shape produced by the operator is similar to the trapezoid shape. After referencing numerous operating trajectories, we designed the trapezoid digging trajectory shown in Fig. 7. By changing the gradient of the trench, different digging objectives can be achieved.

The digging action is typically divided into four different motions: slope penetration, straight dragging, bucket curling and vertical lifting, shown in Fig. 7 as the base trajectory (black line). We would like the robot excavator to be able to excavate a volume of soil in accordance with its specifications. So, each time, the volume of excavated soil was set larger than the bucket volume. Depending on the described volume of earth using the trapezoid shape, the digging depth H and dragging length and the curving start location $x_0 - w_1 - w_2$ of the bucket tip can be determined.

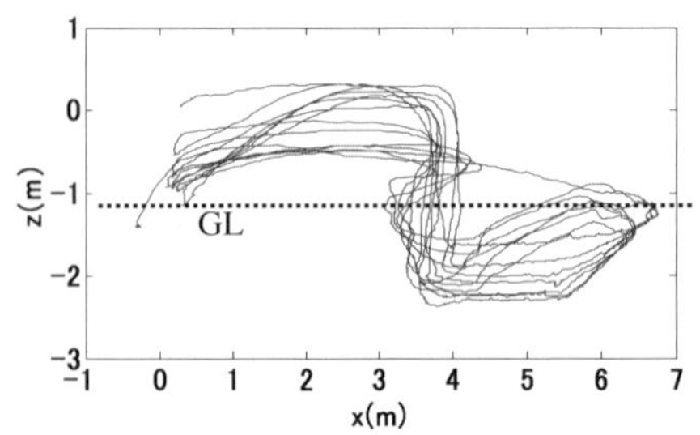

Fig. 6. Skilled operator's digging trajectory

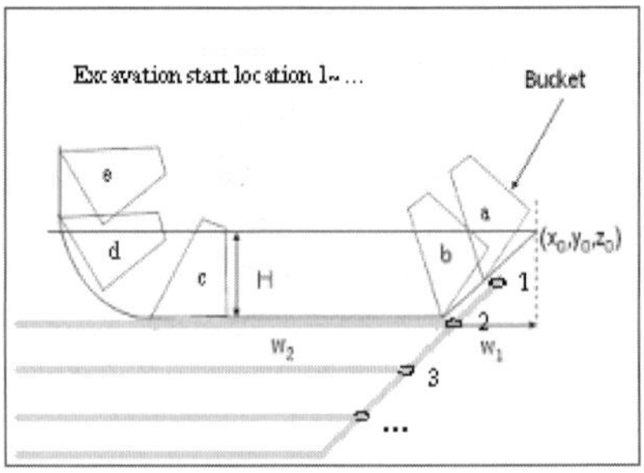

Fig. 7. Excavation planning

To ensure good digging performance of the trapezoid trajectory for the bucket, the consideration must be given to instantaneous orientation control of the bucket from a to e along with a trajectory that ensures that the bucket is filled. The changing pattern of the orientation angle θ_{bucket} following the trapezoid trajectory is shown in Fig. 7, where (x_0, y_0, z_0) is the starting point for digging.

After curling, the orientation angle of the bucket is 180°. The bucket will be directly lifted to a point higher than the location where the earth was left preventing collision between the bucket and the ground, with the orientation angle θ_{bucket} persisting at 180° or more to prevent any earth from falling out of the bucket.

4) Rotation

After finishing Step 3), the bucket is raised and rotated toward the dumping location completing the rotation and decelerating to a stop at the same time. In our case, the rotation angle can be set to any value. In this study, the dumping location is at ground level.

5) Dumping

Due to complete dumping on the ground, this step simply controls the bucket and arm joint so as to implement dumping action at the same time.

6) Moving to the next digging start point

This action is similar to Step 2).

An example of continuous excavation using a trapezoid trajectory is provided. Each digging start point of the continuous excavation process is shown in Fig. 7, and the digging height and width are calculated corresponding to the target requirements and rough digging times.

5 Experiments

The study task of automatic excavation included digging a trench with a slope inclination of 1:1, depth of 1.0 m, bottom length of 2.0 m, with a cross section of the bucket width of the excavator on flat ground (GL is about -1.5 m in the machine coordinate). Therefore, 3–4 times rough digging and 2–3 times finishing digging (shaping) was implemented to realize a cross section of the trench. Since tracking performance is affected by tracking time, we attempted to improve the efficiency of automatic excavation by setting the rough excavation cycle to 22 sec, disregarding digging accuracy. However, in order to satisfy the required accuracy, the shaping action cycle was set to 44 sec. Although a skilled operator can achieve a maximum speed of about 15 sec for one work cycle, with the average speed being about 19–21 sec, these times cannot be continued for long. The automatic excavator, on the other hand, can continue working until the oil tank is empty. Judging from skilled operators' operation data, the average operation circle takes about 2 min 40 sec to complete a task similar to the one mentioned above, and the robot requires only slightly longer, as shown in Table 2. Moreover, for the robot, some of the steps in the work process such as dumping and rotation can be shortened even further; therefore, compared with the time achieved by the skilled operator, the time required to finish one cross section using automatic excavation is not inferior.

Table 2. Action comparison

	Rough digging number	Shaping number	Cycle time for digging one section
Operator	4 times	3 times	2 min 40 sec
Automation	4 times	2 times	2 min 56 sec

5.1 Excavation and Dumping Experiment

Figure 8 (a), (b) shows the planning trajectory for one cycle and the corresponding constraint orientation angle of the bucket. x_r *(dashed line)*, y_r *(solid line)* and z_r *(dotted line)* in the (a) are the bucket end-effect position in the machine coordinate. the_{bucket} *max(dashed line)*, the_{bucket} *min (solid line)* and the_{bucket} *(dotted line)* in the (b) are the maximum orientation angle, the minimum orientation angle and the planned orientation angle. From that we can see that the designed orientation position angle θ_{bucket} along with the changing trajectory is in the range [$\theta_{bucket\_\min}$, $\theta_{bucket\_\max}$]. The excavation results of the trench are shown in Fig. 9 (a), (b), (c). In Fig. 9 (a) the *dotted lines* are the designed trajectories of the bucket tip, the *solid lines* are the bucket tip trajectories in the time axis. From that we can see the data log for digging2, digging3,

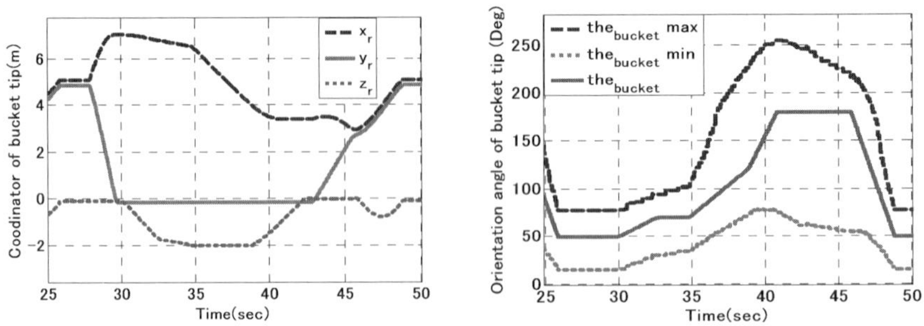

Fig. 8. Planned trajectory and corresponding orientation angle

digging4 and shaping1, 2, where it is a trench excavation there are 4 times rough digging and two times shaping excavation, the data is logged from the second digging. From that we can also see the cycle time of the rough diggings and the cycle time of the shaping excavations are different. From Fig. 9 (b) we can see the cross-section trajectory of the continuous excavation. The shaping error of direction z is smaller than 10 cm. To some extent, we have achieved automatic continuous excavation and dumping, including shaping action with the required accuracy. Figure 9 (c) shows the top view of the backhoe coordinates. In the trenching work process, we did not focus too intensely on accuracy during the lift operation and dumping end in the air space. Figure 10 shows the scenery of excavation and dumping and the finished trench. The scale placed at the bottom of the trench is about 2 m in length.

5.2 Tracking Measurement of Bucket Tip by TS (Total Station)

Total Station is a distance measurement instrument used at civil construction sites. In this study, we used Total Station GTS800 from TOPCON. In order to compare the accuracy of the bucket following the trajectory with the world coordinates, we calculated the position of the bucket tip using the sensor data and measured the position of the bucket tip by TS at the same time, as shown in Fig. 11. O_G is the origin of the world coordinates. O is the origin of the machine coordinates. Based on the adequacy of discussing shaping action performance, TS was set to track the reflection sheet pasted on the side of bucket tip, while moving action was slowly performed in the air space. The sensor data was logged at the same time. After coordinate transformation, the trajectory of the bucket tip calculated by the sensor data in machine coordinates was converted into world coordinates, and then compared with the TS data, wherein the TS data is compensated into the middle location of the bucket tip. The measured results are shown in Fig. 12 (a), (b). Figure 12 (a) is the Gx-Gz plane of the world coordinates, and (b) is the Gy-Gz plane of the world coordinates. From Fig. 12 we can see that the movement accuracy of the position control almost reflects the measurement accuracy under the world coordinates, satisfying the construction requirements. This makes it possible to complete the designed task with required accuracy at construction sites by utilizing 3D terrain information and GPS information.

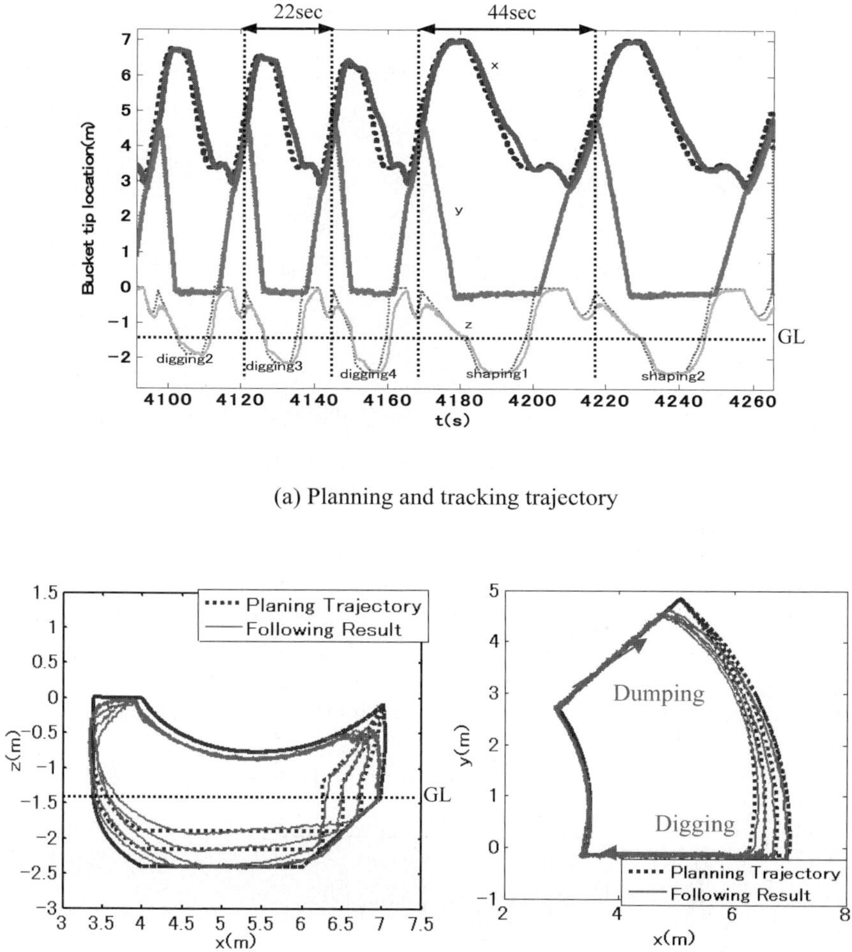

(a) Planning and tracking trajectory

(b) Side view of the bucket trajectory (c) Top view of the bucket trajectory

Fig. 9. Trajectory tracking results of continuous excavation

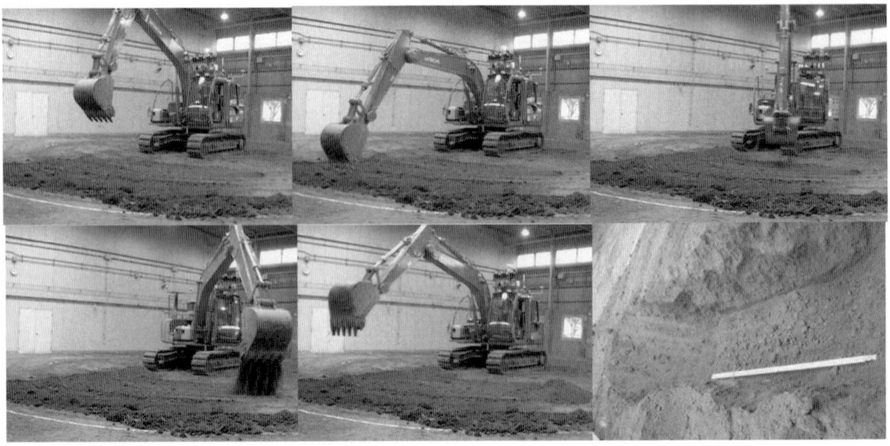

Fig. 10. Excavation and dumping scene: the picture was listed by the turn of initial posture, digging, rotating, dumping, moving to the next excavation location and the trench shape

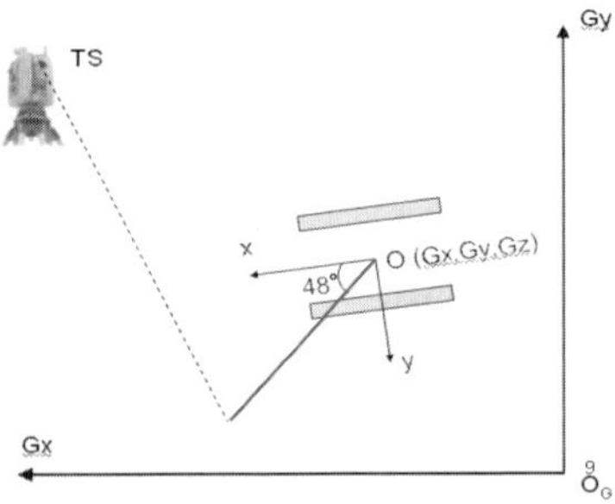

Fig. 11. TS measurement scene

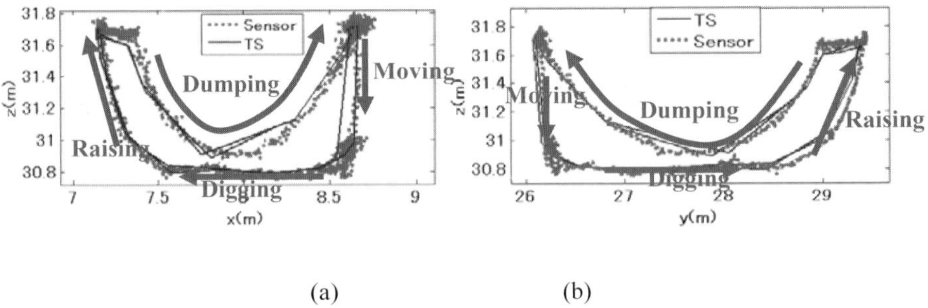

Fig. 12. Results of TS measurement

6 Conclusions

In this study, the continuous automatic digging experiment for the defined objective of trench digging with required accuracy was completed successfully, and the shaping accuracy was nearly satisfied. Throughout the operation process, in order to guarantee both work productivity and work precision, we proposed rough excavation and finishing excavation with similar digging trajectory. The efficiency of the automatic excavator is not inferior to that of skilled operators. In the future, the digging start location, digging depth and length will be generated automatically based on basis of the 3D information, and the numbers of finishing excavation times will be determined by the shaping accuracy. Although the system has not been designed to adapt to an environment with large obstacles, it could complete trench digging tasks regardless of soft or hard soil conditions using 3D information. Our work makes it possible to apply automatic excavation to a civil construction work site not only for simple earthmoving tasks, but also for more complex work. The expected bucket end-effect trajectory would be generated automatically in the future and the excavator is also expected to operate automatically in a random, unstructured environment and automatically become mobile on construction sites.

References

1. Rowe, P.S.: Adaptive Motion Planning for Autonomous Mass Excavation, Ph.D Thesis, Carnegie Mellon University (1999)
2. Singh, S.: Synthesis of Tactical Plans for Robotic Excavation, Ph.D Thesis, Carnegie Mellon University (1995)
3. Bradley, D.A., Seward, D.W., Mann, J.E., Goodwin, M.R.: Artificial Intelligence in The Control and Operation of Construction Plant—The Autonomous Robot Excavator. Automation in construction 2, 217–228 (1993)
4. Quang, N.H.: Robust Low Level Control of Robotic Excavation, Ph.D Thesis, Australian Center for Field Robotics, The University of Sydney (2000)
5. Kimura, N., Inoue, S., Fujioka, A., Kawakami, K.: Examination of practical utility of remotely controlled robots in disasters. In: 23rd ISARC, Tokyo, Japan, pp. 642–647 (2006)
6. Hirabayashi, T., Yamaguchi, T., Yano, H., Iwata, H.: Experiment on Teleoperation of Underwater Backhoe with Haptic Information. In: 23rd ISARC, Tokyo, Japan, pp. 36–41 (2006)
7. Shao, H., Yamaguchi, T., Yamamoto, H.: Bucket Trajectory Planning of Hydraulic Excavator. In: 12th Robotics Symposium, Nagaoka, Japan, pp. 354–359 (2007)
8. Yamamoto, H., Ishimatsu, Y., Yamaguchi, T., Uesaka, K., Aritomi, K., Tanaka, Y.: Introduction to the General Technology Development Project: Research and Development of Advanced Execution Technology by Remote Control Robot and Information Technology. In: 23rd ISARC, Tokyo, Japan, pp. 24–29 (2006)

Accuracy of a Novel Parallel Robot with Orthogonal Chains

Wei Liu[1,2], Feng Gao[3], Kaicheng Qi[1,2], and Jianzheng Zhang[3]

[1] School of Mechanical Engineering & Automation, BeiHang University, Beijing, 100083, China
[2] School of Mechanical Engineering, Hebei University of Technology, Tianjin, 300130, China
[3] State Key Laboratory of Mechanical System and Vibration, Shanghai Jiao Tong University, Shanghai, 200030, China
canglang_1@me.buaa.edu.cn

Abstract. A novel parallel robot with orthogonal chains and redundant actuators was designed for simulator. In order to improve the accuracy of the simulator, a comprehensive error model and a new method of kinematic calibration were studied. Based on the orthogonal feature of the mechanism and the principle of the influence coefficients, the error model was established, which accommodated all possible geometrical errors: the joint manufacturing errors, the installation errors, the actuation errors etc. A sensitivity index was designed to characterize the influence of the error sources on the end precision. Based on the index, error analysis was carried out to decide the major errors that need to be identified in kinematic calibration. Furthermore, a new calibration method based on relative displacement measurement was presented for avoiding the high-cost end pose measurement. Finally, the simulation of the calibration gave the validation of the new method.

Keywords: parallel robot; accuracy; error model; kinematic calibration.

1 Introduction

For several advantages of high rigidity, smaller moving mass and high-speed, the parallel robots now apply in more and more area. Here, a novel parallel robot with orthogonal chains and redundant actuators is designed for simulator.

One of the important issues in using parallel robots is accuracy. In engineering, error analysis and kinematic calibration are used to improve the accuracy of the machines after completing installation, and that error analysis plays an important role to guide the kinematic calibration.

With the method of Denavit-Hartenberg(D-H), Wang[1] and Maurine[2] studied the error models of Stewart and Delta4 platform respectively. T. Ropponen and T. Arai[3] set up the error model using the differential method to analyze the influence of the driving errors and the joints errors on the end effectors. Based on the vector analytical method, Huang[4] studied the error mapping of a class of 3-DOF parallel manipulator and identified the source errors affecting the uncompensable pose error.

C. Xiong et al. (Eds.): ICIRA 2008, Part II, LNAI 5315, pp. 1212–1222, 2008.

Other researchers [5, 6] focused on the effects of joint clearance on the end accuracy. The unsatisfactory of the previous works was the complicated modeling process using the matrix transfer or partial derivation. Furthermore, most error models in previous works did not contain all the possible error sources.

Thanks to the orthogonal feature of the mechanism and the principle of influence coefficients, the error model of the simulator is established without complicated calculation, which taking into account all the 144 possible geometrical errors.

As mentioned above, the most economical and feasible way to enhance the machine accuracy is kinematic calibration. The former researchers have proposed various calibration techniques. The double ball bar systems [7, 8] were used to get the measurement information to identify the kinematic parameters. Other measurement apparatus were also used to calibrate the parallel robots [9~11]. Huang [12] proposed to identify the parameters using a minimum set of pose error measurements.

However, most of the previous researchers got the pose data via the expensive or complex measuring equipment. Few investigations focus on improving the calibration model for identifying the parameters with the low-cost measurement ways. In this paper a new method based on relative displacement errors in single-direction was proposed. With this method, we can only use the common and low-cost measurement instruments to get the 6 relative displacements.

The remainder of this paper is organized as follows. The following section briefly reviews a mechanism of a novel parallel robot with orthogonal chains and redundant actuator and illustrates the coordinate frame systems. Section 3 outlines the error modeling strategy. Error analysis is discussed in section 4. The calibration strategy and the simulation validation are described in section 5 and 6.

2 Description of the Parallel Simulator

As shown in Fig. 1, the simulator is a fully parallel manipulator, for which an upper platform is connected to the base through six kinematic chains which are arranged orthogonally. Every chains consist of three assembled joints: prismatic-spherical-spherical joints. The prismatic is the actuator. To achieve high payload, branched-chain 1 and 6 are double actuated.

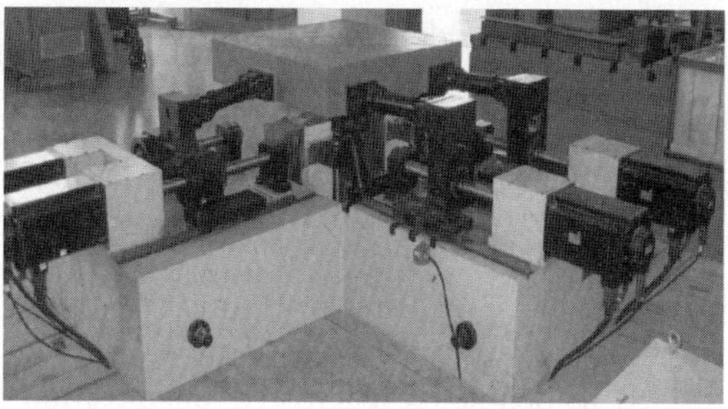

Fig. 1. Six DOF parallel simulator

Fig. 2 illustrates the sketch of the simulator and the coordinate frame systems. $O'-x'y'z'(\{F'\})$ and $O-xyz(\{F\})$ denoted, respectively, the moving and fixed coordinate frames. At the initial pose, the moving and the fixed coordinate system had the same pose.

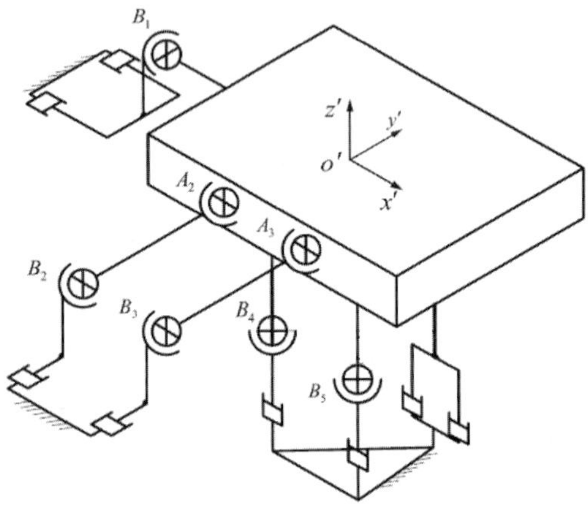

Fig. 2. Sketch of the parallel simulator

3 Error Modeling of the Parallel Simulator

In order to take all geometric errors into account, each kinematic chain is equivalent to the corresponding series mechanism, and described by D-H coordinate system. The universal joint is equivalent to two series revolute joints, and spherical joints to three series revolute joint, which allow the manufacturing and assembling errors of joints to be accommodated in the error model.

Each leg comprises 28 D-H parameters. The prismatic joint is the actuating joint, the universal and spherical joints are the passive joints. If the errors of the passive variable are not considered, the number of error parameters of each leg is 23. In addition, each leg has a driving error δl_i $(i=1,2.....6)$, so, 144 error parameters in total are taken into account in the error models. All the errors are as follows:

$\delta \boldsymbol{a}_i = [\delta a_{i0}, \delta a_{i1}, \delta a_{i2}, \delta a_{i3}, \delta a_{i4}, \delta a_{i5}, \delta a_{i6}]^T$;

$\delta \boldsymbol{\alpha}_i = [\delta \alpha_{i0}, \delta \alpha_{i1}, \delta \alpha_{i2}, \delta \alpha_{i3}, \delta \alpha_{i4}, \delta \alpha_{i5}, \delta \alpha_{i6}]^T$;

$\delta \boldsymbol{d}_i = [\delta d_{i1}, \delta d_{i2}, \delta d_{i3}, \delta d_{i4}, \delta d_{i5}, \delta d_{i6}, \delta d_{i7}]^T$;

$\delta \boldsymbol{\theta}_i = [\delta \theta_{i1}, \delta \theta_{i7}]^T$, δl_i, $(i=1,2.....6)$.

$\boldsymbol{D}_p$ and $\boldsymbol{D}_R$ are defined to denote, respectively, the position error vector and the orientation error vector of the end-effector. According to the method of the influence coefficients, $\boldsymbol{D}_p$ and $\boldsymbol{D}_R$ can be expressed in the form by:

$$\boldsymbol{D}_p = \boldsymbol{G}_{ia}^P \cdot \boldsymbol{\delta a}_i + \boldsymbol{G}_{id}^P \cdot \boldsymbol{\delta d}_i + \boldsymbol{G}_{i\alpha}^P \cdot \boldsymbol{\delta \alpha}_i + \boldsymbol{G}_{i\theta}^P \cdot \boldsymbol{\delta \theta}_i \ . \quad (1)$$

$$\boldsymbol{D}_R = \boldsymbol{G}_{i\theta}^R \cdot \boldsymbol{\delta \theta}_i + \boldsymbol{G}_{i\alpha}^R \cdot \boldsymbol{\delta \alpha}_i \ . \quad (2)$$

Where, $\boldsymbol{G}_{ia}^P, \boldsymbol{G}_{id}^P, \boldsymbol{G}_{i\theta}^P, \boldsymbol{G}_{i\alpha}^P, \boldsymbol{G}_{i\theta}^R$ and $\boldsymbol{G}_{i\alpha}^R$ are error influence coefficients matrixes. In fact, these error influence coefficients matrixes can be obtained directly with the method of reference [13].

Combined eq.(1) and eq.(2) to the following form:

$$\boldsymbol{D}_d = \boldsymbol{G}_{ia}^D \cdot \boldsymbol{\delta a}_i + \boldsymbol{G}_{id}^D \cdot \boldsymbol{\delta d}_i + \boldsymbol{G}_{i\alpha}^D \cdot \boldsymbol{\delta \alpha}_i + \boldsymbol{G}_{i\theta}^D \cdot \boldsymbol{\delta \theta}_i \ . \quad (3)$$

Where $\boldsymbol{D}_d$ is the pose error vector of the end-effector, and:

$$\boldsymbol{G}_{ia}^D = \begin{bmatrix} \boldsymbol{G}_{ia}^P \\ \boldsymbol{0}_{3\times6} \end{bmatrix}, \quad \boldsymbol{G}_{id}^D = \begin{bmatrix} \boldsymbol{G}_{id}^P \\ \boldsymbol{0}_{3\times6} \end{bmatrix}, \quad \boldsymbol{G}_{i\alpha}^D = \begin{bmatrix} \boldsymbol{G}_{i\alpha}^P \\ \boldsymbol{G}_{i\alpha}^R \end{bmatrix}, \quad \boldsymbol{G}_{i\theta}^D = \begin{bmatrix} \boldsymbol{G}_{i\theta}^P \\ \boldsymbol{G}_{i\theta}^R \end{bmatrix}$$

With the help of driving errors, applying eq.(3) to six legs of the simulator, the following expression in matrix form can be obtained:

$$\boldsymbol{D} = \boldsymbol{J} \cdot \boldsymbol{\delta q} + \boldsymbol{G}_a \cdot \boldsymbol{\delta a} + \boldsymbol{G}_\alpha \cdot \boldsymbol{\delta \alpha} + \boldsymbol{G}_d \cdot \boldsymbol{\delta d} + \boldsymbol{G}_\theta \cdot \boldsymbol{\delta \theta} \ . \quad (4)$$

Where : $\boldsymbol{D} = [\delta x, \delta y, \delta z, \delta\alpha, \delta\beta, \delta\gamma]^T$;

$\boldsymbol{\delta q} = [\delta l_1, \delta l_2, \delta l_3, \delta l_4, \delta l_5, \delta l_6]^T$ is the vector of driving error;

$\boldsymbol{J}$ is the Jacobian matrix of the simulator;

$[\boldsymbol{\delta a}]_{42\times1}$, $[\boldsymbol{\delta \alpha}]_{42\times1}$, $[\boldsymbol{\delta d}]_{42\times1}$ and $[\boldsymbol{\delta \theta}]_{12\times1}$ are all the errors to be considered; $[\boldsymbol{G}_a]_{6\times42}$, $[\boldsymbol{G}_\alpha]_{6\times42}$, $[\boldsymbol{G}_d]_{6\times42}$ and $[\boldsymbol{G}_\theta]_{6\times12}$ are all the error influence coefficient matrixes corresponding to the errors.

4 Error Analysis of the Parallel Simulator

Eq. (4) is the error model including 144 errors. Each error has a different impact on the end accuracy. Determining the major errors is significant to kinematics calibration and error compensation.

$$E_{pi} = D_{pi} / D_{p\max} \ . \quad (5)$$

$$E_{Ri} = D_{Ri} / D_{R\max} \ . \quad (6)$$

E_{pi} and E_{Ri} are error sensitivity indexes which are defined to characterize the comprehensive impact of each error on the end accuracy.

D_{pi} and D_{Ri} represent the average of the position and orientation errors of the end platform due to error i in the workspace. $D_{p\max}$ and $D_{R\max}$ show the maximum value of the position and orientation errors of the end platform due to all errors in the workspace. Based on the index, the influence of 144 errors on the end accuracy is studied through numerical simulation.

The major nominal values of the parameters of the simulator are: the dimension of the platform is 1m×1m×0.2m, the length of the bar between the two spherical joint (A_iB_i) is 0.372m, joint A_1 is located at the center of the side of the platform. The distance between two joints A_2 and A_3 is 0.6m, other dimensions are illustrated in reference [14].

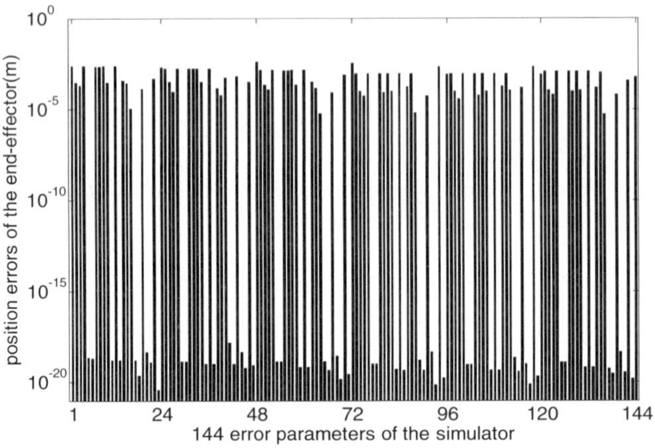

Fig. 3. Position errors of the end-effector due to the 144 errors

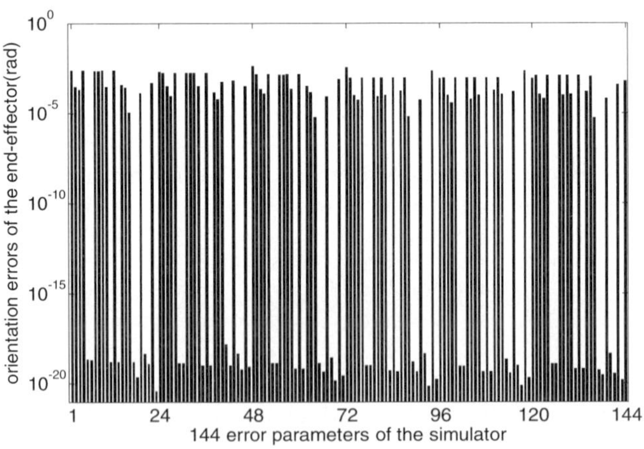

Fig. 4. Orientation errors of the end-effector due to the 144 errors

The aim of the simulation is to study the comprehensive impact of each error on the end accuracy. The desired trajectories are as follows: The end-effector performs along the axes of x, y and z and around the axes of x', y' and z', respectively. The average value of the errors of end-effector in one trajectory is defined to denote the influence on the end accuracy.

To illustrate explicitly, each value of the length error is given 0.002m, and also each angular error is given 1 degree. Then the numerical simulation is performed in Matlab to analysis the 144 error parameters' influence on the end accuracy.

The 144 error parameters' influences on the end position and orientation errors are shown in Fig. 3 and Fig. 4. The serial number of the errors is arranged by the order of the leg, namely, 1~24 belong to the leg 1, 25 ~ 48 belong to the leg 2, and by analogy, 121 ~ 144, belong to the leg 6.

As is clearly shown in fig. 3 and fig. 4, the end errors due to some error parameters are significant and due to others are very small. Anatomizing the simulation result, we find that, in each leg, the number of error parameters which have great influence on the end accuracy is 15. These 15 error parameters are $\delta l_i, \delta a_{i0}, \delta a_{i1}, \delta a_{i2}, \delta a_{i5}$, $\delta a_{i6}, \delta d_{i1}, \delta d_{i2}, \delta d_{i4}, \delta d_{i6}, \delta d_{i7}, \delta\alpha_{i0}, \delta\alpha_{i3}, \delta\alpha_{i6}$ and $\delta\theta_{i7}$ ($i = 1, 2......6$), which denote, respectively, the axis errors of the joint, dimension errors of the fixed length bar and the driving errors.

Now, the error parameters of leg i to be identified in calibration will be confirmed among the 15 errors. Through investigating, we can see that δa_{i0} and δd_{i2} denote the same position error of the joint center, which can be combined to one error, $\delta a_{i2}, \delta a_{i5}, \delta\alpha_{i0}$, $\delta\alpha_{i3}$, $\delta\alpha_{i6}$ and $\delta\theta_{i7}$ are the manufacturing errors of the joint. For the high precision of the standardized parts, the manufacturing errors of the spherical joint will be very small, so it will be ignored in the kinematic calibration. Consequently, 8 errors of leg i are considered in calibration: δl_i, $\delta a_{i0} + \delta d_{i2}$, δa_{i1}, $\delta a_{i6}, \delta d_{i1}, \delta d_{i4}, \delta d_{i6}$ and δd_{i7}. So, 48 errors of the simulator in total are determined to be identified in the calibration.

5 Kinematic Calibration Algorithm

A new calibration model will be set up in this section to identify the parameters with a low-cost measurement method. A vernier caliper will be used to measure the relative displacement of 4 target balls installed to the platform.

It is well-known that the pose of the end-effector can be described by a coordinate frame attached to the platform: the position vector $\left[x, y, z\right]^T$ and the orientation angle α, β and γ (Z-Y-X Euler angles).

As shown in Fig. 5, $\boldsymbol{O'-x'y'z'}$ ($\{F'\}$) is the moving coordinate frame attached to the platform.

The target balls $N_0 \sim N_3$ are accurately installed to ensure the parallelity of vector $\boldsymbol{N_0N_1}, \boldsymbol{N_0N_2}$ and $\boldsymbol{N_0N_3}$ with the corresponding coordinate axis of $\{F'\}$.

Then we can describe the orientation of the upper-platform by the direction cosine of the angle between the three vector $\boldsymbol{N_0N_1}$, $\boldsymbol{N_0N_2}$, $\boldsymbol{N_0N_3}$ and the corresponding axis of the fixed coordinate frame $\{F\}$.

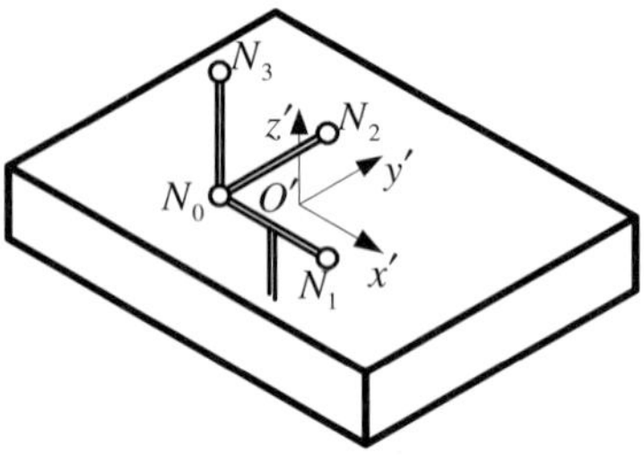

Fig. 5. The target ball and the upper-platform of the simulator

We define that the fixed coordinate frame ($\{F\}$) coincided with the moving one at the initial pose. Therefore, the coordinates of $N_0 \sim N_3$ with repect to $\{F\}$ are:

$$^{o}N_0(0,-m,m)^T,\ ^{o}N_1(m,-m,m)^T,\ ^{o}N_2(0,0,m)^T,\ ^{o}N_3(0,-m,2m)^T$$

where the superscript 'o' denotes the initial pose, 'm' is one of the location parameter of the target ball.

When the end-effector moves to another pose, the coordinates of $N_0 \sim N_3$ are

$$N_0(x_0,-m+y_0,m+z_0)^T;\ N_1(m+x_1,-m+y_1,m+z_1)^T;$$

$$N_2(x_2,y_2,m+z_2)^T;\ N_3(x_3,-m+y_3,2m+z_3)^T.$$

where x_i, y_i and z_i $i=0,1,2,3$ are the single-direction displacements of $N_0 \sim N_3$ compared to the initial pose.

The rotation matrix from $\{F'\}$ to $\{F\}$ can be achieved :

$$^{F}_{F'}R = \begin{bmatrix} A_{11} & A_{12} & A_{13} \\ A_{21} & A_{22} & A_{23} \\ A_{31} & A_{32} & A_{33} \end{bmatrix}$$

where:

$A_{11} = (m + x_1 - x_0)/m$; $A_{12} = (x_2 - x_0)/m$; $A_{13} = (x_3 - x_0)/m$;
$A_{21} = (y_1 - y_0)/m$; $A_{22} = (m + y_2 - y_0)/m$; $A_{23} = (y_3 - y_0)/m$;
$A_{31} = (z_1 - z_0)/m$ $A_{32} = (z_2 - z_0)/m$; $A_{33} = (m + z_3 - z_0)/m$.

Three elements are independent in the rotation matrix. We choose A_{12}、A_{23} and A_{31}, so the other six elements can be described by the three independent ones. And the expressions are unique in the workspace of the simulator [8, 15].

Apparently, A_{12} , A_{23} and A_{31} are determined by 6 relative displacements: x_0 , y_0 , z_0 , x_2 , y_3 and z_1 . Based on this, the position vector can be expressed:

$x=(x_0+x_2)/2+mA_{12}/2-mA_{13}$;

$y=(y_0+y_3)/2-m+mA_{22}-3mA_{23}/2$;

$z=(z_0+z_1)/2+m-mA_{31}/2+mA_{32}-mA_{33}$.

So, the rotation matrix and the position vector of the platform are all described by the 6 relative displacements.

According to the conclusion of section 4 and eq. (4), the relationship between 6 relative displacements errors and the 48 errors to be identified is achieved:

$$\boldsymbol{BD}'=\boldsymbol{J}\cdot\boldsymbol{\delta q}+\boldsymbol{G}_a'\cdot\boldsymbol{\delta a}'+\boldsymbol{G}_\alpha'\cdot\boldsymbol{\delta\alpha}'+\boldsymbol{G}_d'\cdot\boldsymbol{\delta d}'+\boldsymbol{G}_\theta'\cdot\boldsymbol{\delta\theta}' \quad (7)$$

where $\boldsymbol{D}'=[\delta x_0,\delta y_0,\delta z_0,\delta x_2,\delta y_3,\delta z_1]^T$;

$\boldsymbol{B}$ is a transformation matrix between $\boldsymbol{D}$ and $\boldsymbol{D}'$;

$\boldsymbol{\delta a}',\boldsymbol{\delta\alpha}',\boldsymbol{\delta d}'$ and $\boldsymbol{\delta\theta}'$ are the 42 parameter errors to be identified;

$\boldsymbol{G}_a',\boldsymbol{G}_\alpha',\boldsymbol{G}_d'$ and $\boldsymbol{G}_\theta'$ are the error coefficient matrixes corresponding to 42 errors.

Now we find that the residuals of the six relative displacements can be used to identify the kinematic parameters, instead of the residuals of end pose.

Define $\boldsymbol{X}'$ to denote the measurement data of the 6 relative displacements in single-direction:

$\boldsymbol{X}'=[x_0,y_0,z_0,x_2,y_3,z_1]^T$.

The deviation between the $\boldsymbol{X}'$ and the nominal data $\boldsymbol{X}$ is the $\boldsymbol{D}'$

Supposing the driving parameters l_i is accurate, i.e. $\boldsymbol{\delta q}=\boldsymbol{0}$. Then eq.(7) can be re-written in the following form:

$$\boldsymbol{D}'=\boldsymbol{CdE} \quad (8)$$

where

$\boldsymbol{C}=[\boldsymbol{B}^{-1}\boldsymbol{G}_a',\boldsymbol{B}^{-1}\boldsymbol{G}_\alpha',\boldsymbol{B}^{-1}\boldsymbol{G}_d',\boldsymbol{B}^{-1}\boldsymbol{G}_\theta']$; $\boldsymbol{E}=[\boldsymbol{\delta a}',\boldsymbol{\delta\alpha}',\boldsymbol{\delta d}',\boldsymbol{\delta\theta}']$.

6 Measuring Method and Calibration Simulation

As illustrated in Fig. 6, the gauge plate is extraordinary accurate and the three plates are perpendicular each other. It was installed to the base with the pose as shown in Fig. 6. We use the modified vernier calipers to measure the distance between the target balls and the gauge plate. The magnetism of the ball shell ensures the accurate contact and concentricity of the ball and the ball shell. The resolution of the vernier calipers is 10^{-5}m.

Six distances need to be measured at one pose: the distance between N_0 and the plate in x, y and z direction, N_1 in z direction , N_2 in x direction and N_3 in x direction.

First, we should measure the 6 distances at the initial pose, ${}^{o}\boldsymbol{dd}$ denotes the distance vector at initial pose:

$${}^{o}\boldsymbol{dd} = [{}^{o}x_{d0}, {}^{o}y_{d0}, {}^{o}z_{d0}, {}^{o}x_{d2}, {}^{o}y_{d3}, {}^{o}z_{d1}]^{T}$$

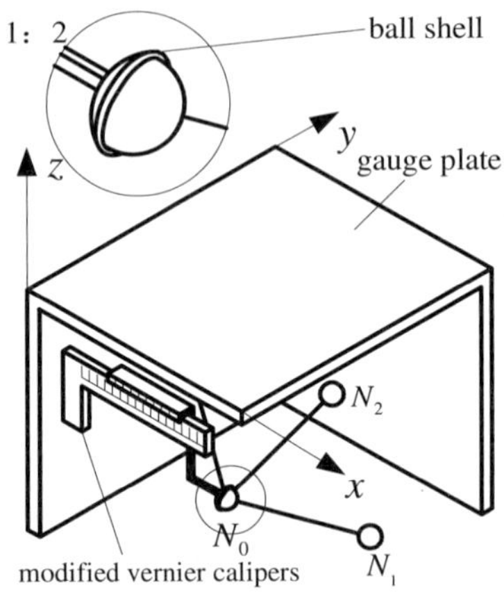

Fig. 6. Measuring method of the displacement

similarly, the distance vector at pose j is:

$${}^{j}\mathbf{dd} = [{}^{j}x_{d0}, {}^{j}y_{d0}, {}^{j}z_{d0}, {}^{j}x_{d2}, {}^{j}y_{d3}, {}^{j}z_{d1}]^{T}$$

Define vector ${}^{j}\boldsymbol{X}'$ to represent the relative displacement of pose j relative to the initial pose:

$${}^{j}\mathbf{X}' = {}^{j}\mathbf{dd} - {}^{o}\mathbf{dd} \tag{9}$$

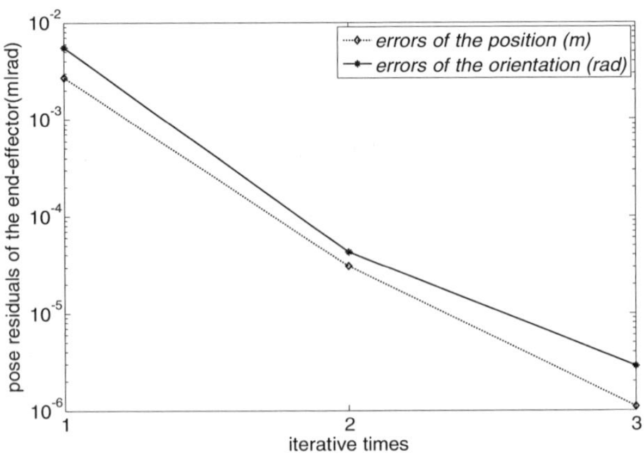

Fig. 7. Relationship between iterative times and pose residuals

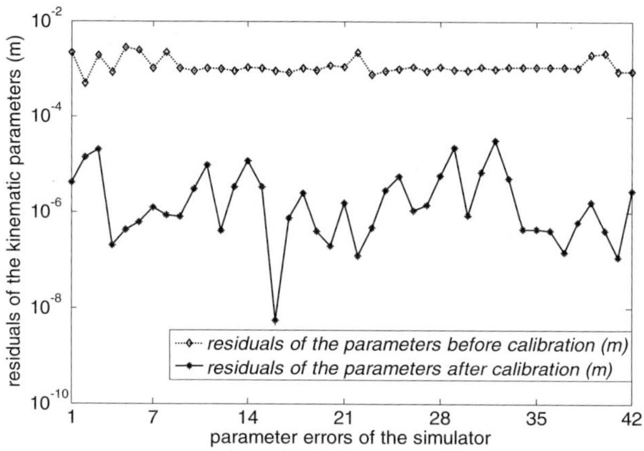

Fig. 8. Residuals of parameters before and after calibration

Then we can choose adequate poses to simulate the calibration process. The least-squares algorithm is used to identify the errors. The simulation is performed in principle without considering the measurement errors of the vernier calipers. The initial errors of the parameters are given about 10^{-3}m. Fig. 7~8 depict the simulation result.

As shown in Fig. 7, this algorithm of calibration is effective and converges rapidly. The pose accuracy of the end-effector improves dramatically. Fig.8 illustrates the comparison of the parameter errors before and after calibration. We can see that all of parameter errors are all identified and reach the precision about 10^{-5}m.

So, avoiding using the expensive measurement instruments to get the pose of the end-effector, we improved the accuracy of parallel simulator to the precision about 10^{-5}m with the low-cost and common measurement tools. In the process of the calibration, only six relative displacements in single-direction of the target balls need to be measured at one pose.

7 Conclusion

We studied the accuracy of a novel parallel robot with orthogonal chains and redundant actuator.

The comprehensive error mode which accommodated all 144 possible geometrical errors is set up without complicated derivation and matrix transfer. Based on the error analysis, the major errors to be identified in the calibration are determined.

A new calibration method was presented to solve the pose measurement problem. With this method, the expression of the functional relation between residuals of six relative displacements of the target ball and the parameter errors of the simulator is set up. So, instead of the end pose measurement, we just need the residuals of the six relative displacements for parameter identification. And the six relative displacements in single-direction can easily obtained with the common tools: the modified vernier calipers and the gauge plate.

Finally, the simulation approved the validity of the new calibration method in principle. Thanks to the common measurement apparatus, this method should have a wide-ranging application field in engineering.

Acknowledgement

This work was supported by the National Key Basic Research Program of China (2006CB705400) and partially by the national Natural Science Foundation of China (60534020).

References

1. Wang, J., Masory, O.: On the Accuracy of a Stewart Platform-Part I: The Effect of Manufacturing Tolerances. In: Proceeding of IEEE International Conference on Robotics and Automation, pp. 114–120 (1993)
2. Maurine, P., Dombre, E.: A calibration procedure for the parallel robot Delta 4. In: Proceedings of IEEE international Conference on robotics and Automation, Minneapolis, pp. 975–980 (1996)
3. Roopponen, T., Arai, T.: Accuracy Analysis of a Modified Stewart Platform. In: Proceeding of IEEE International Conference on. Robotics and Automation, Nagoya, pp. 521–525 (1995)
4. Huang, T., Li, Y., et al.: Error modeling, sensitivity analysis and assembly process of a class of 3-DOF parallel kinematic machines with parallelogram struts. Science in China (Series E) 45(5), 467–476 (2002)
5. Mahir, H., Leila, N.: Design modification of parallel manipulators for optimum fault tolerance to joint jam. Mech. Mach. Theory 40, 559–577 (2005)
6. Wang, J.S., BAI, J.W., et al.: Accuracy analysis of joint-clearances in a Stewart platform. Journal of Tsinghua University 42(6), 758–761 (2002) (in Chinese)
7. Patel, A.J., Ehmann, K.F.: Calibration of a hexapod machine tool using a redundant leg. Int. Mach. Tools Manu. 40(4), 489–512 (2000)
8. Ota, H., Shibukawa, T., Tooyama, T., Uchiyama, M.: Forward Kinematic Calibration Method for Parallel Mechanism Using Pose Data Measured by a Double Ball Bar System. In: Proceedings of the Year 2000 Parallel Kinematic Machines International Conference, Ann Arbor, MI, pp. 57–63 (2002)
9. Zhuang, H., Yan, J., Masory, Q.: Calibration of Stewart Platform and other Parallel Manipulator by Minimizing Inverse Kinematic Residuals. Robotic Syst. 15, 395–405 (1998)
10. Maurine, P., Dombre, E.: A Calibration Procedure for the Parallel Robot delta4. In: Proceedings of IEEE International Conference on Robotics and Automation, pp. 975–980 (1996)
11. Besnard, S., Khalil, W.: Calibration of Parallel Robot Using Two Inclinometers. In: Proceedings of IEEE International Conference on Robotics & Automation, pp. 1758–1763 (1999)
12. Huang, T., Chetwynd, D.G., Whitehouse, D.J., et al.: A general and novel approach for parameter identification of 6-DOF parallel kinematic machines. Mech. Mach. Theory 40, 219–239 (2005)
13. Huang, Z., Kong, L.F., et al.: Mechanism and Control of Parallel Robots[M], pp. 174–179. China Machine Press, Beijing (1997)
14. Liu, W.: Study on Key Techniques of Earthquake Simulator with 3-2-1 Structure Parallel Mechanism [MA. Thesis]. Tianjin: Hebei University of Technology, pp. 16–25 (2004)
15. Zhao, J.B: Research on the macro moving system of chromosome incision equipment: [PhD Thesis]. Tianjin: Hebei University of Technology, pp. 9–26 (2008)

Application of a New Fault Detection Approach to Aerocraft's Closed-Loop Control System

Jing Zhou[1,2] and Xinhan Huang[1]

[1] Department of Control Science and Engineering, Huazhong University of Science and Technology
[2] Department of Mathematics and computer science, Jianghan University
Wuhan Hubei 430074, China
zhou_8132@yahoo.cn

Abstract. The main contributions of this paper is the successful application in the aerocraft's closed-loop control system. As we know, the fault detection approaches proposed before mainly aim at the open-loop system. Meanwhile, a new LMI (linear matrix inequality)-based filter design methodology for fault detection in LTI plants is presented. For fault detection, H_∞ and H- index are used to measure the residual's robustness against disturbances and sensitivity to faults respectively. In this paper, the H- index is transformed to H_∞ norm by using the residual error instead of residual. Eventually, the design scheme is applied in an aerocraft's longitudinal closed-loop system and the advantages of this approach are highlighted.

Keywords: Fault detection filter; Linear matrix inequality(LMI); H_∞ filtering; Multi-objective optimization; Closed-loop.

1 Introduction

The fields of fault detection (FD) have attracted much attention from control engineers, especially in the flight control community during the last 30 years. Various approaches to fault detection based on model-based analytical redundancy techniques have been proposed, see for example([1]-[3]). Model-based FDI schemes could be realized in two steps: firstly, residual generation part which consists in the design of signals that are sensitive to the faults, and secondly, a residual evaluation part that includes a threshold and a decision logic unit ([4]). As we know, fault detection filter have to be robust, i.e., insensitive or even invariant to noise and disturbances. A number of approaches using the H_∞ norm optimization techniques have been developed for the design of robust fault detection filters. One of them is to introduce a performance index and formulate the FD design problem as the indices optimization problems([5] [6]). Another widely used way is to introduce a reference model and formulate the design of residual generator as a standard H_∞ model matching problem[7]. The design objective of this scheme is to minimize the effect of the fault signal, the disturbance and the modeling errors on the fault estimation error, in a H_∞-norm sense[4]. However, this approach may produce a false alarm in no fault

C. Xiong et al. (Eds.): ICIRA 2008, Part II, LNAI 5315, pp. 1223–1232, 2008.

situation. Thus, we propose a new approach based on multi-objective H_∞ optimization method. To indicate the residual's sensitivity to faults, a new H- index was propsed by Hou and Patton [9]. To express the best sensitivity to the fault, the H- index was introduced. The H- index is defined as the minimum nonzero singular value of a transfer matrix[10]. However, this is not a norm. Thus, optimization problems with this index cannot be solved in a systematic way. Therefore, the model-matching problem needs to be introduced to relate the minimum gain from fault to residual with the residual error[11]□then unify the two indices (H- and H_∞) to one index (H_∞). There are many methods which can optimize the H_∞ norm, such as the BRL[12].

Except the filter-designing schemes introduced above, there are also some schemes based on observer-design([13][14]) can be used to approach the RFD problem. A FDI observer scheme combined with a residual weighting matrix. Different indices are set up for the design of the observer gain and the residual weighting factor ([2][15][16]). Recently, a linear matrix inequality(LMI) formulation is proposed to find a robust fault detection filter which optimally approximates, in the H_∞ norm sense, the ideal solution provided by a reference model([17][18]). LMI techniques were also considered in the area of FD to derive a solution of a scaled H_∞ estimation problem for systems subjected to structured linear time varying uncertainties systems and in Ding et al. for time-delay linear systems.

A very interesting application of H_∞ estimation algorithms to aircraft inflight ice detection was given in [19]. A robust failure detection and isolation algorithm based on robust H_∞ estimation filters was presented in [20] and applied to the open-loop pitch dynamics of an underwater vehicle to detect a single actuator fault. Their analyses were based on open-loop LTI responses where the filters were designed for a nominal condition and tested for a second off-nominal LTI plant for robustness analysis. In [21] the H_∞-FDI Ricatti-based approach is used to design fault detection filters for an inverted pendulum. Unfortunately the application was not fully carried out in this case (i.e. no simulations).

The importance of this paper is on the application of the FD filter design approach which based on multi-objective(H_∞ and H-) optimation to a closed-loop control system, a certain type of aircraft, to detect a single actuator fault, where issues of realistic disturbances and robustness have to be accounted for in the design stage.

2 Problem Formulation

2.1 Residual Generation

Let's consider the following continuous linear time invariant system described by(1), we will use the so-called fault detection filter in the following form as (2). The residual r is defined as $r = z - y$. Thus, the robust fault detection filter (RFDF) design problem can be described as designing the filter (A_F, B_F, C_F, D_F). As mentioned in section 1, the residual must be sensitive to faults and insensitive to disturbance, so $\|T_{rf}\|_-$ should be maximized and $\|T_{rd}\|_\infty$ should be minimized. Then applying the

BRL[12], we can get the result $\|T_{rf}\|_{-} > \gamma_f$, $\|T_{rd}\|_{\infty} < \gamma_d$. As already mentioned, $\|\cdot\|_{-}$ is not norm so its optimization is difficult. But, if we use the residual error instead of the residual, the $\|T_{rf}\|_{-}$ can be transformed to $\|T_{\tilde{r}f}\|_{\infty}$. Then applying the BRL, we can get $\|T_{\tilde{r}f}\|_{\infty} < \gamma_f$, $\|T_{rd}\|_{\infty} < \gamma_d$, it equals to obtain $\min \gamma_f$ and $\min \gamma_d$. The residual error is defined as $\tilde{r} = Wf - r = r' - r$ ([4]). Thus, the block diagram for the residual error $\tilde{r}$ with shaping filter W is shown in Fig. 1. The two shaping filters in Fig. 1 is described as Eq. (3). Including the weighting functions W_d and W_F into the model (1) leads to the standard linear-fractional form. By including the filter (2) and using some linear fractional algebra, it can be verified that the closed-loop model $R = (\tilde{P} \times F)$ admits the state space equation described as Eq. (4).

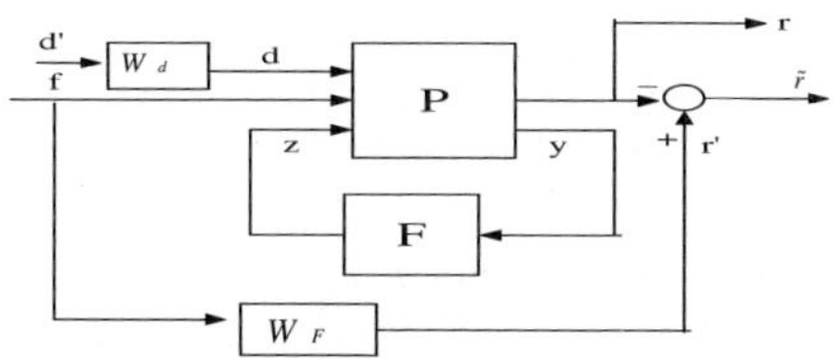

Fig. 1. The block diagram for the FD structure

$$P:\begin{cases}\dot{x} = Ax + B_d d + B_f f \\ y = C_2 x + D_d d + D_f f\end{cases} \tag{1}$$

$$F:\begin{cases}\dot{x}_F = A_F x_F + B_F y \\ z = C_F x_F + D_F y\end{cases} \tag{2}$$

$$W_d:\begin{cases}\dot{x}_d = A_m x_d + B_m d' \\ d = C_m x_d + D_m d'\end{cases}, \quad W_F:\begin{cases}\dot{x}_w = A_w x_w + B_w f \\ r' = C_w x_w + D_w f\end{cases} \tag{3}$$

$$R:\begin{cases}\begin{pmatrix}\dot{x} \\ \dot{x}_d \\ \dot{x}_w \\ \dot{x}_F\end{pmatrix} = \begin{pmatrix}\tilde{A} & 0 \\ B_F\tilde{C} & A_F\end{pmatrix}\begin{pmatrix}x \\ x_d \\ x_w \\ x_F\end{pmatrix} + \begin{pmatrix}\tilde{B}_d \\ B_F\tilde{D}_d\end{pmatrix}d' + \begin{pmatrix}\tilde{B}_f \\ B_F\tilde{D}_f\end{pmatrix}f \\ \tilde{r} = \begin{pmatrix}\tilde{C}_F & -C_F\end{pmatrix}\begin{pmatrix}x \\ x_d \\ x_w \\ x_F\end{pmatrix} + ((I - D_F)\tilde{D}_d)d' + ((I - D_F)\tilde{D}_f + D_w)f\end{cases} \tag{4}$$

$$\tilde{A} = \begin{pmatrix}A & B_d C_m & 0 \\ 0 & A_m & 0 \\ 0 & 0 & A_w\end{pmatrix}, \tilde{B}_d = \begin{pmatrix}B_d D_m \\ B_m \\ 0\end{pmatrix}, \tilde{B}_f = \begin{pmatrix}B_f \\ 0 \\ B_w\end{pmatrix}$$
$$\tilde{C} = (C_1 \quad D_d C_m \quad 0), \tilde{D}_d = D_d D_m, \tilde{D}_f = D_f, \tilde{C}_F = ((I - D_F)C_1 \quad (I - D_F)D_d C_m \quad C_w) \tag{5}$$

$$A_{\tilde{r}d} = A_{\tilde{r}f} = \begin{pmatrix}\tilde{A} & 0 \\ B_F\tilde{C} & A_F\end{pmatrix}, B_{\tilde{r}d} = \begin{pmatrix}\tilde{B}_d \\ B_F\tilde{D}_d\end{pmatrix}, B_{\tilde{r}f} = \begin{pmatrix}\tilde{B}_f \\ B_F\tilde{D}_f\end{pmatrix}, C_{\tilde{r}d} = C_{\tilde{r}f} = \begin{pmatrix}\tilde{C}_F & -C_F\end{pmatrix},$$
$$D_{\tilde{r}d} = (I - D_F)\tilde{D}_d, D_{\tilde{r}f} = (I - D_F)\tilde{D}_f + D_w \tag{6}$$

From the Eq. (4), we can get Eq.(5) and Eq.(6). Then applying the BRL to equation (4) results in the inequalities (7) and inequalities (8) [11]. To proceed further, we'll need to partition the V and P variable as Eq. (9). Using the matrix inequalities (7), (8) and (9), then multiply the matrix (10) both sides, the inEq. (7) and inEq. (8) can be rewrittened as inequation (11) and (12) respectively.

$$\begin{bmatrix} -(V+V^T) & V^T A_{rd}+P & V^T B_{rd} & 0 & V^T \\ A_{rd}{}^T V+P & -\mu P & 0 & C_{rd}{}^T & 0 \\ B_{rd}{}^T V & 0 & -\gamma_d I & D_{rd}{}^T & 0 \\ 0 & C_{rd} & D_{rd} & -\gamma_d I & 0 \\ V & 0 & 0 & 0 & -P/\mu \end{bmatrix} < 0 \tag{7}$$

$$\begin{bmatrix} -(V+V^T) & V^T A_{rf}+P & V^T B_{rf} & 0 & V^T \\ A_{rf}{}^T V+P & -\mu P & 0 & C_{rf}{}^T & 0 \\ B_{rf}{}^T V & 0 & -\gamma_f I & D_{rf}{}^T & 0 \\ 0 & C_{rf} & D_{rf} & -\gamma_f I & 0 \\ V & 0 & 0 & 0 & -P/\mu \end{bmatrix} < 0 \tag{8}$$

$$P=\begin{bmatrix} P_1 & P_3^T \\ P_3 & P_2 \end{bmatrix}, \quad V=\begin{bmatrix} V_{11} & V_{12} \\ V_{21} & V_{22} \end{bmatrix} \tag{9}$$

$$diag\left(I \quad V_{22}^{-1}V_{21} \quad I \quad V_{22}^{-1}V_{21} \quad I \quad I \quad I \quad V_{22}^{-1}V_{21}\right) \tag{10}$$

$$\begin{bmatrix} -(V_{11}+V_{11}^T) & -(S_1^T+S_2^T) & V_{11}^T\tilde{A}+\hat{B}_F\tilde{C}+P_1 & \hat{A}_F+\hat{P}_3^T & V_{11}^T\tilde{B}_d+\hat{B}_F\tilde{D}_d & 0 & V_{11}^T & S_1^T \\ * & -(S_1+S_1^T) & S_2\tilde{A}+\hat{B}_F\tilde{C}+\hat{P}_3 & \hat{A}_F+\hat{P}_2 & S_2\tilde{B}_d+\hat{B}_F\tilde{D}_d & 0 & S_2 & S_1^T \\ * & * & -\mu P_1 & -\mu\hat{P}_3^T & 0 & \tilde{C}_F^T & 0 & 0 \\ * & * & * & -\mu\hat{P}_2 & 0 & -\hat{C}_F^T & 0 & 0 \\ * & * & * & * & -\gamma_d I & \tilde{D}_d^T(I-\hat{D}_F)^T & 0 & 0 \\ * & * & * & * & * & -\gamma_d I & 0 & 0 \\ * & * & * & * & * & * & \frac{1}{\mu}P_1 & \frac{1}{\mu}\hat{P}_3^T \\ * & * & * & * & * & * & * & \frac{1}{\mu}\hat{P}_2 \end{bmatrix} < 0 \tag{11}$$

$$\begin{bmatrix} -(V_{11}+V_{11}^T) & -(S_1^T+S_2^T) & V_{11}^T\tilde{A}+\hat{B}_F\tilde{C}+P_1 & \hat{A}_F+\hat{P}_3^T & V_{11}^T\tilde{B}_f+\hat{B}_F\tilde{D}_f & 0 & V_{11}^T & S_1^T \\ * & -(S_1+S_1^T) & S_2\tilde{A}+\hat{B}_F\tilde{C}+\hat{P}_3 & \hat{A}_F+\hat{P}_2 & S_2\tilde{B}_f+\hat{B}_F\tilde{D}_f & 0 & S_2 & S_1^T \\ * & * & -\mu P_1 & -\mu\hat{P}_3^T & 0 & \tilde{C}_F^T & 0 & 0 \\ * & * & * & -\mu\hat{P}_2 & 0 & -\hat{C}_F^T & 0 & 0 \\ * & * & * & * & -\gamma_f I & \tilde{D}_f^T(I-D_F)^T+D_w^T & 0 & 0 \\ * & * & * & * & * & -\gamma_f I & 0 & 0 \\ * & * & * & * & * & * & \frac{1}{\mu}P_1 & \frac{1}{\mu}\hat{P}_3^T \\ * & * & * & * & * & * & * & \frac{1}{\mu}\hat{P}_2 \end{bmatrix} < 0 \tag{12}$$

Where

$$\begin{aligned} & S_1=V_{21}^T V_{22}^{-T} V_{21} \quad S_2=V_{21}^T V_{22}^{-T} V_{12}^T \quad \hat{B}_F=V_{21}^T B_F \quad \hat{P}_2=V_{21}^T V_{22}^{-T} P_2 V_{22}^{-1} V_{21} \quad \hat{P}_3^T=P_3^T V_{22}^{-1} V_{21} \\ & \hat{A}_F=V_{21}^T A_F V_{22}^{-1} V_{21} \quad \hat{C}_F=C_F V_{22}^{-1} V_{21} \quad \hat{D}_F=D_F \end{aligned} \tag{13}$$

The H_∞ filtering solvability condition is reformulated as feasibility problem of equation (11) and (12) with respect to $\hat{A}_F, \hat{B}_F, \hat{C}_F, \hat{D}_F S_1, S_2, V_{11}, \hat{P}, \gamma_d, \gamma_f$. The filter matrices A_F, B_F, C_F, D_F can be derived by means of the following procedure:
Compute V_{22}, V_{21} by solving the factorization problem as Eq. (14).

$$S_1 = V_{21}^T V_{22}^{-T} V_{21} \tag{14}$$

Compute A_F, B_F, C_F, D_F from Eq. (15).

$$A_F = V_{21}^{-T} \hat{A}_F V_{21}^{-1} V_{22},\ B_F = V_{21}^{-T} \hat{B}_F,\ C_F = \hat{C}_F V_{21}^{-1} V_{22},\ D_F = \hat{D}_F \tag{15}$$

As described before, after unify the two indices to H_∞ norm, the RFD filter (A_F, B_F, C_F, D_F) must satisfy the (16) as below:

$$\min_{\hat{A}_F, \hat{B}_F, \hat{C}_F, S_1, S_2, V_{11}, \hat{P}, \gamma} \{\gamma_d + \gamma_f\},\ \hat{P} > 0 \tag{16}$$

In summary, the RFD filter in the multi-objective H_∞ formulation can be solved if and only if (11) and (12) holds. The minimum value can be found from (16). Also, the filter realization is obtained from (15).

2.2 Residual Evaluation

After designing of residual generation, the remaining important task for FD is the evaluation of the generated residual. One of the widely adopted approaches is to choose a threshold Jth>0 and use the following logical relationship for fault detection: if $\|r\|_\tau > J_{th}$, then alarm the fault, else if $\|r\|_\tau \le J_{th}$, it means no fault. Where the so-called residual evaluation function $\|r\|_\tau$ is determined by Eq. (17).

$$\|r\|_\tau = \sqrt{\frac{1}{\tau} \int_0^\tau r^T r d\tau} \tag{17}$$

Here, [0, T] is the finite-time window. Note that the length of the time window if finite. A major requirement for fault detection is to reduce false alarms. Thus, in the absence of any faults, $\|r\|_\tau$ should be less than the threshold value J_{th}, i.e.,

$$J_{th} = \sup \|r\|_\tau \tag{18}$$

Under fault-free conditions, $\|r\|_\tau$ can be described as([18])

$$r(s) = T_{ru}^0(s)u(s) + T_{rd}^0(s)d(s) \tag{19}$$

The threshold J_{th} can be found as follows:

$$J_{th} \equiv \|r\|_\tau = \|T_{ru}^0 u + T_{rd}^0 d\|_\tau \le \|T_{ru}^0\|_\infty \|u\|_\tau + \|T_{rd}^0\|_\infty \|d\|_\tau = \gamma_u \|u\|_\tau + \gamma_d \|d\|_\tau \tag{20}$$

Where γ_u and γ_d come from the optimization problem (16), and $\|d\|_\tau$ is the worst disturbance acting on the plant. Thus, in (20), $\|d\|_\tau$ is evaluated off-line while u is assumed to be known and $\|u\|_\tau$ is calculated on-line.

3 Aircraft Model

The aircraft LTI model for the longitudinal axis is presented. The nonlinear body-axes longitudinal motion of the certain aerocraft, not including flexible effects, can be described by the following differential equations (21).

$$\begin{aligned} &\ddot{\alpha}+a_4\alpha+a_4'\theta-\dot{\vartheta}=-a_5\delta_{z_1}+a_8Y_f \\ &\ddot{\vartheta}+a_1\dot{\vartheta}+a_1'\dot{\alpha}+a_2\alpha=-a_3\delta_{z_1}+a_6M_{Z_1f} \\ &\theta=\vartheta-\alpha \end{aligned} \tag{21}$$

The dynamics of an aircraft is nonlinear and complex, we linearize equation (21) based on the method of selection of the character point, at which the dynamics of the aircraft is most instable. So, if the FD approach proposed in this paper is effective to the aerocraft's model at the character points, then it can be guanteed effective during the whole time field. Based on this idea, we can get the linear the model of aerocraft as equation (22), and the aerocraft's dynamics parameter in equation (22) can be find in Table 1 (at four character points respectively).

$$\begin{pmatrix}\dot{\alpha}\\ \dot{\omega}_z\\ \dot{\vartheta}\end{pmatrix}=\begin{bmatrix}-a_4 & 1 & 0\\ -a_2 & -a_1 & 0\\ 0 & 1 & 0\end{bmatrix}\begin{pmatrix}\alpha\\ \omega_z\\ \vartheta\end{pmatrix}+\begin{pmatrix}0\\ -a_3\\ 0\end{pmatrix}\delta_{z_1},\quad y=\begin{pmatrix}0 & 1 & 0\end{pmatrix}\begin{pmatrix}\alpha\\ \omega_z\\ \vartheta\end{pmatrix}=\omega_z \tag{22}$$

In equation (22), the longitudinal measurable state-variables are angle of attack α (rad), pitch rate ω_z (rad/s) ($\dot{\vartheta}=\omega_z$), pitch angle ϑ (rad). The elevator deflection δ_{z1} (deg) is the input, and the pitch rate ω_Z (rad/s) is the output of the closed-loop system. The aero-dynamic forces along the X- and Z- axis pitching moment are given by Y_f and M_{Z_1f}, respectively. The influence of the a_1'、a_4'、a_5 and Y_f can be ignored because of their small value.

Table 1. Aerocraft's dynamics parameter table

t	a_1	a_2	a_3	a_4
0.35s	0.1029	0.0536	0.2553	2.9281
8.2s	0.3376	23.39	37.62	0.5894
32.8s	0.3487	29.34	39.12	0.6120
131.2s	0.3701	44.92	42.72	0.7233

4 Simulation

As described in section 3, we can get the aerocraft's longitudinal model at four character points as Eq. (23). In Eq. (23), the dimension is reduced because of the pitch angle ϑ is an independent variable. The closed-loop control system with actuator fault is given as Fig 2.

$$A_1=\begin{bmatrix}-2.9281 & 1\\ -0.0536 & -0.1029\end{bmatrix},\ B_1=\begin{bmatrix}0\\ -0.2553\end{bmatrix},\ C_1=\begin{bmatrix}0 & 1\end{bmatrix}$$
$$A_2=\begin{bmatrix}-0.5894 & 1\\ -23.39 & -0.3376\end{bmatrix},\ B_2=\begin{bmatrix}0\\ -37.62\end{bmatrix},\ C_2=\begin{bmatrix}0 & 1\end{bmatrix}$$
$$A_3=\begin{bmatrix}-0.6120 & 1\\ -29.34 & -0.3487\end{bmatrix},\ B_3=\begin{bmatrix}0\\ -39.12\end{bmatrix},\ C_3=\begin{bmatrix}0 & 1\end{bmatrix} \qquad (23)$$
$$A_4=\begin{bmatrix}-0.7233 & 1\\ -44.92 & -0.3701\end{bmatrix},\ B_4=\begin{bmatrix}0\\ -42.72\end{bmatrix},\ C_4=\begin{bmatrix}0 & 1\end{bmatrix}$$
$$B_f=\begin{bmatrix}0\\ 1\end{bmatrix}\quad B_d=\begin{bmatrix}0.1\\ 0.2\end{bmatrix}\quad D_d=0.05\quad D_f=1$$

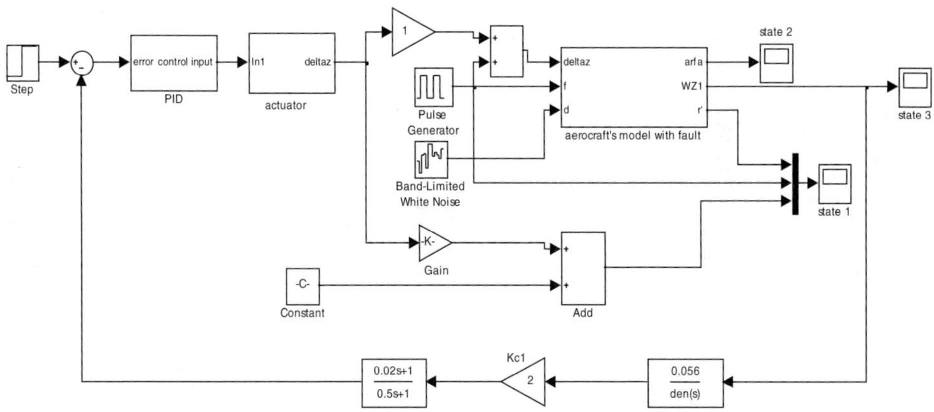

Fig. 2. The simulink figure for the closed-loop system including the LMI-FD approach

The fault signal is simulated as a pulse of unit amplitude that occurs from 30 to 40 seconds and is zero elsewhere. The unknown input d is assumed to be band-limited white noise with power 0.0005 and the upperbound of $\|d\|_\tau$ is given as 0.15. This value is used to calculate J_{th} using Eq. (20). With these conditions, we can get the RFD filter data A_F, B_F, C_F, D_F from Eq. (15). Meanwhile, we want to detect faults in the frequency range between 0 and 2 rand/s with a -20dB/dec roll-off at the higher frequencies, so the weighting functions W_d and W_F is given as $W_d = W_d(s) = \dfrac{0.15s+0.0034}{s+0.02}, W_F = W_F(s) = \dfrac{0.03s+4}{s+20}$.

The simulation results of the output--pitch rate ω_Z of closed-loop system(absence of fault and occurance of fault respectively) at different character points are given as Fig 3. From which, we can see that when the fault occurs from 30 to 40 seconds, ω_Z become unstable during the same pierod, but become stable almost at 48s after the FD approach is included in the system. The simulation result of the FD approach at 0.35s is shown in Fig 4(because of the limit of paper's length, the result figures at other character points are omitted, which are similar to Fig 4), from which, we can see that when the fault occurs at 30s, the residual error exceeds J_{th} at 30.1s, it means with the filter, the residual can detect the fault in time.

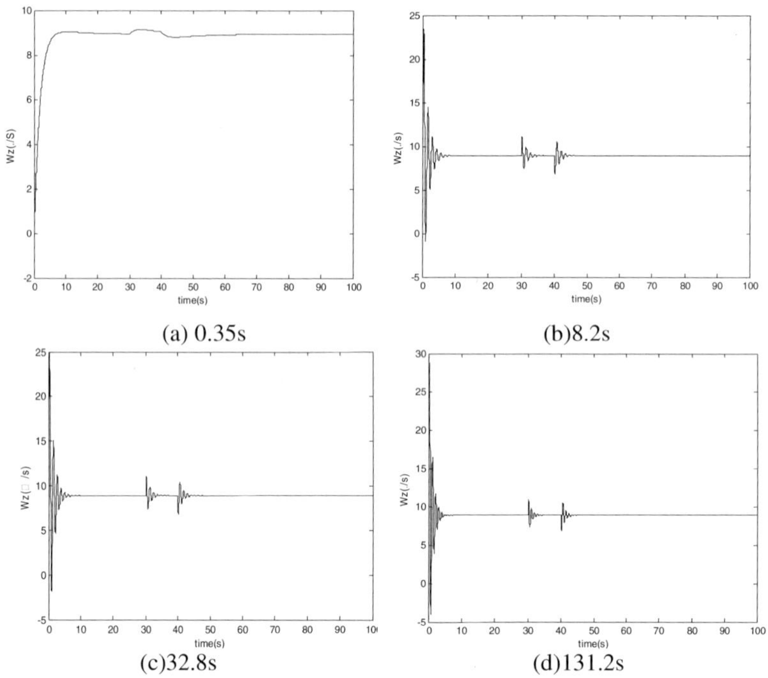

Fig. 3. ω_Z in closed-loop system which includes FD approach at four character points

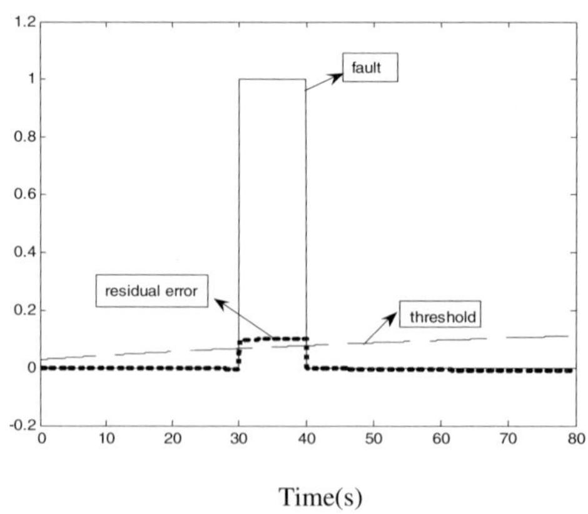

Fig. 4. Residual error output and fault threshold

5 Conclusion

A new LMI-based filter design methodology which can solve the multi-objective optimation problem for fault detection in LTI plants is proposed in this paper The main contributions of our study is the formulation of the FD problem as a filter-based multi-objective optimization problem and the new LMI-based technique as the solution. The reference residual error, which can be used to describe the robustness against disturbances and sensitivity to faults simultaneously, is an optimal solution of the RFDF. The existence of the solution is presented in terms of LMI formulation, which can be obtained conveniently by using Matlab LMI toolbox. Eventually, the approach is used in an aerocraft's closed-loop system, the simulation results have demonstrated that it can detect the fault effectively and the system including the FD approach can become stable rapidly after the actuator fault occurs.

References

1. Basseville, M.: On-board component fault detection and isolation using the statistical local approach. Automatica 34, 1391–1415 (1998)
2. Frank, P.M.: Enhancement of robustness in observer-based fault detection. International Journal of Control 59, 955–981 (1994)
3. Zhong, M.Y., Ye, H., Ding, S.X., Wang, G.Z.: Observer-Based Fast Rate Fault Detection for a Class of Multirate Sampled-Data Systems. IEEE Transactions on automatic control 52, 520–525 (2007)
4. Henry, D., Zolghadri, A.: Design of fault diagnosis filters: A multi-objective approach. Journal of the Franklin Institute 342, 421–446 (2005)
5. Frank, P.M., Ding, X.: Survey of robust residual generation and evaluation methods in observer-based fault detection systems. Journal of Process Control 7, 403–424 (1997)
6. Chen, J., Patton, P.R.: Robust model-based fault diagnosis for dynamic systems. Kluwer Academic Publishers, Boston (1999)
7. Ding, S.X., Zhong, M.Y., Tang, B.Y.: An LMI approach to the design of fault detection filter for time-delay LTI systems with unknown inputs. In: The American control conference, Arlington, VA, pp. 2137–2142 (2001)
8. Frisk, E.: Residual generation for fault diagnosis: Nominal and robust design. Technical Report 739, Department of Electrical Engineering, linkopings Universitet, Linkopings, Sweden (1998)
9. Chen, J., Patton, R.J., Liu, G.P.: Optimal residual design for fault-diagnosis using multiobjective optimization and genetic algorithms. International Journal of Systems Science 27, 567–576 (1996)
10. Liu, J., Wang, J.L., Yang, G.H.: An LMI approach to minimum sensitivity analysis with application to fault detection. Automatica l 41, 1995–2004 (2005)
11. Kim, Y.M., Watkins, J.M.: A New Approach for Robust and Reduced Order Fault Detection Filter Design. In: The 2007 American Control Conference, New York, pp. 11–13 (2007)
12. Wu, F., Lu, B.: Anti-windup control design for exponentially unstable LTI systems with actuator saturation. Systems & Control Letters 52, 305–322 (2004)
13. Wang, J.L., Yang, G.H., Liu, J.: An LMI approach to H– index and mixed H–/H∞ fault detection observer design. Automatica 43, 1656–1665 (2007)

14. Wang, H.B., Wang, J.L., Lam, J.: Robust Fault Detection Observer Design: Iterative LMI Approaches. Dynamic Systems, Measurement and Control 129, 77–82 (2007)
15. Edelmayer, A., Bokor, J., Szigeti, F., Keviczky, L.: Robust detection filter design in the presence of time varying system perturbations. Automatica 33, 471–475 (1997)
16. Chen, J., Patton, R.: Standard h1 filtering formulation of robust fault detection. In: SAFEPROCESS 2000, IFAC, Budapest (2000)
17. Nobrega', E.G., Abdalla, M., Grigoriadis, K.M.: LMI-Based Filter Design for Fault Detection and Isolation. In: The 39th IEEE Conf. on Decision and Control, Sydney (2000)
18. Zhong, M., Ding, X., Lam, J., Wang, H.B.: An LMI Approach to Design Robust Fault Detection Filter for Uncertain LTI Systems. Automatica 39, 543–550 (2003)
19. Melody, J.W., Hillbrand, T., Basar, T., Perkins, W.R.: $H\infty$ parameter identification for inflight detection of aircraft icing: The time-varying case. Control Engineering Practice 9, 1327–1335 (2001)
20. Mangoubi, R.S., Appleby, B.D., Verghese, G.C., Vander, W.E.: A robust failure detection and isolation algorithm. In: 34th IEEE conference on decision and control, New Orleans, pp. 2377–2382 (1995)
21. Felicio, P., Stoustrup, J., Niemann, H., Lourie, P.: Applying parametric fault detection to a mechanical system. In: American control conference, Anchorage, AK (2002)

Design of Dexterous Arm-Hand for Human-Assisted Manipulation

L. Wang, M. Xie, Z.W. Zhong, H.J. Yang, and J. Li

School of Mechanical & Aerospace Engineering, Nanyang Technological University
Singapore 639798

Abstract. Arm-hand subsystem, as the manipulator and end-effecter of a humanoid robot, is important from application point of view since humanoid robot is expected to help people in the future. A powerful arm-hand system can perform as many tasks as human beings do. However, owe to limited space and weight, humanoid robots were usually equipped with simple-structured upper limbs, especially for hand. In this paper, a multi-DOF and dexterous arm-hand module is presented, which owns lightweight and compact structure with incremental encoder, absolute encoder in each joint as well as force/torque sensor to feedback the force information. Moreover, the arm-hand module adopts distributed control system for joint actuators, which is compact and easy to be installed inside.

Keywords: Humanoid Robot, Arm-hand System, Distributed Control System.

1 Introduction

Humanoid robots were developed out with the purpose that they could serve people as elderly, patients [1] and communicate with people in ordinary life. At present, there are several existing prototypes in the world, such as ASIMO, HRP2, HUBO, and QRIO [1-5]. They share several common characteristics as excellent biped walking and friendly appearance. However, they are provided with a preliminary arm-hand system and can only perform simple tasks. For example, ASIMO has a 5-DOF arm and each hand with just one DOF [2], while HRP2 has a 6-DOF arm but only has champ instead [3]. Although HUBO has 6-DOF arm with 5-DOF for one single hand, the thumb is placed opposite to the other fingers [4], which makes the hand less humanlike. Humanoid arm-hand module with limited DOFs is largely restricted the motion and task it can achieve.

Though there are a lot of achievements on industrial robot arm as well as dexterous hand, for example: DLR dexterous hand which has 13 independent degrees of freedom and powerful sensor on the fingers [6]. But the emphasis of humanoid arm-hand differs from them. In contrast with industrial robot, which mainly focuses on mechanical rigidity, precision and high velocity [7], a humanoid upper limb should have humanlike appearance, movable joints that corresponds to human being, and lightweight structure.

This paper gives insight into the development of mechanical structure and control system of the humanoid robot Loch's upper limb, which is desired to have the ability of grasping, pulling, pushing, carrying, throwing and interaction with human.

C. Xiong et al. (Eds.): ICIRA 2008, Part II, LNAI 5315, pp. 1233–1240, 2008.

2 Humanoid Arm-Hand System Design

2.1 Specification

To make a more human-like appearance, the physical parameters of the arm-hand system are decided according to the standard human. However, the mass distribution of the arm-hand system has to be adjusted for mounting actuators and sensors, which take a considerable part of the total weight. Table 1 presents comparison of the dimensions between human being and robot as well as the mass distribution.

Table 1. Arm-hand specification

	Mass (kg)		Length (mm)
	Human being	Robot	
Forearm	1.4×2	2.5×2	280
Upper Arm	2.4×2	3×2	320
Hand	0.6×2	1.8×2	160
Whole Body	75	75~85	1750

The degrees of freedom (DOF) of the arm-hand system are presented in Fig.1. To be more specific, each arm of the robot has six degrees of freedom including three in shoulder, one in elbow and two in wrist. This enables the robot have similar kinematics as human being and do majority of things in the ordinary life. Meanwhile each hand is assigned to have 6 independent degrees of freedom along with four passive ones. Since the limited space of the hand, the passive DOFs with simpler structure enable the hands to approach more functions.

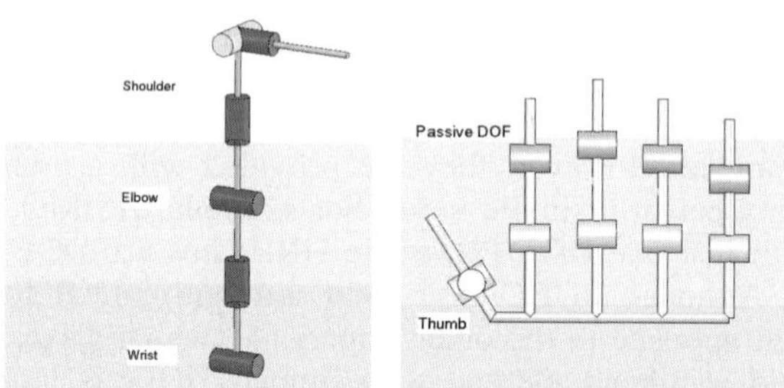

Fig. 1. DOF Distribution on arm-hand system

Movement Range

For movement range of each joint, we designed that to be about the same as that of standard human so that the humanoid robot performs human tasks as well as human. Table 2 shows the data on movable range of upper arm, fore arm and hand with comparison with standard human respectively.

Table 2. Joint movement range

	Joints	Human being	robot
Shoulder	Pitch	-45 deg. to 90 deg.	-180 deg. to 180 deg.
	Roll	- 90 deg. to 30 deg.	- 120 deg. to 30 deg.
	Yaw	-30 deg. to 80 deg.	-180 deg. to 180 deg.
Elbow	Pitch	-140 deg. to 10 deg.	-135 deg. to 0 deg
wrist	Pitch	- 30 deg. to 55 deg.	- 30 deg. to 30 deg.
	Yaw	-180 deg. to 10 deg.	-180 deg. to 180 deg.
Hand	Pitch	0 deg. to 90 deg.	0 deg. to 90 deg.

However, as shown above, some movable ranges of humanoid joints should be adjusted by several reasons. Firstly, some joints' movable range, such as that of shoulder pitch and roll are extended since we require the humanoid robot to perform motions that are impossible for human. While shoulder yaw and wrist yaw movement ranges are enlarged because it is easy for robot to attain wider range that exists in human with current configuration. However, ranges of elbow pitch and wrist pitch are slightly reduced for the constraint of structures.

Appearance Design

The appearance of the robot's upper limb is restricted by three constraints. The first is having the similar profile of that of a human. The second is the consideration of the DOF distribution and installment of actuators. And the last is the arm-hand system should be adequate to its application and some emergency cases. The final exterior of arm and hand is showed in Fig.2.

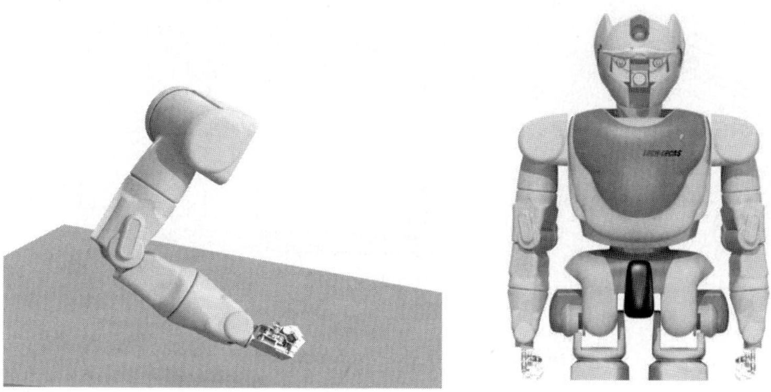

Fig. 2. Appearance of Arm-hand and Upper Body

In the design above, the shoulder roll and pitch motions can easily attain a relative large scope, and the yaw actuator is allocated along the upper arm. Further more, the three axes of the shoulder joint intercross at one point; this would be helpful for the computing of planning in the further research. As to the elbow joint, the movement range of elbow joint is limited and hard to attain that of human being for structural constraint, thus axis offset is made to extend the movement range. The wrist joint has two DOFs, and the wrist yaw movement is allocated along the forearm the same as shoulder yaw. This will help to reduce the distal weight of the arm. The hand has a palm and five fingers, except for the two-DOFs thumb, the other fingers will only have one actuator each for the compact space.

2.2 Structure Design

The structure design focuses on the mechanical modules that realize the objects established above. This will include the actuators, transmission structure, sensor mounting, and wiring.

Joint Structures of Arm

In order to simplify the joint structure, the joint principals are grouped. There are altogether two kinds of structures utilized under the constraints of the dimensions of motors and the space to install the transmission structures. The first one is directly-driven structure (Fig.3), in which the power is transferred from the motor to output shaft through transmission structure such as timing pulley/belt, harmonic gear or worm/worm wheel. In elbow joint, the motor is connected with a set of timing pulley/belt and harmonic gear serially; while in wrist pitch joint, the transmission system is consist of motor and worm/worm gears. After that, the output speed is reduced and the torque is enlarged. There is also a set of absolute encoder mounted on the shaft to detect the real-time position of the joints. This structure is not only compact-sized, easy to install but also capable of structure braking when the motor is out of power.

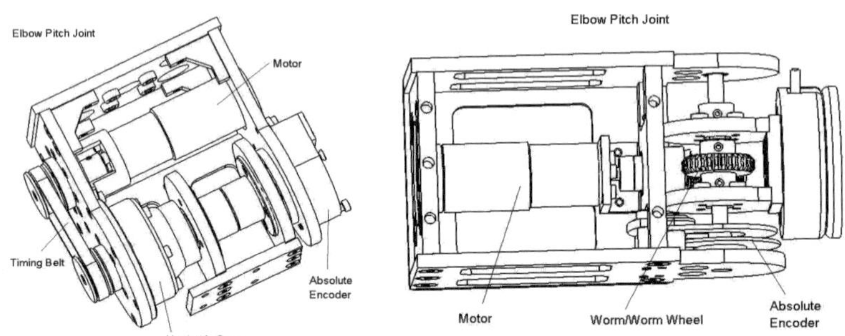

Fig. 3. Directly-driven Structures

The second one is the relative-driven structure. In this structure, the harmonic gear works in a different method as compared with the former one.

Harmonic gear is consisted of three components: circular spline (CS), flexspline (FS) and wave generator (WG) and it has several work modes. Usually CS is fixed and FS is connected with output shaft, however, in relative-driven structure, the roles of CS and FS are exchanged as shown in Fig.4a. This structure is adopted in wrist

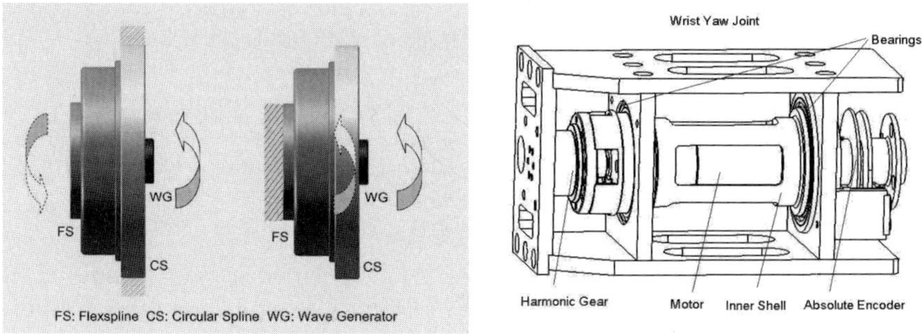

Fig. 4. a. Different Applications of Harmonic Gear**; b.** Wrist Yaw Joint

yaw, shoulder yaw and shoulder roll joints. Fig.4b presents the detailed structure of wrist yaw joint: the output shaft of the motor is connected with wave generator of the harmonic gear, while FS and CS are fixed with outer flame and inner shell separately. Two angular contact bearings are connected with the inner sleeve and outer frame respectively. When the power of motor is on, the inner shell, which works as the output of the structure, will rotate in a reduced speed. The outstanding advantage of this structure is that it can afford large spatial forces; it is useful since the arm works in a unconstructed environment.

Joint Structures of Hand

There are 6 independent DOFs, and 4 passive DOFs for each hand. And the thumb is assigned two independent DOFs while the other four fingers are assigned one independent and one passive DOF.

The structure of the thumb is presented in Fig.5: two DC motors coupled with worm gears drive two bevel gears, which are connected with a cross-axle structure. This mechanism can move in two orthogonal orientations, resulting in a two-DOF structure.

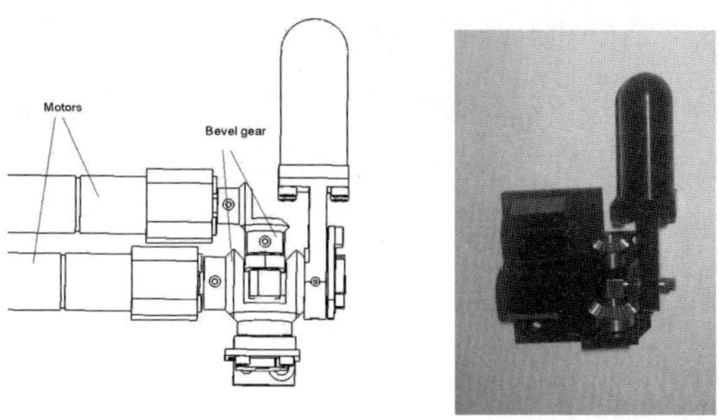

Fig. 5. Mechanical Structure of Thumb and the Prototype

Fig.6 shows the structure for each finger, a DC motor coupled with worm gear converts the rotating movement into the bending motion. A 4-link structure is used between the first and second segments of the finger. With suitable configuration, the two segments can bend with same velocity and position.

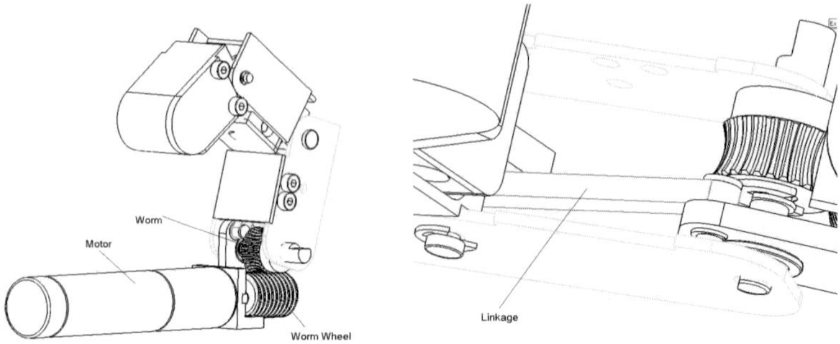

Fig. 6. a. Worm/Worm Wheel Transmission**; b.** 4-link Structure

2.3 Absolute Encode and Force/Torque Sensors

While the robot is performing a task, it is important to know the posture and the force imposed on the joints. Thus, force and position sensors are required to give sensory feedback to the robot. Totally, two kinds of position sensors are chosen according to the requirements of precision and limits of dimension: one is used on the arm, while the other is on the fingers as shown in Fig.7a and Fig.7b.

Moreover, force/torque sensor is utilized as force sensor to provide force and torques data for manipulation in three axis. Fig.7c shows a kind of force/torque sensor from ATI industrial Automation.

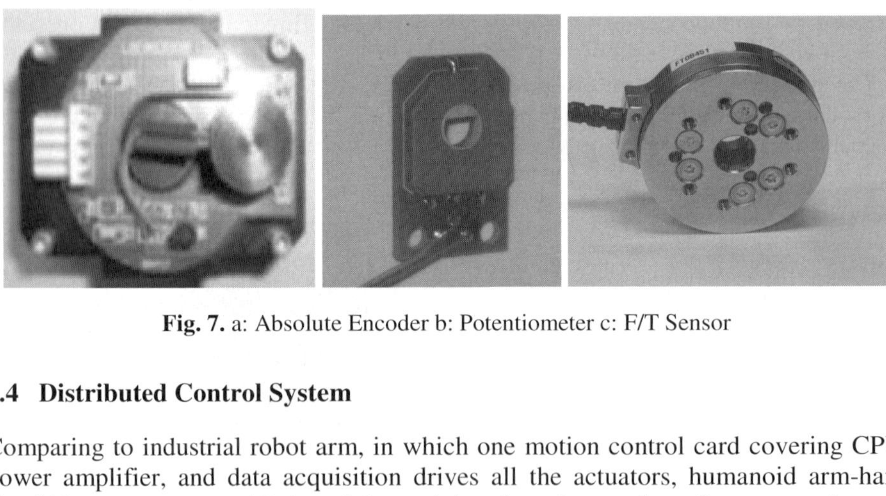

Fig. 7. a: Absolute Encoder b: Potentiometer c: F/T Sensor

2.4 Distributed Control System

Comparing to industrial robot arm, in which one motion control card covering CPU, power amplifier, and data acquisition drives all the actuators, humanoid arm-hand should keep compact and lightweight modules since the number of sensors and actuators is large, or it will make the control system complex and lead problems in wiring and installation. Finally distribute controller system (DCS) is adopted, and the whole control system is consisted of two levels: the high level is in charge of task space planning and organizes the whole system; While the low level control corresponds to the local control unit, which is consisted of local micro-process unit, power amplifier

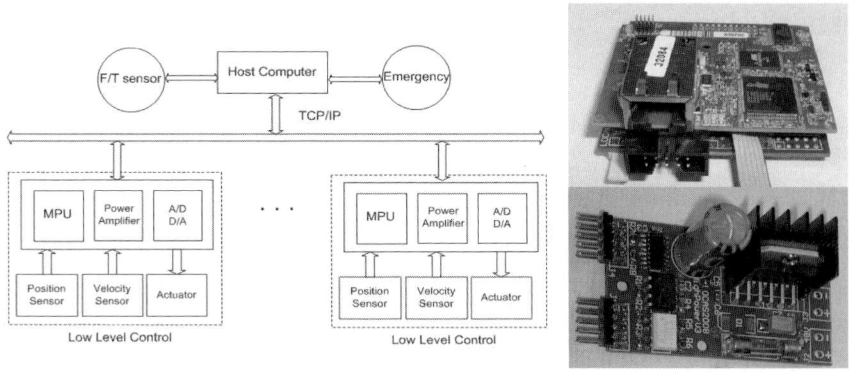

Fig. 8. Arm-hand Control System and One Local Control Unit

and A/D,D/A converter. The two levels communicate through TCP/IP protocol. That is, to some extend, similar to the human nervous system, which is consisted of the central and peripheral nervous system.

3 System Integration and Prototype

The prototype of the arm-hand system is shown as below. It contains all the joints modules and sensors. The total mass of the arm-hand is about 7.0 kg, which is less than the initial assignment and the movement ranges of the joints are quite close to the planned data.

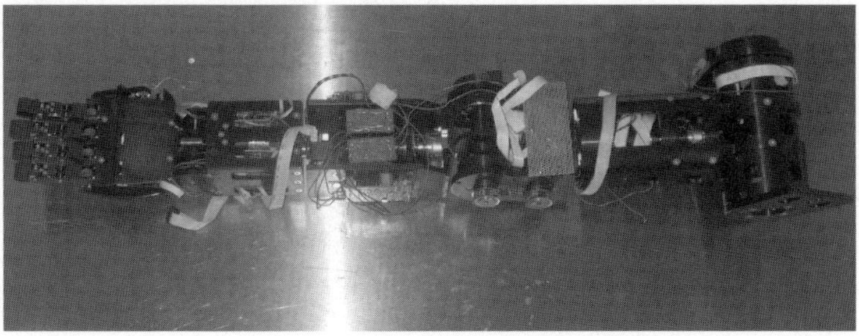

Fig. 9. Prototype of Arm-hand System

4 Conclusion

This paper presented how we developed the advanced arm-hand module for Loch, which is expected to have the ability of grasping, pulling, pushing, following, throwing and other motions. Several compact mechanisms are developed to provide dexterous joints for these tasks, what is more, a distribute control system to manage all the information and drive the joint actuators. Till now, basic functions are tested and more experiments are planned to refine the arm-hand system in the next step.

Acknowledgement

The authors would like to thank the project sponsor. In particular, the guidance and advices from Lim Kian Guan, Cheng Wee Kiang, Ngiam Li Lian and New Ai Peng are greatly appreciated.

References

1. Takashi, N., Hiroshi, H., et al.: Communication Agent embedded in Humanoid Robot. In: SICE Annual Conference in Fukui (2003)
2. Yoshiaki, S., Ryujin, W., et al.: The intelligent ASIMO: System overview and integration. In: Proceedings of the IEEE/RSJ intl. Conference on intelligent Robots and System, Lausanne, Switzerland, pp. 2478–2483 (2002)
3. Kenji, K., Fumio, K., et al.: Design of Prototype Humanoid Robotics Platform for HRP. In: Proceedings of the IEEE/RSJ Intl. Conferences on Intelligent Robots and Systems, Lausanne, Switzerland, pp. 2431–2436 (2002)
4. Ill-Woo, P., Jung-Yup, K., Jungho, L., Jun-Ho, O.: Mechanical Design of Humanoid Robot Platform KHR-3. In: Proceedings of 5th IEEE-RAS International Conference on Humanoid Robots, pp. 321–326 (2005)
5. Kohtaro, S.: Development of Entertainment Robot and Its Future. Digest of Technical Papers. In: 2005 Symposium on VLSI Circuits (2005)
6. Jiang, L., Jin, M., et al.: Multisensory HIT/DLR Dexterous Robot Hand. In: Procedings of IEEE/ASME International Conference on Advanced Intelligent Mechatronics, pp. 76–81 (2003)
7. Albert, A., Sven, B., et al.: Upper Body of a new Humanoid Robot the Design of ARMAR III. In: Proceedings of 6th IEEE-RAS International Conference on Humanoid Robots, pp. 308–313 (2006)

Noise Properties in Spool Valves with Cavitating Flow

Xin Fu, Liang Lu, Xiao-dong Ruan, Jun Zou, and Xue-wen Du

State Key Laboratory of Fluid Power Transmission and Control, Zhejiang University, Hangzhou, 310027, China
{junzou,luliang829}@zju.edu.cn

Abstract. Investigations on cavitation noise in non-circular opening spool valves have been conducted in this paper. The cavitation noise is used as a good sign to cavitation process because of its similar trends in different valves. Cavitation inception is judged from the overall sound levels and the noise spectrums, which show good similarity. However, the characteristics of the cavitation's distribution seem discrepant in valves with different grooves. In the valves with V-grooves, cavitation always grows up by the throttling edges, and in the valves with U-grooves, two grow-up states exist. Moreover, the flow-choking phenomenon has been found in the cases of test valves.

Keywords: Cavitation noise, Inception judgement, Choked flow.

1 Introduction

Cavitation is an undesirable phenomenon in fluid power systems, which not only changes the fluid characteristics like density and compressibility, but also induces vibration, noise and erosion. In oil hydraulic systems, cavitation most frequently occurs in valves, pumps and actuators, inside which the pressure plays an important role in formation and development of cavitation. It is clear that when the local hydrostatic pressure drops below the fluid vapor pressure at the actual temperature, cavitation occurs. Simulation and experimental efforts were conducted to obtain pressure distribution characteristics in the grooves of valves. Gao H. et al. [1] performed numerical researches on cavitation in circular opening poppet valves with commercial software Fluent. The RNG k-ε turbulent model and cavitation model were used in the simulation, and pressure distributions were obtained, which were quite coincident with Oshima's experimental data [2]. Cavitation also appears in rotary machinery like pumps and propellers frequently. Moritz and Sudolf [3] predicted the cavitation in a centrifugal pump impeller using CNS3D-code and compared the simulated void fraction distribution with pictures of the cavitation region on the blade. Further more, vibration characteristics induced by cavitation were revealed by Sato et al. [4], which showed good similarity with the cavitation noise. In Timo KOIVULA's [5] paper, cavitation's noise, vibration and erosion characteristics were studied in both orifices and valves, and the relationships between the bubble inception and flow-choking conditions were illustrated. The threshold of cavitation inception was determined by camera views. In addition, a book written by Christopher [6] referred that, the onset of cavitation was often detected first by noise rather than by visual observation of the bubbles.

C. Xiong et al. (Eds.): ICIRA 2008, Part II, LNAI 5315, pp. 1241–1249, 2008.

As mentioned above, many researches on cavitation in the hydraulic valves and orifices have been conducted, and most of the flow channels are axis-symmetrical. However, the distribution, noise and flow properties in non-circular opening spool valves have not been discussed in detail. In this research, two types of non-circular opening spool valves with U-grooves and V-grooves are studied respectively. Different cavitation distribution states in two type valves are revealed by high-speed camera technology. Similar cavitation noise trends are found, and their relationships with flow properties are presented.

2 Experimental Facility

The test facility (Fig. 1) is composed of a hydraulic circuit to control the experimental pressure and flow rate, a high speed camera system to record the evolution of hydrodynamic cavitation inside the valve and a noise detecting instrument to gain the inside view of the cavitation noise. Two pressure gauges are used to measure the inlet/outlet pressure of the valve. A flowmeter is used to measure the supply flow rate. These signals are acquired by a data acquisition card and processed by a computer. The experiments are conducted in a plexiglass model (Fig. 2), which is the same size as a prototype valve. The visualization apparatus consists of a high-speed video camera (FASTCAM-ultima APX) with a maximal speed of 120,000 frames per second, a non-stroboscopic lamp used for flow field lumination.

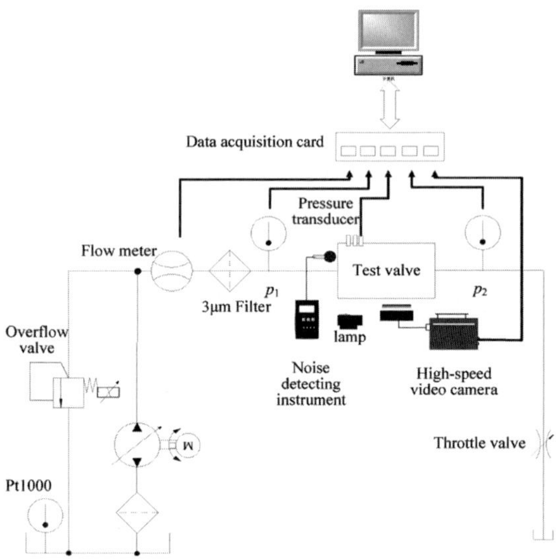

Fig. 1. Experimental set-up

Three spools with two types of grooves, named V02, U01 and U02 respectively, are used for testing. Structural parameters of the grooves are listed in Table 1 (Fig. 3). The only differentia among U-grooves is the grooves' depth. Fig. 3(c) shows the geometrical structures of the non-circular opening spool valves used in.

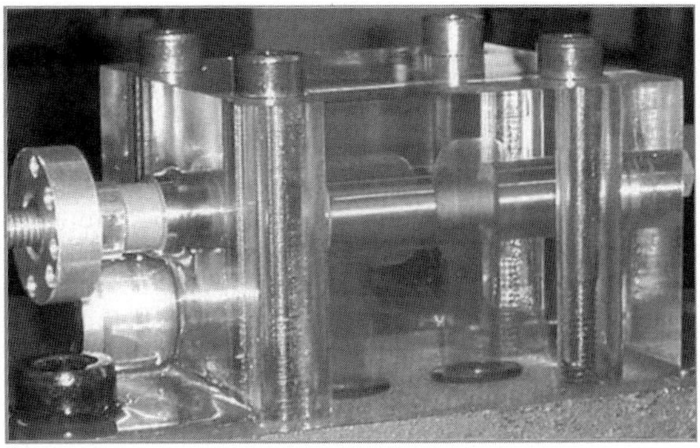

Fig. 2. Plexiglass valve model

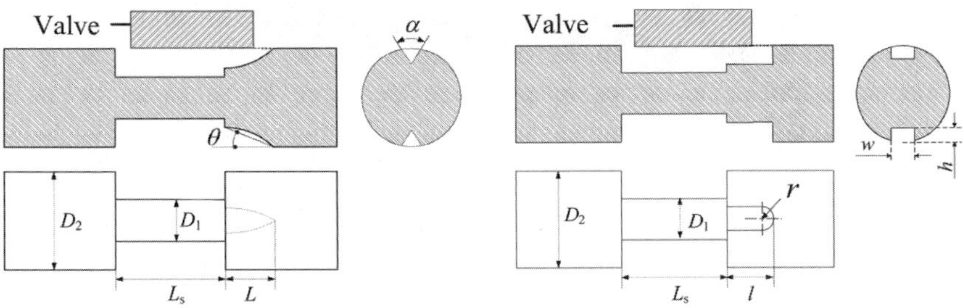

(a) Geometrical structures of V-groove (b) Geometrical structures of U-groove

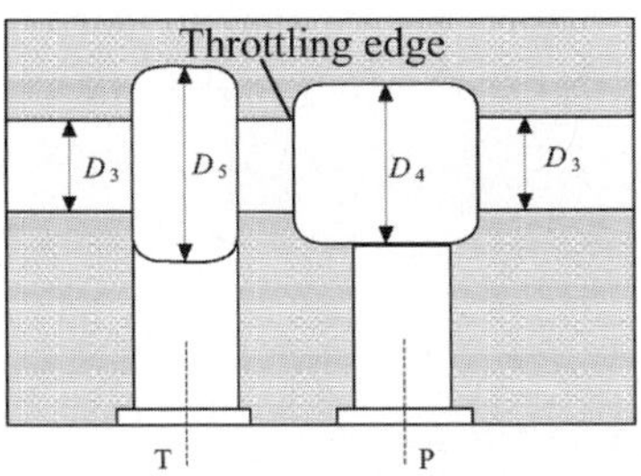

(c) Geometrical structures of the valve body

Table 1 Structural parameters

Type	L(mm)	R(mm)	α(°)	θ(°)
V02	5	12.5	60	17
Type	l(mm)	r(mm)	w(mm)	h(mm)
U01	5	1	2	1.5
U02	5	1	2	2.0

Fig. 3. Structural parameters of test valves

3 Results and Discussion

3.1 Cavitation Inception

Cavitation inception was investigated a lot in various cavitation models and by various ways, and several engineering methods were proposed. As in pump cases, detection of the net positive suction head (*NPSH*) and paint erosion were usually used as direct index for cavitation inception judgement. In some cases, the measurement of static pressures on the volute-casing wall was used as evidences for cavitation distributions. Sound and vibration were mostly used for cavitations' detection. An effective method based on audible sound judgement was obtained by M. ČUDINA [7] in his pump cavitation studies. A discrete frequency tone at the 147 Hz was put forward as a signal to cavitation onset. In our experimental studies, no similar discrete frequency tone was obtained based on the one-third octave bands spectrums. However, the noise spectrums offered a cavitation onset judgement method.

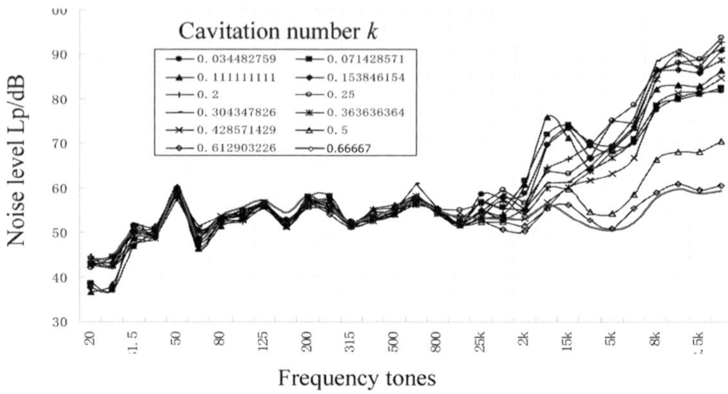

Fig. 4. Noise spectrum of U02-groove with the 4mm opening condition

As we know, a simplified cavitation number k (Formula 2) could be used to describe the cavitation process. That is to say, before the cavitation inception, k describes the likelihood of cavitation inception, and the cavitation degree after cavitation incept.

$$\sigma = \frac{2(P_1 - P_2)}{\rho v^2} \tag{1}$$

$$k = \frac{p_2 - p_v}{p_1 - p_2} = \frac{p_2}{p_1 - p_2} \tag{2}$$

σ : Cavitation number
k : Simplified cavitation number
P_1: Inlet pressure
P_2: Outlet pressure
P_v: Vapor pressure (P_v=0 in oil medium)

The experiments detecting the noise's spectrums with the cavitation number as the variable were conducted. Fig. 4 shows the spectrums obtained from U02 grooves with the 4.0mm opening condition. As we see, the curves raises in high frequencies. Yet curve 1 and 2 keeps close noise levels among all the frequencies, which are defined as non-cavitation conditions. Curve 3 shows a sharp ascending from curve 1 and 2, the noise of which in high frequencies are obviously high than that of low frequencies, which is recon as the remark of cavitation inception. Moreover, with the continued decreasing of the cavitation number, noise levels raises in small ranges. All the curves separate by the frequency tone at the 0.8 kHz, and noises changes few below 0.8 kHz, which are reckon as contributions of mechanical operations. Correspondingly, the high frequency noises are recognized to be generated by cavitations. Same properties of cavitation noise spectrums are observed in all groove type and opening cases. Based on the spectrum curves' distribution properties, it is easily to figure out the cavitation onset condition. The inception thresholds of the cavitation number in U-groove cases are within 0.4~0.6 (Fig. 5), which is accorded with Martin et al.'s [8] studies on spool valves with circular openings. However, in V-grooves cases, the inception cavitation numbers are smaller than that of U-grooves', which means that the structure property of V-grooves is better to restrict cavitations.

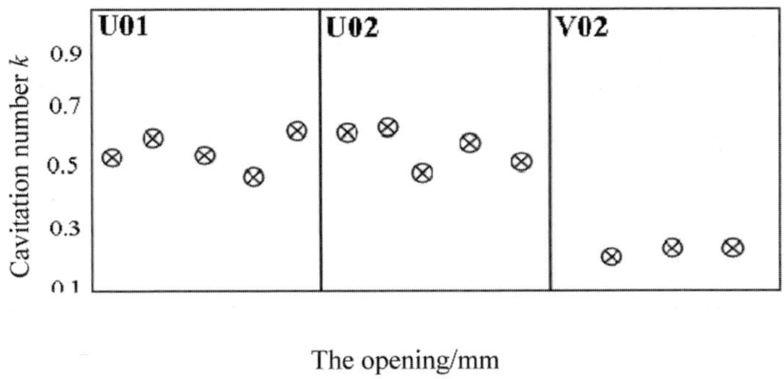

Fig. 5. Cavitation inception thresholds (valve types and openings vs. the cavitation number)

The overall sound pressures were also acquired during the experiments. It is found that the sound pressures have similar trends in different valves and opening cases. One of the curves is selected, as shown in Fig. 6. As we see from the curve, with the decreasing of the cavitation number, the sound pressure experiences a small-range raising process at first. Then, a sharp climb of the curve appears, which denotes the cavitation onset according lots of studies [6] [9]. Moreover, at a certain cavitation number, the sound comes to its maximum level, and then goes to a second peck level before the cavitation number reaches zero. The cavitation inception thresholds σ_i can easily be obtained from the curves (Fig.6) with sharp raisings, and the judgement results of which are quite accorded with the results of spectrum judgement method (Fig. 5).

The cavitation noises are concentrated in high frequencies, which can be easily distinguished from the low frequency environmental noises based on the spectrums. As a result, the spectrum judgement for the cavitation inception is immune from the interference of environmental noise, which makes the spectrum way better compared with the overall sound pressure judgement. When the environmental noises are in high levels, the overall sound pressure curves get raised earlier before cavitation incept.

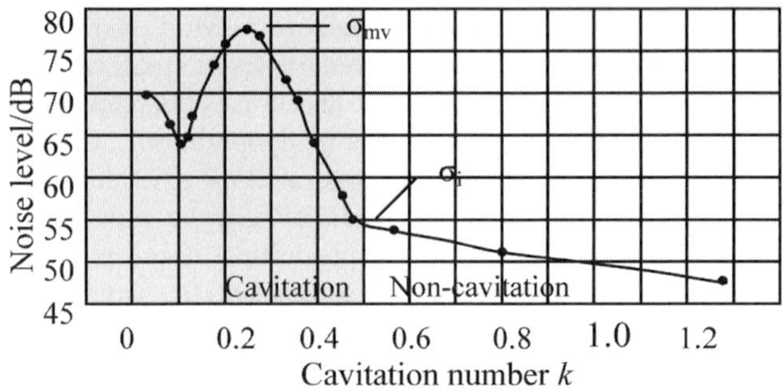

Fig. 6. Typical graph plotting noise vs. cavitation number, obtained from U02-groove with the 4.0mm opening condition

3.2 Cavitation Distribution and Noise Properties

Cavitation distribution properties are illustrated by the assistance of high-speed camera technology. It is found that in small opening conditions of U-grooves, cavitation forms under the bottom of the groove and then transfers to form by the throttling edge with a sudden change as the opening enlarges (Fig.7 (a) and (b)). And in V-grooves, cavitation always incepts by the throttling edge (Fig. 7 (c) and (d)). Cavitation in U-grooves seems quite corporeal since obvious bodies exist. There is obvious interface between cavitation and the oil liquid. Cavitation bubbles always collapse in the downstream of the channel in U-grooves, and the cavitation noise generates. The shedding processes become fiercer in larger opening cases, and the noise levels are correspondingly higher. However, in V-grooves, as cavitation happens, the flow channels are full of flog-like gases (Fig. 7(c) and (d)). There are no visible interfaces between the two phases, and the cavitation bodies are surrounded by small bubbles. The bubbles in V-grooves crumble before they get to the downstream, which makes the collapsing in V-grooves forward and enlarges the collapsing area. This can be the reason for higher noise levels in V-grooves, as shown in Fig.9.

(a) (c)

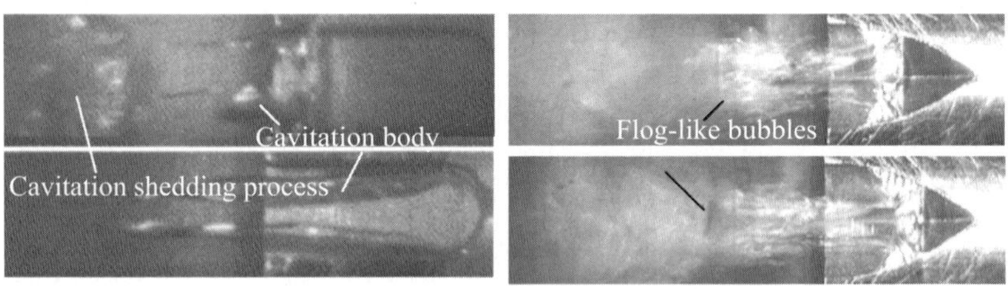

(b) (d)

Fig. 7. Cavitation distribution states in different grooves. All the images are presented in the noises' maximal levels. (a). U01-groove with the 3.0mm opening condition, k=0.43. (b). U01-groove with the 0.5mm opening condition, k=0.36. (c) V02-groove with the 3.0mm opening condition, k=0.20. (d). V02-groove with the 2.0mm opening condition, k=0.15.

Comparing two types of grooves, cavitation seems to be harder to happen in V-grooves, and the cavitation processes in which are short-lived, which may be explained by the good continuity of the groove structure. The effective throttling areas in V-grooves are smaller than that of U-grooves in the same opening conditions. As a result, the average velocity of V-grooves is correspondingly faster, and cavitation bodies are easily demolished into flog-like states. Moreover, three-dimensional simulations are done to validate cavitation states in V-grooves. Commercial simulation code Fluent is employed and RNG *k*-ε turbulent model is used. As we see in Fig. 8, low pressure distributes near the outside area of the throttling edge and the lowest pressure zone is accorded with the throttling edge. It is easy to imagine that cavitation forms by the throttling edges and extends to the outside area of the edge. The cavitation images in Fig. 7(c) and (d) show good coherence with the simulated results (Fig. 8).

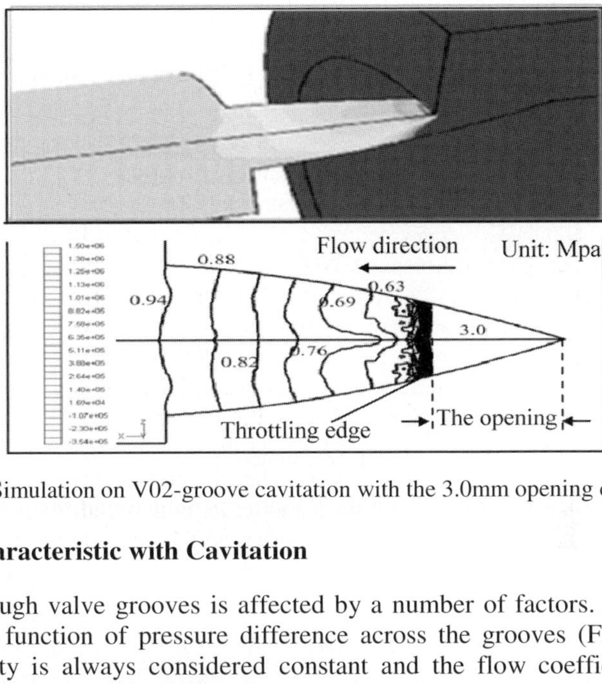

Fig. 8. Simulation on V02-groove cavitation with the 3.0mm opening condition

3.3 Flow Characteristic with Cavitation

Flow rate through valve grooves is affected by a number of factors. First of all, the flow rate is a function of pressure difference across the grooves (Formula 3). The medium density is always considered constant and the flow coefficient is mainly obtained by the geometry of the flow model.

$$Q = C_d A_0 \sqrt{\frac{2\Delta p}{\rho}} \tag{3}$$

It is easy to figure out that the flow rate increases successively with the decreasing of cavitation number based on the experiential formula. However, the real situations seem not so consistent with the calculation results. As we see in Fig. 9, the experimental curves separate from the calculated curves at certain cavitation numbers (σ_1) and kept horizontal from relatively small cavitation number thresholds (σ_2), which are familiar with Timo KOIVULA's findings in orifices, yet not all the same. In Timo's opinion, it assumed that once cavitation happens, the flow gets choked. However, it seems that only when cavitation develops to some extent, like the σ_2 conditions, the flow saturates. When cavitation incepts, the experimental curves separates from calculational ones, but still ascends with the decreasing of the cavitation numbers. It is easy to imagine that the oil flow's continuity and effective throttling areas are affected once cavitation formed, and the ascending trend of the flow rate is restricted. However, there is no uniform explanation for the choking-flow phenomena. Comparing the noise and flow curves in Fig. 9, it is found that the separation thresholds (σ_1) of the flow rates' experimental curves and calculational curves are coincident with the cavitation inception threshold (σ_i) and the flow get choked (σ_2) when the noise got its maximum valve (σ_{mv}).

Fig. 9 shows the properties of the flow and noise of V02 and U02 grooves with the same 2.0mm opening condition. Good reflections between the flow and noise are remarked by the dashed. Similar situations are found in different valve and opening cases. Comparing the two graphs in Fig. 9, it can be found that the V-grooves have larger non-cavitation working ranges while the U-grooves have lower noise levels.

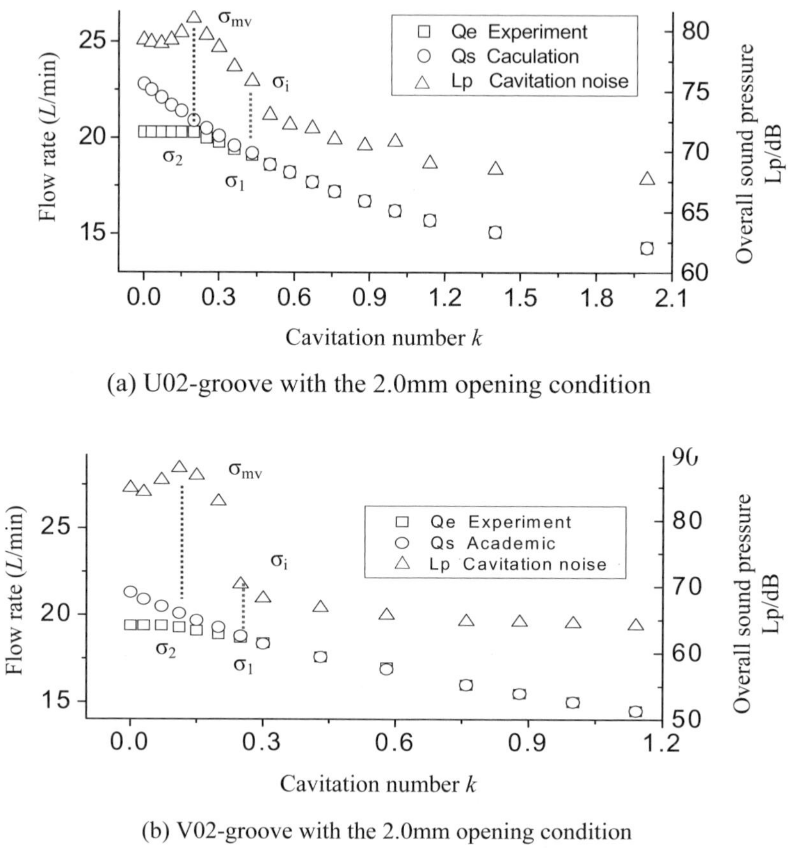

(a) U02-groove with the 2.0mm opening condition

(b) V02-groove with the 2.0mm opening condition

Fig. 9. Good relationships between the cavitation noise and the flow

4 Conclusions

Acoustical signals are used to judge the thresholds of cavitation inception. The interferences from environmental noise can be easily eliminated based on the spectrum method. The cavitation inception numbers are within 0.4~0.6 for U-grooves and 0.2~0.4 for V-grooves. The overall sound pressure has similar trends in different valve and opening cases, comparing with the flow characteristics, it can be found that the experimental flow curve goes beyond from the calculated one when cavitation occurs and the flow gets choked when the overall sound pressure researches its maximum. The cavitation distribution states play an important role on the cavitation noise. In U-grooves, there are obvious interface between cavitation and the oil fluid, while in V-grooves, the flog-like bubbles surrounding the cavitation bodies make the collapsing forward and enlarge the collapsing area, as a result, cavitation noise in V-grooves is relatively higher. Comparing the two types of valves, the V-groove valve has larger non-cavitation working range while U-groove valves have lower cavitation noise.

Acknowledgements

The authors are grateful to the National Basic Research Program (973) of China (No. 2006CB705400) and National Natural Science Foundation of China (No. 50705082) for the financial support.

References

1. Gao, H., Lin, W., Tsukiji, T.: Investigation of Cavitation near the Orifice of Hydraulic Valves. Proceedings of the Institution of Mechanical Engineers, Part G: Journal of Aerospace Engineering 220, 253–265 (2006)
2. Oshima, S., et al.: Effect of cavitation in water hydraulic poppet valves. Int. Fluid Power 1, 5–13 (2001)
3. Moritz, F., Sudolf, S.: Numerical and experimental investigations of the cavitating flow in a centrifugal pump impeller. ASME FED 257, 361–368 (2002)
4. Keiichi, S., Yasuhiro, S.: Unstable cavitation behavior in a circular-cylindrical orifice flow. JSME International Journal, Series B: Fluids and Thermal Engineering 45, 638–645 (2002)
5. Time, K.: On cavitation in fluid power. In: Proc. of 1st FPNI-PhD Symp. Hamburg, 371–382 (2000)
6. Christopher, E.B.: Fundamentals of multiphase flow. Cambridge University Press, Cambridge (2005)
7. ČUDINA, M.: Detection of cavitation phenomenon in a centrifugal pump using audible sound. Mechanical Systems and Signal Processing 17, 1335–1347 (2003)
8. Martin, C.S., et al.: Cavitation inception in spool valves. Journal of Fluids Engineering, Transactions of the ASME 103, 564–576 (1981)
9. Kiesbauer, J., Vnucec, D.: Prediction cavitation damage in control valves. Hydrocarbon Processing, 55–61 (2006)

Author Index

Printing: Mercedes-Druck, Berlin
Binding: Stein+Lehmann, Berlin